OXFORD MEDICAL PUBLICATIONS

Autonomic Failure

Autonomic Failure

A Textbook of Clinical Disorders of the Autonomic Nervous System

FOURTH EDITION

Edited by

Christopher J. Mathias

D. Phil. (Oxon), D. Sc. (Lon.), F.R.C.P.
Professor of Neurovascular Medicine and Consultant Physician
Neurovascular Medicine Unit, Division of Neuroscience and Psychological Medicine,
Imperial College School of Medicine at St Mary's Hospital,
Imperial College of Science, Technology and Medicine, London;
and Autonomic Unit, National Hospital for Neurology and Neurosurgery,
and University Department of Clinical Neurology, Institute of Neurology,
University College London; University of London.

and

Sir Roger Bannister

C.B.E., M.A., M. Sc., D.M. (Oxon), F.R.C.P.
Former Master, Pembroke College, Oxford;
Hon. Consultant Physician, National Hospital for
Neurology and Neurosurgery, London;
Hon. Consultant Neurologist, St Mary's Hospital, London,
Oxford District Health Authority, and
Oxford Regional Health Authority

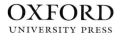

OXFORD
UNIVERSITY PRESS

OXFORD

UNIVERSITY PRESS

Great Clarendon Street, Oxford OX2 6DP

Oxford New York

Athens Auckland Bangkok Bogota Buenos Aires Calcutta
Cape Town Chennai Dar es Salaam Delhi Florence Hong Kong Istanbul
Karachi Kuala Lumpur Madrid Melbourne Mexico City Mumbai
Nairobi Paris São Paolo Singapore Taipei Tokyo Toronto Warsaw

and associated companies in
Berlin Ibadan

Oxford is a trade mark of Oxford University Press

Published in the United States
by Oxford University Press, Inc., New York

First published 1983 (ed. Sir Roger Bannister)
Second edition published 1988 (ed. Sir Roger Bannister)
Third edition published 1992 (ed. Sir Roger Bannister and Christopher J. Mathias)
First published in paperback 1993 (ed. Sir Roger Bannister and Christopher J. Mathias)
Fourth edition published 1999 (ed. Christopher J. Mathias and Sir Roger Bannister)

British Library Cataloguing in Publication Data
Data available

Library of Congress Cataloging in Publication Data
Autonomic failure: a textbook of clinical disorders of the autonomic
nervous system / edited by Christopher J. Mathias and Sir Roger
Bannister. – 4th ed.
(Oxford medical publications)
Includes bibliographical references and index.
1. Autonomic nervous system—Diseases. I. Mathias, C. J.
II. Bannister, Roger.   III. Series.
[DNLM: 1. Autonomic Nervous System—physiopathology. 2. Autonomic
Nervous System Diseases.   WL 600 A939 1999]
RC407.A95   1999   616.8′8—dc21   98–31569

1 3 5 7 9 10 8 6 4 2

ISBN 0 19 2628518

Typeset by EXPO Holdings, Malaysia

Printed in Great Britain on acid free paper by
The Bath Press, Avon

Preface to the Fourth Edition

In this fourth edition we aim to continue to provide, as in previous editions, a comprehensive basis for the diagnosis and treatment of a wide range of autonomic disorders which are being increasingly recognized. This edition incorporates the substantial advances made since 1992. There has been extensive revision of previous chapters with the introduction of 20 new chapters. We are grateful for the wide range of international expertise through our contributors, who come from Europe, the United States, and Australia.

This edition begins with an updated classification of autonomic disorders. This is followed by the history of the autonomic nervous system, which is of particular relevance as it is just 100 years since Langley introduced the term 'autonomic'. Autonomic Units are now an integral part of major hospitals and neuroscience centres, and deal with a wide range of neurological and medical diseases. The scientific basis and clinical background are needed for diagnosis, investigation, and management of autonomic disorders. The first two sections deal with fundamental aspects of autonomic structure, function, and its integration. There are new chapters dealing with the neurobiology of the autonomic nervous system, nerve growth factors, genetic mutations, neural and hormonal control of the cerebral circulation, autonomic innervation of the lung, and pathophysiological mechanisms causing nausea and vomiting. The third section incorporates the many technological advances that have led to effective non-invasive investigation of the autonomic nervous system. Both established and state-of-the-art techniques are described, together with critical interpretation of complex abnormalities related to associated pathology.

The fourth section provides detailed and fresh information on the primary autonomic failure syndromes, and in particular multiple system atrophy, that accounts for approximately 10 per cent of patients previously thought to have Parkinson's disease. It is the most common neurodegenerative disorder affecting the autonomic nervous system. The diagnosis of multiple system atrophy is important because the prognosis is poor, complications are difficult to treat, and interventional approaches such as substantia nigra implantation are more likely to fail than in Parkinson's disease.

The fifth section focuses on the major peripheral autonomic neuropathies, which include common disorders such as diabetes mellitus and rarer disorders such as dopamine β-hydroxylase deficiency and allied hereditary autonomic neuropathies. New chapters on familial dysautonomia and amyloidosis are included. The sixth and final section has undergone considerable expansion as there are many disorders with a substantial autonomic component. New chapters include neurocardiology, neurally mediated syncope, cardiac and rhythm causes of syncope, shock, disorders affecting cutaneous blood flow, migraine, the effects of drugs, chemicals and toxins, and ageing.

Advances in the clinical management of autonomic disorders are critically dependent on the bridge between basic and applied science, and it is intended that different sections of this book will make diagnosis increasingly precise by fully evaluating the underlying anatomical and functional deficits that will lead to more effective treatment. As before, it is intended that this new edition will continue to provide practitioners in different fields, including neurology, cardiology, geriatric medicine, diabetology, and internal medicine, in addition to other disciplines, with a rational guide to aid them in the recognition, evaluation and management of autonomic disorders.

London C.J.M.
Oxford R.B.
May 1999

Acknowledgements

This book owes much to many. We thank our patients, from whom we have learnt much; the many clinical practitioners who have referred patients to us; and, importantly, our families, who have unflinchingly supported us. We wish to acknowledge our gratitude in particular to: Professor Sir Stanley Peart for continuing inspiration and advice; the scientific and clinical staff of the Autonomic and Neurovascular Medicine Units, including Katharine Bleasdale-Barr, Laura Everall, Jeffery Kimber, Lydia Thornley, and Laura Watson; our colleagues at the National Hospital for Neurology and Neurosurgery/Institute of Neurology and St Mary's Hospital/Imperial College School of Medicine; the research fellows from the UK and abroad who have worked in our Units—many are in senior positions in neurology and cardiovascular medicine, and some are directing autonomic departments abroad; the many charitable bodies who have provided support, including the Wellcome Trust (who deserve special mention for their sustained support), the Brain Research Trust, and the Autonomic Disorders Association Sarah Matheson Trust; and Christine Wyke for co-ordinating the many aspects of this edition.

Preface to the First Edition

In the past 10 years the clinical syndromes of autonomic failure have been studied by a wide range of new physiological, pharmacological, pathological, and neurochemical techniques, but the information is scattered in papers in many different journals and is not easily available to the clinician. Much is still to be learnt about these syndromes and their management but it is now possible to review these recent advances.

The presenting symptoms of autonomic failure, such as low blood pressure, may overlie unrecognized disturbances of function which are widespread and involve altered control of many different parts of the body including the heart, the kidneys, the pancreas, the bladder, the gut, and the pupils. Symptoms may therefore lead patients to many different specialists who are unfamiliar with these autonomic syndromes. The cardiologist, for example, sees some of the patients with idiopathic orthostatic hypotension and the neurologist, patients with orthostatic hypotension associated with parkinsonism or multiple system atrophy (Shy–Drager syndrome). The general physician encounters many problems of autonomic failure in association with diseases such as diabetes, alcoholism, or amyloidosis. The geriatrician sees the consequences of failure of body-temperature regulation. The genitourinary surgeon is often presented with a difficult problem of the neurogenic bladder. It would be wrong to think of autonomic failure as a single disease entity but progressive autonomic failure in which pathological lesions are to some degree established provides a model for investigation which can be compared with other diseases in which defective autonomic function is part of a wider picture, as in diabetes.

This book aims to provide clinicians in many fields with a guide to useful tests of differing complexity which are now needed to identify autonomic defects of a particular organ in which they have a special interest and should help them to interpret these tests. Interpretation is as important as knowing how to undertake the tests because the autonomic nervous system includes more subtle variations in response than the somatic nervous system and has many compensating mechanisms for impending failure. The practical tests described in the book are set against the more general background of current advances in physiology and pathology of the autonomic nervous system in order to form a basis for rational management in a field which is generally recognized to be exceedingly difficult.

The book also aims to introduce the clinician to new theoretical concepts of the organization of the autonomic nervous system. The old-fashioned notion of a simple duality of a sympathetic–adrenal system causing rather unselective 'fight or flight' responses and a parasympathetic–cholinergic system providing tonic activity, has given way to a new view of a highly selective autonomic nervous system with an integrative action at least as complex as that of the somatic nervous system. New transmitters and modulators abound and receptors, both pre- and postsynaptic, can be blocked, activated, or modified in their numbers and affinities. New general biological principles have emerged with 'up' and 'down' regulation of receptor numbers and affinities and manipulation pharmacologically of pre- and postsynaptic receptors by transmitter depletion or blockade. These fields provide an exciting prospect for future biological as well as medical research. It is appropriate to end with a quotation from my teacher, the late Sir George Pickering, who also concluded a review of autonomic function with the words that it was 'in fact no more than an overture. The main body of the work is to come'.

London R.B.
September 1982

Contents

Contributors

P. Anand, Academic Department of Neurology, St Bartholomew's and the Royal London School of Medicine and Dentistry, Royal London Hospital, Whitechapel, London E1 1BB, UK

P. L. R. Andrews, Department of Physiology, St. George's Hospital Medical School, Cranmer Terrace, London SW17 0RE

Felicia B. Axelrod, New York University Medical Center, 530 First Avenue, New York, NY 10016, USA

Roger Bannister, Autonomic Unit, National Hospital for Neurology and Neurosurgery, Queen Square, London WC1, UK

Peter J. Barnes, Department of Thoracic Medicine, National Heart and Lung Institute, Dovehouse St., London SW3 6LY, UK

Eduardo E. Benarroch, Department of Neurology, Mayo Clinic, Rochester, MN 55905, USA

Anne E. Bishop, Department of Histochemistry, Division of Diagnostic and Investigative Sciences, Imperial College School of Medicine, Hammersmith Hospital, London W12 ONN, UK

David J. Brooks, MRC Cyclotron Unit, Imperial College School of Medicine, Hammersmith Hospital, London, W12 0NN, UK

Geoffrey Burnstock, Autonomic Neuroscience Institute, Department of Anatomy and Developmental Biology, Royal Free Hospital School of Medicine, Rowland Hill Street, London NW3 2PF, UK

A. John Camm, St George's Hospital Medical School, London, UK

Sudhansu Chokroverty, The Departments of Neurology and Neurophysiology, and the Sleep Laboratory of Saint Vincents Hospital and Medical Center, New York, USA

Jay N. Cohn, Cardiovascular Division, Department of Medicine, University of Minnesota Medical School, Minneapolis, Minnesota 55455, USA

Kenneth J. Collins, Department of Geriatric Medicine, St Pancras Hospital, The University College Hospitals, London NW1 OPE, UK

Susan E. Daniel, Parkinson's Disease Society Brain Research Centre, Institute of Neurology, 1 Wakefield Street, London WC1N 1PJ, UK

William C. de Groat, Department of Pharmacology, School of Medicine, University of Pittsburgh, Pittsburgh, PA 15261, USA

Gerald F. DiBona, Department of Internal Medicine, University of Iowa College of Medicine; and Veterans Administration Medical Center, Iowa City, IA 52242, USA

M. Di Rienzo, La RC Centro di Bioingengeria, Fondazione Pro Juventute, Milan, Italy

Peter D. Drummond, Division of Psychology, Murdoch University, 6150 Western Australia

M. E. Edmonds, Diabetic Department, King's College Hospital, Denmark Hill, London SE5 9RS, UK

Marjorie Ellison, National Hospital for Neurology and Neurosurgery, Queen Square, London WC1 3BG, UK

Robert D. Fealey, Department of Neurology, Mayo Clinic, Rochester, MN 55905, USA

Clare J. Fowler, Department of Uro-Neurology, National Hospital for Neurology and Neurosurgery and University Department of Clinical Neurology, Institute of Neurology, Queen Square, London WC1N 3BG, UK

Gary S. Francis, Cardiovascular Division, Department of Medicine, University of Minnesota Medical School, Minneapolis, Minnesota 55455, USA

Hans L. Frankel, National Spinal Injuries Centre, Stoke Mandeville Hospital, Aylesbury, Bucks HP21 8AL, UK

Derek B.Frewin, Department of Clinical and Experimental Pharmacology, University of Adelaide, Adelaide 5005, Australia

Peter J. Goadsby, Institute of Neurology, The National Hospital for Neurology and Neurosurgery, Queen Square, London WC1N 3BG, UK

Blair P. Grubb, Cardiology, The Medical College of Ohio, 3000 Arlington Ave, Toledo, Ohio 43699, USA

Roger Hainsworth, Institute for Cardiovascular Research, University of Leeds, Leeds LS2 9JT, UK

Robert W. Hamill, Department of Neurology, College of Medicine, University of Vermont, Burlington, Vermont 05401, USA

Juha E. K. Hartikainen, Kuopio University Hospital, Kuopio, Finland

Wilfrid Jänig, Physiologisches Institut, Christian-Albrechts-Universität zu Kiel, Ohlshausenstrasse 40, 24098 Kiel, Germany

Barry Karas, The Medical College of Ohio, 3000 Arlington Ave, Toledo, Ohio 43699, USA

John M. Karemaker, Department of Physiology, Academic Medical Centre, University of Amsterdam, Amsterdam, The Netherlands

Edmund F. LaGamma, Departments of Pediatrics and Neurobiology, University Hospital Medical Center at Stony Brook, Stony Brook, New York 11794-8111, USA

A. J. Lees, Department of Neurology, National Hospital for Neurology and Neurosurgery, Queen Square, London WC1N 3BG, UK

Lewis A. Lipsitz, Hebrew Rehabilitation Center for Aged, 1200 Centre Street, Boston, Massachusetts 02131-1097, USA

Phillip A. Low, Department of Neurology, Mayo Clinic, Rochester, MN 55905, USA

John Ludbrook, University of Melbourne Department of Surgery, Royal Melbourne Hospital, Parkville, Victoria 3050, Australia

Ian A. Macdonald, School of Biomedical Sciences, Medical School, Queen's Medical Centre, Nottingham NG7 2UH, UK

Robert Macfarlane, Department of Neurological Surgery, Addenbrooke's Hospital, Cambridge, UK

Elspeth M. McLachlan, Prince of Wales Medical Research Institute, Randwick, 7 High Street, NSW 2031, Sydney, Australia

J. G. McLeod, Department of Medicine, University of Sydney, Sydney, New South Wales 2006, Australia

G. Mancia, Clinica Medica, University of Milan and Ospedale S. Gerardo, Monza, Italy

Christopher J. Mathias, Neurovascular Medicine Unit, Division of Neuroscience and Physiological Medicine, Imperial College School of Medicine at St Mary's Hospital, Imperial College of Science Technology and Medicine, London W2; and Autonomic Unit, National Hospital for Neurology and Neurosurgery, Queen Square, and University Department of Clinical Neurology, Institute of Neurology, University College, London WC1 3BG, UK

Margaret R. Matthews, Department of Human Anatomy and Genetics, University of Oxford, South Parks Road, Oxford OX1 3QX, UK

Pamela Milner, Autonomic Neuroscience Institute, Department of Anatomy and Developmental Biology, Royal Free Hospital School of Medicine, Rowland Hill Street, London NW3 2PF, UK

John Morgan-Hughes, National Hospital for Neurology and Neurosurgery, Queen Square, London WC1 3BG, UK

Michael A. Moskowitz, Stroke and Neurovascular Regulation, Massachusetts General Hospital, 149 13th Street, Charlestown, MA 02129, USA

Krzysztof Narkiewicz, Cardiovascular Division, Department of Internal Medicine, University of Iowa, 200 Hawkins Drive, Iowa City, IA 52242, USA

Jes Olesen, Department of Neurology, Glostrup Hospital, Nordre Ringvej 57, DK-2600 Glostrup, Denmark

S. Omboni, Instituto Scientifico Ospedale S. Luca, Instituto Auxologico Italiano, Milan, Italy

G. Parati, Instituto Scientifico Ospedale S. Luca, Instituto Auxologico Italiano, Milan, Italy

Stephen J. Peroutka, 1025 Tournament Drive, Barlingame, CA 94010-7429, USA

Julia M. Polak, Department of Histochemistry, Division of Diagnostic and Investigative Sciences, Imperial College School of Medicine, Hammersmith Hospital, London W12 ONN, UK

Ronald J. Polinsky, Clinical Neuropharmacology Section, Clinical Neuroscience Branch, National Institute of Neurological Disorders and Stroke, Bethesda, Maryland 20892, USA

Mary M. Reilly, National Hospital for Neurology and Neurosurgery, Queen Square, London, UK

Martin A. Samuels, Department of Neurology, Brigham and Women's Hospital and Harvard Medical School, 75 Francis Street, Boston, MA 02115, USA

G. D. Schott, The National Hospital for Neurology and Neurosurgery, Queen Square, London WC1N 3BG, UK

J. T. Shepherd, Mayo Clinic and Foundation, Rochester, Minnesota 55905, USA

R. F. J. Shepherd, Mayo Clinic and Foundation, Rochester, Minnesota 55905, USA

Shirley A. Smith, Diabetes Day Centre, St Thomas' Hospital, London SE1 7EH, UK

S. E. Smith, Department of Neuro-Ophthalmology, National Hospital for Neurology and Neurosurgery, Queen Square, London WCIN 3BG, UK

Virend K. Somers, Cardiovascular Division, Department of Internal Medicine, University of Iowa, 200 Hawkins Drive, Iowa City, IA 52242, USA

K. M. Spyer, Royal Free and University College Medical School, Royal Free Campus, Rowland Hill Street, London NW3 2PF, UK

E. M. Tansey, The Wellcome Institute for the History of Medicine, 183 Euston Road, London NW1 2BE, UK

P. K. Thomas, Royal Free Hospital School of Medicine and Institute of Neurology, London, UK

Lars Lykke Thomsen, Department of Neurology, Glostrup Hospital, Nordre Ringvej 57, DK-2600 Glostrup, Denmark

Anne L. Tonkin, Department of Clinical and Experimental Pharmacology, University of Adelaide, Adelaide 5005, Australia

B. Gunnar Wallin, University of Göteborg, Department of Clinical Neuroscience, Section of Clinical Neurophysiology, Sahlgren Hospital, Göteborg, Sweden

P. J. Watkins, Diabetic Department, King's College Hospital, Denmark Hill, London SE5 9RS, UK

Wouter Wieling, Department of Medicine, Academic Medical Centre, University of Amsterdam, Amsterdam, The Netherlands

Christopher S. Wilcox, Division of Nephrology and Hypertension, Georgetown University Medical Center, 3800 Reservoir Road, NW, PHC F6003, Washington, DC 20007, USA

David L. Wingate, Gastrointestinal Science Research Unit, The London Hospital Medical College, London E1 2AJ, UK

P. A. van Zwieten, Departments of Pharmacotherapy and Cardiology, Academic Medical Centre, University of Amsterdam, 1105 AZ Amsterdam, The Netherlands

Abbreviations

AADC	L-amino acid decarboxylase deficiency
ACE	angiotensin-coverting enzyme
ACh	acetylcholine
AChE	acetylcholinesterase
ACTH	adrenocorticotrophic hormone
ADH	vasopressin (antidiuretic hormone)
AF	autonomic failure
AIDS	acquired immunodeficiency syndrome
AII	angiotensin II
AMPA	α-amino-3-hydroxy-5-methyl-4-isoxazole propionic acid
ANP	atrial natriuretic peptide
ANS	autonomic nervous system
AP	amyloid P
Apo A-1	apolipoprotein A-1
APV	2-amino-5-phosphonovalerate
AR	autoregressive modelling method
ARDS	adult respiratory distress syndrome
ARMA	autorepressive moving average method
ATP	adenosine 5′-triphosphate
AV	atrioventricular
AVP	vasopressin
BDNF	brain-derived neurotrophic factor
bHLH	basic helix–loop–helix
BIBP	
BiPAP	bilevel positive airway pressure
BMP	bone morphogenic protein
bnst	bed nucleus of the stria terminals
BP	blood pressure
BPH	benign prostrate hyperplasia
BRS	baroreflex sensitivity
cAMP	cyclic adenosine monophosphate
CAN	central autonomic circuits
CARP I	peripheral complex regional pain syndrome
CASS	composite autonomic scoring scale
CAT	choline acetyl transferase
CAT	computed axial tomography
CBD	corticobasal degeneration
CBF	cerebral blood flow
CCK	cholecystokinin
CDF	cholinergic differentiation factor
CG	ciliary ganglion
CGRP	calcitonin-gene-related peptide
ChAT	choline acetyltransferase
CHF	congestive heart failure
CIDP	chronic inflammatory demyelinating polyradiculopathy
CLQTS	congenital long QT syndrome

CNA	central nucleus of the amygdala
CNQX	6-cyano-7-nitro-quinoxaline-2-3-dione
CNS	central nervous system
CNTF	ciliary neurotrophic factor
CNV	contingent negative variation
COPD	chronic obstructive pulmonary disease
CPAP	continuous positive airway pressure
CRH	corticotrophin-releasing hormone
CRPS	complex regional pain syndrome
CSF	cerebrospinal fluid
CSMG	coeliac–superior mesenteric ganglion
CT	computed tomography
CVC	cutaneous vasoconstrictor
CVLM	caudal ventrolateral medulla
DBH	dopamine β-hydroxylase
DBN	down-beat nystagmus
d.c.	direct current
DDAVP	desmopressin
DHPG	dihydroxyphenylglycol
DIC	disseminated intravascular coagulation
DM	diabetes mellitus
DMPP	dimethylphenylpiperazine
DNP	dinitrophenol
dopa	3,4-dihydroxyphenylalanine
DOPS	dihydroxyphenylserine
DRG	dorsal root ganglion
DTPA	diethylenetriaminepentaacetic acid
DVN	dorsal vagal nucleus
EAN	experimental allergic neuritis
EBV	Epstein–Barr virus
EC	enterochromaffin
ECG	electrocardiograph
ECM	extracellular matrix
ECV	extracellular fluid volume
EDNRB	endothelin-B receptor
EDRF	endothelium-derived relaxant factor
EEG	electroencephalograph
EJP	excitatory junction potential
ELISA	enzyme-linked immunosorbent assay
EMG	electromyogram
ENS	enteric nervous system
EPSC	excitatory postsynaptic current
EPSP	excitatory postsynaptic potential
ERSNA	efferent renal sympathetic nerve activity
ESCN	electrolyte–steroid–cardiopathy with necroses
ESP	
EUS	external urethral sphincter

FAP	familial amyloid polyneuropathy		MED	male erectile dysfunction
FD	familial dysautonomia		MELAS	mitochondrial encephalopathy with lactic acidosis and stroke-like episodes
FDG	2-fluoro-2-deoxy-D-glucose		MEN	multiple endocrine neoplasia
FFA	free fatty acid		MHPG	3-methoxy-4-hydroxyphenylglycol
FFI	fatal familial insomnia		MIBG	meta-iodobenzyl guanidine
FFT	fast Fourier transform		MMC	migrating motor complex
FGF	fibroblast growth factor		MMP-PCR	mismatched primer PCR
			MPTP	1-methyl-4-phenyl-1,2,3,6-tetrahydropyridine
GABA	γ-aminobutyric acid		MR	motility regulating
GAD	glutamic acid decarboxylase		MRI	magnetic resonance imaging
GCI	oligodendroglial cytoplasmic inclusion		MRS	proton magnetic resonance spectroscopy
GDNF	glial-derived neurotrophic factor		MSA	multiple system atrophy
GER	gastro-oesophageal reflux		MSNA	muscle sympathetic nerve activity
GFAP	glial fibrillary acidic protein		MUSE	medicated urethral system for erection
GFR	glomerular filtration rate		MVC	muscle vasoconstrictor
GHRF	growth hormone releasing factor			
GMP	guanosine monophosphate		NAA	N-acetyl aspartate
GRP	gastrin-releasing peptide		NAd	noradrenaline
GTN	glyceryl trinitrate		NANC	non-adrenergic, non-cholinergic
			NC	neural crest
HD	Hirschsprung's disease		NCAM	neural cell adhesion molecule
HDA	hypothalamic defence area		NCSC	neural crest stem cell
5-HIAA	5-hydroxyindoleacetic acid		NEFA	non-esterified fatty acid
HMSN	hereditary motor and sensory neuropathies		NEP	neutral endopeptidase
HR	heart rate		NGF	nerve growth factor
HSAN	hereditary sensory and autonomic neuropathies		NIDDM	non-insulin-dependent diabetes mellitus
5-HT	5-hydroxytryptamine		NKI	neurokinin 1
HVA	homovanillic acid		NKA	neurokinin A
			NMB	neuromedin B
IASP	International Association for the Study of Pain		NMDA	N-methyl-D-aspartate
IBZM	iodobenzamide		NNP	nucleated neuronal profiles
ICD	cardioverter-defibrillator		NO	nitric oxide
IDDM	insulin-dependent diabetes mellitus		NOS	nitric oxide synthase
IFN	interferon		NP	neuronal progenitor
IJP	inhibitory junction potential		NPY	neuropeptide Y
IL	interleukin		NT	neurotrophin
IML	intermediolateral column		NTS	nucleus of the tractus solitarius (solitary tract)
i-NANC	inhibitory non-adrenergic, non-cholinergic			
IP3	inositol trisphosphate		6-OHDA	6-hydroxydopamine
IPD	idiopathic Parkinson's disease		OPCA	olivopontocerebellar atrophy
IPSC	inhibitory postsynaptic current		OSAS	obstructive sleep apnoea syndrome
IPSP	inhibitory postsynaptic potential			
IR	immunoreactive		PACAP	pituitary adenylate cyclase activating peptide
			PAF	pure autonomic failure
KA	kainate		PAG	periaqueductal grey matter
			PCR	polymerase chain reaction
LBNP	lower-body negative pressure		PD	Parkinson's disease
L-glu	L-glutamate		PET	positron emission tomography
LIF	leukaemia inhibitory factor		PEV	posturally evoked vomiting
L-NAME	N^G-nitro-L-arginine methyl ester		PGE_2	prostaglandin E_2
LQTS	long QT syndrome		PHI	peptide with N-terminal histidine and C-terminal isoleucine
LUT	lower urinary tract		PHM	peptide with N-terminal histidine and C-terminal methionine
MANS	membrane-associated neurotransmitter stimulating factor		PHV	
MAO	monoamine oxidase		PI	pulse interval
MCA	middle cerebral artery		PMC	pontine micturition centre
m-CPP	meta-chloro-phenylpiperazine			

PMT	pacemaker-mediated tachycardia	SHR	spontaneously hypertensive rat
PNA	phrenic nerve activity	SIDS	sudden infant death syndrome
PNMT	phenylethanolamine-*N*-methyltransferase	SM	sudomotor
PNS	parasympathetic nervous system	SMP	sympathetically maintained pain
POAH	pre-optic area/anterior hypothalamus and septum	SN	sinus nerve
POTS	postural orthostatic tachycardia sundrome	SNA	sympathetic nerve activity
PPP	pancreatic polypeptide	SND	striatonigral degeneration
PRA	plasma renin activity	SNGFR	single-nephron glomerular filtration rate
PRV	pseudorabies virus	SNPF	single-nephron plasma flow
PSP	progressive supranuclear palsy	SNS	sympathetic nervous system
PV	plasma volume	SP	substance P
PVN	paraventricular nucleus	SPACE	single potential analysis of cavernosus electrical activity
QSART	quantitative sudomotor axon reflex test	SPECT	single photon emission computed tomography
		SPNs	sympathetic preganglionic neurones
RAR	rapidly adapting receptor	SSNA	skin sympathetic nerve activity
RBD	REM behaviour disorder	SSR	sympathetic skin response
RBF	renal blood flow	SUD	sudden unexplained death
rCBF	regional cerebral blood flow		
rCMRGlc	regional cerebral glucose metabolism	TCD	transcranial Doppler ultrasonography
rCMRO$_2$	regional cerebral oxygen metabolism	TDP	torsade de pointes
REM	rapid eye movement	TGF-β	transforming growth factor-β
RET	rearranged transfection proto-oncogene	TH	tyrosine hydroxylase
RGC	retrograde giant contraction	TNC	trigeminal nucleus caudalis
RIA	radioimmunoassay	TNF	tumour necrosis factor
RMP		TOCP	tri-ortho-cresyl phosphate
RSD	reflex sympathetic dystrophy	TP	tracheal pressure
RTPCR	reverse transcriptase polymerase chain reaction	TSS	toxic shock syndrome
RVLM	rostral ventrolateral medulla	TST	thermoregulatory sweat test
		TTR	transthyretin
SAD	sinoaortic denervation		
SAP	serum amyloid P	VIP	vasoactive intestinal polypeptide
SAR	slowly adapting receptor	VLM	ventrolateral medulla
SCG	superior cervical ganglia	VMA	vanillylmandelic acid
SD	standard deviation	VMM	ventromedial medulla
SFO	subfornical organ	VVC	visceral vasoconstrictor
SGA	small for gestational age		
SHH	sonic hedgehog	WGA-HRP	

Introduction and classification of autonomic disorders

Roger Bannister and Christopher J. Mathias

The autonomic nervous system innervates every organ in the body, creating, as Galen suggested, 'sympathy' between the various parts of the body. It has as complex a neural organization in the brain, spinal cord, and periphery as the somatic nervous system, but remains largely involuntary or automatic. Claude Bernard wrote 'nature thought it provident to remove these important phenomena from the capriciousness of an ignorant will'. Langley, who in 1898 first proposed the term 'autonomic nervous system', based his experiments on the blocking action of nicotine at synapses in ganglia. In 1921 Loewi discovered 'Vagusstoff' which was released by stimulation of the vagus nerve and proved to be acetylcholine. In the same year Cannon discovered that 'sympathin', later shown to be noradrenaline, was produced by stimulation of the sympathetic trunk. The basis therefore was laid for Dale's distinction between cholinergic and adrenergic transmission in the autonomic nervous system. A more detailed history of the autonomic nervous system is provided after this chapter.

Peripheral autonomic function

The peripheral autonomic nervous system, an efferent system, is made up of neurons that lie outside the central nervous system and are concerned with visceral innervation. Both sympathetic and parasympathetic systems have preganglionic neurons in the brain and spinal cord arranged as shown in Fig. 1. The afferent limbs of autonomic reflexes may lie in any afferent nerve. The preganglionic sympathetic fibres are myelinated and leave the spinal roots as white rami communicantes and synapse in the ganglia of the sympathetic. Unmyelinated postganglionic fibres rejoin the anterior spinal roots by the arrangement shown in Fig. 2, although some sympathetic fibres traverse the paravertebral ganglia and synapse in more peripheral ganglia.

The transmitter at all preganglionic terminals is acetylcholine, which is not blocked by atropine (the nicotinic effect), whereas the action of acetycholine at the distal end of the cholinergic postganglionic fibres is blocked by atropine (the muscarinic effect). Muscarinic receptors are now subdivided into at least three subtypes. Noradrenaline is the principal transmitter for postganglionic sympathetic nerves, but there are a few areas where there is cholinergic transmission. These exceptions include sudomotor nerves, putative vasodilator fibres to muscle, and the adrenal medulla which is innervated by preganglionic (cholinergic) fibres and which itself secretes both adrenaline and noradrenaline. Noradrenaline is stored in the post-ganglionic nerve terminals and is released by nerve activity or by sympathomimetic drugs, which may act partly indirectly on the

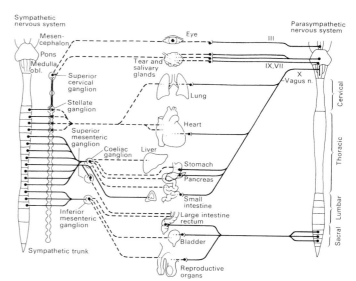

Fig. 1   (From Jänig 1995)

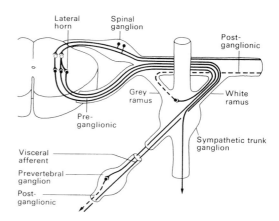

Fig. 2

ganglia or more centrally, e.g. ephedrine and amphetamine, or on the terminals, e.g. phenylephrine or tyramine. The different actions of noradrenaline and adrenaline are caused by relative effects on different receptors. α-adrenoceptors may be either postsynaptic (α1) or presynaptic (α2); the latter when stimulated decrease the release of the transmitter. α2-adrenoceptors are also present at the postsynaptic level and cause vasoconstriction when stimulated with agonists. β-adrenoceptors mediate vasodilatation (especially in skeletal muscles), increase the rate and force of the heart (with a tendency to arrhythmias), and cause bronchial relaxation. They are further subdivided into β1-adrenoceptors, mediating the chronotropic cardiac action of isoprenaline, and β2-adrenoceptors, which are responsible for most of the peripheral effects of β-adrenergic stimulation. Though autonomic sensitivity phenomena were first described more than a century ago, and the research was summarized by Cannon and Rosenblueth in 1949 under the title, *The supersensitivity of denervated structures: a law of denervation*. Attention since then has concentrated on the 'up' and 'down' regulation of receptor function depending on the availability of the transmitter.

The cells of the autonomic nervous system tend to act in conjunction and this is achieved mainly by specialized intercellular junctions at the ganglion cells which have been demonstrated by electron microscopy and freeze fracture techniques. The autonomic ganglia also contain small intensely fluorescent cells ('SIF' cells) which contain many peptides, thought to act as modulators and transmitters at synaptic sites. Substance P, vasoactive intestinal peptide (VIP), encephalins, and somatostatin have all been identified in autonomic ganglia although their precise role in control of nerve transmission is not yet known.

The previously held distinction between cholinergic and catecholaminergic cells, underlying the dual hypothesis of antagonism in the autonomic nervous system, is no longer tenable. Immature ganglion cells in culture contain both acetylcholine and catecholamines. Sympathetic ganglia have about 45 per cent of acetylcholine-containing neurons in which non-adrenergic, non-cholinergic ('NANC') transmission is now accepted. Within any central pathway there is no simple consistency of a single transmitter and some cells have multiple transmitters: posterior root ganglion cells, for example, have been found to have as many as 10 neuropeptides and putative transmitters. After birth, sweat glands change from adrenergic to cholinergic sympathetic innervation, whereas innervation of some gut structures is switched from sympathetic to cholinergic mechanisms. Presynaptic cholinergic endings may affect noradrenergic sympathetic transmission, and noradrenaline may act not only directly as a transmitter but indirectly by modulating the effect of acetylcholine, as has been shown peripherally where small doses of adrenaline and noradrenaline facilitate transmission but larger doses inhibit it.

Central control of the autonomic nervous system

The hypothalamus can be considered the 'highest' level of integration of autonomic function. It remains under the influence of the cortex and the group of structures known as the 'limbic system', which includes the olfactory areas, the hippocampus and amygdaloid complex, the cingulate cortex, and the septal area. These regions of the brain regulate the hypothalamus and are critical for emotional and affective expression. In phylogenetic development the limbic system represents the older or palaeomammalian cortex as opposed to the neomammalian cortex. Its function is thought to be concerned with levels below cognitive behaviour and inductive and deductive reasoning, though it nevertheless is concerned with a feeling of individuality and identity. It analyses the significance of the input of sensation to the organism in relation to the instinctive drives which promote the perpetuation of the individual by satisfying hunger, thirst, and sexual needs.

The hypothalamus is also concerned with maintaining homeostasis against a changing environment and ensures the propagation of the species by sexual and parental drives which can at times override the more selfish self-perpetuating drives of the individual. The essence of its function is choice of patterns of bahaviour based on sensory information. As it overlaps both with sensory and motor systems it is essential for many aspects of memory and learning. The autonomic nervous system and many metabolic functions are under the control of the limbic system by means of nerve centres, many of which are situated in the hypothalamus, lying ventrally to the thalamus and constituting the floor of the third ventricle. The hypothalamus contains a large number of scattered ganglion cells, which have been differentiated into a number of nuclei (Appenzeller and Oribe 1997).

The hypothalamus controls the autonomic nervous system in two ways, by means of the pituitary and hence other endocrine glands and by direct descending nervous pathways. Despite these descending pathways, some regions of the brainstem are to some extent autonomous and function in animals after pontine section of the brainstem. These include cardiac and respiratory function and 'centres' for vomiting and micturition, but under natural circumstances cardiovascular responses never occur in isolation but accompany the processes of exercise, digestion, sexual function, and temperature regulation. The integration of these changes takes place in the hypothalamus. The main course taken by descending sympathetic fibres from the hypothalamus is uncrossed and by way of the lateral tegmentum of the brainstem and lateral medullary formation. Some fibres end directly on the intermediolateral column cells, while others synapse in the reticular formation.

Diseases of the autonomic nervous system

The lesions of the nervous system in autonomic failure, with their widespread consequences, are, in Claude Bernard's terms, 'real experiments by which physicians and physiologists profit'. Some may complain that nature is an imprecise experimentalist! The study of individuals with rare disorders can sometimes throw much light on the subtle and complex integration of the autonomic nervous system. A recent example is the relatively recently described disease with a specific enzyme fault, dopamine β-hydroxylase deficiency (Chapter 40). The syndromes of chronic autonomic failure also offer an example of the system degenerations which are so common in neurology and are yet so baffling. We need to find some common biological basis for this curious selective vulnerability. If we can do this, we shall be closer to finding an effective treatment, not only for these particular diseases but possibly also for a wider range of disabling progressive degenerative diseases of the nervous system.

The systematic application of physiological techniques of study to patients with autonomic failure started in the 1960s. Research interest in postural hypotension, the usual presenting symptom of autonomic failure, was stimulated by its occurrence after the weightlessness of space travel. Since then there have been striking advances in the investigation and classification of the syndromes of autonomic failure which were until recently both confused and confusing.

Peripheral neuropathies with an autonomic component have long been recognized, particularly in diabetes, alcoholism, and amyloidosis. Sharpey-Schafer and Taylor (1960) showed that the sympathetic vasoconstrictor pathway to the hands was intact in diabetic autonomic neuropathy, and they therefore attributed the absence of circulatory reflexes and the postural hypotension to an afferent lesion. Though an afferent lesion could not be excluded, their interpretation was probably incorrect because the sympathetic efferent pathway to resistance vessels is often defective in diabetes and the patchiness of lesions on the efferent side is now appreciated.

A large section of this book is concerned with the chronic or primary neurological disorders in which the autonomic nervous system is selectively involved by both pre- and postganglionic neuronal degeneration (Shy and Drager 1960; Johnson *et al.* 1966; Bannister *et al.* 1967). Some might doubt the worth of such serious attention given to rare diseases but there are many precedents to show that just such studies of rare disease often lead to the recognition of an entirely new group of disorders of which other examples then are found. It is certain that the detailed study of these diseases by the extensive biochemical, physiological and histochemical techniques now available has yielded a rich harvest of knowledge, much of it unexpected, which can now be applied more widely.

The detailed studies of autonomic failure are complemented by the sections of the book which are devoted to particular diseases such as diabetes mellitus (Chapter 39) in which autonomic disturbances occur sooner or later. Diabetes is overwhelmingly more common than other forms of autonomic dysfunction, and rapid advances have been made now such that the methods of testing, most of which were pioneered in relation to autonomic failure, are being applied to the even more complex disturbances in diabetes. There are also other large groups of patients with autonomic symptoms; first, patients with parkinsonian symptoms who may have MSA; second, the elderly; and third, patients on drugs which affect autonomic function.

First symptoms of autonomic failure

Most forms of autonomic failure are insidious in their onset, with mild symptoms which are concealed for years because of autonomic or other compensatory mechanisms. As Cannon (1929) pointed out, this system can respond to many and varied stresses from the internal and external environment in ways which conceal its dysfunction. When man first took it upon himself millions of years ago to stand on his two legs he imposed great strains on the cardiovascular control needed to protect him against the effect of pooling of blood in the lower extremities. Postural hypotension occurring in emotional syncope raises the intriguing teleological question of whether it has evolutionary significance in avoiding danger by a sudden fall into the horizontal position and the simulation of death. However, a true fainting attack such as vasovagal syncope, as opposed to other causes of transient loss of consciousness, requires an intact autonomic nervous system, although persistent postural hypotension is the cardinal feature of autonomic failure. Patients may start with mild symptoms of vague weakness, postural dizziness, or faintness, which can very easily be overlooked, or result in erroneous referral to a psychiatrist or cardiologist. The crux of the diagnosis is the measurement of blood pressure when standing rather than lying, still often neglected, which can, like the tip of an iceberg, reveal a much more complex underlying autonomic disturbance. In certain circumstances postural hypotension may be unmasked by food, alcohol, or exercise (see Chapter 20). The blood pressure control mechanisms at the lower end of the scale are just as elaborate and fascinating as those which cause the more commonly studied problems of hypertension, though the study of these patients with *hypotension* has in fact thrown light on the mechanisms of *hypertension.*

Some patients with autonomic failure first have urinary bladder symptoms or impotence, not postural hypotension. In addition to the group of patients with autonomic failure alone, 'pure autonomic failure', there is a second group of patients that may present with symptoms of autonomic failure but within months also develop other neurological symptoms, usually with parkinsonism or cerebellar manifestations. However, there may be subtle features which suggest that the parkinsonism is atypical, with a predominance of rigidity and akinesis over tremor, or the presence of mild pyramidal signs. Such parkinsonian patients may develop marked postural hypotension when treated with levodopa or may fail to respond to this drug. Some may have additional bulbar involvement. These features raise the possibility of more widespread involvement of the central nervous system and point to the diagnosis of multiple system atrophy.

Classification

In this chapter an historical approach to classification has been followed. Recently this classification and nomenclature of the primary autonomic failure syndromes has been confirmed by a Consensus Panel of international clinicians and scientists convened by the American Autonomic Society and co-sponsored by the American Academy of Neurology, (Consensus statement 1996). It is discussed further in Chapter 31.

Accurate diagnosis is essential for proper management of autonomic failure (AF) but in attempting to classify autonomic disease there is a philosophical point to be borne in mind. As in much of medicine, we use a mixed diagnostic classification. There are localized (Table 1) and more generalized disorders (Table 2); drugs are an important cause of autonomic dysfunction (Table 3). We have a list of diseases of largely known pathology such as diabetes and we make a diagnosis of 'secondary' autonomic failure when abnormal tests in life point to a structural disturbance of autonomic reflexes and pathways in patients with a specific disease. Other patients, without certainly known pathology in common, share certain autonomic symptoms and, from tests in life and observation of similar patients after death, we choose to use the word 'primary' disease (Table 2). In such patients tests can hardly be said to prove a disease but this is the only way we can place patients in different categories and hope, by research to locate the lesions more precisely and hence improve their treatment.

Autonomic fibres are also damaged secondarily in a variety of medical disorders, most commonly in diabetes and alcoholism, but also in a wide range of acute, subacute, and chronic peripheral neuropathies (see Table 2). This is discussed later (Chapter 38).

We can now consider the more complex problem of the classification of the group of patients in whom autonomic failure appears to result from a primary or unexplained selective neuronal degeneration. This may occur in a 'pure' form without any other neurological signs. Or, it may occur in association with two quite different degenerations of the nervous system, multiple system atrophy and Parkinson's disease.

Historically, the first reported cases of autonomic failure were described by Bradbury and Eggleston (1925) as 'idiopathic orthostatic hypotension' because of their presenting feature. This term is misleading because it stresses only one feature of autonomic failure and ignores the more usually associated neurological disturbances of urinary bladder control, sexual function, and sweating, and also because the word 'idiopathic' implies that it is a single disease entity, which though probable is not proven. The term 'pure autonomic failure' (PAF) is now generally accepted for this syndrome.

Two cases now recognized as autonomic failure with multiple system atrophy (MSA) were described by Shy and Drager in 1960 and it is appropriate to quote from their original description.

"The full syndrome comprises the following features: orthostatic hypotension, urinary and rectal incontinence, loss of sweating, iris atrophy, external ocular palsies, rigidity, tremor, loss of associated movements, impotence, the findings of an atonic bladder and loss of rectal sphincter tone, fasciculations, wasting of distal muscles, evidence of a neuropathic lesion in the electromyogram that suggests involvement of the anterior horn cells, and the finding of a neuropathic lesion in the muscle biopsy. The date of onset is usually in the 5th to 7th decade of life."

Though they noted degeneration of the intermediolateral column cells in their pathological report, credit for first specifically linking this with the presenting features of postural hypotension rests with Johnson et al. (1966). At this stage olivopontocerebellar atrophy had not been linked with autonomic failure.

Autonomic failure was also described in patients with otherwise apparently typical Parkinson's disease (PD) (Fichefet et al. 1965; Vanderhaegen et al. 1970). Such cases pathologically had hyaline eosinophilic cytoplasmic neuronal inclusions known as Lewy bodies, also present in PD (see Chapters 33 and 34). It is an important fact that Lewy bodies, some of which may contain, apart from neurofilament proteins and ubiquitin, catecholamine degeneration products, are usually also found in the brains of patients with PAF, without parkinsonian features, but very rarely in patients with MSA. This evidence, discussed below, tends to separate patients with autonomic failure into two groups: first, pathologically proven-MSA without Lewy bodies and second, PAF, and AF with PD, with Lewy bodies.

It must be recognized that at an early stage an accurate prognosis of primary autonomic failure cannot be given. It may remain as PAF for a few years, relatively static, or in time it may also come to be associated either with PD or MSA; with care the earliest features of the other condition may be detected clinically. Conversely, the earliest features of autonomic failure may be detected later in some patients with PD or MSA. For example, Miyazaki (1978) has shown that careful study of cases of non-familial olivopontocerebellar atrophy with significant postural hypotension shows a high incidence of urinary, pyramidal, and extrapyramidal symptoms and signs, whereas familial cases, without postural hypotension, very rarely have these additional features.

There is evidence that virtually all patients with primary autonomic failure as opposed to secondary autonomic failure, studied at

post-mortem, have severe loss of intermediolateral column cells, the final common pathway cell for the sympathetic nervous system (See Chapter 33). It is becoming more probable that the pathological process, whether viral, biochemical, immunological, or of some other kind, that leads to this loss of intermediolateral column cells differs significantly in PAF, (and probably in autonomic failure with PD), from that in autonomic failure with MSA. In PAF there appears to be an additional loss of ganglionic neurons (see Chapter 34) which are relatively intact in MSA. This suggests the existence of a more distal process in PAF than in MSA. The hypothesis that at least one of the lesions in PAF is also more distal accords with the evidence that, in general, plasma noradrenaline levels are lower in PAF than in MSA (see Chapter 20). This view now finds support from recent neuro-endocrine studies (Kimber et al. 1997) and magnetic resonance imaging (MRI) and positron emission tomography (PET) brain scans of patients with PAF which have failed to show evidence of central lesions (see Chapter 32).

When considering the effects of treatment, so that like is compared with like, it is vital to diagnose patients as precisely as possible on the basis of physiological, pharmacological, biochemical, and neuro-imaging findings, even though the ultimate criterion of diagnosis is the post-mortem pathological findings. Moreover, it seems probable that there are a number of different types of sympathetic terminal dysfunction in autonomic failure, which may be the consequence of pathological processes that differ in degree or kind (Nanda et al. 1977; Bannister et al. 1979; Man in't Veld et al. 1987; Mathias et al. 1990). Just as the defects of nicotinic and muscarinic receptors in human disease have proved to be far more complex than ever was expected (Bannister and Hoyes 1981), it is probable that disturbances of sympathetic receptors will also prove at least as complex (Fraser et al. 1981).

The evaluation and accurate diagnosis of the cause of autonomic symptoms is necessary in order to plan treatment. Even if specific treatment is not available this evaluation will make it easier to manage the patient in such a way that the quality of life can be maintained for as long as possible.

Table 1. Examples of localized autonomic disorders*

Holmes—Adie Pupil
Horner's syndrome
Crocodile tears (Bogorad's syndrome)
Gustatory sweating (Frey's syndrome)
Reflex sympathetic dystrophy
Idiopathic palmar/axillary hyperhidrosis
Chagas' disease (*Trypanosomiasis Cruzi*)#
Surgical procedures*   – Sympathectomy—regional   – Vagotomy and gastric drainage procedures in 'dumping syndrome'   – Organ transplantation—heart, lungs

* Surgery may cause some of the disorders listed above (such as Frey's syndrome following parotid surgery).

Listed here as it targets intrinsic cholinergic plexuses in the heart and gut.

Adapted from Mathias (1996)

Table 2. Classification of disorders resulting in autonomic dysfunction*

Primary (Aetiology unknown)
Acute/subacute dysautonomias
    Pure cholinergic dysautonomia
    Pure pandysautonomia
    Pandysautonomia with neurological features

Chronic autonomic failure syndromes
    Pure autonomic failure
    Multiple system atrophy (Shy-Drager syndrome)
    Autonomic failure with Parkinson's disease

Secondary
Congenital
    Nerve growth factor deficiency

Hereditary
    Autosomal dominant trait
        Familial amyloid neuropathy
        Porphyria

    Autosomal recessive trait
        Familial dysautonomia—Riley-Day syndrome
        Dopamine β-hydroxylase deficiency
        Aromatic L-amino acid decarboxylase deficiency

    X-linked recessive
        Fabry's disease

Metabolic diseases
    Diabetes mellitus
    Chronic renal failure
    Chronic liver disease
    Vitamin B_{12} deficiency
    Alcohol-induced

Inflammatory
    Guillain-Barré syndrome
    Transverse myelitis

Infections
    Bacterial—Tetanus
    Viral—human immuno-deficiency virus infection
    Parasitic—Trypanosomiasis Cruzi; Chagas' disease
    Prion—fatal familial insomnia

Neoplasia
    Brain tumours—especially of third ventricle or posterior fossa
    Paraneoplastic, to include adenocarcinomas—lung, pancreas and Lambert-Eaton syndrome

Connective tissue disorders
    Rheumatoid arthritis
    Systemic lupus erythematosus
    Mixed connective tissue disease

Surgery
    Regional sympathectomy—upper limb, splanchnic
    Vagotomy and drainage procedures—'dumping syndrome'
    Organ transplantation—heart, kidney

Trauma
    Spinal cord transection

Table 2. (*continued*)

Neurally mediated syncope
    Vasovagal syncope
    Carotid sinus hypersensitivity
    Micturition syncope
    Cough syncope
    Swallow syncope
    Associated with glossopharyngeal neuralgia

Drugs, chemicals, poisons and toxins
    See Table 3

*Adapted from Mathias (1996)

Table 3. Drugs, chemicals, poisons and toxins causing autonomic dysfunction*

Decreasing sympathetic activity
    Centrally acting
        Clonidine
        Methyldopa
        Reserpine
        Barbiturates
        Anaesthetics

    Peripherally acting
        Sympathetic nerve ending (guanethidine, bethanadine)
        α-adrenoceptor blockade (phenoxybenzamine)
        β-adrenoceptor blockade (propranolol)

Increasing sympathetic activity
    Amphetamines
    Releasing noradrenaline (tyramine)
    Uptake blockers (imipramine)
    Monoamine oxidase-A inhibitors (tranylcypromine)
    β-adrenoceptor stimulants (isoprenaline)

Decreasing parasympathetic activity
    Antidepressants (imipramine)
    Tranquillisers (phenothiazines)
    Antidysrhythmics (disopyramide)
    Anticholinergics (atropine, probanthine, benztropine)
    Toxins (botulinum)

Increasing parasympathetic activity
    Cholinomimetics (carbachol, bethanechol, pilocarpine, mushroom poisoning)
    Anticholinesterases
        Reversible carbonate inhibitors (pyridostigmine, neostigmine)
        Organophosphorus inhibitors (parathion)

Miscellaneous
    Alcohol, thiamine (vitamin B_1 deficiency)
    Vincristine, perhexiline maleate
    Thallium, arsenic, mercury

*Adapted from Mathias (1996). Also see Chapter 54.

References

Appenzeller, O. and Oribe, E. (1997). *The autonomic nervous system* (5th edn). Elsevier, Amsterdam.

Bannister, R., and Hoyes, A. D. (1981). Generalised smooth-muscle disease with defective muscarinic receptor function. *Br. Med. J.* 282, 1015–18.

Bannister, R., Ardill, L., and Fentem, P. (1967). Defective autonomic control of blood vessels in idiopathic orthostatic hypotension. *Brain* 90, 725–46.

Bannister, R., Davies, I. B., Holly, E., Rosenthal, T., and Sever, P. (1979). Defective cardiovascular reflexes and supersensitivity to sympathomimetic drugs in autonomic failure. *Brain* 102, 163–76.

Bradbury, S., and Eggleston, C. (1925). Postural hypotension: a report of three cases. *Am. Heart J.* 1, 73–86.

Cannon, W. B. (1929). Organisation for physiological homeostasis. *Physiol. Rev.* 9, 399–431.

Cannon, W. B., and Rosenblueth, A. (1949). *The supersensitivity of denervated structures: a law of denervation.* MacMillan, New York.

Consensus statement on the definition of orthostatic hypotension, pure autonomic failure and multiple system atrophy. (1996). *Clin. Aut. Res.* 6, 125–6.

Fichefet, J. P., Sternon, J. E., Franken, L., Demanet, J. C., and Vanderhaegen, J. J. (1965). Etude anatomo-clinique d'un cas d'hypotension orthostatique 'idiopathique'. Considerations pathogenique. *Acta Cardiol.* 20, 332–48.

Fraser, C. M., Venter, J. C., and Kaliner, M. (1981). Autonomic abnormalities and auto-antibodies to beta-adrenergic receptors. *New Engl. J. Med.* 305, 1165–70.

Jänig, W. (1995). In *Physiologie des menschen* (Ed. R. F. Schmidt and G. Thews), 26th edn, pp. 340–69, Springer Verlag, Heidelberg, Berlin.

Johnson, R. H., Lee, G. de J., Oppenheimer, D. R., and Spalding, J. M. K. (1966). Autonomic failure with orthostatic hypotension due to intermediolateral column degeneration. *Quart. J. Med.* 35, 276–92.

Kimber, J. R., Watson, L., and Mathias, C. J. (1997). Distinction of idiopathic Parkinson's disease from multiple system atrophy by stimulation of growth hormone release with clonidine. *Lancet* 349, 1877–81.

Man in't Veld, A. J., Boomsa, H., Moleman, P., and Schalekamp, M. A. D. H. (1987). Congenital dopamine-beta-hydroxylase deficiency: a novel orthostatic syndrome. *Lancet* i, 183–7.

Mathias, C. J., Bannister, R., Cortelli, P., Heslop, K., Polak, J. M., Raimbach, S., Springall, D. R., and Watson, L. (1990). Clinical, autonomic and therapeutic observations in two siblings with postural hypotension and sympathetic failure due to an inability to synthesize noradrenaline from dopamine because of a deficiency of dopamine beta hydroxylase. *Quart. J. Med.*, New Series 75, 617–33.

Mathias, C. J. (1995). Autonomic neuropathy—aspects of diagnosis and management. In *Peripheral nerve disorders 2*, (eds. A. K. Asbury and P. K. Thomas), pp. 95–117. Butterworth-Heinemann, Oxford.

Mathias, C. J. (1996). Disorders of the autonomic nervous system. In *Neurology in clinical practice*, (2nd edn), (eds. W. G. Bradley, R. B. Daroff, G. M. Fenichel, and C. D. Marsden), pp. 1953–81. Butterworth-Heinemann, Boston.

Miyazaki, M. (1978). Shy-Drager syndrome-a nosological entity? In *International symposium on spinocerebellar degenerations*. Medical Research Foundation, Tokyo.

Nanda, R. N., Boyle, R. C., Gillespie, J. S., Johnson, R. H., Keogh, H. J. (1977). Idiopathic orthostatic hypotension from failure of noradrenaline release in a patient with vasomotor innervation. *J. Neurol. Neurosurg. Psychiat.* 40, 11–19.

Sharpey-Schafter, E. P., and Taylor, P. J. (1960). Absent circulatory reflexes in diabetic neuritis. *Lancet* i, 559–62.

Shy, G. M., and Drager, G. A. (1960) A neurological syndrome associated with orthostatic hypotension. *Arch. Neurol., Chicago* 3, 5511–27.

Vanderhaegen, J. J., Perier, O., and Sternon, J. E. (1970). Pathological findings in idiopathic orthostatic hypotension: its relationship with Parkinson's disease. *Arch. Neurol., Chicago* 22, 207–14.

Historical perspectives on the autonomic nervous system—with a particular emphasis on chemical neurotransmission

E. M. Tansey

Understanding what we now call the autonomic nervous system, its normal functioning, and the role of its various components, is clearly fundamental to the investigation and treatment of the dysfunction of that system. This chapter will review briefly how our present-day knowledge has developed, focusing particularly on the discovery and impact of chemical neurotransmission in the autonomic nervous system.

First of all, a note about terminology. The creation, and use, of new words, new definitions, and new classifications are proper, and important, parts of scientific endeavour and exemplify the discovery of new facts and the development of fresh concepts. The autonomic nervous system is no exception, indeed the very expression 'autonomic nervous system' was not known before 1898, when, in a paper about the superior cervical ganglion, the Cambridge physiologist J. N. Langley, wrote:

> I propose to substitute the word 'autonomic' [for the word visceral] … The word implies a certain degree of independent action, but exercised under control of a higher power. The 'autonomic' nervous system means the nervous system of the glands and of the involuntary muscle; it governs the 'organic' functions of the body.

The term did not receive immediate or overwhelming acceptance, and for some years other expressions were current—as will be noted

ON THE UNION OF CRANIAL AUTONOMIC (VISCERAL) FIBRES WITH THE NERVE CELLS OF THE SUPERIOR CERVICAL GANGLION. By J. N. LANGLEY, D.Sc., F.R.S., *Fellow of Trinity College, Cambridge.*

CONTENTS.

Title of the article in which the word 'autonomic' was first used, from J. N. Langley (1898) (reproduced, with permission of the Physiological Society, from *Journal of Physiology* 23, 240.)

below the words 'sympathy' and 'sympathetics', often used for the entire autonomic system, have a long history, and 'vegetative' and 'involuntary' were used well into the twentieth century. Throughout the present chapter, unless clearly contraindicated, the expression 'autonomic nervous system' will be used, although its use to refer to the system before 1898 is anachronistic.

Sympathy and the sympathetics

Before the nineteenth century, knowledge about the autonomic nervous system was almost completely derived from anatomical studies of animals, and after the Renaissance increasingly from human dissections. From dissections of apes and pigs, and possibly from observations on the wounded gladiators he attended as a physician, Galen (129–216) described a ganglionic (sympathetic) chain, which he thought arose from the brain, and the white rami communicantes. For over 1000 years his account, rigidly maintained by medical and religious authorities, was accepted. Challenges and additions by later anatomists included those by Thomas Willis (1621–1675), who described the vagus or 'wandering nerves' and named the ganglionic nerves the 'intercostal nerves', and Jacobus Winslow (1669–1760), who agreed with Willis that the ganglia were 'small brains', although he introduced the term 'great sympathetic nerve' instead of the 'intercostal nerves'. The French anatomist François Xavier Bichat (1771–1802) distinguished between the somatic and visceral functions of the nervous system, and also acknowledged the influence of emotions on the visceral system. However, elucidation of the function of these components was patchy: Willis sectioned the vagus of a dog and observed that the heart fluttered; the French surgeon François Poerfour de Petit (1664–1741) noted that cutting the cervical sympathetic nerves affected pupil size and the nictating membrane; and the dedication of his later compatriots to the guillotine permitted Albert Regnard and Paul Loye (1861–1890) to stimulate the vagus of a decapitated criminal and observe the appearance, 45 minutes after execution, of gastric juice on the inner surface of the stomach.

Nerves and nets

By the middle of the nineteenth century more elaborate anatomical and functional studies were under way. The development and informed use of microscopes encouraged the examination of numerous organs and tissues, including those of the autonomic nervous system. Robert Remak (1815–1865) discovered unmyelinated sympathetic fibres, and that nerve fibres arose from ganglion cells, collections of which he found in the heart and bladder; and the laborious quantitative work of Friedrich Bidder (1810–1894) and Alfred Wilhelm Volkmann (1800–1877) revealed that postganglionic fibres were more numerous than preganglionic fibres. Physiological experiments increasingly revealed functional aspects of the system: Bidder showed that curare did not inhibit autonomic control of the heart or intestine; Benedict Stilling (1810–1879) coined the expression 'vasomotor system' for the autonomic fibres to the muscle fibres in vessel walls; and Claude Bernard (1813–1878) produced vasodilation by sectioning the sympathetic nerve, whereas Edouard Brown-Séquard (1817–1894) stimulated the cut end to obtain vasoconstriction. Perhaps more startling were the experiments of Ernst Heinrich Weber (1795–1878) and his brother Eduard (1806–1871), who reported that vagal stimulation stopped the heart, thus introducing into neurophysiology the concept of inhibition.

Critical debates raged, in the final decades of the nineteenth century, about the detailed structure of the nervous system. The Italian anatomist Camillo Golgi (1844–1926) maintained that the nervous system was a complex net-like structure, a reticulum; whereas the Spaniard Santiago Ramon y Cajal (1852–1934) proposed that each nerve cell was an independent unit, the neurone. The two men shared the Nobel Prize for Physiology or Medicine in 1906, both firmly wedded to their irreconcilable views. Improvements in histological techniques produced a mounting body of evidence supporting the neurone theory, which posed problems about the transfer of information between nerve cells, and between nerve and effector cells. The physiological implications of this were clearly recognized by Charles Sherrington (1857–1952), then investigating the reflex activities of the nervous system, and in 1897 he proposed the word 'synapse' to describe the region between functional units of the nervous system. Physiological investigations of the autonomic nervous system were to reveal much about the properties of synapses.

'Like reading an account of the circulation before Harvey'

Just before the Second World War, the eminent neurologist Walter Langdon-Brown (1870–1946) declared that 'to read an account of [the autonomic nervous] system before Gaskell is like reading an account of the circulation before Harvey'. Who then was Gaskell, and what were his contributions? Walter Gaskell (1847–1914) was a Cambridge physiologist whose work elucidated much of the anatomical complexity of the system, his outstanding contribution being the clear delineation, both morphologically and functionally, of the two major nervous outflows, the thoracolumbar (sympathetic) and craniosacral (parasympathetic). In 1886 he wrote, somewhat prophetically,

> The evidence is becoming daily stronger that every tissue is innervated by two sets of nerve fibres of opposite characters so that I look forward hopefully to the time when the whole nervous system shall be mapped out … into two great divisions of the nervous system which are occupied with chemical changes of a synthetical and analytical character respectively, which therefore

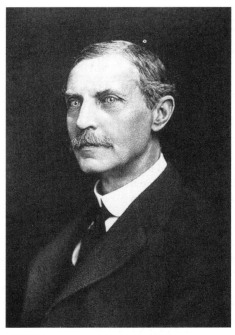

J. N. Langley (1852–1925) (reproduced, with permission of the Physiological Society, from *Journal of Physiology* (1926) **62**, facing p. 1).

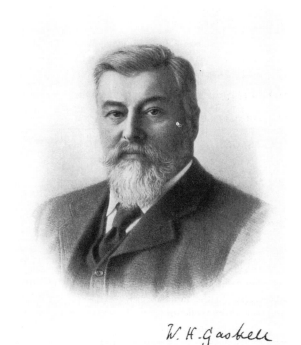

Walter H. Gaskell (1847–1914) (reproduced, with permisson, from Sir Humphrey Rolleston, *The Cambridge Medical School: a biographical history*, Cambridge University Press (1932), facing p. 95).

in their actions must show the characteristic signs of such opposite chemical processes.

His work provided the morphological base for all subsequent studies on what Gaskell himself continued to call the 'visceral' or 'involuntary' nervous system. His close colleague, J. N. Langley (1852–1925), devoted a substantial part of his career to investigating the distribution and function of the system, largely accepting Gaskell's differentiation although he regarded the nerve cells of the gastrointestinal tract's plexuses as a distinct, third, component of the autonomic nervous system, the 'enteric nervous system'.

In 1878 Langley started to use drugs as investigative tools, examining the effects of pilocarpine and atropine on the secretion of saliva from the submaxillary gland. Their opposing effects, stimulating and inhibitory, suggested to him that there was a mutual exclusivity in their action which came about through some form of chemical interaction. He proposed that 'there is some substance or substances in the nerve endings or gland cells with which both atropine and pilocarpine are capable of forming compounds'.

Langley also applied chemicals directly to autonomic ganglia with a paintbrush, and discovered that nicotine caused facilitation of the neural impulse, closely followed by paralysis. This became a useful tool for dissecting out what he was able to distinguish, physiologically, as the preganglionic and postganglionic component parts of the system, and the results accelerated his interest in the specific and selective actions of the drugs *per se*. Langley provided pharmacological confirmation of Gaskell's anatomical divisions of the system, and developed a theoretical account of the interactions between ganglion cells and chemicals. In 1905 he postulated the existence of 'receptive substances' between the nerve and the cell of the effective organ, activated by the arrival of the neural impulse at the nerve ending, thus, Langley argued, making the presynaptic release of specific chemicals unnecessary for the transmission of the neural effect.

From ergot to acetylcholine, via adrenaline

Two of Gaskell and Langley's students, Henry Dale (1875–1968) and Thomas Elliott (1877–1961), made the next important observations, although the significance of their findings were not recognized at the time. Elliott showed that stimulation of the hypogastric nerve could be mimicked by the application of adrenaline, and when, in 1904, he presented his results to the Physiological Society, he suggested 'adrenaline might then be the substance liberated when the nervous stimulus reaches the periphery'. Precisely *what* he meant by this ambiguous statement is unclear, although it has been interpreted as the first definitive proposal of chemical neurotransmission. It can be understood, with the benefit of hindsight, to suggest that adrenaline might be released from the nerve endings in response to the passage of a nervous impulse. At the same time his Cambridge contemporary Henry Dale was at the Wellcome Physiological Research Laboratories, working, at the suggestion of Henry Wellcome, on the pharmacology of extracts of ergot, then used in obstetric practice to reduce post-partum haemorrhage. Doing similar physiological experiments to those of Elliott, Dale observed that his preparation of ergot reversed the effects of splanchnic nerve stimulation *and* reversed the effect of adrenaline. This evidence corroborated Elliott's findings of close sim-

PROCEEDINGS

OF THE

PHYSIOLOGICAL SOCIETY,

May 21, 1904.

On the action of adrenalin. By T. R. ELLIOTT.
(*Preliminary communication.*)

Title of T. R. Elliott's 1904 Communication to the Physiological Society, showing that stimulation of the hypogastric nerve could be mimicked by the application of adrenaline. (Taken with permission of the Physiological Society, from *Journal of Physiology* (1904) **31**).

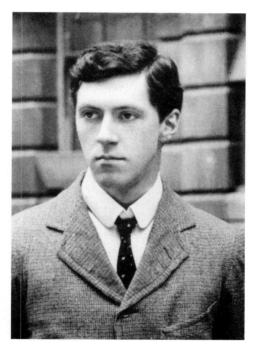

Henry Hallett Dale (1876–1968), aged 27. Reproduced from a photograph of 'The medical firm of Dr Samuel Gee, St Bartholomew's Hospital, 1902' from the archives of the Royal College of Physicians of London, with permission).

ilarities between sympathetic nerve stimulation and the application of adrenaline. Dale recognized that his ergot derivative had, somehow, paralysed 'the structures which adrenaline stimulates', although like Elliott he was unable, or unwilling, to provide a hypothesis to explain the phenomenon. However, the experiments encouraged Dale to investigate the action of chemicals on the autonomic nervous system further, which he continued to do for the rest of his entire scientific career. With the chemist George Barger (1878–1939), he started a detailed chemical and physiological study of chemicals structurally related to adrenaline. Barger synthesized the amines in his lab, and Dale tested their physiological effects. Over a period of nearly 3 years the two men examined more than 50 compounds, for which they invented the word 'sympathomimetic' to indicate mimicry of the effects of stimulation of the sympathetic nervous system. They identified one derivative in particular, called noradrenaline, as a potent sympathomimetic, but failed to investigate it thoroughly, the chemical then being known as merely a laboratory product and not a naturally occurring compound. In 1913 Dale published an elegant dissection, and discussion, of the two major actions of adrenaline— vasoconstriction, the normally predominating effect that accounted for the pressor response, and the contrary effect of vasodilatation when a lower dose was applied—but he was unable to clarify this difference. In private correspondence, Dale referred to this as 'the central mystery' of the sympathetic nervous system, and it was to plague investigators, and investigations, for many years. Efforts to explain how one chemical could bring about such apparently opposite effects gave rise to at least one convoluted theoretical account, the sympathin E and sympathin I story, as will be described below. That paper marked Dale's final major contribution to the study of transmitter candidates in the sympathetic nervous system, and it was his change of research direction, towards the parasympathetic nervous system, especially after the First World War, that was ultimately to provide a substantial body of evidence for chemical neurotransmission.

The stage is set

Dale's personal research work concentrated on the identification of acetylcholine as the chemical neurotransmitter in the parasympathetic system, and later at the neuromuscular junction of the peripheral nervous system. Acetylcholine was first synthesized in 1867, but not until 40 years later was a detailed study made of its pharmacological activities, by Reid Hunt (1870–1948). Hunt investigated choline, which caused a lowering of blood pressure in the experimental animal, and several of its chemical derivatives, and demonstrated that, of a range of 19 synthetic chemicals, acetylcholine had an even more effective depressor activity than choline. Writing in 1906, Hunt suggested:

> [Acetylcholine] is a substance of extraordinary activity. In fact, I think it safe to state that, as regards its effect upon the circulation, it is the most powerful substance known. It is one hundred thousand times more active than choline, and hundreds of times more active than nitro-glycerine; it is a hundred times more active in causing a fall of blood-pressure than is adrenaline in causing a rise.

He never succeeded in isolating the compound from any animal tissue, and, like noradrenaline, acetylcholine was known only as an artificial compound for many years. Even the therapeutic possibilities of using this effective chemical were severely limited because its depressor effects, although profound, were extremely transitory. This problem, of acetylcholine's powerful but evanescent activity, was to cause both experimental and interpretative difficulties for many years.

Naturally occurring acetylcholine was first isolated by Henry Dale in 1913, in what he considered to be one of the luckiest incidents of his career. A sample of an obstetric ergot preparation was sent to Dale

for routine physiological investigation. Injection into the vein of an anaesthetized cat caused immediate and intense inhibition of the heartbeat, from which the animal rapidly recovered. A further demonstration convinced Dale that the ergot was contaminated with an unusual depressor constituent that resembled the effects of muscarine. Muscarine, from the mushroom *Amanita muscaria*, caused slowing of the heart beat, similar to vagal stimulation. But the effects Dale observed were, unlike those of muscarine, very short-lasting and, recalling Hunt's work, Dale suggested to a chemist colleague, Arthur Ewins (1882–1957), that the mystery substance might be acetylcholine. Ewins rapidly confirmed that identification, and isolated acetylcholine from ergot, an important impetus to further work on its actions. Dale himself started a detailed physiological study in which he clearly distinguished the two principal effects of acetylcholine: one that could be reproduced by injections of muscarine, and one imitated by nicotine.

Writing in 1938, Dale summed up the situation just before the First World War:

> Such was the position in 1914. Two substances [adrenaline and acetylcholine] were known, with actions very suggestively reproducing those of the two main divisions of the autonomic nervous system; both, for different reasons, were very unstable in the body, and their actions were in consequence of a fleeting character; and one of them [adrenaline] was already known to occur as a natural hormone. These properties would fit them very precisely to act as mediators of the effects of autonomic impulses to effector cells, if there were any acceptable evidence of liberation at the nerve endings. The actors were named, and the parts allotted; a preliminary hint of the plot had, indeed, been given ten years earlier, and almost forgotten; but only direct and unequivocal evidence could ring up the curtain, and this was not to come till 1921.

The curtain rises

There were two main approaches to the further identification of a likely transmitter candidate: the type of work that Dale and Elliott had performed at the beginning of the century, observing the effects of applied chemicals and noting their correlation with endogenous neural stimulation. The second method was to attempt to recover and characterize a chemical after neural stimulation. Both techniques were adopted by the Austrian pharmacologist Otto Loewi (1873–1961), who, in 1921, reported the results of the experiment that 'could ring up the curtain', now regarded as a classic in the history of neurotransmission. It was seemingly simple: the beating hearts were removed from two frogs, and placed in separate irrigation chambers. Electrical stimulation of the vagal nerves to one heart caused a slowing, then a cessation, of the heart beat. Using a syringe, the fluid bathing the first heart was transferred into the chamber surrounding the second, still beating, heart, causing this also to slow and stop. Loewi claimed that this was strong evidence for the transfer of a chemical substance, released upon neural stimulation of the first heart, into the chamber containing the second heart. Similar experiments, stimulating sympathetic nerves to the first heart, produced a stimulatory effect that was transferable with the surrounding fluid. Loewi proposed the release, by neural stimulation, of two substances *Vagusstoff* (released by vagal, parasympathetic stimulation) and *Acceleransstoff* (released by sympathetic stimulation). These experiments were not, however, uncontroversial, and critics pointed to several inconsistencies and difficulties. Loewi began detailed chemical examinations and gradually the similarity of the *accelerans* substance to adrenaline was recognized, and further evidence was accrued that *vagusstoff* was a choline ester, similar to acetylcholine, rapidly inactivated by a blood-borne esterase. But acetylcholine had still not been identified as a normal constituent of the animal body, and it was to be some time before the positive identification of the postganglionic parasympathetic transmitter as acetylcholine. It was to come from Henry Dale who was searching for histamine.

Dale, working for the Medical Research Council at its National Institute for Medical Research, was, during the 1920s, principally occupied with experiments on the physiology and pharmacology of histamine, another substance not then known to occur naturally. With Harold Dudley (1887–1935), Dale made a determined effort to find histamine, and in so doing, found convincing evidence for the presence of acetylcholine in the mammalian spleen. This important breakthrough stimulated further research on the role of acetylcholine, as Dale and Dudley suggested,

> … there has been a natural and proper reluctance to assume, in default of chemical evidence, that the chemical agent concerned in these effects, or in the humoral transmission of vagus action, was a substance known, hitherto, only as a synthetic curiosity, or as an occasional constituent of certain plant extracts … It appears to us that the case for acetylcholine as a physiological agent is now materially strengthened by the fact that we have now been able to isolate it from an animal organ and thus to show that it is a natural constituent of the body.

The major problem that continued to complicate further research work on acetylcholine was the extreme transiency of its effects. Experiments to show its release after nervous stimulation were unsuccessful—if it was released, it was so quickly hydrolysed by circulating cholinesterases that there was nothing left to measure. In 1933 a new arrival in Dale's laboratory, the pharmacologist Wilhelm Feldberg (1900–1993), a refugee from Nazi Germany, brought with him two valuable techniques: one was to increase the measurable levels of circulating acetylcholine by inhibiting the hydrolysing enzyme with eserine; and second the use of a bioassay, of the ventral muscle of the leech also treated with eserine, to measure acetylcholine. These methods were immediately incorporated into the experiments in Dale's lab, and evidence began to accrue of the role of acetylcholine in ganglionic transmission in the autonomic nervous system, at the parasympathetic postganglionic junction and at the neuromuscular junction of the voluntary nervous system.

One of the most significant developments of the period was not a laboratory finding, but the suggestion by Dale of the words 'cholinergic' and 'adrenergic', to describe nerve fibres by the nature of the chemical that they used, or might use, as a transmitter, rather than by the then accepted anatomical classification of fibres as sympathetic or parasympathetic. Dale's reasoning was straightforward, 'I think', he wrote in 1934, 'such a usage would assist clear thinking, without committing us to precise chemical identifications, which may be long in coming'. The distinction was important, as it acknowledged that chemical neurotransmitters might be 'adrenaline-like' and 'acetylcholine-like' but were not necessarily either of those two chemicals.

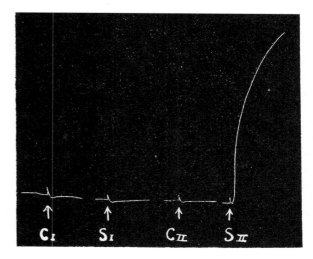

Eserinized leech muscle as a measure of acetylcholine in an experiment to verify the connection between the output of acetylcholine and the transmission of nerve impulses to the sweat glands of an anaesthetized cat. CI and SI are measurements of acetylcholine in the venous outflow from the right foot of the anaesthetized cat, with the hairless pads which contain the sweat glands ligatured; CI being a control period of no stimulation, SI a period of stimulation of the right sympathetic chain. CII is a measurement of a similar control period from the left foot, with the hairless pads intact, and SII from a period of stimulation of the left sympathetic chain, which caused secretion of sweat and also the release of acetylcholine, as shown by the leech muscle response. (Taken with permission of the Physiological Society, from Dale and Feldberg, *Journal of Physiology* (1934) **82**, p. 124, paper in Dale (1965).)

Cannon's sympathins and Ahlquist's receptors

While Dale and his colleagues focused their attention on the parasympathetic nervous system, others were concentrating on the nature of the transmitter in the sympathetic branch. Shortly after Loewi's demonstration of *acceleransstoff* in 1921, the American physiologist Walter Cannon (1871–1945) provided complementary evidence that in adrenalectomized animals stimulation of the hepatic nerve produced a chemical that caused acceleration of the heart beat. The word 'sympathin' was used for this unidentified substance, which was similar to, but not identical with, adrenaline. Further experiments by Cannon and Arturo Rosenblueth (1900–1970) suggested that the different effects observed after sympathetic nervous stimulation indicated the presence of two distinctly separate endogenous sympathin complexes, sympathin E (excitatory) and sympathin I (inhibitory). This theoretical account achieved quite successful currency in contemporary scientific literature, and by the late 1930s and 1940s the theory had almost achieved the status of a 'law', especially in American pharmacology. Cannon and Rosenblueth's major work, *Autonomic neuro-effector systems*, promoted their sympathin theory to the exclusion of all else, and in Britain, where the concept was less well received, one reviewer, John Gaddum (1900–1965), echoed the views of several colleagues when he suggested that it was 'unnecessarily complicated'. A former co-worker of Cannon's, the Belgian pharmacologist Zenon Bacq (1903–1984) went some way to clearing away the confusion sown by Cannon and Rosenblueth, by suggesting that 'sympathin I' was adrenaline and 'sympathin E' could be noradrenaline, although overall he remained sceptical of the sympathin scheme. By this time many other investigators were emphasizing the point made by Barger and Dale in 1910, that noradrenaline was a closer mimic of sympathetic activity than was adrenaline.

Two major boosts to the understanding of the sympathetic nervous system and the chemical identification of its transmitter(s) came shortly after the Second World War. Ulf von Euler (1905–1983) showed that extracts of sympathetic nerves and some of their end organs contained appreciable amounts of noradrenaline. Thus the long-standing objection to noradrenaline because it was not known to occur naturally, was removed. An equally important theoretical contribution was made by Raymond Ahlquist (1914–1983) who resolved, and finally offered an adequate explanation for, some of the apparently paradoxical experimental differences observed by Dale and others. Using a range of different adrenergic agonists, Ahlquist defined two major classes of adrenoceptors, with a range of differential potencies for catecholamines. He postulated α-receptors, which were more sensitive to noradrenaline than to adrenaline and isoprenaline, whereas β-receptors were preferentially sensitive to isoprenaline, then to adrenaline and least responsive to noradrenaline. The awkward results reported by many investigators, including of course Cannon and Rosenblueth's observations but not their theories, of both excitation and inhibition in the sympathetic system, could now be re-interpreted in the light of Ahlquist's scheme.

Consolidation and diversification

The increasing confirmation and acceptance, of chemical transmission, of adrenergic nerves releasing noradrenaline and cholinergic nerves releasing acetylcholine, became, in their turn, codified into a 'law'. This was largely influenced by John Eccles (1903–1997), who believed that the long latency at the terminals of the parasympathetic nervous system, such as those in the heart, contrasted markedly with much shorter latencies at sites such as sympathetic ganglia and the voluntary neuromuscular junction, and so had proposed his alternative scheme, that electrical impulses were solely responsible for these faster responses. After formally announcing his 'conversion' to chemical mechanisms, he formulated what became known as 'Dale's law' which stipulated 'one neurone, one transmitter'. As the concept of chemical neurotransmission achieved widespread acceptance it became the new orthodoxy, and it was widely assumed that only a few specific chemicals, including acetylcholine and noradrenaline, were involved in the process.

The idea of a simple duality, a sympathetic/adrenergic system countered by a parasympathetic/cholinergic system, was gradually modified as evidence of new transmitter candidates and neuromodulaters, emerged. During the 1950s and 1960s it became increasingly obvious that many autonomic nerve fibres were neither adrenergic nor cholinergic. Prime amongst those postulating more complex chemical mechanisms at autonomic neuroeffector junctions was Geoffrey Burnstock (b. 1929) who, in 1963, first suggested that the myenteric plexus of the guinea-pig intestine contained non-adrenergic, non-cholinergic (NANC) neurones, thus providing a pharmacological distinction for the 'enteric nervous system' postulated by Langley at the beginning of the century. By the late 1960s Burnstock and his group had provided extensive evidence for the existence of such neurones, and postulated that ATP (adenosine triphosphate) was the neurotransmitter at these neuronal terminals. This view, challenging contemporary dogma, received little sympathy, as one witness has recalled; 'Burnstock', wrote Michael Rand, 'faced a considerable amount of tough opposition, not always in the spirit of scientific criticism.'

Chemical coding, and into the clinic

During the next decade, however, the hypothesis of ATP, or as Burnstock proposed echoing Dale's classification of 40 years earlier, purinergic transmission, gained considerable support, and in so doing encouraged the investigation of other possible neurotransmitter candidates, including biologically active polypeptides such as somatostatin, vasoactive intestinal polypeptide (VIP), substance P, and neurotensin.

This diversity of chemical mediators stimulated a further revolutionary hypothesis from Burnstock in 1976, that nerve cells might release more than one transmitter. The coexistence and co-release of transmitters from nerves has opened up an entirely new field of research on the autonomic nervous system. Understanding the details of these combinations of transmitters, known as 'chemical coding', has led to detailed physiological and pharmacological investigations into the effects of disease at the autonomic neuroeffector junction, and to the development of sophisticated pharmaceutical responses to those disease processes. Thus, throughout the twentieth century, basic scientific studies of the autonomic nervous system have continued to elucidate functional mechanisms that underlie all nervous system activity and the clinical application of such research has evolved in a variety of directions, as other chapters in this volume will illustrate.

Neuroscience, 1976. Vol. 1, pp. 239–248. Pergamon Press. Printed in Great Britain.

COMMENTARY

DO SOME NERVE CELLS RELEASE MORE THAN ONE TRANSMITTER?

GEOFFREY BURNSTOCK
Department of Anatomy and Embryology, University College. London, WC1E 6BT

Abstract—The concept that each nerve cell makes and releases only one nerve transmitter (widely known as Dale's Principle) has been re-examined. Experiments suggesting that some nerve cells store and release more than one transmitter have been reviewed. Developmental and evolutionary factors are considered. Conceptual and experimental difficulties in investigating this problem are discussed. .It is suggested that the term 'transmitter' should be applied to any substance that is synthesised and stored in nerve cells, is released during nerve activity and whose interaction with specific receptors on the postsynaptic membrane leads to changes in postsynaptic activity. Expressed in this way, it seems likely that while many nerves do have only one transmitter, others in some species, during development or during hormone-dependent cycles, employ multiple transmitters.

Title of Geoffrey Burnstock's 1976 paper, proposing that 'Dale's principle' of 'one neurone, one transmitter' was no longer valid. (Taken, with permission of Elsevier Science, from *Neuroscience* (1976) 1, 239.)

Acknowledgements

I am grateful to Mrs Wendy Kutner for secretarial help, to the Wellcome Photographic Library for supplying the illustrations, and to the Wellcome Trust for financial support.

References and selected further reading

Ackerknecht, E. H. (1974). The history of the discovery of the vegetative (autonomic) nervous system. *Medical History* **18**, 1–8.

Ahlquist, R. P. (1948). A study of the adrenotropic receptors. *Am. J. Physiol.* **153**, 586–99.

Ahlquist, R. P. (1973). Adrenergic receptors: a personal and practical view. *Perspectives in Biol. Med.* **16**, 119–22.

Burnstock, G. (1976). Do some nerve cells release more than one neurotransmitter? *Neuroscience* **1**, 239–48.

Cannon, W. B. and Rosenblueth A. (1937). *Autonomic neuro-effector systems.* Macmillan, New York.

Dale, H. H. (1965). *Adventures in physiology, with excursions into autopharmacology.* The Wellcome Trust, London. (A selection of Dale's papers, annotated by the author, including all the work referred to in this chapter).

Elliott, T. R. (1904). The reaction of the ferret's bladder to adrenalin. *J. Physiol.* **31**, lix.

Euler, U. S. von (1946). A specific sympathomimetic ergone in adrenergic nerve fibres (sympathin) and its relations to adrenaline and noradrenaline. *Acta Physiol. Scand.* **12**, 73–97.

Gaskell, W. H. (1886). On the structure, distribution, and function of the nerves which innervate the visceral and vascular systems. *J. Physiol.* **7**, 1–80.

Gaskell, W. H. (1916). *The involuntary nervous system.* Longmans, Green & Co, London.

Hunt, R. and Taveau, M. (1906). On the physiological action of certain cholin derivatives and new methods for detecting cholin. *BMJ*, ii, 1788–9.

Langley, J. N. (1898). On the union of cranial autonomic (visceral) fibres with the nerve cells of the superior cervical ganglion. *J. Physiol.* **23**, 240–70.

Langley, J. N. (1921). *The autonomic nervous system. Part 1.* Heffer & Sons, Cambridge.

Pick, J. (1970). *The autonomic nervous system. Morphological, comparative, clinical and surgical aspects.* J. B. Lippincott, Philadelphia.

Rand, M. J. and Mitchelson, F. (1986). The guts of the matter: contribution of studies on smooth muscle to discoveries in pharmacology. In *Discoveries in pharmacology, Vol. 3: Pharmacological methods, receptors and chemotherapy,* (ed. M. J. Parham and J. Bruinvels). Elsevier, Amsterdam.

Sheehan, D. (1941). The autonomic nervous system prior to Gaskell. *New Engl. J. Med.* **224**, 457–60.

PART I

Scientific Aspects of Structure and Function

1. Neurobiology of the autonomic nervous system

Wilfrid Jänig and Elspeth M. McLachlan

Introduction

Motor activity and patterned behaviours originating in the brain are only possible when the cells, tissues, and organs of the body are maintained in an optimal environment, so as to enable continuous adjustments to the varying internal and external demands that are placed on the organism, both in the short and long term. Short-term control includes control of blood flow, body fluid volume and osmotic pressure, body temperature, gastrointestinal and pelvic organ function, and metabolism. Long-term control includes the growth and maintenance of body tissues and organs, sleep and wakefulness, protection and defence from the cellular level to the whole organism.

Just as motor actions are controlled by the brain, so are all other body functions. To perform these functions, the brain acts on peripheral target tissues of diverse composition (smooth muscle, cardiac muscle, exocrine and endocrine glands, metabolic tissues, immune cells, etc.). The *efferent systems* are neural (the autonomic nervous system) and hormonal (the neuroendocrine system). The time scales of these controls differ by orders of magnitude: autonomic regulation normally occurs in seconds to minutes whereas neuroendocrine regulation occurs over tens of minutes, hours, or even days. The *afferent signals* that lead to changes in these outputs are neural, hormonal, and humoral (e.g. blood glucose concentration, blood temperature, etc.). As with the somatomotor system, autonomic and endocrine regulation are represented in the brain (in the hypothalamus, brain stem, and spinal cord). Thus the brain contains the 'sensorimotor programmes' for the co-ordinated regulation of the body's tissues and organs as well as its skeletal muscles. There is considerable overlap within the brain, not only between the areas that are involved with the outputs of autonomic and endocrine signals, but also between these and the regions controlling the somatomotor system.

The precision and biological importance of the control of peripheral target organs by the autonomic nervous system become most obvious:

(1) when the autonomic nervous system fails to function (e.g. during severe infectious diseases);

(2) when the peripheral autonomic neurones are damaged, by injury or a metabolic disease (such as diabetic autonomic neuropathy);

(3) when autonomic neurones are inherently absent (such as the Hirschsprung's disease), or when dopamine β-hydroxylase, an enzyme for noradrenaline synthesis, is deficient;

(4) when the spinal cord is lesioned (interrupting supraspinal connections with the autonomic outflow); or

(5) in old age when autonomic systems may decrease in effectiveness.

Under these circumstances, the storage functions of bladder and bowel become poorly controlled. Temperature regulation is inadequate. Even the simplest actions, such as standing up, may become a burden because there are no adjustments to maintain the pressure perfusing the brain, leading to loss of consciousness.

In this article the neuroneal basis for the precise control of the peripheral target organs is described. Ideas of how autonomic neurones in the central nervous system (CNS) and in the periphery are organized and how, in normal health, these neurones integrate and transmit centrally derived signals to their peripheral targets are presented. Understanding the biology of these nerve pathways should lead to a better understanding both of primary disorders of the autonomic nervous system and of autonomic dysfunction which is secondary to various diseases. For the physiology of the various autonomic control systems, we refer the reader to the chapters in this book, and to Loewy and Spyer (1990) and Greger and Windhorst (1996).

Divisions of the peripheral autonomic nervous system

Langley (1921) originally proposed the generic term *autonomic nervous system* to describe the innervation of all tissues and organs except striated muscle fibres. This system has also been called the vegetative nervous system (particularly in Europe). Langley's division of the autonomic nervous system into the sympathetic, parasympathetic, and enteric nervous systems is now universally applied. The definition of the *sympathetic* and *parasympathetic nervous systems* is primarily anatomical. The outflow from the CNS is separated into a tectal, bulbar and sacral system (the craniosacral or parasympathetic system) and a thoracolumbar system (the sympathetic system). These correspond to the somitic levels from which neural crest cells migrate to become parasympathetic/enteric neurones and sympathetic neurones, respectively. The other main feature distinguishing the outflows is their separation by the cervical and lumbar enlargements (supplying the innervation of the limbs). The *enteric nervous system* is intrinsic to the wall of the gastrointestinal tract and consists of interconnecting plexuses along its length. These are responsible for the reflex activity involved in peristalsis and segmentation during transit of food along the bowel.

The sympathetic and parasympathetic systems consist of two populations of neurones in series which are connected synaptically. The final sympathetic and parasympathetic neurones lie entirely outside the central nervous system. Their cell bodies are grouped in *autonomic ganglia*. Their axons are unmyelinated and project from these ganglia to the target organs. These neurones are called *ganglion cells* or *postganglionic neurones*. The efferent *preganglionic neurones* have cell bodies that lie in the spinal cord and brain stem. They send axons from the CNS into the ganglia and form synapses on the dendrites and somata of the postganglionic neurones. Their axons are either thinly myelinated (B fibres, conduction velocity 1–15 m/s) or unmyelinated (C fibres, conduction velocity 0.1–1 m/s).

Organization of preganglionic neurones in the neuraxis

Langley showed, by stimulating individual ventral roots, that the control of each target organ arises from preganglionic neurones in a few adjacent segments of the spinal cord. Within the spinal cord and brainstem, the preganglionic somata are topographically organized and form functionally distinct columns resembling those of the motoneurone pools supplying particular skeletal muscles. Retrograde labelling techniques have been used to demonstrate this, in particular for the dorsal motor nucleus of vagus (Ritter *et al.* 1992) and the lumbar (Jänig and McLachlan 1987) and sacral segments of the spinal cord (see Chapter 19).

Thoracolumbar (sympathetic) system

The cell bodies of the sympathetic preganglionic neurones lie in the spinal cord, extending from segments T1 to the rostral part of L3. They are clustered together in clumps at the edge of the intermediate grey matter, forming the intermediolateral columns. During development, the neurones migrate dorsolaterally from the central canal; a few cells end up in the dorsolateral funiculus (the lateral horn) whereas others remain in bands crossing the midline. The overall arrangement is ladder-like. The neurones receive inputs from interneurones in the dorsal horn and intermediate zone as well as direct projections from the medulla, pons and hypothalamus.

The preganglionic axons project ipsilaterally from the cord via the segmental ventral root and spinal nerve, and thence in the white ramus to the paravertebral chain where they synapse with postganglionic neurones in the same and several adjacent segmental ganglia. Neurones in the upper thoracic segments project rostrally to control targets in the head, whereas many lumbar preganglionic neurones project caudally to regulate targets in the lower trunk and hindlimbs. Some preganglionic axons project across the chain into the splanchnic nerves (major, minor, and lumbar) and synapse in the *prevertebral ganglia* (coeliac, superior mesenteric, and inferior mesenteric) which supply the abdominal and pelvic viscera.

The *paravertebral ganglia* are interconnected to form a chain on either side of the vertebral column, extending from the base of the skull to the sacrum. There is usually one pair of ganglia per segment, except for the superior cervical ganglia (SCG) at the rostral end of the cervical sympathetic trunk and the stellate ganglia at the rostral end of the thoracic sympathetic chain. Paravertebral ganglion cells project to the somatic territories in all parts of the body and innervate blood vessels, pilomotor muscles, and sweat glands. Most of the paravertebral neurones project through the grey rami to their respective spinal nerves and then via peripheral nerve trunks to the effector cells of trunk and limbs. Paravertebral neurones do not project to the extremities along the major blood vessels. Postganglionic neurones in the SCG send their axons in the internal carotid nerve bundles to join the nerves to target organs in the head. At least 50 per cent of SCG neurones are vasoconstrictor and the rest mainly pilomotor, sudomotor or secretomotor to salivary glands. A subpopulation supplies targets in and around the eye and a few innervate the pineal gland. Postganglionic neurones in the stellate ganglion project through branches to the heart and lungs and through grey rami to C4–C8 spinal nerves to supply the neck and upper limbs. Some paravertebral neurones project via the splanchnic nerves (including the pelvic nerves) to the viscera, where they mainly innervate blood vessels.

The *prevertebral ganglia* lie around the base of the large arterial branches from the abdominal aorta and contain neurones that regulate motility and secretion. They project in nerve bundles accompanying the vascular supply to the abdominal organs or in special nerves (e.g. the hypogastric nerves) to the pelvic organs. They receive preganglionic inputs from the midthoracic and upper lumbar segments. Some sympathetic postganglionic cell bodies are also found in the ganglia of the pelvic or hypogastric plexus, which contains both sympathetic and parasympathetic neurones (see below). The sympathetic neurones supply the internal reproductive organs, bladder and, distal bowel.

The effector cells and organs of the sympathetic nervous system are listed in Table 1.1, together with the reactions they effect. Cells in the *adrenal medulla* are ontogenetically homologous to sympathetic postganglionic neurones. When activated by their preganglionic axons, the medullary cells release adrenaline and noradrenaline directly into the circulation.

Craniosacral (parasympathetic) system

The cell bodies of the parasympathetic preganglionic neurones lie in the brain stem and in sacral spinal cord segments S1–S3. In the brainstem they are grouped in distinct nuclei (e.g. dorsal motor nucleus, Edinger-Westphal nucleus) and project via distinct cranial nerves. They pass via III (oculomotor) nerve to the ocular muscles and glands, via VII (facial) and XI (glossopharyngeal) nerves to the nasal and palatal glands, and via X (vagal) nerve to the thoracic and abdominal viscera. In the sacral cord, the preganglionic neurones lie in clusters across the intermediate zone and around the lateral part of the ventral horn, and project via the sacral ventral roots and pelvic splanchnic nerves to supply the pelvic organs. Like the sympathetic preganglionic neurones, they receive inputs from spinal interneurones as well as supraspinal projections (Chapter 9).

Parasympathetic preganglionic neurones project their axons directly to the organs they supply, where the postganglionic neurones are located in small ganglia (often interconnected in a plexus) just outside, or even within the wall of the target organ. *Parasympathetic ganglia* are found only in the head (ciliary ganglia to eye; pterygopalatine ganglia to lachrymal, nasal, and palatal glands; otic and submandibular ganglia to salivary glands) and near or in the wall of various effector organs (heart, airways, pancreas, gall bladder, pelvic organs). The cranial parasympathetic ganglia receive preganglionic innervation from brainstem nuclei and are generally larger aggregations of neurones than the parasympathetic ganglia of the trunk. Preganglionic neurones which project to the gastrointestinal tract synapse with neurones that are part of the enteric nervous system. This may not always be the case as pathways to the colon/rectum also contain a synapse within the pelvic plexus.

The effector cells and organs of the parasympathetic nervous system are listed in Table 1.1, together with the reactions they effect.

Table 1.1. Effects of activation of sympathetic and parasympathetic neurones on autonomic target organs

Organ and organ system	Activation of parasympathetic nerves	Activation of sympathetic nerves
Heart muscle	Decrease of heart rate Decrease of contractility (only atria)	Increase of heart rate Increase of contractility (atria, ventricles)
Blood vessels		
Arteries		
in skin of trunk and limbs	0	Vasoconstriction
in skin and mucosa of face	Vasodilatation	Vasoconstriction
in visceral domain	0	Vasoconstriction
in skeletal muscle	0	Vasoconstriction Vasodilation (cholinergic)
in heart (coronary arteries)		Vasoconstriction
in erectile tissue (helical arteries and sinusoids in penis and clitoris)	Vasodilatation	Vasoconstriction
in cranium	Vasodilatation (?)	Vasoconstriction
Veins	0	Vasoconstriction
Gastrointestinal tract		
Longitudinal and circular muscle	Increase of motility	Decrease of motility
Sphincters	Relaxation	Contraction
Capsule of spleen	0	Contraction
Urinary bladder		
Detrusor vesicae	Contraction	Relaxation (small)
Trigone (internal sphincter)	0	Contraction
Reproductive organs		
Seminal vesicle, prostate	0	Contraction
Vas deferens	0	Contraction
Uterus	0	Contraction Relaxation (depends on species and hormonal state)
Eye		
Dilator muscle of pupil	0	Contraction (mydriasis)
Sphincter muscle of pupil	Contraction (miosis)	0
Ciliary muscle	Contraction (accomodation)	
Tarsal muscle	0	Contraction (lifting of lid)
Orbitale muscle	0	Contraction (protrusion of eye)
Tracheo-bronchial muscles	Contraction	Relaxation (mainly by adrenaline)
Piloerector muscles	0	Contraction
Exocrine glands		
Salivary glands	Copious serous secretion	Weak serous secretion (submandibular gland)
Lacrimal glands	Secretion	0
Nasopharyngeal glands	Secretion	
Bronchial glands	Secretion	?
Sweat glands	0	Secretion (cholinergic)
Digestive glands (stomach, pancreas)	Secretion	Decrease of secretion or 0
Mucosa (small, large intestine)	Secretion	Decrease of secretion or reabsorption
Pineal gland	0	Increase in synthesis of melatonin
Brown adipose tissue	0	Heat production
Metabolism		
Liver	0	Glycogenolysis, Gluconeogenesis
Fat cells	0	Lipolysis (free fatty acids in blood increased)
Beta-cells in islets of pancreas	Secretion	Decrease of secretion
Adrenal medulla	0	Secretion of adrenaline and noradrenaline
Lymphoid tissue	0	Depression of activity (e.g. of natural killer cells)

Most parasympathetic activity increases motility of visceral organs and secretion in mucosae.

The enteric nervous system

Within the wall of the gastrointestinal tract, a complexly interconnected neuronal system extends from the oesophagus to the rectum. Two interconnected plexuses of ganglia are located (1) between the longitudinal and circular muscle layers (myenteric or Auerbach's plexus) and (2) in the submucosa (submucosal or Meissner's plexus). Neurones of the myenteric ganglia project into the external and internal muscle layers, whereas many in submucosal plexus extend into the mucosa. In addition, some neurones of both plexuses have processes that project circumferentially, orally, or anally for up to many centimetres (Furness and Costa 1987; Furness and Bornstein 1995).

Functionally, both plexuses contain afferent (sensory) neurones, interneurones, and efferent neurones which bring about complex reflex changes in motility (peristalsis, segmentation, etc.) via excitatory or inhibitory actions on the smooth muscle layers, and also regulate secretion and absorption by the mucosal epithelial cells. Mechanical and chemical stimuli excite afferent endings in the mucosa or within the muscle. Sets of neurones performing specific reflexes are repeated at regular intervals along the tract, their properties being adapted progressively to the changing functions at different levels. This system, together with the gut tissues, behaves as an effector tissue which is regulated via sympathetic and parasympathetic pathways from the CNS.

Autonomic effector responses to activation of sympathetic and parasympathetic axons

Table 1.1 describes the overall reactions of the peripheral targets to activity in sympathetic and parasympathetic neurones. These responses have been defined by reflex activation or by electrical stimulation of the respective nerves. In some cases, the effects of nerve activity have been deduced by the changes in organ function that follow transection of the nerve supply. The table shows that:

1. Most target tissues react predominantly to only one of the autonomic systems (the pacemaker cells in the heart are one exception).
2. A few target organs react to activity in both autonomic systems (e.g. iris, heart, urinary bladder).
3. Opposite reactions to activity in sympathetic and parasympathetic neurones are more the exception than the rule.
4. Most responses are excitatory, i.e. inhibition (e.g. relaxation of muscle, decrease of secretion) is rare.

The table shows that the idea of antagonism between the parasympathetic and sympathetic nervous systems is largely a misconception. Where there are reciprocal effects on the target cells, it can usually be shown either that the systems work synergistically or that they exert their influence under different functional conditions. For example, in larger mammals, fast changes of heart rate during changes of body position and mental arousal are generated via changes in the activity of parasympathetic neurones to the pacemaker cells; the sustained increase of heart rate during exercise is mainly generated by increased activity of sympathetic neurones. It should be noted that these effects of nerve activity are not necessarily the same as the responses of the effector tissues to the application of exogenous transmitter (see below).

Visceral afferent neurones

About 85 per cent of the axons in the vagus nerve and up to 50 per cent of those in the splanchnic nerves (greater, lesser, least, lumbar, and pelvic) are afferent. These visceral afferents come from sensory receptors in the internal organs. Their cell bodies lie in the ganglia of nerves X and XI and in the dorsal root ganglia of the segments corresponding to the autonomic outflow (spinal visceral afferents). Most visceral afferent axons are unmyelinated, some are thinly myelinated. Spinal visceral afferents project through the *white rami* to the respective spinal segments. It is unlikely that peripheral axons of spinal afferent neurones project along the sympathetic chain and blood vessels to the extremities and to the head; some supply the spinal joints and parietal tissues. Sometimes thoracolumbar and sacral afferents are labelled 'sympathetic' or 'parasympathetic' but this nomenclature is misleading. There is no reason to associate any of these visceral afferent neurones with only one of the autonomic systems.

Vagal and sacral visceral afferents

Visceral afferents from the lungs, cardiovascular system, gastrointestinal tract, evacuative, and reproductive organs project to the nucleus of the solitary tract in the brainstem and to the sacral spinal cord. Most of these afferents react to distension and contraction of the organs. Their activity encodes intraluminal pressure (e.g. arterial baroreceptor afferents, afferents from the urinary bladder) or volume (afferents from the gut, atria, and lungs). Some are chemosensitive (arising from arterial chemoreceptors in the carotid bodies, chemosensors in the gut mucosa, and osmosensors in the liver). Most vagal visceral afferents do not signal noxious events. Pelvic visceral afferents signal noxious events as well as distension and contraction; pain arises during strong contractions and distensions of the pelvic organs as well as after inflammation (Ritter *et al.* 1992; Jänig and Koltzenburg 1993).

Thoracolumbar spinal visceral afferents

The sensory receptors of thoracolumbar visceral afferents are situated in the serosa, the mesenteries, and the walls of some organs. The number of these afferents associated with the pelvic organs is much higher than with the abdominal organs. Most are mechanosensitive and some are active only during tissue inflammation and ischaemia. These afferents are involved (1) in organ-specific spinal reflexes (e.g. cardio-cardiac, reno-renal) and (2) in pain of all visceral organs (Cervero 1994; Jänig 1996a).

Functional autonomic motor pathways

Most individual sympathetic pre- and postganglionic neurones are spontaneously active and/or can be activated or inhibited by appropriate physiological stimuli. This has been shown in anaesthetized animals for neurones of the lumbar sympathetic outflow to skeletal muscles, skin and pelvic viscera, and for neurones of the thoracic sympathetic outflow to the head and neck, as well as in unanaesthetized humans for the sympathetic outflow to skeletal muscles and skin. The reflexes observed correspond to the effector responses which are induced by changes in activity in these neurones. The reflex patterns elicited by stimulation of various afferent input systems are characteristic for each functional sympathetic pathway and therefore represent physiological 'fingerprints' for each pathway (Jänig 1985, 1996*b*; Jänig and McLachlan 1987). Reflex patterns for muscle vasoconstrictor (MVC), visceral vasoconstrictor (VVC), cutaneous vasoconstrictor (CVC), and sudomotor (SM) neurones and for one type of motility regulating (MR) neurone are shown in Figs 1.1–1.3:

1. Discharge patterns in MVC and VVC neurones consist of inhibition by arterial baroreceptors (Fig. 1.2a) but excitation by arterial chemoreceptors, cutaneous nociceptors, and spinal visceral nociceptors (Fig. 1.1a,b).
2. Most CVC neurones are inhibited by stimulation of cutaneous nociceptors, spinal visceral afferents, arterial chemoreceptors, and central warm-sensitive neurones in the spinal cord and hypothalamus (Fig. 1.1).

3. SM neurones are activated by stimulation of Pacinian corpuscles in skin (Fig. 1.1c) and by some other afferent stimuli.
4. MR neurones are excited or inhibited by stimulation of sacral afferents from the urinary bladder, hindgut, or anal canal (Fig. 1.3), but are not affected by arterial baroreceptor activation (Fig. 1.2b). Functionally different types of MR neurones can be discriminated by way of their reflex pattern.

So far 12 different functional groups of postganglionic and preganglionic sympathetic neurones have been identified (Table 1.2). The neurones in eight of these pathways have ongoing activity whereas in four pathways they are normally silent. Experimental studies show (Fig. 1.4) that:

(1) the reflex patterns observed in each group of sympathetic neurones are the result of integrative processes in spinal cord, brainstem, and hypothalamus;

(2) functionally similar preganglionic and postganglionic neurones are synaptically connected in the sympathetic ganglia, probably

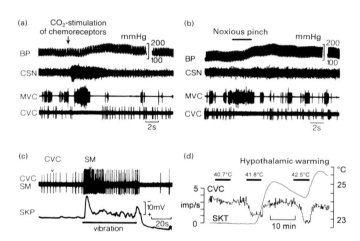

Fig. 1.1. Reflexes in muscle (MVC) and cutaneous (CVC) vasoconstrictor and sudomotor (SM) neurones recorded from postganglionic axons in anaesthetized cats. (a) Stimulation of the carotid chemoreceptors by a bolus injection of CO_2-enriched saline into the carotid artery (at arrow) activated the MVC neurones and inhibited the CVC neurone (recorded simultaneously). Increased afferent activity in the carotid sinus nerve (CSN) was monitored. The increase of blood pressure evoked by chemoreceptor stimulation led to a baroreceptor-mediated inhibition of MVC activity but not of the CVC activity. (b) Stimulation of cutaneous nociceptors by pinching the ipsilateral hindpaw (indicated by bar) also excited the MVC neurones and inhibited the CVC neurones. (c) Simultaneous recording of a single CVC neurone (small signal) and a single SM neurone (larger signal) and the skin potential (SKP) from the central paw pad. Stimulation of Pacinian corpuscles by vibration excited the SM neurone and inhibited the CVC neurone. SM activation was correlated with the changes in the SKP. (d) Inhibition of CVC neurones to warming of the anterior hypothalamus. Note the increase of skin temperature (SKT), on the central paw pad followed the depression of CVC activity. (Data for (a) to (c) from Jänig and Kümmel, unpublished; (d) from Grewe *et al.* (1995). *J. Physiol.* **448**, 139–2. (With permission from Jänig and McLachlan 1992*a*.)

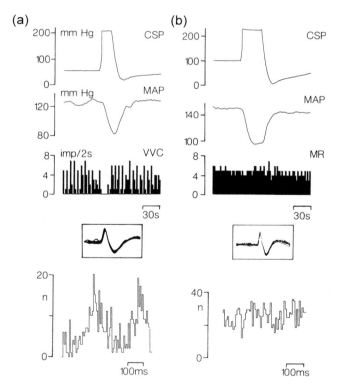

Fig. 1.2. Baroreceptor reflex in sympathetic neurones. Responses of (a) a single preganglionic visceral vasoconstrictor (VVC) neurone, (b) a single preganglionic motility regulating (MR) neurone and blood pressure to isotonic pressure changes at the carotid sinus baroreceptors. Traces (from above, down) show carotid sinus pressure (CSP), mean arterial blood pressure (MAP) and neuronal activity in the VVC neurone and the MR neurone (peristimulus histograms). The activity of the neurones was recorded from the axons isolated from the lumbar splanchnic nerves in anaesthetized cats. Insets show the form of the action potentials of each unit. Post-R-wave histograms (below) from 500 superimposed sweeps over two cardiac cycles show the absence of cardiac rhythmicity in the activity of the MR neurone. (With permission from Michaelis *et al.* (1993). *J. Auton. Nerv. Syst.* **42**, 241–50.)

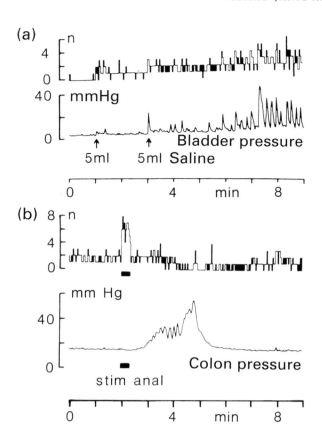

Fig. 1.3. Responses of a preganglionic motility regulating (MR) neurone to stimulation of different groups of pelvic visceral afferents generated by (a) isovolumetric urinary bladder contractions and (b) stimulation of afferents from the anal mucosa by mechanical shearing stimuli as well as contraction of the colon. The activity of the neurone was recorded from axons in a lumbar splanchnic nerve in an anaesthetized cat. The records show excitation during bladder contraction and anal stimulation, and inhibition during colon contraction. Other types of MR neurones show responses which are opposite to those shown here or respond only to anal stimulation. (Modified from Bahr *et al.* (1986). *J. Auton. Nerv. Syst.* **15**, 109–30.)

Table 1.2.   Functional classification of sympathetic neurones based on reflex behaviour *in vivo*[a]

Likely function	Location	Target organ	Likely target tissue	Major identifying stimulus[b]	Ongoing activity
Vasoconstrictor					
Muscle	Lumbar[c]	Hindlimb muscle	Resistance vessels	Baro-inhibition[d]	Yes
	Cervical[e]	Head and neck muscle	Resistance vessels	Baro-inhibition	Yes
Cutaneous	Lumbar	Hindlimb skin vessels	Thermoregulatory vessels	Inhibited by CNS warming	Yes
	Cervical	Head and neck skin	Thermoregulatory vessels	Inhibited by CNS warming	Yes
Visceral	Lumbar splanchnic	Pelvic viscera	Resistance vessels	Baro-inhibition	Yes
Vasodilatator					
Muscle	Lumbar	Hindlimb muscle	Muscle arteries	Hypothalamic stimulation	No
Cutaneous	Lumbar	Hindlimb skin	Skin vasculature	?	No
Sudomotor	Lumbar	Paw pads	Sweat glands	Vibration (in cat)	Yes, some
Pilomotor	Lumbar	Tail	Piloerector muscles	Hypothalamic stimulation	No
Inspiratory	Cervical	Airways?	Nasal mucosal vasculature	Inspiration	Yes
Pupillomotor	Cervical	Iris	Dilator pupillae muscle	Inhibition by light	Yes, some
Motility regulating					
Type 1	Lumbar splanchnic	Hindgut, urinary tract	Visceral smooth muscle	Bladder distension	Yes
Type 2	Lumbar splanchnic	Hindgut, urinary tract	Visceral smooth muscle	Inhibited by bladder distension	Yes
Reproduction	Lumbar splanchnic	Internal reproductive organs	Visceral smooth muscle, other?	?	No

[a] Experimental data from anaesthetized cats (Jänig 1985, 1996*b*; Jänig and McLachlan 1987).

[b] Excitation by stimulus unless inhibition specified.

[c] 'Lumbar' represents preganglionic and postganglionic axons in lumbar outflow.

[d] 'Baro-inhibition' represents inhibition by stimulation of arterial baroreceptors.

[e] 'Cervical' represents preganglionic axons in the cervical sympathetic trunk.

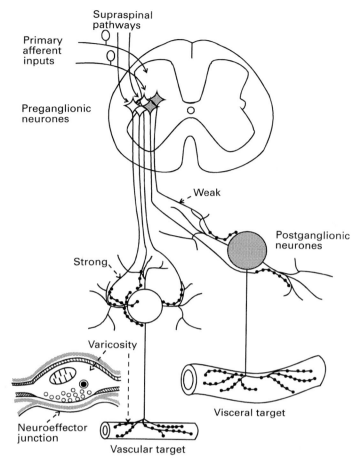

Fig. 1.4. Organization of the sympathetic nervous system into building blocks. Separate functional pathways extend from the CNS to the effector organs. Preganglionic neurones located in the intermediate zone integrate signals decending from brain stem and hypothalamus and arising segmentally from primary afferent fibres. The preganglionic neurones project to peripheral ganglia and converge onto postganglionic neurones. Many preganglionic inputs to postganglionic neurones are always suprathreshold (or strong, see Fig. 1.6). Others are subthreshold (weak) and must summate. The postganglionic axons form multiple neuroeffector junctions with their target cells (see Figs 1.9 and 1.10). (With permission from Jänig and McLachlan 1992a.)

without little or no 'cross-talk' between different peripheral pathways; and

(3) the messages in these functional pathways are transmitted to the autonomic effector cells by distinct neuroeffector mechanisms.

In contrast, relatively few systematic studies have been made on the functional properties of parasympathetic pre- and postganglionic neurones. However, there are good reasons to assume that the principle of organization into functionally discrete pathways is the same as in the sympathetic nervous system, the only difference being that some targets of the sympathetic system are widely distributed throughout the body (e.g. blood vessels, sweat glands, erector pili muscles, fat tissue) (Jänig and McLachlan 1992a,b).

Organization and function of autonomic ganglia

A major function of the peripheral ganglia is to distribute the centrally integrated signals by connecting each preganglionic axon with several postganglionic neurones. The extent of divergence varies significantly, the ratio of pre- to postganglionic axons being, in pathways such as in the ciliary ganglion to the iris and ciliary body, as low as 1 : 4 and in others, such as in the superior cervical ganglion with many vasoconstrictor neurones, as high as 1 : 150. However, it is clear that limited divergence and much divergence, respectively, are not characteristics of the parasympathetic and sympathetic systems (Wang *et al.* 1995). Probably, by analogy with somatic motor units, limited divergence is common in pathways to small targets with discrete functions whereas widespread divergence is a feature of pathways to anatomically extensive effectors that act more or less simultaneously. Such effectors may be innervated by either system (McLachlan 1995).

Sympathetic ganglia

Within sympathetic ganglia, each convergent cholinergic preganglionic axon produces an excitatory postsynaptic potential by activating nicotinic receptor-channels. The amplitude of the potential varies between inputs, ranging from a few millivolts to suprathreshold. In most cases, one or a few inputs has, like the skeletal neuromuscular junction, a high safety factor and always initiates an action potential (Fig. 1.5). Thus the ganglion cell relays the incoming impulses of only a few of its preganglionic inputs. If there are several suprathreshold inputs, then each must have a low firing rate as postganglionic axons with ongoing activity (mostly vasoconstrictor) discharge at only about 1 Hz (Chapter 23; Jänig 1985, 1995). When activity increases during reflex activation or arousal, postganglionic neurones discharge at up to 5–10 Hz, probably more by increased discharge of the few suprathreshold inputs than by summation. The function of the subthreshold synapses in ganglia is not clear.

Muscarinic and peptidergic contributions to ganglionic transmission follow high-frequency activation of preganglionic inputs, e.g. in muscle vasoconstrictor pathways in anaesthetized cats (Jänig 1995), but such effects have not been demonstrated in humans.

Paravertebral (sympathetic) neurones have relatively uniform cell properties. Structurally, they have several dendrites, the number of which is correlated with the number of preganglionic inputs (Purves *et al.* 1986). At least one of these inputs is suprathreshold and relays CNS-derived signals directly. In contrast, *prevertebral (sympathetic) neurones*, at least in experimental animals, do not have uniform properties. Three broad groups differ electrophysiologically (by the K$^+$ channels that control excitability), morphologically (by their size and dendritic branching), and neurochemically (by their neuropeptide content) (Boyd *et al.* 1996). Two groups, like paravertebral neurones, have suprathreshold synaptic connections, but the mode of synaptic transmission in the third group is different. These neurones receive preganglionic inputs that do not necessarily activate them. However, they also receive many nicotinic inputs from mechanosensitive afferents in the intestine. Summation of synaptic potentials from peripheral and preganglionic inputs is necessary to initiate their discharge. These neurones also depolarize slowly when their inputs are activated at high frequency. The slow responses arise from the release of neuropeptides such as vasoactive intestinal polypeptide (VIP) from

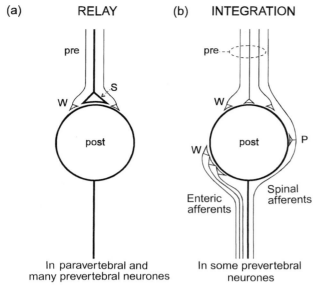

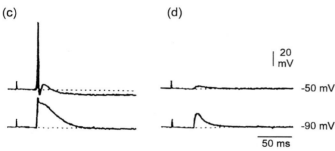

Fig. 1.5. Two types of transmission in autonomic ganglia. (a) Most
ganglion cells receive one or a few preganglionic inputs that, when
activated, produce a suprathreshold ('strong', S) response. Most also
receive several weak (w) convergent inputs that evoke only a subthreshold
synaptic potential. Transmission occurs predominantly via the S input,
which relays its signals directly to the postganglionic neurone.
Summation of weak responses is probably rare. (b) In some prevertebral
sympathetic neurones, the preganglionic inputs are only of the weak type
but other cholinergic inputs that arise in the enteric nervous system also
converge on the cell. Activation occurs by temporal and/or spatial
summation. Peptides released from spinal afferent neurones (P) may
potentiate transmission. (c, d) Synaptic potentials recorded in a ganglion
cell at resting membrane potential (upper traces) and with the membrane
hyperpolarized to block action potential initiation (lower traces). When a
single strong input is stimulated (c), the response is suprathreshold at
resting membrane potential and a large amplitude excitatory synaptic
potential is evoked at –90 mV. In response to stimulation of a single weak
preganglionic axon (d), a small subthreshold excitatory synaptic potential
is evoked that increases in amplitude with hyperpolarization. The
differences in amplitude reflect differences in the number of quanta of
acetylcholine released from each axon.

the enteric afferent projections or substance P (SP) released from
spinal primary afferent neurone collaterals (see Fig. 1.7). These prevertebral neurones therefore depend on temporal and spatial integration of incoming signals, much like neurones within the CNS. The
function of these connections is discussed below.

Parasympathetic ganglia

The structure of many parasympathetic ganglion cells, with few
dendrites, is simpler than that of sympathetic neurones. The preganglionic input is correspondingly simple, often consisting of a
single suprathreshold input. However, many parasympathetic ganglia
in the trunk contain, as well as postganglionic neurones, neurones
that behave as primary afferent and interneurones, i.e. they have the
potential for reflex activity independent of the CNS, like the enteric
system (see above). For example, in the intracardiac ganglia (Edwards
et al. 1995; Fig. 1.6), only a proportion of the ganglion cells receive
input from preganglionic axons and project to cardiac muscle. A subpopulation of neurones that cannot be activated synaptically may
consist of afferent neurones. These cells have intrinsic pacemaker
activity which might be responsible for ongoing synaptic activity
recorded in other neurones within the ganglia. A third group of
smaller neurones receives local synaptic inputs and may also terminate on cardiac muscle. Although both the location of the endings of
the putative afferent neurones and the adequate stimuli that excite
them remain mysteries, these peripheral connections are a feature of
several parasympathetic ganglia (e.g. Mawe 1995). The intramural
ganglia show some similarities to sympathetic ganglia and some to
the enteric system. No evidence of interneurones or pacemaker activity has yet been detected in cranial ganglia.

The pelvic or hypogastric plexuses contain the neurones that
innervate the pelvic organs. Some of these ganglion cells are noradrenergic and are innervated by lumbar preganglionic axons, others
are cholinergic and receive sacral inputs (Keast 1995). A proportion

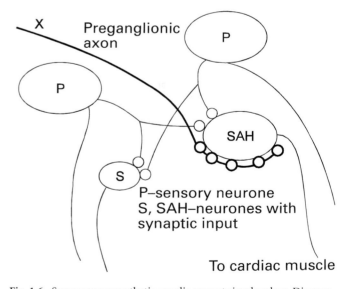

Fig. 1.6. Some parasympathetic ganglia are not simple relays. Diagram
of the component neurones of intracardiac ganglia. Only one neurone
type (SAH, synaptic, afterhyperpolarization) receives vagal synaptic
inputs. SAH cells and another neurone type (S, synaptic) receive synaptic
inputs with ongoing activity arising from the third neurone type which is
spontaneously active (P, pacemaker neurones). P cells may be sensory
neurones with afferent terminals within the heart. (Modified from
Edwards *et al.* 1995.)

of pelvic neurones receive synaptic connections from both hypogastric and pelvic nerves. In bladder ganglia (see Chapter 19), noradrenaline (NAd) from stimulated sympathetic postganglionic terminals can inhibit acetylcholine (ACh) release from preganglionic axons and so depress transmission of sacral signals. NAd does not affect the parasympathetic neurones directly. Neuropeptide Y (NPY) released from sympathetic noradrenergic terminals has a similar inhibitory effect in intracardiac ganglia (Potter 1991).

Peripheral reflexes

Spinal visceral afferent neurones are not only involved in reflexes at spinal and supraspinal levels (see earlier) but probably also in peripheral reflexes that never involve the CNS. In addition, afferent neurones within the enteric nervous system (and possibly other effector tissues) have axons that project back into autonomic ganglia and initiate reflex activity in postganglionic neurones. These latter are known as *peripheral afferents*. Distension activates mechanosensitive endings of enteric neurones that project in the mesenteric nerves back to the prevertebral ganglia (Fig. 1.7). Axons from a considerable length of the intestine converge on each ganglion cell although the majority probably arise in the proximal colon. Summation of the effects of enteric afferents triggers postganglionic discharges and leads to the release of NAd and thus relaxation of the intestine. These peripheral reflexes between different parts of the intestine presumably contribute to the storage function of the large bowel. Further, peptides released in prevertebral sympathetic ganglia from collaterals of spinal visceral afferent neurones can enhance cholinergic synaptic transmission from both preganglionic axons and enteric neurones.

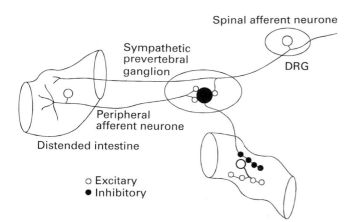

Fig. 1.7. Peripheral reflexes. Distension of the bowel activates afferent terminals of local enteric afferent neurones as well as those of primary afferent neurones with cell bodies in dorsal root ganglia (DRGs). The enteric afferents project only to prevertebral ganglia where they release ACh to activate nicotinic receptors and excite postganglionic neurones projecting to another part fo the bowel. This leads to inhibition of enteric excitatory motoneurones and relaxation. In addition, collateral branches of primary afferent neurones release substance P (SP) in the ganglion, leading to a prolonged depolarization that facilitates discharge by nicotinic inputs.

Transmitter substances in autonomic neurones

The principles of chemical transmission were defined in the autonomic nervous system based on the release of the 'conventional' neurotransmitters, acetylcholine (ACh) and noradrenaline (NAd). However, it is now clear that several chemical substances are often contained within individual autonomic neurones, can be released by action potentials, and can have multiple actions on effector tissues (Furness *et al.* 1989; Morris and Gibbins 1992).

1. ACh is released by all preganglionic axons at their synapses in ganglia, and the effects of nerve activity are antagonized by blockade of nicotinic ACh receptors. Under some experimental conditions, repetitive activation of preganglionic axons can release enough ACh to activate extrasynaptic muscarinic receptors (Jänig 1995).

2. Most sympathetic postganglionic axons release NAd, but sympathetic sudomotor and muscle vasodilator axons are cholinergic. Most, but not all, nerve-mediated effects can be antagonized by blockade of adrenoceptors or muscarinic ACh receptors (see below).

3. Although parasympathetic postganglionic neurones in many tissues release ACh, not all effects of stimulating parasympathetic nerves are blocked by muscarinic antagonists (Table 1.3) and so must be mediated by other transmitters. Although the postganglionic neurones involved have been called non-adrenergic, non-cholinergic (NANC) neurones, recent evidence indicates that all parasympathetic neurones are cholinergic (Keast 1995).

NANC transmission has been studied extensively, e.g. in the enteric nervous system where nitric oxide (NO) and VIP, possibly together with adenosine 5'-triphosphate (ATP), are thought to mediate inhibition of gastrointestinal smooth muscle by enteric neurones. 'Nitrergic' nerves (containing the enzyme neuronal nitric oxide synthase) are vasodilator or relaxant in several tissues (Table 1.3). Currently, various peptides, ATP and NO appear to act as NANC transmitters.

Responses of tissues to nerve-released NAd and ACh usually only follow repetitive activation of many axons. High-frequency stimuli, particularly in bursts, may produce effector responses due to the concomitant release of a neuropeptide. Immunohistochemistry has revealed the presence of many peptides (particularly in the enteric nervous system), although only a few of these have been demonstrated to modify function after release from nerve terminals *in vivo*. Examples are:

1. NPY in sympathetic vasoconstrictor axons potentiates the effects of NAd on the contractile apparatus. In the heart, NPY released by sympathetic activity inhibits vagal slowing (see above).

2. VIP is thought to be the primary *vasodilator* transmitter released from cholinergic vasodilator, sudomotor, and secretomotor axons.

3. There appear to be interactions between autonomic axons and the terminals of primary afferent neurones that express SP and calcitonin-gene-related peptide (CGRP) in the regulation of vasoconstriction in some vascular beds, such as skin and mesentery. CGRP released by axon reflex activation of afferent terminals during inflammation is a potent vasodilator.

Table 1.3. Possible transmitter substances in autonomic neurones

System	Neurone	Transmitter	Co-transmitters
Parasympathetic	Preganglionic	ACh	
	Postganglionic	ACh	VIP and/or NO
Sympathetic	Preganglionic	ACh	
	Postganglionic	NAd,	ATP and/or NPY
		some ACh	VIP and/or NO
Enteric	[Vagal and pelvic inputs	ACh]	
	[Sympathetic inputs	NAd]	
	Intrinsic afferent neurones	Substance P (tachykinins)	
	Interneurones	ACh	Some ATP
	Motor		
	Excitatory	ACh	Substance P (tachykinins)
	Inhibitory	NO/?VIP/PACAP/?ATP	
	Secretomotor	ACh	VIP

ACh, acetylcholine; NAd, noradrenaline; ATP, adenosine 5′-triphosphate; NO, nitric oxide; NPY, neuropeptide Y; VIP, vasoactive intestinal polypeptide; PACAP, pituitary adenylate cyclase-activating peptide.

Mechanisms of neuroeffector transmission

In peripheral tissues, the effects of activity in autonomic nerve terminals can be due to the release of several different compounds. When the effects of nerve activity are not blocked completely by an adrenoceptor or muscarinic antagonist at a concentration that entirely abolishes the response to exogenous transmitter, it may not necessarily be the case that a NANC transmitter is involved. The effects of exogenous transmitter substances on cellular functions are known for many tissues but the consequences of activation of postjunctional receptors by neurally released transmitters have been investigated surprisingly rarely. When they have, the mechanisms of neuroeffector transmission have been found to be diverse. Excitation or inhibition may involve a range of cellular events, including:

1. Brief openings of ligand-gated channels (as at many neuroneal synapses) or slower conductance changes mediated by second messenger systems.
2. The ensuing depolarization may open voltage-dependent Ca^{2+} channels, leading to Ca^{2+} influx.
3. Receptor activation may lead, after G-protein activation, to release from intracellular Ca^{2+} stores or modulation of the Ca^{2+} sensitivity of the contractile/secretory mechanism.
4. β-Adrenoceptors linked to adenylate cyclase modify cell function by changing intracellular levels of cyclic AMP.
5. Inhibition (relaxation) often involves the activation of cyclic GMP-dependent protein kinases.

One important concept has emerged: the mechanism utilized by endogenously released transmitter is often not the same as that activated by exogenous transmitter substances or their analogues (Hirst *et al.* 1996). The following examples illustrate this point.

Innervation of the cardiac pacemaker

Vagal stimulation slows action potential firing in atrial pacemaker cells. During nerve stimulation, the action potentials slow without any change in their configuration and without membrane hyperpolarization (Fig. 1.8). Exogenous ACh, in contrast, slows firing by hyperpolarizing the membrane and reducing the amplitude and duration of the action potentials, consistent with an increase in K^+ conductance (Fig. 1.8). Both responses are blocked by atropine but, as the postreceptor conductance changes clearly differ, the muscarinic receptors activated by vagal ACh cannot be the same as those to which exogenous ACh binds.

Similar data have been obtained for the sympathetic innervation, which increases the rate of pacemaking. Both neurally released and exogenous NAd activate β-adrenoceptors but neural NAd modifies the pacemaker current rather than producing the rise in cyclic AMP that follows application of exogenous NAd. Because both noradrenergic and cholinergic axons form close neuromuscular junctions on cardiac pacemaker cells (Fig. 1.8), it seems likely that neurally released transmitters act on junctional receptors that differ from those at extrajunctional sites. The latter would be most readily activated by exogenous compounds.

Cholinergic innervation of the ileum

The longitudinal muscle of the ileum is innervated by cholinergic neurones that lie in the myenteric plexus. Nerve-evoked contractions and contractions to exogenous ACh are both abolished by atropine. Nerve-evoked contractions are reduced but not abolished by blockade of voltage-dependent Ca^{2+} channels. Depolarizations evoked by nerve stimulation are associated with increases in intracellular Ca^{2+}. Both the depolarizations (and the accompanying contraction) are blocked by antagonists that do not affect the depolarization and contraction produced by exogenous ACh. Figure 1.9 summarizes the cellular mechanisms that seem to be involved in these responses. Close junctions between varicose terminals and smooth muscle also exist in this tissue. These findings suggest that muscarinic receptors involved in transmission from cholinergic nerves to this muscle are restricted to the junctional membrane and differ from those activated by exogenous ACh.

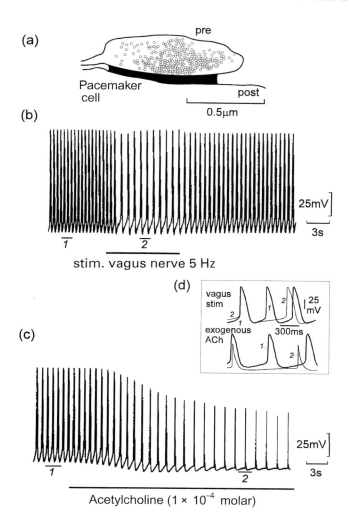

Fig. 1.8. Innervation of the cardiac pacemaker. (a) Tracings of a cholinergic varicosity forming a neuromuscular junction on a cell of the guinea-pig sinoatrial node (from Klemm *et al.* (1992). *J. Auton. Nerv. Syst.* **39**, 139–50; Choate *et al.* (1993). *J. Auton. Nerv. Syst.* **44**, 1–12). Membrane effects of (b) vagally released acetylcholine (ACh) and (c) exogenously applied ACh differ. (d) Nerve-mediated responses show no change in action potential configuration but a reduced slope of the pacemaker potential (upper records in inset), whereas exogenous ACh hyperpolarizes the membrane and shunts the action potential, reducing its amplitude and duration (lower records in inset) (modified from Campbell *et al.* (1989). *J. Physiol.* **415**, 57–68).

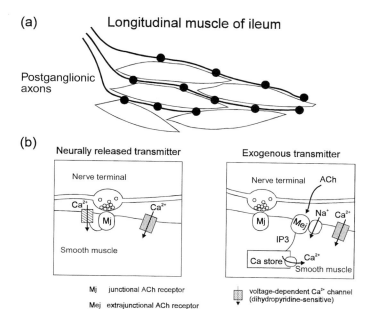

Fig. 1.9. Neuroeffector transmission to the longitudinal muscle of the ileum. (a) The longitudinal muscle of the ileum receives a cholinergic innervation from the enteric plexus which terminates as neuromuscular junctions. (b) The transmitter, acetylcholine (ACh), after release by nerve impulses, activates local junctional muscarinic receptors (Mj) leading to depolarization by influx of cations (including Ca^{2+}) through channels linked to the receptors; this depolarization opens voltage-dependent Ca^{2+} channels. In contrast, ACh applied by superperfusion activates extrajunctional muscarinic receptors (Mej) linked to non-specific cation channels, leading to depolarization and activation of voltage-dependent Ca^{2+} channels. In addition, Ca^{2+} is released from intracellular stores via the inositol trisphosphate (IP3) pathway. Increases in intracellular Ca^{2+} concentration from any of these sources contribute to smooth muscle contraction.

Sympathetic innervation of blood vessels

Most blood vessels constrict when exogenous NAd is applied to them; this pharmacological action is largely mediated by α_1-adrenoceptors and does not depend on the entry of extracellular Ca^{2+} through voltage-dependent channels, i.e. most of the Ca^{2+} triggering vasoconstriction is released from intracellular stores by second messengers. Blood vessels are innervated by terminals containing NAd, and in most cases also NPY. Many of the varicosities on small muscular vessels of less than 0.5 mm diameter form close neuromuscular junctions (Luff and McLachlan 1989), the proportion that do not form junctions varying between vessels at different sites throughout the circulation. In various vessels, nerve stimulation evokes brief depolarizations due to the action of ATP on P_{2X} purinoceptors or of NAd on α_1-adrenoceptors, and in some a slow depolarization reflects the action of NAd on α_2-adrenoceptors (Hirst *et al.* 1996). Constriction of some small arteries during sympathetic nerve activity is abolished by α-adrenoceptor antagonists but is partly dependent on membrane depolarization (Brock *et al.* 1997). In contrast, in some small arterioles, vasoconstriction produced by nerve stimulation is unaffected by α-adrenoceptor blockade (Evans and Surprenant 1992). Thus neural control of constriction can involve different transmitters and both voltage-dependent and voltage-independent mechanisms in different parts of the vascular tree.

NPY can play a neuromodulatory role. When it is released (probably by high-frequency bursts of activity), it can potentiate the contractile response to nerve stimulation in some vessels.

Other effectors

The examples given above indicate the diversity of mechanisms for neuroeffector transmission in different targets. As the responses of other tissues to nerve stimulation are studied, our traditional ideas about the ability of conventional transmitters to mimic the effects of nerve activity must be reconsidered. If the intention is to interfere with ongoing nerve-mediated effects *in vivo*, it is more useful to determine which antagonists reduce or abolish the effects of nerve activity than to know which receptor subtypes are present on the tissue.

Concluding remarks

The autonomic nervous system supplies each target organ and tissue via a separate pathway which consists of sets of pre- and post-ganglionic neurones with distinct patterns of reflex activity. This has been established for the lumbar sympathetic outflow to skin, skeletal muscle and viscera, for the thoracic sympathetic outflow to the head and neck, and probably applies to all autonomic systems. The specificity of the messages that these pathways transmit from the CNS arises from integration within precisely organized pathways in the neuraxis. The messages travel along discrete functional pathways and are transmitted to the target tissues often via organized neuroeffector junctions. Modulation in the periphery can occur within each pathway, both in ganglia and at the level of the effector organs. Much remains to be discovered about the control of the diverse functions of the vasculature, glands, and viscera.

Acknowledgements

The authors were supported by the Deutsche Forschungsgemeinschaft, Germany, the National Health Medical Research Council of Australia and the Max-Planck Gesellschaft.

References

Boyd, H., McLachlan, E. M., Keast, J. R., and Inokuchi, H. (1996). Three electrophysiological classes of guinea pig sympathetic neurone have distinct morphologies. *J. Comp. Neurol.* **369**, 372–87.

Brock, J. A., McLachlan, E. M., and Rayner, S. E. (1997). Contribution of α-adrenoceptors to depolarization and contraction evoked by continuous asynchronous sympathetic nerve activity in rat tail artery. *Br. J. Pharmacol.* **120**, 1513–21.

Cervero, F. (1994). Sensory innervation of the viscera: peripheral basis of visceral pain. *Physiol. Rev.* **75**, 95–138.

Edwards, F. R., Hirst, G. D., Klemm, M. F., and Steele, P. A. (1995). Different types of ganglion cell in the cardiac plexus of guinea-pigs. *J. Physiol.* **486**, 453–71.

Evans, R. J. and Surprenant, A. M. (1992). Vasoconstriction of guinea-pig submucosal arterioles following sympathetic nerve stimulation is mediated by the release of ATP. *Br. J. Pharmacol.* **106**, 242–9.

Furness, J. B. and Bornstein, J. C. (1995). The enteric nervous system and its extrinsic connections. In *Textbook of gastroenterology*, (2nd edn) (ed. T. Yamada), pp. 2–20. J.B. Lippincott, Philadelphia.

Furness, J. B. and Costa, M. (1987). *The enteric nervous system.* Churchill Livingstone, Edinburgh.

Furness, J. B., Morris, J. L., Gibbins, I. L., and Costa., M. (1989). Chemical coding of neurones and plurichemical transmission. *Ann. Rev. Pharmacol. Toxicol.* **29**, 289–306.

Greger, R. and Windhorst, U. (1996). *Comprehensive human physiology. From cellular mechanisms to integration*, Vols 1 and 2. Springer Verlag, Berlin.

Hirst, G. D., Choate, J. K., Cousins, H. M., Edwards, F. R., and Klemm, M. F. (1996). Transmission by post-ganglionic axons of the autonomic nervous system: the importance of the specialized neuroeffector junction. *Neuroscience* **73**, 7–23.

Jänig, W. (1985). Organization of the lumbar sympathetic outflow to skeletal muscle and skin of the cat hindlimb and tail. *Rev. Physiol. Biochem. Pharmacol.* **102**, 119–213.

Jänig, W. (1995). Ganglionic transmission *in vivo*. In *Autonomic ganglia*, (ed. E.M. McLachlan), pp. 349–95. Harwood Academic Publishers, Luxembourg.

Jänig, W. (1996*a*). Neurobiology of visceral afferent neurones: neuroanatomy, functions, organ regulations and sensations. *Biol. Psychol.* **42**, 29–51.

Jänig, W. (1996*b*). Spinal cord reflex organization of sympathetic systems. In *The emotional motor system*, (ed. R. Bandler, G. Holstege, and C. B. Saper). *Prog. Brain Res.* **107**, 43–77.

Jänig, W. and Koltzenburg, M. (1993). Pain arising from the urogenital tract. In *The autonomic nervous system*, (ed. G. Burnstock), Vol. 2 *Nervous Control of the Urogenital System* (ed. C. A. Maggi), pp. 523–76. Harwood Academic Publishers, Chur, Switzerland.

Jänig, W. and McLachlan, E. M. (1987). Organization of lumbar spinal outflow to the distal colon and pelvic organs. *Physiol. Rev.* **67**, 1332–1404.

Jänig, W. and McLachlan, E. M. (1992*a*). Characteristics of function-specific pathways in the sympathetic nervous system. *Trends Neurosci.* **15**, 475–81.

Jänig, W. and McLachlan, E. M. (1992*b*). Specialized functional pathways are the building blocks of the autonomic nervous system. *J. autonom. nerv. Syst.* **41**, 3–14.

Keast, J. R. (1995). All pelvic neurons in male rats contain immunoreactivity for the synthetic enzymes of either noradrenaline or acetylcholine. *Neurosci. Lett.* **196**, 209–12.

Langley, J. N. (1921). *The autonomic nervous system*, part 1. Heffer, Cambridge.

Loewy, A. D. and Spyer, K. M. (ed.) (1990). *Central regulation of autonomic functions*. Oxford University Press, New York.

Luff, S. E. and McLachlan, E. M. (1989). Frequency of neuromuscular junctions on arteries of different dimensions in the rabbit, guinea-pig and rat. *Blood Vessels*, **26**, 95–106.

McLachlan, E. M. (ed.) (1995). *Autonomic ganglia*. Harwood Academic Publishers, Luxembourg.

Mawe, G. M. (1995). Prevertebral, pancreatic and gallbladder ganglia: non-enteric ganglia that are involved in gastrointestinal function. In *Autonomic ganglia*, (ed. E.M. McLachlan), pp. 397–444. Harwood Academic Publishers, Luxembourg.

Morris, J. L. and Gibbins, I. L. (1992). Co-transmission and neuromodulation. In *Autonomic neuroeffector mechanisms*, (ed. G. Burnstock and C.H.V. Hoyle), pp. 33–119. Harwood Academic Publishers, Chur, Switzerland.

Potter, E. K. (1991). Neuropeptide Y as an autonomic neurotransmitter. In *Novel peripheral neurotransmitters*, (ed. C. Bell), pp. 81–112. Pergamon, New York.

Purves, D., Rubin, E., Snider, W. D., and Lichtman, J. (1986). Relation of animal size to convergence, divergence, and neuronal number in peripheral sympathetic pathways. *J. Neurosci.* **6**, 158–63.

Ritter, S., Ritter, R. C., and Barnes, C. D. (ed.) (1992). *Neuroanatomy and physiology of abdominal vagal afferents*. CRC Press, Boca Raton.

Wang, F. B., Holst, M. C., and Powley, T. L. (1995). The ratio of pre- to postganglionic neurones and related issues in the autonomic nervous system. *Brain Res. Rev.* **21**, 93–115.

2. Autonomic nervous system development

Robert W. Hamill and Edmund F. LaGamma

Introduction

Over the past 5 years rapidly accumulating data have expanded substantially our understanding of the mechanisms underlying the fundamental interactions between the forces of 'nature' versus 'nurture' as they sculpt the developing organism. 'Nature' refers to the cell's intrinsic potential, i.e. its genetic make-up, which provides the potential for a neurone's eventual repertoire of cellular processes and adult characteristics. 'Nurture' refers to extrinsic forces that influence the developmental cascade of neural maturation and serve to shape ontogenetic processes and determine the neurone's adult state. As the number of genes, neurotrophic factors, inflammatory and haematolymphopoietic cytokines, extracellular matrix proteins, and inter/ intracellular developmental mechanisms continue to be revealed, the interdependence and integration of 'nature and nurture' are evident as they merge their determinants of the maturation of the organism. It is not only clear that genes and epigenetic factors are the key players in this ontogenetic symphony, but it is also apparent that roles and understandings of mechanisms change almost as frequently as new observations appear. The current chapter will summarize basic aspects of autonomic nervous system (ANS) development and will highlight the advances in molecular genetics, neurotrophin and cytokine biology, the influences of extracellular matrix proteins, and the observations garnered from mutant animals; i.e. 'gene knock-outs'. The embryology and maturation of spinal and peripheral components of the ANS are reviewed briefly, addressing the following areas: stages of development; neural crest, genes, gene knock-outs, neurotrophic factors (neurotrophins, cytokines, haematopoietic factors), and their influence on lineage formation. Developmental disorders related to these ontogenetic principles and the potential relationship of age-related disorders to the processes and factors required to sustain neuronal survival, function, and plasticity during adulthood will be mentioned. Recent reviews of neuronal development include Sommer *et al.* 1995; Henderson 1996; Davies 1997; Gershon 1997; Mehler and Kessler 1997; Mehler *et al.* 1997; Perris 1997. In order to assist in the reading of this chapter, abbreviations used in the text and all illustrations are listed in Table 2.1.

Table 2.1. ANS abbreviations

Classification	Abbreviation	Definition
Cytokines		
Neurotrophins	NGF	Nerve growth factor
	BDNF	Brain-derived neurotrophic factor
	GDNF	Glial-derived neurotrophic factor
	TrkA, B, C	Tyrosine kinase A, B, C
	NT-3, 4, 5, 6	Neutrophins 3, 4, 5, and 6
Neuropoietic factors	ACT A	Activin A
	LIF	Leukaemia inhibitory factor
	LIFR	Leukaemia inhibitory factor receptor
	CNTF	Ciliary Neurotrophic factor
	OM	Oncostatin M
	MANS	Membrane-associated neurotransmitter-stimulating factor
	SGF	Sweat gland factor
Haematopoietic factors	BMP2, 4, 7	Bone morphogenic proteins 2, 4, and 7
	EPO	Erythropoitein
	IL-1, 2, 6, 11	Interleukins
	INFγ	Interferon-gamma
	SCF	Stem cell factor
Growth factors	CT-1	Cardiotrophin 1
	GGF	Glial growth factor
	IGF	Insulin growth factor
	FGF	Fibroblast growth factors, acidic (a), basic (b), and others
	TGF	Transforming growth factors, α and β

Table 2.1. (*continued*)

Classification	Abbreviation	Definition
Neuropeptides	CGRP	Calcitonin gene-related peptide
	CCK	Cholecystokinin
	CRF	Corticotrophin releasing factor
	DYN	Dynorphin
	ENC	Enkephalin
	NPY	Neuropeptide Y
	NT'	Neurotensin
	PACAP	Pituitary adenylate cyclase activity peptide
	SOM	Somatostatin
	SP	Substance P
	VIP	Vasoactive intestinal polypeptide
Neurochemical transmitters	A	Adrenaline
	ACh	Acetylcholine
	APUD	Amine precursor uptake and decarboxylation
	ATP	Adenosine triphosphate
	CA	Catecholamine
	DA	Dopamine
	GABA	Gamma aminobutyric acid
	NA	Noradrenaline
	NO	Nitric oxide
	5-HT	5-Hydroxytryptamine
	SIF	Small intensely fluorescent
Neurone(s)/neural systems	ANS	Autonomic nervous system
	CG	Ciliary ganglion
	CN	Cholinergic neurone
	DBH	Dopamine β-hydroxylase
	ECM	Extracellular matrix
	EDNRB	Endothelium β-receptor
	ENS	Enteric nervous system
	MASH1	Mammalian achaete–scute homolog 1
	M	Melanocyte
	MP	Multipotent Progenitor
	NC	Neural crest
	NCSC	Neural crest stem cell
	NF68	Neurofilament 68
	NF160	Neurofilament 160
	NSE	Neurone-specific enolase
	NP	Neuronal progenitor
	PN	Parasympathetic neurone
	PNS	Parasympathetic nervous system
	SC	Schwan cell
	SCG	Superior cervical ganglion
	SM	Smooth muscle
	SN'	Sensory neurone
	SN	Sensory neuroblast
	SNS	Sympathetic nervous system
	SAN	Sympathoadrenal neuronal progenitor
	SYM	Sympathetic neurone
	SYM'	Sympathetic neuroblast
	TC	Transiently catecholaminergic

Stages of development

Embryonic

Embryologically, ANS ontogeny is related to two main processes: basal plate development within the spinal cord; and neural crest development, migration, and phenotypic expression. In humans, neural development begins during the third week when the ectoderm thickens to form the neural plate. Fusion of the neural folds, which form from the elevated lateral edges of the neural plate, results in the formation of the neural tube; neurulation is completed by approximately 26–28 days of gestation (Kissel *et al.* 1981). Upon closure, neuroepithelial cells become neuroblasts, which form the mantle zone surrounding the neuroepithelial layer. As more neuroblasts accrue, dorsal and ventral thickenings appear, and between the alar and basal plates, progenitors of the dorsal and ventral horns, a smaller collection of neuroblasts form the intermediolateral horn. These early descriptive stages may now be viewed in light of recently accumulating evidence that an expanding subclass of the transforming growth factor-β (TGF-β) superfamily of molecules, called bone morphogenetic proteins (BMPs), directly influence a host of developmental processes including neurulation and the dorsoventral patterning of the neural tube (reviewed by Mehler *et al.* 1997). In fact, a balance between various BMPs and another class of inductive signals, sonic hedgehog (SHH), will lead to the generation of dorsal and ventral cell types within the spinal cord; the BMPs appear to have a prominent role in directing the appearance of dorsal sensory neurones, interneurones, and neural crest stem cells. The interplay of ectoderm-related BMPs and notochord-associated SHH probably underlies the intermediate cell types. In humans the preganglionic neurones and ventral nerve rootlets are apparent by the fifth week of maturation.

During the fifth week of human intrauterine development, midthoracic preganglionic fibres (white rami communicans) appear and subsequently exist along the entire length of the sympathetic chain (Kanerva *et al.* 1974). The grey rami communicans develop from the sixth to the eighth week. During the fifth to seventh week vagal parasympathetic preganglionic fibres are present along the trachea, reach the pulmonary parenchyma as well as the proximal intestinal tract (oesophagus and stomach), and form the cardiac plexus. Fibres appear in the conduction system of the heart and epithelium of the lung during the tenth week, and, as target organ and enteric ganglion development occurs, preganglionic maturation continues in a craniocaudal fashion (Kissel *et al.* 1981).

Neural crest

The peripheral ANS, including the peripheral sympathetic nervous system (SNS), parasympathetic nervous system (PNS), and enteric nervous system (ENS), is derived fully from neural crest (NC) cells. The cellular émigrés that form the ANS originate from the vagal, truncal, and sacral crest, and are under a host of influences from origin to destination. The extraordinary pluripotential nature of these cells is evident by the wide range of neurotransmitter phenotypes that reside within the ANS, all derived from the NC (Table 2.2). Neural crest stem cells (NCSC) are generated by inductive signals that originate from non-neural cells adjacent to the neural tube. NC cells are initially located dorsomedially between the neural tube and the overlying ectoderm, and before neurulation is complete crest cells begin to migrate in a rostrocaudal manner along two distinct paths—dorsolaterally and ventrolaterally. The ventral pathways result in the development of autonomic and sensory neurones, paraganglia, chromatophores (non-neuronal support cells), and adrenal chromaffin cells. NC cells are the progenitors of a wide variety of neuronal and neuroendocrine populations which are distinct in phenotypic and functional characteristics; some of the factors responsible for this complex evolution are illustrated in Fig. 2.1. This cartoon summarizes molecules that are instrumental in NC differentiation and maturation during the following stages of development: lineage restriction; lineage commitment, proliferation, and survival; neuronal differentiation; transmitter and receptor phenotypic expression; axodendritic process outgrowth; and neuronal survival. The ontogeny of NC and neural development in general are the result of combinatorial interactions between and among neurotrophins, haematolymphopoietic (BMPs) and inflammatory cytokines (neurokines), all influencing the genetic substrate of stem cells and neuroblasts. Additionally, these effects may be autocrine (molecules produced by the cell itself), paracrine (molecules produced by adjacent cells), endocrine (molecules arriving via the circulation), or target derived (molecules

Table 2.2. Neuronal derivatives of neural crest

Primitive cell	Adult cell/structure	Neurotransmitters
Bipolar neuroblast	Dorsal root ganglia	

Multipolar neuroblast	Sympathetic neurones
	  Paravertebral ganglia
	  Prevertebral ganglia
	  Terminal ganglia
		NA, CCK, SOM, SP, ENC, ACh, VIP, PACAP,
		5-HT, NPY

	Parasympathetic ganglia
	  Major parasympathetic ganglia
	    Ciliary
	    Sphenopalatine
	    Otic
	    Submandibular/sublingual
	    Pelvic ganglia
	    Terminal parasympathetic ganglia (target tissue)
		ACh, VIP, SP, NO, CAs-SIF, NPY

	Enteric neurones
	  Myenteric plexus (Auerbach's)
	  Submucosal plexus (Meissner's)
	  Enteric ganglia
		GABA, ACh, VIP, 5-HT, SP, ENC, SRIF, SOM, DYN,
		NO, NT', NPY, ATP, CRF, CGRP, CCK
		motilin-like peptide,
		bombesin-like peptide

	Chromaffin cells of adrenal medulla	A, NA, ENC, NPY, APUD
	Paraganglia-chromaffin	5-HT, DA, A
	Small intensely fluorescent (SIF) cells, ganglia	5-HT, DA, A, ENC

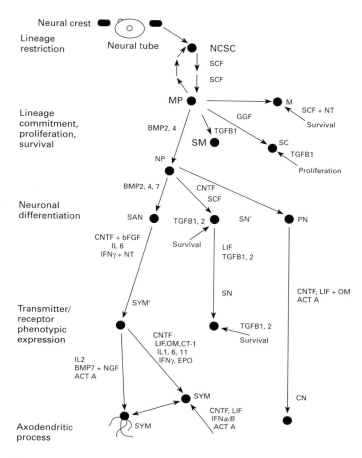

Fig. 2.1. Peripheral autonomic nervous system development: roles of cytokines and neurotrophins (adapted from Mehler and Kessler 1997).

that are transported retrogradely to the neurone cell body after nerve terminal innervation of the target). The transition from lineage restriction to lineage commitment arrives as stem cell populations mature to multipotent progenitor cells that, under the influence of various molecules, evolve to neuronal progenitors (NP) as well as non-neural elements, such as smooth muscle, Schwann cells, and melanocytes. Neural crest-derived lineage commitment is instructive, receiving directions by neuregulins and/or the TGF-β subfamily. The NP is the founding cell for sympathetic, parasympathetic, enteric, and sensory neurones. It is of note that BMPs not only contribute to the cascades profiled in Fig. 2.1 but are also involved in initiating apoptosis (programmed cell death) so that odd-numbered branchiogenic neural crest rhombomeres are removed (the primary BMP is BMP4) (Mehler *et al.* 1997). Review of Fig. 2.1 indicates that the same molecule, or group of molecules, appears along the cascade from early maturation, such as lineage commitment, proliferation, and survival, to the final transition to neurochemical phenotypic characteristics and the ultimate process of establishing neuronal processes and synaptic contact. This schema is not meant to be all inclusive as the role(s) of various molecules are complicated and cannot be fully presented and discussed; key variables such as environmental and interneuronal influences are not represented (see Chapter 2 in Bannister and Mathias 1992).

NC cells participate in a spatiotemporally co-ordinated migratory process such that these pluripotential cells disperse along various paths, some to survive, some to succumb, and it is the physical environment, including the topographical arrangement and relative

expression of many extracellular matrix (ECM) proteins, that influences the ultimate fate of these cells. The ECM proteins are generally viewed as either permissive (widely expressed, promoting motility), non-permissive (scarce or absent from migratory pathways), or inhibitory (restricted, impeding cell motility) molecules (reviewed by Perris 1997). Thus there may be a 'go and stop' set of mechanisms, and the timing of the expression of these ECM proteins may be critical in order for their role to be effected properly; they appear to be involved not only in migration but also in the formation of ganglia. Not surprisingly, migrating NC cells appear to influence their own direction of movement as they express cell surface molecules, such as $\alpha4\beta1$ integrin, that contribute to the condensation of NC cells into ganglia. Accordingly, the theories of NC cell homing must include considerations of a wide range of signals derived from the ECM as well as the phenotype of the migrating NC cells (Perris 1997). Although the exact function of this vast array of ECM proteins is just beginning to emerge, it is interesting to note that the *lethal spotted* (*ls/ls*) and *piebald lethal* (*s'/s'*) mouse mutants, which are pathophysiologically analogous to Hirschsprung's disease in humans, exhibit an ECM mutation that precludes the ability of NC cells to colonize the myenteric and submucosal plexuses, resulting in deficient innervation in the distal colon. As genetic mutants were created we recognized that the endothelin B receptor gene 'knock-out' results in the aganglionic megacolon. The ENS offers a number of unique functional characteristics, including a diversity of CNS neurotransmitters (Table 2.2), implying that the migrating NC cells and developing autonomic neuroblasts are indeed pluripotential. The major NC cells contributing to the ENS originate from vagal and sacral NC and the truncal crest only colonizes the rostral foregut (see Table 2.3).

The timetable of normal human sympathetic development indicates that by the fifth week migrating NC cells coalesce to form the primitive sympathetic chains and during the sixth week the chain extends rostrally into the superior cervical ganglion region and caudally with segmentation (Kanerva *et al.* 1974). Postganglionic fibres also are developing: grey rami appear by the sixth week and axons are growing toward targets shortly after the appearance of the catecholamine transmitters at approximately 8–9 weeks. Enteric ganglia maturation in human occurs rostrocaudally; ganglion cells appear in the gut early in the first trimester, with Auerbach's plexus visible by 9–10 weeks; Meissner's plexus follows at 13–14 weeks. By 24 weeks ganglion cells have reached the rectum.

Noradrenergic fibres innervate the ductus arteriosus very early and by 8–10 weeks of fetal life catecholaminergic fibres are present within the mesentery and gut wall (Kanerva *et al.* 1974). The heart responds to cholinergic stimuli by 4 weeks, adrenergic stimuli by 7 weeks, and the hormones glucagon and triiodothyronine by 11 weeks. Parasympathetic nerves appear by 8 weeks, and sympathetic nerves by 10 weeks, whereas neuroeffector transmission is not present until 11 weeks (cholinergic) and 14 weeks (adrenergic). The heartbeat appears by 4 weeks, is generally auscultated at 18 weeks and changes in fetal heart rate occur by 20 weeks (Walker 1975; Papp 1988). The iris, pineal, and vas deferens are not substantially innervated until after birth (Kanerva *et al.* 1974).

Postnatal

The ANS is at various developmental stages at birth, and postnatal human development is normally gauged by physiological observations. Blood flow, bowel transit, and urinary bladder emptying

Table 2.3. Lineage of the crest-derived cells that form the ENS (adapted from Gershon 1997)

Source: crest cells	Regions colonized	Dependencies	Analogous lineages
Truncal	Rostral foregut; presumptive oesophagus and cardiac stomach	Ret/GDNF-independent MASH1-dependent	Caudal sympathetic ganglia: Ret-independent
Vagal	Caudal foregut, midgut, and hindgut; Presumptive caudal stomach, small intestine, caecum, colon	Ret/GDNF-dependent Two lineages: MASH1-dependent; MASH1-independent	Superior cervical ganglion: affected by Ret/GDNF knock-out, but MASH1-independent. Thyroid parafollicular cells: express, but do not depend on MASH1
Sacral	Postumbilical bowel; presumptive ileum, caecum, colon	Ret/GDNF-dependent MASH1-dependent?	?

depend upon maturation of peripheral neural structures as well as central autonomic control mechanisms. Peripherally, the differentiation of neuroblasts into enteric ganglion cells and mature plexuses is quite delayed; in fact, at birth only approximately one-third of the neuroblasts are differentiated and development continues throughout the first 5 years of life (Kissel *et al.* 1981). Similarly, the development of pelvic autonomic ganglia and the innervation of pelvic structures involved in micturition are delayed. Voluntary control over these functions eventually ensues by 2–3 years of age.

Functional development

Maturation of integrated sympathoadrenal function in humans begins with the appearance of catecholamines in the adrenal medulla by 8–9 weeks' gestation and with reflex release by 10 weeks (Gootman and Gootman 1983; Papp 1988). At the cellular level, the human fetus will release catecholamines from non-innervated paraganglia to a greater extent than from the partially innervated adrenal medulla. These responses mature to become qualitatively similar to adult responses by birth when, for example, hypoxia or head-up tilting results in preferential release of noradrenaline over adrenaline. In contrast, insulin, as in the adult, primarily causes release of adrenaline (Slotkin 1985).

The functional development of thermoregulation and cardiovascular control has been well studied. Although a newborn human infant can initiate vasodilation and panting in response to hyperthermia and releases catecholamines to vasoconstrict and augment thermogenesis during hypothermia, the neonate and infant adapt poorly to temperature stress. In general, cardiovascular control appears more mature than temperature control. Although incomplete vascular responses to thermal stimuli may be present until about 2–3 months of age, cardiovascular responses controlling normal vasomotor tone are present before birth, as early as the end of the second trimester, and the newborn's cardiovascular response to cold stress is normal, implying intact sympathoadrenal responses and baroreceptor mechanisms (Gootman and Gootman 1983). Reflex control of heart rate and integrated distribution of blood flow begins between 10 and 20 weeks of gestation and matures considerably thereafter (Pappano 1977; Papp 1988). Of interest is the slightly earlier appearance of functional parasympathetic reflex responsiveness (Pappano 1977; Papp 1988), i.e. well-developed baroreflex function exists in nearly all viable preterm neonates (> 24 weeks' gestation), but is less sensitive and allows for greater blood pressure and heart rate variability (Gootman and

Gootman 1983; Papp 1988). Studies examining neurotransmitters and their metabolites have revealed that all CA compounds are present at birth, CAs increase rapidly by 5 years, and adult levels of CA are reached during adolescence. Studies in swine and rodents provide detailed reviews of the morphological, physiological, and neurochemical development of autonomic systems involved in cardiovascular control (Gootman and Gootman 1983; Slotkin 1985).

In the broadest sense, the practical issues of neuronal development have achieved a new prominence in perinatal medicine with the survival of increasingly smaller neonates [as early as 24 weeks' (400–500 g) gestation]. Therefore, the clinical urgency for application of information regarding the neurobiology of neuronal development has become critical. For example, these newborns will undergo a four- to fivefold increase in their birth weight while under the direct care of the clinician in the neonatal intensive care unit, prior to becoming mature enough for discharge from the hospital to parents. Consequently, a failure to comprehend, or a lack of appreciation of, the ramifications of environmental influences (e.g. drugs, therapy, etc.) on human neonatal development could have disastrous consequences. This is illustrated by the long-recognized association of autonomic neuronal dysfunction in infants of drug addicts or in those neonates born to women who abuse ethanol in pregnancy (DeCristofaro and LaGamma 1995).

Other aspects of sympathoadrenal function are recognized as critical mediators of the successful adaptation into extrauterine life. For example, in the well-characterized catecholamine system, catecholamine transmitters serve an important function in temperature regulation, brown fat metabolism, glucose homeostasis, blood pressure, heart rate, and distribution of blood flow regulation, as well as in pulmonary surfactant production and release. The physiological mechanisms evoked by stress-responsiveness at the cellular level utilize the same biochemical signals (i.e. transmitters, hormones, growth factors, cell–cell interactions, etc.) as those necessary during development or for regulated expression and function in maturity.

Regulatory phenomena
The problem of complexity

Explaining the process of organization of the nervous system's billions of neurones is a formidable challenge. A remarkable degree of accuracy and precision must exist in order for the schema of neuronal maturation to play out. To accomplish this feat, an impressive array of biological 'cues' is utilized. Broad categorical mechanisms may contain many, possibly 50 mediators each, and the problem of correctly addressing the processes of lineage restriction and commitment, proliferation of precursors, neuronal differentiation, development of neurochemical phenotype, and the structural phenomena of axodendritic processes, connectivity, synapse elimination, and synapse stabilization is clearly mind boggling. In light of the level of complexity, it is not surprising that developmental disorders appear; in fact, it is truly remarkable that such aberrations are relatively uncommon. The following discussion highlights intrinsic and extrinsic mechanisms, and will focus on the newer aspects of molecular genetics and NT; we recognize that knowledge is limited and all important studies cannot be referenced.

Intrinsic influences on peripheral autonomic development ('nature')

Genetic encoding

The explosion in information regarding the role of specific genes in neuronal development is truly remarkable. Although *in vitro* and animal studies have taken the lead in dissecting the potential role of specific genes, the translation of this information to humans is not far behind; for instance, of the 65 000 protein-coding regions in the human genome, almost 50 per cent of them have been sequenced. As the homologous regions of genes are understood from *Drosophila* to humans, new understanding of human development and human diseases and disorders will certainly emerge. Probably in few other areas have the advances made in cell biology and animal research been so fundamental to our understanding of human development. The potential for this critical information to unlock the mystery of human disorders and the accruing benefits to society will be inestimable. Understanding relationships that exist at the molecular level is only beginning, but it seems clear that environmental stimuli and cell responsiveness at the molecular level are intertwined, affecting biological adaptation and phenotypic expression throughout development. Thus, during development a dynamic balance must exist between processes intrinsic to the cell (nature) and epigenetic factors, i.e. extrinsic factors that function as determinants (nurture) of cell outcome. Intrinsic processes require tissue-specific gene control in which factors initiating transcription are critical determinants of function or of choices made during development (Yamamoto 1985). Although many examples might be given, two transcription factors are of particular interest in ANS development: MASH1 and Phox2.

An excellent illustration of the critical role for specific gene expression during development is the MASH1 gene. MASH1 is a basic helix–loop–helix (bHLH) transcription factor that is the mammalian homologue of the proneural protein (*ac-sc*) in *Drosophila*. Targeted mutation in the MASH1 gene indicates that it is required for the generation of the peripheral autonomic nervous system, including sympathetic, parasympathetic, and enteric neurones (Sommer *et al.* 1995). This gene is essential for uncommitted neural crest cells to differentiate into specific autonomic neurones. A model of this specific function is illustrated in Fig. 2.2. These studies revealed that MASH1 is critical for the final passage from autonomic neuronal precursor to autonomic neurone. If there is an absence of MASH1, ANS development does not proceed beyond the neuronal

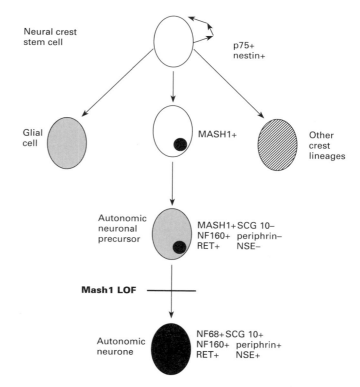

Fig. 2.2. Function of MASH1 in trunk neural crest differentiation (adapted from Sommer *et al.*, 1997).

precursor cell line. Of note, a number of markers (NF160, RET) previously presumed to be specific for terminally differentiated neurones are expressed in the precursor cell. Phenotypes related to MASH1 loss of function are discussed in the section profiling genetic knock-out animals.

Another gene involved in autonomic maturation is the gene for the transcription factor Phox2 (Tiveron *et al.* 1996). This homeodomain protein contributes to the process by which an individual neurone is assigned its fate and may also actually contribute to the establishment of specific circuits with the ANS. For instance Phox2 is expressed in all autonomic ganglia and several groups of neurones in the hindbrain. In the PNS Phox 2 is expressed in the earliest primordia of the sympathetic chain and later in developing adrenal medullary cells and all ganglia, including pelvic and enteric ganglia. Thus, all three divisions of the peripheral ANS express this gene product. Although at early stages of development dopamine β-hydroxylase (DBH) expression is coincident with Phox2 expression, DBH persists only in sympathetic ganglia. Of note, when this molecule is studied in the central nervous system, the expression of Phox2 is linked to neurones that use norepinephrine as a transmitter. For instance *in situ* hybridization in embryos identifies cells along the lateral wall of the rhombencephalon that are progenitors of the locus coeruleus and subcoeruleus. Studies more caudally revealed that Phox2-positive (Phox2+) cells occupied a continuous column in the ventrolateral medulla corresponding to the A1 and C1 group of catecholaminergic neurones. Also, Phox2+ cells were located in areas corresponding to the preganglionic neurones projecting to the salivary and lacrimal glands, as well as a central group of neurones in area X of the spinal cord. These latter neurones are dorsal to the central canal where preganglionic neurones to specific peripheral ganglia have been recognized, although neurones in the traditional intermediolateral preganglionic sympathetic areas were not labelled. This gene product is expressed in virtually all noradrenergic or adrenergic neurones, as identified by the co-localization of the enzyme dopamine β-hydroxylase. Phox2 expression occurs in neuronal populations that subserve a number of autonomic control pathways, including medullospinal reflex control of cardiovascular functions and preganglionic parasympathetic pathways including neurones in dorsal motor neurones on the vagus. The role(s) of the transcription factor Phox2 in promoting the development of autonomic circuits remains to be fully understood, but two hypotheses are presented by Tiveron et al. (1996) They are:

(1) Phox2 may promote the integration of two distant neurones by influencing the expression of molecules involved in pathfinding at a distance; and

(2) Phox2 may influence target selection by controlling the expression of cell–cell adhesion receptors in two interacting cells.

In either scenario, these data indicate that Phox2 plays a clear role in autonomic ontogeny by determining neurotransmitter phenotype and molecular recognition among groups of neurones subserving similar functions and sharing connectivity.

Gene knock-outs

A major advance in understanding the role of specific genes has occurred with the use of genetically engineered animals. These animals develop without the presence of a certain gene or set of genes and the phenotypic character of the animal is studied. Utilizing this strategy, several abnormalities related to ANS development have been recognized. Additionally, specific functional deficits have been recognized and relate to altered central and/or peripheral autonomic function. Deficits in the ENS in genetically altered mice have been reviewed by Gershon (1997). The regions of the gut colonized by migrating neural crest cells are highly dependent on MASH1, and GDNF and its functional receptor Ret. Ret is encoded by the c-ret proto-oncogene, which is expressed transiently by ENS precursors. Rodents with c-ret knocked out have an aganglionic bowel. Similarly, if the gene encoding GDNF is knocked out, the gut will contain no neurones caudal to the oesophagus and cardiac stomach. Truncal neural crest are Ret/GDNF-independent. These studies in knock-out animals have also revealed new information regarding the timing of ENS development. Vagal crest cells have at least two lineages: one that is MASHl-dependent and one that is MASHl-independent. It appears that the early developing subset of enteric neurones is susceptible and completely lost, whereas the late-developing subset of enteric neurones arrives and develops. Furthermore, these studies have revealed that the development of the superior cervical ganglion (SCG) is altered by Ret/GDNF knock-out, but is MASH1-independent suggesting that the SCG follows the caudal ENS which is Ret/GDNF dependent. In contrast, the more caudal sympathetic ganglia, which are independent of Ret, are more similar to the enteric neurones of the oesophagus and cardiac stomach that are derived from the truncal crest. The story that emerges is that two NC lineages may exist:

(1) a sympathoenteric lineage, giving rise to the SCG and vagal-derived enteric neurones; and

(2) a sympathoadrenal lineage that will form the caudal SNS, adrenal medulla, and the rostral foregut enteric neurones.

Further work suggests that the sympathoenteric lineage may have two components and the caudal bowel is populated by MASH1-independent migrating cells that are born late, are never catecholaminergic and become CGRP-containing neurones. The range of ENS abnormalities resulting from a host of gene knock-outs is reviewed in Table 2.4. As indicated, receptors and their identified ligands, and transcription factors, are the most prominent molecules studied to date, revealing a range of deficits, from the loss of specific phenotypically characterized neurones (substance-P- or nitric-oxide-containing neurones) to complete aganglionosis of the colon below the rostral foregut.

The range of deficits, structural and physiological, that appear in the ANS following disruption of the genes responsible for specific protein molecules and their receptors are presented in Table 2.5. Although specific functions are attributed to the removal of these gene products, it is important to point out that interpretation of deficits from knock-out animals is complicated. Undoubtedly, relationships, both developmental and functional, are altered in these animals such that interpretations might be skewed; i.e. some animals reveal no phenotypic alteration despite the deletion of a specific gene. Does that mean the gene is unimportant? Most likely not. For instance, nature has built in critical redundancies to ensure normal maturation. Also, a specific gene mutation may exert its effects via another gene product that is integrally involved with the gene of interest. Thus, combinatorial events may exist that cannot be detected with current methodologies. The evidence that specific gene alterations result in similar phenotypic alterations (e.g. hypotension, enteric dysautonomia, sympathetic neuropathy, see Table 2.5) demonstrates the overlapping functional outcomes ensuing in targeted genetic knock-outs. Nevertheless, the power of these new tools provide the ability to develop new models of disease states and to discern new developmental and functional relationships.

Extrinsic influences on peripheral autonomic development ('nurture')

Neurotrophins

The concept of neurotrophins (NTs), polypeptide molecules that are required for neuronal survival during development and at various stages of adult life, originated from the early observations that target organs influence the development of the innervating neurone. These studies revealed that nerve growth factor (NGF), which is retrogradely transported to the noradrenergic cell bodies in the SCG, is critical for normal growth and development of sympathetic neurones (reviewed by Black 1978; Levi-Montalcini 1987). In turn, sympathetic cells influence target development. Neural crest cells migrating to the embryonic heart contribute to the normal formation of its outlet and influence the intrinsic rate of beating. Removal of these cells prior to migration results in cardiac malformations (Kirby 1987). NGF is the original prototype of a group of NTs that regulate neuronal growth and development, influencing neuronal survival, neuronal growth (neurite outgrowth), and/or neuronal neurochemical phenotype. It is now apparent that the amount of a given NT is in low abundance and the successful competition for NTs by the innervating neurone may indeed determine the survival of the cell. That is, failing to make optimum contact and garner NTs a neurone might enter the process of programmed neuronal cell death; thus the extent and pattern of innervation may be determined by NTs. Over the past 5 years a

Table 2.4.　Gene knock-outs and the development of ENS (adapted from Gershon 1997)

Gene/product	Phenotypes of knock-outs,	Comments
	Global effects	
c-ret	Complete failure of enteric neurones and glia to develop in the entire bowel below the rostral foregut	Encodes Ret, a receptor tyrosine kinase expressed by crest-derived cells that colonize the gut Ret—functional receptor for GDNF
GDNF	Similar to knock-out of c-ret	Essential for development and/or survival of early crest-derived precursors
Mash-1	Aganglionosis—rostral foregut (i.e. oesophagus and cardiac stomach) Absence of the early born TC lineage of enteric neurones in the rest of the bowel	Encodes a transcription factor required by the precursors of serotonergic, but not CGRP-containing, neurones
	Limited effects	
CNTFRα or LIFRβ	Loss of neurones that express substance P or nitric oxide synthase (smooth muscle motor neurones)	Newborn lethal, not mimicked by knock-out of genes encoding the ligands, CNTF or LIF
Endothelin 3 (edn-3)	Aganglionosis—terminal colon Spotted coat color	Selectively activates the EDNRB Naturally mutated in lethal spotted (ls/ls) mice Effects are not crest-autonomous
Endothelin B receptor (ednrb)	Aganglionosis—terminal colon, spotted coat color similar to that seen in edn-3 knock-out, but more severe	Activated with equal potency by endothelins 1, 2, and 3 Naturally mutated in piebald lethal (s′/s′) mice
	Effects expected: not yet detected	
NT-3	Expressed in ENS Causes hyperganglionosis when overexpressed in the gut of transgenic mice	Selectively promotes development and survival of enteric neurones and glia Stimulates neurite extension The preferred ligand for TrkC
TrkC	Expressed in ENS, but not yet studied in detail	Only high-affinity neurotrophin receptor expressed by crest-derived neural and glial precursors in developing bowel (humans express TrkA and B)

Table 2.5.　Gene knock-outs and the development of the ANS (adapted from Fritz and Robertson 1996)

Gene product	Phenotype
Receptor	
α₂-Adrenergic (Adra2c gene)	Defective pressure control
Endothelin B	Aganglionic megacolon
Angiotensin AT-1a	Hypotension
Angiotensin AT-2	Hypertension
Tyrosine kinase (Ret)	Enteric dysautonomia
Neurotrophin TrkA	Sympathetic neuropathy
Neurotrophin TrkB	Sympathetic neuropathy
Matrix; enzymes; neurotrophins	
Endothelin-1	Hypertension
Endothelin-3	Aganglionic megacolon
Dopamine β-hydroxylase	Hypotension
Tyrosine hydroxylase	Hypotension
Nerve growth factor	Sympathetic neuropathy
Neurofibromatosis type I (NF1 gene)	Sympathetic hyperplasia
Neurotrophin-3	Sympathetic neuropathy
Mammalian achaete–scute homolog 1 (MASH1)	Dysautonomia Enteric dysautonomia
Glial-derived neurotrophic factor (GDNF)	Dysautonomia Enteric dysautonomia

number of new growth factors influencing ANS development have been identified: brain-derived neurotrophic factor (BDNF), neurotrophin-3 (NT-3), neurotrophin-4 (NT-4) (also called NT-5 or NT-4/5) and neurotrophin-6 (discovered in fish, no known mammalian counterpart). These molecules are complemented in their actions by members of the neurokine (CNTF) and transforming growth factor (TGF)-β families. The potential interactions of these proteins during various stages of neuronal development are depicted in Table 2.6.

Early studies indicated that NGF is critical for normal prenatal and postnatal sympathetic development (reviewed by see Levi-Montalcini 1987). Neonatal treatment with antibodies directed against NGF results in sympathectomy, and exposure to anti-NGF prenatally, via maternal transfer of antibody, or postnatally, via cross-fostering experiments with immunized mothers, precludes the normal morphological and biochemical development of peripheral ganglia. The clinical relevance of the role of NGF is evident; the immune incompetence associated with the fetal alcohol syndrome may be associated with alcohol-induced perturbation of the normal NGF-influenced noradrenergic regulation of the immune system or the interaction between NGF and other hormonal factors such as thyroid and glucocorticoids (Gottesfeld et al. 1990). In total, NGF exerts regulatory influences on sympathetic systems throughout life. Roles for other NTs in the growth and development of the SNS are

Table 2.6. Neurotrophins and neuronal development (adapted from Henderson 1996)

Stage of neuronal development	Developmental outcome/function	Neurotrophic factors implicated in different systems
Proliferation of precursors	Differentiation	BDNF, NT-3, FGF-2
Target contact by immature neurones	Survival/maturation	BDNF, NT-3, NT-4/5
Programmed cell death	Survival	NGF, NT-3, NT-4/5, BDNF, CNTF, LIF, GDNF, TGF-β_2, TGF-β_3, FGFs, IGFs
Synapse elimination	Sprouting Synapse stabilization	NT-4/5, BDNF CNTF, FGFs, IGFs
Functional maturation	Synaptic efficacy	BDNF, NT-3, NT-4/5, CNTF

now emerging (Fig. 2.1 and Table 2.6). For instance, *in vitro* studies of NT-3 indicate that immature neurones (neuroblasts) during early maturation are supported by NT-3 and not by NGF; failing to be exposed to NT-3, SCG neurones experience increased apoptosis and a reduced number of neurones results. Concordant with these data is the observation that TrkC mRNA is expressed in high levels in early sympathetic ganglia and, in a paracrine fashion, the surrounding non-neuronal cells express high levels of NT-3 mRNA (reviewed by Davies 1997). As development proceeds these neurones become more dependent on NGF as they innervate target organs. Although as more data accrue these interpretations may be revised, it appears that a switch in NT dependence occurs. Such a phenomena is best described in sensory neurones derived from neural crest. These neurones switch from BDNF and NT-3 dependence to NGF during ontogeny, a pattern that recapitulates phylogeny (Davies 1997).

The development of cholinergic neurones of the peripheral parasympathetic nervous system is also dependent on NT for normal maturation. Ciliary ganglion (CG) neurones undergo substantial cell death during normal development; 50 per cent die. Death occurs around the time that synaptic contact with the iris, the target organ of the CG, occurs. CNTF is produced by CG targets and influences CG neuronal survival. Studies utilizing a monoclonal antibody to CNTF suggest that CNTF is critical for normal maturation of cholinergic components of the ANS (Hendry *et al.* 1988). Fibroblast growth factors (FGFs) also appear to have an ability to influence neuronal survival in the CG. Interestingly, CNTF also influences differentiation of sympathetic neurones; the transmitter phenotype in rodent SCG in culture will change from noradrenergic to cholinergic in the presence of CNTF. A new member of the LIF/CNTF family, cardiotrophin-l, promotes the survival of peripheral sympathetic neurones and appears to induce a phenotypic switch from noradrenergic to cholinergic (Henderson 1996).

Other molecules appear to influence the transmitter phenotype of the neurone. For instance, sympathetic neurones in the SCG destined to innervate sweat glands will convert from noradrenergic to cholinergic, and this switch is dependent upon substances derived from the target tissue (Schotzinger and Landis 1988). Factors purified from a number of sources appear to influence transmitter phenotype; cholinergic differentiation factor (CDF), membrane-associated neurotransmitter stimulating factor (MANS), CNTF, and cardiotrophin-l all result in a similar transition from catecholaminergic to cholinergic phenotype (Rao *et al.* 1990; Henderson 1996). In addition to the transmitter switch, receptor systems in cholinergic targets

switch as well. Recent work suggest that innervation-dependent factors are responsible for these changes (Habecker *et al.* 1996).

BDNF regulates the development of the central processes of neural-crest-derived peripheral sensory neurones. Also, trigeminal mesencephalic neurones and brainstem proprioceptive neurones derived from neural crest depend on BDNF, but this NT does not increase the survival of SNS or PNS neurones. Thus, a scenario appears to exist: the maturation of the peripheral components of a dorsal root ganglion neurone may depend on NT-3, NGF, and CNTF as well as other NTs, and the survival and connectivity of centrally coursing fibres may depend on BDNF and such transcription factors as Phox2.

Neurotrophic factors, proto-oncogenes and NT receptors—Trks

Oncogenes were discovered in the process of examining retroviral systems of cell transformation to tumours. These viral-incorporated cellular oncogenes have analogues that are part of normal cells and were designated proto-oncogenes. Transcription of these genes leads to the production of oncogene-encoded proteins that regulate not only transcriptional activity of genes, including their own, but also interact with second messenger systems within the cell. Thus, nuclear and cytoplasmic proto-oncogene proteins exist and appear to be involved in signal transduction from the cell membrane to the nucleus, as well as gene regulation. Not surprisingly, the natural role for these molecules includes a means by which cells respond to extracellular signals involved in growth and development. Identification of the TrkA proto-oncogene as a functional receptor NGF was a major breakthrough in understanding the signal transduction of NTs. Other members of this Trk family of receptor tyrosine kinases that respond to specific NTs exist: TrkB is activated by BDNF and NT-4/5; TrkC is activated by NT-3; NT-3 also will activate TrkA and Trk B, but with less avidity. Earlier in this chapter we reviewed the neurokines/cytokines and BMPs, other burgeoning groups of molecules with neuronotrophic effects. The neurokines CNTF and LIF have specific effects on peripheral autonomic neurones and act at receptors that share (gp130 and LIFRβ) and exhibit specific (CNTFRα) components. Also, the emergence of the TGF-β superfamily—in particular GDNF—as potent NTs for the ANS has expanded the landscape of molecules modulating neuronal maturation.

Proto-oncogenes are key molecules in the neurone's response to other extracellular signals, namely hormonal factors. Neurones in the central nervous system exhibit induction of FOS protein following oestrogen administration and oestrogen activation of the ovalbumin gene involves the *fos jun* proto-oncogene complex. These proto-oncogenes and their protein products are also involved in the regulation of transcriptional activation and inhibition by other steroid hormones, such as glucocorticoids. The glucocorticoid receptor will repress AP-1 (*fos jun* dimer) mediated transcriptional activation. In turn, *jun* inhibits the normal activation of glucocorticoid steroid responsive genes. The field of signal transduction mechanisms has expanded substantially and cannot be reviewed fully here. Undoubtedly, the data accruing will reveal new mechanisms underlying ANS development and lead to new treatment strategies for developmental and adult disorders of the ANS system.

The concept of plasticity

Traditional teachings concerning neuronal plasticity maintained a restricted view in which neuronal tissue was believed to be committed, unresponsive, or immutable. The collective work of many investigators over the past few decades has revealed a remarkable degree of synaptic, transmitter, and receptor plasticity, and, indeed, ongoing neuronal cell division. Most intriguing is the recognition that the fundamental basis of plasticity is the expression of certain proteins. Control of protein synthesis reflects the cell's specificity in control of gene expression. In turn, gene expression results from *trans*-acting DNA-binding proteins functioning in *cis* (LaGamma *et al.* 1991). During adulthood and ageing the concepts of neuroplasticity underlie the ability of the nervous system to adjust and adapt. It is presumed that the more plastic the nervous system, the better it will manage the burdens inflicted by ageing and disease.

Clinical issues

Developmental disorders

ANS developmental disorders, which illustrate potential ontogenetic aberrations of NC, are familial dysautonomia (Riley–Day syndrome) and Hirschsprung's disease. Familial dysautonomia, an autosomal inherited recessive trait, is essentially confined to Ashkenazic Jews, a pattern suggestive of an altered single mutant allele at one gene locus. Patients experience symptom complexes related to disturbances of autonomic and sensory neurones: cardiovascular instability, swallowing and gastrointestinal dysfunction (vomiting crises), tearing and taste bud alterations, and insensitivity to pain and temperature. Since NGF plays a critical role in autonomic development, and since anti-NGF (see above) produces similar pathological changes in animals, a defect in NGF was proposed. Although β-NGF in serum and fibroblasts from these patients was believed to be reduced, recombinant DNA techniques established that the structural gene for β-NGF is not defective. Whether defects in the processing of NGF or in the NGF receptor exist, or whether defects in other NTs or neurokines are present, remains unknown. In the Ashkenazi Jewish population the frequency of carrying this gene is 1 in 30 to 1 in 50. The location of the gene has been identified on the long arm of chromosome 9 (9q31–33). The gene's relationship to known NTs or the Trk receptors is unknown. Isolation of the exact gene remains to be determined and will clarify its role in producing the disease. A maximum lod score of 21.2 with no overlap was achieved with the flanking marker D9S58. The localization of two additional flanking markers, D9S53 and D9S105, should permit genetic testing and assist in isolating the affected gene.

Hirschsprung's disease results from the absence of enteric ganglia from a segment of bowel and presents clinically as intestinal obstruction. Distention of the bowel proximal to the aganglionic section is present and megacolon may result. Hirschsprung's disease occurs in approximately 1 of every 5000–8000 births, and 80 per cent of the patients are male. Initial hypotheses suggested that, since the pathology is most frequently localized to the distal bowel, rectum, and rectosigmoid colon (70–80 per cent of cases), a defect in neural crest migration must exist. However, since other neurocristopathies, such as Waardenburg's syndrome, Marcus Gunn ptosis, and von Recklinghausen's disease, may be associated with Hirschsprung's disease, a primary alteration in the differentiation of neural-crest-derived neuroblasts may occur. A similar disease occurs in animals following overexpression of the *Hox 1.4* gene (Wohlgemuth *et al.* 1989). Also, models of Hirschsprung's disease now exist in 'genetic knock-outs': animals missing the endothelin 3 gene exhibit aganglionosis of the terminal colon whereas c-*ret* deletions demonstrate a complete loss of enteric neurones in the entire bowel below the rostral foregut (Tables 2.3 and 2.4). Alternatively, failure of neuroblasts to survive within the bowel because of a defect in the microenvironment, or failure of specific signalling systems to activate known NTs or their receptors, may be underlying pathophysiological mechanisms. Whether any of these defects occur in humans has yet to be determined. It is important to recognize that data gathered from animal models are not immediately transferable to humans. For instance, TrkA and TrkB are expressed in enteric neurones in humans and not in rats; consequently, different regulatory mechanisms may exist in humans and disease states may develop secondary to unique perturbations relevant only to human development.

There are important observations in the human model where maintenance of the enteric phenotype after maturation requires the 'nurturing' signal of an intact nervous system. For example, in the transplanted human intestine, extrinsic adrenergic and perivascular fibres fail to regenerate yet intrinsic neurones (expressing NPY, CGRP, enkephalin, somatostatin, etc.) sustain a normal distribution, but exhibit reduced density. Motility and digestive functions appear to be maintained despite these changes.

The hereditary sensory and autonomic neuropathies (HSAN) are a group of developmental disorders which also reflect perturbations of ANS maturation. These illnesses include alteration in the perception of pain as well as autonomic function, and certainly may develop from dysfunctional development of NC, but defects in later stages of maturation of Schwann cells, neurones, or the microenvironment may exist. There is evidence that one of these disorders may be transmitted as an X-linked recessive trait whereas others appear to be inherited in an autosomal dominant fashion. The frequency of these disorders are low and the exact genes involved are unknown.

Stress, metabolic adaptation, and the influence of the environment

Endocrine and molecular responses to stress are well studied in the context of a 'fight or flight' response to hypoxaemia, hypoglycaemia, hypothermia, etc. (Udelsman and Holbrook 1994) and observations of failed adrenaline surges in response to repeated exposure to hypoglycaemia in the adult suggest links between these environmental stressors and biological adaptation. Neonatal brown fat is well recognized for its high content of mitochondria that are important in thermoregulation. Extraordinary increases in the levels of circulating catecholamine (unique to the birthing process) are involved in uncoupling oxidative metabolism in this adaptive response to temperature homeostasis. In fact, about 20 per cent of the thermogenic response to food can be attributed to noradrenaline through pharmacological blockade. Similar autonomic mechanisms are believed to modulate neonatal adaptive responses to hypoglycaemia, yet differ from those in adults in that endogenous glucose production provides only about one-third of the glucose needed to prevent hypoglycaemia, and small for gestational age neonates (SGA) fail to mount a ketogenic response or to increase circulating adrenaline. Although evidence linking enteral feeding, diet, and particularly carbohydrate metabolism and insulin resistance to autonomic dysfunctions, are well established in the adult (Reaven *et al.* 1996), these associations have not been well established in the neonate. Nevertheless, based on observations in adults and animal models, one might expect some evidence of dietary environmental influence on the development of autonomic adaptive processes, since the neonatal period is unique in many ways. For example, the bowel of neonates is sterile at birth; they experience an abrupt cessation of sustenance after severing placental functions and are prone to hypoglycaemia and hypoxaemia; they have reduced enteral nutrient intake and then are subsequently exposed to large quantities of carbohydrate as lactose during a period of rapid bacterial colonization of the intestine. Since it is currently recognized that short-chain fatty acids arising from fermented enteral carbohydrates mature brush border epithelial cells and assist in switching liver protein synthesis from α-fetoprotein to albumin after birth, it might not be unreasonable to hypothesize a similar role existing for 'diet' or other perinatal stressors affecting neuronal maturation.

Sudden infant death syndrome (SIDS) has an overall incidence of about 1 in 500 births and has often been implicated as a maladaptive cardiopulmonary response to environmental stress or to developmental influences such as diet, drugs, smoking, infections or gastro-oesophageal reflux. Clear evidence exists for a familial risk, suggesting a genetic predisposition, although this is wholly undefined at the molecular level. Most cases remain classified as 'idiopathic' and some have even been implicated as a form of child abuse. At the moment, the most significant insight into the pathophysiology of this problem has been the observation that prone position during sleep is associated with a higher rate of sudden infant death compared to supine. The prone position showed a decreased variation in behaviour, respiratory rate, an increased heart rate, and increased peripheral skin temperature compared to infants in the supine position—all implicating a role of the autonomic nervous system in modulating responses without any new unifying hypothesis. Nevertheless, these phenomena have obvious practical applications in parent education and in child rearing in the first year of life (Willinger *et al.* 1994).

Developmental issues and their relationship to autonomic failure, including the multiple system atrophies

We hypothesized in the third edition of this book that alterations of the mechanisms involved during development might occur during ageing and disease. Thus, an undoing of NT influences in the broadest sense might underlie neuronal degeneration observed in certain central and peripheral autonomic cell populations. Since NTs clearly appear to influence which cells or groups of cells survive during maturation, they may also assist in helping us to understand why specific cell populations appear uniquely susceptible to disease processes. Relevant questions might include: why do certain chemically defined neuronal populations fail during adulthood; why, during adulthood, do specific components of the ANS exhibit dysfunction, degenerate, and die; why do specific cell groups appear to exhibit functional decline with age?

Over the past 5 years a number of investigators have broached these questions, specifically addressing the potential role(s) of NGF in ageing and neurodegenerative diseases. In a review of whether the neurotrophic hypothesis might explain age-related loss of neuroplasticity and the occurrence of neuronal degeneration, no specific evidence to support a relationship to decreased availability of NGF exists (Gavazzi and Cowen 1996). These studies were largely in rodents (rats) which are not ideal models of ageing, and only focus on one NT–NGF. There is no convincing evidence that a deficit of NGF or Trks exists in neurodegenerative ANS disorders. Nevertheless, it remains quite possible that the postreceptor effects of NGF may be muted, as observed with other ligand–receptor interactions in the ageing SNS, or that NGF up-regulation in response to disease fails to occur, so that vulnerable neurones are lost. As apparent from the combinatorial factors involved in development, the ageing process is probably no less complicated. Thus, future studies will begin to address the interactions of NTs, receptor tyrosine kinases, cytokines, extracellular matrix proteins, interneuronal mechanisms, and other environmental factors during ageing and disease.

Neuropathological studies of the multiple system atrophies (MSAs) have revealed neuronal loss in the intermediolateral cell column of the spinal cord, but only mild morphological changes occur in peripheral ganglia. The main pathology is within the brain, with severe loss of neurones in specific brain-stem and cerebellar nuclei (see Chapter 34). Also, cytoskeletal changes (argyrophilic inclusions) are present in oligodendrocytes and neurones, but it is not clear whether these changes are primary or secondary. The system degeneration suggests that possibly the absence of some trans-synaptic trophic factor or specific neurone-sustaining influence, or the presence of a trans-synaptic life-ending signal (i.e. apoptosis) may be relevant to the pathogenesis of these disorders. These are clearly speculative notions as no data exist to support the idea that similar signals during development might be absent during degeneration.

Another approach to examine human disease is to consider the 'knock-out' models. For instance, the syndrome of isolated DBH deficiency, resulting in orthostatic hypotension, essentially absent noradrenaline levels and elevated dopamine (DA) levels, may be viewed as a 'genetic knock-out', with a specific gene deficit resulting in an inability to make noradrenaline. Genetic aberrations will give us the opportunity to consider specific gene product alterations that might be acquired during life and present as clinical disorders (Table 2.5).

Since cellular processes are on a continuum and mechanisms existing during ontogeny probably exist throughout life—from birth through senescence—the aetiologies of various autonomic syndromes may be viewed in terms of developmental mechanisms. It seems reasonable to hypothesize that, throughout life, many of the intrinsic and extrinsic forces described earlier must continue and provide for normal function as well as survival of autonomic neurones. Dissection of these regulatory issues will undoubtedly lead to new insights into human disease across the life span.

Acknowledgements

These efforts are supported in part by NINCDS Grant NS22103 to R. W. Hamill.

References

Black, I. B. (1978). Regulation of autonomic development. *Ann. Rev. Neurosci.* 1, 183–214.

Davies, A. M. (1997). Neurotrophin switching: where does it stand? *Curr. Opin. Neurobiol.* 7, 1100–18.

DeCristofaro, J. D. and LaGamma, E. F. (1995). Prenatal exposure to opiates. *Ment. Retard. Devel. Disab. Res. Rev.* 1, 177–82.

Fritz, J. and Robertson, D. (1996). Gene targeting approaches to the autonomic nervous system. *J. autonom. nerv. Syst.* 61, 1–5.

Gavazzi, I. and Cowen, T. (1996). Can the neurotrophic hypothesis explain degeneration and loss of plasticity in mature and aging autonomic nerves? *J. auton. nerv. syst.* 58, 1–10.

Gershon, M. (1997). Genes and lineages in the formation of the enteric nervous system. *Curr. Opin. Neurobiol.* 7, 101–9.

Gootman, N. G. and Gootman, P. M. (1983). *Perinatal cardiovascular function.* Marcel Dekker, New York.

Gottesfeld, A., Morgan, B., and Perez-Polo, J. R. (1990). Prenatal alcohol exposure alters the development of sympathetic synaptic components and of nerve growth factor receptor expression selectivity in lymphoid organs. *J. Neurosci. Res.* 26, 308–16.

Habecker, B. A., Malec, N. M., and Landis, S. C. (1996). Differential regulation of adrenergic receptor development by sympathetic innervation. *J. Neurosci.* 16, (1), 229–37.

Hamill, R. W., and La Gamma E. F. (1992). Autonomic nervous system development. In *Autonomic Failure—A textbook of clinical disorders of the autonomic nervous system* (ed R. Bannister and C. J. Mathias) pp. 15–35. Oxford University Press, New York.

Henderson, C. E. (1996). Role of neurotrophic factors in neuronal development. *Curr. Opin. Neurobiol.* 6, 64–70.

Hendry, I. A., Hill, C. E., Belford, D., Watters, D. J. (1988). A monoclonal antibody to a parasympathetic neurotrophic factor causes immunoparasympathectomy in mice. *Brain Res.* 475, 160–3.

Kanerva, L., Hervonen, A., and Hervonen, M. (1974). Morphological characteristics of the ontogenesis of the mammalian peripheral adrenergic nervous system with special remarks on the human fetus. *Med. Biol.* 52, 144–53.

Kirby, M. L. (1987). Cardiac morphogenesis—recent research advances. *Pediat. Res.* 21, (3), 219–24.

Kissel, P., Andre, J. M., and Jacquier, A. (1981). *The neurocristopathies*, pp. 1–15, 165–83, 219–21. Year Book Medical Publishers, Chicago.

LaGamma, E. F., DeCristofaro, J. D., and Weisinger, G. (1991). Cholinergic agonist induced binding of adrenal medullary nuclear proteins to the rat preproencephalin promoter. *Mol. Cell. Neurosci.* 2, December.

Levi-Montalcini, R. (1987). The nerve growth factor 35 years later. *Science* 237, 1154–62.

Mehler, M. F. and Kessler, J. A. (1997). Hematolymphopoietic and inflammatory cytokines in neural development. *Trends Neurosci.* 20, (8), 357–65.

Mehler, M. F., Mabie, P. C., Zhang, D., and Kessler, J. A. (1997). Bone morphogenetic proteins in the nervous system. *Trends Neurosci.* 20, (7), 309–17.

Papp, J. G. (1988). Autonomic responses and neurohumoral control in the human early antenatal heart. *Basic Res. Cardiol.* 83, (1), 2–9.

Pappano, A. J. (1977). Ontogenetic development of autonomic neuroeffector transmission and transmitter reactivity in embryonic and fetal hearts. *Pharmacol. Rev.* 29, 3–34.

Perris, R. (1997). The extracellular matrix in neural crest-cell migration. *Trends Neurosci.* 20, (1), 23–31.

Rao, M. S., Landis, S. C., and Patterson, P. H. (1990). The cholinergic neuronal differentiation factor from heart cell conditioned medium is different from the cholinergic factors in sciatic nerve and spinal cord. *Develop. Biol.* 139, 65–74.

Reaven, G. M., Lithell, H., and Landsberg, L. (1996). Hypertension and associated metabolic abnormalities—the role of insulin resistance and the sympathoadrenal system. *New Engl. J. Med.* 334, 374–81.

Schotzinger, R. and Landis, S. C. (1988). Cholinergic phenotype developed by noradrenergic sympathetic neurons after innervation of a novel cholinergic target *in vivo*. *Nature* 335, 637–9.

Slotkin, T. A. (1985). Development of the sympathoadrenal axis. Endocrine control of synaptic development in the sympathetic nervous system: the cardiac sympathetic axis. In *Developmental neurobiology of the autonomic nervous system*, (ed. P. M. Gootman), pp. 69–96. Humana Press, New York.

Sommer, L., Shah, N., Rao, M., and Anderson, D. (1995). The cellular function of MASH1 in autonomic neurogenesis. *Neuron* 15, 1245–58.

Tiveron, M., Hirsch, M., and Brunet, J. (1996). The expression pattern of the transcription factor Phox2 delineates synaptic pathways of the autonomic nervous system. *J. Neurosci.* 16, (23), 7649–60.

Udelsman, R. and Holbrook, N. (1994). Endocrine and molecular responses to surgical stress. *Curr. Probl. Surg.* 31, 655–720.

Walker, D. (1975). Functional development of the autonomic innervation of the human fetal heart. *Biol. Neonate* 25, 31–43.

Willinger, M., Hoffman, H. J., and Hartford, R. B. (1994). Infant sleep position and risk for sudden infant death syndrome: report of meeting held January 13 and 14, 1994, National Institutes of Health, Bethesda, MD. *Pediatrics* 93, (5), 814–19.

Wohlgemuth, D. J., Behringer, R. R., Mostoller, M. P., Brinster, R. L., and Palmiter, R. D. (1989). Transgenic mice overexpressing the mouse homeobox-containing gene Hox 1.4 exhibit abnormal gut development. *Nature* 27, 464–7.

Yamamoto, K. R. (1985). Steroid receptor regulated transcription of specific genes and gene networks. *Ann. Rev. Genet.* 19, 209–52.

3. Nerve growth factors and the autonomic nervous system

P. Anand

Introduction

A neurotrophic factor may be defined as a substance that plays a role in the development, maintenance, or regeneration of the nervous system. Neurotrophic factors are commonly proteins produced by cells in the target organ, e.g. blood vessels. Trophic factors act via receptors on specific nerve cells to influence their survival and gene expression (Altin and Bradshaw 1993). Nerve cells themselves produce trophic substances, including neuropeptides and neurotrophic factors, which in turn act on cells in the target organ. Abnormalities of these interactions may result in nerve dysfunction, abnormal regeneration, and pain (Anand 1995, 1996).

The best-established neurotrophic factor is nerve growth factor (NGF) (Longo et al. 1993). In adults, it is required for survival of sympathetic neurones and for gene expression, including expression of the neuropeptides substance P and calcitonin-gene-related peptide (CGRP) in sensory fibres (Lindsay and Harmar 1989). NGF is synthesized by cells of the target organ, e.g. vascular smooth muscle cells (Tuttle et al. 1993), and taken up by specific receptors on a subpopulation of sensory fibres (DiStefano et al. 1992). The NGF is then retrogradely transported to the cell body in the dorsal root ganglion, where it induces the expression of CGRP and substance P. NGF deprivation leads to reduced expression of substance P and CGRP: changes in neuropeptide expression thus reflect the activity of neurotrophic factors.

New neurotrophic factors and their receptors have been described, some of which belong to the NGF-superfamily: BDNF, NT-3 and NT-4/5 (Altin and Bradshaw 1993). Subpopulations of primary afferent fibres share the low-affinity NGF receptor (p75^{NGFR}), but have differential expression of the high-affinity receptors (Trks) (DiStefano et al. 1992). NGF is trophic to sympathetic and unmyelinated (nociceptive) neurones via TrkA. Glial cell-line-derived neurotrophic factor (GDNF), a distantly related member of the transforming growth factorβ family (TGF-β), has been recently isolated and cloned from B 49 glial cell lines (Engele et al. 1991; Attisano et al. 1994). It was originally thought to be a specific neurotrophic factor for dopaminergic neurones within the central nervous system (CNS). Since then, rat GDNF mRNA has been found in many peripheral tissues, including kidney, gut, lung, liver, and testis, at different stages of development (Springer et al. 1994). GDNF synthesis has been reported in a distinct subpopulation of embryonic muscle fibres, in Schwann cells, and in the nerve sheath region of the ventral spinal root (Henderson et al. 1994). GDNF has a broad range of neurotrophic actions on CNS and peripheral nervous system (PNS) neurones via a multicomponent receptor (Trupp et al. 1996).

There are several other families of neurotrophic factors and their receptors, whose role in the development and maintenance of the autonomic nervous system is being defined, including evidence from mice lacking, or overexpressing, these factors and receptors. In the subsequent sections of this chapter, key studies that have demonstrated a pathophysiological role for neurotrophic factors in human autonomic disorders will be discussed.

NGF in the urinary bladder

The mechanisms of pain in the human urinary bladder are poorly understood, particularly in idiopathic sensory urgency and interstitial cystitis (Gillenwater and Wein 1988; Frazer et al. 1990). The former presents with suprapubic pain and urinary frequency, and the latter is marked, in addition, by increased numbers of mast cells and suburothelial nerve fibres in the bladder (Feltis et al. 1987). Recent evidence suggests that nerve growth factor (NGF) plays a key role in inflammatory pain (Anand 1995; McMahon 1996; Woolf 1996). The levels of NGF in bladder biopsies from women with idiopathic sensory urgency, interstitial cystitis, and painful chronic cystitis have been studied (Lowe et al. 1997); women with stress incontinence served as controls.

Sensory urgency is a cystometric diagnosis, with a first desire to void at less than 150 ml and a strong desire to void at less than 400 ml. There is no associated rise in detrusor pressure, and often a reduced functional bladder capacity, which may be due to pain or urgency on bladder filling. Known causes of sensory urgency include urinary tract infection. However, there is a group of women with idiopathic sensory urgency in whom all investigations, including bladder capacity under anaesthetic and bladder biopsy, are normal, and treatment is unsatisfactory. Chronic cystitis occurs after persistent or repeated attacks of acute bacterial cystitis. Interstitial cystitis is a chronic debilitating condition which occurs characteristically in middle-aged or elderly women. Cystoscopy reveals a hyperaemic, usually contracted, bladder, which bleeds easily when distended. Microscopically, the mucosa may be infiltrated with inflammatory cells, and there are mast cells in the detrusor muscle. It has been questioned whether women with idiopathic sensory urgency have early interstitial cystitis (Frazer et al. 1990).

There is an increase of NGF levels in the urothelium of the urinary bladder, where sensory fibres terminate, in women with idiopathic sensory urgency, interstitial cystitis, and chronic inflammation (Lowe et al. 1997). There are different histological findings in the urinary bladder in these groups of patients, but they share the clinical features of sensory urgency and pain. Anatomical studies have demonstrated a suburothelial plexus of nerve fibres, which are presumed to be sensory in nature (Dixon and Gilpin 1987). They may convey touch, pain or temperature, or act as stretch receptors, and are stimulated as the bladder fills. There is evidence that the suburothelial innervation includes capsaicin-sensitive sensory fibres, which may act as nociceptors and play a role in the regulation of bladder capacity in humans (Maggi *et al.* 1989); they may also serve an efferent function, by releasing neuropeptides from peripheral terminals. Proliferation of nerve fibres within the suburothelial layers has been demonstrated in interstitial cystitis, although not in chronic cystitis, and a report has suggested that the increased innervation may be of sympathetic origin (Christmas *et al.* 1990, Hohenfellner *et al.* 1992).

It was proposed that the increased NGF is responsible for the mechanical hyperalgesia, even in the absence of inflammation, as in patients with idiopathic sensory urgency. In support of this proposal, there is good evidence that raised endogenous tissue levels of NGF are related to local hyperalgesia in humans and in animal models of skin inflammation (Anand 1995). Urinary bladder inflammation and hypertrophy in animal models are associated with increased NGF levels (Steers *et al.* 1991; Koo *et al.* 1993). Exogenous NGF, at appropriate levels, has been shown to produce injection-site hyperalgesia in human volunteers (Petty *et al.* 1994). NGF may produce hyperalgesia by acting directly on sensory nerve endings, or by increasing the levels of the sensory neuropeptides substance P and CGRP, which mediate some of the peripheral and central effects of inflammation (Lewin and Mendell 1993). A number of the clinical and neurochemical changes in the hypoalgesic neuropathies are the opposite of changes in models of inflammatory pain, e.g. arthritis, sunburn. NGF may produce pain by:

(1) directly sensitizing nociceptors;

(2) increasing levels of substance P and CGRP, which may play a role in central sensitization and neurogenic inflammation; or

(3) local effects such as release of histamine from increased numbers of mast cells.

For example, ultraviolet irradiation of skin produces erythema and pain: it induces NGF mRNA in keratinocytes, and a long-term increase in CGRP levels in the dorsal spinal cord. NGF, therefore, may regulate pain sensation in human diseases.

The reason for the increased NGF levels in the bladder of our patients is not known. As the vast majority of patients with idiopathic sensory urgency are women, it may be relevant to consider that oestrogen up-regulates NGF receptor mRNAs in sensory neurones, and testosterone reduces levels of NGF mRNA in cultured fibroblasts (Siminowski *et al.* 1987; Sohrabji *et al.* 1994). Cytokines such as interleukin-1 and tumour necrosis factor can up-regulate NGF expression in tissue inflammation and nerve injury (Heumann *et al.* 1987), but it is not known whether these particular agents are important in the human urinary bladder. Sympathetic fibres may play a role, as sympathetic agents increase NGF secretion from cultured smooth muscle cells (Tuttle *et al.* 1993), and increased NGF levels, in turn, induce nerve fibre sprouting (Diamond *et al.* 1992). Further studies are necessary to establish whether these mechanisms affect NGF expression and secretion in the bladder, and whether NGF is at least partly responsible for the increased mast cell numbers and degranulation in interstitial cystitis.

Various findings suggest that anti-NGF treatment may be rational and effective in intractable urinary bladder pain syndromes. A synthetic human protein, TrkA–IgG, which sequesters endogenous NGF, may provide such a treatment, although it has not yet been studied in humans. This molecule has been shown to produce a sustained hypoalgesia, and is effective in an animal model of bladder inflammation (McMahon *et al.* 1995). In this rat model of cystitis, a progressive increase in bladder reflex excitability occurs with inflammation, reflecting the sensitivity of sensory fibres. Pretreatment with TrkA–IgG prevents the development of hyperreflexia, suggesting that NGF up-regulation is necessary to produce the sensory changes. This agent, and other measures that decrease NGF synthesis or release, may provide new treatments in human painful urinary bladder syndromes. However, there are a number of questions and potential problems that must be addressed in any clinical trial with such agents, including the dose, mode, and frequency of delivery, avoidance of hypoalgesia/hyporeflexia, objective measures of efficacy, and consideration of the effect of treatment on the original cause.

NGF in cerebral blood vessels

The nerve supply to cerebral blood vessels plays an important role in migraine and cerebral vasospasm, via sympathetic fibres containing the vasoconstrictors noradrenaline and neuropeptide Y (NPY), and sensory fibres containing the vasodilators substance P and CGRP (see Chapter 10). The mechanisms invoked in neurogenic inflammation in migraine are similar to those in skin.

Studies were performed on cerebral vessels, from the circle of Willis that were collected post-mortem from subjects with no known neurological disorder (Anand *et al.* 1997). NGF levels were lower in anterior compared to posterior cerebral vessels in the circle of Willis, with a significant age-related decline. The working hypothesis was that NGF may regulate the presentation of vascular headache, based on the following indirect evidence, which may explain a number of clinical features of migraine:

1. The frequency and severity of migraine declines with age, as do the levels of NGF and its dependent peptides, substance P, CGRP and NPY, in human cerebral vessels (Edvinsson *et al.* 1987).

2. The target organ (i.e. the blood vessel) has been shown to be responsible for the reduced cerebral vessel innervation in aged rats, and NGF infusion can reverse this neuronal atrophy (Gavazzi and Cowen 1993). NGF is produced by vascular smooth muscle cells and fibroblasts, and processes such as atheromatous change may contribute to decreased NGF production in ageing.

3. In a study of cultured vascular smooth muscle cells, the hourly pattern of secretion of NGF was found to be elevated by α-adrenergic receptor activation (Tuttle *et al.* 1993).

4. Genetic factors may set levels of NGF in different target tissues: resistance vessel gene expression of NGF is elevated in young, spontaneously hypertensive rats with vascular noradrenergic hyperinnervation (Falckh *et al.* 1992).

5. Hormonal influences may affect NGF activity by modulation of its receptors: oestrogens/proestrus upregulate NGF receptor mRNA in sensory neurones (Siminowski *et al.* 1987; Sohrabji *et al.* 1994).

6. Biopsies of tender superficial temporal arteries in migraine may show oedema, attributed to local release of substance P, and in

cluster headache show increased mast cells during headache-free intervals: NGF sensitizes nociceptor fibres, produces neurogenic inflammation via substance P and CGRP, and is associated with increased numbers of mast cells (Lewin and Mendell 1993).

7. Corticosteroids help inflammatory vascular headache, as in temporal arteritis, and also reduce NGF synthesis (Siminowski *et al.* 1987).

The relationship of cerebral blood vessels and other pain-sensitive intracranial structures to their nociceptor innervation is regulated by NGF. While raised NGF levels may not be the *cause* of migraine, NGF may determine the *presentation* of migraine, i.e. the set-point. Our current studies of NGF and its receptors in vascular tissues, including inflamed cerebral vessels from patients with vascular head pain, will test our hypothesis.

GDNF in the gastrointestinal system

Glial cell-line-derived neurotrophic factor (GDNF) signals through the product of the *ret* proto-oncogene, which is known to be mutated in Hirschsprung's disease (HD) and other conditions with gut dysmotility (Schuchardt *et al.* 1994; Eng 1996; Bar *et al.* 1997). An age-dependent responsiveness to GDNF of sympathetic, parasympathetic, small and large cutaneous sensory neurones, and enteroceptive cells has been reported. Mice lacking GDNF show complete absence of neural crest-derived neurones in the small and large intestine and total renal agenesis due to failure of growth and arborization of the ureteric bud during early stages of kidney morphogenesis. They also show remarkable similarities to mice defective for the gene encoding Ret, which was recently found to be a component of the GDNF receptor (Schuchardt *et al.* 1994). It has been shown that GDNF binds to its receptor complex (GDNFR-α and Ret), and induces tyrosine phosphorylation (Treanor *et al.* 1996).

Receptor tyrosine kinases play important roles in the control of normal cell growth and differentiation. Molecular alterations such as point mutations and rearrangements result in activation of these genes as oncogenes. Germline mutations of the *ret* proto-oncogene lead either to Hirschsprung's disease (HD) or multiple endocrine neoplasia (MEN) Type 2A and 2B, which are also associated with gut dysmotility, depending on the location and nature of the base substitution (Eng 1996). It has been reported that gain of functional mutations of *ret* exon 10 give rise to MEN 2A, whereas loss of functional mutations in the same domain result in the Hirschsprung's phenotype .

Hirschsprung's disease is a congenital abnormality of the enteric nervous system (ENS), which occurs in approximately 1 in 5000 infants and is characterized by the absence of intrinsic ganglion cells in the submucosal and myenteric plexuses of the hindgut. The neurones and glia of the ENS, which regulate intestinal peristalsis, motility, and fluid absorption/secretion in an autonomous fashion, derive from precursor cells formed at the neural crest. During early gestation, primitive neural crest cells migrate ventrally from their origin to move along the developing intestine, ultimately to form enteric ganglion cells and their supportive enteric glia. The mutation of the *ret* oncogene, resulting in Hirschsprung's disease, seems to interfere with this process of migration, differentiation, and maturation.

In a study of GDNF in the human gastrointestinal system, immunohistochemistry and an immunoassay were used to localize and quantify GDNF in human adult and fetal intestine, and in HD (Bar *et al.* 1997; Fig. 3.1). Since GDNF is a survival factor for sensory and autonomic neurones and has neuroprotective properties, it is likely that Schwann cell-derived GDNF has neurotrophic properties on enteric nerve cells. The temporal presence of neurotrophic factors during development and cell-specific localization of the tyrosine kinase receptors is essential for the differentiation of component cells of the ENS. GDNF expression first appears in mouse gut at E9.0, and subsequently is strongly expressed in the mesenchymal and outer smooth muscle layers along the entire gut; there may thus be early sources of GDNF other than glial cells, particularly as these appear relatively late in ontogeny, and after neurones (which require Ret to be stimulated early in ontogeny) are evident. The presence of GDNF and its receptor component, Ret, in the intestine and during development, and the involvement of the latter in Hirschsprung's disease, reflects the importance of this neurotrophic factor. The presence of strong GDNF and Ret-immunopositivity in adult specimens suggests that its role may not be restricted to development but may, additionally, be associated with neuronal survival in adults.

Ret mutations have been identified in patients with Hirschsprung's disease and a role in pathogenesis is implied. Exactly how Ret contributes to the development of Hirschsprung's disease remains unclear. It has been suggested that disturbances of the cell signalling pathway upstream, downstream, or unrelated to Ret can predispose

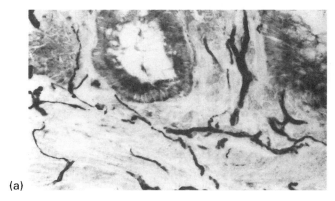

(a)

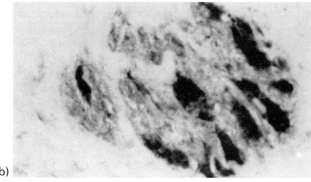

(b)

Fig. 3.1. (a) GDNF immunoreactivity in nerve fibre-like structures in normal human gut, present in Schwann cells. (b) RET immunoreactivity in neuronal cell bodies in the myenteric plexus of normal human gut. (Magnification ×200.)

to Hirschsprung's disease. There is an apparent high expression level of Ret in the hypoganglionic segment in HD, which has been shown to be a feature of the primitive and immature ENS during early hindgut development. In the study by Bar *et al.* (1997), the assay levels and pattern of GDNF immunostaining were similar in normal ganglionic, hypoganglionic, and aganglionic bowel in Hirschsprung's disease. These Hirschsprung's disease bowel samples came from patients with short segment involvement and were of sporadic type, which is associated with a low incidence of Ret mutations. Other associated mutations have been described in this condition, including genes encoding the G-protein coupled endothelin B receptor and its ligands endothelin-3 (Eng, 1996). Recent mutation studies suggest that GDNF is a minor contributor to human HD susceptibility, although in rare instances it may act in tandem with Ret mutations to produce an enteric phenotype. The incidence of GDNFR-α mutations in Hirschsprung's disease, if present, is not known. There is likely to be a complex interaction between the Ret and endothelin B pathways in normal enteric development and in HD, which needs to be addressed in future studies. Further investigations are also required to determine whether differences in GDNF levels exist in different genotypes and phenotypes of Hirschsprung's disease.

The presence of GDNF and its receptor in developing and adult human intestine suggests further studies to elucidate their role in pathogenesis and treatment of gastrointestinal disease.

Conclusion

There is increasing evidence that neurotrophic factors and their receptors play a role in the pathogenesis of human autonomic disorders. Understanding these mechanisms should provide a basis for new rational treatments with recombinant human neurotrophic factors and their modulators in human disease states.

References

Altin, J. G. and Bradshaw, R. A. (1993). Nerve growth factor and related substances: Structure and mechanisms of action. In *Neurotrophic factors* (ed. S. E. Loughlin and J. H. Fallon JH), pp. 129–80. Academic, San Diego.

Anand, P. (1995). Nerve growth factor regulates nociception in human health and disease. *Br. J. Anaesth.* 75, 201–8.

Anand, P. (1996). Neurotrophins and peripheral neuropathy. *Phil. Trans. R. Soc. London, B* 351, 449–54.

Anand, P., Parrett, A., Chadwick, L., and Hamlyn, P. J. (1997). Nerve Growth Factor in human cerebral vessels. *J. Neurol. Neurosurg. Psychiat.* 62, 199–200.

Attisano, L., Wrana, J. L., Lopez-Casillas, F., and Massague, J. (1994). TGF-beta receptors and actions. *Biochim. Biophys. Acta* 1222, 71–80.

Bar, K. J., Facer, P., Williams, N. S., Tam, P., and Anand, P. (1997). Localisation and quantitation of GDNF in human adult and fetal intestine and in Hirschsprung's disease. *Gastroenterology* 112, 1381–5.

Christmas, T. J., Rode, J., Chapple, C. R., Milroy, E. J. G., and Turner-Warwick, R. T. (1990). Nerve fibre proliferation in interstitial cystitis. *Virchows Archiv A Pathol. Anat.* 416, 447–51.

Diamond, J., Holmes, M., and Coughlin, M. (1992). Endogenous NGF and nerve impulses regulate the collateral sprouting of sensory axons in the skin of the adult rat. *J. Neurosci.* 12, 1454–66.

DiStephano, P. S., Friedman, B., Radziejewski, C. *et al.* (1992) The neurotrophins BDNF, NT-3, and NGF display distinct patterns of retrograde axonal transport in peripheral neurons. *Neuron* 8, 983–93.

Dixon, J. S. and Gilpin, C. J. (1987). Presumptive sensory axons of the human urinary bladder, a fine structural study. *J. Anat.* 151, 199–207.

Edvinsson, L., Ekman, R., and Jansen, I. (1997). Peptide-containing nerve fibres in human cerebral arteries: immunocytochemistry, radioimmunoassay and in vitro pharmacology. *Ann. Neurol.* 21, 431–7.

Eng, C. (1996). The ret proto-oncogene in multiple endocrine neoplasia Type 2 and Hirschsprung's disease. *New Engl. J. Med.* 335, 943–51.

Engele, J., Schuber, D., and Bohn, M. C. (1991). Conditioned media derived from glial cell lines promote survival and differentiation of dopaminergic neurons in vitro: role of mesencephalic glia. *J. Neurosci. Res.* 30, 359–71.

Falckh, P. H., Harkin, L. A., and Head, R. J., (1992). Resistance vessel gene expression of NGF is elevated in young spontaneously hypertensive rats. *J. Hypertension* 10, 913–8.

Feltis, J. T., Perez-Marrero, R., and Emerson, L. E. (1987). Increased mast cells in interstitial cystitis: A possible disease marker. *J.Urol.* 138, 42–3.

Frazer, M. I., Haylen, B. T., and Sissons, M. (1990). Do women with idiopathic sensory urgency have early interstitial cystitis? *Br. J. Urol.* 66, 274–8.

Gillenwater, J. Y. and Wein, A. J. (1988). Summary of the National Institute of Arthritis, Diabetes, Digestive and Kidney Diseases Workshop on Interstitial Cystitis, National Institutes of Health, Bethesda, Maryland, August 28–29, 1987. *J. Urol.* 140, 203.

Gavazzi, I. and Cowen, T. (1993). NGF can induce a 'young' pattern of re-innervation in transplanted cerebral blood vessels from ageing rats. *J. Comp. Neurol.* 334, 489–96.

Heumann, R., Korsching, S., Bandtlow, C., and Thoenen, H. (1987). Changes of nerve growth factor synthesis in non-neuronal cells in response to sciatic nerve transection. *J. Cell Biol.* 104, 1623–31.

Henderson, C. E., Phillips, H. S., Pollock, R. A. *et al.* (1994). GDNF: A potent survival factor for motoneurons present in peripheral nerve and muscle. *Science* 266, 1062–4.

Hohenfellner, M., Nunes, L., Schmidt, R. A., Lampel, A., Thuroff, J. W., and Tanago, E. A. (1992). Interstitial cystitis: increased sympathetic innervation and related neuropeptide synthesis. *J. Urol.* 147, 587–91.

Koo, H. P., Santarosa, R. P., Buttyan, R., Shabsigh, R., Olsson, C. A., and Kaplan, S. A. (1993). Early molecular changes associated with streptozotocin-induced diabetic bladder hypertrophy in the rat. *Urol. Res.* 21, 375–81.

Lewin, G. and Mendell, L. M. (1993). Nerve growth factor and nociception. *Trends Neurosci.* 16, 353–9.

Lindsay, R. M. and Harmar, A. J. (1989). Nerve growth factor regulates expression of neuropeptide genes in adult sensory neurones. *Nature* 337, 362–4.

Longo, F. M., Holtzman, D. M., Grimes, M. L., and Mobley, W. C. (1993). NGF: actions in the peripheral and central nervous systems. In *Neurotrophic factors*, (ed. S. E. Loughlin and J. H. Fallon), pp. 209–56. Academic Press, San Diego, USA.

Lowe, E., Anand, P., Terenghi, G., and Osborne, J. (1997). Increased NGF levels in the urinary bladder of women with idiopathic sensory urgency and interstitial cystitis. *Br. J. Urol.* 79, 572–7.

Maggi, C. A., Barbanti, G., and Santicioli, P. (1989). Cystometric evidence that capsaicin-sensitive nerves modulate the afferent branch of the micturition reflex in humans. *J. Urol.* 142, 150–4.

McMahon, S. B. (1996). NGF as a mediator of inflammatory pain. *Phil. Trans. R. Soc. London, B* 351, 431–40.

McMahon, S. B., Bennett, D. L., Priestley, J. V., and Shelton, D. L. (1995). The biological effects of endogenous NGF in adult sensory neurons revealed by a trkA–IgG fusion molecule. *Nature Med.* 1, 774–80.

Petty, B. G., Cornblath, D. R., Adornato, B. T. *et al.* (1994). The effect of systemically administered recombinant human nerve growth factor in healthy human subjects. *Ann. Neurol.* 36, 244–6.

Schuchardt, A., D'Agati, V., Larsson-Blomberg, L., Costantini, F., and Pachnis, V. (1994). Defects in the kidney and enteric nervous system of mice lacking the tyrosine kinase receptor Ret. *Nature* 367, 380–3.

Siminowski, K., Murphy, R. A., Rennert, P., and Heinrich, G., (1987). Cortisone, testosterone, and aldosterone reduce levels of nerve growth factor messenger ribonucleic acid in L929 fibroblasts. *Endocrinology* 121, 1432–7

Sohrabji, F., Miranda, R. C., and Toran-Allerand, C. D. (1994). Estrogen differentially regulates estrogen and NGF receptor mRNAs in adult sensory neurons. *J. Neurosci.* **14**, 459–71.

Springer, J. E., Mu, X., Bergmann, L. W., and Trojanowski J. Q. (1994). Expression of GDNF mRNA in rat and human nervous tissue. *Exp. Neurol.* **127**, 167–70.

Steers, W. D., Kolbeck, S., Creedon, D., and Tuttle, J. B. (1991) Nerve growth factor in the urinary bladder of the adult regulates neuronal form and function. *J. Clin. Invest.* **88**, 1709–15.

Treanor, J. J. S., Goodman, L., de Sauvage, F. *et al.* (1996). Characterisation of a multicomponent receptor for GDNF. *Nature* **382**, 80–3.

Trupp, M., Arenas, E., Fainzilber, M. *et al.* (1996). Functional receptor for GDNF encoded by the c-ret proto-oncogene. *Nature* **381**, 785–9.

Tuttle, J. B., Etheridge, R., and Creedon, D. J. (1993). Receptor-mediated stimulation and inhibition of NGF secretion by vascular smooth muscle. *Exp. Cell Res.* **208**, 350–61.

Woolf, C. J. (1996). Phenotypic modification of primary sensory neurons: the role of nerve growth factor in the production of persistent pain. *Phil. Trans. R. Soc. London, B* **351**, 441–8.

4. Molecular genetic approaches to the autonomic nervous system

Stephen J. Peroutka

Introduction

The Human Genome Project and other efforts to sequence the human genome have resulted in the availability of vast amounts of information concerning the location and sequence, but not necessarily the clinical relevance, of specific genes. Traditional approaches to understanding the genetic basis of disease have been based on the 'physical mapping' of a single clinical phenotype to a specific region of human DNA and, ultimately, to a specific genetic variant. This method has been very successful for a number of rare, clinically distinct disorders such as Huntington's disease, cystic fibrosis, and breast cancer.

Traditional approaches have, however, been less useful in elucidating the complex relationship between the multiple genes or multiple disease phenotypes of disorders such as dysfunction of the autonomic nervous system (ANS). In seeking to understand the genetic influences on ANS function, it is important to remember that data derived from rare cases or isolated populations may lead to the identification of specific genetic variants which are significant in a small number of individuals, but which may or may not be relevant to ANS function in the general population. Alternatively, data derived from small numbers of patients may lead to important insights into the pathophysiology of the ANS. The ability to assess the effects of genetic variants on ANS function is a significant advance in the ability to analyse and understand the ANS.

This chapter reviews current data on the genetic basis of ANS function. The chapter is divided into two major sections: (1) specific mutations causing autonomic dysfunction; and (2) other genetic causes of autonomic dysfunction. Each section is expected to grow exponentially in the years ahead as knowledge derived from the Human Genome Project is applied to the analysis of the ANS. A continually updated listing of molecular genetic data can be obtained via a search of Online Mendelian Inheritance in Man (Internet address: http://www3.ncbi.nlm.gov/omim/searchomim.html).

Specific mutations causing autonomic dysfunction

Dopamine receptor D4 (DRD4) 13-base-pair deletion: autonomic hyperactivity

The DRD4 receptor gene is one of the five known G protein-coupled receptors for which dopamine is the primary neurotransmitter. The gene is located at CHR 11p15.5 and codes for a receptor protein of 387 amino acids (Van Tol *et al.* 1991). At least three common poly-morphic variants of the gene exist in the human population based as a result of known variations in a 48-base-pair sequence in the third cytoplasmic loop of the receptor (Van Tol *et al.* 1992). Variations in this sequence have been reported to be associated with subtle differences in personality traits such as 'novelty seeking' behaviours (Benjamin *et al.* 1996; Ebstein *et al.* 1996).

A 13-base-pair deletion of bases 235–247 in the DRD4 gene has been identified in approximately 2 per cent of the general population (Nöthen *et al.* 1994). The deletion alters the reading frame from amino acid 79 in the receptor and generates a stop codon 20 amino acids downstream, thereby truncating the receptor to an abnormally short 98 amino acids. No major neuropsychiatric disturbances have been observed in heterozygotes with this mutation (Nöthen *et al.* 1994). However, in a single homozygous individual with this mutation, autonomic hyperactivity was observed. Specifically, the 50-year-old (at the time of the study) male reported severe dermatographism and excessive sweating. These symptoms were exacerbated in social gatherings and moderately warm temperatures. The individual denied feeling anxious in these situations but characterized himself as nervous and explosive since early adulthood. He has had severe migrainous headaches since adolescence, successfully treated with a tricyclic antidepressant. He has been obese since adolescence. He had an acoustic neuroma removed at age 38, with a negative family history, and a recurrence removed at age 44. Pulse-rate fluctuations leading to intermittent sinus tachycardia had been treated with beta-blockers since approximately age 40. A consistently reduced body temperature (35.4 °C) was documented (Nöthen *et al.* 1994). The authors speculated that at least some of these autonomic disturbances could be attributed directly to the absence of a functional DRD4 receptor (Nöthen *et al.* 1994).

Neurotrophic tyrosine kinase receptor, type 1 (NTRK1): congenital insensitivity to pain

The NTRK1 gene is located at CHR 1q32–q41 and is believed to be a primary receptor for nerve growth factor (NGF). In three unrelated patients with congenital insensitivity to pain, different mutations within the NTRK1 gene have been identified (Indo *et al.* 1996).

Specifically, a single base C deletion at nucleotide 1726 in exon C causes a frameshift and premature termination of the receptor protein in two individuals with congenital insensitivity to pain. The individuals are homozygous for the mutation. The authors suggested that the clinical symptomatology results from the fact that the NGF–NTRK1 system plays a critical role in the development and function of the peripheral pain and temperature systems (Indo *et al.* 1996).

In two Ecuadorian brothers with congenital insensitivity to pain and anhidrosis, a deletion of exon D (nucleotides 1872–2112) was found on one allele of the NTRK1 gene and part of the same exon was deleted on the other allele. The authors suggested that these changes resulted from splicing errors due to activation of a cryptic splice donor site. The 5' splice site of an intron between exons D and E contained an A-to-C transversion in the third position, a type of mutation that can result in the skipping of the preceding exon (Indo *et al.* 1996).

A third mutation in the NTRK1 gene has also been associated with congenital insensitivity to pain and anhidrosis. A G-to-C transversion at nucleotide 1795 in exon C leads to a G571A substitution. An individual was identified who was homozygous for this mutation and the authors noted that this amino acid is highly conserved in the tyrosine kinase family of receptors (Indo *et al.* 1996).

Rearranged transfection proto-oncogene (RET): Hirschsprung's disease

The RET gene, for a tyrosine kinase receptor, is located at CHR 10q11.2. Mutations in the RET gene exist in 50 per cent of patients with familial Hirschsprung's disease (or aganglionic colon), a congenital disorder characterized by complete absence of the enteric ganglia along a variable portion of the intestine (Edery *et al.* 1994; Attie *et al.* 1995; Pasini *et al.* 1996). Penetrance is greater in males than in females, in keeping with the higher frequency of the disorder in males. Clinically, the disorder results in intestinal obstruction in neonates and severe constipation in infants. A large number of mutations exist throughout the gene in the familial cases as well as in approximately 33 per cent of sporadic cases. Specifically, frameshift and mis-sense mutations disrupt or change the structure of the protein (Romeo *et al.* 1994).

Endothelin-B receptor (EDNRB): Hirschsprung's disease type 2

The endothelins are a family of potent vasoactive peptides whose effects are mediated via G protein-coupled receptors. Mutations within the EDNRB gene are the molecular basis of Hirschsprung's disease type 2 (Puffenberger *et al.* 1994; Attie *et al.* 1995; Kusafuka *et al.* 1996). It has been estimated that EDNRB mutations account for approximately 5 per cent of cases of Hirschsprung's disease (Chakravarti 1996). However, penetrance is not 100 per cent for some of the mutations, even in homozygotes with the mutation (Puffenberger *et al.* 1994). These data suggest that the EDNRB gene may be an important modifier gene for the development of Hirschsprung's disease type 2.

Transthyretin (TTR): amyloid polyneuropathy

Transthyretin is a prealbumin protein of 127 amino acids and is a primary transport protein for thyroxine and retinol (vitamin A). The protein is a common constituent of neuritic plaques and microangiopathic lesions related to amyloid deposition (see Chapter 42). More than 40 different mutations associated with amyloid deposition have been identified within the TTR gene located at CHR 18q11.2–q12.1 (Saraiva 1995). The majority of the mutations result in an amyloid polyneuropathy which involves small, unmyelinated fibres. The neuropathy disproportionately affects pain and temperature sensation. However, significant clinical variation exists between the various mutations.

Other genetic causes of autonomic dysfunction

Dopamine β-hydroxylase (DBH) deficiency: absence of noradrenergic autonomic function

DBH converts dopamine to noradrenaline as is co-released with noradrenaline from postganglionic sympathetic neurones. As a result, plasma DBH levels have been used as an index of peripheral sympathetic activity. The DBH gene is located at CHR 9q34 and is approximately 23 kb in length, consisting of 12 exons (Kobayashi *et al.* 1989). Although a specific causative mutation within this gene has yet to be identified, several patients have been analysed with congenital DBH deficiency (see Chapter 40). The individuals have noradrenergic denervation and adrenomedullary failure, but baroreflex afferents, cholinergic innervation, and adrenocortical function are normal. Noradrenaline, adrenaline, and their breakdown products are not detectable in plasma, urine, and cerebrospinal fluid, but dopamine levels are increased significantly. Physiological and pharmacological stimuli of sympathetic nervous system activity cause increases in dopamine but not noradrenaline.

A consistent clinical syndrome has emerged from the analysis of individuals with DBH deficiency (Robertson *et al.* 1986; Man in't Veld *et al.* 1987; Mathias *et al.* 1990; Thompson *et al.* 1995). DBH-deficient infants have a delay in the opening of the eyes (2 weeks in one case) and ptosis has been observed in almost all DBH-deficient infants. Some of the infants have been reported to be sickly in the neonatal stage and survival is often believed to be unlikely. Hypotension, hypoglycaemia, and hypothermia are present early in life. Postural hypotension is exhibited during exercise in childhood and is marked by an increase in heart rate as the blood pressure falls. Syncopal episodes may be misinterpreted as epilepsy in the children, leading to treatment with anticonvulsants. In general, symptoms worsen during adolescence and severely limit the function of the individual.

Clinical features during adolescence and adulthood include reduced exercise tolerance, skeletal muscle hypotonia, recurrent hypoglycaemia, ptosis of the eyelids, nasal stuffiness, and prolonged or retrograde ejaculation. The severe postural hypotension is attributed to the impairment of sympathetic vasoconstrictor function. Symptoms in DBH deficiency have also been reported to worsen in the morning, after exercise, and in warm weather (Mathias *et al.* 1990). Clinical signs and symptoms relating to excessive dopamine levels include hypoprolactaemia (Man in't Veld *et al.* 1988). No other neurological or psychiatric abnormalities have been reported. A single case report identified an elderly woman with severe orthostatic hypotension and a presumed acquired DBH deficiency of unknown aetiology (Gentric *et al.* 1993).

The symptoms of DBH-deficiency respond well to treatment with D-dihydroxyphenylserine (DOPS) (see Chapter 40). This molecule is converted to noradrenaline by decarboxylation of the terminal carboxyl group. Treatment with DOPS (150–600 mg/day) leads to a reduction in orthostatic hypotension, increased plasma levels of noradrenaline and, in males, the ability to ejaculate. In a brother and sister with congenital DBH deficiency, treatment with DOPS was reported to induce a feeling of confidence and optimism, with a tendency to be argumentative (Mathias *et al.* 1990). No side-effects have been noted with long-term DOPS therapy.

Dopamine receptor D2 (DRD2) *Nco*I C to T polymorphism: migraine with aura

Migraine is a common clinical disorder known to have a strong genetic component (Peroutka 1997) as well as dysfunction of the ANS (Johnson 1978). In a recent study, an *Nco*I polymorphism in the gene encoding the D2 dopamine receptor (DRD2) was evaluated in a group of 250 unrelated individuals (Peroutka *et al.* 1997). The major finding of the study was that susceptibility to migraine with aura is modified by the DRD2 *Nco*I C and T allele at nucleotide 3420 (H313H). The presence of the DRD2 *Nco*I C allele has a significant effect on susceptibility to migraine with aura compared to a control group of non-migraineurs as well as to individuals with migraine without aura. The incidence of migraine with aura was lowest in individuals with the T/T genotype. However, it is also clear that since not all individuals with the DRD2 *Nco*I C/C genotype suffer from migraine with aura, multiple additional genes are involved in the pathogenesis of migraine. Thus, the DRD2 *Nco*I C allele is neither necessary nor sufficient to cause migraine with aura.

Since molecular variations within the DRD2 gene have been associated with variations in dopaminergic function (Noble 1996), these data suggest that alterations in dopaminergic neurotransmission can modulate the clinical susceptibility to migraine with aura. Therefore, these data provide molecular genetic support for the hypothesis that the pathophysiological basis of migraine can be modified by variations in dopamine D2 receptor function. The fact that dopamine plays a significant but unclear role in the postganglionic sympathetic nervous system (Lackovic and Relja 1983) indicates that the known autonomic abnormalities in migraine (Johnson 1978) may be related to peripheral dopaminergic dysfunction.

Familial dysautonomia: Riley–Day syndrome

A clinical syndrome consisting of a congenital lack of tearing, emotional lability, paroxysmal hypertension, increased sweating, cold hands and feet, corneal anaesthesia, erythematous skin blotching, and drooling has been termed the Riley–Day syndrome or hereditary sensory and autonomic neuropathy II (Brunt and McKusick 1970; Chapter 41). The clinical manifestations are variable and may also include absence of fungiform papillae of the tongue, severe scoliosis, and neuropathic joints. The individuals also have an impaired response to pressor agents. Excretion of both dopamine and noradrenaline metabolites is reduced and plasma DBH levels are low. The specific molecular basis of this disorder remains unknown. However, linkage analysis has localized a causative gene to CHR 9q31–q33 (Blumenfeld *et al.* 1993).

Future directions

Molecular genetics allows for an objective diagnostic evaluation of the ANS. Moreover, the molecular genetic data offer the potential to provide immediate therapeutic guidance. For example, the effectiveness of DOPS in congenital DBH deficiency allows for a significant reduction in morbidity. The coupling of molecular genetic diagnoses and rational therapeutic approaches based on these data should have a significant impact on the diagnosis and management of patients with autonomic dysfunction in the near future. The insights gained from the genetic analysis of the ANS should significantly decrease the morbidity from genetically based autonomic dysfunction.

References

Attie, T., Till, M., Pelet, A. *et al.* (1995). Mutation of the endothelin-receptor B gene in Waardenburg–Hirschsprung disease. *Hum Mol Genet.* 4, 2407–9.

Benjamin, J., Li, L., Patterson, C., Greenberg, B. D., Murphy, D. L., and Hamer, D. H. (1996). Population and familial association between the D4 dopamine receptor gene and measures of novelty seeking. *Nature Genet.* 12, 81–4.

Blumenfeld, A., Slaugenhaupt, S. A., Axelrod, F. B. *et al.* (1993). Localization of the gene for familial dysautonomia on chromosome 9 and definition of DNA markers for genetic diagnosis. *Nature Genet.* 4, 160–4.

Brunt, P. W. and McKusick, V. A. (1970). Familial dysautonomia. A report of genetic and clinical studies, with a review of the literature. *Medicine* 49, 343–74.

Chakravarti, A. (1996). Endothelin receptor-mediated signaling in hirschusprung disease. *Hum. Mol. Genet.* 5, 303–7.

Ebstein, R. P., Novick, O., Umansky, R. *et al.* (1996). Dopamine D4 receptor (D4DR) exon III polymorphism associated with the human personality trait of novety seeking. *Nature Genet.* 12, 78–80.

Edery, P., Pelet, A., Mulligan, L. M. *et al.* (1994). Long segment and short segment familial Hirschsprung's disease: variable clinical expression at the RET locus. *J. Med. Genet.* 31, 602–6.

Gentric, A., Fouilhoux, A., Caroff, M., Mottier, D., and Jouquan, J. (1993). Dopamine B hydroxylase deficiency responsible for severe dysautonomic orthostatic hypotension in an elderly patient. *J. Am. Geriatr. Soc.* 41, 550–1.

Indo, Y., Tsuruta, M., Hayashida, Y. *et al.* (1996). Mutations in the TRKA/NGF receptor gene in patients with congenital insensitivity to pain with anhidrosis. *Nature Genet.* 13, 485–8.

Johnson, E. S. (1978). A basis for migraine therapy—the autonomic theory reappraised. *Postgrad. Med. J.* 54, 231.

Kobayashi, K., Kurosawa, Y., Fujita, K., and Nagasu, T. (1989). Human dopamine B-hydroxylase gene: two mRNA types having different 3′-terminal regions are produced through alternative polyadenylation. *Nucleic Acids Res.* 17, 1089–102.

Kusafuka, T., Wang, Y., and Puri, P. (1996). Novel mutations of the endothelin-B receptor gene in isolated patients with Hirschsprung's disease. *Hum. Mol. Genet.* 5, 347–9.

Lackovic, Z. and Relja, M. (1983). Evidence for a widely distributed peripheral dopaminergic system. *Fed. Proc.* 42, 3000–4.

Man int' Veld, A., Boomsma, F., Lenders, J. *et al.* (1988). Patients with congenital dopamine beta-hydroxylase deficiency. A lesson in catecholamine physiology. *Am. J. Hypertens.* 1, 231–8.

Man in't Veld, A. J., Boomsma, F., Moleman, P., and Schalekamp, M. A. (1987). Congenital dopamine-beta-hydroxylase deficiency. A novel orthostatic syndrome. *Lancet*, i, 183–8.

Mathias, C. J., Bannister, R. B., Cortelli, P. *et al.* (1990). Clinical, autonomic and therapeutic observations in two siblings with postural hypotension and sympathetic failure due to an inability to synthesize noradrenaline from dopamine because of a deficiency of dopamine beta hydroxylase. *Q. J. Med.* 75, 617–33.

Noble, E. P. (1996). The gene that rewards alcoholism. *Sci. Med.* 3, 52–61.

Nöthen, M. M., Cicohon, S., Hemmer, S. *et al.* (1994). Human dopamine D4 receptor gene: Frequent occurrence of a null allele and observation of homozygosity. *Hum. Mol. Genet.* 3, 2207–12.

Pasini, B., Ceccherini, I. and Romeo, G. (1996). RET mutations in human disease. *Trends Genet.* **12**, 138–44.

Peroutka, S. J. (1997). Genetic evaluation of migraine, in *Blue books of practical neurology: headache*, (ed. P. J. Goadsby and S. D. Siberstein), Vol. 17, pp. 107–14. Butterworth–Heinemann, Boston.

Peroutka, S. J., Wilhoit, T., and Jones, K. (1997). Clinical susceptibility to migraine with aura is modified by dopamine D2 receptor (DRD2) *Nco*I alleles. *Neurology*, **49**, 201–6.

Puffenberger, E. G., Hosoda, K., Washington, S. S. *et al.* (1994). A missense mutation of the endothelin-B receptor gene in multigenic Hirschsprung's disease. *Cell* **79**, 1257–66.

Robertson, D., Goldberg, M. R., Onrot, J. *et al.* (1986). Isolated failure of autonomic noradrenergic neurotransmission: evidence for impaired beta-hydroxylation of dopamine. *New Engl. J. Med.* **314**, 1494–7.

Romeo, G., Ronchetto, P., Luo, Y., Barone, V., Seri, M., and Ceccherini, I. (1994). Point mutations affecting the tyrosine kinase domain of the RET proto-oncogene in Hirschsprung's disease. *Nature* **367**, 377–8.

Saraiva, M. J. (1995). Transthyretin mutations in health and disease. *Hum. Mutat.* **5**, 191–6.

Thompson, J. M., O'Callaghan, C. J., Kingwell, B. A., Lambert, G. W., Jennings, G. L., and Esler, M. D. (1995). Total norepinephrine spillover, muscle sympathetic nerve activity and heart-rate spectral analysis in a patient with dopamine beta-hydroxylase deficiency. *J. Autonom. Nerv. Syst.* **55**, 198–206.

Van Tol, H. H. M., Bunzow, J. R., Guan, H. C. *et al.* (1991). Cloning of the gene for a human dopamine D4 receptor with high affinity for the antipsychotic clozapine. *Nature* **350**, 610–14.

Van Tol, H. H. M., Wu, C. M., Guan, H. C. *et al.* (1992). Multiple dopamine D4 receptor variants in the human population. *Nature*, **358**, 149–52.

5. Central neurotransmitters and neuromodulators in cardiovascular regulation

Eduardo E. Benarroch

Introduction

The central neural circuits controlling arterial blood pressure (BP), heart rate (HR), and renal function are located at all levels of the neuraxis, have a complex neurochemical organization, and are highly interconnected (Chapter 6: Loewy and Spyer 1990; Dampney 1994; Spyer 1994). These regions integrate central and peripheral commands to maintain a continuous level of activity of cardiovascular effectors; prevent wide variations of BP through compensatory reflexes; and initiate integrated adaptive cardiovascular responses in response to external stimuli or during different behaviours.

Combined application of a variety of anatomical, physiological, and pharmacological techniques has provided a wealth of information about the functional anatomy and neurochemistry of the central pathways controlling cardiovascular function. These techniques include:

(1) mapping of central autonomic pathways using anterograde, retrograde, and transneuronal transport (e.g. pseudorabies virus) methods;

(2) immunocytochemical identification of neurones and fibres containing neuropeptides or specific neurotransmitter-synthesizing enzymes (Benarroch et al. 1995);

(3) mapping of expression of immediate early genes (e.g. c-fos) in specific regions in response to a variety of stimuli;

(4) localization of receptors by autoradiography and, more recently, in situ hybridization to detect mRNA encoding for specific receptor subunits;

(5) detection of endogenous release of neurotransmitters in restricted brain areas by microdialysis;

(6) local microinjection of selective agonists or antagonists, combined with recording of BP, HR, and sympathetic nerve activity; and

(7) intra- and extracellular recordings 'in vivo' and preparations, in vitro to study spontaneous activity, ionic conductances, and neurochemical responses of central 'cardiovascular' neurones (Renaud and Bourque 1991; Sun 1996).

The central autonomic circuits interact via a complex 'chemical coding' provided by two types of signals:

(1) fast (or classical) point-to-point excitation or inhibition mediated by amino acid neurotransmitters; and

(2) slower 'modulation' of neuronal excitability, mediated by amino acids, acetylcholine (ACh), monoamines, neuropeptides, purines, nitric oxide (NO), and steroids.

These substances, their synthesizing enzymes, or their respective receptors have been identified in cell bodies, fibre pathways, and synaptic terminals in different areas involved in the central control of circulation.

The complexity of the chemical coding stems from the coexistence of different neurotransmitters in single neurones, the various receptor subtypes for a given neurotransmitter, the presynaptic and postsynaptic interactions among the various neurochemicals, and the plasticity of neurotransmitter expression or receptor function in response to activity and environmental factors.

Overview of the functional and neurochemical anatomy of central cardiovascular control

Central autonomic control areas

The central areas controlling cardiovascular function are interconnected and distributed throughout the neuraxis. These include the insular, anterior cingulate and ventromedial prefrontal cortices, the central nucleus of the amygdala (CNA)/bed nucleus the stria terminalis (bnst) complex; the paraventricular (PVN) and other nuclei of the hypothalamus; the periaqueductal grey matter (PAG), the parabrachial nucleus, the nucleus of the solitary tract (NTS), the ventrolateral medulla (VLM), the ventromedial medulla, and the lateral tegmental field (Dampney 1994).

The final outputs of these central regulatory circuits are mediated by:

(1) sympathetic preganglionic neurones (SPNs) of the intermediolateral cell column (IML) of the spinal cord;

(2) cardiovagal neurones of the nucleus ambiguus; and

(3) vasopressin (AVP) secreting magnocellular neurones of the hypothalamus.

The insular cortex is the primary viscerosensory cortex and receive inputs from taste and general visceral afferents. The prefrontal and anterior cingulate cortices are the highest-level 'premotor' autonomic regions. The CNA/bnst complex plays a critical role in integration of emotional responses (Amaral et al. 1992). The PVN is an important a site for integration autonomic and neuroendocrine responses to stress. The PAG is a site of integration of autonomic, behavioural, and antinociceptive stress responses (Lovick 1993). The NTS is the first relay station for visceral afferent information (Loewy and Spyer 1990; Lawrence and Jarrott 1996). Its rostral region relays taste inputs to the thalamus; its intermediate region receives topographically organized general visceral afferents and mediates a variety of medullary reflexes; and its caudal region is a site of convergence of viscerosensory inputs and relay of visceral information to the forebrain.

The rostral VLM contains neurones that project massively to the intermediolateral cell column and tonically activate the sympathetic preganglionic neurones (SPNs) controlling cardiovascular effectors (Dampney 1994; Spyer 1994). Rostral VLM neurones mediate reflex and behavioural influences controlling sympathetic activity, including responses to hypoxia. On the other hand, the caudal VLM is a site of integration of medullary depressor reflexes. Both the rostral and caudal VLM relay viscerosensory information to the hypothalamus. The ventromedial medulla, including the caudal raphe nuclei, provides direct inputs to preganglionic sympathetic neurones (Chalmers and Pilowsky 1991).

Chemical signaling in central autonomic pathways

'Classical neurotransmission' is the rapid, point-to-point chemical synaptic transmission of excitatory or inhibitory signals. Excitatory amino acids, such as L-glutamate, and inhibitory amino acids, such as γ-aminobutyric acid (GABA), are involved in rapid transmission within the central autonomic circuits (CAN) via activation of specific ligand-gated (ion channel) receptors. Acetylcholine, monoamines, neuropeptides, and adenosine are involved in modulation of neuronal excitability, via activation of a large variety of GTP-binding (G) protein-coupled receptors. Neuropeptides and monoamines may diffuse through the extracellular fluid to act on targets distant from the site of release. This process is referred to as 'volume transmission'.

Angiotensin II, vasopressin (AVP), natriuretic peptides, opioids, corticotrophin-releasing hormone (CRH) and a variety of cytokines (e.g. interleukin-1) affect central cardiovascular control by acting both as endogenous transmitters in central autonomic pathways and as hormonal systems. As circulating signals they affect peripheral targets and exert important central control by acting via receptors in the circumventricular organs (Ferguson and Wall 1992).

Fast Neurotransmission

Excitatory inputs mediated by L-glutamate (L-glu), or other excitatory amino acids, and inhibitory inputs mediated by GABA control the spontaneous, reflex-mediated, and behaviourally controlled activity of cardiovascular neurones in the NTS, the rostral and caudal VLM, nucleus ambiguus, IML, hypothalamus, and amygdala.

L-Glutamate

L-Glutamate or other excitatory amino acids are considered as the likely transmitters of descending sympathoexcitatory inputs from the rostral VLM to SPNs; baroreceptor afferent inputs to the NTS (Lawrence and Jarrott 1996); inputs from baroreceptive NTS neurones to effector cardiovagal neurones of the nucleus ambiguus and sympathoinhibitory neurones of the caudal VLM (Dampney 1994; Spyer 1994) and descending excitatory inputs from the hypothalamus and other regions to vasomotor neurones of the rostral VLM. Fast excitatory transmission is mediated via three classes of ionotropic receptors: AMPA (α-amino-3-hydroxy-5-methyl-4-isoxazole propionic acid), kainate (KA), and NMDA (N-methyl-D-aspartate) receptors. The AMPA/kainate receptors are permeable to monovalent ions (Na^+, K^+). The NMDA receptor channel is a voltage-dependent cation channel, which is positively modulated by glycine and allows entry of Ca^{2+} in addition to Na^+. The NMDA

receptor Ca^{2+} channel is blocked by Mg^{2+}, and this blockade is inhibited by depolarization.

It is likely that L-glutamate may act via several receptor mechanisms in a given circuit. Increase in intracellular Ca^{2+} ($[Ca^{2+}]_i$) is an important consequence of activation of several subtypes of excitatory amino acid receptors. Rapid increase in $[Ca^2]_i$, following activation of NMDA, AMPA, and metabotropic receptors, results in activation of several Ca^{2+}-dependent enzymatic cascades, including activation of constitutive forms of nitric oxide synthase (NOS) present in neurones, glia, and endothelium. Nitric oxide (NO) is a diffusible messenger molecule that activates cytoplasmic guanylate cyclase. As retrograde messenger, NO may increase presynaptic L-glu release. Neurones containing NOS are identified by its reactivity with NADPH-diaphorase, and include preganglionic sympathetic and other central autonomic neurones (Fig. 5.1) (Benarroch et al. 1995; Smithson and Benarroch 1996).

In addition to L-glutamate, other substances may produce fast excitation in central autonomic circuits, acting via ionotropic cation-channel receptors. These include ACh acting via nicotinic receptors; ATP via P2X purinoceptors; and serotonin via 5-HT3 receptors (see below).

GABA

γ-Aminobutyric acid (GABA), the most abundant inhibitory neurotransmitter in brain, is found mainly in local circuit neurones; these neurones are identified by their immunoreactivity for glutamic acid decarboxylase (GAD). GABA produces both pre- and postsynaptic inhibition, via GABAA and GABAB receptors. GABAA receptor activation leads to opening of a Cl-channel; this produces fast inhibitory

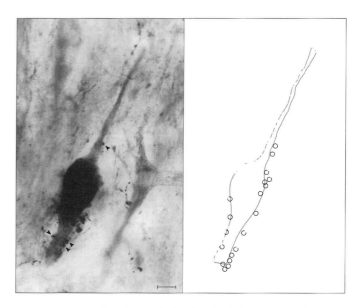

Fig. 5.1. Horizontal section at T8 double stained for NADPH-diaphorase and tyrosine hydroxylase (TH). TH-positive varicosities (arrowheads) appear to contact the NADPH-diaphorase-stained SPN. Right: Diagram of the same SPN with possible points of TH fibre contact marked by a circle. Five different focal planes were captured to visualize clearly the multiple points of contact with the SPN. Bar = 15 μm. (Reprinted with permission from Smithson and Benarroch (1996).)

postsynaptic potentials (fast IPSPs); presynaptic GABAA receptors in primary afferents inhibit neurotransmitter release. GABAA receptors are activated by muscimol, inhibited by bicuculline, and allosterically potentiated by barbiturates and benzodiazepines. The GABAB receptor is a G-protein-coupled receptor; its activation may produce both postsynaptic and presynaptic inhibition, via an increase in K^+ conductance or decrease in Ca^{2+} conductance, respectively. GABA has been implicated in both tonic and reflex inhibition of medullary vasomotor, cardiovagal (Spyer 1994), and hypothalamic (Renaud and Bourque 1991) neurones.

Neuromodulation

Acetylcholine, monoamines, and neuropeptides mediate slower modulatory influences within the central autonomic network, mainly via G (GTP-binding)-protein-coupled receptors.

Acetylcholine

Acetylcholine (ACh) is synthesized by choline acetyl transferase (CAT), a specific marker of cholinergic neurones. It has been identified in preganglionic autonomic neurones and in (possibly local) neurones of the NTS, VLM, and hypothalamus. ACh is the primary neurotransmitter of preganglionic sympathetic and parasympathetic neurones. In addition it has been implicated in stimulation of secretion of AVP; activation of sympathoexcitatory neurones in the rostral VLM, and intermediolateral cell column; regulation of the baroreflex at the level of the NTS; and inspiratory inhibition of cardiovagal neurones of the nucleus ambiguus (Spyer 1994). Acetylcholine acts via central nicotinic and muscarinic receptors.

Catecholamines

Catecholamines in the central nervous system include dopamine, noradrenaline, and adrenaline. Noradrenaline is also the peripheral sympathetic neurotransmitter. Tyrosine hydroxylase (TH) is the biochemical marker of all catecholamine neurones. Dopamine β-hydroxylase (DBH) allows transformation of dopamine into noradrenaline. Phenylethanolamine-N-methyltransferase (PNMT) is a marker of adrenaline neurones. Noradrenaline and adrenaline neurones form two anatomically segregated but functionally integrated systems, the locus coeruleus and the lateral tegmental system. The lateral tegmental system includes neurones of the A5 group in the ventrolateral pons; a ventrolateral (A1/C1) group, close to the ventral medullary surface; and a dorsomedial (A2/C2) group in the region of the NTS (Fig. 5.2) (Guyenet 1991). The A1, A2 and A5 groups synthesize noradrenaline; whereas the C1 and C2/3 (PNMT-positive) groups synthesize adrenaline. Lateral tegmental catecholaminergic neurones have extensive interconnections with areas involved in autonomic and neuroendocrine control, including preganglionic autonomic neurones, autonomic brainstem nuclei, hypothalamus, and amygdala.

Catecholamines have been implicated in both excitatory and inhibitory modulation of preganglionic sympathetic neurones; facilitation of the baroreflex at the level of the NTS, presynaptic inhibition of C1 neurones; and stimulation of AVP and CRH secretion from the hypothalamus. The responses to catecholamines are complex, and involve excitatory and inhibitory, pre- and postsynaptic G-protein receptors. In general, excitatory effects are mediated by α_1- and inhibitory effects by α_2-receptors.

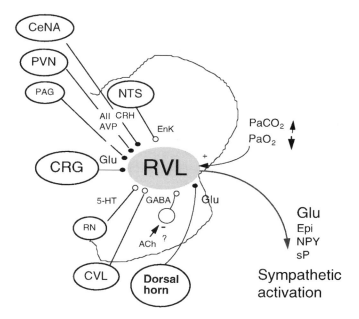

Fig. 5.2. Neurochemical influences on sympathoexcitatory neurones of the rostral ventrolateral medulla (RVL). These neurones release L-glutamate (Glu), adrenaline (Epi), neuropeptide Y (NPY), and substance P (sP) to the intermediolateral cell column. RVL neurones receive inputs from the nucleus of the solitary tract (NTS); central nucleus of the amygdala (CeNA); paraventricular nucleus (PVN); periaqueductal grey (PAG), the central respiratory generator (CRG); raphe nucleus (RN); caudal ventrolateral medulla (CVL); and dorsal horn. Excitatory inputs (filled circles) are mediated by L-glutamate (Glu) vasopressin (AVP), and corticotrophin-releasing hormone (CRH). Inhibitory inputs (open circles) are mediated by GABA, serotonin (5-HT, via 5-HT$_{1A}$ receptors), and enkephalins (EnK). Acetylcholine (ACh), acting via M2 receptors, may disinhibit RVL neurones. RVL neurones are directly excited by hypoxia and hypercapnia.

Serotonin

Serotonin (5-hydroxytryptamine, 5-HT) is synthesized from L-tryptophan by action of tryptophan hydroxylase, a marker of serotonergic neurones, fibres, and terminals within central autonomic pathways (Helke *et al.* 1993). Serotonergic innervation of central autonomic regions arises from the raphe nuclei. Serotonin has been implicated in baroreflex modulation at the level of the NTS (Lawrence and Jarrott 1996), control of paraventricular CRH neurones, and both excitatory and inhibitory control of sympathetic preganglionic neurones (Chalmers and Pilowsky 1991). There is a wide variety of serotonin receptors; in general 5-HT$_1$-type receptors produce inhibition and 5-HT$_2$ (and 5-HT$_3$) receptors produce excitation.

Neuropeptides

Neuropeptides and their receptors have a widespread but heterogeneous distribution in the central autonomic network. The hypothalamus, amygdala, and NTS are among the areas of the brain richest in neuropeptides.

Neuropeptide Y (NPY) coexists with catecholamines in neurones of the A1/C1 and A2/C2 groups, and modulates catecholaminergic neurotransmission both pre- and postsynaptically. It potentiates

α_2-mediated effects in the NTS and the α_1-mediated activation of AVP magnocellular neurones.

Corticotrophin releasing hormone (CRH), produced by the PVN and the amygdala, is a critical mediator of the stress response. It activates the pituitary–adrenal axis, and serves as a neural transmitter in autonomic 'premotor' regions to produce cardiovascular changes typical of stress.

Substance P is present in primary visceral afferents, in pathways from the amygdala and NTS, and in bulbospinal pathways from the raphe and VLM. It acts via depolarizing neurokinin 1 (NK1) receptors and has been implicated in the transmission of excitatory information from baroreceptor afferents to the NTS (Lawrence and Jarrott 1996), and from the ventral medulla to SPNs (Chalmers and Pilowsky 1991).

Opioid peptides have been identified in virtually all central autonomic areas, and have predominantly inhibitory action, both pre- and postsynaptically. The central cardiovascular effects of opiates are complex, and vary with the site of application, receptor, species, and state of consciousness. In general, opioids modulate baroreflex responses and inhibit sympathoexcitatory neurones of the rostral ventrolateral medulla (Lawrence and Jarrott 1996).

Angiotensin II, natriuretic peptides, AVP, endothelins, and cytokines can influence BP and other cardiovascular functions by their direct effects on peripheral target organs; via the circumventricular organs; and as endogenous neurotransmitter/neuromodulators in central autonomic pathways.

Angiotensin II, acting via AT-1 receptors, produces sympathoexcitation, baroreflex inhibition, increase in secretion of AVP and adrenocorticotrophic hormone (ACTH), and stimulation of water intake and salt appetite (Ferguson and Wall 1992). Endogenous AVP mediates some of the central pressor effects of angiotensin II, and is present in projections from the PVN to other central autonomic regions. Its central effects are mediated by V1 receptors and include excitation of rostral VLM and preganglionic sympathetic neurones, and inhibition of the baroreflex. On the other hand, circulating AVP activates the baroreflex (Ferguson and Wall 1992).

Natriuretic peptides and their receptors overlap in their brain distribution with the angiotensin system. Natriuretic peptides oppose the angiotensin II-induced water intake, AVP release, and sympathoexcitation.

Other substances

Purines, including adenosine and ATP; prostaglandins; NO and carbon monoxide (CO); and steroids may all affect neurochemical transmission in central autonomic pathways. Their function in central cardiovascular control is still incompletely understood.

Specific circuits

Sympathetic preganglionic neurones

The SPNs are organized into functionally distinct units controlling the different vascular beds, heart, and adrenal gland. These neurones receive selective innervation from multiple sources and project to target-specific postganglionic neurones. Inputs to SPNs originate from two main sources, segmental (visceral and somatic) afferents and supraspinal pathways.

Table 5.1. Neurochemical influence on preganglionic sympathetic neurones

Source	Transmitter	Receptor	Effect on BP and HR
Primary afferent	Substance P	NK 1	↑
Local interneurone	GABA	GABA$_A$	↓
Rostral ventrolateral medulla (C1)	Glutamate	AMPA/KA NMDA	↑
	Adrenaline	α_1	↑
		α_2	↓
	Substance P	NK1	↑
Raphe/VMM	Serotinin	5-HT$_1$	↓
		5-HT$_2$	↑
	Substance P	NK1	↑
A5 group	Noradrenaline	α_2	↓
Paraventricular nucleus	Vasopressin	V1	↑

Several descending pathways containing a variety of neurotransmitters exert a differential control on SPNs. Important sources include the PVN; the A5 group; the rostral VLM (including the C1 group); and the ventromedial medulla (VMM) and caudal raphe nuclei (Table 5.1; Fig. 5.1). Glutamatergic inputs from the rostral VLM and VMM are thought to be responsible for tonic background excitation of SPNs. Catecholaminergic inputs from the A5 and C1 groups produce both an α_1-receptor-mediated activation and an α_2-receptor-mediated inhibition. Substance P, released from both ventromedullary pathways and primary segmental afferents, activates SPNs via NK1 receptors (Chalmers and Pilowsky 1991); AVP released from PVN projections, exerts similar effects via V1 receptors (Cabot 1990).

Ventrolateral medulla

The rostral VLM includes glutamatergic bulbospinal neurones and the C1 adrenaline neurones, which may co-contain NPY, substance P, and L-glutamate (Chalmers and Pilowsky 1991). Rostral VLM neurones play three major roles in cardiovascular regulation: (1) tonic monosynaptic excitation to SPNs; (2) final common effectors of a variety of reflexes and descending influences affecting sympathetic activity; and (3) 'chemosensors' activated by hypoxia, and mediating sympathoexcitatory and cerebral vasomotor responses to hypoxia–ischaemia (Dampney 1994; Spyer 1994; Sun 1996). In addition to projection neurones, the rostral VLM contains a variety of neurochemically diverse neuronal populations, likely including local and propriobulbar neurones.

The activity of bulbospinal sympathoexcitatory rostral VLM neurones is regulated by a variety of neurotransmitters (Table 5.2; Fig. 5.2). L-Glutamate mediates sympathoexcitatory responses to hypothalamic or somatic nerve stimulation (Sun 1996). GABA mediates both tonic and baroreflex inhibition of rostral by caudal VLM neurones. Activation of β-adrenergic, M2 muscarinic, NPY, substance P, angiotensin II, AVP, and endothelin receptors produces increases in arterial pressure. On the other hand, 5-HT$_1$ serotonergic atrial natriuretic peptide-, opioid- and NO-related mechanisms produce sym-

Table 5.2. Neurochemical control of RVL neurones

Source	Neurotransmitter	Receptor	Effect on BP and HR
Local neurones (?)	L-Glutamate	NMDA non-NMDA	↑
Local neurone	Acetylcholine	M_2	↑
Caudal ventrolateral medulla	GABA	$GABA_A$	↓
Raphe	Serotonin	$5-HT_1$	↓
NTS	Enkephalin	mu	↓
C1/A1; C2/A2, A5?	Noradrenaline/ adrenaline	α_2 (autoreceptor)	↓
	NPY	Y1	↑
Paraventricular nucleus	Vasopressin	V1	↑
Amygdala	CRH		↑
Local ?	Endothelin	ET-1	↑
Local ?	NO		↓
Local ?	Angiotensin II	AT-1	↑
Drugs	Clonidine	I_1	↓
		α_2	↓
	Propranolol	β blockage	↓
	Urapidil	$5-HT_{1A}$	↓

RVL, rostral ventrolateral medulla.

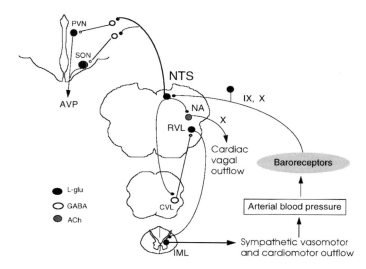

Fig. 5.3. Neurochemistry of the baroreceptor reflex. A current model of the baroreceptor reflex circuit. Baroreceptor afferents release L-glutamate (L-glu) or another excitatory amino acid at their synapse in the nucleus of the solitary tracts (NTS). Baroreceptive NTS neurones initiate three responses: (1) sympathoinhibition, via a projection to GABAergic neurones of the caudal ventrolateral medulla (CVL), that inhibit sympathoexcitatory neurones of the rostral ventrolateral medulla (RVL); (2) activation of vagal cardiac output via connections with the nucleus ambiguus (NA); and (3) inhibition of release of vasopressin (AVP) from magnocellular neurones of the supraoptic (SON) and paraventricular (PVN) hypothalamic nuclei, via activation of GABAergic neurones in the medial septal region. IML, intermediolateral cell column; ACh: acetylcholinie.

pathoinhibition and hypotension (Sun 1996). The sympathoexcitatory response to hypoxia appears to involve direct activation of O_2-sensitive Ca^{2+} channels in rostral VLM bulbospinal neurones, rather than mediation by a local neurotransmitter (Sun 1996).

Nucleus of the solitary tract and baroreflex circuit

The organization of the medullary baroreflex circuit has been investigated extensively (Dampney 1994; Spyer 1994). Baroreceptor-stimulated NTS neurones initiate a feedback loop that ultimately results in excitation of cardiovagal neurones and inhibition of sympathoexcitatory neurones in the rostral VLM. A currently accepted model is that sympathoinhibitory information from barosensitive NTS neurones is relayed through propriospinal neurones in the caudal VLM, which in turn inhibit sympathoexcitatory neurones of the RVL; cardiovagal activation may involve direct excitatory projections from the NTS to the nucleus ambiguus (Fig. 5.3) (Dampney 1994; Spyer 1994).

Baroreceptor afferents release L-glutamate or another excitatory amino acid which may activate NTS neurones via both non-NMDA and NMDA, as well as metabotropic receptors (Van Giersbergen *et al.* 1992; Lawrence and Jarrott 1996). Barosensitive NTS neurones initiate three main responses to an increase in arterial pressure:

(1) they send excitatory (L-glutamate?) projections to propriobulbar GABAergic neurones of the caudal ventrolateral medulla that, in

turn, inhibit sympathoexcitatory neurones of the rostral VLM, via $GABA_A$ mechanisms;

(2) they directly stimulate cardiovagal neurones of the nucleus ambiguus, producing bradycardia; and

(3) they give rise to an ascending projection that leads ultimately to local GABAergic inhibition of AVP-secreting magnocellular neurones of the hypothalamus (Dampney 1994; Spyer 1994).

Several neurochemical influences, arising from primary afferents, local neurones, or other autonomic regions, may act at the level of the NTS to affect arterial pressure or baroreflex responses (Table 5.3; Fig. 5.4) (Van Giersbergen *et al.* 1992; Lawrence and Jarrott 1996).

Barosensitive neurones of the NTS, caudal VLM, and nucleus ambiguus appear to be tonically inhibited by local GABAergic mechanisms. The NTS contains abundant GABAergic neurones, and activation of local $GABA_A$ receptors inhibits barosensitive neurones and results in an increase of arterial pressure and heart rate. This is thought to be a mechanism through which descending influences from 'defence' areas of the brain inhibit baroreflex responses during adaptation to stress (Spyer 1994). The role of $GABA_B$ receptor mechanisms in the NTS is undetermined: baclofen, a $GABA_B$ agonist, decreases arterial pressure when administered into the NTS; this may reflect presynaptic inhibition of release of GABA, and thus disinhibition of NTS neurones (Lawrence and Jarrott 1996).

Table 5.3. Neurochemical influences on NTS neurones

Source	Transmitter	Receptor	Effect on ABP and HR
Baroreceptor afferent	Glutamate	AMPA/KA	↓
		NMDA	↓
		Metabotropic	↓
	NO		↓
	Substance P	NK1	↓
Local neurones	GABA	$GABA_A$	↑
		$GABA_B$	↑
	Glycine		↑
Local ?	Acetylcholine	M_1	↓
Raphe	Serotonin	$5-HT_1$	↑
		$5-HT_3$	↓
A1/A2/A5	Noradrenaline	α_2	↓
	NPY	Y2	↓
Paraventricular nucleus	Vasopressin	V1	↑
Circulation	Vasopressin	V2	↓
	Angiotensin II	AT-1	↑
	Atriopeptin		↓
Local (?)	Adenosine	A1	↑
		A2	↓

NTS, nucleus of the solitary tract; ABP, arterial blood pressure.

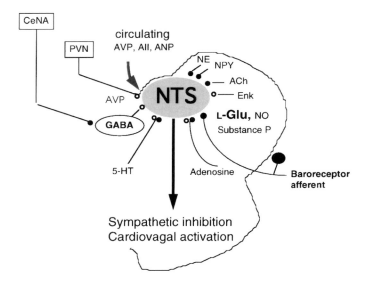

Fig. 5.4. Neurochemical influences on baroreceptive neurones of the nucleus of the solitary tract (NTS). Primary baroreceptor afferents excite (filled circles) NTS neurones via release of L-glutamate (L-Glu); these effects are potentiated by nitric oxide (NO), produced by Glu-triggered cascades, and substance P, co-released by the afferent. Baroreceptor responses are facilitated by noradrenaline (NE) and neuropeptide Y (NPY), and inhibited (open circles) by locally released GABA and vasopressin (AVP). Serotonin (5-HT) and adenosine may excite or inhibit these neurones, via different receptor subtypes. PVN, paraventricular nucleus; CeNA, central nucleus of the amygdala; ANP, atrial natriuretic peptide; AII, angiotensin II.

Primary baroreceptor afferents release substance P, which may stimulate barosensitive NTS neurones both directly and by potentiating the excitatory effects of L-glutamate. Nitric oxide, produced in response to glutamate-receptor-triggered, Ca^{2+}-dependent activation of NOS, may also facilitate the baroreflex (Lawrence and Jarrott 1996). The NTS receives noradrenergic innervation, from A2, A1, and A5 regions (Lawrence and Jarrott 1996). Noradrenaline facilitates baroreflex responses via activation of local α_2-receptors; lesions or pharmacological blockade affecting noradrenergic mechanisms in the NTS produces chronic lability of arterial pressure. Neuropeptide Y and galanin coexist with noradrenaline in NTS neurones and afferents, and may modulate the baroreflex both directly and via interactions with adrenergic mechanisms (Lawrence and Jarrott 1996). The NTS receives endorphin-containing inputs from the hypothalamus, and contains enkephalin-producing neurones. Activation of opioid receptors in the NTS may inhibit baroreflex responses (Lawrence and Jarrott 1996).

Vasopressin (AVP), angiotensin II, natriuretic peptides, and endothelins may modulate baroreflex responses by acting either as circulating signals affecting receptors of the area postrema or as endogenous neurochemical mediators in intrinsic neurones and pathways innervating the NTS. The circulating and endogenous peptides may exert similar or opposite effects on baroreflex responses. Both circulating and endogenous angiotensin II inhibit, and atrial natriuretic factor potentiate, baroreflex responses. On the other hand, circulating AVP potentiates the baroreflex, whereas endogenous AVP (presumably released from PVN projections to the NTS) inhibits it (Lawrence and Jarrott 1996).

Paraventricular nucleus and integrated responses to stress

The PVN is thought to play a critical role in the co-ordination of neuroendocrine, autonomic, and behavioural responses to stress. It contains magnocellular neurones producing AVP and oxytocin; parvicellular neurones producing CRH and other regulatory hormones controlling the anterior pituitary; and neurones that project to autonomic regions of the brain stem and spinal cord.

The afferent control of the PVN is very complex, and includes four main types of inputs:

(1) ascending projections from the NTS, VLM, and parabrachial nucleus, that relay viscerosensory information and contain a variety of neurochemicals, including catecholamines, NPY, galanin, and somatostatin;

(2) inputs from the subfornical organ (SFO), a circumventricular organ that contains receptors for circulating angiotensin II and atrial natriuretic peptides, and that projects to the hypothalamus to influence AVP secretion and central sympathetic output;

(3) projections from the limbic system via the bed nucleus of the stria terminalis; and

(4) intrahypothalamic projections, including those from the suprachiasmatic nucleus, involved in circadian rhythms, and the dorsomedial nucleus, which has been implicated in responses to stress.

Projections from limbic structures and other hypothalamic nuclei contain a variety of neuropeptides.

The reflex control of AVP secretion by magnocellular neurones and PVN (and supraoptic nucleus) and the activation of the CRH–adrenocortical axis are integral components of the central mechanisms of cardiovascular regulation.

Catecholaminergic and GABAergic mechanisms are thought to play an important role in reflex regulation of AVP release. The A1 noradrenergic neurones of the caudal VLM receive cardiopulmonary, baroreceptor, and chemoreceptor inputs, both directly and via the NTS. Stimulation of the caudal VLM or local administration of noradrenaline excite AVP-secreting neurones, via α_1-mediated receptors. Other co-transmitters, including NPY, ATP, and NO, may contribute to these effects. This pathway appears to mediate the stimulating effects of chemoreceptors on AVP release. On the other hand, AVP release is tonically inhibited by baroreceptors and cardiopulmonary receptors. This pathway involves a relay in the NTS and the hypothalamus, and ultimately results in GABAergic inhibition of the magnocellular neurones (Day 1989).

Clinical correlations

Tetraplegia

Interruption of supraspinal inputs to SPNs produces severe abnormalities in control of sympathetic function in tetraplegic patients. Interruption of the tonic glutamatergic inputs from the VLM and perhaps ventromedial medulla may explain the low levels of supine blood pressure, circulating catecholamines, and sympathetic nerve activity, and the profound orthostatic hypotension in response to tilt with no compensatory increase in sympathetic activity.

Interruption of descending monoaminergic and peptidergic modulatory influences accounts for the exaggerated pressor response to AVP and other pressor agents; and for the unpatterned, generalized sympathetic activation triggered by somatic or visceral stimuli below the lesion in chronic tetraplegics. This phenomenon, referred to as autonomic dysreflexia, is characterized by acute hypertension, vasomotor changes, and bradycardia, together with other manifestations of autonomic hyperactivity.

Patients with chronic tetraplegia have intact supraspinal reflex circuits controlling cardiovagal outflow and AVP release. They have a marked increase in AVP secretion in response to hypotension induced by tilt, and have exaggerated pressor responses to circulating AVP.

Multiple system atrophy

Catecholaminergic inputs to the hypothalamus are thought to be important for reflex stimulation of release of AVP (e.g. in response to hypotension) and CRH (e.g. in response to hypoglycaemia). In humans, there are abundant A1/C1 neurones in the medulla and α_1-receptors in the hypothalamus. Depletion of medullary catecholaminergic neurones and catecholamine markers in the hypothalamus occur in patients with MSA. These patients, unlike those with tetraplegia, fail to increase AVP release in response to tilt-induced hypotension, yet they have a normal AVP response to increased osmolarity. Catecholaminergic denervation of the hypothalamus may account, at least in part, for the inability of these patients to increase ACTH and β-endorphin release in response to hypoglycaemia, and an impaired growth hormone response to the α_2-agonist, clonidine.

Patients with MSA have reduced levels of substance P, as well as catecholamine, 5-HT, and ACh markers in cerebrospinal fluid. Patients with Parkinson's disease, a condition commonly associated with autonomic failure, have reduced numbers of C1 adrenergic neurones (Gai et al. 1993).

Hypertension

Several neurochemical abnormalities in central cardiovascular circuits have been described in the spontaneously hypertensive rat (SHR), a model of human essential hypertension.

Several antihypertensive drugs used clinically are thought to act on vasomotor neurones of the rostral VLM. Clonidine, a centrally active antihypertensive drug, stimulates both α_2- and imidazoline (I_1) receptors in this region. Rilmenidine and moxonidine, two I_1 antagonists that lack α_2-agonist activity, produce hypotension when administered to the rostral VLM. Agmatine, a derivative of arginine, is an endogenous ligand of the I_1 receptor, and is present in the brain. Urapidil is an antihypertensive drug that acts in part by stimulating 5-HT1A receptors in the rostral VLM (Helke et al. 1993); and the effects of propranolol have been attributed to blockade of β-receptors in this region. Losartan, an angiotensin AT-1 receptor antagonist, may block the pressor effects of angiotensin II at the levels of both the hypothalamus and rostral VLM.

References

Amaral, D. G., Price, J. I., Pitkanen, A., and Charmichael, S. T. (1992). Anatomical organization of the primate amygdaloid complex. In *The amygdala: neurobiological aspects of emotion*, (ed. J. P. Aggleton), pp. 1–66. Wiley-Lyss, New York.

Benarroch, E. E., Smithson, I. L., and Low, P. A. (1995). Localization and possible interactions of catecholamine- and NADPH-diaphorase neurones in human medullary autonomic regions. *Brain Res.* **684**, 215–20.

Cabot, J. B. (1990). Sympathetic preganglionic neurons: Cytoarchitecture, ultrastructure, and biophysical properties. In *Central regulation of autonomic functions*, (ed. A. D. Loewy and K. M. Spyer), pp. 44–67. Oxford University Press, New York.

Chalmers, J. and Pilowsky, P. (1991). Brainstem and bulbospinal neurotransmitter systems in the control of blood pressure. *J. Hypertension*, **9**, 675–94.

Dampney, R. A. (1994). Functional organization of central pathways regulating the cardiovascular system. *Physiol. Rev.* **74**, 323–64.

Day, T. A. (1989). Control of neurosecretory vasopressin cells by noradrenergic projections of the caudal ventrolateral medulla. *Prog. Brain Res.* **81**, 303–17.

Ferguson, A. V. and Wall, K. M. (1992). Central actions of angiotensin in cardiovascular control: multiple roles for a single peptide. *Can. J. Physiol. Pharmacol.* **70**, 779–85.

Gai, W. P., Geffen, L. B., Denoroy, L., and Blessing, W. W. (1993). Loss of C1 and C3 epinephrine-synthesizing neurons in the medulla oblongata in Parkinson's disease. *Ann. Neurol.* **33**, 357–67.

Guyenet, P. G. (1991). Central noradrenergic neurons: the autonomic connection. *Prog. Brain Res.* **88**, 365–80.

Helke, C. J., McDonald, C. H., and Phillips, E. T. (1993). Hypotensive effects of 5-HT$_{1A}$ receptor activation: ventral medullary sites and mechanisms of action in the rat. *J. autonom. nerv. Syst.* **42**, 177–88.

Lawrence, A. J. and Jarrott, B. (1996). Neurochemical modulation of cardiovascular control in the nucleus tractus solitarius. *Prog. Neurobiol.* **48**, 21–53.

Loewy, A. D. and Spyer, K. M. (1990). *Central regulation of autonomic functions.* Oxford University Press, Oxford.

Lovick, T. A. (1993). Integrated activity of cardiovascular and pain regulatory systems: role in adaptive behavioural responses. *Prog. Neurobiol.* **40**, 631–44.

Renaud, L. P. and Bourque, C. W. (1991) Neurophysiology and neuropharmacology of hypothalamic magnocellular neurons secreting vasopressin and oxytocin. *Prog. Neurobiol.* **36**, 131–69.

Smithson, I. L. and Benarroch, E. E. (1996). Organization of NADPH-diaphorase-reactive neurons and catecholaminergic fibers in human intermediolateral cell column. *Brain Res.* **723**, 218–22.

Spyer, K. M. (1994). Annual Review Prize Lecture: Central nervous mechanisms contributing to cardiovascular control. *J. Physiol.* **474**, 1–19.

Sun, M. (1996). Pharmacology of reticulospinal vasomotor neurons in cardiovascular regulation. *Pharmacol. Rev.* **48**, 465–94.

Van Giersbergen, P. L., Palkovits, M., and de Jong, W. (1992). Involvement of neurotransmitters in the nucleus tractus solitarii in cardiovascular regulation. *Physiol. Rev.* **72**, 789–824.

6. Central nervous control of the cardiovascular system

K. M. Spyer

Introduction

The anatomical features of the integrative network that exists within the brainstem that is responsible for the control of the autonomic outflows to the cardiovascular system have been identified. These provide a basis for understanding the role of the central nervous system in homeostatic regulation and in the changes that occur in developing major changes in cardiovascular function that accompany, and support, behavioural activities. The present chapter will build on this information and highlight progress that has been made in understanding the underlying physiological processes and their pharmacology.

Innervation of autonomic preganglionic neurones

In considering the central nervous regulation of the cardiovascular system it is necessary to note that the preganglionic vagal and sympathetic neurones are the final common pathway within the central nervous system through which this control is exerted. Sympathetic preganglionic neurones are localized within the intermediolateral cell column of the thoracic and upper lumbar spinal cord (for a detailed review see Gilbey 1997). 'Vasomotor' neurones are distributed throughout the extent of the column, but those sympathetic neurones that influence cardiac activity, both chronotropic and inotropic, are restricted to the upper thoracic segments of the cord (T1–T4). The vagal preganglionic neurones that affect cardiac control are located within the nucleus ambiguus of the ventrolateral medulla (VLM) and the dorsal vagal nucleus: this localization is highly species-selective (Izzo and Spyer 1997). It is not as yet resolved whether individual vagal preganglionic neurones subserve chronotropic, inotropic, and dromotropic function (Izzo and Spyer 1997). However, considerably more is known of the details of central nervous function in heart rate control than of its influence on cardiac dynamics and action potential conduction through the myocardium.

Sympathetic neurones

There is an extensive literature indicating the pattern of innervation of these groups of autonomic neurones from studies using conventional neuroanatomical approaches with various retrograde and anterograde traces (reviewed by Loewy 1990). The more recent development of retrograde trans-synaptic viral traces has added much to this knowledge (Loewy 1990; Janssen *et al.* 1995). With regard to sympathetic neurones innervating the adrenal medulla, a particularly

clear picture has been provided using these methods (Fig. 6.1). Secretions from the adrenal medulla have profound cardiovascular influences. These data are consistent with an earlier report from Loewy and his colleagues, using more conventional approaches (Loewy 1990), and indicate that a range of descending pathways

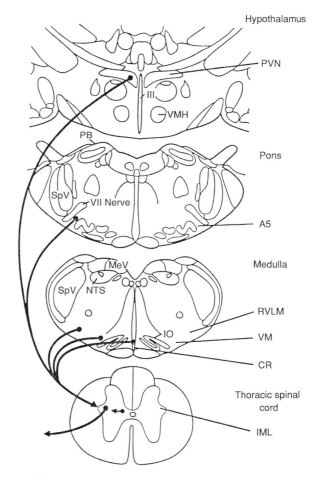

Fig. 6.1. Illustration of the innervation of preganglionic sympathetic neurones. PVN, paraventricular nucleus: A5, A5 group of noradrenergic neurones: RVLM, rostroventrolateral medulla: VM, ventromedial medulla; CR, caudal raphe nuclei; IML, intermediolateral cell column: III, third ventricle, VMH, ventromedial hypothalamus; PB, parabrachial nucleus, SpV, spinal trigeminal nucleus; MeV medial vestibular nucleus; NTS, nucleus tractus solitarius; IO, inferior olivary nucleus. (Reproduced with permission from Spyer (1989).)

innervate these sympathetic preganglionic neurones. They arise from hypothalamic, midbrain, pontine, and medullary cell groups. These include cell groups that have been shown, using immunocytochemistry, to contain particular amines and peptides. In this regard, it is notable that more than 20 putative neurotransmitter substances have been located within the immediate vicinity of preganglionic sympathetic neurones, and include glutamate, GABA, glycine, noradrenaline, adrenaline, dopamine, serotonin, substance P, encephalin, oxytocin, vasopressin, and numerous other neuropeptides and purines, many of which may be co-localized (reviewed by Chalmers and Pilowsky 1991). For the purpose of the current discussion, information concerning the pharmacology of the innervation of a sympathetic preganglionic neurone that arises from the adrenaline and noradrenaline neurones of the ventrolateral medulla and A5 pontine noradrenergic neurones will be reviewed, as well as reference to the input that these neurones receive from the raphe complex. Indeed, physiological significance may residue in the pattern of innervation of individual sympathetic neurones from these various central cell groups but this is, as yet, unproven (Chalmers and Pilowsky 1991). The belief would be that neurones of a particular class, for example vasomotor to skeletal muscle, would have a distinctive pattern of innervation, distinguishing them from, say, a sympathetic preganglionic neurone destined to influence other vascular beds or gastrointestinal function.

This physiological role of brainstem cell groups innervating the intermediolateral cell column, excitatory or inhibitory, and particularly those arising from the medulla, has been assessed using a range of electrophysiological techniques by Gebber and his colleagues (Gebber 1990). A major attempt has been made to assess the temporal relationships between the firing of brainstem neurones and sympathetic pre- or postganglionic activity neurones as a basis for connectivity. To this have been added studies, using antidromic mapping techniques, to determine the specific projections of individual brainstem neurones. Neurones in the rostral ventrolateral medulla (RVLM), including those of the adrenaline-containing neurones of the C1 group, have been shown to innervate the intermediolateral cell column and the intermediate regions of the spinal cord (discussed by Sun 1996). Complementary evidence has now been obtained at ultrastructural level for direct monosynaptic connections of RVLM neurones with both the soma and dendrites of sympathetic neurones (Bacon et al. 1990). Similar evidence exists for connections from the raphe complex, in particular the raphe magnus and pallidus, and these are implicated in the 5-hydroxytryptamine (5-HT) innervation of the intermediolateral cell column (Zagon and Bacon 1991).

With regard to the RVLM projection to the spinal cord, Guyenet and others (Gebber 1990; Guyenet 1990; Sun 1996) have indicated that these bulbospinal neurones have properties indicative of a sympathoexcitatory function (Fig. 6.2). They have a strong cardiac rhythm in their ongoing discharge, and this rhythm appears to depend on inhibitory input from the arterial baroreceptors. In the rat, they fire at around 20 Hz, and the magnitude of their discharge is directly related to the level of arterial blood pressure (Fig. 6.2). More recent evidence from an intracellular recording study in the rat (Zagon and Spyer 1996) indicates that the RVLM also contains a significant population of neurones that have physiological properties indicative of a sympathoinhibitory function. This is consistent with other data that demonstrated significant projections on to sympathetic preganglionic neurones from the RVLM make synaptic con-

nections that were indicative of an inhibitory function; i.e. the synaptic specializations were of the symmetrical configuration as seen at the electron microscope (Zagon and Smith 1993). Another dispersed group of medullary neurones, located in the lateral tegmental field, shows a temporal relationship to sympathetic discharge that, when compared with the equivalent relationship between RVLM neurones and sympathetic discharge, suggests that they feed an excitatory input on to RVLM neurones (Gebber 1990). Equally, it appears that many brainstem neurones affect sympathetic discharge in a manner that can be independent of baroreceptor input. Gebber and his colleagues have demonstrated intrinsic rhythms in both medullary and hypothalamic neurones that are also represented in sympathetic discharge in the absence of baroreceptor input. This implies that sympathetic 'tone' is generated by widely distributed neuronal groups distributed throughout the brainstem but that a prominent factor in vasomotor tone is the activity of RVLM sympathoexcitatory neurones.

With regard to raphe spinal connections, there are indications that these may mediate both excitatory and inhibitory control of sympathetic neurones (Gebber 1990; Gilbey and Spyer 1993a, b). A proportion of raphe spinal neurones have small myelinated axons that are known to contain 5-HT. 5-HT, when delivered by ionophoresis on to lumba sympathetic neurones, evokes excitation in a majority of cases but inhibition in a small number (Gilbey 1997). This prevalence of excitation confirms earlier observations in thoracic sympathetic neurones. The studies of Bacon et al. (1990) have now provided convincing evidence that raphe neurones make monosynaptic connections with those sympathetic preganglionic neurones that innervate the adrenal medulla. These observations go further in indicating the potential functional implications of such an innervation. Those lumbar sympathetic neurones that were excited by 5-HT were invariably inhibited by noxious input, whereas those few that were inhibited by 5-HT were excited by the equivalent noxious input. The basis for these actions may be related to the specialization of raphe spinal connections with regard to function (see earlier), and the heterogeneity of 5-HT receptor subtypes located in the intermediolateral column of the spinal cord. Whichever explanation is correct, these connections appear to be important in patterning sympathetic activity in regard to noxious inputs and, presumably, to the cardiovascular adjustments that accompany these inputs.

In an analogous manner, there is evidence for both α_1- and α_2-adrenergic receptors within the intermediolateral column, and evidence that both noradrenergic and adrenergic fibres project from the brainstem to this region. The actions of adrenergic ligands on the activity of sympathetic neurones have been controversial. Both excitatory and inhibitory effects have been seen, and there are considerable differences in the literature between observations made in vivo and those made using in vitro preparations. From in vitro studies there is now good evidence that α_1-mediated effects are largely excitatory whereas α_2-mediated effects are inhibitory, and that, on occasions, both actions can be identified on individual preganglionic neurones (Sun 1996). Recent studies by Gilbey and his co-workers have provided a basis for the in vivo α_2-mediated excitatory response (Marks and Gilbey 1992). However, these observations cannot be taken as support for a role of the C1 group of neurones in evoking largely excitatory control of sympathetic neurones through the release of adrenaline. This results from observations in another in vitro study using a brainstem–spinal cord preparation of the neonatal rat (Deuchers et al. 1995). In that study, activating the RVLM either

47

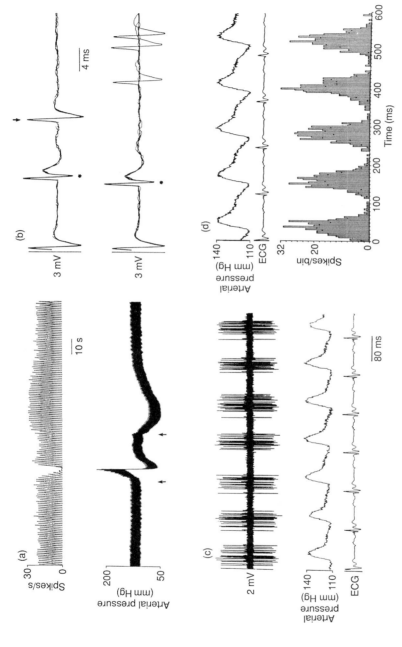

Fig. 6.2. Characteristics of the identified rostral ventrolateral spinal 'vasomotor' neurones. (a) Effect of change in arterial pressure on the neuronal discharge rate. Neuronal activity is represented in the form of an integrated rate histogram. Arterial pressure was elevated via descending aortic constriction (started at the first arrow and stopped when the neurone become silent) and reduced by intravenous injection of 0.1–0.2 mg sodium nitroprusside (at the second arrow). (b) Spinal projection of the neurone. The evoked antidromic spikes (arrow) by the spinal cord stimulation (asterisks) collided with spontaneously occurring spikes and failed to occur at recording site when the stimulation was applied within a critical period after spontaneously occurring spikes (bottom trace). (c) Pulse-synchronous discharge of the rostral ventrolateral spinal 'vasomotor' neurone. The arterial pressure trace (middle) and ECG signal (bottom) represent a single sweep, whereas the trace of neuronal discharge represents 12 consecutive sweeps, all triggered on ECG signals. (d) ECG-triggered time histograms of the neuronal activity (300 sweeps, 3 ms/bin). The top and middle traces represent averaged arterial pressure and ECG signals, respectively (50 sweeps each). (Reproduced with permission from Sun and Spyer (1991).)

electrically or with the application of excitant amino acids resulted in the monosynaptically evoked excitatory postsynaptic potentials (EPSPS) in sympathetic preganglionic motoneurones that were mediated by both non-NMDA- and NMDA-type receptors, indicating that glutamate is the primary transmitter. This confirms earlier indications that the descending pathway may act through a local release of glutamate in the spinal cord (discussed by Guyenet 1990), but leaves open the possibility that adrenaline, or other putative transmitters or modulators, may be co-released with glutamate (discussed by Chalmers and Pilowsky 1991).

Of particular interest was the observation that when the actions of glutamate are antagonized pharmacologically, a monosynaptic inhibitory postsynaptic potential (IPSP) was evoked by RVLM stimulation (this was sometimes discernable without blockade of the excitatory input) and this was mediated by GABA acting at $GABA_A$ receptors (Deuchars et al. 1997). The apparent monosynaptic inhibitory input is consistent with the in vivo observations of Zagon and Spyer (1996) that the RVLM contains a significant population of sympathoinhibitory neurones.

Medullary premotor sympathetic or 'vasomotor' neurones

As indicated above, there is convincing evidence that some neurones in the RVLM provide significant excitatory input to sympathetic preganglionic neurones. These neurones appear to form a relatively discrete group of cells in close proximity to the facial nucleus. Indeed, there is a belief that these neurones, which include a subclass defined as the C1 adrenaline-containing neurones, represent the classical 'vasomotor' centre (Guyenet 1990). This conclusion has resulted, in part, from a demonstration that their destruction, or inhibition, by the topical application of glycine to the ventral medullary surface, results in a fall of blood pressure to a level that is associated with that seen in an acute spinal preparation. More recent studies have indicated that the acute effects seen in both cat and rat are not apparent under more chronic situations, and previous data reviewed would seem to add emphasis to the importance of multiple descending pathways in affecting sympathetic activity. These RVLM neurones do, however, have a pivotal role since they have properties that indicate that they integrate inputs from several reflex pathways and also from the output of regions of the central nervous system that have been shown to be involved in cardiovascular control. In addition, suggestions have been made that they have intrinsic pacemaker properties, since they are rhythmically active in an in vitro slice preparation and this discharge is not silenced in the presence of kynurate, the nonselective antagonist of glutamate (Guyenet 1990). However, Lipski et al. (1996) have provided a contrary view with regard to rhythm generation, questioning the absence of synaptic drive as a basis for rhythmic activity.

RVLM sympathoexcitatory neurones receive a powerful inhibitory input from the arterial baroreceptors that is mediated by GABA acting at a $GABA_A$ receptor (see Fig. 6.4), an excitatory input from the arterial chemoreceptors, and variable influences from vagal afferents. They often exhibit a respiration-related discharge, largely showing heightened activity during inspiration, and evidence of a pulmonary stretch afferent input. Numerous regions of the CNS which are concerned with different behavioural activities and associated with large changes in the cardiovascular system, such as the hypothalamic defence area, when activated produce marked changes in the discharge of RVLM bulbospinal neurones. Equally, variable inputs to these neurones have been described when activating regions of the cerebellum, pons, and midbrain and, more recently, a powerful biphasic influence from the area postrema has been shown (Sun 1996). In addition, they are affected powerfully by noxious inputs delivered to the limbs and tail in the anaesthetized rat, and their pattern of response to these inputs is consistent with a major role in the expression of the cardiovascular responses in nociception (Sun and Spyer 1991).

Other studies have shown that, aside from those RVLM neurones with spinally projecting axons, there are numerous cells in the same general area that receive varying patterns of peripheral and central input concerned with cardiovascular regulation, and that intermixed within them there are also sympathoinhibitory neurones (see above; Zagon and Spyer 1996). This implies that this area may have a major, yet not exclusive, role in cardiovascular control, since the inputs to this area, both central and peripheral, are distributed to other cell groups located in the lower brainstem, which equally well may have powerful connections on to sympathetic neurones of the spinal cord.

The source of the inhibitory input to RVLM sympathoexcitatory neurones that is evoked by the arterial baroreceptors is considered to be a group of GABA-containing neurones in the caudal ventrolateral medulla (CVLM) that project to the RVLM and are the target of an efferent projection from the NTS (Izzo and Spyer 1997). Recent studies from Sawchenko's laboratory may, however, indicate an alternative route for the action of the baroreceptors (for example, Chan and Sawchenko 1995). Regions of the NTS that receive a monosynaptic input from the arterial baroreceptors do not appear to project to the CVLM but give a distinct projection to the RVLM in the rat (Chan and Sawchenko 1996). Presumably this input provides a direct excitation of sympathoinhibitory neurones in the RVLM that may make local inhibitory synaptic connections within the RVLM.

Vagal preganglionic cardiomotor neurones

Vagal cardioinhibitory neurones (with B-fibre axons) have been shown to be located primarily within the ventrolateral subdivision of the nucleus ambiguus (Loewy and Spyer 1990). This localization places them within close apposition to the premotor sympathetic neurones of the RVLM described above. In addition, they share input with these neurones from numerous regions of the forebrain hypothalamus and amygdala as well as lower brainstem. The nucleus ambiguus has been shown to receive afferents from at least 13 different regions of the brain in the rat, including:

(1) the bed nucleus of the stria terminalis;

(2) the substantia innominata;

(3) the central nucleus of the amygdala;

(4) the paraventricular hypothalamic nucleus;

(5) the dorsomedial hypothalamic nucleus;

(6) the lateral hypothalamic area;

(7) the zona incerta;

(8) the posterior hypothalamus;

(9) the mesencephalic central grey;

(10) the mesencephalic reticular formation;

(11) the parabrachial nucleus, including the Kölliker–Fuse nucleus;

(12) the nucleus of the tractus solitarius (NTS); and

(13) the medullary reticular formation.

All of these innervate the RVLM. A particularly powerful source of afferent input to the nucleus ambiguus arises from the caudal NTS (cNTS), and recent ultrastructural studies, using the anterograde transport of biocytin, have shown monosynaptic connections being made from the NTS on to vagal neurones of the nucleus ambiguus (reviewed by Izzo and Spyer 1997). Similarly, evidence has been derived to show that cardiomotor neurones are contacted by synaptic boutons containing 5-HT. As yet, the source of this input is unknown but, interestingly, many vagal neurones, other than cardiomotor neurones of both the nucleus ambiguus and dorsal vagal motonucleus, also show a marked 5-HT innervation.

While emphasis has been placed on the role of those vagal moto-neurones located in the nucleus ambiguus, recent data have revived interest in the role of those vagal motoneurones that are located in the dorsal vagal nucleus (DVN) (Izzo and Spyer 1997). It is now clear that these neurones relay to the cardiac ganglia with C-fibre axons in most species; in the rabbit B fibres also arise from vagal moto-neurones localized within the DVN. Also there is convincing evidence that when activated they produce cardiac slowing but with a smaller effect than activating B-fibre axons that originate in the nucleus ambiguus and with a different time course and pharmacology of action within the cardiac ganglion (Jones et al. 1994). These neurones receive a powerful excitatory input from vagal afferents with endings in the pulmonary vascular bed that are sensitive to phenylbiguanide and appear to participate in a C-fibre reflex pathway.

Reflex control of cardiovascular control

It is well documented that several groups of peripheral receptors contribute to the reflex control of circulation. These include the arterial baroreceptor and chemoreceptors, and receptors within the heart as well as the airways and lungs (Spyer 1990, 1994).

The primary site of interaction of these afferents within the central nervous system is at the level of the NTS (reviewed by Spyer 1994). Neurophysiological studies have shown that specific areas of the NTS receive innervation from the arterial baroreceptors (Fig. 6.3), and that these same regions of the nucleus receive a variable innervation from other vagal afferents and the arterial chemoreceptors. In particular, the dorsolateral and dorsomedial regions of the NTS at levels rostral to the obex have been shown, using an anti-dromic mapping technique, to receive an input from both myelinated and unmyelinated carotid sinus baroreceptor afferents, and also from aortic baroreceptors (Spyer 1990). Since the NTS receives a patterned input from afferents arising from receptors that reflexly affect both the cardiovascular and respiratory systems (Fig. 6.4), and also receives inputs from many regions of the central nervous system, it is a potential site of cardiorespiratory integration (discussed by Richter and Spyer 1990). Accordingly, interest has been aroused in determin-

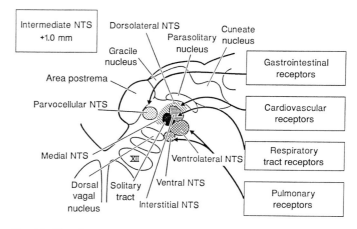

Fig. 6.3. The viscerotropic pattern of innervation of the nucleus of the tractus solitarius (NTS). This drawing illustrates the nucleus of the tractus solitarius of the cat in the transverse plane and the number given indicates the distance from the obex. The nomenclature used follows that presented by Loewy and Burton (1978). (Reproduced with permission from Loewy (1990).)

ing the synaptic mechanisms underlying the processing of barorecep-tor inputs. The importance of these considerations resides in the fact that, while sinoaortic denervation leads to a lability in arterial blood pressure, destruction of the NTS leads acutely to fulminating hyper-tension with concomitant pulmonary oedema, and chronically to maintained hypertension.

There is now strong evidence that NTS neurones that are excited by stimulation of the arterial baroreceptors also receive convergent excitatory inputs form other reflex inputs that exert qualitatively similar efferent effects (Dawid-Milner et al. 1995). Furthermore, many NTS neurones that are excited by baroreceptor stimulation are inhibited by chemoreceptor afferent inputs (Silva-Carvalho et al. 1995b). This implies a functional organization of neurones within the NTS, and their control by other inputs from central structures may have particular significance for the expression of cardiorespiratory control, both in homeostasis and in adjustment of this control in relation to behavioural activity.

The NTS itself makes extensive connections with regions of the lower brainstem, including the nucleus ambiguus, CVLM and RVLM, and with the various pontine nuclei that are concerned with cardiorespiratory regulation, and with forebrain regions. Details of the connections from the NTS to the nucleic ambiguus and, in partic-ular, on to cardiomotor neurones, have been referred to above. The mechanisms, and pathways, that mediate baroreceptor control of RVLM 'sympathoexcitatory' neurones remain to be resolved (for dis-cussion see above). The ascending pathways from the NTS may well play an additional role in mediating baroreceptor and other reflexes, and control of neuroendocrine function, although their relative importance in cardiovascular regulation seems to be fully assessed. The present discussion would seem to indicate that the basic reflex is accomplished within the medulla (Fig. 6.4) and involves, not merely the cardiomotor neurones of the nucleus ambiguus and the neurones of the RVLM, but, presumably, baroreceptor actions at the level of other neurones where baroreceptor-mediated influences have been demonstrated (Gebber 1990).

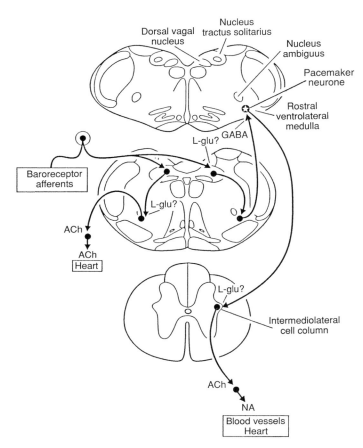

Fig. 6.4. A model of the neural circuitry involved in the baroreflex. Incoming baroreceptor afferents terminate in the nucleus tractus solitarius. These first-order neurones have their cell bodies in the ganglia of the IXth and Xth cranial nerves. The transmitter involved is unknown, but may be L-glutamate (L-glu) or a related chemical. Second-order neurones in the nucleus tractus solitarius project to two sites in the medulla oblongata: cardiac preganglionic neurones (shown on left) and GABA-containing neurones in the region near the nucleus ambiguus (shown on right). The latter are thought to project to pace-maker neurones in the rostral ventrolateral medulla. The pace-maker neurones may project directly to the sympathetic preganglionic neurones and use L-glutamate or a related chemical as a transmitter. The transmitters used at each central synapse remain speculative because the full requirements needed for proof that a particular chemical is acting as a transmitter have not been fulfilled. ACh, acetylcholine; NA, noradrenaline; GABA, γ-aminobutyric acid. (Reproduced with permission from Guyenet (1990).)

Cardiorespiratory interactions

The role of the cardiovascular system in homeostasis can only be achieved adequately if there is integration of cardiovascular and respiratory function. This is well evidenced in terms of the parallel changes in cardiac output and respiratory minute volume that occur in relation to changes in the level of activity and metabolic demand. There is also a large body of evidence indicating that extensive interactions occur between those reflexes that provide moment-by-moment regulation of the cardiovascular and respiratory systems

(Daly 1997). Indeed, the influences exerted by these reflex inputs are explained by algebraic summation of their individual effects, but must involve a complex, and as yet unresolved, set of interactions at different levels within the central nervous system.

Recently, neurophysiological studies have gone some way to explaining the underlying central mechanisms that are responsible for this integration, at least with regard to cardiac control. From studies in several laboratories it is clear that the NTS is not a major site of respiratory modulation of reflex function (see discussion in Spyer 1994; Daly 1997). However, as long ago as the 1930s Anrep and his colleagues (discussed by Richter and Spyer 1990; Daly 1997) demonstrated that sinus arrhythmia was the consequence of a respiratory control of the vagal outflow to the heart. They identified two distinct factors that were responsible for the generation of this respiratory arrhythmia. The first was central in origin; the second a consequence of reflexes evoked during respiratory movements.

Electrophysiological studies in the cat have now shown that the central mechanism involves a direct synaptic regulation of cardiac vagal motoneurones exert by a subset of those brainstem neurones that are responsible for generating the respiratory rhythm (Richter and Spyer 1990). Vagal preganglionic motoneurones are actively hyperpolarized during inspiration by a wave of chloride-dependent inhibitory postsynaptic potentials (Fig. 6.5). This results in a fall of membrane input resistance that shunts the excitatory influences of the arterial baroreceptors. Hence, any influence that increases inspiratory drive will lead, by this process, to both a suppression of vagal efferent discharge and a reduced sensitivity of these neurones to other excitatory inputs, whether central or reflex in origin (Fig. 6.6). The outcome is a tachycardia in inspiration sinus arrhythmia.

The pattern of discharge of vagal motoneurones during the respiratory cycle indicates that they have close similarities to one of the subsets of respiratory neurones, the postinspiratory neurones that are involved in modulating the discharge and timing of activity in other

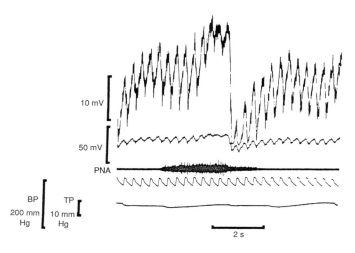

Fig. 6.5. Respiratory modulation of pulse-rhythmic excitatory postsynaptic potentials recording in a cell in which inhibitory postsynaptic potentials have been versed previously by Cl⁻ Injection (3 nA for 5 min). Further details in text. Traces from above: high- and low-gain d.c. recordings of membrane potential, phrenic nerve activity (PNA), femoral arterial blood pressure (BP), and tracheal pressure (TP). (Reproduced with permission from Gilbey et al. (1984).)

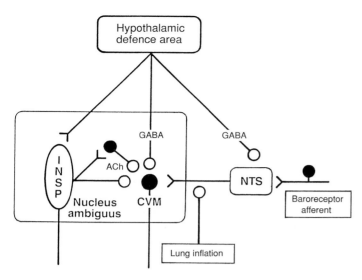

Fig. 6.6. The diagram illustrates the control exerted on vagal cardioinhibitory neurones (CVM) by baroreceptor afferent input, inspiratory neurones (INSP), and the hypothalamic defence area. Excitatory inputs are shown as solid lines with forked endings; inhibitory inputs as lines ending in open circles. (NTS, nucleus tractus solitarius, ACh, acetylcholine: GABA, γ-aminobutyric acid. See text for details. (Reproduced with permission from Spyer (1989).)

subsets of the respiratory generator (Richter and Spyer 1990). The vagal outflow to the heart and postinspiratory neurones are most susceptible to reflex inputs during stage I of expiration, when there is maintained, yet declining, activity in the phrenic outflow. This respiratory patterning of vagal outflow is also mirrored by similar changes in the excitability of sympathetic preganglionic motoneurones (Richter and Spyer 1990). Studies in the rat and cat have shown that sympathetic preganglionic neurones show distinct phases of activity correlating with the central respiratory cycle, as well as being modulated by pulmonary stretch inputs. More recent intracellular studies have indicated that this is imprinted on the discharge of sympathetic neurones, at least as regards inspiration-related activity, by descending excitatory drive. As mentioned earlier, there is evidence that neurones in the RVLM that project to the intermediolateral cell column have their activity modulated by respiratory activity, but it remains a possibility that at least a portion of the respiratory discharge of sympathetic neurones is also mediated by classical respiratory pathways (discussed by Richter and Spyer 1990).

The suppressive action of lung inflation inputs on reflexly evoked bradycardia has been well characterized by Daly (1997), but the central site at which slowly adapting vagal lung stretch afferents act has yet to be discerned. Detailed neurophysiological studies have not revealed an action of this input on baroreceptor or chemoreceptor inputs at the level of the NTS (see above), although there is no doubt that lung inflation modulates the sensitivity of vagal preganglionic motoneurones to these reflex inputs. It is notable that the effects of lung inflation inputs are not of similar magnitude on all reflexes. Reflex activation of those pulmonary receptors excited by phenyl-biguanide is much less affected by lung inflation than are either baroreceptor, chemoreceptor, or cardiac afferent inputs (Daly 1997). The possibility that DVN vagal motoneurones might be a target for

lung stretch inputs has been considered but recent studies by Jones (1993) have failed to substantiate this notion.

Although the site of action of lung inflation inputs remains to be resolved, it is clear that changes in respiratory state will exert an enormous direct influence on the sensitivity of both vagal and sympathetic neurones to other inputs. As yet, we have a limited knowledge of the mechanisms by which respiration affects the sympathetic outflow, and this has yet to be correlated directly to the functional role of individual sympathetic preganglionic motoneurones. These influences, however, indicate a potential source of hazard for any input that produces a period of apnoea. At this time, cardiac vagal motoneurones are highly sensitive to other concomitant excitatory inputs, and so apnoea is a state during which the potential for fatal bradycardia is enhanced (Daly 1997). Aside from providing a plausible explanation for sudden unexplained bradycardia, the apparently tight coupling of cardiac control to respiratory activity ensures a moment-by-moment matching of cardiac output to respiratory minute volume in diverse physiological situations, such as exercise and breath-holding diving. The underlying neural processes so far considered, will thus provide a framework on which to base further studies into the central nervous basis of cardiorespiratory homeostasis.

Supramedullary control of the cardiovascular system

The cardiovascular system has a major role in homeostasis. it achieves this largely by adjusting the blood supply to different vascular beds in proportion to the level of their activity. Basically, the nervous system achieves this by maintaining arterial pressure within relatively fine limits in consequence of changes in afferent input. The net effect is to regulate cardiac output in the face of different behavioural demands through the interplay of these reflex inputs (see above) and central drives. In order to achieve this regulation, the discharge of the autonomic outflows are patterned, and these patterns are highly specific for the different repertoire of responses that can be made by the organism. From studies in man and experimental observations in a range of vertebrates, much has now been learned of the cardiovascular responses that accompany sleep, exercise, and emotional responses, yet it is only with respect to affective behaviour that we have a detailed description of the central structures and neural pathways that are involved in mediating these complex autonomic changes (Jordan 1990; Spyer 1994). The investigations on the defence reaction of the cat by Hilton and his colleagues (reviewed by Jordan 1990), and the playing-dead or freezing response of the rabbit, have shed considerable light on the role of the amygdala and hypothalamus in organizing these responses. These two distinct animal models of behaviour may have provided information of considerable significance in understanding the human adaptations to environmental and emotional stress.

The defence reaction

With regard to the organization of affective behaviour, the hypothalamus has long been seen to play a major role (Jordan 1990). Indeed, the activation of the perifornical region of the hypothalamus, either directly by electrical stimulation through microelectrodes or by activation of other brain areas or general afferent excitation, has been seen to induce patterns of behaviour and autonomic change that are typical of the alerting stage of the defence reaction. The cardiovascular pattern of response accompanying the defence reaction has been shown to involve a rise in heart rate and aortic blood flow (and hence cardiac output), a widespread vasoconstriction, but a characteristic withdrawal of vasoconstrictor tone of the vasculature of skeletal muscle and, in the cat, to an activation of sympathetic cholinergic vasodilator fibres in this particular bed (Spyer 1989; Jordan 1990, Fig. 6.7). In all species, vasodilatation in skeletal muscle is enhanced by an increased outpouring of catecholamines from the adrenal medulla. Cutaneous, renal, and mesenteric blood flow is diminished, and arterial pressure and pulse pressure rise dramatically. Further, under appropriate experimental conditions, a similar pattern of response can be elicited on electrical stimulation of the central nucleus of the amygdala in the cat, and there is good evidence that at least a part of the forebrain control of behaviour is mediated via the amygdala, which is itself afferent to the hypothalamus (discussed by Jordan 1990). Recent studies have questioned the importance of the hypothalamus in the integration of this response, since it has proved difficult to elicit the defence reaction by using chemical means to activate neurones in this region of the hypothalamus. However, in the baboon, Smith *et al.* (1980) describe low lesions in

the periformical region abolished the cardiovascular component but spared the behavioural component of conditioned adverse responses. The main focus of attention has moved to the amygdala (see above) and to the midbrain periaqueductal grey, where both electrical and chemical stimulation are effective in eliciting the characteristic cardiovascular response (Jordan 1990).

Playing-dead response

While stimulation in the periformical region of the rabbit hypothalamus may evoke similar cardiovascular responses to those seen in other species, affective behaviour in this species is usually associated with a bradycardia and hypotension and a suppression of motor activity—freezing or playing dead (Applegate *et al.* 1983). This is accompanied by rapid, shallow breathing. This is the characteristic response that can also be evoked by stimulation of the central nucleus of the amygdala in both anaesthetized and conscious preparations (Cox *et al.* 1987).

Efferent pathways for affective behaviour

The role of the central nucleus of the amygdala and the hypothalamic defence area in patterning the cardiovascular and respiratory responses in affective behaviour has been described. Considerable evidence is now available indicating that the connections of the central nucleus of the amygdala that mediate these affects involve parallel descending pathways influencing several cell groups within the midbrain, including the central grey, the pontine Kölliker–Fuse and parabrachial nuclei, and, within the medulla, the nucleus of the tractus solitarius, dorsal vagal nucleus, nucleus ambiguus, and also the rostroventrolateral medulla (Fig. 6.8). In many instances reciprocal connections can be shown between these cells groups and the central nucleus. The descending connections of the hypothalamic defence area, which have been mapped electrophysiologically, include many of the same regions of midbrain, pons, and medulla. Indeed, there is now plentiful evidence that activating the hypothalamic defence area and the periaqueductal grey exerts relatively direct control of neurones in the rostral VLM (Guyenet 1990). These descending pathways are likely to represent the major means by which both sympathetic and vagal neurones are influenced, but other direct connections between the hypothalamus and spinal cord have also been shown (Loewy 1990).

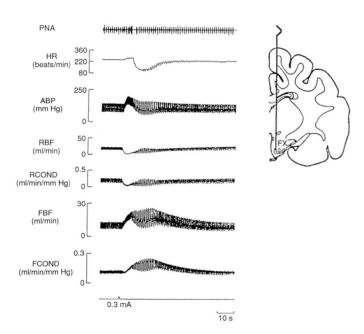

Fig. 6.7. Cardiovascular and respiratory responses to electrical stimulation in the periformical region of the hypothalamus of the althesin-anaesthetized cat. The diagram on the right illustrates the electrode position on a hemicoronal section (FX, fornix). The stimulus was a 4 s train of 0.5 ms pulses delivered at 100 Hz, initiated at the time shown in the lower trace on the polygraph record shown on the left-hand side. Traces from top to bottom: PNA, phrenic nerve activity; HR, heart rate: ABP, arterial blood pressure; RBF, renal blood flow; RCOND, renal vascular conductance: FBF, femoral blood flow; FCOND, femoral vascular conductance. RBF and FBF were recorded using electromagnetic flow probes. (Reproduced with permission from Spyer (1989).)

Reflex modification

One of the most striking features of the defence reaction elicited on electrical stimulation of either the hypothalamus or the amygdala in the cat, is the concomitant rise in arterial blood pressure and heart rate (see Fig. 6.7). This has been taken to suggest a central suppression of the baroreceptor reflex (Hilton 1966). In part, this resetting could be seen as a consequence of increased inspiratory activity, which, on the basis of our review, would be expected to exert a profound inhibition of cardiac vagal efferent activity. However, both vascular and cardiac components of the reflex appear to be affected. In

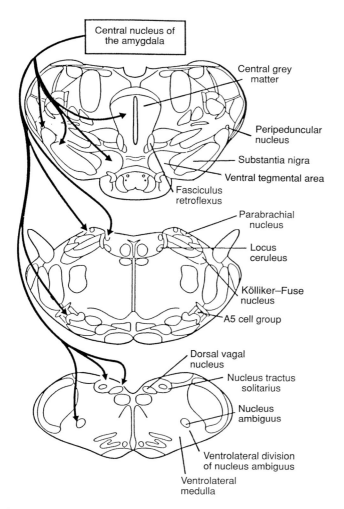

Fig. 6.8. Series of drawings showing the descending projections from the central nucleus of the amygdala that innervate the brain stem. (Reproduced with permission from Loewy (1990).)

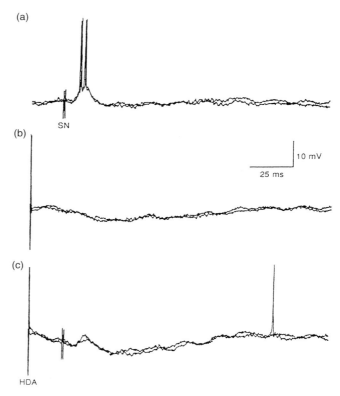

Fig. 6.9. Inhibitory actions of the hypothalamic defence area (HDA) within the NTS. (a) Intracellular recording (membrane potential, −62 mV) from a cell that responded to sinus nerve (SN) stimulation (2 pulses, 0.1 ms, 1 kHz, 10 V given at 1 Hz) with an EPSP and action potential discharge. (b) an IPSP evoked by the stimulation of the HDA (5 pulses, 0.1 ms, 500 Hz, 50 μA given at 1 Hz) is shown; only the last HDA pulse is illustrated. (c) When the sinus nerve SN stimulation was preceded by HDA stimulation (interval, 20 ms) the IPSP evoked by HDA stimulation shunts the response to SN stimulation. Each panel shows two superimposed traces. (Reproduced with permission of Silva-Carvalho et al. (1995a).)

contrast, in the rabbit the bradycardia and hypotension resulting from stimulation in the central nucleus of the amygdala appear to involve a facilitatory modulation of the baroreceptor reflex (Cox et al. 1986). Since the descending output from both amygdala and hypothalamus appears to target the NTS (Fig. 6.8), it is probable that this is the site of major interaction between reflex and central drives. In the cat, evidence has now been obtained to show that those NTS neurones that are excited by baroreceptor stimulation receive an inhibitory input on stimulating within the hypothalamic defence area (Fig. 6.9). The inhibitory action is mediated by GABA acting at GABA$_A$ receptors and may be antagonized by the iontophoretic application of bicuculline (Spyer 1990, 1994). The descending pathways are likely to converge on intrinsic GABAergic neurones of the NTS, since there is no evidence that descending GABAergic pathways are involved (Silva-Carvalho et al. 1995a). These same intrinsic NTS neurones may also be influenced by descending input from the various pontine nuclei involved in cardiorespiratory control (Fig. 6.10b). The paradigm of electrical stimulation does not distinguish between fibres with different functions and it is now clear that efferent pathways from, or relaying through, the hypothalamus can

evoke different changes in reflex function. For instance, in some circumstances stimulation in the hypothalamus has been shown to facilitate baroreceptor inputs on to NTS neurones (Silva-Carvalho et al. 1995a). Similarly, when the central nucleus of the amygdala is activated in the rabbit, NTS neurones receiving baroreceptor input are facilitated. This suggests that two distinct mechanisms may be activated on diencephalic stimulation—the one more prevalent in the cat, involving an inhibition, the other more prevalent in the rabbit, exerting facilitation, but both expressed to a degree in each species. The significance of this set of observations is that these two distinct mechanisms may represent simple operating principles by which the complex forms of behaviour that are associated with stress can express themselves in subtle or gross changes in cardiovascular activity. The powerful actions at the NTS that may be elicited from stimulation in regions of the diencephalon may be enhanced by the action of descending pathways acting at other levels within the brainstem. The inhibitory effects exerted by defence area stimulation in the cat at the level of the NTS, which will remove inhibitory control over medullary premotor sympathetic neurones (i.e. disinhibition) will be

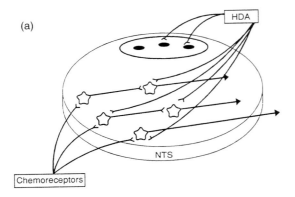

(a)

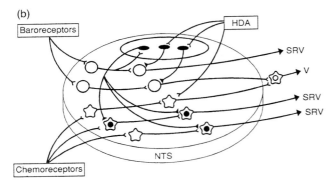

(b)

Fig. 6.10. Schemes of NTS interactions. Schematic diagram of the connections within the nucleus tractus solitari (NTS) that mediate arterial chemoreceptor inputs and interactions with the arterial baroreceptors. (a) Basic scheme of NTS connections mediating chemoreceptor reflex excitatory connections, shown as ⌁. Intrinsic GABA-containing neurones are shown as filled ovals. Descending inputs from the hypothalamic defence area (HDA) impinge on these, and NTS neurones, which receive, directly or indirectly, input from the arterial chemoreceptors (further details in the text). (b) Inputs to NTS from baroreceptors, chemoreceptors, and HDA are shown. Exclusively baroreceptor-sensitive neurones are shown as ○; chemoreceptors are ⬠. Excitatory inputs are shown as ⌁ and inhibitory as ⌁. Neurones receiving convergent baroreceptor and chemoreceptor inputs are shown as combined symbols: ⬟ when baroreceptor influence is excitatory, ⬟ when inhibitory. Further details in the text. R, respiratory; S, sympathetic; V, vagal. (Reproduced with permission from Silva-Carvalho *et al.* (1995*b*).)

reinforced by the more directly distributed excitatory input that RVLM neurones receive simultaneously. Such inhibitory control is not directed exclusively to baroreceptor inputs since many of the NTS neurones that are excited by baroreceptor inputs are also affected by inputs from other receptors. In particular, a recent study has shown that laryngeal mechanoreceptor afferent inputs converge on to NTS neurones that are excited by baroreceptor inputs (Dawid-Milner *et al.* 1995). The reflex cardiorespiratory effects of laryngeal mechanoreceptor stimulation are also inhibited on hypothalamic defence area (HDA) stimulation.

In other studies it has been shown that the arterial chemoreceptor reflex is facilitated by hypothalamic stimulation, and that activating

this particular reflex may also provoke the autonomic features of the defence response. Neurophysiological studies have shown that this interaction between chemoreceptor inputs and the defence response involves a synaptic action of a descending input at the level of the NTS (Silva-Carvalho *et al.* 1995*b*). NTS neurones that are excited by specific chemoreceptor activation are also excited by HDA stimulation (Fig. 6.10*a*). Such neurones also receive inhibitory inputs from the arterial baroreceptors (Fig. 6.10*b*).

These data provide an insight into the neural substrate through which the effectiveness of the baroreceptor and chemoreceptor reflexes are modified in affective responses. Equally, similar neural interactions may play a role in promoting the parallel changes in the cardiovascular and respiratory systems that accompany other forms of behaviour, such as the response to exercise.

Conclusions

In endeavouring to provide a relatively contemporary analysis of the central nervous control of the cardiovascular system, this review has assessed the neural pathways by which the excitability of both vagal and sympathetic preganglionic motoneurones is regulated. Emphasis has been placed on understanding the reflex and, particularly, the baroreflex control of these two groups of autonomic neurones. Further, attempts have been made to identify the central neural mechanisms by which these reflex inputs are modulated during affective behaviour. It appears that certain simple neural principles dictate the patterns of these interactions, and a fundamental design principle appears to involve a coupling of respiratory and cardiovascular regulation.

These observations indicate that the central nervous system exerts its control over autonomic, and specifically cardiovascular, function in a manner analogous to the way in which motor activities are controlled. In particular, the modification of reflex action, which can be exerted by rostral brainstem and subcortical areas, may provide an indication of potential mechanisms whereby stress and emotion can cause profound changes in the cardiovascular system. Whether the acute, and clearly reversible, changes of the type reviewed in this discussion may be converted, on repetition, to prolonged and irreversible alterations remain to be investigated.

Acknowledgements

The financial support of the British Heart Foundation and the Wellcome Trust is gratefully acknowledged.

References

Applegate, C. D., Kapp, B. S., Underwood, M. D., and McNall, C. L. (1983). Autonomic and somatomotor effects of amygdala central nucleus stimulation in awake rabbits. *Physiol. Behav.* **31**, 353–60.

Bacon, S. J., Zagon, A., and Smith, A. D. (1990). Electron microscopic evidence of a monosynaptic pathway between cells in the caudal raphe nuclei and sympathetic preganglionic neurons in the rat spinal cord. *Exp. Brain Res.* **79**, 589–602.

Chalmers, J. P. and Pilowsky, P. M. (1991). Brainstem and bulbospinal neurotransmitter systems in the control of blood pressure. *J. Hypertension* **9**, 675–94.

Chan, R. K. W. and Sawchenko, P. E. (1998). Organization and transmitter specificity of medullary neurons activated by sustained hypertension; implications for understanding baroreceptor reflex circuitry. *J. Neurosci.* **181**, 371–87.

Cox, G. E., Jordan, D., Moruzzi, P., Schwaber, J. S., Spyer, K. M., and Turner, S. A. (1986). Amygdaloid influences on brainstem neurones in the rabbit. *J. Physiol. London* **381**, 135–48.

Cox, G. E., Jordan, D., Paton, J. F. R., Spyer, K. M., and Wood, L. M. (1987). Cardiovascular and phrenic nerve responses to stimulation of the amygdala central nucleus in the anaesthetised rabbit. *J. Physiol.* **389**, 541–56.

Daly, M. de B. (1997). Peripheral arterial chemoreceptors and respiratory–cardiovascular integration. *Monographs of the Physiological Society*, Vol. 46. Clarendon Press, Oxford.

Dawid-Milner, M. S., Silva-Carvalho, L., Goldsmith, G. E., and Spyer, K. M. (1995). Hypothalamic modulation of laryngeal reflexes in the anaesthetized cat; role of the nucleus tractus solitarii. *J. Physiol.* **487.3**, 739–49.

Deuchars, S. A., Morrison, S. F., and Gilbey, M. P. (1995). Medullary stimulation elicits EPSPs in neonatal rat sympathetic preganglionic neurones *in vitro*. *J. Physiol.* **487.2**, 453–63.

Deuchars, S. A., Spyer, K. M., and Gilbey, M. P. (1997). Stimulation within the rostral ventrolateral medulla can evoke monosynaptic GABAergic IPSPs in sympathetic preganglionic neurons *in vitro*. *J. Neurophysiol.* **77**, (1), 229–35.

Gebber, G. L. (1990). Central determinants of sympathetic nerve discharge. In *Central regulation of autonomic functions*, (ed. A. D. Loewy and K. M. Spyer), pp. 126–44. Oxford University Press, New York.

Gilbey, M. P. (1997). Fundamental aspects of the control of sympathetic preganglionic neuronal discharge. In *Central nervous control of autonomic function. Series: The autonomic nervous system*, Vol. 11 (ed. D. Jordan), pp. 1–28. Harwood Academic Publishers, The Netherlands.

Gilbey, M. P. and Spyer, K. M. (1993*a*). Essential organization of the sympathetic nervous system. In *Ballière's clinical endocrinology and metabolism; catecholamines*, (ed. K. G. M. M. Aberti, G. M. Besser, J. R. Bierich, H. G. Burger, P. Franchimont, and R. Hall), Vol. 7, pp. 259–78. Baillière Tindall, London.

Gilbey, M. P. and Spyer, K. M. (1993*b*). Physiological aspects of autonomic nervous system function. *Curr. Opin. Neurol. Neurosurg.* **6**, 518–23.

Gilbey, M. P., Jordan, D., Richter, D. W., and Spyer, K. M. (1984). Synaptic mechanisms involved in the inspiratory modulation of vagal cardio-inhibitory neurons in the cat. *J. Physiol., London* **356**, 65–78.

Guyenet, P. G. (1990). Role of the ventral medulla oblongata in blood pressure regulation. In *Central regulation of autonomic functions*, (ed. A. D. Loewy and K. M. Spyer), pp. 145–67. Oxford University Press, New York.

Hilton, S. M. (1966). Hypothalamic regulation of the cardiovascular system. *Br. Med. Bull.* **22**, 243–8.

Izzo, P. N. and Spyer, K. M. (1997). The parasympathetic innervation of the heart. In *The autonomic nervous system*, Vol. 11, (ed. G. Burnstock), Harwood Academic Publishers, The Netherlands.

Jansen, A. S. P., Nguyen, X. V., Karpitskiy, V., Mettenleiter, T. C., and Loewy, A. D. (1995). Central command neurons of the sympathetic nervous system: Basis of the fight-or-flight response. *Science*, **270**, 644–6.

Jones, J. F. X. (1993). The central control of the pulmonary chemoreflex. Ph.D Thesis, University of London.

Jones, J. F. X., Wang, Y., and Jordan, D. (1994). Activity of cardiac vagal preganglionic neurones during the pulmonary chemoreflex in the anaesthetized cat. In *Arterial chemoreceptors cell to system: advances in experimental medicine and biology*, Vol. 360, (ed. R. G. O'Regan, P. Nolan, D. S. McQueen and D. J. Paterson), pp. 301–3. Plenum Press, New York.

Jordan, D. (1990). Autonomic changes in affective behaviour. In *Central regulation of autonomic functions*, (ed. A. D. Loewy and K. M. Spyer), pp. 349–66. Oxford University Press, New York.

Lipski, J., Kanjhan, R., Kruszewska, B., and Rong, W. (1996). Properties of presympathetic neurones in the rostral ventrolateral medulla in the rat: an intracellular study *in vivo*. *J. Physiol.* **490**, 729–44.

Loewy, A. D. (1990). Central autonomic pathways. In *Central regulation of autonomic functions*, (ed. A. D. Loewy and K. M. Spyer), pp. 88–103. Oxford University Press, New York.

Loewy, A. D. and Burton, H. (1978). Nuclei of the solitary tract; efferent projection to the lower brainstem and spinal cord of the cat. *J. Comp. Neurol.* **181**, 421–50.

Loewy, A. D. and Spyer, K. M. (1990). Vagal Preganglionic Neurones. In *Central regulations of autonomic functions*. (ed. A. D. Loewry and K. M. Spyer), pp. 68–87. Oxford University Press, New York.

Marks, S. A. and Gilbey, M. P. (1992). Effect on inferior cardiac nerve activity of microinjecting phenylephrine into the intermediolateral cell column of the upper thoracic spinal cord of the anaesthetized cat. *J. Physiol.* **453**, 185–95.

Richter, D. W. and Spyer, K. M. (1990). In *Central regulation of autonomic functions*, (ed. A. D. Loewy and K. M. Spyer), pp. 189–207. Oxford University Press, New York.

Silva-Carvalho, L., Dawid-Milner, M. S., and Spyer, K. M. (1995*a*). The pattern of excitatory inputs to the nucleus tractus solitarii evoked on stimulation in the hypothalamic defence area of the cat. *J. Physiol.* **487.3**, 727–37.

Silva-Carvalho, L., Dawid-Milner, M. S., Goldsmith, G. E., and Spyer, K. M. (1995*b*). Hypothalamic modulation of the arterial chemoreceptor reflex in the anaesthetized cat: role of the nucleus tractus solitarii. *J. Physiol.* **487.3**, 751–60.

Smith, O. A., Asley, C. A., De Vito, J. L., Stein, J. M., and Walsh, K. E. (1980). Functional analysis of the hypothalamic control of the cardiovascular responses accompanying emotional behaviour. *Fed. Proc.* **39**, 2487–94.

Spyer, K. M. (1989). Neural mechanisms involved in cardiovascular control during affective behaviour. *Trends Neurosci.* **12**, 506–13.

Spyer, K. M. (1990). The central nervous organisation of reflex circulatory control. In *Central regulation of autonomic functions*, (ed. A. D. Loewy and K. M. Spyer), pp. 168–88. Oxford University Press, New York.

Spyer, K. M. (1994). Annual Review Prize Lecture: Central nervous mechanisms contributing to cardiovascular control. *J. Physiol.* **474**, 1–19.

Sun, M.-K. (1996). Pharmacology of reticulospinal vasomotor neurons in cardiovascular regulation. *Pharmacological Reviews*, **48**, (4), 465–94.

Sun, M.-K. and Spyer, K. M. (1991). Nociceptive inputs into rostral ventrolateral medulla-spinal vasomotor neurones in rats. *J. Physiol., London* **436**, 685–700.

Zagon, A. and Bacon, S. J. (1991). Evidence of monosynaptic pathway between cells of the ventromedial medulla and the motoneuron pool of the thoracic spinal cord in rat: electron microscopic analysis of synaptic contacts. *Eur. J. Neurosci.* **3**, 55–65.

Zagon, A. and Smith, A. D. (1993). Monosynaptic projections from the rostral ventrolateral medulla oblongata to identified sympathetic preganglionic neurons. *Neuroscience* **54**, (3), 729–43.

Zagon, A. and Spyer, K. M. (1996). Stimulation of the aortic nerve evokes three different response patterns in neurons of the rostral ventrolateral medulla of the rat. *Am. J. Physiol.* **271**, (*Regulatory Integrative Comp. Physiol.* 40), R1720–8.

7. Adrenergic and cholinergic receptors

P. A. van Zwieten

Introduction

Since the discovery of the neurohumoral phenomena associated with the autonomic nervous system there has been a great deal of interest in the receptors that are the targets of the endogenous neurotransmitters, in particular noradrenaline/adrenaline in the sympathetic nervous system and acetylcholine in the parasympathetic nervous system. This field is of particular interest in a variety of physiological and pathophysiological processes. Much of our present, detailed knowledge of autonomic receptors has been obtained using pharmacological methods resulting from the availability of a large number of experimental compounds, which are more or less selective agonists or antagonists with respect to the numerous receptor subtypes associated with the autonomic nervous system. Conversely, the more detailed knowledge of the various receptor types has also allowed the discovery of new and specific therapies for a variety of diseases, predominantly those involving the cardiovascular system. Traditionally, the adrenergic system and its receptors have been studied with great intensity, and a wealth of valuable information has been obtained during the past 2–3 decades. More recently, the field of cholinergic receptors has received a new, strong impetus from the discovery that muscarinic receptors are heterogeneous and therefore should be subdivided into different subtypes with different spectra of biological functions and agonists/antagonists. Both adrenergic and cholinergic receptors are of particular importance and will be discussed in this chapter.

Adrenoceptors (adrenergic receptors)

Subdivision and classification

Adrenoceptors are the primary targets of the endogenous neurotransmitters noradrenaline and adrenaline, in mediating sympathetic activation to peripheral organs, thus causing well-documented effects such as increased cardiac activity (heart rate and contractile force), vasoconstriction, and a rise in plasma glucose levels. In addition, the various adrenoceptors are also important as targets of several synthetic drugs, which can be used to mimic the effects of catecholamines or, conversely, to decrease their actions.

Ahlqvist (1948) postulated that the adrenoceptors are different in various organs and he proposed the subdivision into α- and β-subtypes, a classification which is now widely accepted. There has since been further subdivision into β_1/β_2- and α_1/α_2-adrenoceptors (Lands *et al.* 1967). More recently, evidence has been put forward for the existence of a distinct β_3-adrenoceptor. Subsequently, a more

sophisticated subdivision of α_1-adrenoceptors into α_{1A}, α_{1B}, α_{1D}, and possibly other subtypes, has been derived from radioligand binding studies. Similarly, the more refined subdivision of α_2-adrenoceptors into $\alpha_{2A}/\alpha_{2B}/\alpha_{2C}$ has been proposed. The subdivision and classification into α/β, β_1/β_2 and α_1/α_2 are based upon functional pharmacological data, as reflected by a particular preference for certain agonists and antagonists at postsynaptic (postjunctional) sites with respect to the postganglionic sympathetic neurones and their adjacent synapses. Most of the α- and β-adrenoceptor subtypes have been isolated and their chemical structures (amino acid sequences) have been analysed by molecular biological techniques. The distinction between the various subtypes, based upon functional studies with agonists and antagonists has been largely confirmed by the determination of receptor structures by means of cloning techniques.

The concept of *pre- and postsynaptic* receptors, which is not unique for α-adrenoceptors, was developed and substantiated in the 1970s predominantly by Langer, Starke, and their co-workers (Langer 1981; Starke 1981). The terminology pre/postsynaptic (or pre/postjunctional) refers to the anatomical position of the receptors and does not necessarily coincide with their functional pharmacological profile. Accordingly, presynaptic adrenoceptors belong to the α_2- and β_2-types, whereas in most blood vessels both α_1- and α_2-, but only β_2-adrenoceptors are found at postsynaptic sites. Postsynaptic adrenoceptors, located in the end organs (see Fig. 7.1) are the targets of neurotransmitters and synthetic drugs, and their stimulation or blockade will be translated into a variety of physiological and pharmacological effects. Presynaptic receptors are located at the membranes of the presynaptic vesicles which are the stores of noradrenaline. The stimulation (or blockade) of presynaptic adrenoceptors modulates the release of noradrenaline from its vesicular storage (Fig. 7.1).

It is widely accepted that adenosine triphosphate (ATP) and neuropeptide Y (NPY) are important co-transmitters, which are released from the nerve endings simultaneously with noradrenaline.

The subdivision into α_1/α_2- or $\beta_1/\beta_2/\beta_3$-adrenoceptors implies that all sympathomimetic and sympatholytic drugs should be defined more precisely with respect to their receptor profile (Tables 7.1 and 7.2).

The endogenous catecholamines, noradrenaline and adrenaline, are rather unselective since they can stimulate several receptor subtypes simultaneously. From a teleological, speculative point of view this seems plausible—the activation of a large number of different receptor subtypes can thus be realized by means of one or two neurotransmitters only, and there is no necessity for numerous different release systems for a large variety of humoral (neurotransmitter) systems. Conversely, there are now several synthetic compounds available which are selective stimulants or antagonists with respect to one particular adrenoceptor subtype.

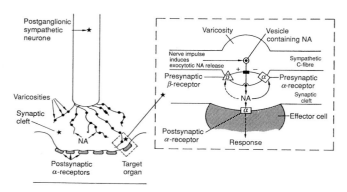

Fig. 7.1. Adrenergic synapse. Nerve activity releases the endogenous neurotransmitter noradrenaline (NA) and also adrenaline from the varicosities. Noradrenaline and adrenaline reach the postsynaptic α- (or β-) adrenoceptors on the cell membrane of the target organ by diffusion. Upon receptor stimulation, a physiological or pharmacological effect is initiated. Presynaptic α_2-adrenoceptors on the membrane (see insertion), when activated by endogenous noradrenaline as well as by exogenous agonists, induce an inhibition and blockade a facilitation of the amount of transmitter noradrenaline released per nerve impulse. Conversely, the stimulation of presynaptic β_2-receptors enhances noradrenaline release from the varicosities. Once noradrenaline has been released, it travels through the synaptic cleft and reaches both α- and β-adrenoceptors at postsynaptic sites, thus causing physiological effects such as vasoconstriction or tachycardia.

Table 7.2. β-Adrenoceptor agonists and antagonists: characterization with respect to their selectivity for β_1- and β_2-adrenoceptors.

Agents	Receptors stimulated or blocked
Agonists	
Noradrenaline (neurotransmitter)	$\beta_1 + \alpha_1 + \alpha_2$
Adrenaline (neurotransmitter)	$\beta_1 + \beta_2 + \alpha_1 + \alpha_2$
Dobutamine	$\beta_1 > \beta_2 + \alpha_1$
Isoprenaline	$\beta_1 + \beta_2$
Orciprenaline	$\beta_1 + \beta_2$
Fenoterol	$\beta_2 \gg \beta_1$
Pirbuterol	$\beta_2 \gg \beta_1$
Rimiterol	$\beta_2 \gg \beta_1$
Ritodrine	$\beta_2 \gg \beta_1$
Salbutamol	$\beta_2 \gg \beta_1$
Terbutaline	$\beta_2 \gg \beta_1$
BRL 37344	$\beta_3 > \beta_1$ and β_2
Antagonists	
Propranolol	
Alprenolol	
Pindolol	and various other
Oxprenolol	non-selective $\quad \beta_1 + \beta_2$
Timolol	β-blockers
Sotalol	
Atenolol	$\beta_1 > \beta_2$
Metoprolol	$\beta_1 > \beta_2$
Bisoprolol	$\beta_1 \gg \beta_2$
ICI 118,551	$\beta_2 > \beta_1$
Carazolol	$\beta_3 > \beta_1$ and β_2

Table 7.1. α-Adrenoceptor agonists and antagonists: characterization with respect to their selectivity for α_1- and α_2-adrenoceptors

Agents	Receptor stimulated or blocked
Agonists	
Nordrenaline (neurotransmitter)	$\alpha_1 + \alpha_2 + \beta_1$
Adrenaline (neurotransmitter)	$\alpha_1 + \alpha_2 + \beta_1 + \beta_2$
Phenylephrine	$\alpha_1 > \alpha_2$
Clonidine (Catapres, Catapresan)	$\alpha_2 > \alpha_1$
Guanfacine	$\alpha_2 > \alpha_1$
Azepexole (B-HT 933)	α_2
B-HT 920	α_2
UK-14,304	α_2
Antagonists	
Phentolamine (Regitine)	$\alpha_1 + \alpha_2$
Tolazoline	$\alpha_2 > \alpha_1$
Prazosin (Minipress)	α_1
Doxazosin	α_1
Terazosin	α_1
Trimazosin	α_1
Tamsulosin	α_{1A}
Labetalol	$\alpha_1 + \beta_1 + \beta_2$
Corynanthine	α_1
Rauwolscine (diastereoisomers)	α_2
Yohimbine	α_2
Idazoxan	α_2

α-Adrenoceptors

α-Adrenoceptors are found in particular in blood vessels and to a less important degree in the heart, as well as in other tissues and organs such as thrombocytes, the vas deferens, the kidney, urethra, prostate, and the central nervous system. As a result of the development of cloning techniques much has been learned over the past few years concerning the structures (amino acid sequence) of the various α-adrenoceptor subtypes. For most of the α_1- and α_2-adrenoceptor subtypes the amino acid sequence has now been elucidated, like so many receptors the various α-adrenoceptor subtypes appear to contain seven transmembrane helices. A great deal of information has also been obtained with respect to the processes of signal transduction subsequent to α-adrenoceptor stimulation. All adrenoceptors appear to be G-protein coupled. With respect to the α_1-adrenoceptor, a G_1-protein mediates the activation of phospholipase Cβ. The α_2-adrenoceptor, when activated, will mediate the inhibition of adenylyl cyclase via a G_i-protein. The α_2-adrenoceptor is also coupled to ion channels, and therefore involved in the regulation of Ca^{2+}- and K^+-ion fluxes.

In blood vessels the postsynaptic α-adrenoceptors are of both the α_1- and α_2-subtypes. Their stimulation with an appropriate agonist causes vasoconstriction; this is so for both α_1- and α_2-adrenoceptor stimulation. Conversely, the blockade of both α_1- and α_2-adrenoceptors at postsynaptic sites causes vasodilatation. The stimulation of presynaptic α_2-adrenoceptors with an agonist induces the inhibition of noradrenaline from its vesicular stores, whereas α_2-adrenoceptor blockade enhances the release of noradrenaline. Since presynaptic

α-adrenoceptors are virtually only of the α_2-type, the selective stimulation or inhibition of α_1-adrenoceptors does not interfere with the presynaptic release of noradrenaline. (Reviewed by Starke (1981); van Zwieten and Timmermans (1984); Insel (1996).)

Stimulation of myocardial α_1-adrenoceptors increases contractility which, at least in the human heart, is much weaker than that caused by β_1-adrenoceptor excitation. Platelet aggregation is enhanced by stimulation of the α_2-adrenoceptors. Stimulation of α_2-adrenoceptors in certain CNS regions, such as the nucleus tractus solitarii, vagal nucleus, and vasomotor centre, will cause a hypotensive response due to the reduction of peripheral sympathetic nervous activity. This mechanism is the basis of the antihypertensive activity of clonidine and α-methyldopa (via its active metabolite α-methylnoradrenaline), which are α_2-adrenoceptor stimulants. Recently it has been discovered that clonidine also owes an important part of its central antihypertensive activity to the stimulation of imidazoline (I_1) receptors in the rostral ventrolateral medulla. Moxonidine and rilmenidine are somewhat more selective I_1-receptor stimulants, which have been introduced as centrally acting antihypertensives with a possibly lower incidence of adverse reactions such as sedation and dry mouth, which are known to be mediated by central α_2-adrenoceptors (Reviewed by van Zwieten et al. 1984; van Zwieten 1997). The α_2-adrenoceptors in the brain are similar to, or possibly identical with, peripheral vascular α_2-receptors, both in radioligand-binding experiments and with respect to their preference for known selective agonists and antagonists (van Zwieten and Chalmers 1994).

The further subdivision of α_1-adrenoceptors into α_{1A}, α_{1B}, α_{1D}, and possible further subpopulations has so far not led to important functional insights or therapeutic improvements. It may be mentioned that the α_{1A}-adrenoceptor seems to be the functionally predominant subtype in urethral and prostate tissues, whereas its density and functional relevance in blood vessels appear to be much lower.

α-Adrenoceptor changes associated with disease

Hypertensive disease in an established phase has been reported to be associated with an increased density of α_2-adrenoceptors in thrombocytes, although this may be a secondary phenomenon. Changes in α_1-adrenoceptor density in hypertensives are usually very small and not relevant as a potential cause of hypertension. Several authors have established that there exists an exaggerated response to both α_1- and α_2-adrenoceptor agonists in hypertensives, which is probably not related to changes in α-receptor characteristics but rather the reflection of vascular hypertrophy.

Congestive heart failure is characterized by a decreased density of cardiac β-adrenoceptors, thus causing a relatively enhanced sensitivity of cardiac α_1-receptors.

α-Adrenoceptor agonists and antagonists as therapeutic agents

Vasoconstriction via α_1/α_2-adrenoceptor stimulation is an important physiological and pathophysiological principle, although it is of modest therapeutic interest, as in the use of nasal and ophthalmic decongestants or the addition of adrenaline or noradrenaline to local anaesthetic agents. α-Adrenoceptor antagonists (α-blockers) are the major example of therapeutic agents that owe their efficacy (and most of their side-effects) to their interaction with α-adrenoceptors. Prazosin and related selective α_1-adrenoceptor antagonists (e.g. doxazosin or terazosin) appear to be preferable to non-selective ($\alpha_1 + \alpha_2$)-

blockers such as phentolamine. The non-selective α-blockers enhance the release of endogenous noradrenaline as a result of presynaptic α_2-receptor blockade, and they cause pronounced reflex tachycardia. These problems are not encountered during the use of selective α_1-blockers, which do not interfere with the α_2-receptor-mediated presynaptic mechanisms. Prazosin and related drugs are used as antihypertensives, and occasionally as vasodilators in the treatment of congestive heart failure. Vasodilatation, based on α_1-adrenoceptor blockade, readily explains the therapeutic efficacy of these compounds. Orthostatic hypotension, their major adverse reaction, is also caused by rapid vasodilatation, predominantly in the venous vascular bed. Owing to its slower onset of action, the newer compound doxazosin causes less orthostatic hypotension and reflex tachycardia, and therefore seems to be preferable to prazosin, also because in hypertensives a once-daily dose is sufficient for adequate control of hypertension (van Zwieten et al. 1984; van Zwieten 1995).

Selective α_1-adrenoceptor antagonists have been introduced recently in the treatment of impaired micturition, associated with prostate hyperplasia. Tamsulosine, a rather selective α_{1A}-adrenoceptor antagonist enhances micturition in patients with benign prostate hyperplasia (BPH), with a relatively much weaker effect on blood vessels, and, therefore, a reduced risk of orthostatic hypotension when compared with prazosin.

The older antihypertensive, α-methyldopa, owes its antihypertensive activity (via its active metabolite α-methylnoradrenaline) to the stimulation of α_2-adrenoceptors in the central nervous system. Clonidine exerts peripheral sympathoinhibition and central antihypertensive activity due to the stimulation of both α_2-adrenoceptors and imidazoline (I_1) receptors in the brainstem. The central α_2-adrenoceptors are probably very similar to their peripheral counterparts, although small differences may exist.

β-Adrenoceptors

β-Adrenoceptors are found in various cardiac tissues, in most blood vessels, in the bronchi and intestine, on lymphocytes, adipocytes, and in the central nervous system. Stimulation of postsynaptic β-adrenoceptors will cause a variety of physiological and pharmacological effects, as outlined in Table 7.3. β-Receptor blockade by β-adrenoceptor antagonists (β-blockers) suppresses these effects and this is the basis of their therapeutic efficacy and also of most of their adverse reactions. The molecular structure of β-receptors in several tissues and systems has been elucidated. As established for many receptor types, the structure of β-adrenoceptors is characterized by seven transmembrane helices, with particular areas/regions that are required for the combination with agonists and antagonists (in the extracellular part) or with coupling proteins at intracellular sites.

As for the α-adrenoceptors, much information has become available concerning the signal transduction processes that are triggered by β-adrenoceptor stimulation with appropriate agonists. β-Adrenoceptors are also G-protein coupled. Accordingly, β-receptor stimulation is associated with the activation of a G_s-protein, and, subsequently adenylylcyclase. At postsynaptic sites, both β_1- and β_2-adrenoceptors are found, as summarized in Table 7.3.

β-Adrenoceptors at presynaptic sites are predominantly of the β_2-type. Their stimulation with an agonist causes enhanced release of endogenous noradrenaline from its vesicular stores. Conversely, the blockade of β_2-adrenoceptors with an appropriate antagonist will

Table 7.3. Effects on the stimulation and blockade by β_1-, β_2- and β_3-adrenoceptors by means of appropriate agonists and antagonists

Receptor type	Tissue/organ	Stimulation (agonist)	Blockade (antagonist)
β_1	Cardiac pacemaker cells	Heart rate $\uparrow$	Heart rate $\downarrow$
	AV node	AV conduction $\uparrow$	AV conduction $\downarrow$
	Myocardium	Contractility $\uparrow$	Contractility $\downarrow$
	Intestine	Relaxation	—
β_2	Bronchi	Relaxation	Constriction
	Myocardium ($\beta_2 < \beta_1$)	Contractility $\uparrow$	Contractility $\downarrow$
	Blood vessels	Dilatation	Constriction
	Intestine	Relaxation	—
	Adenylcyclase	Hyperglycaemia	Hypoglycaemia
		Free fatty acids $\uparrow$	Free fatty acids $\downarrow$
β_3	Adipose tissues	Lipolysis	?
		Thermogenesis	

reduce the rate of release of endogenous noradrenaline from pre-synaptic storage sites. β-Adrenoceptors are present in various structures of the central nervous system, but their functional role and potential basis as a therapeutic target remain uncertain. They are probably similar to their peripheral counterparts, as indicated by radioligand-binding experiments.

More recently, a great deal of information concerning the β_3-adrenoceptor has become available. β_3-Adrenoceptors are found in brown adipose tissue, intestinal smooth muscle, and blood vessels. The role of these receptors in humans has not been defined in detail, but it has been demonstrated that when stimulated they enhance lipolysis and the generation of heat in fatty tissues.

β-Adrenoceptor changes associated with disease

With respect to the influence of disease on the characteristics of β-adrenoceptors, the most convincing results have been obtained in congestive heart failure (CHF). Various types of CHF, caused by severe coronary heart disease and valvular disease, are associated with a significant degree of down-regulation of both β_1- and β_2-adrenoceptors, as reflected by a reduction in the density of both receptor subtypes in the myocardium. In the myocardial tissue of patients with dilated cardiomyopathy the down-regulation remains limited to β_1-adrenoceptors, without changes in the density of β_2-adrenoceptors. The reduced density of β-adrenoceptors is most probably explained by the elevated plasma levels of noradrenaline reported in patients with advanced stages of CHF. The lowered density of cardiac β-receptors in CHF readily explains the well-known tachyphylaxis towards β-adrenoceptor agonists, which may be used in the treatment of CHF. β-Receptor down-regulation may be reversed by treatment with β-blockers in very low doses and this may be the basis of the observation that low-dose β-blocker therapy may be beneficial in CHF, despite the risk of negative inotropic effects. More recently it has been shown that in congestive heart failure β_2-adrenoceptors are uncoupled, possibly as a result of an increase in G-protein receptor kinases. Reports on changes in β-adrenoceptor density (in particular the β_2-receptors on lymphocytes) in hypertension are controversial: increased, decreased, or unchanged β_2-receptor densities on lymphocytes from essential hypertensives, have all been described.

β_3-Adrenoceptor changes may be involved in certain types of obesity, in particular those associated with non-insulin-dependent diabetes (NIDDM), as found in the Pima Indians, for example.

β-Adrenoceptor agonists and antagonists as therapeutic agents

β-Adrenoceptor agonists may be used to increase contractile force in patients with CHF, or as bronchodilators in patients with asthma or other types of obstructive airways disease. The use of β-agonists in CHF is associated with various side-effects: these inotropic agents may cause tachycardia, with an increased risk of tachyarrhythmias. None of the β-adrenoceptor agonists so far available can be used orally, making intravenous administration unavoidable. Chronic administration of these compounds leads to down-regulation and desensitization of β-adrenoceptors and hence to tachyphylaxis. Of the drugs available at present, dobutamine is used most frequently. Its use is limited to infusions of a few days' duration, and its beneficial effect is no more than palliative.

Salbutamol, salmeterol, terbutaline, and fenoterol are selective β_2-adrenoceptor stimulants. They are well-known bronchodilators, which have replaced non-selective $\beta_1 + \beta_2$-agonists, such as iso-prenaline and orciprenaline. These latter compounds cause a greater degree of tachycardia (as a result of their β_1-component) than observed for the selective β_2-receptor stimulants.

β_2-Adrenoceptor stimulants, such as ritodrine, are frequently used in obstetrics, with the aim to postpone premature parturition, via relaxation of uterus smooth muscle.

β_3-Adrenoceptor agonists can be thought of as anti-obesity drugs, especially in patients with NIDDM, although clinical data on this potential treatment are hardly available.

β-Adrenoceptor antagonists (β-blockers) have obtained widespread therapeutic application, especially in the treatment of essential hypertension and angina pectoris. Their therapeutic efficacy is caused by the blockade of β_1-adrenoceptors, and so are most of their adverse reactions. This important subject has been reviewed extensively (Fitzgerald 1991).

The use of low-dose β-blockers in congestive heart failure has been mentioned. The beneficial effect in this condition is probably caused by a reduction of tachycardia (an expression of sympathetic hyperactivation in patients with congestive heart failure), and possibly also by the partial reversal of β-adrenoceptor down-regulation in the hearts of such patients.

Cholinergic receptors

Traditionally, cholinergic receptors have been subdivided into nicotinic and muscarinic subtypes, based predominantly on the classical work in this field by Sir Henry Dale and his co-workers in the 1930s. The nicotinic receptors are located in the autonomic ganglia (both sympathetic and parasympathetic) and in neuromuscular junctions. Muscarinic receptors are located in all target organs of the parasympathetic nervous system. More recently, muscarinic receptors have also been demonstrated in certain structures of peripheral sympathetic (adrenergic) neurones. The central nervous system also contains muscarinic receptors, which are involved in cognitive processes, extrapyramidal functions, and probably also in the central regulation of blood pressure and heart rate.

The distinction between nicotinic and muscarinic receptors is based solely upon differential pharmacodynamic effects and preferences for agonists and antagonists. Modern molecular biological techniques have confirmed the different structures and amino acid sequences of both types of cholinergic receptors. As in numerous other receptors, both the nicotinic and muscarinic receptors contain the well-known pattern of seven helices. Both nicotinic and muscarinic cholinergic receptors are G-protein coupled.

Nicotinic cholinergic receptors

Nicotinic receptors are known to play an important role in neurohumoral transmission in all autonomic ganglia (parasympathetic and sympathetic) as well as in neuromuscular junctions. It has been proposed that different subtypes of nicotinic receptors may exist but this hypothesis has not been as fully substantiated as for the muscarinic receptors.

Both agonists and antagonists for nicotinic receptors have been developed and a few of these are clinically useful. Nicotine (in low doses) and dimethylphenylpiperazine (DMPP) are classical stimulants of nicotinic receptors, both in the sympathetic and parasympathetic autonomic ganglia. Succinylcholine (suxamethonium) is an agonist, particularly with respect to the nicotinic receptors in neuromuscular junctions. Its muscle relaxant action, frequently used in anaesthesiology, is based upon the permanent depolarization it causes, thus abolishing the process of neurotransmission.

All inhibitors of the enzyme cholinesterase, such as neostigmine, fysostigmine, pyridostigmine, and tacrine, but also the polyalkylphosphates such as fluostigmine, parathion, and sarin (nerve gas), will cause the accumulation of endogenous acetylcholine, which is a non-specific agonist for both nicotinic and muscarinergic cholinergic receptors. The beneficial effect of neostigmine and related drugs in myasthenia gravis and related disorders of neuromuscular transmission is based upon the stimulation of nicotinic receptors in the neuromuscular junction. Their major side-effects are caused by stimulation of parasympathetic muscarinic receptors. The polyalkylphosphates (some of them nerve gases or insecticides) are only of toxicological interest. Their extremely high toxicity is based predominantly upon a general activation of all cholinergic receptors (including those in the central nervous system) by accumulated endogenous acetylcholine.

Antagonists to nicotinic receptors in the autonomic ganglia are the ganglioplegic agents or ganglion blockers. Examples of these are pentolinium, hexamethonium, or trimetaphan. These compounds were among the first drugs used to treat hypertension. Their antihypertensive activity is based upon the blockade of transmission in sympathetic ganglia. These compounds were effective antihypertensives, but at present are unacceptable because of their severe adverse reactions, which are largely based upon the simultaneous blockade of both sympathetic and parasympathetic ganglia. Trimetaphan is still used occasionally by anaesthetists to lower blood pressure for short periods during surgery.

A second group of nicotinic receptor antagonists are the compounds related to tubocurarine, such as gallamine, pancuronium, vecuronium, and rocuronium. They are muscle relaxants, widely used in anaesthesiology. Their beneficial effect is based upon blockade of transmission in the neuromuscular junction as a result of competitive antagonism at the level of nicotinic receptors.

Muscarinic cholinergic receptors

Muscarinic receptors are intricately linked to the parasympathetic nervous system as targets of the endogenous neurotransmitter acetylcholine. Recent studies indicate that muscarinic receptors in various organs and tissues are heterogeneous. There are at least four subtypes (M_1, M_2, M_3, and M_4) and possibly more. As in the sympathetic system, the existence of presynaptic muscarinic receptors in addition to those at postsynaptic sites has been demonstrated.

Furthermore, the classification of muscarinic receptor subtypes requires a more precise designation of receptor agonists/antagonists with respect to their preference for the various classes of muscarinic receptors. As these developments are recent, the receptor classification is less firmly established than that for adrenoceptors. A major problem is the limited availability of highly selective agonists and antagonists, which are suitable as tools in the pharmacological analysis of the muscarinic receptor subtypes.

Subdivision and classification

The subdivision of muscarinic receptors into at least four subtypes is based predominantly upon radioligand-binding studies because of the availability of appropriate ligands and selective M-receptor antagonists. These four subtypes, M_1, M_2, M_3, and M_4, and the antagonists used are listed in Table 7.4, which also shows the tissues where these receptor subtypes can be demonstrated to exist. The introduction of pirenzepine, a selective antagonist to M_1 receptors, has been a major breakthrough in the modern classification of M receptors. The concept of M_1, M_2, and M_3 receptors was formulated originally by Doods et al. (1987). Apart from these three well-established subtypes, a fourth type (M_4) has been identified recently. The radioligand-binding studies that have been pivotal to the subclassification of M receptors are being followed up slowly by functional experiments, the results of which are globally in line with the findings of the binding data. Table 7.4 shows the functional aspects of stimulation/blockade of the M-receptor subtypes. (Reviewed by Eglen 1995; Lambrecht et al. 1995).

Molecular biological cloning techniques have led to the identification of at least five different muscarinic receptor species, the amino acid sequence and structure of which have been elucidated. Again, the model of seven transmembrane helices appears to underlie the structure of these receptor species. These five muscarinic receptor

Table 7.4. Various types of muscarinic receptors in different tissues. The effects of receptor stimulation and blockade by appropriate agonists and antagonists are also shown

Receptor type	Tissue/organ	Stimulation (agonist)	Blockade (antagonist)
M_1	Neurones	Excitation	Depression
	Ganglia (sympathetic)	Noradrenaline release ↑	Noradrenaline release ↓
M_2	Heart	Bradycardia	Tachycardia
		Contractility ↓	Contractility ↑
	Smooth muscle	Contraction	Relaxation
M_3	Glands	Secretion ↑	Secretion ↓
	Ileum	Contraction	Relaxation
M_4	Striatum	No functional data available	
	Lungs		

species have been denominated as m_1, m_2, m_3, m_4, and m_5, respectively. The m_1, m_2, m_3, and m_4 types broadly coincide with the M_1-, M_2-, M_3-, and M_4-receptor subtypes established by means of radioligand-binding techniques (Table 7.4). The functional role of the m_5 species so far remains unknown (Bonner 1987).

Biochemical studies have indicated that muscarinic receptors are coupled to adenylyl cyclase via G-proteins. In contrast to β-adrenoceptors, the influence of muscarinic receptor stimulation is inhibitory (involving a G_i-protein), thus causing a decrease in the cellular concentration of cAMP. Few data are available concerning possible changes of muscarinic receptor density associated with disease and no clear picture has as yet emerged.

Muscarinic receptor agonists and antagonists: potential therapeutic agents

Acetylcholine, the endogenous neurotransmitter in the parasympathetic nervous system, is a non-selective agent that stimulates muscarinic receptors of the three subtypes, M_1, M_2, and M_3, in addition to nicotinic cholinergic receptors. Most of the classical synthetic muscarinic receptor agonists are non-selective with respect to the various muscarinic receptor subtypes. This lack of selectivity is known for muscarine, aceclidine, pilocarpine, bethanechol, carbachol, and arecoline. Carbachol and arecoline also stimulate ganglionic nicotinic receptors in addition to their agonistic effect on muscarinic receptors.

Methacholine appears to possess some selectivity towards the vascular muscarinic receptors, which may be of the M_2 or the M_3 type, depending on the vascular bed and animal species investigated. The experimental compounds McN-A 343 and xanomeline appear to display selectivity towards M_1 receptors, particularly those present in the brain and at the sympathetic ganglia. Virtually all other muscarinic receptor agonists available are non-selective with respect to the various M-receptor subtypes. In fundamental pharmacology the development of highly selective agonists for the three (or more) muscarinic receptor subtypes would be most valuable.

Special attention should be paid to the role of muscarinic receptors in the release of the endothelium-derived relaxant factor (EDRF) from vascular endothelium. Stimulation of vascular M_3 receptors with acetylcholine (ACh) enhances the release of EDRF, now widely assumed to be identical with nitric oxide (NO), an important endogenous vasodilator agent. Consequently, the vasodilator action

of ACh is an indirect effect, mediated by NO. In endothelium-denuded vessels ACh causes vasoconstriction, as a result of the stimulation of M-receptors on vascular smooth muscle. Atropine is a non-selective antagonist with a high affinity for the various muscarinic receptor subtypes. Pirenzepine is a selective M_1-receptor antagonist, with a much lower affinity for M_2 or M_3 receptors. AF-DX 116 is a cardioselective antagonist for M_2 receptors, as is methoctramine. 4-DAMP shows some selectivity for M_3-receptors as do hexahydro-sila-difenidol and related compounds. Tropicamide and himbacine show moderate selectivity for the M_4 receptor.

The present muscarinic receptor classification is predominantly based upon the series of antagonists and agonists mentioned above. Since the number of experimental compounds is rapidly increasing, the receptor classification may well be subject to important future changes.

Therapeutic applications

Muscarinic receptor stimulants have traditionally been used for activation of the smooth muscle of the intestine and/or urinary bladder and for lowering elevated intraocular pressure in glaucoma. Carbachol and bethanechol, which are used to stimulate smooth muscle, are examples of the former. They display a modest selectivity towards intestinal and urinary bladder smooth muscle as compared to that of the cardiovascular system. Adverse reactions are related to stimulation of the peripheral parasympathetic nervous system. Pilocarpine, when applied locally to the eye, causes miosis and a reduction of intraocular pressure, as in glaucoma treatment. Systemic side-effects do not usually occur, although the ocular adverse reactions are substantial.

Therapeutic applications of selective muscarinic receptor agonists are currently a matter of speculation. Highly cardioselective M_2-receptor agonists may be used to reduce heart rate in the treatment of angina pectoris or supraventricular tachycardia. M_1-receptor stimulation in the CNS has been proposed as a potential therapeutic approach to treat Alzheimer's disease.

The cholinesterase inhibitor, tacrine (tetrahydro-amino-acridine), has recently been demonstrated to somewhat retard the deterioration of cognitive functions in Alzheimer's disease.

Of the muscarinic receptor antagonists, pirenzepine is a selective M_1-agonist which has been introduced in the treatment of peptic ulcer. It appears to have fewer side-effects on the cardiovascular system, the eye, and the exocrine glands.

Various non-selective M-receptor antagonists may be used in ophthalmology to provoke mydriasis. Scopolamine may be used as a potent centrally acting anti-emetic agent.

On theoretical grounds cardioselective M_2-receptor antagonists may benefit patients with impaired atrioventricular (AV) conduction in the period before a pacemaker is implanted, and may also be useful in conditions such as the sick sinus syndrome, digitalis intoxication, or arrhythmia caused by torsade de pointes (TDP). None of these therapeutic options has been explored clinically on a sufficiently large scale (Goyal 1989). Finally, coronary spasm may involve a cholinergic component in certain patients and the beneficial effects of atropine have been demonstrated. A highly selective antagonist of vascular M_2 (or M_3) receptors, which appears to be involved in this type of spasm, may be preferable to a non-selective agent such as atropine.

References

Ahlqvist, R. P. (1948). A study of the adrenotropic receptors. *Am. J. Physiol.* **153**, 586–91.

Bonner, T. I. (1989). The molecular basis of muscarinic receptor diversity. *Trends Neurosci.* **12**, 148–51.

Doods, H. N., Mathy, M.-J., Davidesko, D., van Charldorp, K. J., de Jonge, A., and van Zwieten, P. A. (1987). Selectivity of muscarinic antagonists in radioligand and *in vivo* experiments for the putative M_1, M_2 and M_3 receptors. *J. Pharmacol. exp. Ther.* **246**, 929–34.

Eglen, R. M. (1995). Muscarinic M_2 and M_3 receptors in smooth muscle. *Exp. Opin. Invest. Drugs* **4**, 1167–71.

Fitzgerald, J. D. (1991). The applied pharmacology of beta-adrenoceptor agonists (beta blockers) in relation to clinical outcomes. *Cardiovasc. Drugs Ther.* **5**, 561–76.

Goyal, R. K. (1989). Muscarinic receptor subtypes. Physiology and clinical implications. *New Engl. J. Med.* **321**, 1022–8.

Insel, P. A. (1996). Adrenergic receptors—evolving concepts and clinical implications. *New Engl. J. Med.* **334**, 580–5.

Lambrecht, G., Gross, J., Hacksell, U. *et al.* (1995). The design and pharmacology of novel selective muscarinic agonists and antagonists. *Life Sci.* **56**, 815–22.

Lands, A. M., Arnold, A., McAuliff, J. P., Lunduena, F. P., and Brown, R. G. (1967). Differentiation of receptor systems activated by sympathomimetic amines. *Nature* **214**, 597–8.

Langer, S. Z. (1981). Presynaptic regulation of the release of catecholamines. *Pharmacol. Rev.* **32**, 337–62.

Starke, K. (1981). α-Adrenoceptor subclassification. *Rev. Physiol. Biochem. Pharmacol.* **88**, 199–236.

Van Zwieten, P. A. (1995). Alpha-adrenoceptor blocking agents in the treatment of hypertension. In *Hypertension: pathophysiology, diagnosis and management*, (ed. J. H. Laragh and B. M. Brenner), 2nd edn, pp. 2917–35, Raven Press, New York.

Van Zwieten, P. A. (1997). Central imidazoline (I_1) receptors as targets of centrally acting antihypertensives. *J. Hypertension*, **15**, 117–25.

Van Zwieten, P. A. and Chalmers, J. P. (1994). Different types of centrally acting antihypertensives and their targets in the central nervous system. *Cardiovasc. Drugs Ther.* **8**, 787–99.

Van Zwieten, P. A. and Timmermans, P. B. M. W. M. (1984). Central and peripheral α-adrenoceptors. Pharmacological aspects and clinical potential. *Adv. Drug Res.* **13**, 209–54.

Van Zwieten, P. A., Timmermans, P. B. M. W. M., and van Brummelen, P. (1984). Role of alpha-adrenoceptors in hypertension and in antihypertensive treatment. *Am. J. Med.* **77**, 17–25.

8. Structural and chemical organization of the autonomic nervous system with special reference to non-adrenergic, non-cholinergic transmission

Geoffrey Burnstock and Pamela Milner

Introduction

The versatility of the autonomic nervous system can be attributed to the structural characteristics of autonomic neuroeffector junctions and the multiplicity of neurotransmitters and receptors that are involved in autonomic neurotransmission. Neuromodulation and co-transmission are features of non-adrenergic, non-cholinergic (NANC) neurotransmission in sympathetic, parasympathetic, and sensory–motor nerves and in intrinsic ganglia. There are thus many levels at which autonomic failure can operate. Recent advances in the study of autonomic neurotransmission include the cloning of purine receptor subtypes, which has reinforced the concept of purinergic neurotransmission, and the realization that nitric oxide (NO) is a transmitter in some autonomic nerves as well as an endothelium-derived relaxing factor. The plasticity of autonomic nerves, even in adult animals, offers the potential for therapy in disease.

The autonomic neuroeffector junction

The autonomic neuroeffector junction between autonomic nerve fibres and smooth muscle cells differs in several ways from the neuromuscular junction in skeletal muscle and from the synapses in the central and peripheral nervous systems (Burnstock 1986a). The autonomic effector is a muscle bundle rather than a single cell and low-resistance pathways between individual muscle cells allow electrotonic spread of activity within the effector bundle. Morphologically, the sites of electrotonic coupling are represented by areas of close apposition between the plasma membranes of adjacent muscle cells which can be identified under the electron microscope as gap junctions or nexuses. These gap junctions vary in size from punctate junctions to junctional areas of more than 1 μm in diameter. Gap junctions are composed of integral membrane proteins which form groups of hemichannels, two hemichannels from adjacent cells aligning to form an intercellular channel. The hemichannel is a hexameric structure of connexin protein subunits. Several different connexin genes have been cloned; connexins 43 and 40 are expressed in vascular smooth muscle. Little is known about the quantity and arrangement of gap junctions in effector bundles relative to the density of autonomic innervation. Thus, within an effector muscle bundle only a certain percentage of cells are directly innervated, the remainder being coupled to these cells via gap junctions.

Another characteristic of the autonomic neuromuscular junction is that it is not a synapse with a well-defined structure and pre- and postjunctional specializations like the skeletal muscle motor end plate. Unmyelinated, highly branched, postganglionic autonomic nerve fibres reaching the effector smooth muscle become beaded or varicose (Fig. 8.1). These varicosities are not static in their relationships to

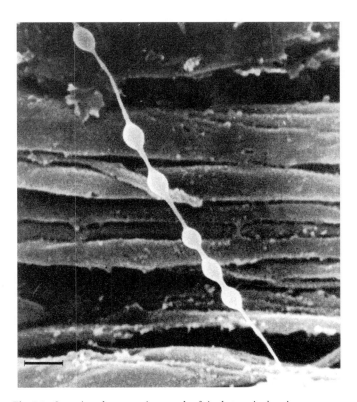

Fig. 8.1. Scanning electron micrograph of single terminal varicose nerve fibre lying over smooth muscle of the small intestine of a rat. Intestine was pretreated to remove connective tissue components by digestion with trypsin and hydrolysis with HCl. Bar, 3 μm. (From Burnstock 1988.)

smooth muscle, consistent with the lack of postjunctional specialization. They are 0.5–2 μm in diameter and about 1 μm in length and are packed with vesicles and mitochondria. Neurotransmitters from autonomic nerve fibres are released from these varicosities, which occur at intervals of 5–10 μm along axons. The distance of the cleft between the varicosity and smooth muscle varies considerably depending on the tissue, from 20 nm in densely innervated structures such as the vas deferens to 1–2 μm in large elastic arteries. Neurotransmitter is released *en passage* from varicosities during conduction of an impulse along an autonomic axon; however, it has been shown that a single impulse will evoke release from only a small percentage of the terminal varicosities.

Release of neurotransmitter causes a transient change in membrane potential of the postjunctional cell. If the result of a single pulse is a depolarization, the response is called an excitatory junction potential (EJP). EJPs sum and facilitate with repetitive stimulation and upon reaching sufficient amplitude, the threshold for generation of an action potential is reached, resulting in a mechanical contraction. If the result of a single pulse of neurotransmitter release is a hyperpolarization, the response is called an inhibitory junction potential (IJP). IJPs prevent action potential discharge in spontaneously active smooth muscle and thus cause relaxation.

The multiplicity of neurotransmitters in the autonomic nervous system

The classical view of autonomic nervous control as antagonistic actions of noradrenaline (NAd) and acetylcholine (ACh) causing either constriction or relaxation, depending on the tissue, was changed in the early 1960s when clear evidence of a non-adrenergic, non-cholinergic (NANC) system was presented (see Burnstock 1986*b*). IJPs blocked by tetrodotoxin were recorded, using the sucrose-gap technique, in intestinal smooth muscle during stimulation of guinea-pig enteric nerves in the presence of adrenergic- and cholinergic-blocking agents. At about the same time, other researchers showed that relaxation of the cat stomach following vagal stimulation was resistant to adrenergic and cholinergic blockade. Similar observations were consequently made on a wide variety of tissues, including urinary bladder, lung, oesophagus, seminal vesicles, trachea, and blood vessels.

Purinergic neurotransmission

The first substance that was found to best satisfy the criteria for a neurotransmitter in NANC nerves in the intestine and urinary bladder was the purine nucleotide, adenosine 5'-triphosphate (ATP). Subsequently, the purinergic nerve hypothesis was formulated (Burnstock 1972) which suggested that: ATP synthesized in nerve terminals is stored in large opaque vesicles; after its release and activation of purinergic receptors in the postjunctional membrane, ATP is rapidly broken down by magnesium-activated ATPase and 5'-nucleotidase to adenosine; adenosine is taken up by a high-affinity uptake system, converted to ATP, and reincorporated into physiological stores; any adenosine not taken up this way is broken down by adenosine deaminase to inosine which is inactive and leaks into the circulation.

Based on the relative potencies of purine nucleosides and nucleotides on a variety of tissues, two major types of purine receptor have been distinguished (Burnstock 1996*a*). P1 receptors are most sensitive to adenosine, are competitively blocked by methylxanthines, and occupation leads to changes in levels of intracellular cyclic AMP. P2 receptors are most sensitive to ATP, are not blocked by methylxanthines nor act via an adenylate cyclase system, and their occupation may lead to prostaglandin synthesis. Pharmacological, biochemical, receptor binding and more recently, cloning studies, have enabled subdivision of these two types of receptor. P1 receptors are generally of the A_1, A_{2A}, A_{2B} or A_3 subtypes: A_1 receptors are preferentially activated by N^6-substituted adenosine analogues and their occupation leads to decreased cyclic AMP levels, whereas A_2 receptors show preference for 5'-substituted compounds and cyclic AMP levels are increased; occupation of A_3 receptors does not lead to changes in adenylate cyclase. Selective agonists and antagonists for these P1-receptor subtypes have been identified (Jacobson and Suzuki 1996). Following expression cloning, transduction mechanism studies, and the use of newly synthesized agonists and antagonists, it has been proposed by Abbracchio and Burnstock (1994) that, in keeping with other neurotransmitters, P2 receptors should be divided into two major families, a P2X receptor family which are ligand-gated ion-channel receptors mediating fast transmission and a P2Y receptor family which are G-protein-coupled receptors mediating slower responses. Currently seven P2X ($P2X_{1–7}$) subclasses and six P2Y ($P2Y_{1–4,6,8}$) subclasses have been recognized. These incorporate the receptors that respond to the pyrimidine derivative UTP as well as to ATP and also receptors that respond to adenine dinucleotide polyphosphates (Burnstock 1996*a*). The recent molecular biological approaches to identify the molecular structures for P2X and P2Y receptors have greatly reinforced the concept of purinergic neurotransmission (see Burnstock 1996*b*).

Peptidergic neurotransmission

Hints that there were in fact more than three different neurotransmitters in the autonomic nervous system came from ultrastructural studies of the enteric nervous system in the 1960s which revealed at least nine distinguishable types of axon profile (see Burnstock 1986*a*). The use of immunohistochemical techniques subsequently led to a rapid expansion in our knowledge of the diversity of the autonomic neurotransmitters since it allowed the identification of several different biologically active peptides and transmitter synthesizing enzymes in neural elements (Furness and Costa 1987). The following neuropeptides have now been proposed as neurotransmitters in the mammalian autonomic nervous system: enkephalin/endorphin, vasoactive intestinal polypeptide (VIP) and peptide histidine methionine (PHM), substance P (SP) and neurokinins A and B, gastrin releasing peptide/bombesin, somatostatin, neurotensin, pituitary adenylate cyclase-activating protein, cholecystokinin (CCK)/gastrin, neuropeptide Y (NPY) and pancreatic polypeptide, galanin, angiotensin, vasopressin, adrenocorticotrophic hormone, and calcitonin-gene-related peptide (CGRP). It is quite likely that advances in the techniques of molecular cloning and gene expression will lead to the identification of other new bioactive peptides which play a role in autonomic neurotransmission.

By virtue of their structure, the mode and site of synthesis of neuropeptide transmitters differs from other neurotransmitters. Neuropeptides are cleaved from larger precursor molecules synthesized in the nerve cell body and transported along the nerve fibre to the site of release, a mechanism quite different from the reuptake and/or synthesis of other neurotransmitters that occurs at the axon terminal. Neuropeptides may thus act in a modulatory capacity and mediate long-term events, rather than as rapidly acting neurotransmitters. As there is no known reuptake mechanism for removal of neuropeptides from the site of action, it is likely that their action is terminated mainly by metabolism by proteolytic enzymes. A few key ectoenzymes, including endopeptidase 24.11 and angiotensin-converting enzyme, are now thought to account for the degradation of most neuropeptides.

Neuropeptides act on specific receptors which, in turn, activate second messenger systems or G proteins, a mechanism of action similar to that for the classical neurotransmitters. There are relatively few useful antagonists available to block neuropeptide transmitter actions; however, in the past few years, use of new selective non-peptide antagonists has aided characterization of receptor sub-types. Many neuropeptide receptor subtypes have now been cloned (Dockray 1994).

Nitrergic neurotransmission

Nitric oxide (NO), first identified as the endothelium-derived relaxing factor (EDRF), is now known to play an important role as a primary messenger in transmitting information from nerves to smooth muscles in specific tissues (Rand 1992; Lincoln et al. 1997). NO is formed by oxidation of a terminal nitrogen atom of L-arginine, a reaction catalysed by nitric oxide synthase (NOS). Immunohistochemical studies have confirmed, amongst other locations, a neural localization of this enzyme in several tissues, including myenteric neurones of the gut and nerve fibres innervating cerebral arteries. NO is atypical as a neurotransmitter in several ways: it is not stored in vesicles but appears to be synthesized in the cytoplasm on demand; it is released by simple diffusion, not exocytosis; and, rather than acting on membrane receptor proteins, its receptor target is iron in the active centre of the enzyme, guanylyl cyclase, inside the cell. By binding to iron, NO initiates a three-dimensional change in the shape of the enzyme which increases its activity and consequently the production of cyclic GMP. The original criteria for defining a neurotransmitter have now been re-evaluated to encompass the roles of neurally released substances, such as NO, which act on cells close to the site of release, are inactivated endogenously, and mimic the process of transmission. Agents that potentiate or inhibit the action of NO affect the process of transmission in the same way (Lincoln et al. 1997).

Other non-adrenergic, non-cholinergic neurotransmitters

Serotonin (5-hydroxytryptamine; 5-HT), dopamine, and γ-aminobutyric acid are also known to be autonomic neurotransmitters (see Burnstock 1986a,b).

Mechanisms of co-transmission and neuromodulation

The coexistence of more than one neurotransmitter within a single nerve terminal is now well documented (Burnstock 1996c). Peptides, purine nucleotides, and NO (identified by localization of NOS) are often found together with the classic neurotransmitters, NAd and ACh (Fig. 8.2). In fact, the majority, if not all, of nerve fibres in the

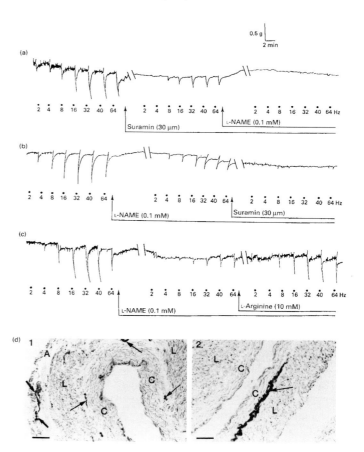

Fig. 8.2. Relaxations of the rabbit portal vein to neurogenic transmural stimulation for 10 s (2–64 Hz, 0.7 ms, 100 V) at 5 min intervals. Guanethidine (3.4 μM) and atropine (0.114 μM) were present throughout to block adrenergic and cholinergic neurotransmission, respectively. Tone was induced with ergotamine (8.6 μM). Panel (a) shows that pre-incubation with a P2 receptor antagonist, suramin (30 μM) for 20 min reduced the nerve-mediated relaxations compared with controls, and that suramin-resistant neurogenic relaxations were abolished 20 min after the addition of an NOS inhibitor, N^G-nitro-L-arginine methyl ester (L-NAME, 0.1 mM). Panel (b) shows that neurogenic relaxations remaining after 20 min pretreatment of the tissue with L-NAME (0.1 mM) were abolished 20 min after the addition of suramin (30 μM). In (c), the effect of adding L-NAME (0.1 mM) to the tissue is shown; there was an additional rise in tone and inhibition of the response to nerve stimulation after a 20 min incubation period. The subsequent treatment of tissues with L-arginine (10 mM) for 20 min reversed this effect. Panel (d) shows the histochemical localization of NADPH-diaphorase (a marker of NOS-containing nerves) in the rabbit portal vein. (d1) NADPH-diaphorase reaction was seen in nerve fibres between the inner circular (C) and the outer longitudinal (L) muscle coats (thin black arrows). Note also the NADPH-diaphorase-positive nerves in adventitia (A) (thick black arrows). Tangentional section. (d2) NADPH-diaphorase reaction seen in a dense nerve plexus between the inner circular (C) and outer longitudinal (L) muscle coats of the portal vein (thin black arrow). Transverse section. The calibration bar for d1 and d2 is 30 μM. Each of the traces in (a), (b), and (c) is representative of similar results in six separate experiments. (From Brizzolara et al. (1993).)

autonomic nervous system contain a mixture of different neurotransmitter substances that vary in proportion in different tissues and species and during development and disease.

It should be noted that immunohistochemical evidence of coexistence should not necessarily be interpreted as evidence of co-transmission, since in order for substances to be termed co-transmitters it is essential to show that postjunctional actions to each substance occur via their own specific receptors. Some substances stored and released from nerves do not have direct actions on effector muscle cells but alter the release and/or the actions of other transmitters; these substances are termed neuromodulators. Many other substances are neuromodulators in that they modify the process of neurotransmission, for example, circulating neurohormones, locally released agents such as prostanoids, bradykinin, histamine, and endothelin, and neurotransmitters from nearby nerves. Many substances that are co-transmitters are also neuromodulators.

The wide and variable cleft characteristic of autonomic neuroeffector junctions makes them particularly amenable to the mechanisms of neural control mentioned above. There are many different ways in which co-transmitters and neuromodulators interact to effect neurotransmission (Fig. 8.3):

1. Autoinhibition: a transmitter, in addition to its postjunctional effects, reduces its own release via prejunctional receptors; release of co-transmitters may also be inhibited.

2. Cross-talk: a neuromodulator may act on closely juxtaposed terminals.

3. Synergism: each of two transmitters, either from different nerve terminals or co-transmitters have the same postjunctional effect so that there is a reinforcement of their individual effects.

4. Opposite actions: occasionally, a transmitter may have opposite actions in different postjunctional effector cells; sensitivity of the responses of co-transmitters depends on the tone of the effector cell.

5. Prolongation of effect: a neuromodulator may act on degradative enzymes, for example, peptidases responsible for removal of neuropeptides from the junctional cleft, to prolong the time course of their effect.

6. Trophic effects: a neurotransmitter may effect the expression of another transmitter or receptor within a population of neurones (for example in ganglia) at the level of gene transcription.

All these mechanisms of control of neurotransmission reflect the versatility of the peripheral components of the autonomic nervous system.

Neurotransmission at the sympathetic neuroeffector junctions: evidence for co-release and roles of NAd, ATP, NPY, and opioids

There is plenty of evidence to show that NAd and ATP are co-transmitters in the sympathetic nervous system in many species , including man (Burnstock 1995). There is considerable variation in the proportions of ATP and NAd released, depending on the tissue

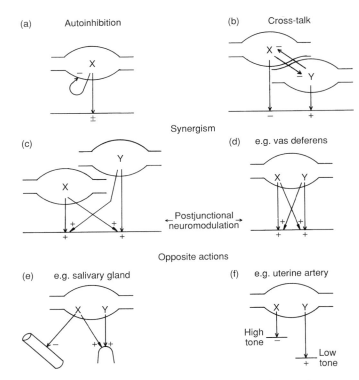

Fig. 8.3. Schematic representation of different types of interactions between two nominal vascular neurotransmitter substances (X and Y). (a) A diagram depicting the process of autoinhibition where, in addition to the neurotransmitter (X) acting postjunctionally to either contract (+) or relax (−) the muscle, it acts on prejunctional receptors (usually of a different subclass) to form a negative feedback system that inhibits release of transmitter. (b) A diagram depicting the process of cross-talk. Transmitters X and Y, contained in separate varicosities, not only act on receptors in the muscle (usually producing opposite actions), but also on prejunctional receptors on each other's nerve terminals to modulate transmitter release. (c) A diagram showing that transmitter X and transmitter Y, contained in separate nerve varicosities, have the same contractile (+) action on the muscle cell. They potentiate each other's action by the process of postjunctional neuromodulation. This is an example of synergism occurring in another type of cross-talk. (d) A diagram showing X and Y, released as co-transmitters from a single varicosity, acting synergistically on the postjunctional effector cell. (e) A diagram showing how the co-transmitters X and Y can have opposite actions on different effector cell sites, although they again act synergistically on the one effector cell type. (f) A diagram showing how the co-transmitters X and Y express opposite actions depending on the tone of the vessel: in high-tone situations, X produces vasodilatation (−), while in low-tone preparations, transmitter Y dominates, producing vasoconstriction. (From Burnstock (1987).)

and species in question, for example rabbit saphenous and mesenteric arteries have a substantial purinergic component, whereas in the rabbit ear artery the purinergic component is relatively small. The relative contribution of each compound to neurogenic contractions is dependent on the parameters of stimulation; short bursts (1 s) at low frequency (2–5 Hz) particularly favour the purinergic component, whereas longer periods of nerve stimulation (30 s or more) favour the adrenergic component. In submucosal arteries the responses to sympathetic nerve stimulation are mediated solely by ATP with NAd acting as a prejunctional modulator via α_2-adrenoceptors causing depression of transmission (Evans and Surprenant 1992). NPY is also stored in, and is released from, most sympathetic nerves, including cardiac and perivascular nerves in many vascular beds in man; NPY release is optimal with high frequency, intermittent stimulation. In most tissues, including vas deferens and most blood vessels, NPY does not act as a genuine co-transmitter, having little direct postjunctional effect, but rather acts as a neuromodulator, often by prejunctional reduction of the release of NAd and ATP and postjunctional potentiation of the adrenergic and purinergic components of sympathetic nerve responses. Although mainly neuromodulatory in sympathetic nerves, NPY does have direct vasoconstrictor effects on certain blood vessels, for example those of the spleen, kidney, heart, and brain in many species. In humans, NPY induces a direct vasoconstrictor response in some vessels which is characteristically slow in onset and long-lasting. A dense plexus of perivascular NPY-containing nerve fibres has been described in many vessels, including human omental, mesenteric, skin, spinal, pulmonary, renal, gastric, splenic, coronary, and cerebral vessels (Mione *et al.* 1990). Because of its distribution and constrictor effects, this component of the sympathetic nervous system has been implicated in the development of hypertension and is also a contender for one of the vasospasmic agents responsible for the delayed ischaemic deficit that occurs after subarachnoid haemorrhage.

Opioid peptides are also widely distributed in sympathetic neurones where their functional role appears to be related to their prejunctional inhibitory effects on sympathetic transmission.

Some preganglionic postganglionic sympathetic neurones contain NOS; however, as yet, a co-transmitter role for NO in these neurones has not been established. In contrast to parasympathetic ganglia, few postganglionic neurones in sympathetic prevertebral or paravertebral ganglia contain NOS.

Sympathetic nerves can interact with both sensory–motor and parasympathetic nerves in close proximity. The activity of sensory–motor nerves is subject to prejunctional inhibitory neuromodulation by the sympathetic co-transmitters, NAd and NPY, and by adenosine, following breakdown of released ATP. Opioids also elicit inhibitory effects on sensory–motor nerves. Prejunctional inhibitory effects of NPY on cholinergic neurotransmission may explain the prolonged attenuation of the action of the vagus in controlling heart rate following sympathetic stimulation.

Neurotransmission at the parasympathetic neuroeffector junctions: the atropine-resistant components of parasympathetic neurotransmission

The neuropeptide most frequently associated with parasympathetic neurotransmission is VIP. An elegant series of experiments by Lundberg in 1981 on the cat exocrine salivary gland with reference to the involvement of VIP and ACh in the control of secretion and blood flow, showed that VIP and ACh were stored in separate vesicles in the same nerve terminal, and were both released upon transmural nerve stimulation but with different stimulation parameters. ACh was released during low-frequency stimulation to increase salivary secretion from acinar cells and to elicit some minor dilatation of blood vessels in the gland, whereas at high stimulation frequencies, VIP was released to produce marked dilatation of the blood vessels in the gland and to act as a neuromodulator postjunctionally on the acinar gland to enhance the actions of ACh, and prejunctionally on the nerve varicosities to enhance the release of ACh. ACh was also found to have an inhibitory action on the release of VIP. VIP has since been shown to have a direct vasodilatory action in the human submandibular gland. Recent studies extend the complexity of parasympathetic co-transmission by the demonstration that NOS and NPY are also co-localized in parasympathetic neurones of the submandibular salivary gland (Modin 1994).

VIP has been co-localized with the ACh synthesizing enzyme, choline acetyltransferase, in many perivascular nerve fibres, where it is localized mainly in large vesicles. NOS is often co-localized with these neurotransmitters in parasympathetic nerves innervating blood vessels and urinogenital smooth muscle; NO and VIP have been proposed as the fast and slow components, respectively, of neurogenic vasodilatation of the uterine artery, acting as co-transmitters. Recent evidence for NO enhancement of sympathetic neurotransmission opens up the possibility of parasympathetic modulation of sympathetic activity.

Parasympathetic co-transmission involving NO and VIP may be particularly important in cerebral vessels where VIP- and NOS-containing nerve fibres originate from the cranial parasympathetic ganglia, in particular from the sphenopalatine ganglion (Nozaki *et al.* 1993). The anterior vessels of the circle of Willis receive a more dense innervation of VIP-containing nerve fibres than those in the posterior circulation (Mione *et al.* 1990). VIP acts as a direct vasodilator in several blood vessels. A peptide found in human tissue, PHM (peptide with N-terminal histidine and C-terminal methionine), which is derived from the same pre-pro-molecule as VIP (the animal form is PHI, C-terminal isoleucine), has a similar distribution pattern to VIP and also has vasodilator properties, although it is less potent than VIP. Perivascular nerves displaying VIP/PHM immunoreactivity tend to occur more frequently around vessels in regional vascular beds than in association with larger conducting vessels. In addition, small arterioles are generally more sensitive to VIP/PHM than larger vessels.

VIP is thought to play a role in parasympathetic neurotransmission in the urinogenital tract since postganglionic nerves from the pelvic ganglia containing VIP and ACh project to the urethra, colon, and penis. NOS is co-localized with VIP in some postganglionic parasympathetic nerves. Both VIP and NO are implicated in the mechanism of penile erection. Numerous immunohistochemical studies have demonstrated VIP in autonomic nerves in the penile artery and penile tissues from a variety of species, including man. NOS has been localized to neurones of the major pelvic ganglion, axons of the penile cavernous nerve, and in neuronal plexuses in the adventitial layer of penile arteries. Electrical stimulation of pelvic nerves induces vasodilatation of penile blood vessels and increases blood flow to the cavernous tissue. This action may be mediated by co-release of VIP and NO. Administration of either substance leads to increased penile volume, relaxation of the corpus cavernosum, corpus spongiosum smooth muscle and blood vessels. VIP is increased in the venous effluent of the penis during psychogenic-, drug-, or electrically induced erection. Furthermore, in diabetic impotence in man, there is a dramatic reduction of VIP-immunoreactive nerve fibres in penile vessels.

The human bladder body receives a dense parasympathetic innervation comprised predominantly of ACh-containing nerves. It is widely accepted that ATP is a co-transmitter utilized by excitatory nerves supplying the rodent urinary bladder; however, pharmacological studies have demonstrated only a small purinergic component in response to electrical field stimulation in humans; P2X receptors have also been localized in the human bladder (Bo and Burnstock 1995). There are marked regional variations in the distribution of the atropine-resistant component in human bladder and, indeed, ATP responses and receptors are dense in the trigone region but very low or absent in the tip of the bladder dome. The physiological significance of these responses may be of greater importance in the functionally disturbed bladder. Of particular interest is the report that in women with interstitial cystitis, about 50 per cent of the reponse of the bladder to parasympathetic nerve stimulation is purinergic (Palea et al. 1993).

There are now several reports that some cranial, ciliary, and paracervical parasympathetic ganglia that supply VIP/ACh-containing nerves to cerebral arteries, iris, and uterine artery also contain NPY (Mione et al. 1990). Dopamine β-hydroxylase, dynorphin, and somatostatin have also been localized in guinea-pig paracervical ganglia.

Neurotransmission at sensory–motor neuroeffector junctions: the roles of SP, CGRP, and ATP

The phenomenon of antidromic vasodilatation, such that antidromic impulses pass down collateral branches of primary afferent sensory nerves, resulting in the release of neurotransmitter and thus causing vasodilatation in the skin, the 'axon reflex' concept, was originally proposed by Lewis in 1927. More recently, interest has been aroused in the dual sensory–efferent functions mediated by sensory neurones in many other tissues. The neurotransmitters essentially involved in sensory–motor neurotransmission are SP and CGRP and, in some cases, ATP (Rubino and Burnstock 1996). The sensory origin of SP- and CGRP-containing nerve fibres has been substantiated by using the selective neurotoxin, capsaicin. Chronic treatment with this drug leads to degeneration of small afferent nerves and a marked loss of SP- and CGRP-containing nerves from most tissues of the cardiovascular system, urinogenital system, and airways. SP and CGRP coexist in large granular vesicles in sensory neurones and perivascular nerves in the guinea-pig; however, in the rat, CGRP immunoreactivity appears to occur in two populations of sensory neurones. In the trigeminal ganglion, small to medium-sized vesicles contain SP and are sensitive to capsaicin, while larger vesicles contain no SP and are resistant to capsaicin. In addition to its role as a neurotransmitter, CGRP may modulate the action of SP by inhibiting its degradation. In the vasculature, unlike CGRP, SP does not appear to act directly on receptors of the vascular smooth muscle, but rather acts via occupation of receptors on endothelial cells at the lumen to bring about

NO release and consequent vasodilatation. This action of neurally released SP may be particularly important in the microvasculature, but access of neurally released SP to the endothelium in large vessels is questionable where it is largely released from endothelial cells (Burnstock and Ralevic 1994). There are increasing examples in the literature of cross-talk between sensory–motor, sympathetic and parasympathetic nerves. In the heart, SP has excitatory effects on cardiac parasympathetic innervation, in contrast to CGRP which is inhibitory (Fig. 8.4; Rubino et al. 1996).

In humans, SP and other tachykinins have been shown to coexist with CGRP in sensory neurones. Activation of the trigeminal cerebrovascular system may be a mechanism involved in cerebrovascular spasm following subarachnoid haemorrhage, since the vasoconstriction induced by subarachnoid blood is markedly prolonged following trigeminovascular pathway lesion but not after trigeminal nerve section. In addition, CGRP levels in middle cerebral arteries are reduced 7–10 days after subarachnoid haemorrhage in man. CGRP and SP levels are also reduced in human cerebrospinal fluid following subarachnoid haemorrhage. Indeed, altered functioning of capsaicin-sensitive sensory neurones may be involved in the pathogenesis of several human diseases, including skin disease, rheumatic disease, asthma and bronchial hyper-reactivity, and in the unstable bladder. In the human urinary bladder, VIP, cholecystokinin (CCK), and

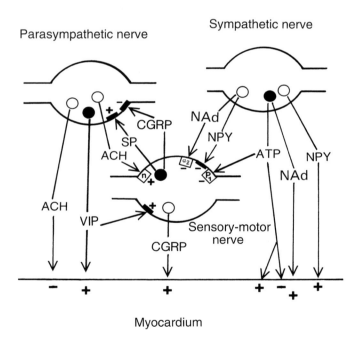

Fig. 8.4. Schematic representation of different interactions of sensory–motor nerves with sympathetic and parasympathetic innervation of the heart. Classical and NANC neurotransmitters exert cardioexcitatory (+) or inhibitory (−) activity. In addition, the sympathetic transmitters NAd, NPY and ATP have neuromodulatory actions on sensory–motor nerve activity by inhibiting (−) release of neuropeptides. ACh (via nicotinic mechanisms) and its co-transmitter, VIP, both activate sensory–motor nerves, while CGRP inhibits (−) parasympathetic neurotransmission at a prejunctional site. In contrast, SP, co-released with CGRP from sensory–motor nerves, has excitatory effects (+) on parasympathetic innervation. (From Rubino et al. (1996).)

dynorphins are present together with SP and CGRP in the afferent projections to the lumbosacral spinal cord. The reduction in innervation by VIP, SP and CGRP, but not NPY-containing nerve fibres, in the unstable bladder with urinary outflow prostatic obstruction indicates possible afferent dysfunction resulting from the prostatic obstruction . VIP has been localized in other sensory neurones, those of the dorsal root and trigeminal ganglion of several species.

ATP is established as a co-transmitter with peptides in small primary sensory nerves mediating mechanical and/or nociceptive signals (Burnstock and Wood 1996).

NOS has been localized in populations of primary sensory neurones of trigeminal and dorsal root ganglia, where its functional role is yet to be elucidated.

Neurotransmission involving intrinsic neurones: special reference to neurotransmitters localized in nerve cell bodies in the heart, bladder, intestine, and lung

Intrinsic neurones are numerous throughout the autonomic nervous system. They have been demonstrated by persistence after extrinsic denervation and by tissue culture techniques in the heart, bladder, lung, and alimentary tract . The intrinsic neurones of the myenteric and submucous plexuses of the gastrointestinal tract have been analysed extensively (Furness and Costa 1987). These enteric neurones contain a variety of neuroactive substances, sometimes up to six different neuropeptides existing in a single neurone. It is likely that these substances act as neuromodulators and/or trophic factors rather than neurotransmitters. ATP is still a main contender as a neurotransmitter responsible for the inhibitory junction potentials that predominate from the stomach to the rectum, probably co-released with NO and VIP, albeit in different proportions in different regions of the gut (Burnstock 1996c).

The projections and connections of enteric neurones containing specific neuropeptides have been defined in an elaborate series of surgical manipulations (Furness and Costa 1987). Some enteric neurones project from the intestine to innervate the mesenteric arteries and arterioles of the colon; however, most form a complex network of interconnections between the two major plexuses and the mucosa. With such an integrated system, it is easy to see how an imbalance in the level of just one neuropeptide could lead to disordered intestinal motility, for example, VIP levels are altered in the distal colon in man in two such disorders, being reduced in patients with idiopathic constipation and increased in diverticular disease.

There are many intrinsic neurones in the heart, particularly in the right atrium where guanethidine sympathectomy leads to a depletion of only 46 per cent of NPY. Tissue-culture studies on newborn guinea-pig atria have shown immunostaining for NPY, 5-HT, and NOS in subpopulations of intrinsic cardiac neurones (Hassall et al. 1992). Projections of these intrinsic neurones form perivascular plexuses in small coronary vessels but do not innervate large coronary arteries. NOS-positive perivascular nerves have been localized in arterioles of the atria (Sosunov et al. 1995). Intrinsic neurones have been reported to express receptors for ACh, NAd,

purines, and several neuropeptides and amino acids. The range of interactions between extrinsic sympathetic, parasympathetic, and sensory–motor fibres and intracardiac neurones illustrates the high degree of complexity of these neurones and their possible importance in the modulation of extrinsic nervous input to the heart (Rubino et al. 1996).

Intrinsic ganglia in the bladder wall consist of sophisticated circuitry to allow integration of activities in the bladder and urethra. These ganglia have been shown to contain both NPY and somatostatin. Intramural ganglia containing NPY and VIP have been identified in the human urethra.

Information is unfolding regarding the electrophysiological characteristics of intramural ganglia within the tracheobronchial tree of the airways. Two extreme types of firing behaviour have been identified in intramural paratracheal neurones, short, high-frequency bursts of action potentials at regular intervals in response to prolonged stimulation, and no burst firing activity but firing tonically at low frequencies for the duration of the applied stimulus. The high degree of electrophysiological specialization displayed by these neurones suggests that they may act as sites of integration and/or modulation of the input from extrinsic nerves, or permit some local control of aspects of airway function by local reflex mechanisms. The interconnections of intramural ganglia within the respiratory tract and their projections to airway smooth muscle, submucosal glands and bronchial arteries are only now beginning to be understood. There is recent evidence that a substantial number of paratracheal ganglia express NOS.

Plasticity of the autonomic nervous system: some examples of altered expression of neurotransmitters/ neuromodulators in autonomic nerves during development, ageing, following trauma, surgery, chronic exposure to drugs and in disease

Neurones possess the genetic potential to produce many neurotransmitters. The particular combination and quantity that results is partly pre-programmed and partly determined by 'trophic' factors that trigger the expression or suppression of the appropriate genetic machinery. A number of studies have demonstrated the plasticity of the autonomic nervous system in development and ageing, following trauma, surgery, and chronic exposure to drugs, and in disease (Burnstock 1990b; Milner and Burnstock 1994).

The pattern of innervation of blood vessels by sympathetic nerves with age is known to vary considerably from one vessel to another. Studies of the development of peptide-containing perivascular nerves show that even peptides that are co-localized within the same nerve fibre do not show the same innervation pattern during development. In cerebral vessels of the ageing rat, there is a decrease in the expression of the vasoconstrictor neurotransmitters, NAd and 5-HT, but an increase in the expression of the vasodilator neurotransmitters, VIP, and CGRP. In humans, a decrease in the levels of NPY, VIP and SP in cerebral vessels has been reported between the ages of 1 and 46 years, consistent, in terms of relative life span, with the changes reported in rat. During pregnancy, the expression of NPY in perivascular nerves of the uterine artery increases while NAd levels fall, an event unrelated to systemic progesterone treatment.

In patients with bladder areflexia following lower motor spinal lesion there is increased innervation by VIP, NPY, and NAd-containing nerve fibres to the striated muscle of the intrinsic external urethral sphincter, which may indicate a regulatory mechanism via the intrinsic ganglia and/or the somatic nervous system to help overcome this type of bladder dysfunction.

An example of plasticity of expression of co-transmitters in parasympathetic nerves supplying the human urinary bladder is seen in patients with interstitial cystitis when there is an increase in the ratio of purinergic to cholinergic components of excitatory transmission (Palea *et al.* 1993). A greater co-transmitter role for ATP compared with NAd in the vasculature of spontaneously hypertensive rats has also been reported (see Burnstock 1986*b*).

Sympathectomy produces remarkable changes in the innervation of tissues, for example: unilateral removal of the superior cervical ganglion results in the reinnervation of the denervated cerebral vessels by sprouting nerves from the contralateral ganglion; surgical ganglionectomy leads to increased SP levels in the iris and ciliary body, increased CGRP in pial vessels, and increased expression of NPY in *parasympathetic* neurones supplying cerebral vessels (Mione *et al.* 1990); and long-term guanethidine sympathectomy of both neonate and adult rats results in a drastic increase in the innervation of tissues by the sensory neuropeptide, CGRP, probably due to increased availability to nerve growth factor for which sensory and sympathetic neurones compete (Fig. 8.5, Aberdeen *et al.* 1992). In the myenteric plexus of the ileum, NA levels and catecholamine fluorescent nerve fibres from a non-sympathetic source reappear several months after complete guanethidine sympathectomy (Milner *et al.* 1995). Following parasympathetic denervation of the cat bladder, there is a reorganization of sympathetic preganglionic connections such that there is a conversion of sympathetic inhibitory pathways to excitatory pathways in the denervated bladder. Further, after extrinsic denervation of human respiratory tract by heart–lung transplantation, the intrinsic parasympathetic neurones that persist express an NAd-synthesizing enzyme and NPY, substances normally found in sympathetic nerves. Chronic stimulation of sympathetic nerves induces structural neuromuscular changes and alters the expression of neurotransmitters in related ganglia.

During the course of experimentally induced diabetes there are marked changes in the expression of neurotransmitters/neuromodulators in nerves supplying the bowel. While there are degenerative changes in VIP and NAd-containing nerves early on in the development of the disease, the expression of 5-HT, SP, and CGRP in nerve fibres changes at different times during the progression of the disease. Patients with autonomic neuropathy, including alcoholic and diabetic neuropathy, have reduced levels of SP in their sural nerves, while the change in NAd levels is specific to diabetic neuropathy.

These are just a few examples of altered expression of neurotransmitter substances in the autonomic nervous system, some reflecting damage to nerves, some compensatory, and some appearing to lead to an altered neural control of the tissue in question. Knowledge of the factors controlling the expression of these neurotransmitters/neuromodulators may aid manipulation of the autonomic nervous system in disease to encourage beneficial compensatory changes and hence offers an enormous potential for therapy.

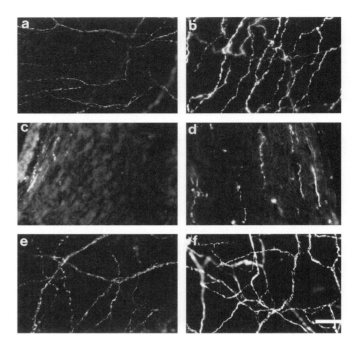

Fig. 8.5. Representative fluorescence micrographs showing the effect of long-term guanethidine sympathectomy of adult rats on CGRP-containing nerve fibres in the mesenteric vein (a,b), the prostatic end of the vas deferens (c,d), and the mesenteric artery (e,f). Left-hand panels are control tissues (a,c,e) and right-hand panels (b,d,f) are treated tissues. CGRP-immunoreactive fibres increased markedly in density and in immunofluorescence intensity in each of these tissues after guanethidine treatment. CGRP-immunoreactive fibres were increased in density in both ends of the vas deferens. Scale bar = 50 μm for all plates. (From Aberdeen *et al.* (1992).)

Conclusions

A combination of the variety of neurotransmitters involved in autonomic neurotransmission and the interactions between sympathetic, parasympathetic and sensory–motor nerves, and those arising from intrinsic ganglia, via mechanisms of co-transmission and pre- and postjunctional neuromodulation, indicate the complexity of peripheral autonomic control and the variety of ways by which autonomic dysfunction can occur. Recent advances in the unravelling of these mechanisms, together with molecular identification of specific receptor subtypes and localization and characterization of their expression, and of the long-term effects of dysfunction, will bring advances towards the design of treatment regimes to combat autonomic failure.

References

Abbracchio, M. P. and Burnstock, G. (1994). Purinoceptors: are there families of P2X and P2Y purinoceptors? *Pharmacol. Ther.* **64**, 445–75.

Aberdeen, J., Milner, P., Lincoln, J., and Burnstock, G. (1992). Guanethidine sympathectomy of mature rats leads to increases in calcitonin gene-related peptide and vasoactive intestinal polypeptide-containing nerves. *Neuroscience* **47**, 453–61.

Bo, X. and **Burnstock, G.** (1995). Characterization and autoradiographic localisation of [³H] α β methylene ATP binding sites in human urinary bladder. *Br. J. Urol.* **76**, 297–302.

Brizzolara, A. L., Crowe, R., and **Burnstock, G.** (1993). Evidence for the involvement of both ATP and nitric oxide in non-adrenergic, non-cholinergic inhibitory neurotransmission in the rabbit portal vein. *Br. J. Pharmacol.* **109**, 606–8.

Burnstock, G. (1972). Purinergic nerves. *Pharmacol. Rev.* **24**, 509–81.

Burnstock, G. (1986*a*). Autonomic neuromuscular junctions: current developments and future directions. *J. Anat.* **146**, 1–30.

Burnstock, G. (1986*b*). The changing face of autonomic neurotransmission. (The First von Euler Lecture in Physiology). *Acta Physiol. Scand.* **126**, 67–91.

Burnstock, G. (1987). Mechanisms of interaction of peptide and nonpeptide vascular neurotransmitter systems. *J. Cardiovasc. Pharmacol.* **10** (Suppl. 12), S74–S81.

Burnstock, G. (1988). Autonomic neural control mechanisms. In *Neural regulation of the airways in health and disease,* (ed. M. Kaliner and P. Barnes), pp. 1–22. Marcel Dekker, New York.

Burnstock, G. (1995). Noradrenaline and ATP: cotransmitters and neuro-modulators. *J. Physiol. Pharmacol.* **46**, 365–84.

Burnstock, G. (1996*a*). P2 purinoceptors: historical perspective and classification. In *P2-Purinoceptors: localization, function and transduction mechanisms,* Ciba Foundation Symposium198, pp. 1–34. John Wiley & Sons, Chichester.

Burnstock, G. (guest editor) (1996*b*). Purinergic neurotransmission. *Semin. Neurosci.* **8**, 171–257.

Burnstock, G. (1996*c*). Cotransmission with particular emphasis on the involvement of ATP. In *Molecular mechanisms of neuronal communication. A tribute to Nils-Åke Hillarp,* (ed. K. Fuxe, T. Hökfelt, L. Olson, D. Ottoson, A. Dahlström, and A. Björklund), pp. 67–87. Pergamon Press, Oxford.

Burnstock, G. and **Ralevic, V.** (1994). New insights into the local regulation of blood flow by perivascular nerves and endothelium. *Br. J. Plast. Surg.* **47**, 527–43.

Burnstock, G. and **Wood, J. N.** (1996). Purinergic receptors: their role in nociception and primary afferent neurotransmission. *Curr. Opin. Neurobiol.* **6**, 526–32.

Dockray, G. J. (1994). Physiology of enteric neuropeptides. In *Physiology of the gastrointestinal tract,* (3rd edn), (ed. L.R. Johnson), pp 169–209. Raven Press, New York.

Evans, R. J. and **Surprenant, A.** (1992). ATP mediates fast synaptic transmission in mammalian neurons. *Nature* **357**, 503–5.

Furness, J. B. and **Costa, M.** (1987). *The enteric nervous system.* Churchill Livingstone, Edinburgh.

Hassall, C. J. S., Saffrey, M. J., Belai, A. *et al.* (1992). Nitric oxide synthase immunoreactivity and NADPH-diaphorase activity in a subpopulation of intrinsic neurones of the guinea-pig heart. *Neurosci. Lett.* **143**, 65–8.

Jacobson, K. A. and **Suzuki, F.** (1996). Recent developments in selective agonists and antagonists acting at purine and pyrimidine receptors. *Drug Dev. Res.* **39**, 289–300.

Lincoln, J., Hoyle, C. H. V., and **Burnstock, G.** (1997). *Nitric oxide in health and disease.* Cambridge University Press, Cambridge.

Lundberg, J. M. (1981). Evidence for coexistence of vasoactive intestinal polypeptide (VIP) and acetylcholine in neurones of cat exocrine glands. Morphological, biochemical and functional studies. *Acta Physiol. Scand. Suppl.* **496**, 1–57.

Milner, P. and **Burnstock, G.** (1994). Trophic factors in the control of smooth muscle development and innervation. In *Airways smooth muscle: development and regulation of contractility,* (ed. D. Raeburn and M. A. Giembycz), pp. 1–39. Birkhäuser Verlag, Basel, Switzerland.

Milner, P., Lincoln, J., Belai, A., and **Burnstock, G.** (1995). Plasticity in the myenteric plexus of the rat ileum after long-term sympathectomy. *Int. J. Dev. Neurosci.* **13**, 385–92.

Mione, M. C., Ralevic, V., and **Burnstock, G.** (1990). Peptides and vasomotor mechanisms. *Pharmacol. Ther.* **46**, 429–68.

Modin, A. (1994). Non-adrenergic, non-cholinergic vascular control with reference to neuropeptide Y, vasoactive intestinal polypeptide and nitric oxide. *Acta Physiol. Scand. Suppl.* **622**, 1–74.

Nozaki, K., Moskowitz, M. A., Maynard, K. I., *et al.* (1993). Possible origins and distribution of immunoreactive nitric oxide synthase-containing nerve fibres in cerebral arteries. *J. Cereb. Blood Flow Metab.* **13**, 70–9.

Palea, S., Artibani, W., Ostardo, E., Trist, D. G., and **Pietra, C.** (1993). Evidence for purinergic neurotransmission in human urinary bladder affected by interstitial cystitis. *J. Urol.* **150**, 2007–12.

Rand, M.J. (1992). Nitrergic transmission: nitric oxide as a mediator of non-adrenergic, non-cholinergic neuro-effector transmission. *Clin. Exp. Pharmacol. Physiol.* **19**, 147–69.

Rubino, A. and **Burnstock, G.** (1996). Capsaicin-sensitive sensory–motor neurotransmission in the peripheral control of cardiovascular function. *Cardiovasc. Res.* **31**, 467–79.

Rubino, A., Hassall, C. J. S., and **Burnstock, G.** (1996). Autonomic control of the myocardium: non-adrenergic non-cholinergic (NANC) mechanisms. In *The autonomic nervous system,* Vol. 9: *Nervous control of the heart,* (ed. J. T. Shepherd and S. F. Vatner; series ed. G. Burnstock), pp. 139–77. Harwood Academic Publishers, Switzerland.

Sosunov, A. A., Hassall, C. J. S., Loesch, A., Turmaine, M., and **Burnstock, G.** (1995). Ultrastructural investigation of nitric oxide synthase-immunoreactive nerves associated with coronary blood vessels of rat and guinea-pig. *Cell Tiss. Res.* **280**, 575-82.

9. Control of blood pressure and the circulation in man

R. F. J. Shepherd and J. T. Shepherd

Introduction

The mechanisms that regulate the arterial blood pressure are complex indeed, involving peripheral sensors, centres in the nervous system, cardiovascular nerves, and endothelial and humoral factors. This brief review will focus on the importance of the regulation of the sympathetic nerves to the systemic resistance blood vessels, their neurotransmitters, the nitrergic nerves, and endothelium-derived nitric oxide.

Sympathetic nerves

In 1946, Von Euler showed that noradrenaline was formed and released from the sympathetic nerves. Since then adenosine triphosphate and neuropeptide Y, a 36-amino-acid peptide, have been identified as co-transmitters (Burnstock 1993; Burnstock and Ralevic 1996). The relative release of these transmitters may depend on the pattern and relative frequency of the action potentials (Stjärne *et al.* 1993). In the smooth muscle of the systemic vessels, noradrenaline excites α_1- and α_2-adrenoceptors, adenosine triphosphate, P_{2x} purinoceptors, and neuropeptide Y, Y_1 receptors to cause vasoconstriction (Fig. 9.1). By contrast in the coronary arteries, the simultaneous activation of β-adrenoceptors and P_{2y} receptors results in their dilatation. Neuropeptide Y also enhances the activity of noradrenaline and adenosine triphosphate on their receptors (Westfall *et al.* 1995). α_2-Adrenoreceptors and neuropeptide Y_2 receptors also are present on the sympathetic nerve varicosities. If these are activated, there is a decrease in the output of norepinephrine and adenosine triphosphate. Also, if adenosine triphosphate is metabolized to adenosine in the synaptic cleft, the latter, by activating a P_1 receptor on the nerve endings, could contribute to the decrease in neurotransmitter release (Fig. 9.1).

In healthy humans, part of the vasoconstrictor action of angiotensin II on forearm resistance vessels is sympathetically mediated, either by activation of angiotensin II receptors on the sympathetic nerve varicosities with resultant increased output of noradrenaline, or by enhancing the actions of noradrenaline on the smooth muscle (Lyons *et al.* 1995).

Reflex control of sympathetic nerve activity

Continuous measurements over a 24-hour period during which normal activities are pursued have shown that, in healthy individuals, arterial blood pressure varies widely as a consequence of continuous

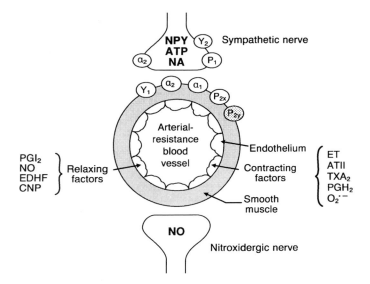

Fig. 9.1. Regulation of systemic resistance blood vessels by perivascular neurotransmitters and endothelium-derived vasoactive factors. The neurotransmitters released from the sympathetic nerves, noradrenaline (NA), adenosine triphosphate (ATP), and neuropeptide Y (NPY), cause contraction of the arterial resistance vessels by NA activating α_1- (α_1) and α_2- adrenoceptors (α_2), ATP activating P_{2X} receptors, and NPY activating Y_1 receptors. Some of the ATP may activate a vasodilator P_{2Y} receptor, but the vasoconstriction predominates. Some of the NA can activate an α_2-adrenoceptor (α_2) on the endothelial cells. The resultant release of NO can attenuate the vasoconstriction. The release of NO from nitroxidergic nerves will cause vasorelaxation. The normal resting endothelial cells continuously release NO to relax the underlying smooth muscle. The other entothelium-derived relaxation factors are prostacyclin (PGl_2), endothelium-derived hyperpolarizing factor (EDHF), and C-type natriuretic peptide (CNP). The endothelial cells also have the potential to release vasoconstrictor substances. These are endothelin-1 (ET), angiotensin II (ATII), thromboxane A_2, (TxA_2), and oxygen-derived free radicals (O_2).

changes in the activity of the nerves to the systemic resistance blood vessels. These changes originate directly from centres in the brain and also from the reflexogenic zones in the systemic circulation. They provide the body with the perfusion pressure appropriate to meet, in conjunction with the local regulation of the resistance blood vessels, the changing metabolic requirements of the organs and tissues of the body in response to the many stresses to which the cardiovascular system is subjected. Systolic and diastolic pressures move in the same direction over the 24-hour cycle, so that there is little change in pulse pressure.

Patients with autonomic failure who exhibit postural hypotension have, like normal subjects, a circadian variation in arterial pressure; however, this is the inverse of the normal pattern, with the highest pressures being at night and the lowest in the morning.

Changes in sympathetic outflow are governed by arterial baroreceptors and chemoreceptors, cardiopulmonary mechanoreceptors, and receptors in skeletal muscles activated by muscular contraction. Changes in sympathetic outflow can also occur form primary changes in the activity of particular centres in the brain. To meet the various stresses to which the body is subjected, the sympathetic outflow occurs in a differentiated pattern. Thus, in response to reflex or central stimuli, the efferent sympathetic activity varies between the different organs and tissues and, in the same organ or tissue, can vary between resistance and capacitance vessels. In some instances, it may increase in some organs and decrease in others.

The carotid and aortic baroreflexes

The primary role of the arterial baroreflexes is the rapid adjustment of arterial blood pressure around the existing mean pressure (Saunders *et al.* 1988). This is accomplished by changes in heart rate, stroke volume, cardiac contractility, total systemic vascular resistance, and venous capacitance in response to changes in activity of the stretch receptors in the carotid sinus and ascending aorta. This is done on a beat-to-beat basis and in the absence of these reflexes the blood pressure is much more labile. Since the adjustments in arterial pressure in humans are not impaired by combined β-adrenergic and parasympathetic blockade, they are due primarily to changes in total systemic vascular resistance rather than to changes in cardiac output.

Mechanical deformation of the baroreceptor sensory endings determines their afferent nerve activity, with an increase when the pressure rises and a decrease when it falls. Resetting of these receptors can occur rapidly in response to different stresses, thus permitting adjustment of their set-point and/or operating range to a higher or lower level. This can be caused by changes in the activity of the vasomotor centres, or by changes in the activity of their stretch receptors. Modulation of this latter activity can occur through ionic mechanisms and by neurohumoral and paracrine factors released from endothelial cells and platelets that act directly on the baroreceptor nerve endings (Chapleau and Abboud 1994). For example stretch-activated ion channels are present on carotid baroreceptor nerve endings, and the opening of these channels during increases in carotid sinus pressure is involved in the basic cellular mechanism of activation of the arterial baroreceptors (Hajduczok *et al.* 1994). Also, in the vascularly isolated carotid sinus of rabbits, nitric oxide (NO) and the related nitrosothiol compound, *S*-nitrosocysteine, released from the endothelial cells, suppress baroreceptor activity by a mechanism independent of guanylate cyclase activation and vascular relaxation, and that endogenous NO released by chemical activation suppresses baroreceptor activity (Matsuda *et al.* 1995).

In obesity there is a marked sympathetic activation, possibly because of reduced distensibility of the arterial walls where the arterial stretch receptors are located, with a resultant impairment of reflex sympathetic restraint (Grassi *et al.* 1995). Patients with obstructive sleep apnoea have high sympathetic activity when awake, with further increases in blood pressure and sympathetic activity during sleep. While part of this may be explained by obesity, the main reason for the high sympathetic discharge is unclear (Somers *et al.* 1995). Concerning the pathophysiology of carotid sinus syndrome, two theories have been proposed. One is a lesion of the nucleus tractus solitarius and the other abnormalities of the neuromuscular structures surrounding the carotid sinus baroreceptors. At this time, the latter is favoured (Tea *et al.* 1996). Ageing is also associated with a decrease in baroreflex activity (Folkow and Svanborg 1993).

Cardiopulmonary reflexes

Like the arterial baroreceptors, the cardiopulmonary receptors with unmyelinated vagal afferents act continuously to inhibit the vasomotor centre. Studies in dogs demonstrate that receptors in the atria, ventricles, and lungs each contribute to this tonic inhibition. When humans change from the supine to the upright position, there is a gravitational shift of blood from the cardiopulmonary region to the dependent parts. This results in a decrease in the activity of the cardiopulmonary and arterial mechanoreceptors. There follow an increase in heart rate, a decrease in stroke volume, a reflex constriction of muscle, splanchnic, and renal resistance vessels, and an increase in plasma renin activity and in plasma noradrenaline (Shepherd and Mancia 1986). In addition, the capacitance vessels, chiefly the veins, contribute by helping to maintain the mean circulatory filling pressure. This is accomplished by a reflex constriction, principally of the splanchnic venous bed. Thus, the cardiopulmonary receptors have an important role in maintaining a sustained increase in sympathetic outflow in response to reductions in central blood volume. In patients with vasovagal syndrome there is evidence of reduced cardiopulmonary baroreceptor sensitivity (Thomson *et al.* 1997). With muscular exercise, in addition to reflex splanchnic venoconstriction, there is a passive decrease in venous capacity caused by compression of the limb veins by the active muscles and by reflex constriction of the precapillary vessels (Janicki *et al.* 1996).

Ergoreflexes

A strong static contraction of the skeletal muscles or rapid powerful rhythmic contractions cause a marked increase in arterial blood pressure, the so-called blood pressure-raising reflex. This increase helps to oppose the reduction in blood flow to the muscles resulting from the mechanical compression. The evidence indicates that this rise is due majorly to products of muscle metabolism activating chemosensitive endings in the muscles, the so-called muscle metaboreceptors (Kaufman and Forster 1996). The afferent fibres involved are the small myelinated (group III) and unmyelinated (group IV). The former are active during the early seconds of muscle contraction, whereas the latter remain active (Rowell *et al.* 1996). These afferent fibres synapse with ascending tracts in the dorsal horn of the spinal cord. A muscle contraction causes a release of substance P at this site which is directly related to the tension developed. Also somatostatin is released (Mitchell and Shepherd 1993). The pressor response, which is caused by increased sympathetic outflow to the circulation, is proportional to the degree of ischaemia in the exercising muscles and to the mass of the ischaemic muscle. Mechanoreceptors stimulated by muscle contraction apparently contribute little (Ray and Mark 1995). This is consistent with a predominantly mechanosensitive role for group III, and a predominantly chemosensitive role for group IV, afferents. Human studies show that the sympathetic outflow is increased to both exercising and non-exercising muscles. In the former this modulates local vasodilator mechanisms to permit maximal oxygen extraction from the blood and regulates precapillary to postcapillary resistance to prevent excessive loss of fluid to the interstitial spaces (Mellander and Björnberg 1992). At the onset of exercise, whether dynamic or static, the arterial baroreflexes are reset. The operating point (set-point) is elevated progressively as the severity of the exercise is increased, while the shape of the stimulus response curve is unchanged. This allows the arterial pressure to increase while permitting changes in pressure around the new operating point to be buffered effectively (Rowell et al. 1996).

Role of nitric oxide in circulatory control

Endothelium

In the endothelial cells, the constitutive enzyme nitric oxide synthase (NOS) converts L-arginine to L-citrulline with a release of nitric oxide (NO). A cofactor, tetrahydrobiopterin, is required for activation of NOS (Cosentino and Katusic 1995). NO activates soluble guanylate cyclase in the underlying smooth muscle and the resultant increase in cyclic guanosine monophosphate (cGMP) causes its relaxation. The NO is inactivated in a few seconds by superoxide anions. There are numerous receptors in the endothelial cells which, if activated, cause a release of NO. Some of the noradrenaline released when the sympathetic nerves are activated stimulates α_2-adrenoceptors on the endothelial cells. The resultant release of NO attenuates the vasoconstriction (Miller and Vanhoutte 1985). Of major importance is that NO is released from these cells as a consequence of the increased shear stress associated with increased blood flow (Davies 1995); the earliest mechanochemical signal transduction is activation of specific G-proteins in the endothelium within a second of flow-induced signalling (Gudi et al. 1996).

NO forms complexes with various biomolecular carriers, such as nitrosothiol (RS–NO), that retain biological activity. Studies on the forearm resistance vessels of normal humans indicate that RS–NO contributes to vascular smooth muscle relaxation (Creager et al. 1997). Other endothelium-derived relaxing factors are prostacyclin, C-type natriuretic factor (Suga et al. 1993), and endothelium-derived hyperpolarizing factor (Cohen and Vanhoutte 1995) (Fig. 9.1).

Nitroxidergic or nitrergic nerves

These nerves have a constitutive neuronal isoform of NO synthase. They cause vasodilatation by releasing nitric oxide (Fig. 9.1), and have been identified in the cerebral, coronary, gastrointestine, renal, and penis arteries (Okamura et al. 1995; Rand and Lie 1995; Toda and Okamura 1996). Since NO is a labile free radicle, unlike other transmitters it is not stored in synaptic vesicles and is not released by exocytosis, but diffuses from the nerve terminals into adjacent cells.

NOS also is present in many regions of the brain and NO may play a role in the development of the nervous system. It also has been implicated as a mediator of neurotoxicity (Zhang and Snyder 1995). Here it decreases sympathetic outflow (Togashi et al. 1992). In rats this may be due mainly to inhibition of renal sympathetic nerve activity caused by a depressor effect on the nucleus tractus solitarius and the rostral ventrolateral medulla (Tseng et al. 1996).

Nitric oxide and arterial blood pressure

The importance of NO in regulating blood pressure is apparent from the observation that inhibition of NOS causes a rapid and sustained increase in pressure. It is suggested that this is due mainly to a suppression of the release of NO from the nitroxidergic nerves rather than an impairment of the basal release of NO from the endothelium (Toda et al. 1993). Offspring of hypertensive patients have a defect in the NO pathway, suggesting that an impairment of NO production precedes the onset of essential hypertension (Taddei et al. 1996). Also there is evidence that part of the hypertension caused by blockade of NO formation is sympathetically mediated (Sander et al. 1995).

The endothelial cells also have the capacity to synthesize the vasoconstrictor substances angiotensin II, endothelin-1, thromboxane A_2, prostaglandin H_2 and superoxide anions (Fig. 9.1). Of these, endothelin has a potency about 10 times that of angiotensin II. It has the potential to contribute to blood pressure control by contraction of vascular smooth muscle, potentiation of α-adrenergic vasoconstriction, and activation of angiontensin-converting enzyme (Rubanyi and Polokoff 1994). Circulating endothelin might suppress the activity of the stretch receptors in the carotid sinus and aortic arch (Chapleau and Abboud 1994).

The perivascular nerves have a trophic influence on vascular endothelial cells. Long-term sympathectomy causes a decrease in endothelial NOS and an increase in endothelin-1 immunoreactivity in the thoracic aortic endothelium of the rat (Aliev et al. 1996).

Of interest is the demonstration that activation of receptors on the venous endothelium, which result in endothelium-dependent relaxation in the arterial system, causes endothelium-dependent contraction of the veins (De Mey and Vanhoutte 1982). While the precise mechanisms of the venoconstriction remain to be determined, from the physiological viewpoint it is advantageous to reduce the capacity of the venous system in circumstances when the systemic vascular resistance is decreased, so that the filling pressure of the heart is maintained.

In conclusion, with the continuing advances in knowledge of the complexity of the nervous, local, and humoral factors regulating the circulation, the interactions between them, and the changes caused by disease, it is obvious that there is no lack of challenges for those concerned with the control of blood pressure and the circulation in man.

References

Aliev, G., Ralevic, V., and **Burnstock, G.** (1996). Depression of endothelial nitric oxide synthase but increased expression of endothelin-1 immunoreactivity in rat thoracic aortic endothelium associated with long-term, but not short-term, sympathectomy. *Circ. Res.* 79, 317–23.

Burnstock, G. (1993). Introduction. Changing face of autonomic and sensory nerves in circulation. In *Vascular innervation and receptor mechanisms,* (ed. L. Edvinsson and R. Uddman), *New Perspectives,* pp. 1–22. Academic Press, New York.

Burnstock, G. and Ralevic, V. (1996). Cotransmission. In *The pharmacology of smooth muscle*, (ed. C. J. Garland and J. Angus). Oxford University Press, Oxford.

Chapleau, M. W. and Abboud, F. M. (1994). Modulation of baroreceptor activity by ionic and paracrine mechanisms: an overview. *Brazilian J. Med. Biol. Res.* 27, 1001–15.

Cohen, R. A. and Vanhoutte, P. M. (1995). Endothelium-dependent hyperpolarization. Beyond nitric oxide and cyclic GMP. *Circulation* 92, 3334–49.

Cosentino, F. and Katusic, Z. (1995). Tetrahydrobiopterin and dysfunction of endothelial nitric oxide synthase in coronary arteries. *Circulation* 91, 139–44.

Creager, M. A., Roddy, M.-A., Boles, K., and Stamler, J. S. (1997). *N*-acetylcysteine does not influence the activity of endothelium-derived relaxing factor *in vivo. Hypertension* 29, 668–72.

Davies, P. F. (1995). Flow-mediated endothelial mechanotransduction. *Physiol. Rev.* 75, 519–60.

De Mey, J. G. and Vanhoutte, P. M. (1982). Heterogeneous behavior of the canine arterial and venous wall: importance of the endothelium. *Circ. Res.* 51, 439–47.

Folkow, B. and Svanborg, A. (1993). Physiology of aging. *Physiol. Rev.* 73, 725–64.

Grassi, G., Seravalle, G., Cattaneo, B. M. *et al.* (1995). Sympathetic activation in obese normotensive subjects. *Hypertension* 25 (part 1), 560–3.

Gudi, S. R. P., Clark, C. B., and Frangos, J. A. (1996). Fluid flow rapidly activates G proteins in human endothelial cells. *Circ. Res.* 79, 834–9.

Hajduczok, G., Chapleau, M. W., Ferlic, R. J., Mao, H. Z., and Abboud, F. M. (1994). Gadolinium inhibits mechanoelectrical transduction in rabbit carotid baroreceptors. Implications of stretch-activated channels. *J. Clin. Invest.* 94, 2392–6.

Janicki, J. S., Sheriff, D. D., Robotham, J. L., and Wise, R. A. (1996). Cardiac output during exercise: contributions of the cardiac, circulatory, and respiratory systems. In *Exercise: regulation and integration of multiple systems*, (ed. L. B. Rowell and J. T. Shepherd), Section 12, pp. 649–704. Published for the American Physiological Society by Oxford University Press, New York.

Kaufman, M. P. and Forster, H. V. (1996). Reflexes controlling circulatory, ventilatory and airway responses to exercise. In *Exercise: regulation and integration of multiple systems* (ed L. B. Rowell and J. T. Shepherd), Section 12, pp. 381–447. Published for the American Physiological Society by Oxford University Press, New York.

Lyons, D., Webster, J., and Benjamin, N. (1995). Angiotensin II. Adrenergic sympathetic constrictor action in humans. *Circulation* 91, 1457–60.

Matsuda, T., Bates, J. N., Lewis, S. J., Abboud, F. M., and Chapleau, M. W. (1995). Modulation of baroreceptor activity by nitric oxide and S-nitrosocysteine. *Circ. Res.* 76, 426–33.

Mellander, S. and Björnberg, J. (1992). Functional organization of vascular smooth muscle and capillary pressure regulation. *News Physiol. Sci.* 7, 113–19.

Miller, V. M. and Vanhoutte, P. M. (1985). Endothelial α_2-adrenoceptors in canine pulmonary and systemic blood vessels. *Eur. J. Pharmacol.* 118, 123–9.

Mitchell, J. H. and Shepherd, J. T. (1993). Control of the circulation during exercise. In *Exercise—the physiological challenge*, (ed. P. McN. Hill), pp. 55–85. Conference Publishing, Auckland, New Zealand.

Okamura, T., Yoshida, K., and Toda, N. (1995). Nitroxidergic innervation in dog and monkey renal arteries. *Hypertension* 25, 1090–5.

Rand, M. J. and Lie, C. G. (1995). Nitric oxide as a neurotransmitter in peripheral nerves: nature of transmitter and mechanism of transmission. *Ann. Rev. Physiol.* 57, 659–82.

Ray, C. A. and Mark, A. L. (1995). Sympathetic nerve activity to nonactive muscles of the exercising and nonexercising limb. *Med. Sci. Sports Exerc.* 27, 183–7.

Rowell, L. B., O'Leary, D. S., and Kellogg, D. L., Jr (1996). Integration of cardiovascular control systems in dynamic exercise. In *Handbook of physiology. Exercise: regulation and integration of multiple systems*, (ed. L. B. Rowell and J. T. Shepherd), Section 12, pp. 770–838. American Physiological Society, Oxford University Press, New York.

Rubanyi, G. M. and Polokoff, M. A. (1994). Endothelins: molecular biology, biochemistry, pharmacology, physiology, and pathophysiology. *Pharmacol. Rev.* 46, 328–415.

Sander, M., Hansen, P. G., and Victor, R. G. (1995). Sympathetically mediated hypertension caused by chronic inhibition of nitric oxide. *Hypertension* 26, 691–5.

Saunders, J. S., Ferguson, D. W., and Mark, A. L. (1988). Arterial baroreflex control of sympathetic nerve activity during elevation of blood pressure in normal man: dominance of aortic baroreflexes. *Circulation* 77 (2), 279–88.

Shepherd, J. T. and Mancia, G. (1986). Reflex control of the human cardiovascular system. *Rev. Physiol. Biochem. Pharmacol.* 105, 1–99.

Somers, V. K., Dyken, M. E., Clary, M. P., and Abboud, F. M. (1995). Sympathetic neural mechanisms in obstructive sleep apnea. *J. Clin. Invest.* 96, 1897–904.

Stjärne, L., Bao, J.-X., Gonon, F. G., Msghina, M., and Stjärne, A. (1993). A nonstochastic string model of sympathetic neuromuscular transmission. *News Physiol. Sci.* 8, 253–60.

Suga, S., Itoh, H., Komatsu, Y. *et al.* (1993). Cytokine-induced C-type natriuretic peptide (CNP) secretion from vascular endothelial cells—evidence for CNP as a novel autocrine/paracrine regulator from endothelial cells. *Endocrinology* 133, 3038–4041.

Taddei, S., Virdis, A., Mattei, P., Ghiadoni, L., Sudano, I., and Salvetti, A. (1996). Defective L-arginine–nitric oxide pathway in offspring of essential hypertensive patients. *Circulation* 94, 1298–303.

Tea, S. H., Mansourati, J., L'Heveder, G., Mabin, D., and Blanc, J.-J. (1996). New insights into the pathophysiology of carotid sinus syndrome. *Circulation* 93, 1411–16.

Thomson, H. L., Wright, K., and Frenneaux, M. (1997). Baroreflex sensitivity in patients with vasovagal syncope. *Circulation* 95, 393–400.

Toda, N. and Okamura, T. (1996). Nitroxidergic nerve: regulation of vascular tone and blood flow in the brain. *J. Hypertension* 14, 423–34.

Toda, N., Kitamura, Y., and Okamura, T. (1993). Neural mechanisms of hypertension by nitric oxide synthase inhibition in dogs. *Hypertension* 21, 3–8.

Togashi, H., Sakuma, I., Yoshioka, M. *et al.* (1992). A central nervous system action of nitric oxide in blood pressure regulation. *J. Pharmacol. exp. Ther.* 262, 343–7.

Tseng, C.-J., Liv, H.-Y., Lin, H.-C. *et al.* (1996). Cardiovascular effects of nitric oxide in the brain stem nuclei of rats. *Hypertension* 27, 36–42.

Westfall, T. C., Yang, C. L., and Cunfman-Falrey, M. (1995). Neuropeptide Y–ATP interactions at the vascular sympathetic neuroeffector junction. *J. Cardiovasc. Pharmacol.* 26, 682–7.

Zhang, J. and Snyder, S. H. (1995). Nitric oxide in the nervous system. *Ann. Rev. Pharmacol. Toxicol.* 35, 213–33.

10. Autonomic and neurohumoral control of the cerebral circulation

Michael A. Moskowitz and Robert Macfarlane

Introduction

There is considerable evidence to support the notion that the sensory and autonomic innervation to the cranium can influence cerebral blood flow under a variety of pathological conditions, and that perivascular sensory nerves play a pivotal role in the development of certain types of head pain, including migraine and cluster headache. This chapter will explore current knowledge of the neural control of the cerebral circulation, and the circumstances under which modulation of the activity of these nerves may be of therapeutic benefit.

The vascular hypothesis of migraine

A vascular aetiology for migraine was first proposed in the 1930s. Accentuated pulsation was observed in the superficial temporal artery during the headache phase of migraine, and treatment with the vasoconstrictor ergotamine both relieved the headache and appeared to diminish the arterial pulsation. Subsequent studies elicited that stimulation of dural arteries at craniotomy provoked throbbing ipsilateral head pain, and that several other drugs efficacious in treating migraine were also vasoconstrictors. The fact that dilatation of cerebral arteries induced by either pharmacological means (e.g. trinitrate or histamine administration) or by mechanical distension (e.g. balloon angioplasty) results in head pain, and that sumatriptan, an effective antimigraine drug that has no known analgesic properties, reduces middle cerebral artery calibre, adds further weight to a direct association between cerebral vasodilatation and headache. Indeed, having identified that cerebral blood vessels contain 5-HT$_{1\beta}$ receptors that mediate constriction, sumatriptan was developed specifically as a selective agonist for this receptor, and has been shown to be efficacious in the treatment of migraine. Yet, compelling though the vascular hypothesis may at first sight appear, the link between vasodilatation and head pain cannot be that simple. Subarachnoid haemorrhage is a potent cause of headache yet is associated with vasoconstriction not vasodilatation, and a doubling of cerebral blood flow (CBF) by carbon dioxide inhalation is not painful at all. Furthermore, single photon emission computed tomography (SPECT) studies of regional cerebral blood flow have failed to show a consistent relationship between headache and hyperaemia during the acute phase of migraine headache. The same holds true for countless other studies spanning more than 50 years, which have been designed to validate cerebral vasodilatation as the fundamental basis for the headache in migraine.

The sensory innervation to the cranium is central to the appreciation of head pain. As such, the trigeminal nerve, its associated neuro-transmitters, and the pain-sensitive structures within the cranium are a logical focus for study in search of a better understanding of the pathophysiological basis for headache. Furthermore, pial sensory and autonomic nerve endings contain potent vasoactive neuropeptides that may influence cerebral blood flow under a variety of other circumstances. One recent report documents the occurrence of sensitization and intracranial mechanical hypersensitivity following chemical stimulation of dura mater with inflammatory mediators (Strassman *et al.* 1996). It has been proposed that these properties contribute to mechanical hypersensitivity and the throbbing pain of migraine.

The autonomic and sensory innervation of the cerebral vasculature: neurogenic influences on cerebral blood flow

Autonomic

Sympathetic

The sympathetic innervation to the cerebral vasculature is largely via the superior cervical ganglion. In addition to the catecholamines, sympathetic nerve terminals contain another potent vasoconstrictor, neuropeptide Y (NPY). This 36-amino-acid neuropeptide is found in abundance in both the central and peripheral nervous systems.

Only minor (5–10 per cent) reductions in cerebral blood flow accompany electrical stimulation of sympathetic nerves; far less than that seen in other vascular beds. Although feline pial arterioles vasoconstrict in response to topical noradrenaline and the response is blocked by the α-blocker phenoxybenzamine, application of the latter alone at the same concentration has no effect on vessel calibre. This and other observations from denervation studies indicate that the sympathetic nervous system does not exert a significant tonic influence on cerebral vessels under physiological conditions. Neither does the sympathetic innervation contribute to CBF regulation under conditions of hypotension or hypoxia. However, sympathetic stimulation does produce a profound fall in CBF if cerebral vessels have been dilated by hypercapnia. From this observation came the 'dual control' hypothesis, proposing that the cerebral circulation is comprised of two resistances in series. Extraparenchymal vessels are thought to be regulated largely by the autonomic nervous system, while intraparenchymal vessels are responsible for the main resistance under physiological conditions, and are governed primarily by intrinsic metabolic and myogenic factors.

As well as exerting a significant influence on cerebral blood volume, the sympathetic innervation has been shown to protect the brain from the effects of acute severe hypertension. When blood pressure rises above the limits of autoregulation, activation of the sympathetic nervous system attenuates the anticipated rise in CBF, and reduces the plasma protein extravasation that follows breakdown of the blood–brain barrier. The autoregulatory curve is 'reset' such that both the upper and lower limits are raised. This is an important physiological mechanism by which the cerebral vasculature is protected from injury during surges in arterial blood pressure. Although cerebral vessels escape from the vasoconstrictor response to sympathetic stimulation under conditions of normotension, this does not occur during acute hypertension.

Sympathetic nerves are also thought to exert trophic influences upon the vessels that they innervate. Sympathectomy reduces the hypertrophy of the arterial wall that develops in response to chronic hypertension. Denervation has been shown to increase the susceptibility of stroke-prone spontaneously hypertensive rats to bleed into the cerebral hemisphere that has been sympathectomized (Mueller and Heistad 1980).

Parasympathetic

The cerebrovascular parasympathetic innervation derives from multiple sources, including the sphenopalatine and otic ganglia, and small clusters of ganglion cells within the cavernous plexus, Vidian, and lingual nerves. Vasoactive intestinal polypeptide (VIP), a potent 28-amino-acid polypeptide vasodilator that is non-EDRF dependent, has been localized immunohistochemically within parasympathetic nerve endings, as has nitric oxide synthase, the enzyme that forms nitric oxide from L-arginine. The multiple sources of innervation and the lack of a suitable VIP antagonist have for some time hampered investigation of the role of the parasympathetic innervation on the cerebral circulation. However, lesioning experiments are now possible following identification of unique parasympathetic anatomy in the rat, where the fibres enter the cranium from the orbit via the ethmoidal foramen.

Although stimulation of parasympathetic nerves does elicit a rise in cortical blood flow, there is, like the sympathetic nervous system, little to suggest that cholinergic mechanisms contribute significantly to CBF regulation under physiological conditions. Nor are parasympathetic nerves involved in the vasodilatory response to hypercapnia. However, chronic parasympathetic denervation increases infarct volume by 37 per cent in rats subjected to permanent middle cerebral artery occlusion, primarily because of a reduction in CBF under situations when perfusion pressure is reduced (Kano et al. 1991). This suggests that parasympathetic nerves may help to maintain cerebral perfusion at times of reduced blood flow, and may in part explain why patients with autonomic neuropathy, such as diabetics, are at increased risk of stroke.

Sensory

The sensory innervation to the brain and meninges is largely via unmyelinated nerve fibres, and has been studied with axonal tracing techniques using wheatgerm agglutinin and horseradish immunoperoxidase. The basic anatomy is remarkably similar in different mammalian species. The sensory innervation is confined to the dura mater, particularly the dural arteries and venous sinuses, and to the larger intracranial arteries (>50 μm diameter). Structures within the supratentorial compartment and rostral third of the posterior fossa are supplied by the ophthalmic division of the trigeminal nerve, supplemented by a small contribution from the maxillary division in primates. The more caudal elements in the posterior fossa are innervated by the C1–2 dorsal roots. The distribution is ipsilateral, with the exception of midline structures that receive a dual innervation. Each individual ganglion cell projects multiple axon collaterals that innervate both the larger branches of the circle of Willis and the overlying dura mater. The extracranial trigeminal innervation is distinct, and no individual neurone supplies both intra- and extracranial structures. Centrally, however, there is convergence, with somatic afferents (innervating the extra-calvarial structures) and visceral afferents (innervating the meninges and cerebral vessels) synapsing onto single interneurones within the trigeminal nucleus caudalis.

The sensory C fibres form a fine network on the adventitial surface of cerebral vessels, and at the junction between adventitia and media. The nerve endings are naked, and contain multiple vesicles which are in close proximity to vascular smooth muscle.

The trigeminovascular system

Contained within vesicles in the naked nerve endings are many different neuropeptides. The most important include the tachykinins, substance P (SP) and neurokinin A (NKA), together with calcitonin-gene-related peptide (CGRP), one of the three products of the calcitonin gene. SP and CGRP are co-localized within nerve terminals. All three, particularly CGRP, are vasodilators, whereas SP and NKA also promote plasma protein extravasation within dura mater (reviewed by Limmroth et al. 1996). Unlike the tachykinins, CGRP inhibits the vasoconstrictor response to sympathetic stimulation and shortens the constrictor response to noradrenaline.

Neurotransmitter release may follow either orthodromic or antidromic mechanisms. Electrical stimulation of the trigeminal ganglion elicits neurogenic vasodilatation in the facial skin and dura mater, and an increase in CGRP levels in the superior sagittal sinus. The cutaneous vasodilatation which accompanies reperfusion of a limb after a period of arterial occlusion is associated with an increase in venous SP, is diminished by chronic sensory denervation, and mimicked by intra-arterial infusion of substance P. The molecules released in response to tissue injury are likely to provide the stimulus for sensory depolarization during ischaemia.

Electrical stimulation of trigeminal afferents elicits a relatively small (17 per cent) and short-lived increase in CBF. Denervation studies, primarily in cats and rats, have demonstrated that perivascular sensory nerves do not have a significant role to play in CBF regulation under physiological conditions. Basal CBF and the vasodilatory response to hypercapnia are unaffected by neurotransmitter depletion. This is in keeping with the nature of these neuropeptides, which have relatively long-lasting effects on the cerebral circulation, and are therefore unsuited for moment-to-moment regulation. However, trigeminal ganglionectomy diminishes the increase in CBF (around 30 per cent) that accompanies acute severe hypertension or seizures in cats, and diminishes the extravasation of radiolabelled albumin that results from disruption of the blood–brain barrier (Sakas et al. 1989). Chronic sensory denervation also attenuates the increase in blood flow that occurs during the early phase of bacterial meningitis (Weber et al. 1996). The hyperaemic response to transient global cerebral ischaemia is reduced by around 50 per cent in cortical grey matter following chronic sensory denervation, but not in the white matter or deep grey matter of the same vascular territory, both of which have a sparse sensory innervation (Moskowitz *et al.* 1989; Sakas *et al.* 1989). The pial arteriolar constrictor response to topical noradrenaline is also prolonged by trigeminal ganglionectomy. A number of putative substances have been implicated in sensory nerve fibre activation during these pathological processes, including bradykinin, potassium, hydrogen ions, adenosine, prostaglandins, leucotrienes, and arachidonate metabolites.

None of the changes in blood flow described above occur acutely after nerve section, i.e. before the nerve endings have been depleted of their neurotransmitters. Nor do they occur after section of the trigeminal nerve proximal to the Gasserian ganglion. The latter will block central transmission, but will not promote Wallerian degeneration as will sectioning of the distal nerve. This indicates that neurotransmitters are released in response to antidromic stimulation independent of central control, i.e. via axon reflex-like mechanisms.

There are several circumstances under which sensory nerve-mediated vasodilatation may be beneficial. It has been suggested that one role may be to provide a protective mechanism to enhance CBF early after subarachnoid haemorrhage, when there is excessive vasoconstriction of large arteries. Several days after subarachnoid haemorrhage there is depletion of neurotransmitters from sensory nerve endings and, in some experimental models, this coincides with the development of cerebral vasospasm. Recent experiments in the monkey have shown that instillation of CGRP into the basal cisterns significantly attenuates the development of delayed vasospasm after subarachnoid haemorrhage (Inoue *et al.* 1996). Secondly, the postocclusive hyperaemia mediated by the trigeminovascular system may help to re-establish perfusion after a period of ischaemia, thereby reducing the risk that some areas of the brain will fail to reperfuse at all—the 'no-reflow' phenomenon (see Macfarlane *et al.* 1991). Thirdly, CGRP has been shown to have a trophic effect on cultured endothelial cells, suggesting a possible role for sensory nerves in angiogenesis (Haegerstrand *et al.* 1990).

Neurogenic inflammation and head pain

Neurogenic inflammation is thought to be an important immediate endogenous defence mechanism in tissue injury (the nocifensor system). The inflammatory response is thought to sensitize the nerve endings, thereby perpetuating the pain after the injurious stimulus has been removed.

Cephalic blood vessels contain a number of nociceptive molecules, including histamine, serotonin, bradykinin, and prostaglandins. Intravenous infusion of SP and NKA, or electrical stimulation of the trigeminal ganglion, results in vasodilatation, platelet aggregation, mast cell degranulation, the formation of endothelial microvilli and vesicles in postcapillary venules, and an increase in plasma protein extravasation in the ipsilateral dura.

Mast cells are found in abundance in the dura mater, and are in close proximity to SP-containing nerve fibres. Unilateral sensory stimulation results in mast cell degranulation, indicating that neural mechanisms may play one important part in the development of neurogenic inflammation. Not only do mast cells secrete many vasoactive, nociceptive, and chemoactive substances, but these in turn are able to stimulate SP release from sensory nerves, thereby amplifying the process. Perivascular oedema, plasma protein extravasation, mast cell degranulation, platelet aggregation, and vasodilatation have all been observed microscopically in the dura following both electrical sensory stimulation and in response to noxious chemical irritation (Dimitriadou *et al.* 1991). In the dura mater, neurogenic inflammation is blocked by drugs efficacious in treating migraine, including sumatriptan, the ergot alkaloids, indomethacin, aspirin, chronic administration of corticosteroids, and some nonsteroidal anti-inflammatory agents (Buzzi *et al.* 1989).

There is good evidence to suggest that serotonin receptors within the dura are a site of action for a number of antimigraine drugs. To date 14 receptor subtypes have been identified, with marked species variability. Trigeminovascular axons innervating the dura mater possess $5-HT_{1D}$-like receptors, of which there are at least six receptor subtypes (reviewed by Moskowitz and Waeber 1996). The antimigraine drugs sumatriptan and the ergot alkaloids are $5-HT_{1B/D}$ agonists, and have been shown both to block neurogenic inflammation in response to trigeminal ganglion stimulation and to attenuate the concomitant increase in CGRP within the superior sagittal sinus. Pretreatment with the $5-HT_{1D}$ receptor antagonist GR-127,935 blocks the effects of sumatriptan on leakage of plasma protein in dura mater. The mechanism must occur via prejunctional mechanisms because the inflammatory response to exogenous SP and NKA is unaffected by sumatriptan, the sumatriptan analogue CP-122,288, or by dihydroergotamine. Neither can the mechanism of action of the antimigraine drugs be the result of vasoconstriction of meningeal arteries, since neither angiotensin nor phenylephrine are able to diminish neurogenic inflammation in the same animal model. A strain of knockout mice, deficient in the expression of the $5-HT_{1B}$ receptor, have helped to confirm the importance of this receptor subtype for the actions of sumatriptan, dihydroergotamine, and other $5-HT_1$ receptor agonists in this species (Yu *et al.* 1996). In rats, not only do the antimigraine drugs diminish plasma protein extravasation and attenuate CGRP levels within the superior sagittal sinus, but they reduce the ultrastructural changes seen in the endothelium, platelets, and mast cells as a result of sensory fibre stimulation. Most recently, the importance of the $5-HT_{1F}$ receptor subtype for inhibition of the plasma extravasation response within the meninges has been documented. $5-HT_{1F}$ receptors are expressed in meningeal vascular smooth muscle, but are not coupled to vasoconstriction. Clinical trials using agonists to the $5-HT_{1F}$ receptor for treatment of migraine are now under way.

The trigeminovascular system and headache

The anatomy of the cranial sensory innervation accounts for a number of the characteristics of headache which, in many respects, are no different to the types of pain experienced with inflammation in other organs. As well as the strictly unilateral distribution of some headaches, the convergence of trigeminal somatic and intracranial nerves onto single interneurones accounts for referral of pain to the forehead (or cervico-occipital region in the case of the caudal elements within the posterior fossa innervated by C1–2) and for the accompanying tension in the frontalis, temporalis, and cervico-occipital musculature (analogous to referred pain and muscle rigidity in cholecystitis or appendicitis, for example). Because the innervation is sparse and with large receptive fields, the pain is poorly localized. Central projections to the nucleus of the tractus solitarius account for the autonomic responses (sweating, tachycardia, hypertension, and vomiting) that may accompany it. Following experimental subarachnoid haemorrhage, a potent cause of headache, peptide and messenger RNA synthesis increase within the trigeminal ganglion, and is consistent with elevated metabolic and neuronal activity. Clinically, an increase in levels of CGRP can be detected in the jugular vein of patients with migraine and subarachnoid haemorrhage, suggesting enhanced release from sensory nerves. Agents that either destroy sensory nerve fibres (e.g. neonatal capsaicin), block action potentials (local anaesthetics), or inhibit neuropeptide release (5-HT$_{1D}$-like agonists), all inhibit neurogenic inflammation in the dura mater. Elevated CGRP levels in the superior sagittal sinus in both animals and humans are decreased by treatment with the serotonin agonist sumatriptan (Goadsby and Edvinsson 1991).

Interactions between sensory and autonomic nerves

Neuropeptide receptors (found, amongst other places, in postganglionic sympathetic fibres innervating the dura mater) have been identified on trigeminovascular afferents, and NPY receptor agonists suppress plasma protein extravasation in response to trigeminal ganglion stimulation via prejunctional mechanisms (Yu and Moskowitz 1995, 1996).

Sensory and parasympathetic nerves may have synergistic effects on the meningeal plasma protein extravasation response. The GABA transaminase activator valproic acid (another drug useful for the prophylactic treatment of migraine), and the GABA$_A$ receptor agonist, muscimol, block neurogenic plasma extravasation. The GABA receptor does not reside on trigeminovascular fibres (Lee et al. 1995). Instead, its action depends upon the integrity of parasympathetic fibres emanating from the sphenopalatine ganglion (Cutrer et al. 1995). The potential therapeutic relevance of this will be discussed later.

Central neurogenic mechanisms

The central connections of the trigeminovascular system beyond the trigeminal nuclear complex are poorly understood, but relays project to the medial, ventral, posterior medial, and interlaminar nuclei of the thalamus and thence to the cerebral cortex. Some circumstantial evidence for central trigeminal activation has become available from studies using antisera directed against the product of the early immediate response gene, c-fos. The expression of this gene has been used widely as a marker of neural activation. Following meningeal stimulation by either experimental subarachnoid haemorrhage or chemical irritation, postsynaptic cells within rexed laminae I and II$_0$ of the trigeminal nucleus caudalis (a region analogous to the dorsal horn of the spinal cord and involved in the processing of nociceptive information) express the protein antigen in a dose-dependent fashion (Nozaki et al. 1992a). This response can be blocked by either sensory denervation or treatment with antimigraine drugs, as well as with analgesics such as morphine. However, sumatriptan does not decrease the c-fos response induced when a noxious stimulus is applied to the nasal mucosa, a trigeminally innervated structure which does not possess 5-HT$_1$-like receptors. If sumatriptan were acting as an analgesic per se, both the response to noxious meningeal and nasal stimulation should be blocked.

Clinical implications
Neural mechanisms in migraine

The initiating event in migraine and the mechanisms by which the trigeminovascular system might be activated are unclear. Cortical spreading depression has been postulated as the initiating event in migraine, in which a wave of depolarization spreads across the hemisphere at a rate of approximately 2–6 mm min, and is followed by neuronal inhibition. A number of substances are capable of inducing this phenomenon in animals, although it has not been well documented in the human brain in vivo. Spreading depression can be elicited experimentally by the microapplication of potassium chloride to the pial surface of the cortex. Moskowitz et al. (1993) have shown that spreading depression is capable of activating the trigeminovascular system, as evidenced by an increase in c-fos immunoreactivity within the trigeminal nucleus caudalis. Both chronic trigeminal denervation and the antimigraine drug sumatriptan suppress c-fos expression in the trigeminal nucleus caudalis in response to spreading depression, but do not inhibit spreading depression per se. Even if spreading depression proves not to be the initiating event in migraine, this study is important in establishing that endogenous neurophysiological events within the cerebral cortex are capable of activating trigeminovascular fibres innervating the meninges and cortical vessels.

A unifying hypothesis for migraine

Although there is no direct evidence for neurogenic inflammation in human meninges, nor has it been observed during migraine, experimental headache in humans induced by histamine injection does not occur after trigeminal nerve section. We believe that some as yet unidentified trigger (likely to be a neurophysiologically driven ionic or metabolic mechanism within the brain) is responsible for depolarizing trigeminal perivascular sensory afferents on the surface of the cortex during migraine. Hydrogen ions, potassium, arachidonate metabolites, serotonin, histamine, and nitric oxide are all possible candidates for sensitizing unmyelinated nerve endings.

Because of the anatomical arrangement of the trigeminal nerve fibres (see above), axon collaterals are also depolarized in the ipsilateral dura mater. Perivascular release of neuropeptides results in vasodilatation, while in the dura mater there follows neurogenic inflammation. The latter sensitizes the nerve endings, hence perpetuating the headache. Central projections are responsible for the vegetative symptoms that accompany the headache. Antimigraine drugs are effective not by directly altering vessel calibre, but by their prejunctional activity which blocks nerurotransmitter release and neurotransmission. The effect is to suppress neurogenic inflammation and central transmission, thereby alleviating the headache. It follows that vasodilatation is a corollary of migraine headache, not the aetiology of the pain, thus accounting for the sometimes paradoxical association between the two. Vasodilatation might modulate pain, but not if the meningeal vessels are not already sensitized. Furthermore, the antimigraine drugs do not address the source of the head pain but act on the final common pathway, namely trigeminovascular activation within the dura mater. The action of 5-HT$_{1D}$ agonists on receptor targets in brainstem remains a distinct possibility, although preclinical data remain unclear as to the extent of their CNS penetration. The possibility that there is a migraine 'generator' within the brainstem deserves further scrutiny. In this instance, ascending projecting fibres might modulate the threshold for cortical events or affect vascular tone as a mechanism for initiating an attack.

Pharmacological strategies for treating head pain

There are important benefits to be gained from a better understanding of the pathophysiology of migraine and of the precise mechanism of action of drugs beneficial in alleviating headache. The first is to develop an agent that is specific for the appropriate receptor subtype, thereby improving potency and reducing unwanted actions. Although sumatriptan is an effective antimigraine drug, it has significant unwanted vascular side-effects. These occur largely through postjunctional receptor activity mediating vasoconstriction, particularly in the coronary circulation. This effect on vascular smooth muscle can be particularly important in certain circumstances, for example subarachnoid haemorrhage, where vasoconstriction or hypotension may exacerbate cerebral ischaemia. Recent studies using reverse transcriptase polymerase chain reaction (RTPCR) and specific probes for $5H$-HT_{1D} and 5-$HT_{1\beta}$ gene sequences have established that although 5-HT_{1D} can be amplified selectively from human trigeminal ganglion, 5-HT_{1D} messenger RNA was not expressed within vascular smooth muscle of pial arteries in one study, but was expressed in another (Bouchelet *et al.* 1996) but not coupled to vasoconstriction. This raises the possibility that drugs can be developed which will activate prejunctional receptors in the dura mater without also causing pial or coronary artery vasoconstriction (Rebeck *et al.* 1994). Moreover, if sumatriptan and the ergot alkaloids are acting on the final common pathway in headache, rather than the aetiology, they may help to alleviate pain caused by meningeal irritation from a variety of conditions, such as meningitis, head injury, or subarachnoid haemorrhage. This has been explored experimentally by looking at c-*fos* immunoreactivity within the trigeminal nucleus caudalis (TNC) after experimental subarachnoid haemorrhage and chemically induced meningitis. Both surgical sensory deafferentation and sumatriptan suppressed the c-*fos* response (Nozaki *et al.* 1992*a*, *b*) in the TNC. The potential benefit of new drugs over conventional analgesics is their effectiveness in alleviating severe headache without depressing conscious level, impairing respiration, or compromising cerebral blood flow.

The $GABA_A$ receptor is another avenue of potential therapeutic importance. Although agonists of this receptor complex (such as valproate, neurosteroids, and benzodiazepines) block neurogenic plasma extravasation, the receptor complex cannot reside on trigeminovascular fibres because valproate remains effective in animals treated neonatally with capsaicin (which permanently depletes their C fibres). Instead, it requires the integrity of parasympathetic fibres emanating from the sphenopalatine ganglion; presumably those innervating the meninges. Hence, unlike the 5-HT_1-like family, this receptor complex lies outside the blood–brain barrier, probably acting through postjunctional receptors within the meninges (Lee *et al.* 1995). Modulators of this receptor may therefore prove to be useful in the development of selective therapeutic drugs for the treatment of vascular headaches.

A further avenue of exploration is the tachykinin receptor complex. To date, three receptors have been identified (NK_1, NK_2, and NK_3). The NK_1 receptor is located on the endothelium and is coupled to the release of nitric oxide. Nitric oxide synthase inhibitors suppress plasma protein extravasation, suggesting that an NK_1 receptor antagonist could also be of benefit in the treatment of headache. However, early reports from clinical trials do not support this assertion.

Concluding remarks

Although much remains to be discovered about the neurophysiological basis for migraine, molecular pharmacology is contributing greatly to knowledge of neuropeptides and neurotransmitter receptors. Further drug discoveries may be possible even without full knowledge of the underlying pathophysiological mechanisms. The triggers for migraine, its neurophysiological basis, and the dissociation of vessel calibre from headache and its treatment, are important issues to be resolved over the next decade.

Acknowledgement

MAM is the recipient of the Bristol-Meyers Unrestricted Research Award in Neuroscience. National Institutes of Health, (1P01NS35611–01), Migraine Program Project, Michael Moskowitz, P.I.

References

Bouchelet, I., Cohen, Z., Case, B., Seguela, P., and Hamel, E. (1996). Differential expression of sumatriptan-sensitive 5-hydroxytryptamine receptors in human trigeminal ganglia and cerebral blood vessels. *Mol. Pharmacol.* **50**, 219–23.

Buzzi, M. G., Sakas, D. E., and Moskowitz, M. A. (1989). Indomethacin and acetylsalicylic acid block neurogenic plasma protein extravasation in rat dura mater. *Eur. J. Pharmacol.* **165**, 251–8.

Cutrer, F. M., Limmroth, V., Ayata, G., and Moskowitz, M. A. (1995). Attenuation by valproate of c-*fos* immunoreactivity in trigeminal nucleus caudalis induced by intracisternal capsaicin. *Br. J. Pharmacol.* **116**, 3199–204.

Dimitriadou, V., Buzzi, M. G., Moskowitz, M .A., and Theoharides, T. C. (1991). Trigeminal sensory fibre stimulation induces morphological changes reflecting secretion in rat dura mater mast cells. *Neuroscience* **44**, 97–112.

Goadsby, P. J. and Edvinsson, L. (1991). Sumatriptan reverses the changes in CGRP seen in the headache phase of migraine. *Cephalgia* **11**, (Suppl. 3).

Goadsby, P. J. and Edvinsson, L. (1993). The trigeminovascular system and migraine: studies characterizing cerebrovascular and neuropeptide changes seen in humans and cats. *Ann. Neurol.* **33**, 48–56.

Haegerstrand, A., Dalsgaard, C. J., Jonzon, B., Larsson, O., and Nilsson, J. (1990). Calcitonin gene-related peptide stimulates proliferation of human endothelial cells. *Proc. Natl Acad. Sci. USA* **87**, 3299–303.

Inoue, T., Shimizu, H., Kaminuma, T., Tajima, M., Watabe, K., and Yoshimoto, T. (1996). Prevention of cerebral vasospasm by calcitonin gene-related peptide slow-release tablet after subarachnoid hemorrhage. *Neurosurgery* **39**, 984–90.

Kano, M., Moskowitz, M. A., and Yokota, M. (1991). Parasympathetic denervation of rat pial vessels significantly increases infarction volume following middle cerebral artery occlusion. *J. Cereb. Blood Flow Metab.* **11**, 628–37.

Lee, W. S., Limmroth, V., Cutrer, F. M., Waeber, C., and Moskowitz, M. A. (1995). Peripheral GABAa receptor mediated effects of sodium valproate on dural plasma protein extravasation to substance P and trigeminal stimulation. *Br. J. Pharmacol.* **116**, 1661–7.

Limmroth, V., Cutrer, F. M., and Moskowitz, M. A. (1996). Neurotransmitters and neuropeptides in headache. *Curr. Opin. Neurol.* 9, 206–10.

Macfarlane, R., Moskowitz, M. A., Sakas D. E. *et al.* (1991). The role of neuroeffector mechanisms in hyperperfusion syndromes. *J. Neurosurg.* 75, 845–55.

Moskowitz, M. A. and Waeber, C. (1996). Migraine enters the molecular era. *Neuroscientist* 2, 191–200.

Moskowitz, M. A., Sakas, D. E., Wei, E. P., Buzzi, M. G., Ogilvy, C., and Kontos, H. A. (1989). Postocclusive hyperemia in feline cortical grey matter is mediated by trigeminal sensory axons. *Am. J. Physiol.* 257, H1736–9.

Moskowitz, M. A., Nozaki, K., and Kraig, R. P. (1993). Neocortical spreading depression provokes the expression of c-*fos* protein-like immunoreactivity within trigeminal nucleus caudalis via trigeminovascular mechanisms. *J. Neurosci.* 13, 1167–77.

Mueller, S. M. and Heistad, D. D. (1980). Effect of chronic hypertension on the blood–brain barrier. *Hypertension* 2, 809–12.

Nozaki, K., Boccalini, P., and Moskowitz, M. A. (1992*a*). Expression of c-*fos*-like immunoreactivity in brainstem after meningeal irritation by blood in the subarachnoid space. *Neuroscience* 49, 669–80.

Nozaki, K., Moskowitz, M. A., and Boccalini, P. (1992*b*). CP-93,129, sumatriptan, dihydroergotamine block c-*fos* expression within rat trigeminal nucleus caudalis caused by chemical stimulation of the meninges. *Br. J. Pharmacol.* 106, 409–15.

Rebeck, G. W., Maynard, K. I., Hyman, B., and Moskowitz, M. A. (1994). Selective 5-HT$_{1D\alpha}$ receptor gene expression in trigeminal ganglia: implications for anti-migraine drug development. *Proc. Natl Acad. Sci. USA* 49, 669–80.

Sakas, D. E., Moskowitz, M. A., Wei, E. P., Kontos, H. A., Kano, M., and Ogilvy, C. (1989). Trigeminovascular fibers increase blood flow in cortical grey matter by axon reflex-like mechanisms during acute severe hypertension and seizures. *Proc. Natl Acad. Sci. USA* 86, 1401–5.

Strassman, A. M., Raymond, S. A., and Burnstein, R. (1996). Sensitization of meningeal sensory neurons and the origin of headaches. *Nature* 834, 560–4.

Weber, J. R., Angstwurm, K., Bove, G. M. *et al.* (1996). The trigeminal nerve and augmentation of regional cerebral blood flow during experimental bacterial meningitis. *J. Cereb. Blood Flow Metab.* 16, 1319–24.

Yu, X.-J. and Moskowitz, M. A. (1995). Neuropeptide Y inhibits neurogenic plasma extravasation in rat dura mater via prejunctional neuropeptide Y$_2$ receptor coupled to pertussis toxin-sensitive G protein. *Cephalgia* 15, (Suppl. 14), 103.

Yu, X.-J. and Moskowitz, M. A. (1996). Neuropeptide Y Y$_2$ receptor-mediated attenuation of neurogenic plasma extravasation acting through pertussus toxin-sensitive mechanisms. *Br. J. Pharmacol.* 119, 229–32.

Yu, X.-J., Waeber, C., Castanon, N. *et al.* (1996). 5-carboxamido-tryptamine, CP-122,288 and dihydroergotamine but not sumatriptan, CP-93,129, and serotonin-5-*O*-carboxymethyl-glycyl-tyrosinamide block dural plasma protein extravasation in knockout mice that lack 5-hydroxytryptamine$_{1B}$ receptors. *Mol. Pharmacol.* 49, 761–5.

PART II

Physiology and Pathophysiology Relevant to Autonomic Failure

11. Autoregulation and autonomic control of the cerebral circulation: implications and pathophysiology

Peter J. Goadsby

Introduction

Autoregulation of the cerebral circulation and the various autonomic neuronal influences upon brain blood flow form an important part of the normal control of cerebral perfusion (Mraovitch and Sercombe 1996). The fact that the cerebral circulation regulates its own flow in considerable measure has long been recognized. Neural control or neurogenically mediated changes in cerebral blood flow are a relatively recently accepted concept, although the observation that nerves exist on the vessels dates to Thomas Willis in 1664. The classical view of the cerebral circulation has been that blood flow and cerebral metabolism are tightly coupled under the influence of substances, such as H^+, adenosine, and K^+, that ensure a rapid and matched supply of blood when required without neural influence (Kuschinsky 1989; Purves 1972). Autoregulation in physiological terms is the very specific phenomenon that brain blood flow remains constant in the face of changing perfusion pressure over a remarkable range of pressures. In this chapter currently accepted views of autoregulation and the effects of the neural innervation are set out based largely on data from experimental animals.

The innervation of the cerebral circulation can be divided conveniently into intrinsic and extrinsic systems. The intrinsic systems originate within the central nervous system and, without exiting the brain, innervate cerebral parenchymal vessels (Hartman *et al.* 1980). They are not strictly autonomic in the classical sense of the word, although as their function is better understood such a distinction may eventually be useful. They have been reviewed well and extensively elsewhere. The extrinsic systems are those that commence within the central nervous system but exit and have an extra-axial synapse before innervating the cerebral vessels. The autonomic innervation of the cerebral circulation is a subset of these extrinsic nerves (Table 11.1), the sympathetic and parasympathetic nerves. The other component of the extrinsic innervation, the trigeminovascular system, has been covered elsewhere in this volume (Chapter 10).

Autoregulation

Autoregulation is that property of a vascular bed maintaining a constant blood flow in the face of changes in perfusion pressure. It is not confined to the brain but the discussion in this section relates to the phenomenon as it affects cerebral blood flow (Fig. 11.1). The perfusion pressure for the brain is the difference between the arterial blood pressure and either the venous or cerebrospinal fluid pressure, dependent on which is greater. Autoregulation is achieved by alterations in vessel calibre so that when perfusion pressure drops, flow

Table 11.1. Extrinsic cerebrovascular innervation

System	Ganglion	Transmitter
Autonomic innervation		
Parasympathetic	Pterygopalatine[a]	Vasoactive intestinal polypeptide (VIP)
	Otic	Peptide histidine methionine (PHM)[b]
	Carotid mini	Helodermin
		Helospectin I and II
Sympathetic	Superior cervical	Noradrenaline
		Neuropeptide Y (NPY)
Sensory innervation		
Trigeminal	Trigeminal	Calcitonin-gene-related peptide (CGRP)
		Substance P
		Neurokinin A
		Pituitary adenylate cyclase activating peptide (PACAP)

[a] Sphenopalatine in experimental animals.

[b] Peptide histidine isoleucine (PHI) in experimental animals.

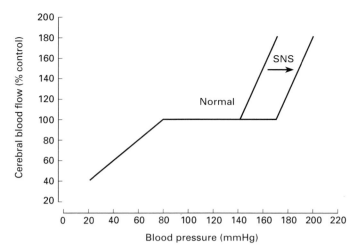

Fig. 11.1. Classical autoregulation of the cerebral circulation is illustrated as the maintainance of cerebral blood flow in the face of change in arterial blood pressure over a range of pressures. It is currently considered that the sympathetic nervous system (SNS) when stimulated acts to extend this range, as indicated by the arrow, thus having an essentially protective effect.

is maintained, and when it elevates there is no excess of flow in comparison to brain requirements. Experimental data suggest that both small cerebral arterioles and large-calibre vessels contribute to cerebral autoregulation. Autoregulation has a time constant in seconds so that Fig. 11.1 represents the steady-state situation with passive changes being observed during the initial portion of any sudden change in blood pressure. This phenomenon is considered to be a property of vessels and is influenced by the neural innervation, particularly the sympathetic nerves, but locally determined by either myogenic or metabolic mechanisms. The most convincing data explain autoregulation as a myogenic mechanism, such that stretch-dependent vasoconstriction or vice versa maintain a constant blood flow. Such a mechanism would be a response to changes in transmural pressure that probably includes an endothelial component and involves calcium entry into endothelial cells during stretch. There is evidence that at lower blood pressures local changes in adenosine may contribute to maintaining cerebral blood flow. It is perhaps of surprise that despite the relatively simple nature of the response and its consistency the precise mechanisms involved in autoregulation remain to be elucidated.

Autonomic neural influences on cerebral autoregulation

Of the currently understood role and effects of the autonomic innervation of the cerebral circulation, the interaction with cerebral autoregulation is by far the best documented. It has been established for some time that stimulation of the sympathetic nerves during hypertension will extend the upper limit of autoregulation. Thus, for a higher blood pressure cerebral blood flow remains constant. It is of interest then that chronic denervation does not alter the limits of autoregulation, so the process is an active one. This has the important clinical implication that in degenerative nervous system diseases involving the autonomic nervous system, autoregulatory dysfunction

is not related to shifts in the normal autoregulatory curve for the cerebral vessels but to disease processes that alter the perfusion pressure. The therapeutic application is that if perfusion pressure is maintained, the patient will experience fewer symptoms. It is considered that the shift in the autoregulatory curve seen with sympathetic activation is a protective phenomenon against cerebral damage that can be caused by excessive pressure. Both noradrenaline and neuropeptide Y (NPY; see below) seem to be involved in this protective process. A similar mechanism is thought to be activated to modulate intracranial pressure. Certainly, sympathetic nerve stimulation can alter intracranial pressure. The regulation of venous capacitance and the dense innervation of the choroid plexus by adrenergic nerves is likely to have an important influence upon intracranial pressure and is the subject of ongoing research.

Parasympathetic influences on the cerebral circulation

The parasympathetic innervation of the cerebral circulation represents the most powerful of the neural vasodilator influences upon that bed and its influence cannot be overlooked in any pathophysiological situation. The parasympathetic system is basically vasodilator in nature and is capable of altering brain blood flow independently of the prevailing metabolic demand and perfusion pressure. It is a potential reserve system that is well characterized in experimental animals but still lacks detailed analysis in humans.

Anatomy

The parasympathetic system is that system arising from the superior salivatory nucleus and passing out of the brain in the facial (VIIth cranial) nerve, distributing fibres through the pterygopalatine (sphenopalatine) and otic ganglia and carotid miniganglia to dilate vessels, almost certainly by way of a peptidergic transmitter (Fig. 11.2). The terms pterygopalatine and sphenopalatine imply the same structure, with the former being the correct term in humans because of its

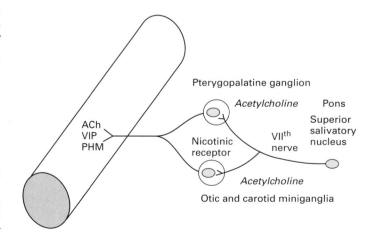

Fig. 11.2. The elements of the parasympathetic innervation of the cerebral circulation. The cell bodies of origin lie in the superior salivatory nucleus of the pons and project from the facial (VIIth) nerve to autonomic ganglia before innervating the vessels.

relationship to the pterygopalatine fossa. Pharmacologically the system is characterized by the presence of one or more substances, such as acetylcholine, vasoactive intestinal polypeptide (VIP), and peptide histidine methionine (isoleucine in the rat, thus PHI).

Origin

Chorobski and Penfield (1932) were the first to describe in detail the anatomy of the facial nerve dilator pathway that runs from the medulla via the greater superficial petrosal to the pial vessels of the cat and monkey. Initially studies examining the parasympathetic innervation of the cerebral vessels did so by defining them as cholinergic. This led to considerable confusion as, although these nerves have cholinergic markers useful for anatomical studies, there was no apparent vasomotor function for the acetylcholine putatively stored in these nerves. It was thus concluded that they had no physiological effect when, in fact, the data, as they were, only demonstrated that acetylcholine plays no immediate role in the effect of activation of parasympathetic nerves. Careful studies using histochemical techniques have shown acetylcholinesterase on the large cerebral vessels. Biochemical and histochemical evidence of choline acetyltransferase (ChAT) activity and the presence of a high-affinity choline uptake system on the vessels have also been useful surrogate markers of the parasympathetic system. Ultrastructural studies have noted a small number of agranular vesicles that store non-adrenergic transmitters. The innervation with cholinergic nerves is regionally variable anterior to posterior and the concentration of nerves along any vessel varies, with the densest innervation being at branching points, particularly in the pial vessels. In the cat and the rat, where detailed studies are available using acetylcholinesterase as a marker, the densest innervation is that of the anterior vessels. Notable variations in ChAT activity are seen between species, with the middle cerebral artery density being less than the basilar in the cat, and other variables such as age being recognized.

The facial/greater superficial petrosal nerve pathway courses to the ipsilateral sphenopalatine and otic ganglia and thence loops back via the ethmoidal nerve to enter the cranial cavity. Ablation of the sphenopalatine ganglion leads to a marked reduction in cholinesterase fibre density in the anterior vessels of the circle of Willis, and it has been shown by direct means that nerves in the posterior circulation innervating the basilar artery also course to the sphenopalatine

ganglion. Furthermore, using the transganglionic tracer, pseudorabies virus, it has been established that the central nucleus for these fibres is in the superior salivatory nucleus of the pons.

Transmitters and modulators

The parasympathetic system contains a number of transmitter or neuromodulator substances which are often co-localized in the same neurones. All the substances known to exist in the parasympathetic nerves are vasodilator (Table 11.2) but their precise role and, in particular, relationship to one another remains unclear. Whether these anatomical subgroups with one, two, three, or even four co-localized transmitters have functional correlates remains to be established.

Acetycholine

The cerebral vessels in isolation bind tritiated cholinergic ligands and thus various muscarinic receptors have been shown to exist on them. Acetylcholine dilates most of the cerebral vessels either *in vitro* or *in vivo* by an atropine-sensitive receptor, an effect that is mediated via the release of an endothelium-derived relaxing factor, nitric oxide. Local application of a cholinomimetic (carbachol) into the cerebrospinal fluid causes pial vessel dilatation, which is again antagonized by atropine. Parenteral administration of acetylcholine increases cerebral blood flow, an effect again inhibited by atropine. Curiously, then, it will be seen below that nicotinic antagonists are completely ineffective when tested during parasympathetic stimulation. The role of acetylcholine in these nerves remains unresolved.

Vasoactive intestinal polypeptide

The characterization of neuropeptides, particularly over the past two decades, has led to a substantial re-evaluation of virtually all neuronal systems with respect to transmitter content. Potent vasodilator peptides have been characterized and identified in the parasympathetic nerves of the cranium, particularly vasoactive intestinal polypeptide (VIP) and, coexistent with it, peptide histidine methionine (PHM). VIP is a 28-amino-acid basic polypeptide that was first isolated from the porcine duodenum. It belongs to a structural superfamily of peptides along with glucagon, secretin, and gastrin inhibitory peptide. The family is characterized by helodermin/helospectin-like peptides that are distributed in the central nervous system and in endocrine

Table 11.2. Transmitters of the parasympathetic system

Level	Structure	Transmitter	Antagonist
Brainstem (pons) course	Superior salivatory nucleus	Glutamate	?
	Facial nerve[b]		
Peripheral ganglion	Pterygopalatine, otic, carotid miniganglia	Acetylcholine	Hexamethonium-sensitive nicotinic receptor
End-organ	Cerebral blood vessels	VIP	None available
		PHI	
		Nitric oxide	Nitric oxide synthase inhibitors
		Helospectin-related[a]	

[a] Helodermin, Helospectin I and II.

[b] The fibres traverse the facial nerve, passing through but not synapsing in the geniculate ganglion and emerging as the greater superficial petrosal nerve.

VIP, vasoactive intestinal polypeptide; PHI, peptide histidine isoleucine (methionine); ?, unknown.

See also Table 11.1.

cells, such as the C cells of the thyroid. It has been shown that each of helodermin and the helospectins I and II are vasodilator in the cerebral circulation. There are as yet no data that address the inter-relationship of these transmitters, although they can have added effects.

It has been established clearly that the large cerebral vessels and cortical pial vessels have a rich VIPergic innervation that can be immunohistochemically identified and measured by radioimmuno-assay. Indeed, using ultrastructural techniques it can be seen that vasoactive intestinal polypeptide is found in large, dense-core neuronal vesicles in perivascular nerve terminals on the vessels. Two important features characterize this innervation: first, it is predominantly in the anterior segments of the circle of Willis, and, secondly, the fibres may be seen to follow the vessels and penetrate into the parenchyma. However, it has been shown that VIP-immunoreactive nerves that innervate the pial vessels may arise, at least in part, from intracortical neurones. The pattern of innervation of the vessels has further been characterized as having a spiral distribution with respect to the lumen and, importantly, this innervation is seen in human vessels. The origin of the nerves is essentially as it is for the cholinergic system.

Peptide histidine methionine (isoleucine)

The third major marker for the parasympathetic system is peptide histidine methionine (PHM). This is cleaved from the same pre-pro-peptide as VIP and there is at least a 50 per cent sequence homology. PHM and PHI (peptide histidine isoleucine) are almost identical, with a difference in two amino acid residues (92, lysine for arginine; 107, methionine for isoleucine), with the latter being the rodent peptide. Immunohistochemical studies have confirmed the existence of PHI(M)-like immunoreactivity on cerebral vessels, and the distribution is essentially parallel to that of VIP. PHI(M) elicits a less potent dose-dependent vasodilatation than VIP *in vitro* and *in vivo*. Microapplication of PHI(M) dilates both arteries and veins *in situ*.

Nitric oxide

The most recent addition to the transmitters or modulators that are involved in parasympathetic cerebrovascular actions is nitric oxide (NO). A short-lived, highly reactive molecule, whose physiology is dealt with elsewhere in this volume, NO is capable of dilating cerebral vessels. The effect of blockade of NO production on non-neural responses, such a hypercapnia, remains somewhat controversial in terms of quantity, while its role in parasympathetic responses seems clearer. Blockade of NO synthesis reduces the effect of parasympathetic stimulation in the cerebral circulation (Goadsby *et al.* 1996). This observation is important because NO can be both deleterious and pro-tective during cerebral ischaemia, thus providing an avenue by which the parasympathetic nervous innervation might mediate protective neurovascular dilatation in the cerebral circulation (Kano *et al.* 1991).

Physiological effects

Effect of parasympathetic blockade

Given that the cranial parasympathetic outflow to the cerebral vessels via the facial nerve is marked by many neurotransmitters or neuro-modulators (acetylcholine, VIP, NO, and PHI(M)), what is the effect of blocking this outflow? The responses that characterize normal cerebral blood flow (CBF) are the hypercapnic vasodilator response, the autoregulatory response to changes in blood pressure, and the hypoxic vasodilator response.

Resting CBF and autoregulation

Few experiments have addressed the question of the facial nerve and its role in autoregulation. Sectioning the facial nerve does not alter autoregulation in the cat, while resting cerebral blood flow or glucose utilization are also unaffected.

Hypercapnia and hypoxia

Studies in the baboon, cat, dog, rat, and rabbit all demonstrate no effect of sections of the facial nerve on either hypercapnic or hypoxic vasodilatation. Similarly, Seylaz and colleagues have demonstrated that the main parasympathetic outflow ganglia, the sphenopalatine ganglion, may be ablated without any alteration of hypercapnic vasodilatation.

Stimulation of the parasympathetic nerves

Local nerve stimulation

To further characterize the relationship between anatomically defined parasympathetic nerves and their transmitters, studies have examined carefully the release of the various marker substances of this system *in vitro*. Incubation of cerebral vessels from either cat or rabbit with labelled choline chloride, a precursor in the synthesis pathway for acetylcholine, permits measurement of labelled acetylcholine when nerves surrounding the vessels are stimulated. This response may be blocked if calcium is removed from the buffer or tetrodotoxin added, suggesting an active neural process. The method of transmural nerve stimulation has been employed in isolated vessel preparations to examine the possible role of identified putative transmitters. Except in porcine vessels, relaxation is only seen if the vessels are pre-contracted. Transmural nerve stimulation leads to contraction of rabbit, goat, and human pial vessels, in contrast to relaxation in those of the cat, dog, and pig. For the cat and pig it is clear that a non-adrenergic, non-cholinergic dilator mechanism is operating and available data suggest that the mediator is VIP. Similar studies have also been used to determine the substances that are released when cerebral nerves are stimulated directly *in vitro*. VIP is released when cerebral arterial nerves are stimulated. Indeed, although no anta-gonist to VIP is available, specific VIP antiserum has been used to inhibit non-cholinergic, non-adrenergic dilator responses in the cranial circulation resulting from both direct and distant nerve stim-ulation. Finally, an *in vivo* study has demonstrated local cortical release of VIP with facial nerve stimulation. This release is blocked by hexamethonium, demonstrating release of VIP in the context of activation of a classical nicotinic autonomic ganglion in the cerebral circulation.

Effect of direct parasympathetic stimulation on cerebral blood flow

Facial nerve stimulation

Direct stimulation of the facial nerve in humans leads to an increase in total cranial blood flow, as does facial nerve nucleus stimulation in the monkey or stimulation of an area just dorsal to it in the cat. In primates and in cats, stimulation of the nerve with its proximal end intact (that is, attached to the brainstem) reduces cerebral blood flow, while stimulation of the sectioned distal segment will increase it. In the baboon, using the ^{133}Xe clearance method, it has been shown that facial nerve stimulation increases cerebral blood flow, and a similar effect is seen in the dog, rat, and rabbit. It has been demonstrated in cats, using iodoantipyrine or laser Doppler flowmetry, that such stimulation can increase cerebral blood flow. Clearly, stimulation of the facial nerve increases cerebral blood flow without altering metabolic activity, as reflected by stable glucose utilization and sagittal sinus oxygen content. These responses are meditated through a classical parasympathetic ganglion as they can be blocked by hexamethonium, and probably use vasoactive intestinal polypeptide as the major transmitter of the system.

Sphenopalatine (pterygopalatine) ganglion

Studies of the peripheral ganglion mediating facial nerve vasodilatation have included peripheral reflex (trigeminal ganglion) and central structure (locus coeruleus) stimulation. It is clear that effects mediated by the facial nerve can be blocked by sphenopalatine ganglion removal and that this same response is VIP mediated. Indeed, using at least three different methods of measurement of cerebral blood flow, stimulation of the sphenopalatine ganglion in the cat and rat has been shown to produce strong frequency-dependent cerebral vasodilator responses. Importantly, cerebral glucose utilization and tissue P_{O_2} are not affected and the response is thus truly neurogenic.

In summary, the cranial parasympathetic pathway to the cerebral vessels arises in the superior salivatory nucleus in the pons; it traverses the facial nerve, joining the greater superficial petrosal nerve to be distributed to the vessels after synapsing chiefly in the sphenopalatine or otic ganglia. A variable small number of fibres in different species (including humans) have this peripheral synapse located in microganglia on the wall of the internal carotid artery, particularly near the carotid siphon. The transmitters contained in this system are acetylcholine, VIP, PHM(I), nitric oxide, and helospectin-related peptides. The ganglionic transmission in the periphery is mediated by a classical parasympathetic nicotinic ganglion, while current data would suggest that VIP is the major neuroeffector substance at the nerve–smooth muscle junction. The pathway does not play a role in either hypercapnic or hypoxic vasodilator responses or autoregulatory responses to changes in arterial perfusion pressure. The system can be activated by either direct stimulation or via connections with other important central neural vasoactive nuclei to increase cerebral blood flow independent of cerebral metabolic needs.

Role and clinical implications

Although there have been considerable advances in understanding the basic capabilities and connectivity of the parasympathetic innervation of the cerebral circulation, these data have not indicated a clear physiological role for the system. The nerves are not involved directly in the most basic cerebrovascular responses, such as hypoxic or hypercapnic vasodilatation, nor do they appear to play a role in autoregulation. Their effects are, however, independent of direct metabolic intervention. This latter fact suggests a role in times of threat, such as during ischaemia or in vasospastic conditions such as subarachnoid haemorrhage (Table 11.3). The parasympathetic system is ideally placed to be engaged to increase cerebral blood flow when ordinary metabolic driving factors are impaired. This protection may, however, be regionally variable since the posterior circulation innervation with VIP is much less than that seen anteriorly. This finding may have implications in situations where predominantly posterior changes are reported, such as migraine. As yet this question has not be adequately addressed. There are, as yet, no studies in

Table 11.3. Clinical conditions in which parasympathetic activation may be implicated

Stroke
Subarachnoid hemorrhage
Migraine*
Cluster headache**
Chronic paroxysmal hemicrania***

* Goadsby *et al.* 1990; ** Goadsby and Edvinsson 1994;
*** Goadsby and Lipton 1997

human autonomic failure to determine whether there is cranial cerebrovascular parasympathetic dysfunction. The first step will be post-mortem studies to address the anatomical question of whether the nerves are present in usual numbers, while animal physiologists pursue the pathophysiological implications of parasympathetic dysfunction. It may be too narrow a perspective to consider only a vasomotor function for these nerves as there is evidence that cholinergic mechanisms can alter capillary permeability, including the movement of amino acids. Whatever their function is ultimately revealed to be, it is now clear that the evidence for the existence of the parasympathetic innervation of the cerebral vessels is beyond question.

Sympathetic influences upon the cerebral circulation

The sympathetic innervation of the cerebral circulation was the first to be characterized, with the development of the Falck–Hillarp histofluorescence technique in the early 1960s. The sympathetic innervation of the brain circulation has thus been studied longer and is better understood than that of the parasympathetic system (Fig. 11.3).

Anatomy

The sympathetic nervous innervation of the cerebral circulation arises in the hypothalamus as first-order neurones and projects to the intermediolateral cell column of the spinal cord. Second-order neurones arise from the sympathetic chain and proceed to synapse with

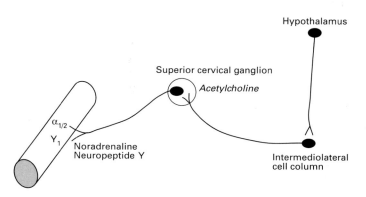

Fig. 11.3. The elements of the sympathetic innervation of the cerebral vessels, including the receptor populations ($\alpha_{1/2}$ and Y_1).

third-order neurones in the superior cervical ganglion. The innervation is lateralized and largely respects the midline, with subsequent projection to the cerebral vessels being provided by sympathetic nerves that run rostral with the carotid artery. There is a dense innervation, particularly of more proximal large arteries, which follows vessels out to the pia and along the brain surface but generally only follow penetrating vessels for a short distance into the cerebral parenchyma. The largest part of the adrenergic supply of the intra-parenchymal vessels is supplied by the locus coeruleus. The sympathetic nerve terminals are often located close to smooth muscle cells in the outer media. The terminals are characterized electron microscopically as small, electron-dense vesicles. The sympathetic innervation of the cerebral vessels accounts for about half the nerves observed in the vessels walls. The innervation is most dense anteriorly, with a relatively sparser supply in the vertebrobasilar territory that is considered to arise largely from the stellate ganglion.

Transmitters and neuromodulators

Noradrenaline

The main transmitter of the sympathetic innervation is the classical autonomic amine transmitter, noradrenaline. Extirpation of the superior cervical ganglion results in a mainly ipsilateral reduction in adrenergic fibres from the vessels. In addition, sympathetic nerve stimulation can cause perivascular release of noradrenaline, while labelled noradrenaline is taken up into the nerves. The effect of noradrenaline release is to constrict the vessels through activation of α-adrenoceptors in the vessels. In humans the predominant receptor subtype is the α_1-adrenoceptor, while in some experimental animals α_2-adrenoceptors can be seen. These receptors mediate vasoconstriction. Of the commonly used experimental species, only the pig cerebral circulation is dominated by dilatory β-adrenoceptors, although all species have dilatory β-adrenoceptors that are unmasked by α-blockade. In humans both β_1- and β_2-adrenoceptors are located on cerebral vessels.

Peptides

In addition to the classic constrictor aminergic transmitter, sympathetic nerves release the vasoconstrictor peptide neuropeptide Y (NPY). NPY is widely distributed in the brain and peripheral nervous system. Fibres that contain NPY form a dense network around cerebral arteries and veins and double stain for noradrenaline (Edvinsson et al. 1983). Retrograde tracing studies have shown NPY-positive fibres that have cell bodies in the superior cervical ganglion, and these fibres are substantially reduced by sympathectomy. Furthermore, NPY co-localizes with dopamine β-hydroxylase in cell bodies in the superior cervical ganglion, demonstrating that the peptide exists in cells that synthesize noradrenaline. NPY is potent constrictor of cerebral vessels at the NPY Y_1 receptor. This receptor has been identified on cerebral vessels using PCR for the human NPY Y_1 receptor and constriction can be mimicked by the agonist NPY_{13-36} and blocked by the Y_1 antagonist BIBP.

Physiological effects

Stimulation

Direct stimulation of the cervical sympathetic nerves in experimental animals results in large vessel constriction but no change to small calibre vessels. The effect is more prominent on the cerebral veins and

is blocked by α_1-adrenoceptor blockade. Consistent with these data, microapplication of noradrenaline reduces local vessel diameter. The details of this system have been further studied using local transmural nerve stimulation although, because of species variation in nerve supply, the results have not always been consistent.

Physiological roles

The influence of the sympathetic innervation of the cerebral circulation is discussed above under 'Autoregulation' and this is by far its best described effect. There are some data to suggest that hypercapnic vasodilatation is influenced by the sympathetic innervation, such that the response is enhanced, but this requires further study.

Trophic effects

There are excellent data that have established a role for the sympathetic nerves in development, particularly of the muscular layer of the wall of cerebral vessels (Dimitriadov et al. 1988). The trophic effects of the sympathetic nerves deserve further investigation.

Summary

Current understanding of the action of the autonomic innervation of the cerebral circulation is detailed, at least in experimental animals. The challenge for the next decade is to turn that knowledge into practical applications for patients with disease of the autonomic nervous system. The tools are now available in the form of functional imaging techniques so that we can anticipate advances in pathophysiological understanding in this field.

Acknowledgements

The author acknowledges the valuable collaboration of H. Kaube, K. Hoskin and, Y. Knight in the conduct of some of the studies reviewed here. The work of the author reported herein has been supported by the Wellcome Trust and the Migraine Trust. PJG is a Wellcome Senior Research Fellow.

Bibliography

Chorobski, J. and Penfield, W. (1932). Cerebral vasodilator nerves and their pathway from the medulla oblongata. Arch. Neurol. Psychiatry 28, 1257–89.

Dimitriadou, V., Aubineau, P., Taxi, J., and Seylaz, J. (1988). Ultrastructural changes in the cerebral artery wall induced by long-term sympathetic denervation. Blood Vessels 25, 122–43.

Edvinsson, L., Emson, P., McCulloch, J., Tatemoto, K., and Uddman, R. (1983). Neuropeptide Y: cerebrovascular innervation and vasomotor effects in the cat. Neurosci. Lett. 43, 79–84.

Edvinsson, L., MacKenzie, E. T., and McCulloch, J. (1993). Cerebral blood flow and metabolism. Raven Press, New York.

Goadsby, P. J. and Edvinsson, L. (1994). Human in vivo evidence for trigeminovascular activation in cluster headache. Brain 117, 427–34.

Goadsby, P. J. and Lipton, R. B. (1997). A review of paroxysmal hemicranias, SUNCT syndrome and other short-lasting headaches with autonomic features, including new cases. Brain 120, 193–209.

Goadsby, P. J., Edvinsson, L., and Ekman, R. (1990). Vasoactive peptide release in the extracerebral circulation of humans during migraine headache. Ann. Neurol. 28, 183–7.

Goadsby, P. J., Uddman, R., and Edvinsson, L. (1996). Cerebral vasodilatation in the cat involves nitric oxide from parasympathetic nerves. *Brain Res.* **707**, 110–18.

Hartman, B. K., Swanson, L. W., Raichle, M. E., Preskorn, S. H., and Clark, H. B. (1980). Central adrenergic regulation of cerebral microvascular permeability and blood flow; anatomic and physiologic evidence. The cerebral microvasculature. *Adv. Exp. Med. Biol.* **131**, 113–26.

Kano, M., Moskowitz, M. A., and Yokota, M. (1991). Parasympathetic denervation of rat pial vessels significantly increases infarction volume following middle cerebral artery occlusion. *J. Cereb. Blood Flow Metab.* **11**, 628–37.

Kuschinsky, W. (1989). Coupling of blood flow and metabolism in the brain—the classical view. In *Neurotransmission and cerebrovascular function*, (ed. J. Seylaz and R. Sercombe), Vol. 2, pp. 331–42. Elsevier Science Publishers, Amsterdam.

Mraovitch, S. and Sercombe, R. (1996). *Neurophysiological basis of cerebral blood flow control: an introduction.* John Libbey and Sons, London.

Purves, M. J. (1972). *The physiology of the cerebral circulation.* Cambridge University Press, Cambridge.

12. Temperature regulation and the autonomic nervous system

Kenneth J. Collins

Introduction

Homeothermy, the constancy of body temperature, expresses a pattern of temperature regulation in which variations in core temperature are maintained within arbitrarily defined limits of ±2 °C despite much larger changes in ambient temperature. In humans, homeothermia is achieved by the complex co-ordination of autonomic, metabolic, and behavioural responses which involves integration of multiple loop systems within the central nervous system. Heat loss is regulated by sympathetic nervous control of vasomotor and sudomotor activity, while thermogenesis depends partly on the sympathetic and sympathoadrenal-medullary control of metabolism. One effect of behavioural reactions to heat is to modify the relationship between the organism and its environment and thereby alter the need for autonomic thermoregulation. This sparing action does not, however, necessarily imply that there is central nervous co-ordination between behavioural and autonomic thermoregulation.

Through experiment and analysis, a large body of knowledge has been built up to describe the role of the autonomic nervous system in temperature regulation, and new physiological, anatomical, and neurochemical insights are being added constantly. It is the purpose of this chapter to review some of the more recent findings; firstly, on normal central and peripheral control and, secondly, on autonomic disorders in human thermoregulation leading to the abnormal states of hypothermia, hyperthermia, and poikilothermia.

Central autonomic control

Body temperature is regulated by a hierarchical neuronal network of thermoregulatory pathways extending from the hypothalamus and limbic system to the lower brainstem, reticular formation, spinal cord, and sympathetic pathways (Boulant 1991). The POAH region (preoptic area/anterior hypothalamus and septum) is the predominant site for integration of central and peripheral information for control of thermoregulatory effector responses through the autonomic nervous system. Various converging excitatory and inhibitory peripheral influences on the control centres markedly change the relation between activities of core temperature sensors and thermoregulatory responses, thereby inducing temporary alteration in temperature thresholds of the effector mechanisms. Hypothalamic thermoregulation processing can be affected by higher cerebral activities, as demonstrated by changes in thermoregulatory responses during sleep and mental stress (Ogawa and Low 1993). A schematic diagram of human temperature regulation is shown in Fig. 12.1. The controlled variable is an integrated value of multiple temperatures rather than the tem-

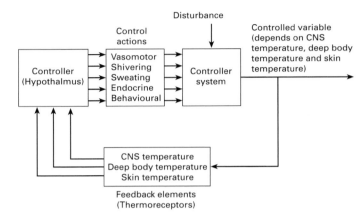

Fig. 12.1. Schematic diagram of the feedback control of body temperature with the controlled variable an integrated value of multiple body temperatures. (From Hensel (1981), with kind permission of Academic Press.)

perature of a limited body area such as the body core. In a multi-loop system such as the thermoregulatory control system, there is an unknown number of closed loops that will counteract the displacement of temperature by setting up feedback signals, and this makes it difficult to measure 'open loop gain' (the change in core temperature divided by the corresponding temperature change at the sensor).

In a proportional control system such as that for thermoregulation, the control action (e.g. autonomic response) is proportional to the difference between the feedback signal and the set-point of the system. Any thermal load, therefore, will necessarily lead to a corresponding deviation of body temperature, or load error. The higher the gain of the control system, the smaller the load error. The set-point of a proportional control system can be defined as that value of the controlled variable (e.g. a function of various body temperatures) at which the control action is zero. However, the set-point temperatures for different control actions, such as heat production, cutaneous vasomotor activity, sweating, and behavioural thermoregulation, need not necessarily be identical. An important property of the set-point mechanism is that it is adjustable. Normal set-point displacement occurs in the diurnal temperature rhythm, sleep, and the menstrual cycle. Abnormally it occurs in fever.

Interaction with other central regulatory mechanisms

Control of thermoregulation is not exclusively mediated by the various thermal inputs. For example, POAH neurones send axons to and receive projections from the ventromedial and lateral hypothalamus, pathways that affect feeding behaviour. A rise in POAH temperature facilitates the activity of glucoreceptive neurones in the ventromedial hypothalamus and inhibits those in the lateral hypothalamus. Stimulation of the ventromedial hypothalamus has been shown to increase non-shivering thermogenesis. Hypothalamic control of thermoregulatory responses is considerably affected by other biological responses, such as changes in fluid and electrolyte balance, hypercapnia, etc. Control loops sharing a common output with thermoregulation are likely to involve the possibility of competition between biological systems.

Behavioural thermoregulation

Autonomic thermoregulatory responses are principally directed to achieve a virtually constant core temperature. In contrast, the primary purpose of thermoregulatory behaviour is to keep the skin temperature at a point of thermal comfort. In humans with thermoregulatory disorders, adequate compensatory behavioural thermoregulation can hinder recognition of autonomic failure. Behavioural thermoregulation is co-ordinated by the hypothalamic centres and the cerebral cortex. Dysfunction of these structures or loss of peripheral thermosensitivity can seriously jeopardize inherent or learned behavioural thermoregulation and thereby maintenance of a relatively stable core temperature (see also the section on poikilothermia).

Central neurotransmission

Following the discovery that the hypothalamus contains relatively large concentrations of noradrenaline and 5-hydroxytryptamine (5-HT), it was proposed that the intrahypothalamic release of these two monoamines controlled normal thermoregulation. Intraventricular injections of 5-HT in cats and primates caused peripheral vasoconstriction, shivering, and huddling, leading to a raised body temperature. Noradrenaline, in contrast, activated processes leading to a fall in body temperature. Quite different responses have, however, been reported in other species, such as sheep, rabbits, and rats. Apart from prostaglandin E, which plays a crucial role in the genesis of fevers, no putative neurotransmitter or mediator has had the same effect in all mammals tested.

Acetylcholine is an obvious transmitter candidate in hypothalamic pathways, and there is evidence indicating the presence of nicotinic receptors in heat loss pathways and muscarinic receptors in heat conservation pathways. Microinjection experiments show that cholinoceptive sites are widely scattered between the levels of the optic chiasma and the mamillary bodies, in contrast to the restricted sites in the POAH for noradrenaline and 5-HT.

A number of hypothalamic neuropeptides have been identified, and many are reported to be important in normal central thermoregulatory control. For many peptides, the information available is insufficient to establish their role (e.g. cholecystokinin, luteinizing hormone-releasing hormone, neurotensin), but for some (e.g. ACTH, α-melanocyte-stimulating hormone, arginine vasopressin) there is good evidence that they may participate as thermolytic substances acting within the brain to reduce fever (Hellon et al. 1991). Endogenous opioids such as β-endorphin and met-enkephalin appear to participate in change in body temperature evoked by stress. The coexistence of so many peptides that alter temperature suggests that there must be a hierarchy of relationships between peptides and

temperature in specific brain tissues, with some specifically involved in hypothalamic pathways and others more important for autonomic functions influencing temperature secondarily.

Thermoregulatory effector mechanisms

Interaction of thermal drives

Three main sympathetic thermoregulatory effectors contribute to adjustment of heat gain and heat loss mechanisms: metabolic, vasomotor, and sudomotor. These regulations have profound effects on core temperature and skin temperature in humans and depend on intact neuronal control with multiple afferent and efferent links. At constant afferent flow from cutaneous thermoreceptors, i.e. at constant skin temperature, a decrease in core temperature leads to a linear increase in metabolic heat production by shivering and non-shivering thermogenesis (Fig. 12.2a). If skin temperature is decreased, there is an increase in the sensitivity of metabolic heat production induced by lowering core temperature. This change of slope (Fig. 12.2a) signifies that the effects of peripheral and central thermosensors on thermogenesis are multiplicative in nature. Alteration of skin temperature, however, shifts the quantitative relationship between core temperature and sweating (Fig. 12.2b) and core temperature and cutaneous vasomotor responses (Fig. 12.2c) in parallel to the right or left, which suggests an additive relationship in the neural processing of these parameters.

Local temperature of the skin has a modifying influence on the responses of sweat glands and cutaneous blood vessels. The local temperature effects are strictly limited to the area affected by the temperature change, and amplify the thermoregulatory effects exerted by the central controller. Thus, lowering the skin temperature locally reduces the sudomotor drive (Fig. 12.2b) and increases the activity of vasoconstrictor neurones, leading to a reduction of convective heat transfer at the skin (Fig. 12.2c). The changing slopes of the curves express a multiplicative interaction between local temperature and the sweating and vasoconstrictor thermal drive. However, local temperature changes in the physiological range have virtually no effect on the response of autonomic effector organs in the skin after denervation. Local temperature appears to affect neuroglandular transmission and the responsiveness of the vascular smooth muscle to neurotransmitters.

Sympathetic control of thermogenesis

Shivering and non-shivering thermogenesis are both forms of so-called facultative or optional thermogenesis, which also includes diet-induced and exercise-induced thermogenesis (Himms-Hagen 1990). The ultimate role of shivering is heat production in order to maintain internal body temperature in cold conditions. Shivering is mainly controlled by somatic motor innervation with a primary motor centre in the dorsomedial portion of the posterior hypothalamus. It can be inhibited consciously and voluntarily by muscle contractions. Sympathetic regulation of thermogenesis is basically directed, therefore, to the control of non-shivering thermogenesis. Non-shivering thermogenesis occurs predominantly in cold-acclimatized animals and in neonates, where significant amounts of brown adipose tissue

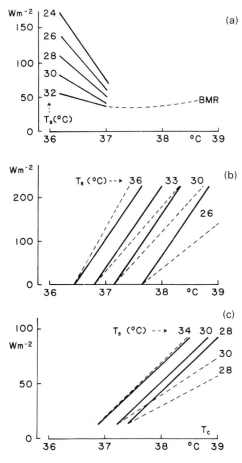

Fig. 12.2. Interaction of core and skin thermal drives on effector mechanisms. Ordinate scales are metabolic heat production (a), evaporative heat loss (b), and convective heat transfer (c) from the skin, in relation to core temperature (T_c, abscissa scales) and skin temperature (T_s). Hatched lines represent the effects of changes in local skin temperature on the sweat glands (b) and blood vessels (c). (From Loewy and Spyer (1990), reprinted by permission of Oxford University Press.)

are found. This specialized tissue is innervated by adrenergic sympathetic nerve fibres and stimulates heat production through a β-adrenergic mechanism with a regulating centre in the POAH.

Non-shivering thermogenesis may also be produced in the adult human by the calorigenic action of catecholamines and other hormones acting on other tissues, including muscles. In subjects exposed to air at 12 °C for 8 hours daily, electromyographic activity due to shivering, and oxygen consumption, both decline with successive exposures. Oxygen consumption, however, declines less than muscle activity, and this has been interpreted as evidence for the development of non-shivering thermogenesis. Outdoor workers such as lumberjacks are reported to develop deposits of brown adipose tissue around the carotid arteries, while indoor workers of the same age do not. The inference is that those who spend much time exposed to cold may develop brown adipose non-shivering thermogenesis as a cold defence mechanism in addition to catecholamine non-shivering thermogenesis. Thyroxine may play a part as an endogenous transmitter (mediator) for non-shivering thermo-

genesis. Evidence is lacking that stimulation of thyroid activity is a pre-requisite for the development of cold adaptation. In humans, there is no consistent thyroid stimulating hormone response to acute cooling. Thyroid hormone, however, causes the response to adrenergic stimulation to increase, in part by increasing the number of β-receptors (Loewy and Spyer 1990). Patients with pathological elevations of calorigenic hormones, e.g. in thyrotoxicosis and phaeochromocytoma, often have an associated hyperthermia. In a severe thyroid crisis, the body temperature can rise quite rapidly to levels observed in heat stroke.

Vasomotor and sudomotor efferents

It is generally assumed that most sympathetic pre-ganglionic neurones are located in the intermediolateral cell column. However, sympathetic preganglionic neurones are distributed throughout the whole intermediate zone of the thoracolumbar spinal cord, extending from the white matter to the central canal, but with the highest concentration of neurones in the intermediolateral cell column. The postganglionic neurones in the paravertebral ganglia, including those supplying the skin, have only a relay function. Despite considerable convergence of preganglionic axons onto any one postganglionic neurone, it is likely that very few preganglionic axons determine the output of the paravertebral neurones (Jänig 1990). It appears that the descending vasoconstrictor and sudomotor pathways lie essentially within the same area, though they do not exactly overlie each other.

Vasomotor neurones

The largest group of sympathetic neurones supplying the skin is probably that of the noradrenergic vasoconstrictor neurones. They contribute to the typical reflex pattern involving thermal stimulation of afferents from the skin surface and the body core. At rest in normal ambient temperatures, spontaneous cutaneous sympathetic activity consisting of bursts of impulses have been recorded intraneurally in peripheral nerves (see Chapter 23) which appear to represent centrally entrained bursts of vasoconstrictor activity.

Vasodilatation is brought about by the effects of locally released metabolites, by inhibition of vasoconstrictor tone, by release of co-localized transmitters from cholinergic sudomotor nerves, and possibly by putative active vasodilator neurones. In order to determine active cutaneous vasodilator responses in the human forearm and finger, skin blood flow has been determined before and after musculocutaneous and median nerve blockade during whole-body heating or cooling (Saumet et al. 1992). The experiments appear to show that an active vasodilator system plays an important role in the timing and amplitude of the cutaneous vasodilation in the forearm but not in the finger. At thermal neutrality, vasoconstrictor tone is high in the finger but not in the forearm. Vasoconstrictor responses to cooling occurred only in the finger. Indirect experimental evidence in animals indicates that the skin is supplied with a separate population of vasodilator neurones but the evidence in humans remains controversial and interpretation must take account of the coincidence between sweating and vasodilatation in warm conditions.

Sudomotor neurones

Efferent nerve fibres originating from the POAH descend through the ipsilateral brainstem and synapse in the intermediolateral cell columns without crossing. The sympathetic sudomotor neurones to the skin of the upper limbs are supplied by T2–T9; the face by T1–T4, the trunk by T4–T12, and the lower limbs by T10–L2 (Sato *et al.* 1993). Sudomotor nerves surrounding the eccrine sweat glands are composed of non-myelinated class C fibres which react strongly in tests for cholinesterase. Together with predominant cholinergic sympathetic neurones, the innervation around the secretory cells contains a few adrenergic terminals. Developmental studies of glands in the footpads of rodents show that, in early stages of development, sudomotor nerves appear to be adrenergic. During development, however, noradrenergic axons lose their store of endogenous catecholamines, but not their capacity for uptake and storage on exposure to catecholamines as they elaborate an axonal plexus in the maturing glands. It is proposed that this is evidence of neurotransmitter plasticity as sudomotor neurones appear to undergo transition from noradrenergic to cholinergic function during development *in vivo*, similar to that described in cell cultures (Landis and Keefe 1983).

Some of the most striking features of neurotrophic actions between nerves and target organs are shown in the ageing sudomotor neuroglandular system. Immunohistochemical studies on forearm skin biopsies from young adult and 80-year-old subjects demonstrate marked regression of secretory coil morphology with age, accompanied by a significant decrease in the number of immunoreactive nerve varicosities and nerve bundles (Fig. 12.3). Only traces of normally strongly acetylcholinesterase-positive sudomotor nerve fibres are found in old age, together with a diminished content of vasoactive intestinal polypeptide (VIP) and calcitonin-gene-related peptide (CGRP)-like immunoreactivity (Abdel-Rahman *et al.* 1992). Several neuropeptides in the sudomotor postganglionic sympathetic nerve fibre terminals surrounding the eccrine sweat glands, including VIP, CGRP, ANP (atrial natriuretic peptide), and substance P, have been identified as possible co-transmitters. Recent findings suggest that CGRP enhances cholinergic sweating and substance P inhibits it (Kumazawa *et al.* 1994).

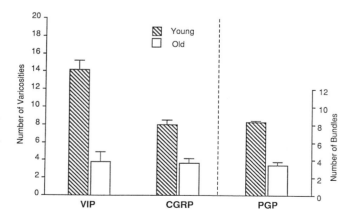

Fig. 12.3. Histogram showing the number of varicosities in sudomotor nerves around each secretory coil of the sweat glands for VIP and CGRP (mean ± SD), and the number of nerve bundles for PGP (the neuronal marker protein gene product) (mean ± SD) for young and old subjects. (From Abdel-Rahman *et al.* (1992), with kind permission of Elsevier Science.)

Thermoregulatory and cardiovascular reflex interactions

In many naturally occurring situations there may be considerable interference between thermoregulatory and other reflex pathways, especially where autonomic reflex systems share a common output, such as in energy production, water metabolism, or the cutaneous circulation. This may involve competition between various reflexes and, in many instances, thermoregulation proves to be a powerful drive, e.g. a high rate of sweat secretion maintained in the face of dehydration, or failure of blood pressure regulation resulting in heat syncope when there is excessive heat-induced vasodilatation.

Skin sympathetic nerve activity (SSNA) responds to acute heat stress to bring about increased heat loss by cutaneous vasodilatation and sweating. In addition, the vasomotor supply to muscles is essential for blood pressure regulation by controlling vascular resistance in muscles. In the resting state, heat stress produces redistribution of blood from the core to the skin by skin vasodilatation and muscle vasoconstriction. The increased muscle sympathetic nerve activity (MSNA) has been recorded by microneurography from the tibial nerve in resting subjects exposed to heat (Niimi *et al.* 1997). Muscle vasodilatation occurs, however, together with SSNA, during exercise, though through increased cardiac venous return and restraint of arterial baroreflexes blood pressure is maintained. Investigations have been made on the influence of baroreceptor unloading (by lower body negative pressure) on cutaneous vasodilatation during heat stress and dynamic exercise (Mack *et al.* 1995). The time course and rapidity with which baroreceptor unloading modulates thermoregulatory control of skin blood flow suggests that the interaction between these two homeostatic mechanisms is primarily neurally mediated. The ability of baroreceptor activity to modulate skin blood flow and sweating suggests a common site of interaction more proximal than the effector organs.

The presence of an autonomic rhythm consisting of sympathetic vasoconstrictor impulses to skin arteriovenous anastomoses is shown to be connected with reciprocal sympathetic and vagal impulses to the heart. This is indicated in power spectral analyses of thermoregulatory fluctuations in cardiovascular responses (Lossius *et al.* 1994). The rhythmic changes in skin blood flow, heart rate, and mean arterial pressure are suppressed in a cool environment. Facial cooling evokes powerful cardiovascular reflexes in which receptors in the face and nasal mucosa innervated by the trigeminal nerve initiate a bradycardia and an increase in total peripheral resistance. Facial cooling differs form the cold pressor response that is evoked from cold and/or pain receptors and which leads to increased MSNA, tachycardia, and increased arterial blood pressure. Interactions between facial cooling and lower body negative pressure (Collins *et al.* 1996) demonstrate a resultant algebraic effect on blood pressure and heart rate while reinforcing the cutaneous vasoconstrictor actions (Fig. 12.4).

Disorders of thermoregulation

Autonomic disorders, including central primary autonomic failure, pre- and postganglionic neuronal degeneration, and peripheral autonomic neuropathies, are frequently associated with thermoregulatory dysregulation. Thermoregulatory tests are valuable for investigating the integrity of the sympathetic system, based on core temperature

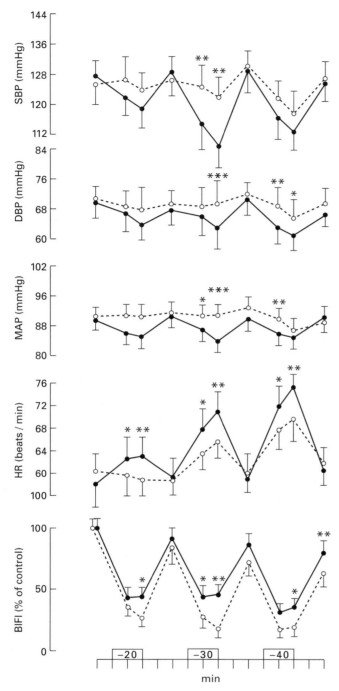

Fig. 12.4. The effect of a progressive lower body negative pressure test (LBNP) at –20, –30, and –40 mmHg (●), and LBNP combined with facial cooling (○) on cardiovascular responses in young (n = 10) healthy subjects (mean ± SEM). Comparisons are between LBNP with and without facial cooling (*, P < 0.05; **, P < 0.01; ***, P < 0.001). SBP, systolic blood pressure; DBP, diastolic blood pressure; MAP, mean arterial pressure; HR, heart rate; BlFI, finger blood flow. (From Collins *et al.* 1996, with kind permission of The Biochemical Society and Portland Press.)

control and assessment of vasomotor and sudomotor function. A crucial step in any such test is to ascertain whether the primary cause of autonomic dysfunction could be due to failure of the target organ,

e.g. a reduction in blood vessel compliance due to atherosclerosis, or a failure of sweating due to morphological changes in the skin. In clinical practice it is also important to establish whether an abnormal autonomic response might be based on the effects of any of a wide range of drugs that enhance or interfere with autonomic nervous function. Disorders of thermoregulation that help to characterize autonomic involvement often destabilize core temperature, resulting in poikilothermia, hypothermia, or hyperthermia.

Poikilothermia

Poikilothermia, the lack of regulated constancy of body temperature, diagnosed by abnormal fluctuation in core temperature of more than 2 °C due to changes in ambient temperature (MacKenzie 1996). The condition usually relates to a lack of central thermoregulatory control even under normal temperature conditions, but it should be noted that in extremes of hypothermia or hyperthermia, central nervous damage can occur and poikilothermia subsequently ensues. Although there appears to be a heterogeneity of brain lesions responsible for the condition, it is claimed that poikilothermia in humans is caused principally by lesions in the posterior hypothalamus and midbrain. Depending on the extent and position of the lesions, symptoms include loss or diminution of thermal comfort sensations (which should be distinguished from temperature sensations), and of autonomic and behavioural thermoregulation.

Under thermal challenge, poikilothermic patients demonstrate varying degrees of deficiency in peripheral vasomotor, shivering, sweating, and metabolic responses. Bilateral lesions of the efferent thermoregulatory pathways below the hypothalamus, e.g. spinal cord injuries, are well known to cause partial poikilothermia (see also Chapter 51). Relative poikilothermia, usually in the absence of acquired hypothalamic disease, is frequently encountered in the newborn, particularly when premature, and in old age. The thermo-lability in these groups can be due to inadequate autonomic responses to abnormal core temperatures or thermal stress. Frequently, lack of thermal discomfort or failure of behavioural thermoregulation plays an important role by failing to compensate for autonomic thermoregulatory failure.

Concurrent endocrine and non-endocrine manifestations of hypothalamic and brainstem disorders are also observed. In the study of MacKenzie (1996) on human poikilothermia, the results of tests of cardiovascular reactivity excluded marked generalized autonomic failure as there was no orthostatic hypotension, and during hypothermia the blood pressure response to Valsalva manoeuvre and head-up tilting was intact.

Hypothermia

Hypothermia, defined as a deep-body temperature below 35 °C, most commonly arises as the result of accidental and excessive exposure to cold, in the elderly, neonates and in undernutrition, and in multiple clinical settings involving dysfunction of central, peripheral, and metabolic autonomic control. Lesions in the region of the hypothalamus can cause either hypothermia or hyperthermia. Frequently, the thermoregulatory disorder is accompanied by endocrine changes or by non-endocrine disorders of consciousness and sleep, cognition, and autonomic, energy, and osmolar balance.

Persistent hypothermia due to thermoregulatory dysfunction with associated hypothalamic damage is well recognized. Acute central nervous dysfunction with hypothalamic involvement but with transient hypothermia has also been described. Periodic hypothermia has been observed with agenesis of the corpus callosum (Shapiro's syndrome), with central nervous abnormalities affecting structures related to thermoregulation, and, rarely, without an associated systemic disease or obvious brain lesion. Most of the latter cases appear to defend a lowered temperature set-point by active body heat dissipation through vasodilatation and sweating, and by decreasing heat generation by behavioural mechanisms. These dramatic hypothermic episodes have been described as 'spontaneous periodic hypothermia' (Kloos 1995).

Secondary hypothermia, in which low body temperature is associated with an existing pathological condition such as diabetes mellitus or with the effects of drugs, is by far the most common presentation (Table 12.1). Hypothermia occurs when there is a marked deterioration of vital functions, especially when associated with serious illness, malnutrition or infections. It is paradoxical that infections may be linked to hypothermia as well as febrile responses. In the course of an infectious disease endogenous pyrogens appear to be able to alter the setting of the hypothalamic control system to cause either high or low deep body temperature.

Fever and hyperthermia

During an immune response leading to fever, phagocytic cells including macrophages release cytokines (endogenous pyrogens), such as interleukin-1, interferons, and tumour necrosis factor, that act on neurones or glial cells at the organum vasculosum of the lamina terminalis, situated in the anterolateral tip of the third ventricle (Hellon

et al. 1991; Cooper 1995). The parenchyma of the organum vasculosum responds to cytokines by releasing prostaglandin E_2, which is believed to diffuse into the medial preoptic area of the hypothalamus, elevating the temperature 'set-point' and producing fever and some of the endocrine and metabolic changes that accompany it. The core temperature is actively defended at the febrile level by intact autonomic and behavioural mechanisms. At the beginning of fever, physiological responses to cold appear, and the core temperature rises to a new level at which thermal neutrality is achieved. As the fever abates, regulatory processes appear that are opposed to excess warming and as a result the core temperature falls to a normal level again.

Fever is distinguished from hyperthermia by the fact that the regulatory processes are hardly burdened at all in fever, whereas in hyperthermia they are working near the limit of their capacity. Any physical injury to the brain cells that allows the entry of macrophages or activates microglial cells to produce cytokines induces a febrile response. Hence fever may occur after cranial trauma or surgery, cerebral haemorrhage, or infection. Fever is also a common manifestation of many malignancies, which may be linked to the production and release of cytokines.

In humans, elevation of rectal temperature above 38.4 °C is arbitrarily considered as hyperthermia or fever. Heat stroke is characterized by a core temperature of 41 °C or more, accompanied by central nervous disturbances leading to convulsions and coma, and anhidrosis, which is often present but is not pathognomonic (Collins 1996). Heat-related deaths during urban heat waves are, however, generally not due to primary thermoregulatory failure but to existing cardiovascular disease combined with heat strain (Semenza et al. 1996). Central nervous dysfunction leading to hyperthermia originates from many of the lesions reported for hypothermia (Table 12.1) and depends on the site of the lesion in the thermoregulatory neuraxis. Conditions in which thermogenesis is stimulated, such as in hyperthyroidism and phaeochromocytoma, often involve hyperthermia. Cardiovascular diseases and sweat gland disorders also generate heat intolerance. Many of the drugs specified in Table 12.1 as inducing hypothermia exhibit a dual action, e.g. alcohol, antidepressants, psychotropics, anaesthetics, and are capable of producing either hypothermia or hyperthermia depending on the dose used and the prevailing ambient temperature conditions. Anticholinergic drugs that interfere with the sweating mechanism are particularly prone to produce hyperthermia in hot ambient conditions.

Neuroleptic malignant syndrome is a rare but potentially lethal complication of medication with neuroleptic agents such as phenothiazines and butyrophenones, particularly in combination with lithium. Symptoms usually progress rapidly over 1–3 days and include hyperthermia, rigidity and tremor, impaired consciousness, and autonomic dysfunction resulting in tachycardia, sweating, and labile blood pressure (Ingall 1993). Although the cause of the syndrome is not known, there is good evidence implicating disturbed dopaminergic function. Another syndrome, malignant hyperthermia, is due to a rare hereditary disorder that presents during anaesthesia with rapid onset hyperthermia, acidosis, and skeletal muscle rigidity. It can be triggered by inhalation of general anaesthetics and by succinylcholine in susceptible individuals. Unexplained autonomic cardiovascular disturbances occur, including ventricular arrhythmia, tachycardia, sweating, and falling blood pressure, and these may herald a hyperthermic crisis. The malignant hyperthermia reaction appears to be due to a sudden rise in the concentration of calcium in

Table 12.1 Causes of secondary hypothermia

Metabolic	Skin disorders
Hypothyroidism	Erythroderma
Hypopituitarism	Extensive burns
Hypoglycaemia	
Diabetic ketoacidosis	Infections
Protein calorie malnutrition	
Uraemia	Drug-induced
Adrenocortical insufficiency	Alcohol
	Anaesthetics
Central nervous dysfunction	Hypnotics
Cerebrovascular accident	Vasodilators
Brain tumour	Psychotropics
Head injury	Tranquillizers
Wernicke's encephalopathy	Hypoglycaemics
Spinal cord lesions	Antithyroids
Multiple sclerosis	Ganglion-blocking agents
Parkinson's disease	
Confusional states	Other
Dementia	Steatorrhoea
	Paget's disease
Cardiovascular	Malignant disease
Myocardial infarction	Osteoarthritis
Congestive cardiac failure	Rheumatoid arthritis
Shock	Systemic lupus erythematosis
Severe haemorrhage	
Peripheral vascular disease	

muscle cytoplasm (reviewed by Britt 1992). An important development in hyperthermia biology occurred when it was demonstrated that certain time-raised body temperature levels could cure tumours in mice but did not permanently damage normal cells. Inactivation of mammalian cells whose normal temperature is around 37 °C starts at 40–41 °C, and becomes exponential at temperatures above 43 °C. In humans, local, regional, and systemic hyperthermia is now used clinically to potentiate radiotherapy and chemotherapy in the treatment of cancer. Hyperthermia treatment requires accurate total body temperature measurement and this has stimulated the search for non-invasive methods of thermometry, such as techniques involving microwave thermometry, acoustic radiometry, and nuclear magnetic resonance computed tomography.

References

Abdel-Rahman, T. A., Collins, K. J., Cowen, T., and Rustin, M. (1992). Immunohistochemical, morphological and functional changes in the peripheral sudomotor neuro-effector system in elderly people. *J. auton. nerv. syst.* **37**, 187–98.

Boulant, J. A. (1991). Thermoregulation. In *Fever: basic mechanisms and management*, (ed. P. A. Mackowiak), pp. 1–22. Raven Press, New York.

Britt, B. A. (1992). Malignant hyperthermia: a review. In *Thermoregulation: pathology, pharmacology and therapy*, (ed. E. Schönbaum and P. Lomax), pp. 179–292. Pergamon Press, New York.

Collins, K. J. (1996). Heat stress and associated disorders. In *Manson's tropical diseases*, (20th edn), (ed. G. C. Cook), pp. 421–32. W. B. Saunders, London.

Collins, K. J., Abdel-Rahman, T. A., Easton, J. C., Sacco, P., Ison, J., and Doré, C. J. (1996). Effects of facial cooling on elderly and young subjects: interactions with breath holding and lower body negative pressure. *Clin. Sci.* **90**, 485–92.

Cooper, K. E. (1995). *Fever and antipyresis*. Cambridge University Press, Cambridge.

Hellon, R., Townsend, Y., Laburn, H. P., and Mitchell, D. (1991). Mechanisms of fever. In *Thermoregulation: pathology, pharmacology and therapy*, (ed. E. Schönbaum and P. Lomax), pp. 19–54. Pergamon Press, New York.

Hensel, H. (1981). *Thermoreception and temperature regulation*, Monographs of the Physiological Society, No. 38, p. 11. Academic Press, New York.

Himms-Hagen, J. (1990). Brown adipose tissue thermogenesis: role in thermoregulation, energy regulation and obesity. In *Thermoregulation: physiology and biochemistry*, (ed. E. Schönbaum and P. Lomax), pp. 327–414. Pergamon Press, New York.

Ingall, T. J. (1993). Hyperthermia and hypothermia. In *Clinical autonomic disorders*, (ed. P. A. Low), pp. 713–29. Little, Brown and Co., Boston.

Jänig, W. (1990). Functions of the sympathetic innervation of the skin. In *Central regulation of autonomic function*, (ed. A. D. Loewy and K. M. Spyer), pp. 334–49. Oxford University Press, Oxford.

Kloos, R. T. (1995). Spontaneous periodic hypothermia. *Medicine*, **74**, 268–80.

Kumazawa, K., Sobue, G., Mitsuma, T., and Ogawa, T. (1994). Modulatory effects of calcitonin gene-related peptide and substance P on human cholinergic sweat secretion. *Clin. Auton. Res.* **4**, 319–22.

Landis, S. C. and Keefe, D. (1983). Evidence for neurotransmitter plasticity *in vivo*: developmental changes in properties of cholinergic sympathetic neurones. *Develop. Biol.* **98**, 349–72.

Loewy, A. D. and Spyer, K. M. (1990). *Central regulation of autonomic functions*. Oxford University Press, Oxford.

Lossius, K., Eriksen, M., and Walloe, L. (1994). Thermoregulatory fluctuations in heart rate and blood pressure in humans: effect of cooling and parasympathetic blockade. *J. auton. nerv. system* **47**, 245–54.

Mack, G., Nishiyasu, T., and Shi, X. (1995). Baroreceptor modulation of cutaneous vasodilator and sudomotor responses to thermal stress in humans. *J. Physiol.* **483**, 537–47.

MacKenzie, M. A. (1996). *Poikilothermia in man: pathophysiological aspects and clinical implications*. Nijmegen University Press, Njimegen.

Niimi, Y., Matsukawa, T., Sugiyama, Y. *et al.* (1997). Effect of heat stress on muscle sympathetic nerve activity in humans. *J. auton. nerv. syst.* **63**, 61–7.

Ogawa, T. and Low, P. A. (1993). Autonomic regulation of temperature and sweating. In *Clinical autonomic disorders*, (ed. P. A. Low), pp. 79–91. Little, Brown and Co., Boston.

Sato, K., Ohtsuyama, M., and Sato, F. (1993). Normal and abnormal eccrine sweat gland function. In *Clinical autonomic disorders*, (ed. P. A. Low), pp. 93–104. Little, Brown and Co., Boston.

Saumet, J. L., Degoute, C. S., Saumet, M., and Abraham, P. (1992). The effect of nerve blockade on forearm and finger skin blood flow during body heating and cooling. *Int. J. Microcircn. Clin. Exp.* **11**, 231–40.

Semenza, J. C., Rubin, C. H., Falter, K. H. *et al.* (1996). Heat-related deaths during the July 1995 heat wave in Chicago. *New Engl. J. Med.* **335**, 84–90.

13. Pain and the sympathetic nervous system: pathophysiological mechanisms

Wilfrid Jänig

Introduction

The sympathetic nervous system can be associated with pain in two ways (Fig. 13.1). First, it shows both generalized and specific localized reactions in response to noxious, tissue-damaging events. The generalized reactions are organized in the mesencephalon, hypothalamus, and suprahypothalamic brain structures and are best understood as components of the different patterns of defence behaviour, such as 'confrontational defence', 'flight', and 'quiescence' (Bandler and Shipley 1994; Jänig 1995). Confrontational defence and flight are typical of an active defence strategy when animals encounter threatening stimuli which are potentially injurious for the body; confrontational defence leading potentially to fight, and flight leading to forward avoidance. Both patterns are represented in the lateral periaqueductal grey of the mesencephalon, activated from the body surface, and associated with endogenous non-opioid analgesia, hypertension, and tachycardia. Quiescence is similar to the natural reactions of mammals to serious injury and chronic pain and is associated in particular to the deep and visceral body domains. It is represented in the ventrolateral periaqueductal grey, activated from the deep body domains, and associated with an endogenous opioid analgesia, hyporeactivity, hypotension, and bradycardia. These stereotyped pre-programmed elementary behaviours and their association with the endogenous control of analgesia enable the organism to cope with dangerous situations which are always associated with pain or impending pain.

There are also more localized and selective reactions of the sympathetic nervous system which are organized within the spinal cord and in the periphery, i.e. somato-sympathetic, viscero-sympathetic, and viscero-visceral reflexes. The hypothalamo-mesencephalic and the spinal level of integration are presumably protective under normal biological conditions and are associated with activation of the adrenocortical system by the hypothalamo-hypophyseal axis (Jänig 1995; Jänig and Häbler 1995).

Secondly, tissue damage in the extremities with and without any overt nerve lesion is sometimes followed by diffuse burning pain and hyperalgesia which can sometimes be relieved by blockade of the (efferent) sympathetic activity to the affected extremity. Spontaneous pain and hyperalgesia may be correlated with changes of blood flow and sweating, tissue oedema, changes of posture and movements, including an increase in physiological tremor, and trophic changes of tissues. These changes are thought to be, directly or indirectly, associated with the sympathetic nervous system and they may be, like the pain, alleviated by blockade of sympathetic activity. Therefore, it is believed that the *efferent* sympathetic nervous system can be actively involved in the generation of pain.

The sympathetic nervous may be causally involved in other pain states, such as hyperalgesia during inflammatory processes in tissues (Levine and Taiwo 1994; Jänig *et al.* 1996) and possibly even visceral pain (e.g. irritable bowel syndrome, non-ulcer dyspepsia, interstitial cystitis, angina pectoris; see Jänig and Häbler 1995).

This chapter will concentrate on possible mechanisms by which the sympathetic nervous system may contribute to pain after traumatic injury to the extremities.

Clinical background and general hypothesis

Complex regional pain syndrome (CRPS) and related disorders

That the sympathetic nervous system may be involved in the generation and maintenance of pain states has been particularly documented for disorders that were previously generically called reflex sympathetic dystrophy (RSD), causalgia, and related disorders that follow trauma, affecting particularly deep tissues with and without obvious nerve lesions, sometimes visceral diseases and sometimes even central lesions (for literature see Bonica 1990; Blumberg and Jänig 1994; Jänig and Stanton-Hicks 1996). To avoid the mechanistic implications of such terminology, clinical and basic researchers have made efforts to define the clinical phenomenology using purely descriptive terms (Merskey and Bogduk 1994; Stanton-Hicks *et al.* 1995). Disorders previously considered to be RSD and causalgia were classified under the neutral umbrella term *complex regional pain syndrome* (CRPS) which is based entirely on clinical criteria. The

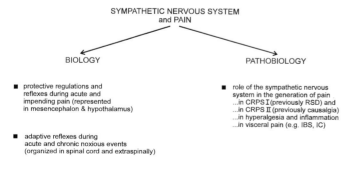

Fig. 13.1. Aspects of 'sympathetic nervous system and pain'. CRPS, Complex regional pain syndrome. IBS, irritable bowel syndrome; IC, interstitial cystitis. For explanation see text. (Modified from Jänig *et al.* (1996).)

inclusion criteria under this overall CRPS syndrome are the presence of regional pain (spontaneous and evoked) and other sensory changes following a noxious event. The pain is associated with changes in skin colour, skin temperature, abnormal sweating, oedema, and sometimes motor abnormalities. Two types of CRPS have been recognized: CRPS type I, corresponding to RSD, and CRPS type II, corresponding to what was formerly considered as causalgia. Table 13.1 summarizes the characteristics of CRPS I and II. The term 'sympathetically maintained pain' (SMP) was not considered as a separate disorder but as a description of a type of pain that can be found in a variety of pain disorders, including CRPS I and CRPS II (Stanton-Hicks *et al.* 1995; Jänig and Stanton-Hicks 1996).

Definition of CRPS I and II may undergo changes and further differentiation. The patients may be subclassified into those with touch-evoked allodynia and those without (Price *et al.* 1989). Furthermore, it is advisable to discriminate patients according to the duration of CRPS (e.g. patients ≤10 days after the initiating event from those who have their CRPS for months or longer; Blumberg and Jänig 1994). This division may not only have considerable diagnostic and therapeutic consequences, but may be relevant as far as the underlying pathophysiological mechanisms are concerned.

It is commonly, yet not universally, recommended to treat many patients with CRPS by sympathetic blocks and by physiotherapy (Bonica 1990). It is irrelevant in the present context (albeit important from the practical point of view) whether the sympathetic blocks are successful in all cases or not, and whether temporary blocks may not lead in some cases to permanent relief of pain. It is important to note that intravenous injection of guanethidine (which displaces noradrenaline from its stores) into the affected and cuffed extremity distal to the occlusion and intravenous injection of an α-adrenoreceptor antagonist (used as a diagnostic tool; Arnér 1991) may abolish the pain. Both procedures correlate quite well with the effects of sympathetic blocks by local anesthetics and strongly support the view that the sympathetic noradrenergic neurones are involved. However, it is poorly understood why temporary sympathetic blocks mostly produce long-lasting if not permanent relief of pain.

A general hypothesis

The clinical phenomenology favours the notion that the (efferent) sympathetic nervous system is an important component in the generation of CRPS. A general hypothesis which explains several clinical phenomena observed in patients with CRPS is sketched in Fig. 13.2. The main clinical observations (see Table 13.1) are double framed; the initiating events are at the top, the most important one being trauma with and without nerve lesion. This expanatory hypothesis consists of several components (see numbers in Fig. 13.2). Some components are fully or partially supported by experiments on animals, some by experimental investigations on humans and some are still hypothetical (Blumberg and Jänig 1985; Jänig 1988; Jänig and Koltzenburg 1991*a*, *b*; Jobling *et al.* 1992; Blumberg *et al.* 1994; Devor 1994; Koltzenburg *et al.* 1995; Jänig *et al.* 1996):

1. The afferent neurones with small-diameter fibres in the affected territory, in particular the nociceptive ones, may be sensitized as a consequence of the trauma. They generate ongoing activity and react abnormally to mechanical, thermal, or chemical stimulation. Lesioned afferent axons may generate ectopically spontaneous and evoked impulse activity.

2. Noradrenergic postganglionic neurones are coupled in some abnormal way to the peripheral afferent neurones generating or enhancing the abnormal afferent impulse traffic to the spinal cord. This coupling may occur at various sites of the afferent neurones in the lesioned and unlesioned tissue.

3. The decoding of nociceptive and non-nociceptive afferent information by neurones in the dorsal horn, including the control of transmission of nociceptive information by supraspinal systems, is changed. Neurones of the central nociceptive pathways are sensitized by the continuous afferent input originating from the primary lesioned as well as the unlesioned tissues.

4. The discharge pattern in the neurones of the sympathetic outflow to the affected extremity may be changed as a consequence of the changes of nociceptive impulse transmission in the spinal cord.

Table 13.1. Criteria for differential diagnosis of complex regional pain syndrome (CRPS) types I and II (from Baron *et al.* in Jänig and Stanton–Hicks 1996)

	CRPS I	CRPS II
Aetiology	Any kind of lesion	Partial nerve lesion
Localization	Distal part of extremity Independent from site of lesion	Any peripheral site of body Mostly confined to the territory of affected nerve
Spreading of symptoms	Obligatory	Obligatory
Spontaneous pain	Common Mostly deep and superficial Orthostatic component	Obligatory Predominantly superficial
Mechanical allodynia	Many patients with spreading tendency	Obligatory
Autonomic symptoms	Distally generalized with spreading tendency	Related to nerve lesion plus distally generalized
Motor symptoms	Distally generalized	Related to nerve lesion plus distally generalized
Sensory symptoms	Distally generalized with spreading tendency	Relative to nerve lesion plus distally generalized
Frequency	Common	Rare
Recommended therapies	Sympathetic block, physiotherapy	Sympathetic block, physiotherapy

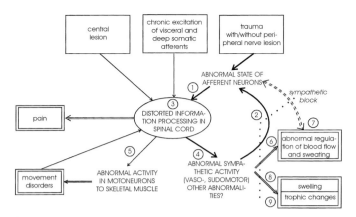

Fig. 13.2. General hypothesis about the neural mechanisms of generation of CRPS I and II following peripheral injury with and without nerve lesions, chronic stimulation of visceral afferents (e.g. myocardial infarction) and deep somatic afferents and, rarely, central trauma. The clinical observations are double framed. Note the vicious circle (arrows in bold black). An important component of this circle is the excitatory influence of postganglionic sympathetic axons on primary afferent neurones in the periphery. This influence leads to orthodromic afferent impulse activity. But it may also induce antidromically conducted impulses in unmyelinated afferents to the periphery which may contribute to the trophic changes (i.e. by release of substances due to antidromic invasion of axon terminals which leads to vasodilation and plasma extravasation). These trophic changes may in turn influence the coupling between postganglionic axons and afferent axons (see interrupted double arrow). Another important component that is not emphasized in this diagram may be that the neurovascular transmission is impaired and that the blood vessels develop hyper-reactivity to circulating catecholamines and to nerve impulses. The numbers refer to the text. (Modified from Jänig 1990; Blumberg and Jänig (1994).)

5. The discharge pattern in α- and γ-motoneurones may also be changed as a consequence of the sensitization of spinal neurones.

6. In the case of nerve lesions, the regulation of small blood vessels by vasoconconstrictor neurones (neurovascular transmission) may be changed following regeneration of lesioned postganglionic axons. Blood vessels may develop hyper-reactivity to circulating catecholamines and to impulses in the vasoconstrictor neurones.

7. Blood vessels in skin and deep somatic tissues (e.g. joint capsule) are also under afferent control. Activation of polymodal nociceptors generates precapillary vasodilatation and (in some tissues) postcapillary plasma extravasation. Both may be enhanced or reduced following trauma.

8., 9. Swelling and trophic changes are thought to be related to sympathetic and afferent neurones.

This complex concerto of events may establish a vicious circle that is interrupted by blocking the sympathetic impulse traffic to the affected territory.

This hypothesis is not testable as such. The prevalence of the different components varies for the generation of CRPS and may help to explain the variable clinical phenomenologies. This chapter will now mainly concentrate on the mechanisms of components 2, 4, 6, and 8 which are the key issues in pain states in which the sympathetic

nervous system might be involved. Table 13.2 lists possible pathobiological mechanisms in which the sympathetic nervous system may be involved. Components 1 and 3 are discussed elsewhere. Components 5, 7, and 9 will not be discussed because there is almost nothing known about their mechanisms.

Coupling between sympathetic postganglionic neurones and primary afferent neurones following peripheral trauma

Physiological conditions

Under physiological conditions there exists almost no influence of sympathetic activity on sensory neurones projecting to skin and deep somatic tissues in mammals. The effects that have been measured under experimental conditions on receptors with myelinated and unmyelinated axons were weak and can, in part, be explained by changes of the effector organs induced by the activation of sympathetic neurones. These rather negative results do not rule out that nordrenaline or co-localized substances released by the postganglionic terminals have secondary long-term effects on the excitability of sensory receptors (Jänig and Koltzenburg 1991a).

Pathophysiological conditions

Under pathophysiological conditions, which develop after peripheral injury, sympathetic noradrenergic neurones may influence afferent neurones in several ways. This is illustrated schematically in Fig. 13.3. Various types of experiments on animal models of nerve injury have shown that the coupling may occur at, or close to, the lesion site, as well as remote from the lesion site.

Coupling between lesioned postganglionic and afferent nerve terminals

Coupling may occur between sympathetic fibres and afferent terminals in a neuroma, following nerve cut or ligation. Some myelinated as well as unmyelinated nerve fibres in the neuroma can be excited following electrical stimulation of the sympathetic supply or by noradrenaline and adrenaline injected systemically. The coupling has been observed in young neuromas and less so in old ones weeks and months after nerve lesion. This is compatible with clinical experience showing that neuroma pain is usually not dependent on sympathetic activity. It is also compatible with histological observations that catecholamine-containing axon profiles are rare within the neuroma and for several centimeters proximal to it, many weeks after cutting and ligating the nerve. Thus, this coupling is chemical and occurs via noradrenaline acting on α-adrenoceptors, although other mediator substances may also be involved. Ephaptic coupling between sympathetic fibres and afferent fibres has so far not been observed in a neuroma (Jänig and Koltzenburg 1991a).

The situation is different when afferent and sympathetic fibres are allowed to regenerate to the target tissue. This has been shown experimentally for the chronic situation more than a year after cross-union of nerves (proximal stump of the sural nerve to the distal stump of the tibial nerve, in the cat) and after reinnervation of appropriate and

Table 13.2. Peripheral and central pathobiological mechanisms that are possibly associated with the sympathetic nervous system and may contribute to the generation of the complex regional pain syndrome (CRP, in particular type I) after peripheral injury with nerve lesions[a]

1. Retrograde cell reactions: interruption of transport of neurotrophic factors from periphery to sympathetic ganglia; shrinkage of axons and cell bodies, death of postganglionic neurones.

2. Anterograde cell reactions: regeneration of postganglionic axons and postganglionic-target organ mismatch after axon lesion; collateral sprouting of postganglionic axons in the dorsal root ganglion and in the periphery.

3. Change and failure of synaptic transmission from preganglionic to postganglionic neurones in sympathetic ganglia.

4. Development of influence of postganglionic sympathetic fibres on primary afferent neurones (at lesion site; remote from lesion site, e.g. in dorsal root ganglion): chemical (by release of noradrenaline); ephaptic (unlikely); indirect via influence on vascular and other non-neural cells, indirect by change of micromilieu.

5. Development of hyper- and hyporeactivity of autonomic effector organs after degeneration and regeneration of their postganglionic innervation; abnormal vascular responses to neural impulses, substances released locally, circulating substances, and external influences (e.g. changes in environmental temperature).

6. Abnormal regulation of blood flow through skin and subcutaneous tissues due to mismatch of vasoconstrictor activity to different sections of vascular beds.

7. Increase of filtration pressure in capillary beds with subsequent chronic formation of oedema due to imbalance of pre- to postcapillary constriction; increase in venular permeability due to release of vasoactive substances (e.g. from primary afferents or local cells) or due to other processes.

8. Activation of local immune-competent and related cells (macrophages, T and B lymphocytes, polymorphonuclear leucocytes, mast cells) in the microenvironment of primary afferent and noradrenergic fibres. Neuroimmune interaction in sustaining nociceptive impulse activity and inflammatory reactions. Participation of histamine, arachidonic acid derivatives (prostaglandins, leucotrienes), cytokines (e.g. interleukins 1 and 2, tumor necrosis factor), growth factors (e.g. nerve growth factor).

9. Development of abnormal discharge properties and abnormal reflexes in sympathetic neurones supplying the affected extremity (skin, deep somatic tissues, etc.) as a consequence of central changes.

[a] Some mechanisms are supported experimentally, some are hypothetical (see Jänig 1990; Jänig and Koltzenburg 1991a; Devor 1994; Jänig and McLachlan 1994; Koltzenburg et al. 1995; Jänig et al. 1996).

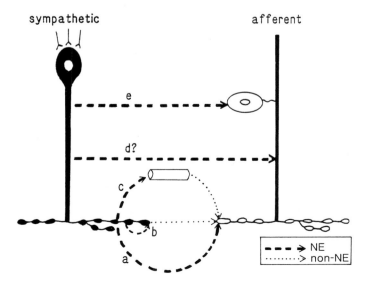

Fig. 13.3. Possible ways of coupling between sympathetic postganglionic neurones and afferent neurones under pathological conditions. (a) Noradrenergic (NE) and possibly also non-noradrenergic (non-NE) chemical coupling between peripheral endings. This may occur preferentially after nerve lesions. (b) Indirect chemical coupling: as believed by Levine and co-workers (Levine and Taiwo 1994), noradrenaline acts prejunctionally at postganglionic varicosities via α_2-adrenoceptors, triggering the release of other substances (e.g. prostaglandins). This may be relevant during states of chronic inflammation. (c) Indirect coupling via the vascular bed (change of neurovascular transmission, development of hyper-reactivity of the vascular bed). This may occur after various forms of trauma with or without nerve lesion. (d) Interaction along the nerve. This may occur after nerve lesions during regeneration and sprouting in the nerve. (e) Noradrenergic coupling in the dorsal root ganglion. This may occur after a remote nerve lesion. (Summary scheme composed from Jänig and Koltzenburg (1991a) and Jänig et al. (1996).)

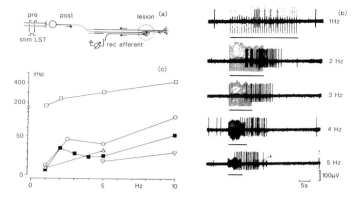

Fig. 13.4. Excitation of unmyelinated afferent units by electrical stimulation of sympathetic fibres following nerve injury. Unmyelinated primary afferents were recorded in cats 11–20 months following a nerve lesion. The central cut stump of a cutaneous nerve innervating hairy skin had been imperfectly adapted to the distal stump of a transected mixed nerve. This preparation was designed to mimic the consequences of a mixed nerve lesion. There was a 'neuroma-in-continuity' at the site of the lesion and cutaneous nerve fibres had regenerated into skin and deep somatic tissue supplied by the mixed nerve. (a) Experimental set-up. Pre, preganglionic; Post, postganglionic; LST, lumbar sympathetic trunk. (b) Record from a single unmyelinated afferent unit (conduction velocity 1.3 m/s). Supramaximal stimulation of the LST with trains of 30 pulses at 1–5 Hz (trains and stimulation artefacts indicated by bars). Note that the afferent unit had some low rate of ongoing activity (impulses before the trains at 1 and 4 Hz) and that a second unit was recruited at 5 Hz (marked by *). (c) Stimulus response curve for the single unit (■) and four filaments containing 2–3 (○, ▽, △) and more than 5 (□) afferent units. Ordinate scale is the total number of impulses exceeding ongoing activity in response to variable stimulation frequency of the LST. (Modified from Häbler *et al.* (1987).)

inappropriate target tissues. Now unmyelinated afferent fibres may be vigorously excited by electrical low-frequency stimulation of the sympathetic supply (Häbler *et al.* 1987). Also this excitation is adrenoceptor-mediated (Fig. 13.4).

Coupling between unlesioned postganglionic and afferent nerve terminals following partial nerve lesion

Intact C-fibre polymodal nociceptors in skin may develop adrenosensitivity following partial nerve injury. Sympathetic nerve stimulation and noradrenaline may excite the polymodal nociceptors or sensitize them for heat stimuli. This activation and sensitization is already seen 4–10 days after partial nerve lesion and is maintained for at least 150 days. This sympathetic–afferent coupling apparently involves the non-lesioned polymodal nociceptive afferent axons that still projected through the lesion site, and non-lesioned postganglionic axons. It is assumed that the unlesioned unmyelinated afferents develop some sort of hyper-reactivity to catecholamines following degeneration of the sympathetic postganglionic axons. Expression of adrenoceptors in afferent fibres may be triggered by collateral sprouting of both afferent fibres and postganglionic fibres in the target tissue (Sato and Perl 1991).

Coupling in the dorsal root ganglion and collateral sprouting following peripheral nerve lesion

A possibility of chemical sympathetic–afferent coupling following peripheral nerve lesion (e.g. cutting and ligating the sciatic nerve in rats) may occur a long way proximally to the injury site, such as in the proximal part of the nerve or in the dorsal root ganglion (DRG; Fig. 13.3). Sympathetic postganglionic fibres reach the spinal nerves via grey rami. Most of these fibres project distally to peripheral target cells, others project proximally (e.g. to the DRG) and are normally found along blood vessels. This situation changes after an experimental nerve lesion (e.g. transection and ligation of the sciatic nerve). Now many perivascular fine catecholamine-containing axons of the unlesioned proximally projecting neurones start to penetrate the DRGs which contain somata with lesioned axons (Fig. 13.5). The extent of this novel *collateral* sprouting increases with time after the nerve lesion. Several weeks after the nerve lesion some somata are partially or almost completely surrounded by varicose catecholaminergic terminals; the frequency of these catecholamine-fluorescent structures increases for more than 70 days after the nerve lesion. The noradrenergic axons sprout preferentially in DRGs which contain somata of lesioned neurones, and here preferentially to large-diameter neurones which are lesioned.

Neurophysiological experiments on rats with the same nerve lesion show that afferent neurones projecting in the lesioned nerve can be affected via the DRG by sympathetic stimulation and by catecholamines (Fig. 13.6). Afferent neurones with myelinated fibres are preferentially involved; the afferent neurones are preferentially excited in the first weeks after lesion and predominantly inhibited in their activity at later times when the catecholaminergic sprouting in the DRG is more prominent (McLachlan *et al.* 1993; Devor *et al.* 1994; Michaelis *et al.* 1996).

Interestingly, the same type of nerve lesion has also been shown to induce sprouting of large-diameter afferent neurones into lamina II of the dorsal horn (Woolf *et al.* 1992). Thus, after a peripheral nerve lesion, mechanosensitive large-diameter afferents may have access to the central nociceptive system, and activity in these afferents may be induced or enhanced by sympathetic activity.

The mechanism leading to the collateral sprouting in the DRG is possibly related to some trophic signal generated by afferent cells with lesioned axons in the DRG or their surrounding Schwann cells. Whether these aberrant pathological connections might account for spontaneous pain and allodynia in some patients after peripheral nerve lesions awaits further investigations (for discussion see Jänig *et al.* 1996).

Adrenoceptors involved in chemical sympathetic–afferent coupling

Excitation and depression of lesioned primary afferent neurones (in the DRG and at their lesioned terminals in the neuroma), or of unlesioned collaterally sprouting primary afferents generated by activation of the sympathetic innervation, is mimicked by systemic injection of noradrenaline and adrenaline and blocked by phentolamine application. Thus both excitation and depression are suggested to be mediated by α-adrenoceptors. The cellular mechanisms underlying the increased sensitivity are unknown. Novel expression or up-regulation of adrenoceptors occurs; alternatively, normally present adrenoreceptors which are not functional become uncovered and effective during the response

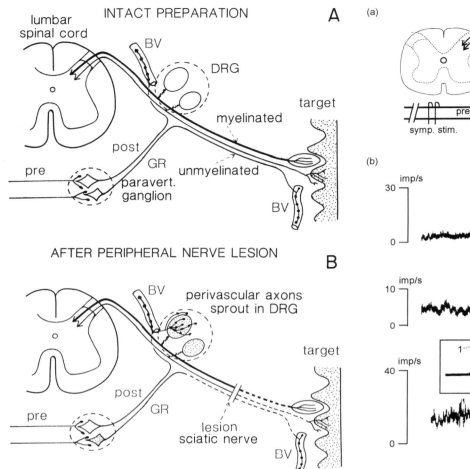

Fig. 13.5. Relation between afferent neurones, sympathetic postganglionic neurones and their projections in the lumbar outflow under physiological and pathophysiological conditions. (a) Myelinated and unmyelinated afferent neurones and postganglionic neurones form separate projections to the periphery and to the spinal cord and do not interact under normal conditions. (b) After ligating and cutting the sciatic nerve, noradrenergic perivascular axons sprout in the dorsal root ganglia and form basket-like structures preferentially around cell bodies of large-diameter axotomized sensory neurones. Repetitive stimulation of the sympathetic supply can activate such neurones; note that many postganglionic sympathetic fibres which projected into the sciatic nerve and which have been axotomized by the lesion, may degenerate (stippled). Moreover, as a consequence of the nerve lesion, sensory neurones with myelinated axons affected by the peripheral lesion may form new spinal branches sprouting into lamina II which gain access to the central nociceptive system (see Woolf et al. 1992). BV, blood vessel; GR, grey ramus; pre/post, pre-/postganglionic. (Modified from Jänig and McLachlan (1994).)

to damage. The subtype of α-adrenoreceptor being involved in the sympathetic–afferent coupling in the different rat models is predominantly α_2. Knowledge about the subtypes of adrenoceptor following nerve trauma may turn out to be useful in the design of more specific treatment modalities for neuropathic pain conditions involving sympathetic efferent activity (Chen et al. 1996; Jänig et al. 1996).

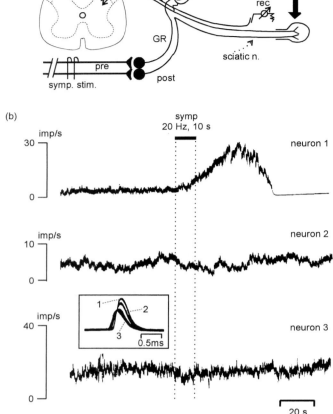

Fig. 13.6. Excitation of primary afferent neurones via the dorsal root ganglion (DRG) by electrical stimulation of sympathetic fibres following nerve injury. (a) Experimental set-up with stimulation and recording electrodes: The sciatic nerve was ligated and cut in the lower popliteal fossa 4–171 days before the experiments. Centrally connected afferent fibres were isolated from the sciatic nerve proximal to the neuroma and identified by stimulation of the dorsal roots L4 and L5 (aff. stim.). The sympathetic supply was excited by electrical stimulation either of the preganglionic axons (pre) in the ventral roots T13 and L1 or L1 and L2 or the lumbar sympathetic trunk (symp. stim.). Dorsal and ventral roots were cut proximally to the stimulation electrodes. GR, grey ramus. (b) Responses of afferent neurones with myelinated axons to electrical stimulation of sympathetic preganglionic efferents in the ventral roots T13 and L1 (symp; 20 Hz stimulation for 10 s). Activity was recorded simultaneously from the axons of these neurones each with spontaneous background activity. Neuron 1 exhibited strong sympathetic excitation followed by after-suppression. Neuron 2 showed a weak suppression to sympathetic stimulation. Neuron 3 showed no response. Inset: superimposed action potentials recorded from the axons. Eight days after sciatic nerve lesion. (Modified from Devor et al. (1994).)

Synopsis

Peripheral trauma, with or without nerve injury, may lead to sensitization and activation of nociceptive and activation of other primary afferent neurones. These processes depend on and are maintained by the sympathetic nervous system. Several ways of coupling between sympathetic postganglionic neurones and primary afferent neurones are possible and have been worked out experimentally on animal models with controlled nerve lesions, showing that there may be intimate relationships between sympathetic neurones and afferent neurones under pathophysiological conditions (Fig. 13.7):

1. The postganglionic sympathetic neurone may develop chemically mediated interactions with primary afferent neurones. Whether this occurs probably depends on the time after nerve lesion as well as on the type of nerve lesion (partial, complete).

2. This interaction is mediated by noradrenaline, but additonal mediator substances are possible.

3. Following peripheral nerve lesion, remote collateral sprouting of unlesioned postganglionic fibres occurs in the dorsal root ganglion, preferentially toward the large-diameter cells. Collateral sprouting of unlesioned postganglionic fibres may also occur in the peripheral target tissue (in particular after partial nerve lesion). The signal(s) intiating this sprouting probably derive from primary afferent neurones and/or Schwann cells and may be neurotrophic substances.

4. Primary afferent neurones express functional adrenoceptors. The type of adrenoceptor involved is preferentially α_2 in the animal models. Signal(s) that initiate the functional expression of adrenoceptors may be related to a decrease of density of noradrenergic innervation (i.e. relative or complete denervation), to activity in the sympathetic neurones, or to neurotrophic signals that derive from the Schwann cells or other cells.

5. Plastic changes of primary afferent and sympathetic postganglionic neurones following peripheral trauma with nerve lesion may explain some of the clinical sensory phenomena in patients with sympathetically maintained pain in CRPS, particularly type II. Whether it can explain the development of pain and associated changes in many patients with CRPS I (previously reflex sympathetic dystrophy) awaits further investigations, particularly on newly designed animal models.

Indirect coupling between noradrenergic nerve terminals and nociceptors in the periphery

Nociceptive afferents are embedded in a complex micromilieu (Fig. 13.8). The state of this micromilieu surrounding the receptive terminals depends on mediator substances that are released during inflammatory processes following trauma from non-neural cells such as mast cells, polymorphonuclear leucocytes, macrophages, fibroblasts, endothelial cells, or other cells. The microcirculation is under neural control of sympathetic vasoconstrictor neurones. Moreover, activation of nociceptive primary afferents not only causes orthodromic impulse traffic but also arteriolar (precapillary) vasodilation and (in some tissues) venular plasma extravasation by the release of neuropeptides from the receptive terminals (e.g. substance P and calcitonin-gene-related peptide (CGRP)) initiating neurogenic inflammation. Thus there are possibilities for indirect coupling between sympathetic and afferent nerve terminals (see Fig. 13.3a, c): first, vascular perfusion of the micromilieu surrounding the nociceptors after nerve trauma may change as consequences of denervation and reinnervation by postganglionic vasoconstrictor neurones and afferent nociceptive neurones and the development of hyper-reactivity of blood vessels (Jobling et al. 1992; Koltzenburg et al. 1995); second,

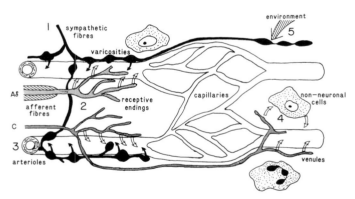

Fig. 13.8. The micromilieu of nociceptors. The microenvironment of primary afferents is thought to affect the properties of the receptive endings of myelinated ($A\delta$) and unmyelinated (C) afferent fibres. This has been particularly documented for inflammatory processes, but one may speculate that pathological changes in the direct surroundings of primary afferents may contribute to other pain states as well. The micromilieu depends on several interacting components. Neural activity in postganglionic noradrenergic fibres supplying blood vessels (1) causes vasoconstriction and the release of noradrenaline and possibly other substances. Excitation of primary afferents (2) causes vasodilatation in precapillary arterioles ($A\delta$- and C-fibres) by the release of CGRP and substance P and plasma extravasation in postcapillary venules (C-fibres only) by the release of substance P and possibly other vasoactive compounds. Some of these effects may be mediated by non-neuronal cells such as mast cells (4). Other factors that affect the control of the microcirculation are the myogenic properties of arterioles (3) and more global environmental influences (5) such as a change of the temperature and the metabolic state of the tissue. (With permission from Jänig and Koltzenburg (1991a).)

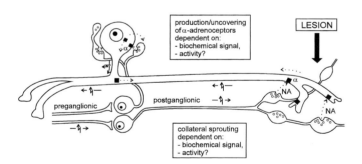

Fig. 13.7. Relation between afferent neurones and sympathetic neurones following peripheral nerve lesion. Collateral sprouting of unlesioned sympathetic neurones in the dorsal root ganglion and in the peripheral target tissue. Up-regulation or uncovering of functional adrenoceptors by afferent neurones after nerve lesion. It is unclear in which way these processes are related to the biochemical signals (e.g. neurotrophins) synthesized by neurones, Schwann cells, and other cells in the DRG and the expression of their receptors. In which way are these processes dependent on activity in the afferent neurones, on the presence/absence of postganglionic noradrenergic neurones or on the activity in the postganglionic neurones? (Taken with permission from Jänig et al. (1996).)

nociceptors may be sensitized by substances such as prostaglandins which are released by noradrenergic nerve terminals or from non-neuronal cells of the micromilieu.

Changes of neurovascular transmission and development of hyper-reactivity of blood vessels

Neural control of blood vessels can change dramatically after trauma with nerve lesions, but possibly also after trauma without lesions of nerves (Jänig and McLachlan 1994; Koltzenburg et al. 1995):

1. Cutaneous blood vessels which are reinnervated after a nerve lesion might exhibit stronger than normal vasoconstrictions to impulses in sympathetic neurones.

2. The sympathetically reinnervated cutaneous blood vessels may show stronger than normal vasoconstrictions to systemic catecholamines and appear to be hyper-reactive.

3. The blood vessels may exhibit changes in vasodilatation to antidromic activation of reinnervated unmyelinated afferents.

The reinnervated blood vessels may therefore be under stronger than normal vasoconstrictor influence which can no longer be counteracted by an afferent-mediated vasodilatation. In vitro investigation of the rat tail artery has shown that the functional recovery of neurovascular transmission may remain permanently disturbed after a nerve lesion (Jobling et al. 1992).

The altered neural and non-neural control of blood vessels will contribute to abnormal regulation of microcirculation following trauma due to nerve lesions. These changes can contribute to the abnormal regulation of blood flow through skin and deep somatic tissues and possibly to the trophic changes (including the oedema) which are seen in patients with CRPS. They may furthermore be a permissive factor in the generation of afferent nociceptive impulse activity and therefore in the sensitization of nociceptors and in the generation of pain.

Finally, it is sometimes believed that skin temperature changes during painful neuropathies (e.g. in CRPS I or II) reflect changes in neural vasoconstrictor activity. Thus, cold skin may then be associated with a high level of activity in the sympathetic cutaneous vasoconstrictor neurones and warm skin with a low level of their activity. This is probably a misconception, and there is no proof at all that the relation between skin temperature and activity in sympathetic neurones holds under these pathophysiological conditions. Therefore, it is also not correct to conclude, only on the basis of cold feet or hands of these patients, that there is a 'high sympathetic tone' or 'hyper-sympathetic' activity.

Indirect influence of sympathetic efferents on afferent impulse traffic by changing the micromilieu of the nociceptors

As already mentioned above, the micromilieu of the nociceptors in skin and deep somatic tissues is dependent on the activity of several types of non-neural cells (Fig. 13.8) and on substances produced by these cells (trophic factors, cytokines, arachidonic acid derivatives, histamine, see Table 13.2). The interaction of these cells with the primary afferent terminal is complex. It leads to a sensitization of nociceptors and therefore to an enhanced afferent impulse traffic to

the CNS. It may furthermore enhance the development and maintenance of trophic changes observed in patients with CRPS and of chronic inflammatory disorders (Levine and Taiwo 1994; Jänig et al. 1996).

How is the sympathetic nervous system involved, except by its putative permissive effect via the control of the vascular bed? A compelling possibility has recently been explored by pharmacological experiments in animal models (Jänig and Koltzenburg 1991a; Levine and Taiwo 1994). Rats were rendered hyperalgesic by repetitive chloroform treatment of the skin or by cutaneous injections of algesic chemicals. The reduction of the threshold for the flexion reflex elicited by paw pressure was used as an indicator for the presence of hyperalgesia and its modification was measured following various pharmacological treatments.

In normal control animals intradermal injection of noradrenaline and α-antagonists into the paw does not significantly change the flexion reflex threshold. This is in agreement with previous neurophysiological results showing that sympathetic efferents have little influence on nociceptive afferents under physiological conditions. In hyperalgesic rats, however, intradermal injections of noradrenaline led to a further drop of the threshold, suggesting that sympathetic activity could aggravate hyperalgesia. Conversely, an increase of the flexion reflex threshold was noted after blockade of α_2-adrenoceptors, but not of α_1-adrenoceptors. The hyperalgesic effect of noradrenaline injections was absent in animals that had been chronically sympathectomized. This led to the hypothesis that catecholamines would not directly sensitize primary afferents but might act on presynaptic α_2-adrenoceptors of postganglionic fibres, thereby releasing other compounds that may subsequently affect the properties of afferent neurones (Fig. 13.3d). As the cyclo-oxygenase inhibitor, indomethacin, could also counteract the hyperalgesic effect of noradrenaline, it was suggested that prostaglandins could be involved. The mechanisms postulated by this exciting hypothesis may be relevant in chronic inflammatory conditions (such as rheumatoid arthritis, for example) and further experimental support is needed.

Changes of the reflex pattern in sympathetic neurones

Changes of the activity of and reflexes in the sympathetic nervous system may also contribute to the disturbed neural control of blood vessels and sweat glands in patients with CRPS I. Many patients with CRPS I can no longer thermoregulate with their affected extremity; furthermore the skin of the affected extremity is usually warmer than on the contralateral side in the early stage of CRPS I and colder later on (Blumberg and Jänig 1994). Thus, in addition to a disturbed neurovascular transmission and the development of hyper-reactivity of blood vessels, the activity in vasoconstrictor neurones may change after trauma caused by nerve lesions in patients with CRPS I. This idea is based primarily on observations of autonomic effector organ responses (changes of blood flow and sweating) in patients with CRPS I, and would imply that the activity or activity pattern in sympathetic neurones to blood vessels and sweat glands has changed.

In neurophysiological experiments tests have been performed to detemine whether the reflex pattern in vasoconstrictor neurones to skin and skeletal muscle of the cat hindlimb changes 6 days to 18 months after various types of nerve lesion (cutting and ligating a skin nerve, connecting the central stump of a skin nerve to the distal stump of a muscle nerve, cross-union of skin and mixed nerve). Following the nerve lesions, the reflex pattern elicited by stimulation of nociceptors, arterial chemoreceptors, and arterial baroreceptors may change in many cutaneous vasoconstrictor neurones, leading to inappropriate effector responses; however, those in muscle vasoconstrictor neurones do not change. The differentiation between cutaneous and muscle vasoconstrictor neurones tends to disappear, although the changed reflexes are rather variable. The qualitative change of the reflex pattern in cutaneous vasoconstrictor neurones is particularly prominent in animals with a cross-union of nerves, and is sustained in this preparation long after regeneration of the nerve fibres to the inappropriate target tissue has occurred (for details and discussion see Blumberg and Jänig 1985, Jänig and Koltzenburg 1991*b*).

This type of experiment illustrates that lesions of nerves can entail long-term changes of reflex activity in sympathetic neurones supplying blood vessels. It appears likely that these changes are due to a reorganization in the spinal cord or brainstem, or both. They may reflect the plasticity of the central organization of the sympathetic nervous system. It may be speculated that activity in muscle vasoconstrictor neurones is normally under predominant control of the medulla oblongata, and activity in cutaneous vasoconstrictor neurones under predominant control of the hypothalamus, resulting in the differentiated reflex patterns which are observed in these neurones. After the nerve lesion, both systems may be under predominant control of the medulla oblongata. These results, which were obtained in anaesthetized cats, correspond to findings in patients with CRPS I, showing that thermoregulation via skin of the affected extremity is disturbed (see Baron *et al.* in Jänig and Stanton-Hicks 1996).

These central changes add to the distorted regulation of the sympathetic effector organs: now a changed centrally generated signal in the sympathetic neurones contributes to the peripheral abnormalities (altered neurovascular transmission, development of hyper-reactivity of blood vessels, impairment of neurogenic vasodilatation mediated by unmyelinated afferents). At present the contribution of the central disturbance of sympathetic function to the development of CRPS and related pain syndromes in patients is unclear.

Conclusion

In healthy individuals, tissue-damaging stimuli in the periphery are encoded by nociceptive afferent neurones. The nociceptive impulse activity is transformed in the spinal cord and faithfully transmitted to the thalamocortical system and to other supraspinal brain centres, leading to perception, appropriate control of the spinal transmission of nociceptive information, and appropriate somatomotor, autonomic, and endocrine reactions. This concerted action of the central nervous system may become disturbed under pathological conditions such as CRPS and related states of neuropathic pain. Peripheral injury (trauma with and without obvious nerve lesions; chronic inflammation) leads to nociceptor sensitization and ectopically generated afferent impulse traffic to the CNS. The peripheral changes

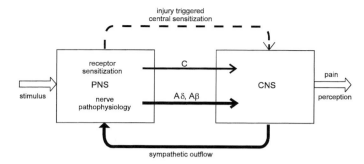

Fig. 13.9. Schematic diagram showing the components that may be important for an understanding of neuropathic pain following peripheral injury, which is dependent on a positive feedback loop via the sympathetic nervous system. Peripheral injury leads to sensitization of nociceptors, afferent impulse activity from lesioned nerve fibres, and slow biochemical changes in the periphery (see Jänig 1988). This in turn produces central changes (generally described as central sensitization) with an abnormal activity in the neurones of the sympathetic outflow. The sympathetic loop feeds directly or indirectly back to the afferent impulse generators, this coupling being the consequence of the peripheral injury. PNS, peripheral nervous system; CNS, central nervous system.

entail changes of central neurones (globally described here as 'central sensitization'), resulting in distorted sensations and distorted autonomic, somatomotor, and endocrine reactions.

In consequence, the sympathetic outflow to the affected peripheral part of the body may be actively involved in the generation of pain and associated processes by way of a positive feedback loop (Fig. 13.9). Stimuli which normally are non-painful may now elicit excessively painful reactions which are dependent on an intact sympathetic innervation. Several pathophysiological mechanisms may be involved in this process:

(1) abnormal coupling of noradrenergic postganglionic fibres to primary afferent neurones;

(2) disturbance of the micromilieu of afferent receptors by changes of neurovascular transmission and by development of hyper-reactivity of blood vessels;

(3) disturbance of the micromilieu of nociceptors by interference of noradrenergic fibres with non-neural inflammatory and immune-competent cells;

(4) changes of the impulse pattern in neurones of the sympathetic outflow, possibly as a consequence of the central changes.

The complexity of the somatosensory and autonomic abnormalities observed in patients with neuropathic pains that may be, in some way or another, associated with the sympathetic nervous system, indicates that several pathobiological processes operate in parallel, on the sensory as well as on the efferent site, and that the actual clinical phenomenology may be dependent on the predominance of one type of pathological mechanism.

Acknowledgement

This work was supported by the Deutsche Forschungsgemeinschaft.

References

Arnér, S. (1991). Intravenous phentolamine test: diagnostic and prognostic use in reflex sympathetic dystrophy. *Pain* **46**, 17–22.

Bandler, R. and Shipley, M. T. (1994). Columnar organization in the midbrain periaqueductal gray: modules for emotional expression? *Trends Neurosci.* **17**, 379–89.

Blumberg, H. and Jänig, W. (1985). Reflex patterns in postganglionic vasoconstrictor neurones following chronic nerve lesions. *J. auton. nerv. Syst.* **14**, 157–80.

Blumberg, H. and Jänig, W. (1994). Clinical manifestations of reflex sympathetic dystrophy and sympathetically maintained pain. In *Textbook of pain*, (3rd edn), (ed. P. D. Wall and R. Melzack), pp. 685–97. Churchill Livingstone, Edinburgh.

Blumberg, H., Hoffmann, U., Mohadjer, M., and Scheremet, R. (1994). Clinical phenomenology and mechanisms of reflex sympathetic dystrophy: Emphasis on edema. In *Proceedings of the 7th World Congress on Pain: progress in pain research and management*, Vol. 2, (ed. G. F. Gebhart, D. L. Hammond, and T. S. Jensen), pp. 455–81, IASP Press, Seattle.

Bonica, J. J. (1990). Causalgia and other reflex sympathetic dystrophies. In *The management of pain*. (2nd edn), (ed. J. J. Bonica), pp. 220–43. Lea & Febinger, Philadelphia.

Chen, Y., Michaelis, M., Jänig, W., and Devor, M. (1996). Adrenoceptor subtype mediating sympathetic-sensory coupling in injured sensory neurons. *J. Neurophysiol.* **76**, 3721–30.

Devor, M. (1994). The pathophysiology of damaged peripheral nerves. In *Textbook of pain*, (3rd edn) (ed. P. D. Wall and R. Melzack), pp. 79–100. Churchill Livingstone, Edinburgh.

Devor, M., Jänig, W., and Michaelis, M. (1994). Modulation of activity in dorsal root ganglion (DRG) neurons by sympathetic activation in nerve-injured rats. *J. Neurophysiol.* **71**, 38–47.

Häbler, H.-J., Jänig, W., and Koltzenburg, M. (1987). Activation of unmyelinated afferents in chronically lesioned nerves by adrenaline and excitation of sympathetic efferents in the cat. *Neurosci. Lett.* **82**, 35–40.

Jänig, W. (1988). Pathophysiology of nerve following mechanical injury. In *Pain research and clinical management: Proceedings of the VIth World Congress on Pain*, Vol. 3 (ed. R. Dubner, G. F. Gebhart, and M. R. Bond), pp. 89–109. Elsevier Science Publishers, Amsterdam.

Jänig, W. (1990). The sympathetic nervous system in pain: physiology and pathophysiology. In *Pain and the sympathetic nervous system*, (ed. M. Stanton-Hicks), pp. 17–89. Kluwer Academic Publishers, Boston.

Jänig, W. (1995). The sympathetic nervous system in pain. *Eur. J. Anaesthesiol.* **12**, (Suppl. 10), 53–60.

Jänig, W. and Häbler, H.-J. (1995). Visceral–autonomic integration. In *Visceral pain. Progress in pain research and management*, (ed. G. F. Gebhart), Vol. 5, pp. 311–48. IASP Press, Seattle.

Jänig, W. and Koltzenburg, M. (1991a). What is the interaction between the sympathetic terminal and the primary afferent fibre? In *Towards a new pharmacotherapy of pain*, (ed. A. I. Basbaum and J. M. Besson), Dahlem Workshop Reports, pp. 331–52. John Wiley & Sons, Chichester.

Jänig, W. and Koltzenburg, M. (1991b). Plasticity of sympathetic reflex organization following nerve lesion in the adult cat. *J. Physiol.* **436**, 309–23.

Jänig, W. and McLachlan, E. M. (1994). The role of modifications in noradrenergic peripheral pathways after nerve lesions in the generation of pain. In *Pharmacological approaches to the treatment of pain: new concepts and critical issues. Progress in pain research and management*, (ed. H. L. Fields and J. C. Liebeskind), Vol. 1, pp. 101–28. IASP Press, Seattle.

Jänig, W. and Stanton-Hicks, M. (ed.) (1996). *Reflex sympathetic dystrophy—a reappraisal*, Vol. 6, IASP Press, Seattle.

Jänig, W., Levine, J. D., and Michaelis, M. (1996). Interaction of sympathetic and primary afferent neurons following nerve injury and tissue trauma. *Prog. in Brain Res.* **112**, 161–84.

Jobling, P., McLachlan, E. M., Jänig, W., and Anderson, C. R. (1992). Electrophysiological responses in the rat tail artery during reinnervation following lesions of the sympathetic supply. *J. Physiol. London* **454**, 107–28.

Koltzenburg, M., Häbler, H.-J., and Jänig, W. (1995). Functional reinnervation of the vasculature of the adult cat paw by axons originally innervating vessels in hairy skin. *Neuroscience* **67**, 245–52.

Levine, J. and Taiwo, Y. (1994). Inflammatory pain. In *Textbook of pain*, (3rd edn) (ed. P. D. Wall and R. Melzack), pp. 45–56. Churchill Livingstone, Edinburgh.

McLachlan, E. M., Jänig, W., Devor, M., and Michaelis, M. (1993). Peripheral nerve injury triggers noradrenergic sprouting within dorsal root ganglia. *Nature* **363**, 543–6.

Merskey, H. and Bogduk, N. (1994). *Classification of chronic pain: descriptions of chronic pain syndromes and definition of terms*. IASP Press, Seattle.

Michaelis, M., Devor, M., and Jänig, W. (1996). Sympathetic modulation of activity in rat dorsal root ganglion neurons changes over time following peripheral nerve injury. *J. Neurophysiol.* **76**, 753–63.

Price, D. D., Bennett, G. J., and Rafii, A. (1989). Psychophysical observations on patients with neuropathic pain relieved by a sympathetic block. *Pain* **36**, 273–88.

Sato, J. and Perl, E. R. (1991). Adrenergic excitation of cutaneous pain receptors induced by peripheral nerve injury. *Science* **251**, 1608–10.

Stanton-Hicks, M., Jänig, W., Hassenbusch, S., Haddox, J. D., Boas, R., and Wilson, P. (1995). Reflex sympathetic dystrophy: changing concepts and taxonomy. *Pain* **63**, 127–33.

Woolf, C. J., Shortland, P. and Coggeshall, R. E. (1992). Peripheral nerve injury triggers central sprouting of myelinated afferents. *Nature*, **355**, 75–8.

14. Autonomic control of the airways

Peter J. Barnes

Introduction

Airway nerves regulate the calibre of the airways and control airway smooth muscle tone, airway blood flow, and mucus secretion. They may also influence the inflammatory process and play an integral role in host defence.

Overview of airway innervation

Neural control of airway function is more complex than previously recognized. Many neurotransmitters are now identified and these act on a multitude of autonomic receptors. Three types of airway nerve are recognized.

(1) parasympathetic nerves which release acetylcholine (ACh);

(2) sympathetic nerves which release noradrenaline; and

(3) afferent (sensory nerves) whose primary transmitter may be glutamate.

In addition to these classical transmitters, multiple neuropeptides have now been localized to airway nerves and may have potent effects on airway function (Barnes *et al.* 1991). All of these neurotransmitters act on receptors which are expressed on the surface of target cells in the airway. It is increasingly recognized that a single transmitter may act on several subtypes of receptor which may lead to different cellular effects mediated via different second messenger systems.

Several neural mechanisms are involved in the regulation of airway calibre, and abnormalities in neural control may contribute to airway narrowing in disease (Fig. 14.1). Neural mechanisms may be involved in the pathophysiology of airway diseases, such as asthma and chronic obstructive pulmonary disease (COPD), contributing to the symptoms and possibly to the inflammatory response (Barnes 1986; Barnes 1990). There is a close inter-relationship between inflammation and neural responses in the airways, since inflammatory mediators may influence the release of neurotransmitters via activation of sensory nerves leading to reflex effects and via stimulation of prejunctional receptors that influence the release of neurotransmitters (Barnes 1992). In turn, neural mechanisms may influence the nature of the inflammatory response, either reducing inflammation or exaggerating the inflammatory response.

Neural interactions

Complex interactions between various components of the autonomic nervous system are now recognized. Adrenergic nerves may modulate cholinergic neurotransmission in the airways and sensory nerves may influence neurotransmission in parasympathetic ganglia and at post-ganglionic nerves. This means that changes in the function of one neural pathway may have effects on other pathways.

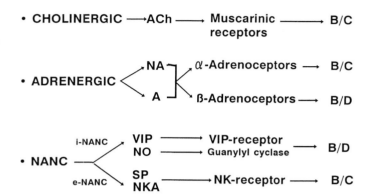

Fig. 14.1. Autonomic control of airway smooth muscle tone. There are neural mechanisms resulting in bronchoconstriction (B/C) and bronchodilatation (B/D). ACh, acetylcholine; NA, noradrenaline; A, adrenaline; VIP, vasoactive intestinal peptide; NO, nitric oxide; i-NANC, inhibitory non-adrenergic, non-cholinergic nerves; e-NANC, excitatory non-adrenergic, non-cholinergic nerves; NK, neurokinin.

Co-transmission

Although it was once the dogma that each nerve has its own unique transmitter, it is now apparent that almost every nerve contains multiple transmitters (Fig. 14.2). Thus airway parasympathetic nerves, in which the primary transmitter is ACh, also contain the neuropeptides vasoactive intestinal polypeptide (VIP), peptide

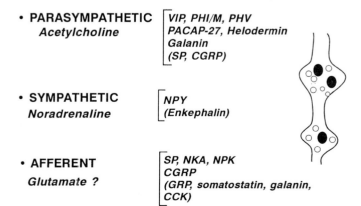

Fig. 14.2. Co-transmission in airway nerves.

histamine isoleucine/ methionine (PHI/M), pituitary adenylate cyclase activating peptide (PACAP), helodermin, galanin, and nitric oxide (NO) (Fig. 14.3). These co-transmitters may have either facilitatory or antagonistic effects on target cells, or may influence the release of the primary transmitter via prejunctional receptors. Thus VIP modulates the release of ACh from airway cholinergic nerves. Sympathetic nerves, which release noradrenaline, may also release neuropeptide Y (NPY) and enkephalins, whereas afferent nerves may contain a variety of peptides including substance P (SP), neurokinin A (NKA), calcitonin-gene-related peptide (CGRP), galanin, VIP, and cholecystokinin.

The physiological role of neurotransmision may be in 'fine tuning' of neural control. Neuropeptides may be preferentially released by high-frequency firing of nerves, and their effects may therefore only become manifest under condition of excessive nerve stimulation. Neuropeptide neurotransmitters may also act on different target cells from the primary transmitter, resulting in different physiological effects. Thus in airways ACh causes bronchoconstriction, but VIP which is co-released may have its major effect on bronchial vessels, thus increasing blood flow to the airways. In chronic inflammation the role of co-transmitters may be increased by alterations in the expression of their receptors or by increased synthesis of transmitters via increased gene transcription.

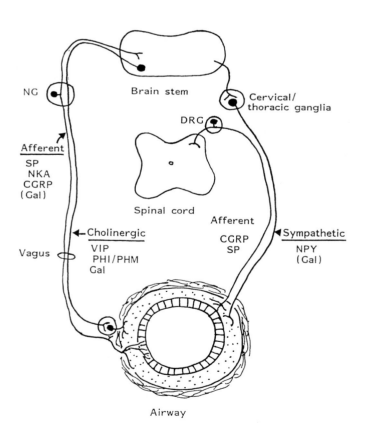

Fig. 14.3. Neurotransmitters and co-transmitters in airway nerves. SP, substance P; NKA, neurokinin A; CGRP, calcitonin-gene-related peptide; Gal, galanin; VIP, vasoactive intestinal peptide; PHI/PHM, peptide histidine isoleucine/methionine; NPY, neuropeptide Y; DRG, dorsal root ganglion; NG, nodose ganglion.

Afferent nerves

The sensory innervation of the respiratory tract is mainly carried in the vagus nerve. The neuronal cell bodies are localized to the nodose and jugular ganglia and input to the solitary tract nucleus in the brainstem. A few sensory fibres supplying the lower airways enter the spinal cord in the upper thoracic sympathetic trunks, but their contribution to respiratory reflexes is minor and it is uncertain whether they are represented in humans. There is a tonic discharge of sensory nerves that has a regulatory effect on respiratory function and also triggers powerful protective reflex mechanisms in response to inhaled noxious agents, physical stimuli, or certain inflammatory mediators.

Laryngeal innervation

The larynx is richly supplied with sensory nerves that are derived from the superior laryngeal nerve. There are numerous sensory arborizations with the appearance of mechanoreceptors. Electrophysiological studies indicate that many afferents function like rapidly adapting (irritant) receptors in the lower respiratory tract (Karlsson et al. 1988). This rich sensory innervation allows the larynx to function as the first-line defence of the lower airways.

Laryngeal afferents are activated by both hypotonic and hypertonic fluids, although the former are a more potent stimulus. These afferents are particularly sensitive to water and some of these fibres respond primarily to an absence of chloride ions. This sensitivity to low chloride ions appears to be confined to the larynx and upper trachea, and may be important in the coughing response to citrate and bicarbonate aerosols in humans.

Laryngeal afferents are also stimulate by mechanical stimulation and by inhaled particulate matter. A wide variety of chemical irritants stimulate laryngeal afferents, including ammonia, cigarette smoke, and CS riot gas. There is a limited sensitivity to capsaicin, which may reflect the paucity of unmyelinated fibres in the larynx. Interestingly, there are also specific cold receptors that appear to be simulated by l-menthol, and may be involved in reflex responses to cold air, including cough.

Laryngeal reflexes

A major function of laryngeal sensory endings is to trigger defence reflexes in the airways, including bronchoconstriction and mucus secretion, to protect the lower respiratory tract against the harmful effects of inhaled foreign agents. Aspiration of fluids or chemical irritants is associated with ventilatory changes, including cough, inhibition of breathing and swallowing. In immature animals the apnoeic response is predominant and, although evolved to prevent inspiration of fluids into the lungs, it has been implicated in cot deaths in human infants. Laryngeal stimulation elicits an increase in tracheal mucus secretion and this effect is due to reflex cholinergic stimulation.

A laryngeal reflex bronchodilatation has been demonstrated recently in animals and humans, but only becomes apparent when cholinergic reflexes are blocked (Lammers et al. 1992). This appears to be mediated by inhibitory non-adrenergic, non-cholinergic (i-NANC) nerves that release NO. It is unlikely that this reflex is important in airway defence as the cholinergic constrictor reflex predominates, but if i-NANC mechanisms become defective, as might occur in chronic inflammation of the airways, then this would lead to exaggerated laryngeal reflex bronchoconstriction.

Lower airway innervation

At least three types of afferent fibre have been identified in the lower airways (Karlsson *et al.* 1988; Coleridge and Coleridge 1997) (Fig. 14.4). Most of the information on their function has been obtained from studies of anaesthetized animals. It has been difficult to apply electrophysiological techniques to humans, so it is difficult to know how much of the information obtained from anaesthetized animals can be extrapolated to human airways.

Slowly adapting receptors

Myelinated fibres associated with smooth muscle of proximal airways are probably slowly adapting (pulmonary stretch) receptors (SARs), that are involved in reflex control of breathing. Activation of SARs reduces efferent vagal discharge and mediates branchodilatation. During tracheal constriction the activity of SARs may serve to limit the bronchoconstrictor response (Karlsson *et al.* 1988). SARs may play a role in the cough reflex since when these receptors are destroyed by high concentrations of SO_2 the cough response to mechanical stimulation is lost.

Rapidly adapting receptors

Myelinated fibres in the epithelium, particularly at the branching points of proximal airways, show rapid adaptation. Rapidly adapting receptors (RARs) account for 10–30 per cent of the myelinated nerve endings in the airways. These endings are sensitive to mechanical stimulation and to mediators such as histamine. The response of RARs to histamine is partly due to mechanical distortion consequent on bronchoconstriction, although if this is prevented by pre-treatment with isoprenaline the RAR response is not abolished, indicating a direct stimulatory effect of histamine. It is likely that mechanical distortion of the airway may amplify irritant receptor discharge.

RARs with widespread arborizations are very numerous in the area of the carina, where they have been termed 'cough receptors' as cough can be evoked by even the slightest touch in this region. RARs respond to inhaled cigarette smoke, ozone, serotonin, and prostaglandin $F_{2\alpha}$, although it is possible that these responses are secondary

to the mechanical distortion produced by the bronchoconstrictor response to these irritants. Neurophysiological studies using an *in vitro* preparation in guinea-pig trachea and bronchi show that a majority of afferent fibres are myelinated and belong to the $A\delta$-fibre group. Although these fibres are activated by mechanical stimulation and low pH, they are not sensitive to capsaicin, histamine, or bradykinin (Fox *et al.* 1993).

C fibres

There is a high density of unmyelinated (C fibres) in the airways and they greatly outnumber myelinated fibres. In the bronchi of cats, C fibres account for 80–90 per cent of all afferent fibres. C fibres play an important role in the defence of the lower respiratory tract (Coleridge and Coleridge 1997). C fibres contain neuropeptides, including SP, NKA, and CGRP, that confer a motor function on these nerves (Maggi and Meli 1988). Bronchial C fibres are insensitive to lung inflation and deflation, but typically respond to chemical stimulation. *In vivo* studies suggest that bronchial C fibres in dogs respond to the inflammatory mediators histamine, bradykinin, serotonin, and prostaglandins (Coleridge and Coleridge 1997). They are selectively stimulated by capsaicin given either intravenously or by inhalation and are also stimulated by SO_2 and cigarette smoke. Since these fibres are relatively unaffected by lung mechanics, it is likely that these agents act directly on the unmyelinated endings in the airway epithelium. In the *in vitro* guinea-pig trachea preparation C fibres are stimulated by capsaicin and by bradykinin, but not by histamine, serotonin, or prostaglandins (with the possible exception of prostacyclin) (Fox *et al.* 1993).

Both RARs and C fibres are sensitive to water and hyperosmotic solutions, with RARs showing a greater sensitivity to hypotonic and C fibres to hypertonic saline. In the *in vitro* guinea-pig trachea preparation $A\delta$ fibres and C fibres are stimulated by water and by hyperosmolar solutions; a small proportion of $A\delta$ fibres are also stimulated by low chloride solutions, as are the majority of C fibres.

Pulmonary C fibres, which are activated via the pulmonary circulation, appear to have different properties to bronchial C fibres. Lobeline, which stimulates pulmonary but not bronchial C fibres, causes cough when perfused through the pulmonary circulation, suggesting that pulmonary C fibres may be involved in the cough reflex.

Defence reflexes

Afferent nerves play a critical role in defence of the airways. Powerful protective reflexes are evoked by stimulation of afferent nerve endings on the surface of the larynx, which serve to limit access of noxious agents to the gas-exchanging surface. If this line of defence is breached, additional defensive reflexes are activated within the lower respiratory tract. These reflexes include changes in the pattern of breathing (rapid shallow breathing or, in infants, apnoea), constriction of the airways, increased airway secretions, and increased blood flow in the tracheal and bronchial circulations. These responses comprise a co-ordinated response which limits the access of the noxious agent to the delicate gas-exchanging surface of the lung in order to preserve oxygenation.

Cough

Cough is an important defence reflex which may be triggered from either laryngeal or lower airway afferents. It is characterized by

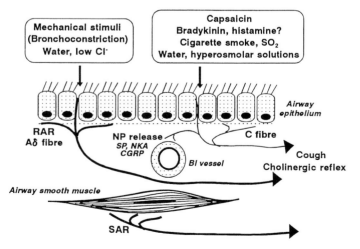

Fig. 14.4. Afferent nerves in airways, Slowly adapting receptors (SAR) are found in airway smooth muscle, whereas rapidly adapting myelinated (RAR) and unmyelinated C fibres are present in the airway mucosa.

violent expiration which provides the high flow rate needed to expel foreign particles and mucus from the lower respiratory tract. There is still debate about which are the mot important afferents for initiation of cough, and this may be dependent on the stimulus. Thus RARs are activated by mechanical stimuli (e.g. particulate matter), bronchoconstrictors, and hypotonic saline and water, whereas C fibres are more sensitive to hypertonic solutions, bradykinin, and capsaicin. In normal humans, inhaled capsaicin is a potent tussive stimulus and this is associated with a transient bronchoconstrictor reflex that is abolished by an anticholinergic drug. It is not certain whether this is due to stimulation of C fibres in the larynx, but as these are very sparse it is likely that bronchial C fibres are also involved. Citric acid is commonly used to stimulate coughing in experimental challenges in human subjects; it is likely that it produces cough by a combination of low pH (which stimulates C fibres) and low chloride (which may stimulate laryngeal and lower airway afferents). Inhaled bradykinin causes coughing and a raw sensation retrosternally, which may be due to stimulation of C fibres in the lower airways. Bradykinin appears to be a relatively pure stimulant of C fibres (Fox *et al.* 1993). Prostaglandins E_2 and $F_{2\alpha}$ are potent tussive agents in humans and also sensitize the cough reflex. This may be relevant to airway defences, since noxious agents may stimulate the release of prostaglandins (particularly PGE_2) from airway sensory nerves, and this may lead to enhanced sensitivity of the cough reflex and thus a greater likelihood of expelling the noxious agent if it persists. Bronchoconstriction and increased mucus secretion are often caused by the same stimuli and provoke cough, thereby increasing the efficiency of the cough reflex.

Cholinergic nerves

Cholinergic nerves are the major neural bronchoconstrictor mechanism in the human airway, and are the major determinant of airway calibre.

Cholinergic control of airways

Cholinergic nerves fibres arise in the nucleus ambiguous in the brainstem and travel down the vagus nerve to synapse in parasympathetic ganglia which are located within the airway wall (Barnes 1986). From these ganglia short postganglionic fibres travel to airway smooth muscle and submucosal glands (Fig. 14.5). In animals, electrical stimulation of the vagus nerve causes release to ACh from cholinergic nerve terminals, with activation of muscarinic cholinergic receptors on smooth muscle and gland cells, which results in bronchoconstriction and mucus secretion. Prior administration of a muscarinic receptor antagonist, such as atropine, prevents vagally induced bronchoconstriction.

Four subtypes of muscarinic receptor have now been identified by binding studies and pharmacologically in lung (Barnes 1993). The muscarinic receptors that mediate bronchoconstriction in human and animal airways belong to the M_3-receptor subtype, whereas mucus secretion appears to be mediated by M_1- and M_3-receptors. Muscarinic receptor stimulation results in vasodilatation via activation of M_3-receptors on endothelial cells which release NO. M_1-receptors are also localized by parasympathetic ganglia, where they facilitate the neurotransmission mediated via nicotinic receptors (Fig. 14.6).

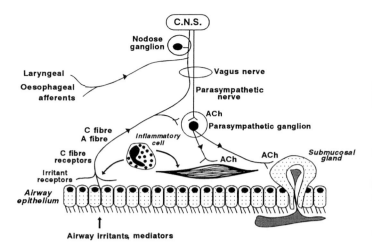

Fig. 14.5. Cholinergic control of airway smooth muscle. Preganglionic and postganglionic parasympathetic nerves release acetylcholine (ACh) and can be activated by airway and extrapulmonary afferent nerves.

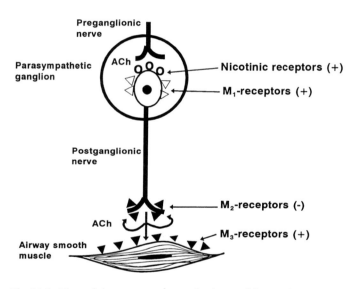

Fig. 14.6. Muscarinic receptor subtypes in airways. M_2-receptors on postganglionic cholinergic nerve terminals inhibit the release of acetylcholine (ACh), thus reducing the stimulation of postjunctional M_3-receptors which constrict airway smooth muscle.

Inhibitory muscarinic receptors (autoreceptors) have been demonstrated on cholinergic nerves of airways in animals *in vivo* and in human bronchi *in vitro* (Barnes 1993). These prejunctional receptors inhibit ACh release and may serve to limit vagal bronchoconstriction. Autoreceptors in human airways belong to the M_2-receptor subtype, whereas those on airway smooth muscle and glands belong to the M_3-receptor subtype. Drugs such as atropine and ipratropium bromide, which block both prejunctional M_2-receptors and postjunctional M_3-receptors on smooth muscle with equal efficacy therefore increase ACh release, which may then overcome the postjunctional blockade. This means that such drugs will not be as effective against vagal bronchoconstriction as against cholinergic agonists, and it may be necessary to re-evaluate the contribution of cholinergic nerves when drugs which are selective for the M_3-receptors are developed for clinical use. The presence of muscarinic autoreceptors has been demonstrated in human subjects *in vivo*. A cholinergic agonist, pilocarpine, which selectively activates M_2-receptors, inhibits cholinergic reflex bronchoconstriction induced by sulphur dioxide in normal subjects, but such an inhibitory mechanism does not appear to operate in asthmatic subjects, suggesting that there may be dysfunction of these autoreceptors. Such a defect in muscarinic autoreceptors may then result in exaggerated cholinergic reflexes in asthma, since the normal feedback inhibition of ACh release may be lost. This might also explain the sometimes catastrophic bronchoconstriction that occurs with β-blockers in asthma which, at least in mild asthmatics, appears to be mediated by cholinergic pathways. Antagonism of inhibitory β-receptors on cholinergic nerves would result in increased release of ACh, which could not be switched off in the asthmatic patient (Fig. 14.7). This explains why anticholinergic drugs block β-blocker-induced asthma. The mechanisms that lead to dysfunction of prejunctional M_2-receptors in asthmatic airways are not certain, but it is possible that M_2-receptors may be more susceptible to damage by oxidants or other products of the inflammatory response in the airways. Experimental studies have demonstrated that influenza virus infection and eosinophils in guinea-pigs may result in a selective loss of M_2-receptors compared with M_3-receptors, resulting in a loss of autoreceptor function and enhanced cholinergic bronchoconstriction.

Cholinergic innervation is greatest in large airways and diminishes peripherally, although in humans muscarinic receptors are localized to airway smooth muscle in all airways. In humans, studies that have tried to distinguish large and small airway effects have shown that cholinergic bronchoconstriction involves predominantly larger airways, whereas β-agonists are equally effective in large and small airways. This relative diminution of cholinergic control in small

airways may have important clinical implications, since anticholinergic drugs are likely to be less useful than β-agonists when bronchoconstriction involves small airways.

In animals, there is a certain degree of resting bronchomotor tone caused by tonic parasympathetic activity. This tone can be reversed by atropine, and enhanced by administration of an inhibitor of acetylcholinesterase (which normally rapidly inactivates ACh released from nerve terminals). Normal human subjects also have resting bronchomotor tone, since atropine causes bronchodilatation and inhalation of the acetylcholinesterase inhibitor, edrophonium, results in bronchoconstriction.

Cholinergic reflexes

Many stimuli are able to elicit reflex cholinergic bronchoconstriction through activation of sensory receptors in the larynx or lower airways. Activation of cholinergic reflexes may result in bronchoconstriction and an increase in airway mucus secretion through the activation of muscarinic receptors on airway smooth muscle cells and submucosal glands. Cholinergic reflexes may also increase airway blood flow, particularly in proximal airways. Stimulation of the vagus nerve in animals results in vasodilatation in proximal airways that is partially reduced by atropine, suggesting a cholinergic component. The residual component is likely to be due to release of neuropeptides (such as VIP and CGRP) and NO. Cigarette smoke inhalation results in an increase in airway blood flow in the pig, through the effects of exogenous NO contained in cigarette smoke, but also via release of endogenous NO from airway nerves. Cholinergic reflexes may also increase mucociliary clearance, presumably via an effect of ACh on ciliated epithelial cells.

Several inhaled irritants have been found to activate cholinergic reflexes in human airways, resulting in bronchoconstriction. These include SO_2, metabisulphite, and bradykinin. Both water (fog) and hypertonic saline also produce cough and bronchoconstriction in asthmatic patients, although the role of cholinergic reflexes in the bronchoconstrictor responses has not been fully evaluated. The activation of cholinergic reflexes by airway irritants is clearly part of a defensive reflex, since the bronchoconstriction serves to reduce the penetration of the noxious substance and increases the efficiency of the cough mechanism, the increase in mucus secretion and increased mucociliary clearance result in more efficient removal of the irritant, and the increase in airway blood flow may serve to bring in inflammatory cells.

Cholinergic reflexes may also be activated from extrapulmonary afferents and these reflexes may also contribute to airway defences. Oesophageal reflux may be associated with bronchoconstriction in asthmatic patients. In some patients this may be due to aspiration of acid into the airways, in other cases acid reflux into the oesophagus activates a reflex cholinergic bronchoconstriction (the 'reflux reflex'). Presumably this reflex evolved to prevent aspiration of stomach contents. There are also reflexes that may be activated by stimulation of sensory receptors in the nose, resulting in bronchoconstriction and laryngeal narrowing. This may serve as an early warning system so that noxious agents inhaled through the nose are prevented from inhalation.

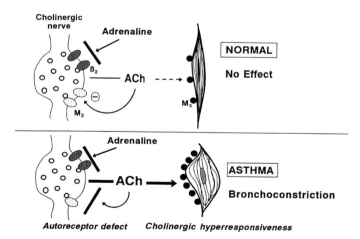

Fig. 14.7. Possible mechanism of β-blocker-induced asthma. Blockade of prejunctional β_2-receptors on cholinergic nerves in normal individuals results in increased release of acetylcholine (ACh), but this is compensated by stimulation of prejunctional muscarinic M_2-receptors to inhibit any increase in ACh. In patients with asthma, prejunctional M_2-receptors are dysfunctional, so that there is a net release of ACh, and ACh also has a greater bronchoconstrictor effect on the airways due to airway hyperresponsiveness.

Neurogenic inflammation

Pain, heat, redness, and swelling are the cardinal signs of inflammation. Sensory nerves may be involved in the generation of each of these signs. There is now considerable evidence that sensory nerves participate in inflammatory responses. This 'neurogenic inflammation' is due to the antidromic release of neuropeptides from C fibres, via an axon reflex. The phenomenon is well documented in several organs, including skin, eye, gastrointestinal track, and bladder (Maggi and Meli 1988). There is also increasing evidence that neurogenic inflammation occurs in the respiratory tract (Barnes 1995; Joos *et al.* 1995). It may contribute to the inflammatory response in asthma and chronic obstructive pulmonary disease (COPD) and may have evolved as an airway defence mechanism.

Activation of airway C fibres may release several neuropeptides, including tachykinins (SP, NKA) and CGRP. In some populations of C fibres other neuropeptides, such as galanin, VIP, and NPY, are also present. These peptides have potent effects on airway function and may lead to a chronic inflammatory state with narrowing of the airways (Fig. 14.8). This presumably evolved as a mechanism of defence against invading organisms and as a mechanism to repair the airway damaged by noxious agents in the respiratory tract.

Tachykinins

SP and NKA, but not neurokinin B, are localized to sensory nerves in the airways of several species. SP-immunoreactive nerves are abundant in rodent airways, but are sparse in human airways. SP-immunoreactive nerves in the airway are found beneath and within the airway epithelium, around blood vessels and, to a lesser extent, within airway smooth muscle. SP-immunoreactive nerves fibres also innervate parasympathetic ganglia, suggesting a sensory input which may modulate ganglionic transmission and so result in ganglionic reflexes. SP in the airways is localized predominantly to capsaicin-sensitive unmyelinated nerves, but chronic administration of capsaicin only partially depletes the lung of tachykinins, indicating the presence of a population of capsaicin-resistant SP-immunoreactive nerves, as in the gastrointestinal tract. Similar capsaicin denervation studies are not possible in human airways, but after extrinsic denervation by heart–lung transplantation there appears to be a loss of SP-immunoreactive nerves in the submucosa.

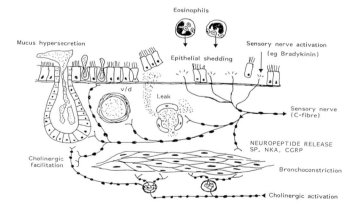

Fig. 14.8. Axon reflex mechanisms. Possible neurogenic inflammation in asthmatic airways via retrograde release of peptides from sensory nerves via an axon reflex. Substance P (SP) causes vasodilatation, plasma exudation, and mucus secretion, whereas neurokinin A (NKA) causes bronchoconstriction and enhanced cholinergic reflexes, and calcitonin-gene-related peptide (CGRP) causes vasodilatation.

Tachykinins have many different effects on the airways, which are mediated via NK$_1$-receptors (preferentially activated by SP) and NK$_2$-receptors (activated by NKA). Tachykinins constrict smooth muscle of human airways *in vitro* via NK$_2$-receptors. The contractile response to NKA is significantly greater in smaller human bronchi than in more proximal airways, indicating that tachykinins may have a more important constrictor effect on more peripheral airways, whereas cholinergic constriction tends to be more pronounced in proximal airways. *In vivo* SP does not cause bronchoconstriction or cough, whereas NKA causes bronchoconstriction in asthmatic subjects. Mechanical removal of airway epithelium potentiates the bronchoconstrictor response to tachykinins, largely because the ecto-enzyme neutral endopeptidase (NEP, E.C. 3.4.24.11), which is a key enzyme in the degradation of tachykinins in airways. SP also stimulates mucus secretion from submucosal glands and goblet cells, stimulates plasma extravasation, and increases airway blood flow, effects that are mediated via NK$_1$-receptors.

Tachykinins are metabolized by NEP, and inhibition of NEP by phosphoramidon or thiorphan markedly potentiates bronchoconstriction and mucus secretion in animal and human airways. The activity of NEP in the airways appears to be an important factor in determining the effects of tachykinins; any factors that inhibit the enzyme or its expression may be associated with increased effects of exogenous or endogenously released tachykinins. Several of the stimuli known to induce bronchoconstrictor responses in asthmatic patients have been found to reduce the activity of airway NEP (Nadel 1991).

Calcitonin-gene-related peptide

CGRP is co-stored and co-localized with SP in afferent nerves. CGRP is a potent vasodilator, which has long-lasting effects. It is an effective dilator of bronchial vessels *in vitro* and produces a marked and long-lasting increase in airway blood flow in anaesthetized animals. Receptor mapping studies have demonstrated that CGRP receptors are localized predominantly to bronchial vessels rather than to smooth muscle or epithelium in human airways. It is likely that CGRP is the predominant mediator of arterial vasodilatation and increased blood flow in response to sensory nerve stimulation in the bronchi. CGRP is a bronchoconstrictor, largely due to the release of spasmogens, such as endothelin-1.

Neurogenic inflammation in human airways

Although there is clear evidence for neurogenic inflammation in rodent airways, it has been difficult to study these mechanisms in human airways. There are few SP-immunoreactive airways in human airways, as discussed above, but there is an apparent increase in patients with asthma, although this has not been confirmed in other studies. The role of neurogenic inflammation in response to inhaled irritants in normal individuals is likely to be minimal or absent. While capsaicin induces bronchoconstriction and plasma exudation in rodents, inhaled capsaicin causes cough and a *transient* bronchoconstriction in humans, suggesting that neuropeptide release does not occur in human airways. Bradykinin is a potent bronchoconstrictor and tussive agent in asthmatic patients, the action of which is reduced by a tachykinin antagonist. Since normal subjects fail to constrict to bradykinin, although it induces cough, this provides some evidence that neurogenic inflammation may be enhanced in asthma but is not present under normal conditions. NEP inhibitors potentiate the bronchoconstrictor response to inhaled NKA in normal and asthmatic subjects, but there is no effect on baseline lung function in asthmatic patients, indicating that there is unlikely to be any basal release of tachykinins. It is possible that NEP may become dysfunctional after viral infections or exposure to oxidants and airway irritants such as cigarette smoke, but this has not yet been investigated in humans.

Tachykinin antagonists are effective in a variety of animal models of asthma (Solway and Leff 1991), but so far there is little evidence that they are efficacious in human airway disease.

Bronchodilator nerves

Neural bronchodilator mechanisms exist in airways and there are considerable species differences.

Sympathetic nerves

Sympathetic innervation of human airways is sparse and there is no functional evidence for innervation of airway smooth muscle, in contrast to the sympathetic bronchodilator mechanisms that exist in other species (Barnes 1986; Fig. 14.9). Sympathetic nerves may regulate bronchial blood flow and to a lesser extent mucus secretion. Sympathetic nerve may also influence airway tone indirectly through a modulatory effect on parasympathetic ganglia; sympathetic nerve profiles have been observed in close proximity to parasympathetic ganglia and postganglionic cholinergic nerve terminals in human airways.

Circulating catecholamines

In the absence of sympathetic nerves, circulating adrenaline may play a role in regulating airway tone. β-Adrenergic blockade causes bronchoconstriction in asthmatic patients, but not in normal subjects, implying an increased adrenergic drive in asthma. This might be provided by circulating adrenaline in asthma. However, circulating concentrations of adrenaline, even in acute exacerbations of asthma, are normal. The mechanism whereby β-blockers may cause bronchoconstriction in asthma is still not completely understood, but may be due to blockage of prejunctional β_2-receptors on cholinergic nerves in the airways, resulting in increased ACh release in asthma, in which, as discussed above, the normal autoreceptor feedback via prejunctional M_2-receptors may be defective (Fig. 14.7).

i-NANC nerves

There are bronchodilator nerves in human airways that are not blocked by adrenergic blockers and are therefore described as i-NANC. The neurotransmitters for these nerves in some species, including guinea-pigs and cats, are VIP and related peptides. The i-NANC bronchodilator response is blocked by α-chymotrypsin, an enzyme which degrades VIP very efficiently, and by antibodies to VIP. However, although VIP is present in human airways and VIP is a potent bronchodilator of human airways *in vitro*, there is no evidence that VIP is involved in neurotransmission of i-NANC responses in human airways, and α-chymotrypsin, which completely blocks the response to exogenous VIP, has no effect on neural bronchodilator responses. It is likely that VIP and related peptides may be more important to neural vasodilatation responses and may result in increased blood flow to bronchoconstricted airways.

The predominant neurotransmitter of human airways is NO. NO synthase inhibitors, such as N^G-L-arginine methyl ester, virtually abolish the i-NANC response (Belvisi *et al.* 1995). This effect is more marked in proximal airways, consistent with the demonstration that nitrergic innervation is greatest in proximal airways. NO appears to be a co-transmitter with ACh, and NO acts as a 'braking' mechanism for the cholinergic system by acting as a functional antagonist to ACh at airway smooth muscle (Ward *et al.* 1993) (Fig. 14.10).

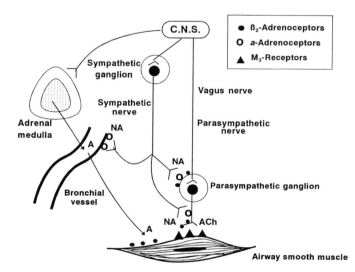

Fig. 14.9. Adrenergic control of airway smooth muscle. Sympathetic nerves release noradrenaline (NA), which may modulate cholinergic nerves at the level of the parasympathetic ganglion or postganglionic nerves, rather than directly at smooth muscle in human airways. Circulating adrenaline (A) is more likely to be important in adrenergic control of airway smooth muscle.

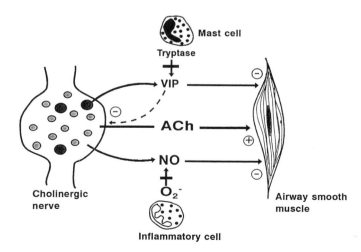

Fig. 14.10. Nitric oxide (NO) and vasoactive intestinal peptide (VIP) may modulate cholinergic neural effects mediated via acetylcholine (ACh). In inflammation NO may be removed by superoxide anions (O_2^-), generated from inflammatory cells, and VIP by mast cell tryptase, therefore diminishing their 'braking' effects, resulting in exaggerated cholinergic bronchoconstriction.

Neural control of airways in disease

Autonomic control of airways may be abnormal, thus contributing to the pathophysiology in several airway diseases.

Asthma

There is compelling evidence that neural mechanisms contribute to the pathophysiology of asthma (Barnes 1995). It has long been proposed that there is an imbalance in autonomic control in asthma, with a preponderance of bronchoconstrictor mechanisms (muscarinic, α-adrenergic) or a deficit in bronchodilator mechanisms (β-adrenergic). While there is no convincing evidence for a primary defect in autonomic control in asthma, several abnormalities arise as a consequence of the disease.

Activation and sensitization of airway sensory nerves may result in the symptoms of cough and chest tightness that are so unpleasant in asthmatic patients. Cholinergic reflex bronchoconstriction may be important, particularly during exacerbations of asthma, when anticholinergic drugs are relatively effective. The defective function of prejunctional M_2-receptors may contribute to exaggerated reflex bronchoconstriction. Furthermore, loss of neuronally produced NO by the action of superoxide anions, generated from inflammatory cells, may leave the cholinergic neural bronchoconstriction unopposed. Whether neurogenic inflammation is present in asthmatic airways is uncertain, but is favoured by the possible loss of NEP in asthma, by increased synthesis of SP, and by increased expression of NK_1-receptors. On the other hand, the clinical response to tachykinin antagonists, which are very effective in animal models of asthma, has been disappointing.

Chronic obstructive pulmonary disease

The airways are structurally narrowed in COPD, which means that the normal vagal cholinergic tone has a relatively greater effect on calibre than in normal airways, purely for geometric reasons. This explains why anticholinergics are as, or more, effective than inhaled β_2-agonists as bronchodilators in these patients. Neural mechanisms may explain the mucus hypersecretion seen in cigarette smokers, and irritants in cigarette smoke may activate axon reflex mechanisms, resulting in the release of tachykinins, which have a potent effect on mucus secretions.

References

Barnes, P. J. (1986). Neural control of human airways in health and disease. *Am. Rev. Respir. Dis.* **134**, 1289–1314.

Barnes, P. J. (1990). Neural control of airway function: new perspectives. *Mol. Aspects Med.* **11**, 351–423.

Barnes, P. J. (1992). Modulation of neurotransmission in airways. *Physiol. Rev.* **72**, 699–729.

Barnes, P. J. (1993). Muscarinic receptor subtypes in airways. *Life Sci.* **52**, 521–8.

Barnes, P. J. (1995). Is asthma a nervous disease? *Chest* **107**, 119S–124S.

Barnes, P. J., Baraniuk, J., and Belvisi, M. G. (1991). Neuropeptides in the respiratory tract. *Am. Rev. Respir. Dis.* **144**, 1391–9.

Belvisi, M. G., Ward, J. R., Mitchell, J. A., and Barnes, P. J. (1995). Nitric oxide as a neurotransmitter in human airways. *Arch. Int. Pharmacodyn. Ther.* **329**, 111–20.

Coleridge, H. M. and Coleridge, J. C. G. (1997). Afferent nerves in the airways. In *Autonomic control of the respiratory system*, (ed. P. J. Barnes), pp. 39–58. Harwood, London.

Fox, A. J., Barnes, P. J., Urban, L., and Dray, A. (1993). An *in vitro* study of the properties of single vagal afferents innervating guinea-pig airways. *J. Physiol.* **469**, 21–35.

Joos, G. F., Germonpre, P. R., and Pauwels, R. A. (1995). Neurogenic inflammation in human airways: is it important? *Thorax* **50**, 217–19.

Karlsson, J., Sant'Ambrogio, G., and Widdicombe, J. G. (1988). Afferent neural pathways in cough and reflex bronchoconstriction. *J. Appl. Physiol.* **65**, 1007–23.

Lammers, J. W. J., Barnes, P. J., and Chung, K. F. (1992). Non-adrenergic, non-cholinergic airway inhibitory nerves. *Eur. Respir. J.* **5**, 239–46.

Maggi, C. A. and Meli, A. (1988). The sensory efferent function of capsaicin sensitive sensory nerves. *Gen. Pharmacol.* **19**, 1–43.

Nadel, J. A. (1991). Neutral endopeptidase modulates neurogenic inflammation. *Eur. Resp. J.* **4**, 745–54.

Solway, J. and Leff, A. R. (1991). Sensory neuropeptides and airway function. *J. Appl. Physiol.* **71**, 2077–87.

Ward, J. K., Belvisi, M. G., Fox, A. J. *et al.* (1993). Modulation of cholinergic neural bronchoconstriction by endogenous nitric oxide and vasoactive intestinal in human airways *in vitro*. *J. Clin. Invest.* **92**, 736–43.

15. The gut and the autonomic nervous system

Anne E. Bishop and Julia M. Polak

Introduction

Although under the overriding control of the central nervous system, the gastrointestinal tract is capable of carrying out its function of food passage, storage, digestion, and absorption after all central connections are severed. Thus, sympathetic denervation has only a transient effect on gut function; denervation of the parasympathetic nervous system usually reduces the tone and degree of peristaltic activity but this is eventually compensated for by increased intrinsic excitability of the enteric plexuses. This autonomy of the gastrointestinal tract has been the subject of much interest and speculation and terms such as 'minibrain' have been used to describe the gut's intrinsic innervation; some indication of the size and importance of the intramural innervation can be gained from the observation that the number of neurones in the human gut is similar to that in the spinal cord (Furness and Costa 1987). Increased interest has centred largely on the recognition that, far from using only the classical autonomic neurotransmitters, acetylcholine and noradrenaline, the nervous system of the gut employs a myriad of substances, including amines, γ-aminobutyric acid, adenosine triphosphate, nitric oxide, and a variety of peptides, to relay information. The neuropeptides are probably the most abundant neurotransmitter type in the gut and are found singly or in combinations with other peptides or neuroactive substances.

This chapter describes the general anatomy of the autonomic nervous system of the gut with particular reference to the peptidergic innervation in normal and disease states and during development.

General anatomy

Sympathetic innervation

Preganglionic fibres from T8 to L3 of the spinal cord pass through the sympathetic chains to synapse with postganglionic neurones in the coeliac and superior and inferior mesenteric ganglia. The postganglionic fibres spread from these ganglia to innervate all parts of the gut. The fibres either innervate their effector organ (i.e. muscle layers, blood vessels, or epithelium) directly or synapse with neurones of the main ganglionated (myenteric or submucous) plexuses.

Parasympathetic innervation

The parasympathetic innervation of the gut is either cranial or sacral in origin. Cranial parasympathetic fibres run mostly in the vagus nerves, whereas sacral nerves originate from S2–S4 of the spinal cord and pass through the nervi erigentes to innervate the lower bowel.

The fibres synapse in the intramural plexuses and postganglionic fibres radiate to effector organs, including other cells in the plexuses.

Intramural plexuses

Most of the fibres that innervate the gut arise from the intramural plexuses. These plexuses form a complex, heterogeneous part of the autonomic nervous system, as was recognized very early in the work of Langley (1898). There are two main ganglionated plexuses—the myenteric (or Auerbach's), which lies between the longitudinal and circular muscle coats, and the submucous (or Meissner's), lying between the circular muscle and the muscularis mucosae. The myenteric plexus contains most of the intrinsic nerve cell bodies of the gut. It can be subdivided into three parts: the primary, secondary, and tertiary plexuses. The primary plexus is composed of the neuronal cells and bundles of fibres running between them, i.e. the core of the plexus. The secondary component is formed by fibres running from ganglia or connecting branches of the primary plexus, which pass to the muscle, whereas the fine fibres that run between the ganglia and branches of the primary plexus are known as the tertiary plexus. The submucous plexus has sometimes been described as having two components, one by the muscularis mucosae, known as Meissner's plexus, and the other against the circular muscle, called Henle's plexus. However, the lack of apparent functional and structural differentiation between the two means that they are unified in most of the relevant literature. The intramural ganglia supply fibres that either synapse with cells in the same or other ganglia, or innervate a range of effector organs in the gut, as well as sending afferents to the central nervous system.

Neurochemistry

Several functionally different neuronal types have been identified in the intramural plexuses of the gut, mainly on the basis of electrophysiology, and attempts have been made to relate the function and morphology of the cells. The work of Dogiel (1899) describing three morphologically and, he hypothesized, functionally distinct types of gut neurones has been shown subsequently, by the investigation of morphofunctional correlations, to be remarkably prescient. In particular, this has been achieved by injection of dye into cells previously characterized electrophysiologically (reviewed by Furness and Costa 1987). Table 15.1 summarizes the current knowledge of the neurones of Dogiel's classification, as studied in the guinea-pig small intestine. There has been much controversy over the value of Dogiel's work but this classification remains a useful basis for neuronal identification. However, it must be noted that not all gut neurones have been found to fit into the classification.

Table 15.1. Dogiel's classification[a]

Type	Axons	Dendrites	Function	Electrophysiology[b]	Products[c,d]
I	Project through other ganglia to muscle	4–20; short, end within ganglia	Motor	S	Substance P, dynorphin, NO, enkephalin, VIP, GRP, CCK
II	Project to other ganglia	3–10; long	Sensory	AH	Somatostatin, substance P, CCK
III	Termination not traced	2–10; short, end within ganglia	?	S	Somatostatin, VIP, dynorphin, CGRP, NPY, CCK

[a] Dogiel (1899).

[b] S, fast excitatory postsynaptic potentials (cholinergic); AH, prolonged after hyperpolarizations.

[c] Furness and Costa (1987); Costa *et al* (1992).

[d] NO, nitric oxide; VIP, vasoactive intestinal peptide; GRP, gastrin-releasing peptide (or bombesin); CCK, cholecystokinin; CGRP, calcitonin-gene-related peptide; NPY, neuropeptide Y.

Many different substances have been identified, by pharmacological, physiological, or morphological means, in the autonomic nervous system of the mammalian gut. Not all of these substances have been shown as yet to satisfy all the criteria used to identify neurotransmitters. However, it is clear that a highly complex, heterogeneous transmitter system exists with subtypes of neurones chemically coded by the presence of a specific substance or combination of substances. Different combinations of the same substances can be found in functionally and morphologically distinct neurones (see Table 15.1, for example). For brevity, Table 15.2 provides a list of the main established and candidate transmitters that have been identified in enteric nerves. Acetylcholine and noradrenaline have long been known to be neurotransmitters in the gut and their excitatory and inhibitory influences on gut function are well described. What has emerged in recent years is the realization that these 'classical' neurotransmitters often coexist with other substances in the gut innervation. For example, in the guinea-pig the peptides cholecystokinin, somatostatin, neuropeptide Y, and substance P, have been localized to cholinergic neurones, identified by immunostaining of the acetylcholine-synthesizing enzyme choline acetyltransferase (Furness and Costa 1987). Similarly, neuropeptide Y has been demonstrated in postganglionic sympathetic neurones supplying the stomach and colon of several species (Ekblad *et al.* 1984; Su *et al.* 1987).

Table 15.2. Neurochemicals identified in the innervation of the human gut

Acetylcholine (ACh)

Adenosine triphosphate (ATP)

Dopamine

γ-Aminobutyric acid (GABA)

Nitric oxide

Noradrenaline

Peptides

Serotonin (5-hydroxytryptamine (5-HT))

Although adenosine triphosphate (ATP) has been put forward as the main transmitter in inhibitory gastrointestinal neurones it seems, at present, that it is more widely accepted as also being present in other types of neurones and acting as some kind of co-transmitter (Burnstock 1981). Dopamine, a precursor to noradrenaline, has been found in gastrointestinal nerves, but is likely to be related to the sympathetic nerves rather than existing as a separate neurotransmitter (Furness and Costa 1987). α-aminobutyric acid (GABA) appears to cause differential modulation of gastrointestinal motility by stimulating cholinergic neurones via $GABA_A$ receptors or reducing cholinergic contractions via the $GABA_B$ subtype (Ong and Kerr 1983). The amine has been identified in the myenteric plexus in neurones that seem to innervate other ganglion cells (Jessen *et al.* 1979).

Serotonin (5-hydroxytryptamine) has long been known to act as a transmitter in the central nervous system but its presence in gastrointestinal nerves was a matter of debate prior to the advent of specific antibodies to the amine. A major problem with evaluation of serotonin as a neurotransmitter is its relatively high concentration in endocrine cells in all areas of the gastrointestinal mucosa. Serotonin has been localized to the intramural plexuses (Furness and Costa 1987) where it has been suggested to contribute to slow potentials in prolonged after hyperpolarization neurones.

NANC innervation: nitric oxide

The major inhibitory innervation of the mammalian gut comes from intrinsic nerves and plays an essential role in most gastrointestinal reflexes. The term NANC (non-adrenergic, non-cholinergic) was coined to describe these nerves, as the neurotransmitter/s they contain remained unknown for many years despite extensive investigation. However, now there is a wealth of morphological, physiological, and pharmacological evidence that the inhibitory transmitter in the gut of a variety of species, including man, is nitric oxide (Bult *et al.* 1990; Toda *et al.* 1990; Sanders and Ward 1992; Stark and Szurszewski 1992; Keef *et al.* 1993; Fig. 15.1). This free-radical gas is a major regulatory factor in the mammalian body and is produced by a variety of cells in addition to nerves, such as endothelium, epithelium, and macrophages (Moncada *et al.* 1991). Nitric oxide is unique among neuroactive substances in that it is a gas with no known storage mechanisms and is very labile with a half-life of a few

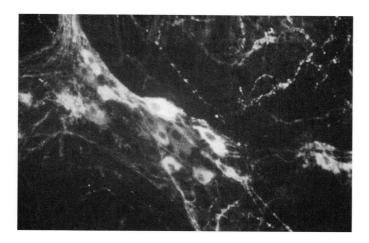

Fig. 15.1. Type I (neuronal) nitric oxide synthase (NOS), immunostained using indirect immunofluorescence in a whole mount preparation of the myenteric plexus of guinea-pig stomach and visualized using a confocal laser microscope. The projections of the immunoreactive fibres in three dimensions have been incorporated into a two-dimensional image. The NOS-immunoreactive ganglion cells have type I Dogiel morphology. (NB The image was captured from a monitor screen.)

adult and developing tissues. One of the best characterized is neural cell adhesion molecule (NCAM), which mediates the initial interaction between nerve and muscle and acts in subsequent stages of synapse development and stabilization (Reiger *et al.* 1985) and maintenance of the neuromuscular system (Thiery 1982; Cunningham 1991). Recent study of the human intestine has shown that NCAM expression can be detected on both muscle and nerves from 8 weeks of gestation, the earliest stage examined (Romanska *et al.* 1996*a*). By 20 weeks of gestation, strong expression was seen on all nerves but only on the muscularis mucosae and the inner edge of the circular muscle. At birth, NCAM was confined to nerves. Thus, muscular expression of NCAM in the human intestine is high during development of the neuromuscular system but tails off once maturation occurs. However, as with skeletal muscle (Covault and Sanes 1985; Cashman *et al.* 1987; Walsh *et al.* 1987, 1988), the levels of NCAM seen on the smooth muscle of the intestine can increase in disease conditions such as Hirschsprung's disease, where strong expression of NCAM is seen on the muscularis mucosae (Romanska *et al.* 1993; Fig. 15.2). The presence of NCAM on muscle in aganglionic bowel is unlikely to be the result of the intractable constipation that occurs as it is not found in bowel taken from individuals with idiopathic constipation and normal-appearing, ganglionic intestine (Romanska *et al.* 1996*b*).

seconds. Instead of interacting with a cell surface receptor, it diffuses across membranes. Once in the cell, it binds to and activates soluble guanylate cyclase, thereby increasing cyclic guanosine monophosphate levels, although it may have other modes of action.

Nitric oxide is synthesized from the terminal guanidino nitrogen of L-arginine by the enzyme known as nitric oxide synthase (NOS), which exists in three main forms: type I (neuronal) NOS and type III (endothelial) NOS are expressed constitutively and are calcium- and calmodulin-dependent whereas type II (inducible) NOS is calcium- and calmodulin-independent (Moncada *et al.* 1991). The nature and short half-life of nitric oxide preclude its localization in tissues but the distribution of the type I enzyme has been studied in several species and it has been found to occur mainly in type I cells of the Dogiel classification, which fits with a role for nitric oxide in the control of motor function in the gut (Costa *et al.* 1992; Springall *et al.* 1992; Ward *et al.* 1992; Young *et al.* 1992; Desai *et al.* 1994). Reduced expression of type I NOS and nitric oxide activity has been described in a number of gastrointestinal dysmotility syndromes, including oesophageal achalasia (Mearin *et al.* 1993), congenital aganglionosis (Hirschsprung's disease) (Vanderwinden *et al.* 1993; Bealer *et al.* 1994; O'Kelly *et al.* 1994; Larsson *et al.* 1995; Tomita *et al.* 1995; Guo *et al.* 1997), and hypertrophic pyloric stenosis (Vanderwinden *et al.* 1992; Abel *et al.* 1998). Interestingly, mice that have had the gene for type I NOS removed by homologous recombination live and reproduce normally and have no demonstrable abnormality of the central nervous system (Huang *et al.* 1993). However, the major pathological feature they do display is gross gastric enlargement with pyloric sphincter hypertrophy.

Neural cell adhesion molecule

A range of cell surface molecules has been studied extensively and shown to contribute to cell-to-cell recognition processes in normal

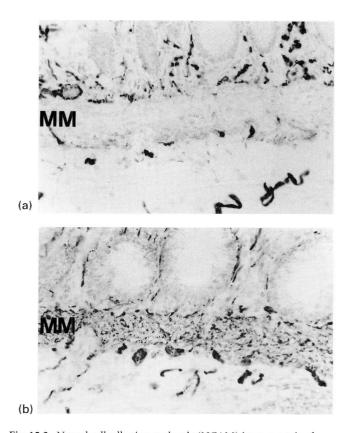

(a)

(b)

Fig. 15.2. Neural cell adhesion molecule (NCAM) immunostained using the avidin-biotin complex method in (a) normal large bowel from a neonate, immunoreactivity for NCAM is confined to the nerves (MM, muscularis mucosae); (b) large bowel from a child with congenital aganglionosis, NCAM is present not only on nerves but also on the muscularis mucosae (MM).

Morphological studies of gut neuropeptides

The most widespread and abundant transmitters in the mammalian gut are the neuropeptides. As yet, not all of them satisfy the classical criteria for neurotransmitters, but they do represent a relatively new discovery in the peripheral nervous system; their numbers are continuously expanding and our understanding of them increasing. The rest of this chapter describes current knowledge of this heterogeneous group of substances, with emphasis on the contribution of morphological investigations.

For brevity, a list of the major peptides currently identifiable in the innervation of the mammalian gut is given in Table 15.3, together with information on their origins, known actions, and number of amino acids. The information in the table is based on data derived from human and experimental animal (mainly rat and guinea-pig) tissues.

Localization of neuropeptides: immunocytochemistry

Most of the literature on the localization of neuropeptides in the gut concerns the application of immunocytochemistry at light or electron microscopical levels. Several immunocytochemical techniques exist and those for light microscopy can be divided broadly into transmitted light methods or fluorescent labelling (reviewed by Polak and Van Noorden 1997). Of the former, the unlabelled antibody enzyme (peroxidase antiperoxidase) or avidin–biotin complex methods are the most widely used. Fluorescence labelling usually employs an indirect method with fluorescein, rhodamine, or some other fluorescent compound coupled to the secondary antibody. The method of choice is

often a matter of personal preference but immunostains visible on transmitted light are permanent and therefore more widely used where long-term storage of preparations is required. Immunostains of neuropeptides can be made on tissue sections or on whole-mount preparations of intact layers of the gut, e.g. intramural plexuses (Figs 15.1 and 15.3) or muscle layers. Co-localization of neuropeptides is achieved using serial sectioning through ganglion cells or by administering anti-

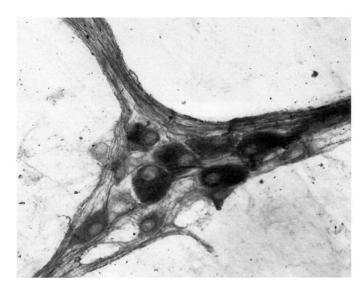

Fig. 15.3. Vasoactive intestinal peptide immunostained using the peroxidase antiperoxidase method in a whole-mount preparation of the submucous plexus of the human colon. Both ganglion cells and nerve fibres show dense immunoreactivity.

Table 15.3. Major gut neuropeptides

Peptides*	No. of amino acids	Main actions	Main origin(s)
Bombesin (GRP)	27	Multiple stimulatory effects, e.g. gastrin release	Local
CGRP	37	Gastric acid secretion, muscle constriction	Local and sensory
CCK8	8	Not known	Local
Dynorphin	17	Opiate effects	Local
Endothelin-1	21	Vasoconstriction	Local
Galanin	29	Muscle constriction	Local
Leu-enkephalin	5	Opiate effects	Local
Met-enkephalin	5	Opiate effects	Local
Neuromedin U	8 or 25	Muscle constriction, vasoconstriction	Local
NPY	36	Vasoconstriction	Local and sympathetic
PACAP	38	Adenylate cyclase activation	Local
PHM	27	Muscle relaxation, secretion	Local
Somatostatin	28	Multiple inhibitory effects e.g. gastrin inhibition	Local
Substance P	11	Vasodilatation, muscle constriction	Local and sensory
VIP	28	Vasodilatation, muscle relaxation, secretion	Local

* CGRP, calcitonin gene-related; GRP, gastrin-releasing peptide; NPY, neuropeptide Y; PACAP, pituitary adenylate cyclase activating peptide; PHM, peptide histidine methionine; VIP, vasoactive intestinal polypeptide.

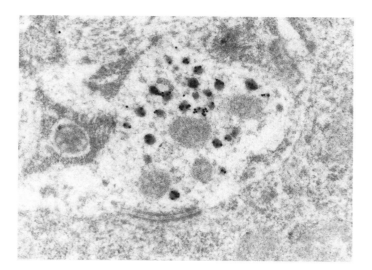

Fig. 15.4. Immunoreactivity for substance P demonstrated in granules in a nerve terminal in guinea-pig colon using the indirect immunogold method and visualized using a transmission electron microscope.

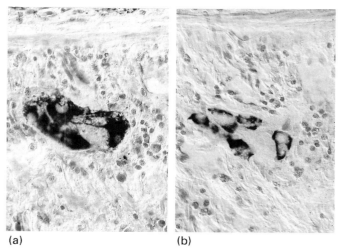

(a)　　　　　　　　　　　　　(b)

Fig. 15.5. Serial sections of inflamed human colon showing the submucous plexus. In (a), the section has been immunostained for vasoactive intestinal polypeptide (VIP) and in (b) *in situ* hybridization with a digoxygenin-labelled riboprobe shows the expression of VIP mRNA in the same cells.

bodies to separate neuropeptides, labelled with different colours, to the same section. The unravelling of the complexity of the enteric nervous system has been aided in recent years by the advent of confocal laser microscopy, which allows quantitative, three-dimensional analysis of immunofluorescent tissue preparation (Matsumoto and Kramer 1994; Fig. 15.1).

Similarly, for electron microscopy a number of methods exist for immunostaining of vesicles containing neuropeptides (and other antigens), the most popular of which are those that employ gold-labelled antibodies. Colloidal gold adsorbs onto the Fc portion of the IgG molecule and is electron-dense. The immunogold staining technique is a straightforward indirect method (De Mey *et al.* 1981; Fig. 15.4) that has been adapted to allow immunostaining of multiple antigens in a single tissue section by the use of antibodies labelled with gold particles of different sizes.

Localization of neuropeptide gene expression: *in situ* hybridization

Immunocytochemistry localizes the final products of gut nerves but information on the sites, rates, and control of neuropeptide gene expression can now be derived from histological preparations using *in situ* hybridization of DNA or RNA species directing neuropeptide synthesis (reviewed by Polak and McGee 1990). This technique utilizes the capacity of labelled complementary nucleic acid sequences to form stable hybrids with endogenous DNA or mRNA. The complementary sequences, in the form of single-stranded DNA or RNA, double-stranded DNA, or synthetic oligodeoxyribonucleotides, can be labelled with isotopes (e.g. ^{32}P, ^{35}S, ^{3}H, etc.) and localized by autoradiography or with substances subsequently localized by immunocytochemistry (e.g. biotin, digoxigenin) (Fig. 15.5).

Neural origins

The nature and projections of neuropeptide-containing gut nerves have been studied extensively in experimental animals. Chemical

manipulations in combination with immunocytochemistry can help to identify particular nerve types containing neuropeptides. For example, immunostaining of neuropeptide Y (NPY) in rats treated with 6-hydroxydopamine shows a loss of NPY-immunoreactive fibres from around gut blood vessels, suggesting that these are noradrenergic sympathetic nerves (Su *et al.* 1987). Similarly, destruction of primary sensory afferents by administration of capsaicin (8-methyl-*N*-vanillyl-5-nonenamide) removes a proportion of calcitonin-gene-related peptide (CGRP)- and substance P-immunoreactive fibres from the rat gut, indicating their sensory nature (Su *et al.* 1987).

Analysis of the origin and projection fields of neuropeptide-containing innervation of the gut requires further manipulations, in the form of surgical interruption of nerve pathways or retrograde tracing using dyes. Interruption of pathways has been a useful way of establishing nerve origins. To continue with the example of NPY-containing nerves, sympathectomy by removal of the coeliac ganglion and plexus and the superior mesenteric ganglion reduces the population of nerves in the rat gut in a similar way to administration of 6-hydroxydopamine (Su *et al.* 1987). Lesioning of pathways can also be used to study neural projections within the gut wall. Myotomy, myectomy, and homotopic autotransplants, with immunocytochemical identification of nerve types, have been used successfully to provide detailed information on the projections of neuropeptide-immunoreactive nerves in certain species, and the most complete analysis of neuronal circuitry of the mammalian gut has been achieved by application of these methods in the guinea-pig small intestine (reviewed by Furness and Costa 1987). However, a less invasive method is retrograde tracing of neuronal pathways, which has the major advantage of being applicable in specimens of human gut, thereby yielding information with direct relevance to clinical gastroenterology. Retrograde tracing uses the ability of nerves to transport dyes retrogradely to their perikarya and consists of injection, *in vivo* to the terminal region of interest, of a suitable chemical (e.g. horseradish, peroxidase, radiolabelled amino acids, fluorescent dyes), which is taken up and labels the cell of origin (reviewed by Su and Polak 1987). This is then identified by neuropeptide immunocytochemistry. In this way, sympathetic, NPY-immunoreactive nerves supplying, for example, the rat stomach have been shown to arise from perikarya in the coeliac and inferior mesenteric ganglia, whereas sensory CGRP-immunoreactive fibres are supplied by bilateral dorsal root ganglia at levels T8–T11 (Su *et al.* 1987). A refinement of this technology has been to apply it *in vitro* to study human enteric neural pathways. Injection of a fluorescent dye, Fluorogold, into human colon maintained *in vitro*, combined with fluorescein immunofluorescence on whole-mount preparations, was used to study the projection field of vasoactive intestinal polypeptide (VIP)-containing nerves in three dimensions (Domoto *et al.* 1990) and, thus, provide a new means by which to study human gut neuroanatomy (Fig. 15.6).

Neuropeptides in the developing human gut

Few studies have been made of neuropeptides in human fetal gut. A comprehensive immunocytochemical study of the ontogeny of major neuropeptides in the human oesophagus revealed their appearance in fibres at 11 (VIP, NPY, gastrin-releasing peptide [GRP]), 13 (galanin, substance P), 15.5 (somatostatin, met-enkephalin), and 18 weeks (CGRP) (Hitchcock *et al.* 1992). Some investigation has been made of the way in which the peptide-containing nerves infiltrate the developing human gut. Traditionally, colonization of the human gut by nerves is considered to occur in a craniocaudal direction, with subsequent passage of neuronal precursors through the muscle to form the major ganglionated plexuses although, in other species, bidirectional migration of neuronal precursors has been detected. Using immunocytochemistry and *in situ* hybridization in combination, the appearance of VIP-containing nerves has been examined in developing human gut (Facer *et al.* 1992). At the earliest

stage examined (8 weeks' gestation) nerve cells, demonstrated by immunostaining of the general nerve marker protein gene product 9.5, were found throughout the length of the gut, but not transversely. Ganglion cells were first found in both myenteric and submucous plexuses at 9 weeks' gestation. VIP immunoreactivity was seen in fibres from 9 weeks' gestation but could not be found in perikarya until 18 weeks' gestation. With *in situ* hybridization, VIP gene expression in cells was detected much earlier, from 9 weeks' gestation, and its temporal appearance was consistent with craniocaudal, transmural neuronal colonization and/or migration.

Neuropeptides in gastrointestinal diseases

Marked abnormalities of the neuropeptide-containing innervation of the gut have been observed in a number of diseases. In view of the rapid breakdown of most neuropeptides, alterations in circulating levels are rare and most changes have been observed on the basis of morphological investigations, sometimes coupled with radioimmunological measurement of peptide concentrations in affected tissues.

Chagas' disease

Severe disturbance of the normal pattern of neuropeptide-containing nerves has been reported in Chagas' disease, an example of acquired aganglionosis. This disease is a common result of long-standing infection with the flagellate protozoan, *Trypanosoma cruzi*. Ganglionitis occurs in the intramural plexuses with subsequent destruction of cells leading to denervation and distension of gut segments, most commonly manifesting as megaoesophagus and/or megacolon. Comparison with both normal controls and patients with multiple system atrophy (Shy–Drager syndrome) has revealed a reduction in both VIP- and substance P-immunoreactive nerves and tissue content of these neuropeptides only in Chagas' disease (Long *et al.* 1980). Thus the neuropeptides appear to be affected by intrinsic but not extrinsic autonomic neuropathy, indicating that VIP and substance P have mainly intrinsic origins in the human bowel. A similar reduction in neuropeptides was found in an equine disease, grass sickness, which is in many ways analogous to human Chagas' disease in being acquired aganglionosis, although the pathogenic agent has yet to be identified (Bishop *et al.* 1984).

Idiopathic constipation

The pathogenesis of idiopathic, slow-transit constipation has yet to be clearly defined and, at present, colectomy is often used to treat the condition. Some changes in the morphology of intramural neurones have been noted and a recent study has examined the morphology and concentrations of the three major gut neuropeptides, VIP, substance P, and NPY, in affected bowel (Milner *et al.* 1990). It seems that substance P- and NPY-containing nerves are not altered in the colon of individuals with severe chronic idiopathic constipation, in comparison with normal control bowel. However, VIP content was reduced in the intramural plexuses of the colon, although no consistent alteration of VIP-immunoreactive nerves was seen on immunocytochemistry.

Hirschsprung's disease

In Hirschsprung's disease, or congenital aganglionosis, the neuronal lesions do not appear to be confined to an absence of intramural

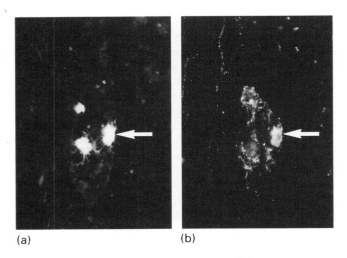

(a)   (b)

Fig. 15.6. (a) Fluorogold-labelled neurones in a whole-mount preparation of the submucous plexus of the human colon after injection of the dye into the submucous layer. (b) Vasoactive intestinal peptide (VIP) immunostained by indirect immunofluorescence in the same specimen. One cell (arrow) is labelled with the dye and also shows immunoreactivity for VIP. Differential visualization of the dye and immunostain in the same cells was achieved by altering the wavelength of observation light.

ganglion cells. Hypertrophied nerve bundles can be observed, often in the serosa or between the longitudinal and circular muscle layers. In addition, alterations of specific nerve types have been noted, including increased adrenergic- and cholinesterase-positive nerves and loss of intrinsic serotonin-containing nerves. For the neuropeptides, a mixed pattern of changes are seen in aganglionic bowel. VIP- (and its related molecule, peptide histidine methionine), substance P-, met-enkephalin-, somatostatin-, and CGRP-immunoreactive nerves are reduced in aganglionic segments, possibly reflecting their mainly intrinsic origin in the human large bowel (Ehrenpreis and Pernow 1953; Tafuri *et al.* 1974; Bishop *et al.* 1981; Hamada *et al.* 1987). In contrast, fibres containing NPY immunoreactivity show a marked increase in aganglionic bowel, particularly in the circular muscle where few such fibres are normally found (Hamada *et al.* 1987; Fig. 15.7). As described earlier, NPY-immunoreactive fibres in the gut have a dual origin from intramural ganglion cells and extrinsic noradrenergic nerves and the latter innervate mainly the vasculature and myenteric plexus (Ekblad *et al.* 1984; Su *et al.* 1987). This change in NPY nerves may thus reflect the reported hyperplasia of aminergic fibres in Hirschsprung's disease.

Diabetic neuropathy

Specific alterations of peptide-containing nerves are seen in the enteric neuropathy associated with streptozotocin-induced diabetes mellitus in rats. It has been reported that VIP nerve immunoreactivity increases, whereas that of CGRP nerves decreases, while substance P- and NPY-immunoreactive nerves remain unchanged (Belai and Burnstock 1990; Belai *et al.* 1993).

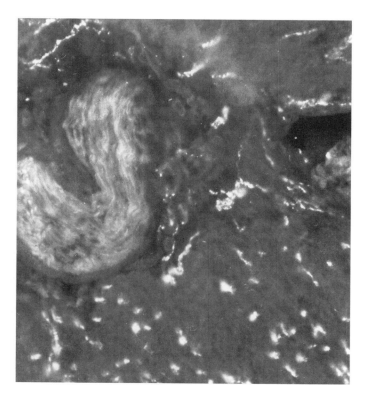

Fig. 15.7. Hyperplastic, numerous neuropeptide Y-immunoreactive fibres demonstrated by indirect immunofluorescence in large bowel from a child with Hirschsprung's disease.

Inflammatory bowel disease

Neuronal abnormalities have long been known to occur in Crohn's disease (regional enteritis) and take the form of general nerve proliferation, sometimes termed neuromatous hyperplasia (Davis *et al.* 1955), but their significance remains unknown. Such changes are not characteristic of ulcerative colitis, and it is possible that the transmural inflammatory process that occurs in Crohn's disease stimulates the neural proliferation, as such a stimulus would be absent from all but the most severe cases of ulcerative colitis. No agreement has been reached on the pathology of peptide-containing nerves in inflammatory bowel disease and a variety of different findings has been published (reviewed by Bishop and Polak 1990). The first study reported that VIP-immunoreactive fibres and the tissue content of VIP is increased in Crohn's disease (ileitis and colitis), in comparison with both ulcerative colitis and normal controls (Bishop *et al.* 1980; O'Morain *et al.* 1984). No evidence has been obtained that these hyperplastic VIP nerves are functional, but it is tempting to speculate that the peptide's potent stimulation of gut secretion and inhibition of motility may contribute to the symptoms of the disease. In contrast, a separate group of researchers reported a reduction of both VIP and substance P nerves in Crohn's disease (Sjolund *et al.* 1983), while another study described loss of VIP from the mucosa/submucosa in Crohn's and ulcerative colitis and an increase in substance P nerves in ulcerative colitis (Koch *et al.* 1987). More recently, increased immunoreactivity for not only VIP but also nitric oxide synthase was described in Crohn's disease, in nerves and inflammatory cells, leading to the suggestion that neural–immunological interactions occur (Belai *et al.* 1997).

Conclusions

The intramural plexuses of the mammalian gut have long been known to form a major part of the autonomic nervous system, but their importance has only been recognized comparatively recently with the discovery of their complex neurochemistry and wide range of actions. The application of new techniques for the investigation of nerves allows delineation of the neuroanatomy of the gut and is revealing pathological alterations which may provide the basis for future therapeutic measures.

References

Abel, R. M., Bishop, A. E., Dore, C. J., Spitz, L., and Polak J. M. (1998). A quantitative study of the morphological and histochemical changes within nerves and muscle in infantile hypertrophic pyloric stenosis. *J. Pediatr. Surg.* **33**, 682–7.

Bealer, J. F., Natuzzi, E. S., Buscher, C. *et al.* (1994). Nitric oxide synthase is deficient in the aganglionic colon of patients with Hirschsprung's disease. *Pediatrics* **93**, 647–51.

Belai, A. and Burnstock, G. (1990). Changes in adrenergic and peptidergic nerves in the submucous plexus of streptozotocin-diabetic rat ileum. *Gastroenterology* **98**, 1427–36.

Belai, A., Facer, P., Bishop, A. E., Polak, J. M., and Burnstock, G. (1993). Effect of streptozotocin-diabetes on the level of VIP mRNA in myenteric neurones. *NeuroReport* **4**, 291–4.

Belai, A., Boulos, P. B., Robson, T., and Burnstock, G. (1997). Neurochemical coding in the small intestine of patients with Crohn's disease. *Gut* **40**, 767–74.

Bishop, A. E. and Polak, J. M. (1990). Gut endocrine and neural peptides. *Endocrinol. Pathol.* 1, 4–24.

Bishop, A. E., Polak, J. M., Bryant, M. G., Bloom, S. R., and Hamilton, S. (1980). Abnormalities of vasoactive intestinal polypeptide-containing nerves in Crohn's disease. *Gastroenterology* 79, 853–60.

Bishop, A. E., Polak, J. M., Lake, B. D., Bryant, M. G., and Bloom, S. R. (1981). Abnormalities of the colonic regulatory peptides in Hirschsprung's disease. *Histopathology* 5, 679–88.

Bishop, A. E., Hodson, N. P., Major, J. H. *et al.* (1984). The regulatory peptide system of the large bowel in equine grass sickness. *Experientia* 40, 801–6.

Bult, H., Boeckxstaens G. E., Pelckmans, P. A., Jordaens, F. H., Van Maercke Y. M., and Herman, A. G. (1990). Nitric oxide as an inhibitory non-adrenergic, non-cholinergic neurotransmitter. *Nature* 345, 346–7.

Burnstock, G. (1981) Neurotransmitters and trophic factors in the autonomic nervous system. *J. Physiol.* 313, 1–35.

Cashman, N. R., Covault, J., Wollman, R. L., and Sanes, J. R. (1987). Neural cell adhesion molecule in normal, denervated and myopathic human muscle. *Ann. Neurol.* 21, 481–9.

Costa, M., Furness, J. B., Pompolo, S. *et al.* (1992). Projections and chemical coding of neurons with immunoreactivity for nitric oxide synthase in the guinea pig small intestine. *Neurosci. Lett.* 148, 121–5.

Covault, J. and Sanes, J. R. (1985). Neural cell adhesion molecule (NCAM) accumulates in denervated and paralysed skeletal muscle. *Proc. Natl. Acad. Sci. USA* 82, 4544–8.

Cunningham, B. A. (1991). Transaction of the ninth annual meeting of The American Gynecological and Obstetrical Society. *Am. J. Obstet. Gynecol.* 164, 939–48.

Davis, D.R., Dockerty, M. B., and Mayo C. W. (1955). The myenteric plexus in regional enteritis: a study of ganglion cells in the ileum in 24 cases. *Surg. Gynaecol. Obstet.* 101, 208.

De Mey, J., Moeremans, M., Geuens, G., Nuydens, R., and De Brabander, M. (1981). High resolution light and electron microscopic localization of tubulin with the IGS (immunogold staining) method. *Cell Biol. Int. Rep.* 5, 889–99.

Desai, K. M., Warner, T. D., Bishop, A. E., Moncada, S., Polak, J. M., and Vane, J. R. (1994). Nitric oxide but not VIP is the main neurotransmitter of vagally-induced relaxation of the guinea pig stomach. *Br. J. Pharmacol.* 113, 1197–202.

Dogiel, A. S. (1899). ueber den bau der Ganglien in den Gefiechten des Darmes und der Gallenblase des Menschen und der Sdugetiere. *Arch Anat. Physiol. Leipzeig, Anat. Abt.*, 130–58.

Domoto, T., Bishop, A. E., Oki, M., and Polak, J. M. (1990). An *in vitro* study of the projections of enteric VIP-immunoreactive neurones in the human colon. *Gastroenterology* 98, 819–27.

Ehrenpreis, T. and Pernow, B. (1953). On the occurrence of substance P in the rectosigmoid in Hirschsprung's disease. *Acta Physiol. Scand.* 27, 380–8.

Ekblad, E., Wahlstedt, C., Ekelund, M., Hakanson, R., and Sundler, F. (1984). Neuropeptide Y in the gut and pancreas. Distribution and possible vasomotor function. *Frontiers Horm. Res.* 12, 85–90.

Facer, P., Bishop, A. E., Moscoso, G. *et al.* (1992). Vasoactive intestinal peptide gene expression in the developing human gastrointestinal tract. *Gastroenterology* 102, 47–5.

Furness, J. B. and Costa, M. (ed.) (1987). *The enteric nervous system.* Churchill Livingstone, Edinburgh.

Guo, R., Nada, O., Suita, S., Taguchi, T., and Masumoto, K. (1997). The distribution and co-localization of nitric oxide synthase and vasoactive intestinal polypeptide nerves of the colon with Hirschsprung's disease. *Virchows Archiv* 430, 53–61.

Hamada, Y., Bishop, A. E., Federici, G., Rivosecchi, M., Talbot, I. C., and Polak, J. M. (1987). Increased neuropeptide Y-immunoreactive innervation of aganglionic bowel in Hirschsprung's disease. *Virchows Archiv* A411, 369–77.

Hitchcock, R. J. I., Pemble, M. J., Bishop, A. E., Spitz, L., and Polak, J. M. (1992). The ontogeny and distribution of neuropeptides in the human fetal and infant oesophagus. *Gastroenterology* 102, 840–8.

Huang, P. L., Dawson, T. M., Bredt, D. S., Snyder, S. H., and Fishman, M. C. (1993). Targeted disruption of the neuronal nitric oxide synthase gene. *Cell* 75, 1273–86.

Jessen, K. R., Mirsky, R., Dennison, M. E., and Burnstock, G. (1979). GABA may be a neurotransmitter in the vertebrate peripheral nervous system. *Nature* 281, 71–4.

Keef, K. D., Du, C., Ward, S. M., McGregor, B., and Sanders, K. M. (1993). Enteric inhibitory neural regulation of human colonic circular muscle: role of nitric oxide. *Gastroenterology* 105, 1009–16.

Koch, T. R., Carney, J. A., and Go V. L. W. (1987). Distribution and quantification of gut neuropeptides in normal intestine and inflammatory bowel disease. *Dig. Dis. Sci.* 32, 369–76.

Langley, J. N. (1898). On the union of cranial autonomic (visceral) fibres with the nerve cells of the superior cervical ganglion. *J. Physiol.* 23, 240–70.

Larsson, L. T., Shen, Z., Ekblad, E., Sundler, F., Alm, P., and Anderson, K. E. (1995). Lack of neuronal nitric oxide synthase in nerve fibres of aganglionic intestine: a clue to Hirschsprung's disease. *J. Pediatr. Gastroenterol. Nutr.* 20, 49–53.

Long, R. G., Bishop, A. E., Barnes, A. J. *et al.* (1980). Neural and hormonal peptides in rectal biopsy specimens from patients with Chagas' disease and chronic autonomic failure. *Lancet* i, 559–62.

Matsumoto, B. and Kramer, T. (1994). Theory and applications of confocal microscopy. *Cell Vision* 1, 190–8.

Mearin, F., Mourelle, M., Guarner, F. *et al.* (1993). Patients with achalasia lack nitric oxide synthase in the gastro-oesophageal junction. *Eur. J. Clin. Invest.* 23, 724–8.

Milner, P., Crowe, R., Kamm, M. A., Lennard-Jones, J. E., and Burnstock, G. (1990). Vasoactive intestinal polypeptide levels in sigmoid colon in idiopathic constipation and diverticular disease. *Gastroenterology* 99, 666–75.

Moncada, S., Palmer, R. M. J., and Higgs, E. A. (1991). Nitric oxide: physiology, pathophysiology and pharmacology. *Pharmacol. Rev.* 43, 109–42.

O'Kelly, T. J., Davies, J. R., Tam, P. K., Brading, A. F., and Mortensen, N. J. (1994). Abnormalities of nitric oxide-producing neurons in Hirschsprung's disease: morphology and implications. *J. Pediatr. Surg.* 29, 294–9.

O'Morain, C., Bishop, A. E., McGregor, G. P. *et al.* (1984). Vasoactive intestinal peptide concentrations and immunocytochemical studies in rectal biopsies from patients with inflammatory bowel disease. *Gut* 25, 57–61.

Ong, J. and Kerr, D. I. B. (1983). GABA$_A$- and GABA$_B$-receptor-mediated modification of intestinal motility. *Eur. J. Pharmacol.* 86, 9–17.

Polak, J. M. and McGee, J. O'D. (ed.) (1990). *In situ hybridization.* Oxford University Press, Oxford.

Polak, J. M. and Van Noorden, S. (1997). *Introduction to immunocytochemistry,* (2nd edn). Bios. Scientific Publishers, Oxford.

Rieger, F., Grumet M., and Edelman G. M. (1985). N-CAM at the vertebrate neuromuscular junction. *J. Cell Biol.* 101, 285–93.

Romanska, H. M., Bishop, A. E., Brereton, R. J., Spitz, L., and Polak, J. M. (1993). Increased expression of muscular neural cell adhesion molecule in congenital aganglionosis. *Gastroenterology* 105, 1104–9.

Romanska, H. M., Bishop, A. E., Moscoso, G. *et al.* (1996a). Neural cell adhesion molecule expression in the nerves and muscle of developing human large bowel. *J. Pediatr. Gastroenterol. Nutr.* 22, 351–8.

Romanska, H. M., Bishop, A. E., Lee, J. C., Walsh, F. S., Spitz, L., and Polak, J. M. (1996b). Idiopathic constipation is not associated with increased neural cell adhesion molecule expression on intestinal muscle. *Dig. Dis. Sci.* 41, 1298–302.

Sanders, K. M. and Ward, S. M. (1992). Nitric oxide as a mediator of non-adrenergic, non-cholinergic (NANC) neurotransmission. *Am. J. Physiol.* 262, G379–92.

Sjolund, K., Schaffalitzky De Muckadell, O. B., Fahrenkrug, J., Hakanson, R., Peterson, B. G., and Sundler, F. (1983). Peptide-containing nerve fibres in the gut wall in Crohn's disease. *Gut* 24, 724–33.

Springall, D. R., Suburo, A., Bishop, A. E. *et al.* (1992). Distinct localization of nitric oxide synthase(s) immunoreactivity in human vasculature and nerves using separate antisera. *Histochem.* **98**, 259–66.

Stark, M. E. and Szurszewski, J. H. (1992). Role of nitric oxide in gastrointestinal and hepatic function and disease. *Gastroenterology* **103**, 1928–49.

Su, H. C. and Polak, J. M. (1987). Combined axonal transport tracing and immunocytochemistry for mapping pathways of peptide-containing nerves in the peripheral nervous system. *Experientia* **43**, 761–7.

Su, H. C., Bishop, A. E., Power, R. F., Hamada, Y., and Polak, J. M. (1987). Dual intrinsic and extrinsic origins of CGRP- and NPY-immunoreactive nerves of rat gut and pancreas. *J. Neurosci.* **7**, 2674–87.

Tafuri, W. L., Maria, T. A., Pittella, J. E., and Bogliolo, L. (1974). An electron microscopic study of the Auerbach's plexus and determination of substance P of the colon in Hirschsprung's disease. *Virchows Archiv* **A362**, 41–50.

Thiery, J. P. (1982). Cell adhesion molecules in early chicken embryogenesis. *Proc. Natl Acad. Sci. USA* **79**, 6737–41.

Toda, N., Baba, H., and Okamura, T. (1990). Role of nitric oxide in non-adrenergic, non-cholinergic nerve-mediated relaxation in dog duodenal longitudinal muscle strips. *Jap. J. Pharmacol.* **53**, 281–4.

Tomita, R., Munakata, K., Kurosu, Y., and Tanjoh, K. (1995). A role of nitric oxide in Hirschsprung's disease. *J. Pediatr. Surg.* **30**, 437–40.

Vanderwinden, J. M., Mailleux, P., Schiffmann, S. N., Vanderhaeghen, J. J., and De Laet, M. H. (1992). Nitric oxide synthase activity in infantile hypertrophic pyloric stenosis. *New Engl. J. Med.* **327**, 511–15.

Vanderwinden, J. M., De Laet, M. H., Schiffmann, S. N. *et al.* (1993). Nitric oxide synthase distribution in the enteric nervous system of Hirschsprung's disease. *Gastroenterology* **105**, 969–73.

Walsh F. S., Moore, S., and Lake, B. (1987). Cell adhesion molecule NCAM is expressed by denervated myofibres in Werding–Hoffman and Kudgelbuerg–Welander type of spinal muscular atrophies. *J. Neurol. Neurosurg. Psychiatry* **50**, 539–42.

Walsh, F. S., Moore, S., and Dickson J. (1988). Expression of membrane antigens in myotonic dystrophy. *J. Neurol. Neurosurg. Psychiatry* **51**, 136–8.

Ward, S. M., Xue, C., Shutleworth, C. W. R., Bredt, D. S., Snyder, S. H. and Sanders, K. M. (1992). NADPH diaphorase and nitric oxide synthase co-localization in enteric neurons of the canine proximal colon. *Am. J. Physiol.* **263**, G277–284.

Young, H. M., Furness, J. B., Shutleworth, C. W. R., Bredt, D. S., and Snyder, S. H. (1992). Co-localization of nitric oxide synthase immunoreactivity and NADPH diaphorase staining in neurons of the guinea-pig intestine. *Histochem.* **97**, 375–8.

16. Nausea, vomiting, and the autonomic nervous system

P. L. R. Andrews

Introduction

Nausea and vomiting are amongst the most common symptoms of disease. The autonomic nervous system plays a major role in the emetic reflex. Visceral afferents, principally in the abdominal vagus are one of the main triggers for emesis. The nucleus tractus solitarius in the brainstem is one of the major nuclei involved in processing visceral information and serves to integrate much of the reflex. The autonomic motor nuclei (e.g. dorsal motor vagal nucleus, nucleus ambiguus, the pre-sympathetic neurones) provide the motor changes which particularly involve the gastrointestinal tract and cardiovascular system. In addition to its role in the emetic reflex, autonomic disorders also result in nausea and vomiting. For example, brainstem turmours involving the nucleus tractus solitarius cause nausea and vomiting as may disordered gastric motility secondary to damage to the extrinsic or enteric innervation of the upper gut. Although nausea and vomiting are often encountered in a clinical context, a fact recognized by Hippocrates and other early physicians, it is important to appreciate that they evolved as components of the body's defensive system, which serve to protect it against accidentally ingested toxins. This 'biological' role has long been recognized, as elegantly illustrated by Robert Boyle in 1686: 'tis profitable for man that his stomach should nauseate and reject things that have a loathsome taste or smell'.

This chapter examines the links between nausea and vomiting and the autonomic nervous system from several aspects: the motor components of nausea and vomiting; the pathways by which they are induced, and the mechanism by which autonomic disorders and drugs used to treat them may induce nausea and vomiting. The chapter concludes with an introduction to the pharmacology of anti-emetics.

Nausea

Nausea is far less well understood than vomiting and yet is considered by patients to be far more of a problem because of its prolonged and debilitating nature. The study of nausea is difficult because it is a subjective sensation relying on the patient to report, describe, and characterize his or her experience in the light of previous experiences. In addition, because it is a subjective sensation it is impossible to study in animals, although the behaviour of animals in the pre-expulsion period can be quantified and can be argued to be correlates, equivalents, or surrogates of the sensation.

Nausea is described variously as 'a feeling that vomiting is about to take place', 'an unpleasant sensation of being about to vomit', 'the imminent desire to vomit', "a vague discomfort in the epigastric region

with 'queasiness' or 'sick-to-the-stomach sensations'" (Koch 1997). In addition to the sensory aspects of nausea, a number of endocrine (ACTH, cortisol, growth hormone, endorphin), autonomic changes (sweating), and somatic (light-headedness, lassitude, and weakness) responses occur. One of the problems in identifying the mechanisms by which the sensation is generated is separating which of these changes are a response to the stressful nature of nausea and which are a component of the mechanism. This issue is far from resolved.

It appears that many, if not all, of the autonomic changes that occur in the pre- and peri-emetic period are either components of the 'vomiting motor programme' or are responses to the 'stress' of nausea. Thus they are not responsible for the genesis of nausea and many of them can be induced independently without being accompanied by nausea. It has been reported that all the autonomic signs of motion sickness have been observed in a decorticate person on an aeroplane (Borison and McCarthy 1983).

Studies, predominantly of motion sickness in man, have identified two consistent responses (elevated vasopressin and gastric dysrhythmias) which appear to be intimately linked to nausea, although a causal relationship has not yet been established (Koch 1997). They will be described briefly.

Vasopressin

An elevation in plasma vasopressin may be expected as a response to the fluid loss involved in vomiting. However, it is difficult to reconcile this function with the very high levels of vasopressin measured during nausea and vomiting in man and animals as these levels are far in excess of those required for anti-diuresis. Studies in man have shown a close temporal correlation between the onset of nausea and the increase in vasopressin levels (Koch 1997). Infusions of vasopressin can induce nausea and bloating but not vomiting (Caras et al. 1997) and gastric dysrhythmias. However, despite this circumstantial evidence, proof of a causal link has remained elusive. In addition, patients with diabetes insipidus incapable of raising vasopressin levels have nausea and vomiting when given apomorphine or oral ipecacuanha (Nussey et al. 1988). It is possible that vasopressin represents the predominant mechanism but when it is absent other substances can fulfill a similar role. Plasticity in the emetic reflex has been reported in animals where removal of one pathway may lead to the induction or expression of an additional mechanism (Andrews and Davis 1995).

Gastric dysrhythmias

These are abnormalities in the frequency of the gastric muscle slow wave or pacesetter potential outside the normal range of 2.4–3.6 cycles/min. Dysrhythmias, often an increase in frequency, have been reported in subjects exposed to motion and in patients with symptomatic diabetic gastroparesis, idiopathic gastroparesis, functional dyspepsia, pregnancy sickness, visceral neuropathy, and after gastric surgery (Koch 1993). As with vasopressin, the question is whether dysrhythmias cause symptoms.

In both cases, if they are involved in the genesis of nausea then how do they generate the sensation? Both stimuli must access pathways which eventually lead to activation of cortical neurones. Recent studies using magnetic source imaging have implicated the inferior frontal gyrus (Miller *et al.* 1996). Studies in animals have provided evidence that the insular cortex may be a visceral sensory area receiving inputs (indirect) from the nucleus tractus solitarius. Vasopressin could activate the nucleus tractus solitarius via the area postrema and the gastric dysrhythmias via motility by activating abdominal afferents projecting to the nucleus tractus solitarius.

Vomiting

Motor components of the emetic reflex (Fig. 16.1)

The motor components of the emetic reflex can conveniently be divided into three phases. Each will be described together with the pathways that mediate the response.

Pre-expulsion

The phase prior to the onset of retching and vomiting is associated with nausea and responses suggestive of autonomic arousal. While the latter coexist with nausea, there is no evidence that they are responsible for the sensation of nausea. It is likely that they are either a part of the emetic motor programme or, perhaps more likely, an indication of generalized autonomic arousal occurring in response to the stressful nature of nausea. Each will be briefly described.

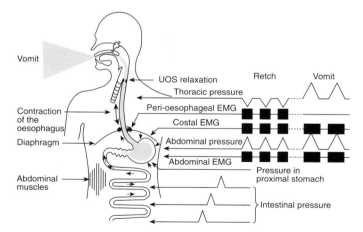

Fig. 16.1. A summary of the major gastrointestinal and somatic motor changes that occur in association with retching and vomiting. Note that retching does not begin until the retrograde contraction in the intestine has reached the stomach and that the stomach relaxes prior to the initiation of this contraction. The main difference between retching and vomiting is in the motor activity of the two parts of the diaphragm. EMG: electromyogram; UOS: upper oesophageal sphincter. Adapted from Andrews and Davis (1995).

Salivation

Salivation, often accompanied by repetitive swallowing, is a clear prodromal sign of emesis in animals, particularly dogs, and is due to activation of the parasympathetic nerves. However, salivary secretion is reduced during each burst of retching and may be absent between bursts (Furukawa and Okada 1994). In addition, salivation could also be evoked by oesophageal distension and gastric mucosal stimulation. It has been argued that the increase in secretion may buffer the acidic nature of the vomitus which could lead to dental erosion. Hypertrophy of the salivary glands is reported in patients with bulimia.

In humans increased salivation is reported to occur prior to emesis, particularly when induced by motion. However, this is based almost exclusively on subjective reports. A study measuring salivary secretion in subjects sick at sea showed that there was a decrease in unstimulated and stimulated salivary flow in 80 per cent of the subjects (Gordon *et al.* 1989). Eight of the 13 subjects reported an increase in salivation, although in six there was a decrease. This and other studies, which attempt to demonstrate a correlation between salivary secretion and subjective symptoms, highlight the difficulty of extrapolating physiological mechanisms from subjective reports. The subject's perception of increased salivation could be due to a reduction in spontaneous swallowing, perhaps allowing an accumulation of saliva in the mouth. Alternatively, it is possible that there is heightened sensitivity of the oral cavity which can be considered one of the early lines of defence against ingested toxins. This would appear to make sense teleologically when the warning, protective, and learning roles of nausea are considered.

Tachycardia

An increase in heart rate is often reported prior to the onset of retching and vomiting. However, the magnitude of the tachycardia does not appear to correlate with the severity of symptoms in response to a motion stimulus (Koch 1993). The mechanism is increased sympathetic drive and a reduction in vagal tone. Once retching and vomiting commence the cardiovascular changes are modulated by the marked oscillations in intrathoracic pressure which modify venous return.

Cutaneous vasoconstriction

Vasoconstriction is presumably due to increased activation of sympathetic adrenergic vasoconstrictor fibres to the skin and gives rise to the characteristic pallid appearance associated with nausea. However, a role for high concentrations of vasopressin cannot be excluded (see above).

Sweating

The pathway for sweating is again sympathetic, although involving cholinergic mechanisms. In association with nausea it appears to be particularly prominent on the face. When there is simultaneous activation of the vasoconstrictor and sudomotor fibres 'cold sweating' occurs, a condition associated with mental stress. Both changes are reflected in an increase in skin conductance.

Pupillary dilatation

The pupil is reported to dilate in the prodromal phase, although it has not been formally characterized. Dilation is another indication of a reciprocal change in the balance of sympathetic and parasympathetic activity, with the former predominating. Ambulatory pupilometry may provide useful insights into the time course of the changes in autonomic activity which occur in the prodromal phase.

Peri-expulsion and expulsion

The basic mechanism by which vomiting occurs due to contraction of the diaphragm and abdominal muscles was identified by the classical studies of Magendie in 1813 who replaced the stomach in a dog with a pig's bladder and demonstrated that the contents of the bladder could be expelled when the animal as given an emetic. More recent studies have revealed many and subtle additional features of the process by recording electromyographic activity from a number of skeletal muscles and the gut. The description below is based mainly on studies in the dog (Lang *et al.* 1993), although the more limited human studies indicate that the mechanism is comparable.

The main activity occurring during the peri-expulsion period is in the gastrointestinal tract whereas the expulsive phase involves the diaphragm and abdominal muscles.

Gastrointestinal tract

Several specific changes occur in the gut prior to the onset of retching and vomiting and the major ones are described below. It must be emphasized that these events are not the cause of nausea but are components of the motor response leading to expulsion, with each event having a function.

The initial event appears to be relaxation of the proximal stomach (De Ponti *et al.* 1990) and while this may occur prior to the onset of emesis to reduce the emptying of an ingested toxin, animal studies have shown that relaxation occurs as a specific component of the emetic reflex. The relaxation allows the stomach to receive the material returned from the intestine prior to retching (see below) and may place the stomach in an anatomically more favourable position for compression by the diaphragm and abdominal muscles. In addition, if the stomach wall is flaccid, the intra-abdominal pressure changes are more likely to be transmitted than if there is a high tone. The mechanism of relaxation is by vagal efferent activation of the intramural non-adrenergic, non-cholinergic inhibitory neurones, using nitric oxide and vasoactive intestinal polypeptides as neurotransmitters. The lower oesophageal sphincter relaxes at this time, again under the influence of the vagus.

When the stomach is relaxed, a single, large amplitude (approximately 1.5 times the amplitude of phase III of the migrating motor complex, MMC) contraction termed the retrograde giant contraction (RGC) originates in the mid-portion of the small intestine and propagates retrogradely to the gastric antrum. The speed of propagation is about 10 cm/s in the dog. This contraction is under vagal control and can be blocked by atropine and hexamethonium but not by phentolamine and propranolol.

The RGC is proposed to have two functions:

(1) to return any contaminated gastric contents to the stomach for expulsion;

(2) to carry alkaline pancreatic and intestinal secretions to the stomach to buffer gastric contents and hence reduce damage to the teeth and oesophagus.

The RGC also carries bile with it, accounting for its frequent presence in vomitus. Studies of the gallbladder and sphincter of Oddi during vomiting have revealed that the gallbladder contracts during retching and the sphincter may undergo transient inhibition, although this usually disappeared before peak contraction of the gallbladder. Thus there appears to be little emptying of the gallbladder during emesis (Qu *et al.* 1995).

The RGC is a key event in the sequencing of the emetic reflex as retching does not begin until the RGC has reached the stomach. Other events occurring in the period immediately before retching include: relaxation of the peri-oesophageal diaphragm (inhibition of a subpopulation of phrenic motor neurones) and tonic contraction of the cricopharyngeus (the upper oesophageal sphincter) and cervical oesophagus (in a longitudinal direction) (Lang *et al.* 1993). This pulls the abdominal oesophagus and the proximal stomach orad. The net effect is to eliminate the abdominal portion of the oesophagus and to cause funnelling of the stomach—both events will facilitate the expulsion of material. Retching begins shortly after the longitudinal pharyngoesophageal contraction.

Retches occur by synchronous rhythmic contraction of the diaphragm, anterior abdominal muscles, and the external intercostal muscles, leading to an increase in intra-abdominal pressure and a concomitant decrease in intrathoracic pressure, generating a pressure gradient between the stomach and the oesophagus. The lower oesophingeal sphincter is relaxed at this time and therefore gastric contents can enter the oesophagus during retching. Between retches the gastric contents return to the stomach and therefore during a burst of retches gastric contents oscillate between the stomach and oesophagus. As mentioned above, retching may be away of 'testing' whether material is sufficiently liquid to be expelled and, in addition, as the force build up during a chain of retches it may also increase momentum in the semi-fluid vomitus to facilitate expulsion. The factors that regulate the number of retches in a burst are under investigation and include gastric volume and end-tidal P_{CO_2}. Also of interest is what determines when a retch is converted into a vomit? Curiously, although material may reach the cervical esophagus and the upper oesophageal sphincter relaxes during each retch, material is not expelled until a vomit is produced.

The vomit is usually a single event at the end of a chain of retches and they are most readily differentiated by the forceful oral expulsion of material, often containing undigested food residue. The underlying motor events also differ in several subtle but critical ways:

1. The contraction of the diaphragmatic dome muscles and the rectus abdominis is maximal.

2. The muscle of the peri-oesophageal diaphragm relaxes, removing another pressure barrier between the stomach and the thoracic oesophagus.

3. During a retch intra-abdominal pressure undergoes positive oscillations coincident with negative oscillations in the intrathoracic pressure, whereas during a vomit both pressures a positive. The intra-abdominal pressure is greater than 100 mmHg and continence appears to be preserved by increased discharge in the pudendal nerve.

4. There is a retrograde contraction of the muscle of the cervical esophagus and the upper oesophageal sphincter is further opened by contraction of the geniohyoideus muscle.

Thus at this stage all barriers to expulsion are removed and the force generated by the compression of the stomach by the diaphragm and abdominal muscles is exerted on the vomitus to propel it in a single stream up the oesophagus where its exodus is facilitated by retrograde contraction of the cervical esophagus.

Post-expulsion

Immediately after the vomit swallowing usually occurs in animals, often accompanied by profuse licking. Relatively little information is available from humans as studies are usually stopped before emesis is induced and as catheters inserted into the gut to monitor activity are usually expelled. During vomiting, one study in which vomiting was recorded showed that about 3 min after the vomit a burst of aborally migrating contractions typical of phase III of the migrating motor complex occurred, originating in the duodenum. Also of note was that the increase in skin conductance, which peaked at the time of the onset of the RGC and vomit, took 10–15 min to return to pre-emesis levels, suggesting that some of the autonomic changes may be sustained (Thompson and Malagelada 1982).

Two questions are of particular interest regarding this phase:

1. What determines whether and when the next episode of retching and vomiting will occur?

2. Why does vomiting produce a sense of relief? Is this due to the removal of a stimulus or is it contributed to by the release of an endogenous opiate?

Pathways by which the emetic mechanism can be activated (Fig. 16.2a)

The section below describes the main pathways by which nausea and vomiting can be activated. These pathways provide a framework within which the mechanisms by which the spectrum of clinical conditions and treatments evoking these symptoms can be considered.

Visceral afferents

From a purely 'biological' perspective, the abdominal vagal afferents are the most important input by which nausea and vomiting can be triggered. Vagal afferents supply the gastrointestinal tract, possibly as far as the first third of the colon with the information projected predominantly to the nucleus tractus solitarius in the brainstem (Grundy *et al.* 1991). Two major types of vagal afferent have been described:

1. 'In series' tension receptors signalling distension and contraction of the muscle of the oesophagus, stomach, and small intestine. The physiological role of these afferents is in vago-vagal reflexes and, in particular, those regulating aspects of motility, such as storage of food in the proximal stomach an probably contributing to the sensation of comfortable fullness or satiety. These afferents are most likely to be responsible for nausea and vomiting induced by gastric stasis (e.g. diabetic gastroparesis), dysrhythmias (see above), or overdistension, particularly in regions such as the gastric antrum which have little receptive capacity. Vagal mechanoreceptors are also the most likely candidates for mediating the emetic response to intestinal obstruction.

2. Mucosal afferents are the second type of abdominal vagal afferent. These afferents monitor features of the luminal environment in the stomach and small intestine, such as shearing of luminal contents against the mucosa and the chemical nature of luminal contents (e.g. osmolarity, pH). They are involved in vago-vagal reflexes regulating the gut but the nature of the sensations they signal is far from clear, although it is likely that they can induce nausea. The emetic response to orally administered hypertonic solutions (e.g. such as may enter the duodenum in dumping syndrome) and

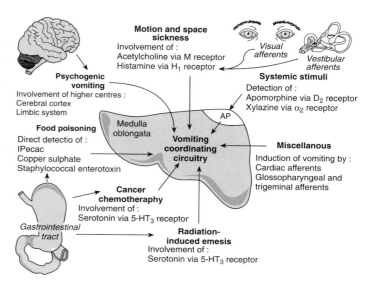

Fig. 16.2a. Diagrammatic summary of different trigger inputs for vomiting. Vomiting coordinated circuitry is located within the medulla oblongata of the brainstem. Area postrema (AP) is thought to contain a chemoreceptor trigger zone for vomiting. Neurotransmitters and receptor subtypes of major importance for eliciting vomiting are indicated for various inputs. D_2, dopamine type 2 receptor; H_1, histamine type 1 receptor; M, muscarinic cholinoreceptor; α_2, alpha type 2 adrenoceptor; $5-HT_3$, 5-hydroxytryptamine type 3 receptor (Modified from Grelot and Miller 1994).

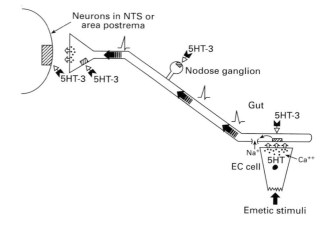

Fig. 16.2b. The relationship between a vagal afferent supplying the intestinal mucosa and a 5-hydroxytryptamine (5-HT) containing mucosal enterochromaffin cell (EC). The location of the ligand gated ion channel $5-HT_3$ receptors is shown. It is proposed that some emetic stimuli (e.g. cytotoxic drugs, radiation, food toxins, mucosal inflammation) induce exocytoxic release of 5-HT via an influx of calcium ions. The 5-HT is proposed to act locally to activate the $5-HT_3$ receptors (blocked by granisetron and ondansetron) evoking an intense afferent discharge which in turn activates the central components of the emetic pathway in the NTS (see text for details). From Andrews (1994).

copper sulphate is mediated by these afferents. Studies of the mechanism by which cytotoxic drugs (e.g. cisplatin) and radiation induce emesis as a side-effect of their antitumour action have provided important insights into a population of these mucosal afferents. It is proposed that these stimuli induce the formation of free radicals in 5-hydroxytryptamine-containing enterochromaffin (EC) cells, leading to an influx of calcium, resulting in an exocytotic release of 5-hydroxytryptamine. The 5-hydroxytryptamine acts on 5-HT$_3$ receptors located on vagal afferents terminating in close proximity to the EC cell (Andrews 1994). Blockade of these 5-HT$_3$ receptors is the main site of action of the 5-HT$_3$ receptor antagonists used to treat the acute emetic effects of anticancer therapy (reviewed by Andrews 1994). Although the weight of evidence supports a predominantly peripheral site of action for 5-HT$_3$ receptor antagonists, this does not exclude a contribution from central 5-HT$_3$ receptors located in the nucleus tractus solitarius (Fig. 16.2b). It is important to recognize that 5-HT$_3$ receptor antagonists are not universal anti-emetics. Although they do have some efficacy against other stimuli (e.g. post-operative emesis), they are not as effective as against the emesis induced by cytotoxic drugs, suggesting that they are not targetting a critical site. However, as 5-HT$_3$ receptor antagonists do not block the emetic response to other stimuli acting via mucosal afferents (e.g. hypertonic saline, copper sulphate), it is likely that substances other than 5-hydroxytryptamine are also involved, either alone or in combination with 5-hydroxytryptamine. The most likely candidates include substance P and cholecystokinin.

The gut is also supplied by splanchnic afferents which signal information about noxious stimuli to the spinal cord and hence the brainstem. Stimulation of the splanchnic afferents does not invoke emesis but nausea is associated with intense pain (Desbiens et al. 1997). There is convergence between vagal and splanchnic afferents in the nucleus tractus solitarius which could provide a substrate for interactions, with activation of the splanchnic afferents perhaps lowering the threshold for vagal afferents to induce emesis.

Emesis may also be evoked by vagal afferents from two other sites: the heart and the auditory meatus. In the cat, stimulation of ventricular vagal afferents induced relaxation of the proximal stomach and vomiting (Abrahamsson and Thoren 1973). These afferents are candidates for inducing the sensation of nausea that may accompany myocardial infarct as well as some of the related circulatory changes. They have also been implicated in the initiation of vaso-vagal syncope. Vomiting may be induced by stimulation of Arnold's nerve (sometimes called Alderman's nerve) the auricular branch of the vagus supplying part of the pinna and the posterior part of the external auditory meatus. The mechanism is not known but could be due to direct activation of the brainstem pathway or secondary to a vaso-vagal attack which can be evoked by this nerve.

Area postrema

The role of the area postrema in emesis is one of controversy (reviewed by Borison 1989; Miller and Leslie 1994). The area postrema is located at the caudal extremity of the fourth ventricle. The presence of fenestrated capillaries means that the blood–brain barrier is incomplete in this and other circumventricular organs. Ablation studies implicated the area postrema in the detection of emetic agents in the bloodstream, a role consistent with its morpho-

logical characteristics, and hence led to it being called 'the chemoreceptor trigger zone for emesis'. While ablation of the area postrema can abolish the emetic response to a range of experimental stimuli (e.g. dopamine and opiate receptor agonists), it now appears likely that the site of action is on dendrites from the nucleus tractus solitarius (within the blood–brain barrier) projecting into the area postrema. The role of the area postrema and nucleus tractus solitarius in mediating the emetic response to some drugs (apomorphine, morphine) is not in question and it is likely that peptides or other agents released from the gut mucosa could act here to induce nausea and vomiting, or perhaps sensitize the emetic system to other inputs. However, it should not be assumed that all substances in the circulation use this pathway. Studies of the mechanism by which cytotoxic anticancer drugs and radiation induce nausea and vomiting have implicated abdominal vagal afferents (reviewed by Andrews and Davis 1995) rather than the area postrema.

The interpretation of the effects of lesions directed at the area postrema is complicated because abdominal vagal afferents project to the area postrema and the subjacent region of the nucleus tractus solitarius. It is inevitable that ablation of the area postrema will cause collateral damage to these afferents. Thus if a systemic emetic agent had a peripheral site of action (e.g. in the gut mucosa) and activated vagal afferents, then a lesion directed at the area postrema could abolish the emetic response leading to the erroneous conclusion that the emetic agent was acting on the area postrema. It is important that the effects of area postrema ablation and abdominal vagotomy are both investigated before drawing conclusions about the site of action of an emetic agent.

Vestibular system

The vestibular system is essential for the genesis of motion sickness, which is due to a 'mismatch' between vestibular, visual, and proprioceptive systems. Care must be taken in distinguishing between vestibular (vertigo) and non-vestibular types of dizziness (Baloh 1993), particularly as nausea and vomiting are common symptoms of the former but not the latter. Non-vestibular dizziness, often described as 'light-headedness', is more likely to be associated with autonomic disorders as it can be induced by diffuse cerebral ischaemia. It is estimated that only 50 per cent of patients complaining of dizziness have vertigo (Baloh 1993).

Disorders affecting vestibular system function and leading to vertigo include benign positional vertigo (due to inner ear disease), Menière's syndrome, viral neurolabyrynthitis, vertebrobasilar insufficiency, and posterior fossa migraine (Baloh 1993).

Higher inputs

The involvement of the higher areas of the brain in triggering the emetic reflex is poorly understood, although the existence of phenomena, such as anticipatory emesis to anticancer therapy and vomiting to horrific sights or unpleasant smells, illustrate that the cerebral cortex is capable of activating brainstem mechanisms. In view of the growing evidence of the extent of central nervous system damage in autonomic disorders, an understanding of these higher inputs is likely to be of increasing importance in understanding symptoms. In addition, careful investigation of nausea and vomiting in such patients may provide insights into the pathways in man.

The higher regions of the brain have a modulatory effect on the brainstem pathways which are capable of generating the somatic motor responses of retching and vomiting and, as far as has been investigated, the autonomic responses (e.g. proximal gastric relaxation). The level of arousal determines the threshold for activation of the emetic reflex, as indicated by marked suppression of the emetic reflex by general anaesthesia. Emesis is usually preceded by arousal, particularly from sleep, and incomplete arousal (e.g. due to alcohol) increases the change of aspiration of vomitus. Activation of the cough reflex is also linked to the level of arousal.

Integration of the emetic reflex

The inputs capable of inducing nausea and vomiting converge in the brainstem with the nucleus tractus solitarius and the parvicellular reticular formation being the most likely regions involved in processing the information and co-ordinating the outputs. Based upon studies of motion sickness where the stimulus intensity can be readily controlled, the normal sequence appears to be that 'low' intensity stimulation induces nausea (a 'warning') and continued activation at 'higher' intensities induces retching and vomiting. The threshold for the latter must be very carefully regulated to prevent 'accidental' activation by a sudden head movement or a large gastric contraction producing an intense vagal afferent discharge. Studies using electrical stimulation of the vagal afferents suggest that the duration of activation is a factor in addition to the intensity.

At some point in the processing the nausea and vomiting pathways must diverge. The signal for the genesis of the sensation of nausea and the release of vasopressin travels rostrally (cortex, hypothalamus) and the signal for retching and vomiting going to the autonomic (e.g. dorsal motor vagal nucleus, nucleus ambiguus, and pre-sympathetic nuclei) and somatic (Bötzinger complex, phrenic nucleus) nuclei to initiate the motor components. Within the motor components the temporal co-ordination is impressive, with retching not beginning until the RGC has reached the stomach.

A knowledge of the central processing is of more than academic interest as an anti-emetic should block both nausea and vomiting. However, unless the drug blocks transmission before the pathways diverge, it is possible that vomiting could be blocked without affecting nausea or vice versa. Animal studies have shown that neurokinin$_1$-receptor antagonists are 'universal' anti-emetics, blocking the retching and vomiting response to vagal afferent, area postrema, and vestibular inputs (Watson et al. 1995) but it is not yet known whether these agents block nausea as effectively. The answer to this important question awaits clinical trials, but whatever the outcome these agents have shown that it is possible to identify broad-spectrum anti-emetics.

Nausea, vomiting and disorders of the autonomic nervous system

The preceding sections have provided a framework within which two aspects of autonomic disorders can be discussed. First, how nausea and vomiting may be induced as symptoms of autonomic disorders, such as diabetes mellitus, and, secondly, the mechanism by which pharmacological treatments (e.g. L-Dopa) for disorders involving the autonomic nervous system may induce nausea and vomiting.

Nausea and vomiting as symptoms of autonomic disorders

Diabetic gastroparesis

Gastroparesis (see Chapter 39) is common in patients with diabetic autonomic neuropathy and particularly in those who are insulin-dependent. The incidence is not known as it is likely that many patients may have impaired gastric emptying without being symptomatic. The pathophysiological mechanisms leading to the severe retention of gastric contents is unclear, but vagal degeneration has been implicated, although this is not a universal finding (Yoshida et al. 1988). The assessment of the extent of vagal damage is difficult because of the lack of simple tests of abdominal vagal integrity and function (approximately 90 per cent of the fibres are afferent), the paucity of histological material, and the high proportion of unmyelinated fibres which can only be adequately assessed by electron microscopy.

Immunohistochemical studies of substance P and calcitonin-gene-related peptide may be helpful in identifying damage to the afferents, as these peptides have been used as markers of vagal afferents. The key question relates to how gastroparesis induces nausea and vomiting.

The incidence of vomiting in patients with diabetic gastroparesis is unclear and may reflect experiences of populations with disease of differing severity, duration, and glycaemic control. In addition, little effort appears to have been made to distinguish nausea from vomiting, although the former is usually of greater concern to patients because of its sustained nature.

In the section on nausea above, the link (not necessarily causal) between nausea and gastric dysrhythmias was noted. Such dysrhythmias have been reported to occur in patients with diabetic gastroparesis. Acute hyperglycaemia in healthy individuals induces gastric dysrhythmias which could be prevented by indomethacin, implicating prostaglandins in the mechanism (Hasler et al. 1995).

Breaking the cycle of impaired gastric emptying and dramatic swings in blood glucose levels is therefore of considerable relevance in some of these patients. This is also important as hypoglycaemia can occur with erratic gastric emptying. Studies with the toxin hypoglycin A have shown that hypoglycaemia can rapidly induce vomiting. The mechanism is unclear, although area postrema ablation affected the acute emetic response (Tanaka 1979). One possibility is that the hypoglycaemia induces a release of adrenal catecholamines and these act on the area postrema to induce nausea and vomiting via activation of α-adrenoceptors (mainly α_2) that have been implicated in emesis at this site (Hikasa et al. 1991).

An excess glucose or fat load in the small intestine will delay gastric emptying, but if the load in the gut lumen is particularly hypertonic, 'dumping' syndrome may result. The mechanism in part appears to involve release of 5-hydroxytryptamine from enterochromaffin cells (see above) and activation of abdominal vagal afferents leading to activation of emetic pathways. In addition, vagal glucoreceptors present in the hepatic portal vein could also contribute an emetic signal, although this has not been formally investigated. Plasma glucose levels influence gastric emptying, with pronounced hypoglycaemia causing acceleration and hyperglycaemia slowing. A study in normal subjects and patients with insulin-dependent diabetes mellitus showed that emptying of a mixed meal is modulated in both groups by the 'physiological hyperglycaemia' following a meal (Schvarcz et al. 1997).

Neurally mediated syncope

Nausea (but usually not vomiting) is a symptom in some patients with vaso-vagal syncope, together with other features, such as light-headedness, dizziness (see also vertigo), blurred vision, weakness, and cognitive impairment. These symptoms may be followed by fainting. Several mechanisms could contribute but these have not been formally investigated:

1. The sensory disturbances may induce a sensation of illusory self-motion, a very effective experimental nauseogenic stimulus (Koch 1993), producing a vestibulo-visual conflict sufficient to cause mild activation of the motion sickness pathways.

2. The gradual reduction in cerebral perfusion which eventually leads to fainting may be sufficient to induce a degree of ischaemia-induced firing of neurones in a sensitive site in the emetic pathway, such as the area postrema, the nucleus tractus solitarius, the vestibular system, or inferior frontal gyrus (see above).

3. Activation of ventricular cardiac afferents can induce nausea and vomiting in humans and vomiting in cats, and these afferents are thought to be responsible for the occurrence of nausea in myocardial infarct patients (Abrahamsson and Thoren 1973). Activation of these receptors also produces reflex gastric relaxation which could contribute to the genesis of nausea. The physiological role of the ventricular receptors is still under investigation but they do provide a potential mechanism by which reduced ventricular filling could induce nausea. They have been implicated in the genesis of the vaso-vagal syndrome which Barcroft and Swan (1953) noted shared a likeness to the response to apomorphine, a dopamine D_2-receptor agonist, inducing emesis via a central action.

4. A fall in blood pressure will reduce the activation of the arterial baroreceptors which provide a tonic inhibitory input to the magnocellular neurones secreting vasopressin. Vasopressin levels will increase, but whether these are sufficient to induce nausea is unclear.

Nausea and the occasional vomiting associated with neurally mediated syncope should be distinguished from posturally evoked vomiting which is associated with posterior fossa lesions.

Disordered dopamine and adrenaline metabolism

Dopamine, adrenaline, and noradrenaline are capable of inducing nausea and vomiting by a direct action on the area postrema (see above) and it is likely that they may also act via delaying gastric emptying.

These substances may be secreted in excess by phaeochromocytomas in which nausea and vomiting may occur, although they are not major symptoms. While attention correctly focuses on the catecholamines as the most likely cause of nausea and vomiting, neuropeptide Y is also released and may be of significance as it can induce emesis and activate area postrema neurones (Carpenter 1990). Ischaemic enterocolitis is a pathological complication of phaeochromocytoma and vomiting can occur in patients with acute mesenteric ischaemia. The mechanism is not known but is presumably via activation of gut afferents due to ischaemia-induced release of local neuroactive mediators.

A pseudo-phaechromocytoma has been described in which there were hypertensive episodes, flushing, nausea, epigastric discomfort, and polyuria (Kuchel 1996). He drew attention to the importance of measuring sulphated as well as free plasma dopamine, as the former has a half-life 60 times that of dopamine.

Dopamine β-hydroxlation deficiency, in which there is a marked increase in plasma dopamine levels, does not appear to induce nausea and vomiting (see Chapter 40).

Familial dysautonomia (Riley–Day syndrome)

Vomiting is a feature of this syndrome (see Chapter 41), with the episodes being triggered by emotional crises. Although this disorder is characterized by a reduction in noradrenaline synthesis, during the emotional crisis plasma noradrenaline and dopamine levels are markedly elevated and whilst the vomiting is reported to be correlated with the dopamine levels, both agents are capable of inducing emesis via an action on the area postrema (see above) with dopamine D_2, and α-$_1$ and α_2-adrenoceptors implicated. The treatment is aimed at the emotional crisis. Diazepam is used which sedates the patient and thus has an indirect action to alleviate the vomiting, but this does not exclude a direct anti-emetic action.

Alcoholic neuropathy

Although nausea and vomiting are not particularly features of alcoholic neuropathy, chronic alcohol intake blunts the emetic reflex. The evidence emerges from studies of patients with head and neck cancer in which alcohol is implicated in the aetiology. In response to the cytotoxic drug cisplatin (a potent emetogen) such patients have little or no vomiting and less nausea than would be expected. The mechanism has not been investigated but it could indicate damage to the enterochromaffin–vagal afferent system or the dorsal brainstem complex (area postrema, nucleus tractus solitarius).

Brainstem tumours and related lesions

Nausea and vomiting may be early symptoms of tumours located in or impacting on the fourth ventricle (North and Reilly 1990). The reason for this is that the tumour itself, or the resulting raised intracranial pressure, or both (i.e. in posterior fossa tumours) compresses the area postrema or, more likely, the subjacent nucleus tractus solitarius, inducing neuronal firing and activation of the emetic pathways, although this has never been demonstrated experimentally. The vagus has a meningeal branch to the dura covering the posterior fossa. It is conceivable that afferents in this branch are implicated in the emesis induced by raised intracranial pressure but this requires experimental investigation. The possibility that neuroactive agents released into the cerebrospinal fluid and acting on the area postrema may contribute should not be excluded.

Vomiting may be induced by postural changes (posturally evoked vomiting, PEV) without the presence of concomitant nystagmus or vertigo, when it is often an indication of a posterior fossa lesion.

Projectile vomiting has been reported in a patient with a solitary metastasis involving the lateral pontine tegmentum and middle cerebellar peduncle without hydrocephalus. In this case it appeared likely that the trigger for emesis was involvement of pathways to or from the 'vomiting centre' (Baker and Bernat 1985).

Nausea and vomiting, together with a constellation of other symptoms, are a feature of acute brainstem lesions such as those seen in Wallenberg's syndrome (lateral medullary stroke). In this syndrome there is an ischaemic attack affecting the brainstem. The ischaemic insult may cause neuronal discharge directly by release of excitatory amino acids, by permeabilizing capillaries, or indirectly by producing localized oedema which may activate the nucleus tractus solitarius by mechanical deformation.

Nausea and vomiting as a side-effect of treatment for autonomic disorders

Bethanecol

The muscarinic receptor agonists carbachol and bethanecol are carbamoyl esters of choline, resistant to the activity of both specific and non-specific cholinestereases (Broadley 1996). They exert relatively selective effects on the gastrointestinal tract and bladder, with both effects being ascribed to an action on muscarinic M_3-receptors, and they have been used in the treatment of urinary retention and markedly delayed gastric emptying and paralytic ileus. Nausea and vomiting are recognized side-effects of both. The mechanism is unclear as it is the muscarinic M_1 and nicotinc cholinoceptors in the dorsal medulla which are most implicated in emesis. Carbachol does have some nicotinic activity but bethanecol has little or none.

Both agents act by stimulating the muscarinic M_3-receptors located on the smooth muscles. In the gastrointestinal tract other approaches are available, such as using the substituted prokinetic benzamides (e.g. metoclopramide and cisapride) which have their prokinetic effect by the release of acetylcholine from myenteric neurones via a 5-HT_4 agonist effect. However, if the myenteric plexus is damaged by autonomic disease then such an approach, although working initially, may not continue to be effective as the disease progresses.

L-Dopa and other anti-Parkinsonian drugs

Oral laevo-dopa (L-dopa) is used in conjunction with a decarboxylase inhibitor (e.g. benserazide, carbidopa) to alleviate the bradykinesia and rigidity of Parkinson's disease. The decarboxylase inhibitor is given to prevent the breakdown of L-dopa to dopamine in the periphery. This is possible as, in contrast to L-dopa, the decarboxylase inhibitors do not cross the blood–brain barrier. It is argued that reducing the conversion of L-dopa to dopamine outside the brain reduces the side-effects of nausea and vomiting. This appears to be supported by clinical experience, with a vomiting frequency of 80 per cent with oral L-dopa in the initial stages of treatment compared to 15 per cent when combined with a decarboxylase inhibitor (Parkes 1986). It is perhaps surprising that the site of the emetic effect of L-dopa is not known with certainty. The most likely site would appear to be the area postrema which is located outside the blood–brain barrier (see above), as dopamine D_2-receptors and ablation or domperidone abolishes the emetic response to dopamine receptor agonists, such as apomorphine, which is used for 'off' episodes in Parkinson's patients refractory to other treatments. Although decarboxylase inhibitors do not cross the blood–brain barrier they would be expected to act in the area postrema which is outside the blood–brain barrier. However, the possibility of a peripheral (gastrointestinal) effect of L-dopa cannot be excluded even when co-administered with a decarboxylase inhibitor, as there is some peripheral conversion to dopamine and dopamine receptors are present in the gut with activation leading to a delay in gastric emptying. In a few patients who had a vagotomy for pyloric stenosis and who were subsequently given L-dopa, no 'sickness' was reported (Parkes 1986). This unique anecdotal observation is suggestive of a peripheral contribution and perhaps this accounts for the residual

nausea and vomiting in patients treated with L-dopa and decarboxylase inhibitors.

Anti-parkinsonian drugs with different mechanisms of action, such as selegiline (monoamine oxidase inhibitor often used in combination with L-dopa), lysuride, and pergolide (D_2-receptor agonist), also have nausea and vomiting as a prominent side-effect, consistent with an involvement of catecholamine receptors in the emetic response.

There is growing evidence for gastrointestinal dysfunction in parkinsonian patients, involving both the vagus and the enteric nervous system (Kaneoke et al. 1995). Such motor disorders may sensitize these patients to the effects of the above drugs, particularly if they lead to further disruption of motility.

One intriguing aspect that does require study is the basis of the tolerance to the emetic effects of most anti-parkinsonian's drugs, which occurs within 1–6 months (Parkes 1986).

Carbamazepine

Epileptic seizures may occasionally be induced by very low cerebral perfusion due to low blood pressure as a result of autonomic failure. Nausea and vomiting are side-effects of the anti-epileptic drug, carbamazepine, acting via blockade of a population of sodium channels.

Clonidine

This is an α_2-adrenoceptor agonist, used in the treatment of hypertension. Occasionally nausea is a side-effect of clonidine and is likely to be due to an action on central α_2-receptors in the area postrema or nucleus tractus solitarius. In addition to acting at α_2-adrenoceptors, clonidine may have an action at another binding site, identified as 'imidazoline receptors/binding sites' (Broadley 1996) of which two subtypes are proposed: I_1 and I_2. The I_1 sites preferentially bind clonidine and idazoxan and are located in the brainstem and kidney, whereas the I_2 receptors have a greater affinity for idazoxan over clonidine and are found in kidney, liver, adipocytes, platelets, urethra, pancreatic B cells, adrenal chromaffin cells, and CNS astrocytes (Reis and Regunathan 1996). The possible role of I_1 and I_2 receptors in the genesis of nausea induced by clonidine has not been investigated. Drugs acting at this class of receptor are of particular interest to clinicians dealing with autonomic disorders as some imidazolines (e.g. efaroxan) enhance insulin secretion. Some evidence has been presented for an endogenous ligand for I receptors which has been identified and is called 'clonidine displacing substance'.

Insulin

Insulin may activate neurones in the area postrema of the dog and the emesis induced within 1 min by systemic insulin administration can be abolished by area postrema ablation (Carpenter and Briggs 1986).

Octreotide

This is a stable analogue of somatostatin used to reduce hormone secretion from tumours, postparandial hypotension, and orthostatic hypotension due to autonomic failure (see Chapter 29). Nausea, vomiting, and abdominal cramps are major side-effects. The site of the emetic effect has not been investigated and although systemic somatostatin is capable of inducing vomiting in dogs, it failed to activate area postrema neurones when applied directly (Carpenter 1990). This could be taken as a very preliminary indication for a peripheral emetic action but requires direct investigation.

The pharmacology of anti-emetics

The 'perfect' anti-emetic agent should be capable of blocking both nausea and vomiting from any cause. At present such an agent is not available clinically (except for general anaesthesia), although several approaches have been identified from preclinical studies. The pharmacology and proposed sites of action of some of the current anti-emetics will be discussed. Until the perfect anti-emetic is available some consideration should be given to the cause of the emesis when deciding which anti-emetic to use. For example, if the cause of the emesis is delayed due to inappropriate activation of vestibular pathways, then an agent acting on appropriate receptors (e.g. histamine$_1$, muscarinic M_3) in the pathway is relevant.

There are four main pharmacological classes of anti-emetic.

Dopamine-receptor antagonists

Several compounds (e.g. domperidone, metoclopramide, and phenothiazines such as prochloperazine, chlorpromazine, trifluorperazine) are classed as 'dopamine-receptor antagonists' but this is not necessarily the only pharmacological action they possess or the mechanism by which they exert their anti-emetic effect.

Domperidone (a benzimidazole derivative) is an antagonist at the dopamine D_2 receptor. Its prokinetic effect, particularly in the stomach and the small intestine, may be the mechanism by which it alleviates nausea and vomiting secondary to delayed gastric emptying (e.g. diabetic gastroparesis). The 'direct' anti-emetic effects of domperidone are still a matter of controversy. At conventional doses, domperidone penetrates the blood–brain barrier poorly and this explains why extrapyramidal reactions are rare. However, it should not be assumed that poor penetration of the blood–brain barrier means that the drug does have a central effect. The area postrema is outside the blood–brain barrier and this is a site at which D_2-receptor agonists e.g. apomorphine, L-dopa, lisuride) can induce emesis, most probably via an action on receptors of nucleus tractus solitarius dendrites projecting into the area postrema. Of note is that domperidone does not block hiccup or yawning produced by L-dopa (Parkes 1986). Furthermore, sufficient drug may reach a critical site in the emetic pathway (e.g. the nucleus tractus solitarius) to exert an effect if the structure is adjacent to a circumventricular organ (e.g. area postrema).

Metoclopramide is a substituted benzamide and unravelling its pharmacology led directly to the development of 5-HT$_3$-receptor antagonists and 5-HT$_4$-receptor agonists (Andrews 1994). Metoclopramide is a D_2-receptor antagonist and it was originally thought that this accounted for its anti-emetic and prokinetic effects. However, subsequent studies of the pharmacology revealed that an agonist action at 5-HT$_4$ receptors on myenteric neurones, leading to a release of acetylcholine, makes a major contribution to the prokinetic effects. At usual therapeutic doses the D_2-receptor antagonism and 5-HT$_4$-receptor agonism account for the clinical effects, but at high doses metoclopramide also acts as a 5-HT$_3$-receptor antagonist. It is this latter action which accounts for its improved anti-emetic efficacy against anticancer therapy-induced emesis when given at high doses (Andrews 1994).

The phenothiazines, exemplified by prochloperazine, have the most complex pharmacology of the 'dopamine' antagonists with antagonist effects at D_1, D_2, H_1 α_1, and cholinergic receptors. Although the anti-emetic effect is most often attributed to dopamine receptor blockade, the presence of histaminic and muscarinic receptors in the motion sickness pathway should not be overlooked. It is possible that by reducing the tonic input to the brainstem from the vestibular system the threshold for activation of the emetic mechanism from other causes is also reduced and this could explain the 'general' anti-emetic effects of prochloperazine. The sedative effects of prochloperazine (and other agents) may also contribute to the anti-emetic effect by reducing arousal.

Muscarinic receptor antagonists

Scopalamine (hyoscine), a plant alkaloid, is perhaps the best known of the antimuscarinic agents but it is unclear exactly which of the five muscarinic receptor subtypes is responsible for the effect. Muscarinic receptors are present in the area postrema and nucleus tractus solitarius. This class of agent is particularly useful in treating emesis involving activation of the labyrinthine system.

Histamine-receptor antagonists

Histamine$_1$-receptor antagonists, such as cinnarizine, promethazine, and dimenhydrinate, are particularly useful in the treatment of labyrinthine disorders and motion sickness. The exact site of action is unclear, although H_1 receptors are present in the vestibulocerebellar pathway and in the nucleus tractus solitarius. The sedative effect of the H_1 antagonists may also contribute to their anti-emetic action.

5-HT$_3$-receptor antagonists

This is the newest class of anti-emetic drug and includes granisetron, ondansetron, and tropisetron. They are all highly selective and potent antagonists of the 5-HT$_3$ receptor which is to date unique amongst the many 5-HT receptor subtypes in being a ligand-gated ion channel. The principle locations of 5-HT$_3$ receptors relevant to the anti-emetic action are on the peripheral and central terminals of abdominal vagal afferent neurones, neurones in the nucleus tractus solitarius, and probably the 5-HT-containing enterochromaffin cells in the gut mucosa. Activation of the receptor leads to depolorization of neurones. Activation of 5-HT$_3$ receptors has been implicated in the emetic response to radiation and cytotoxic anticancer drugs (e.g. cisplatin, cyclophosphamide). It is proposed that these stimuli induce emesis via the release of 5-HT (perhaps together with other neuroactive substances) from the gut mucosal enterochromaffin cells, the 5-HT acts on 5-HT$_3$ receptors located on the peripheral terminals of vagal afferents terminating in close proximity to the basolateral surface of these cells. The resulting intense activation of the vagal afferents which project to the nucleus tractus solitarius constitutes the emetic stimulus. The main site of the anti-emetic effect of the 5-HT$_3$ receptors antagonists is considered to be peripheral on the vagal 5-HT$_3$ receptors but there may be some contribution from blockade of the receptors in the nucleus tractus solitarius and the proposed autoreceptors on the enterochromaffin cells.

It must be emphasized that the 5-HT$_3$-receptor antagonists are not universal anti-emetics. For example, their demonstrated clinical efficacy is limited to emesis induced by radiation and cytotoxic drugs and perhaps postoperative emesis. However, they are ineffective against motion and centrally acting emetics, such as apomorphine and morphine. In addition, they do not block the emetic effect of all experimental stimuli acting via the vagus, suggesting that there are different peripheral transduction mechanisms and that blockade of the 5-HT$_3$ receptors in the nucleus tractus solitarius is insufficient to block emesis.

The universal anti-emetic

Because it is often difficult to identify the precise cause of the nausea and vomiting and the pathways involved in triggering the response to many emetic stimuli have not been investigated, a 'universal' anti-emetic would be of considerable clinical utility. The ideal agent should be able to block emesis induced by peripheral inputs, such as the vagus, as well as central inputs from the area postrema and the labyrinthine system. In animal models agonists at the 5-HT$_{1A}$ and μ opioid receptor appear to have such effects, although they also have a number of behavioural side-effects. Recent studies in several animal species (Watson *et al.* 1995) have demonstrated that blockade of the neurokinin$_1$ receptor (the preferred receptor for the peptide substance P) can markedly reduce or abolish the emetic response to motion and stimuli such as opiates and apomorphine acting at the area postrema and cisplatin and copper sulphate acting via the abdominal vagal afferents. Clinical results with this class of compound are awaited to determine if they are capable of blocking both vomiting and nausea. If a 'universal' anti-emetic is identified, it will provide useful symptomatic relief while the underlying cause of the emesis is identified and treated.

References

Abrahamsson, H. and Thoren, P. (1973). Vomiting and reflex vagal relaxation of thestomach elicited from heart receptors in the cat. *Acta Physiol. Scand.* 88, 433–9.

Andrews, P. L. R. (1994). 5-HT$_3$ receptor antagonists and antiemesis. In *5-Hydroxytryptamine-3 Receptor Antagonists*, Ch. 12, 255–317.

Andrews, P. L. R. and Davis, C. J. (1995). The physiology of emesis induced by anti-cancer therapy. In *Serotonin and scientific basis of anti-emetic therapy*, (ed. D. J. M. Reynolds, P. L. R. Andrews, and C. J. Davis), Ch. 2, 25–49. Oxford Clinical Communications, Oxford.

Baker, P. C. H. and Bernat, J. I. (1985). The neuroanatomy of vomiting in man: association of projectile vomiting with a solitary metastasis in the lateral tegmentum of the pons and the middle cerebellar peduncle. *J. Neurol. Psychiat.* 48, 1165–8.

Baloh, R. W. (1993). Diagnosis and management of vertigo. In *The handbook of nausea and vomiting*, (ed. M. H. Sleisenger), pp. 27–42. Parthenon Publishing Group, New York.

Barcroft, H. and Swan, H. J. C. (1953). *Sympathetic control of human blood vessels*. Edward Arnold, London.

Borison, H. L. and McCarthy, L. E. (1983). Neuropharmacologic mechanisms of emesis. In *Antiemetics and cancer chemotherapy*, (ed. J. Laszlo), Ch. 2, pp. 6–20. Williams and Wilkins, Baltimore.

Borison, H. L. (1989). Area postrema: Chemoreceptor circum ventricular organ of the medulla oblongata. *Prog. Neurobiol.* 32, 351–90.

Broadley, K. J. (1996). *Autonomic pharmacology*, Taylor and Francis, London, UK.

Caras, S. D., Soykan, I., Beverly, V., Lin, Z., and McCallum, R. W. (1997). The effect of intravenous vasopressin on gastric myoelectrical activity in human subjects. *Neurogastroent. Motility* 9, 151–6.

Carpenter, D. O. and Briggs, D. B. (1986). Insulin excites neurons of the area postrema and causes emesis. *Neurosci. Lett.* 68, 85–9.

Carpenter, D. O. (1990). Neural mechanisms of emesis. *Can. J. Physiol. Pharmacol.* 68, (2), 230–6.

DePonti, F., Malagelada, J. R., Azpiroz, F., Yaksh, T. L., and Thomforde G. M. (1990). Variations in gastric tone associated with duodenal motor events after activation of central emetic mechanisms in the dog. *J. Gastrointest. Motility* 2, 1–11.

Desbiens, N. A., Mueller-Rizner, N., Connors, A. F. and Wenger, N. S. (1997). The relationship of nausea and dyspnea to pain in seriously ill patients. *Pain* 71, 149–56.

Furukawa, N. and Okada, H. (1994). Canine salivary secretion from the submaxillary glands before and during retching. *Am. J. Physiol.* 267, G810–817.

Gordon, C. R., Ben-Aryeh, H., Szargel, R., Attias, J., Rolnick, A., and Laufer, D. (1989). Salivary changes associated with seasickness. *J. Autonom. nerv. Syst.* 26, 37–42.

Grelot, L. and Miller, A. J. (1994). Vomiting—its ins and outs. *News in Physiological Science*, 9, 142–7.

Grundy, D., Blackshaw, A., and Andrews, P. L. R. (1991). Neural correlates of the gastrointestinal motor changes in emesis. In *Brain gut interactions*, (ed. Y. Tache and D. Wingate), pp. 325–38. CRC Press, Boca Raton, FL.

Hasler, W. L., Soudah, H. C., Dulai, and Owyang, C. (1995). Mediation of hyperglycaemia evoked slow-wave dysrhythmias by endogenous prostaglandins. *Gastroenterol.* 108, 727–36.

Hikasa, Y., Ogasawara, S., and Takase, K. (1991). Alpha adrenoceptor subtypes involved in the emetic action in dogs. *J. Pharmacol. Exp. Ther.* 261, 746–54.

Kaneoke, Y., Koike, Y., Sakurai, N. *et al.* (1995). Gastrointestinal dysfunction in Parkinson's disease detected by electrogastroenterography. *J. Autonom. Nerv. Syst.* 50, 275–81.

Koch, K. L. (1993). Motion sickness. In *The handbook of nausea and vomiting*, ed. M. H. Sleisenger), pp. 43–60. Parthenon Publishing Group, New York.

Koch, K. L. (1997). A noxious trio: nausea, gastric dysrhythmias and vasopressin. *Neurogast. Motil.* 9, 141–2.

Kuchel, O. (1996). Disorders of dopamine metabolism. In *Primer on the autonomic nervous system*. (Ed. D. Robertson, P. A. Low and R. J. Polinsky) pp. 212–216. Academic Press Inc., San Diego.

Lang, I. M., Sarna, S. K., and Dodds, W. J. (1993). Pharyngeal, esophageal, and proximal gastric responses associated with vomiting. *Am. J. Physiol.* 265, G963–972.

Miller, A. D., and Leslie, R. A. (1994). The area postrema and vomiting. *Frontiers in Neuroendocrin.* 15, 1–20.

Miller, A. D., Rowley, H. A., Roberts, T. P. L., and Kucharczyk, J. (1996). Human cortical activity during vestibular- and drug-induced nausea detected using MSI. *Ann. New York Acad. Sci.* 781, 670–2.

North, B., and Reilly, P. (1990). *Raised intracranial pressure. A clinical guide.* Heinemann Medical Books, pp. 30–1. Heinemann, New York.

Nussey, S. S., Hawthorn, J., Page, S. R., Ang, V. T. Y., and Jenkins, J. S. (1988). Responses of plasma oxytocin and arginine vasopressin to nausea induced by apomorphine and ipecacuanha. *Clin. Endocrinol.* 28, 297–304.

Parkes, J. D. (1986). A neurologist's view of nausea and vomiting. Introduction: vomiting is common in neurological disorders. In *Nausea and vomiting: mechanism and treatment*, (ed. C. J. Davis, G. V. Lake-Bakaar, and D. G. Grahame-Smith), pp. 160–6. Springer-Verlag, Berlin.

Qu, R., Furukawa, N., and Fukuda, H. (1995). Changes in extrahepatic biliary motilities with emesis in dogs. *J. Autonom. Nerv. Syst.*, 56, 87–96.

Reis, D. J. and Regunathan, S. (1996). Imidazoline receptors and their native ligands. In *Primer on the Autonomic Nervous System* (ed. D. Robertson, P. A. Low and R. J. Polinsky) pp. 107–8. Academic Press Inc., San Diego.

Schvarcz, E., Palmer, M., Aman, J., Horowitz, M., Stridsberg, M., and Berne, C. (1997). Physiological hyperglycemia slows gastric emptying in normal subjects and patients with insulin-dependent diabetes mellitus. *Gastroenterology* 113, 60–6.

Tanaka, K. (1979). Jamaican vomiting sickness. In *Handbook of clinical neurology*, (ed. P. J. Vinken and G. W. Bruyn), Vol. 37, Chapter 17, pp. 511–39. North Holland Publishing Company, Amsterdam.

Thompson, D. G. and Malagelada, J. R. (1982). Vomiting and the small Intestine. *Dig. Dis. Sci.* 27, 1121–5.

Watson, J. W., Nagahisa, A., Lucot, J., and Andrews, P. L. R. (1995). The role of NK-1 receptor in emetic responses. In *Serotonin and the scientific basis of anti-emetic therapy*, (ed. D. J. M. Reynolds, P. L. R. Andrews, and C. J. Davis) pp. 233–9. Oxford Clinical Communications, Oxford.

Yoshida, M. M., Schuffler, M. D. and Sumi, S. M. (1988). There are no morphologic abnormalities of the gastric wall or abdominal vagus in patients with diabetic gastroparesis. *Gastroenterology* 94, 907–14.

17. The influence of the autonomic nervous system on metabolic function

Ian A. Macdonald

Introduction

The effects of the autonomic nervous system as demonstrated in many systems in this book, are mediated mainly through the postganglionic noradrenergic and cholinergic innervation of peripheral tissues. Such innervation is important in the regulation of metabolism, but there is also a key role for catecholamines released from the adrenal medulla. This chapter will deal with the influences of both autonomic (mainly sympathetic) postganglionic nerves and plasma catecholamines on metabolism. These effects can occur either through direct actions of catecholamines within metabolically active tissue, or as a consequence of alterations in the major hormones which regulate metabolism. There is now substantial evidence that changes in metabolic or nutritional status can affect the autonomic nervous system (in particular the sympathoadrenal component), and these effects will be considered. The mechanisms by which diabetes mellitus has profound effects on the autonomic and sensory nervous system are not fully understood. However, it is well established that the pathological consequences of this neuropathy for sympathetic function are extremely serious with regard to the postural control of blood pressure and the regulation of sweating. The implications of such diabetic neuropathy on the control of metabolism will be described.

Control of metabolism

There are numerous intracellular biochemical processes which may be under sympathoadrenal regulation. This chapter will focus on the metabolism of the three main components of the diet (carbohydrate, fat, and protein), concentrating on effects that have been established through *in vivo* studies (mainly in humans). Consideration will also be given to overall energy metabolism—assessing the effects of the sympathoadrenal system on resting energy expenditure (thermogenesis). Detailed reviews include those by Young and Landsberg (1977), Macdonald *et al.* (1985), Clutter *et al.* (1988), Niijima (1989), and Webber and Macdonald (1993).

Direct sympathoadrenal control of metabolism

Carbohydrate metabolism (Fig. 17.1)

The maintenance of an adequate supply of glucose to neural tissue is a fundamental component of homeostasis. The carbohydrate component of food is stored in the liver and skeletal muscle as glycogen, under the influence of insulin released from the β-cells of the islets of

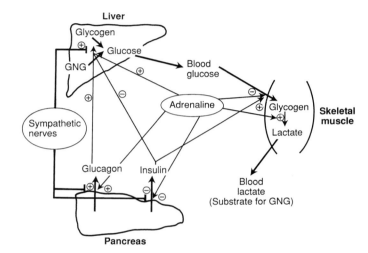

Fig. 17.1. Effects of sympathetic nerves and plasma adrenaline on carbohydrate metabolism. Both direct effects on liver and muscle metabolism and indirect effects via alterations in insulin and glucagon release are illustrated. GNG, gluconeogenesis; +, stimulated; –, inhibited.

Langerhans in the pancreas. During the intervals between meals, or in periods of prolonged starvation, the stored liver glycogen is used to produce free glucose which maintains an adequate blood glucose concentration, thus sustaining neural function. During short periods of starvation (less than 24 h), blood glucose is maintained mainly by the breakdown of the liver glycogen store (the process of glycogenolysis), and partly by the synthesis of glucose (gluconeogenesis) in the liver. This hepatic glycogenolysis is regulated in part by glucagon released from the α-cells of the pancreatic islets, but it is now clear that adrenaline stimulation of glycogenolysis is also important.

In humans, adrenaline stimulates glycogenolysis mainly via activation of β-adrenoceptors, but this does not make a major contribution during short periods of fasting. There is evidence that a small component of hepatic glycogenolysis after an overnight fast is due to stimulation of α-adrenoceptors, probably through the sympathetic innervation of the liver. After more prolonged fasting (i.e. several days), adrenaline contributes to the maintenance of glucose homeostasis although glucagon still has the primary role at this time (Boyle *et al.* 1989).

With more prolonged periods of starvation, the synthesis of glucose (gluconeogenesis), from precursors such as lactate, alanine, and glycerol, is of major importance as the liver glycogen store will be depleted after 2 days of starvation. This gluconeogenesis occurs mainly in the liver (although the kidneys do contribute) and is stimulated by glucagon and adrenaline. In addition to this direct effect on hepatic gluconeogenesis, adrenaline is one of the main stimuli for increasing muscle glycogenolysis in the resting state. By contrast to the liver, muscle glycogen cannot be broken down to free glucose, but instead lactate is produced and passes into the blood. This lactate is a substrate for hepatic gluconeogenesis and thus muscle glycogen can indirectly contribute to the maintenance of blood glucose (the Cori cycle).

The liver has a sympathetic innervation which has been studied extensively by Lautt (1980). Stimulation of the hepatic sympathetic supply leads to increased glycogenolysis and glucose release. There is no direct evidence that these nerves are involved in the regulation of carbohydrate metabolism under normal conditions. For example, applications of local anaesthetic to the coeliac ganglion (preventing sympathetic activation of the liver) has no effect on the increase in release of glucose from the liver during exercise (Kjaer et al. 1993). Denervation of the liver, such as with transplantation, does not produce any gross abnormalities of carbohydrate metabolism, with transplant recipients having the same hepatic glucose production responses to exercise to those seen in healthy subjects (Kjaer et al. 1995). However, with liver transplantation it would be rather difficult to identify more subtle alterations, given the previous metabolic disease and post-transplant immunosuppression. It is more likely that hepatic sympathetic nerves are of importance in severe hypoglycaemia or when the other mechanisms are defective.

Fat metabolism (Fig. 17.2)

The major direct metabolic effects of the sympathoadrenal system are in the control of fat metabolism. The storage of fatty acids as triacylglycerols in adipose tissue is regulated by insulin, which stimulates the storage process and inhibits the breakdown of triacylglycerol to non-esterified fatty acids (NEFA or FFA). This breakdown process (lipolysis) increases if plasma insulin levels fall, but the major stimulation is achieved by several hormones, including adrenaline, and by the sympathetic innervation of the adipose tissue. With short periods of starvation (up to 20 h), there appears to be little involvement of sympathoadrenal stimulation of lipolysis, with the fall in plasma insulin and rise in plasma cortisol being the likely stimuli for an increase in NEFA release from adipose tissue (Samra et al. 1996). More prolonged starvation, and a variety of other stressors, lead to

increased lipolysis via sympathoadrenal stimulation. The sympathoadrenal stimulation of lipolysis occurs via β-adrenoceptor-mediated processes. By contrast, the stimulation of α-adrenoceptors in adipose tissue inhibits lipolysis. This may prevent the occurrence of excessive rates of lipolysis during periods of starvation, as there is evidence that such a state is accompanied by a fall in β-adrenoceptor density and a rise in α-adrenoceptor density in adipose tissue.

The sympathetic innervation of white adipose tissue mainly supplies the vasculature, but in some depots there is a direct innervation of the adipose tissue cells. There is histological evidence that neurotransmitters released from the sympathetic nerves may also stimulate non-innervated adipose tissue cells, thus providing a key role for the sympathetic nervous system in the regulation of adipose tissue blood flow and metabolism (Fredholm 1985). During conditions such as orthostasis, there are transient reductions in human adipose tissue blood flow, mediated by sympathetic nervous innervation of vascular smooth muscle. However, these blood vessels also contain β-adrenoceptors which mediate vasodilatation in response to an increase in plasma adrenaline, or possibly due to diffusion of noradrenaline from the sympathetic neuroeffector junctions. Thus, prolonged sympathetic nervous stimulation to white adipose tissue is accompanied by a type of vasoconstrictor escape, while a rise in plasma adrenaline levels products active vasodilatation (Hjemdahl and Linde 1983). Furthermore, the stimulation of lipolysis by the sympathetic nerves, or plasma adrenaline, leads to a rise in adipose tissue blood flow through metabolic effects—facilitating the transport of fatty acids to other tissues in the body (reviewed by Frayn and Macdonald 1996).

Brown adipose tissue has a more dense vascular supply and innervation than white adipose tissue. Furthermore, many more brown adipose tissue cells are sympathetically innervated directly. The vascular innervation appears to be predominantly vasodilator, with the released noradrenaline acting on β-adrenoceptors. The stimulation of lipolysis in brown adipose tissue is accompanied by a marked increase in the oxygen consumption of the tissue (brown adipose tissue thermogenesis). This metabolic event is mediated by β-adrenoceptors which appear to be somewhat atypical, and have been designated β_3 (Arch et al. 1984). In humans brown adipose tissue is important as a site of thermogenesis in the newborn, but is of limited significance in the adult (see below).

Protein metabolism

There is no evidence of a direct effect of the sympathetic nervous system on protein metabolism. However, it appears that adrenaline is able to decrease the rate of breakdown of body protein. This is based on observations of the effects of adrenaline infusion (Miles et al. 1984) and the physiological and clinical significance are not established.

Indirect autonomic effects on metabolism

The main indirect effect on metabolism is through the modulation of insulin and glucagon release from the pancreas. Stimulation of the sympathetic innervation of the β-cell leads to α-adrenoceptor mediated inhibition of insulin release. Evidence from in vitro studies suggests plasma catecholamines inhibit insulin release through activation of α_2-adrenoceptors, but is not known whether these also mediate the sympathetic nervous effects. The pancreatic β-cells also contain β_2-adrenoceptors, although it is uncommon for these to be stimulated by

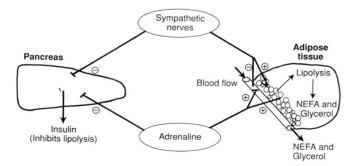

Fig. 17.2. Effects of sympathetic nerves and plasma adrenaline on fat metabolism. Both direct effects on adipose tissue blood flow and metabolism and indirect effects through inhibition of insulin release are illustrated. NEFA, non-esterified fatty acids; +, stimulated; −, inhibited.

plasma adrenaline under physiological conditions—the stimulation of α-adrenoceptors seems to predominate. However, β_2-adrenoceptor agonists such as salbutamol will stimulate insulin release.

An important physiological role of the autonomic nervous system in the control of insulin release is the stimulatory effect of the vagus supply to the pancreas. Stimulation of the parasympathetic innervation of the β-cells leads to insulin release, and is an important component of the cephalic and gastric phases of feeding. Thus, the sight, smell, and taste of food, and its presence in the stomach, will elicit an insulin secretory response, which primes the liver to maximize glucose retention when the food is absorbed. Once nutrient absorption occurs, further insulin release is due to direct effects of glucose and amino acids (and of gastrointestinal hormones) on the β-cells. Stimulation of the parasympathetic nerve supply to the pancreas also gives rise to the secretion of the hormone pancreatic polypeptide. The functions of this hormone are unclear, but its release in response to a variety of stimuli (including food and hypoglycaemia) provides a marker of pancreatic vagal function.

The pancreatic α-cells are stimulated by both their sympathetic innervation and by plasma catecholamines. Glucagon release results from activation of β-adrenoceptors, although such release has not been demonstrated in all studies of the effects of the infusion of adrenaline.

One of the consequences of pancreatic transplantation is to produce a denervated pancreas. However, this cannot readily be used to judge the overall importance of the innervation, as the transplant recipients are patients with insulin-dependent diabetes mellitus (IDDM) who also have severe diabetic complications such as end-stage renal failure. Such pancreatic transplantation is judged to be successful if the patient no longer needs to inject insulin (although this is only achieved with continued immunosuppression). The transplanted pancreas is capable of controlling postprandial blood glucose satisfactorily, and releases glucagon in response to hypoglycaemia. However, it is not known whether the effectiveness of the pancreas in regulating metabolism is compromised by its lack of autonomic innervation.

One of the most important indirect effects of the sympathoadrenal system on metabolism is to reduce the sensitivity of the peripheral tissues to insulin. Thus, under conditions of sympathetic activation or increased adrenal medullary secretion (such as in trauma or after a myocardial infarction) there is a reduction in the effectiveness of insulin to stimulate glucose uptake and utilization in adipose tissue and skeletal muscle. These peripheral effects of the catecholamines seem to be mediated through activation of β_2-adrenoceptors and thus are also produced by drugs such as salbutamol, ritodrine, and terbutaline. Such drugs are commonly used to prevent premature labour. If used in pregnant women with IDDM, these drugs lead to a marked increased in the insulin requirements for achieving adequate control of blood glucose. The latter is of major importance in preventing the occurrence of macrosomia in the fetus. Large doses of these β_2 agonists can stimulate adipose tissue lipolysis and pancreatic glucagon secretion, leading to increased ketone production which may develop into diabetic ketoacidosis. In such conditions of possible premature labour, steroids are sometimes given intravenously to the woman to stimulate the fetal lung maturation process, and in patients with IDDM these high doses of steroids will increase the likelihood of occurrence of diabetic ketoacidosis.

In summary, physiologically the predominant effects of the sympathoadrenal system are to raise blood glucose concentration through direct effects on glycogenolyis and gluconeogenesis and indirectly through reducing insulin release, decreasing insulin sensitivity, and possibly stimulating glucagon release. Of equal, if not greater, importance is the effect of the sympathoadrenal system on the regulation of lipolysis. The sympathetic innervation to adipose tissue and plasma catecholamines both stimulate lipolysis, an effect that is enhanced if there is also a catecholamine-mediated suppression of insulin release. The parasympathetic innervation of the pancreatic β-cell can stimulate insulin release, and is of importance in the early stages of food ingestion.

Thermogenesis

Given the profound effects of the catecholamines on metabolism described above, it would be surprising if there was not also an effect on energy metabolism. It was demonstrated over 60 years ago that the infusion of adrenaline into humans (in amounts that we now know produce plasma adrenaline levels in the physiological range) caused an increase in whole-body energy metabolism, as well as stimulating heart rate and respiration (Cori and Buchwald 1930). This effect is now known as adrenaline (catecholamine)-induced thermogenesis (the stimulation of energy metabolism above resting, baseline levels) and does not involve an increase in physical activity, although adrenaline will, of course, increase skeletal muscle tremor. The existence of this catecholamine-induced thermogenesis has been confirmed many times, and may be of physiological importance in the control of energy balance and of body temperature.

The infusion of noradrenaline also stimulates thermogenesis, mainly through an increase in lipolysis and oxidation of free fatty acids (as is the case with adrenaline), although the amounts that have to be used are somewhat larger than for adrenaline. In fact, the plasma adrenaline threshold for increasing thermogenesis is toward the lower end of the physiological range. Higher plasma levels of noradrenaline are needed to stimulate thermogenesis, indicating that under physiological conditions, it is more likely that direct stimulation of thermogenesis by noradrenaline occurs due to activation of the sympathetic nerves rather than through an effect of plasma noradrenaline.

When the human neonate is exposed to a cool environment, its total heat production increases (cold-induced thermogenesis) to maintain body temperature. It seems most probable that this cold-induced thermogenesis is mediated through the sympathetic nervous system activating thermogenesis in brown adipose tissue—as also seen in cold-adapted rodents and hibernating mammals. Thus, catecholamine-induced thermogenesis is of major importance in neonatal thermoregulation. Studies in adult humans also indicate that cold-induced thermogenesis occurs in the absence of muscle contraction (Jessen et al. 1980) and it has been suggested that this is also stimulated by catecholamines. However, the normal human adult has insufficient brown adipose tissue to contribute significantly to heat production in the cold, and it seems more probable that the splanchnic region and skeletal muscle are the major sites of such thermogenesis. Nevertheless, such non-shivering thermogenesis would be of minor importance in the regulation of body temperature in most situations (this is considered further in Chapter 12).

There is an increasing volume of evidence that sympathoadrenal effects on thermogenesis may be of importance in the overall regulation of energy metabolism. It has been apparent for many years that experimental animals (e.g. rats, pigs), and in some cases humans, can regulate overall thermogenesis to maintain energy balance over a wide range of energy intake. Studies in the rat by Rothwell and Stock (1981) indicated that the consumption of excessive amounts of a varied, palatable diet did not produce the expected degree of weight gain, because of a profound increase in energy expenditure. This increased energy expenditure was not due to physical activity, but was a result of increased sympathetic nervous stimulation of brown adipose tissue and of an increased mass of this tissue. Attempts to make similar observations in adult humans foundered because of the small amounts of this tissue. However, there have now been several demonstrations of marked sympathoadrenal effects on overall energy metabolism.

The first of these demonstrations relates to the effects of insulin and glucose in normal humans. If one raises plasma insulin levels by exogenous infusion, but then infuses glucose to maintain a constant blood glucose, the amount of glucose infused matches the glucose taken up by the tissues and is a measure of the sensitivity of the individual to insulin (the glucose clamp method). In healthy subjects, the glucose taken up by the tissues is either oxidized, or stored as glycogen. Acheson and colleagues demonstrated that this combined infusion of insulin and glucose stimulated thermogenesis (increasing resting energy expenditure by 10–20 per cent), and that the observed increase was substantially greater than the expected increase required to provide the necessary energy for the amount of glycogen being synthesized. The demonstration that this extra energy expenditure could be suppressed by administration of a β-adrenoceptor antagonist led to the proposition that part of the observed glucose-induced thermogenesis was due to sympathoadrenal activation (Acheson 1988).

Further support for a link between glucose metabolism, the sympathoadrenal system and thermogenesis comes from the studies of Astrup and colleagues. They demonstrated an increase in thermogenesis in resting skeletal muscle, approximately 4 h after ingestion of a glucose load, coincident with an increase in plasma adrenaline levels. Subsequent studies by this group showed that the ingestion of a mixed meal has a similar effect, and that in both cases this delayed stimulation of thermogenesis can be prevented by β-adrenoceptor blockade (Astrup et al. 1990). In the same review, these authors provided a useful analysis of previous studies which indicated that β-blockade only reduced meal-induced thermogenesis in the later stages and when there was a high carbohydrate content of the ingested food.

Work by Schwarz and colleagues has shown a positive correlation between the increase in thermogenesis seen after consuming a mixed meal and the stimulation of the sympathetic nervous system (assessed by measuring plasma noradrenaline turnover). Furthermore, the administration of clonidine, to suppress central sympathetic outflow, reduced both the sympathetic stimulation and the thermogenic response to the meals (Schwarz et al. 1988).

In summary, the sympathoadrenal system can stimulate thermogenesis, and there are a number of physiological conditions in which this effect may operate. The final part of this chapter will consider whether disorders of such effects are involved in the aetiology of obesity, or in disturbances of thermoregulation.

Metabolic and nutritional effects on the sympathoadrenal system

In addition to the sympathoadrenal system being important in the regulation of metabolism, it is apparent that alterations in metabolic or nutritional status can affect the activity of the sympathoadrenal system. Some of these effects would be entirely predictable on the basis of the regulation of metabolism discussed above. The best example of this is the effect of an acute reduction in blood glucose concentration producing hypoglycaemia, which leads to adrenaline release from the adrenal medulla and altered sympathetic nervous system activity. However, there are a variety of other metabolic and nutritional effects on the sympathoadrenal system which are considered below.

Dietary effects on the sympathetic nervous system: animal studies

The possibility that the amount and composition of the diet may affect the sympathetic nervous system has been addressed by the studies of Landsberg, Young, and colleagues (Landsberg and Young 1985). They assessed the activity of the sympathetic nervous system by measuring the rate of turnover of the neurotransmitter noradrenaline in specific organs and tissues of rats and mice. These studies have shown that starvation suppresses and overfeeding enhances sympathetic activity, with an increased dietary carbohydrate content being a particularly potent stimulus. This effect of carbohydrate to stimulate the sympathetic nervous system appears to involve an action of insulin in the hypothalamus. This has led to a series of studies on the effects of insulin on the sympathetic nervous system in humans which will be discussed below.

There are impressive correlations between increased noradrenaline turnover and thermogenesis in brown adipose tissue during both excess dietary intake and cold adaptation in rodents. Thus, it would appear that there is an important functional role for diet-induced changes in sympathetic activity. This is supported by the demonstration that a reduced energy intake leads to a fall in sympathetic activity and in blood pressure in spontaneously hypertensive rats.

Human studies

Assessing the activity of the sympathetic nervous system in humans is restricted to intraneural recordings in superficial nerves (Chapter 23), measuring plasma noradrenaline turnover (Esler et al. 1990) or measuring plasma or urinary catecholamine concentrations (Chapter 24). Each of these techniques has some limitations, and caution must be exercised when interpreting any results obtained, especially if there are no associated functional measurements. Alterations in dietary intake in humans are accompanied by changes in sympathetic activity (assessed by plasma noradrenaline turnover and plasma and urinary levels) which are qualitatively similar to the effects seen in animals. A reduced energy intake is accompanied by evidence of reduced sympathetic activity and decreased supine blood pressure, with increased energy intake being associated with opposite changes. Although these effects are modest, they may be of some functional significance and are considered further below (p. 140–1).

Metabolic effects on the sympathoadrenal system

Hypoglycaemia

The most potent metabolic disturbances affecting the sympathoadrenal system relate to alterations in glucose metabolism, or in plasma insulin concentrations. In healthy, adult humans an overnight fast produces blood glucose concentrations of 4–5 mmol/l. Acute reduction of blood glucose to approximately 3.5 mmol/l (with insulin) is followed within 10 minutes by the secretion of adrenaline from the adrenal medulla. More severe hypoglycaemia is associated with progressively increasing adrenaline responses (Fig. 17.3). This release of adrenaline at a relatively high blood glucose level is part of the early endocrine response which opposes the effect of insulin and occurs before any detectable impairment in cerebral function caused by the fall in blood glucose.

More profound hypoglycaemia (blood glucose 2–3 mmol/l) is accompanied by an increase in plasma noradrenaline concentrations, the rate of appearance of noradrenaline in plasma, and by an increase in muscle and skin nerve sympathetic activity (measured by microneurography) (reviewed by Heller and Macdonald 1991). The effect on muscle sympathetic activity is interesting as this appears to be occurring in vasoconstrictor fibres, yet muscle vasodilatation occurs in hypoglycaemia. The latter is not due to the effects of insulin (see below) as it occurs when hypoglycaemia is induced with relatively low plasma insulin levels (below 120 mU/l) whereas the effect of insulin to produce vasodilatation in skeletal muscle does not occur until insulin levels exceed 140 mU/l. It is far more likely that the muscle vasodilatation in hypoglycaemia is due to the increased plasma adrenaline levels as it can be prevented by β-adrenoceptor antagonism. The muscle blood flow response to hypoglycaemia illustrates the need to assess sympathetically mediated function as well as sympathetic nervous system activity.

Such hypoglycaemia occurs most commonly in patients with IDDM. When these patients first develop diabetes, their responses to hypoglycaemia are the same as in non-diabetic subjects. However, within 5 years of the onset of IDDM, most patients lose the ability to release glucagon in response to hypoglycaemia (although not in

response to other stimuli). Such patients are then dependent on an adequate adrenaline response, and on the disappearance of the injected insulin, for blood glucose recovery after hypoglycaemia (unless they eat). When such diabetic patients develop autonomic neuropathy of such a severity that they fail to release adrenaline from the adrenal medulla, they will then be at risk of developing prolonged, severe hypoglycaemia if their insulin dose and food intake are poorly matched.

The symptomatic responses and physiological disturbances that occur with hypoglycaemia are reduced when patients experience regular episodes of low blood glucose. This phenomenon is not well understood, but an episode of hypoglycaemia on one day reduces the adrenomedullary response to the same degree of hypoglycaemia the next day. This reduced response is not due to an adrenal medullary defect, as the plasma adrenaline response to postural change or to mental arithmetic is unaffected by antecedent hypoglycaemia (Robinson *et al.* 1995).

Hyperglycaemia and insulin

A rise in blood glucose concentration is often accompanied by an increase in plasma noradrenaline, heart rate, and blood pressure consistent with stimulation of the sympathetic nervous system. This is confirmed by the demonstration of increased muscle sympathetic nerve activity after glucose ingestion (Berne *et al.* 1989). The effect of glucose can be explained at least partly by an action of insulin on the sympathetic nervous system. The technique of insulin and glucose infusion (glucose clamping) described above leads to a rise in plasma noradrenaline, heart rate, and systolic blood pressure in normal humans. Studies with microneurography have shown increased muscle sympathetic (vasoconstrictor) nerve activity, but again it is interesting to note that forearm (predominantly muscle) blood flow increases in these circumstances (Scott *et al.* 1988*a*). This raises the possibility that insulin may have direct effects on the vascular smooth muscle (or the sympathetic nerve terminals) to produce vasodilatation which leads to reflex activation of the sympathetic nervous system.

A disturbance of the balance between vasodilator effects of insulin and sympathetic nervous system activation may contribute to the falls in blood pressure seen after high carbohydrate meals in the elderly. The normal muscle vasoconstrictor responses to high-fat meals are converted into vasodilator responses (with a fall in blood pressure) by the infusion of insulin to produce plasma concentrations similar to those seen after carbohydrate-rich meals (Kearney *et al.* 1998).

Changes in sympathoadrenally regulated processes during metabolic/nutritional disturbances

Acute (48 h) starvation in healthy humans is accompanied by functional changes consistent with altered sympathoadrenal activity. The regulation of body temperature during cold exposure is impaired with an inadequate increase in thermogenesis and reduction in limb blood flow contributing to a fall in core temperature (Macdonald *et al.* 1984). In addition, there is no increase in thermogenesis during insulin and glucose infusion in starvation. As the latter response is normally mediated by the sympathetic nervous system, this is consistent with reduced sympathetic activity in starvation. Further evidence

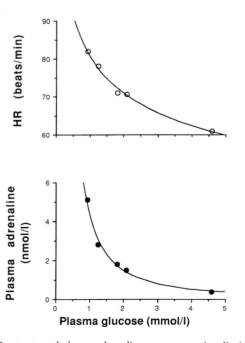

Fig. 17.3. Heart rate and plasma adrenaline responses to insulin-induced hypoglycaemia. In both cases there is a curvilinear relationship with more profound hypoglycaemia having a progressively greater effect.

of functional impairment of sympathetic control during starvation is provided by the falls in arterial blood pressure on standing seen after 48 h starvation in young men with normal orthostatic responses in the fed state (Bennett *et al.* 1984). These functional impairments seen in acute starvation are not due to the inability to respond to catecholamines, as the cardiac and thermogenic responses to infused adrenaline are actually enhanced after 48 hours' starvation.

These demonstrations of functional impairments consistent with reduced sympathetic activity are not restricted to acute starvation. Severe weight loss in human babies (due to inadequate food intake) and adults (with Crohn's disease, coeliac disease, or postoperative fistulas) is accompanied by impaired thermoregulation, particularly with reduced or absent thermogenic responses, which is reversed by weight gain. Impaired thermoregulation also occurs in anorexia nervosa, although it is not clear whether these changes are also reversible. It seems most unlikely that weight loss in anorexia nervosa is contributed to by enhanced thermogenic responses to food or to catecholamines, which would increase overall energy expenditure, producing the opposite effect to that which may occur in obesity (see below). However, the weight loss associated with chronic respiratory disease is accompanied by increases in resting energy expenditure and urinary catecholamine excretion, providing further evidence of an effect of the sympathoadrenal system on energy metabolism.

Many studies have also shown poor orthostatic tolerance during chronic undernutrition, although this may of course be due to disturbances of fluid and electrolyte balance rather than to nutritional effects on the sympathetic nervous system.

Obesity

The role of the sympathoadrenal system in controlling substrate mobilization and thermogenesis, and the links between nutritional factors and the sympathetic nervous system, have led to the proposition that reduced sympathetic activity contributes to the development or maintenance of obesity. It is now clear that in several animal models of obesity reduced sympathetic nervous stimulation of thermogenesis is a contributory factory to the development of the obese state. The genetically obese *ob/ob* mouse cannot produce the peptide leptin in its adipose tissue, and becomes obese through excessive eating and low rates of thermogenesis. Administration of leptin to these animals lowers food intake and increases sympathetic nervous stimulation of brown adipose tissue thermogenesis, causing the animals to lose weight.

In obese humans, some investigators have shown reduced catecholamine-induced thermogenesis, and others have observed altered plasma catecholamine kinetics. However, there have been many conflicting reports, and it seems most probable that human obesity is not due to a single metabolic defect, but has varied aetiologies. However, there is no doubt that if an individual fails to respond to increased carbohydrate intake by activating thermogenesis (possibly through the sympathetic nervous system) then he or she will have a greater tendency to develop obesity than someone who does increase thermogenesis. This is illustrated by studies on Pima Indians and other groups with a high susceptibility to develop obesity, where altered metabolism and low sympathetic activity are risk factors for subsequent weight gain (Astrup and Macdonald 1998).

There have now been several studies of already obese patients which revealed minor impairments of autonomic function associated with obesity (Peterson *et al.* 1988). Most of these changes were in the parasympathetic nervous system (analogous to the early stages of autonomic neuropathy in diabetes mellitus). There is also evidence of abnormal regulation of platelet α-adrenoceptors in obesity, although there is little disturbance of β-adrenoceptor sensitivity unless such patients are underfed (Berlin *et al.* 1990).

Sympathoadrenal dysfunction

The main consequences of sympathoadrenal dysfunction are considered in other sections of this book (Chapters 20 and 24), but it is worth noting here that patients with autonomic failure are frequently insulin resistant and can have impaired glucose tolerance. However, this is likely to result mainly from their low levels of physical activity, and possibly reduced carbohydrate intake, rather than from defects in the autonomic nervous system. The other two clinical situations in which one might expect altered control of metabolism are in adrenal insufficiency (either Addison's disease or post-adrenalectomy) or in diabetic autonomic neuropathy.

Addison's disease is characterized by adrenocortical degeneration and loss of corticosteroids, but the adrenal medulla is usually preserved. However, the enzyme phenyl-ethanolamine N methyl transferase (PNMT), involved in the conversion of noradrenaline to adrenaline, is only produced in the presence of cortisol. Thus, in untreated Addison's disease there would be a deficiency of adrenaline which would contribute to the problems of hypoglycaemia and intolerance of other stresses that characterize this condition. Once the patients are given glucocorticoid replacement therapy there should be normal production of adrenaline, provided the adrenal medulla is preserved.

There is little evidence of impaired thermoregulation or other aspects of metabolism in adrenalectomized patients, although there have been few studies of such patients using the more sensitive methods now available. The fact that adrenalectomy does not produce serious metabolic disturbances (provided that corticosteroid replacement therapy is adequate) is not too surprising as the sympathetic innervation of blood vessels (to regulate heat loss in thermoregulation) and of the metabolically active tissues and endocrine glands, are probably more important than the effects of circulating adrenaline. The major exception is the prevention of hypoglycaemia during exercise, starvation, or in the presence of excess insulin. The primary factor acting to raise blood glucose under these conditions is glucagon, with adrenaline providing a secondary role. Obviously, the absence of a glucagon response in an adrenalectomized patient would then lead to serious problems in the defence of blood glucose concentration. Such an occurrence is likely to be rare, as (apart from the failure to release glucagon in IDDM as mentioned above) the only circumstances likely to affect glucagon release are the infusion of somatostatin or its analogues, and of course, pancreatectomy.

The problems of impaired responses to hypoglycaemia in diabetic autonomic neuropathy were considered above (p. 138). However, diabetic autonomic neuropathy has other implications for metabolism, as these patients have impaired thermoregulatory responses to cold exposure. Such patients have less vasoconstriction in the feet and legs when exposed to the cold, and are more likely to shiver than diabetic patients without such complications. Furthermore, the rate of resting energy expenditure under thermoneutral conditions of the neuropathic patients who shivered was higher than in non-neuropathic patients who did not shiver when cooled (Scott *et al.* 1988*b*). This indicates that inadequate control of the peripheral circulation through impaired sympathetic function is likely to lead to increased heat loss, which requires an elevated resting metabolic rate to maintain thermal balance.

Concluding remarks

The parasympathetic nervous system has a minor role in the regulation of metabolism, via effects on insulin release. Impaired parasympathetic activity is seen in obesity, but the effects are not as marked as in diabetes. By contrast, the sympathoadrenal system is an important regulator of metabolism, and an essential feature of homeostasis is the activation of the sympathoadrenal system when tissue fuel supplies are compromised (e.g. the adrenaline response to hypoglycaemia). However, there does appear to be a more fundamental link between nutritional status and the sympathetic nervous system which may have important implications for the development/maintenance of obesity.

References

Acheson, K. J. (1988). Nutrient induced thermogenesis. In *Clinical progress in nutrition research*, (ed. A. Sitges-Serra, A. Sitges-Creus, and S. Schwartz-Riera), pp. 255–64. Karger, Basel.

Arch, J. R. S., Ainsworth, A. T., and Cawthorne, M. A. (1984). Atypical β-adrenoceptor on brown adipocytes as target for antiobesity drugs. *Nature* 309, 163–5.

Astrup, A. and Macdonald, I. A. (1998). Sympathoadrenal system and metabolism. In *Handbook of obesity*, (ed. G. A. Bray, C. Bouchard, and W. P. T. James), pp. 491–511. Marcel Dekker, New York.

Astrup, A., Christensen, N. J., Simonsen, L., and Bulow, J. (1990). Effects of nutrient intake on sympathoadrenal activity and thermogenic mechanisms. *J. Neurosci. Methods* 34, 187–92.

Bennett, T., Macdonald, I. A., and Sainsbury, R. (1984). The influence of starvation on the cardiovascular responses to lower body subatmospheric pressure or to standing in man. *Clin. Sci.* 66, 141–6.

Berlin, I., Berlan, M., Crespo-Laumonier, B. *et al.* (1990). Alterations in β-adrenergic sensitivity and platelet α_2-adrenoceptors in obese women: effect of exercise and calorie restriction. *Clin. Sci.* 78, 81–7.

Berne, C., Fagius, J., and Niklasson, F. (1989). Sympathetic response to oral carbohydrate administration. Evidence from micro-electrode recordings. *J. Clin. Invest.* 84, 1043–9.

Boyle, P. J., Shah, S. D., and Cryer, P. E. (1989). Insulin, glucagon and catecholamines in prevention of hypoglycemia during fasting. *Am. J. Physiol.* 256, E651–E661.

Clutter, W. E., Rizza, R. A. Gerich, J. E., and Cryer, P. E. (1988). Regulation of glucose metabolism by sympathochromaffin catecholamines. *Diabetes/Metab. Rev.* 4, 1–15.

Cori, C. F. and Buchwald, K. W. (1930). Effects of continuous injection of epinephrine on the carbohydrate metabolism, basal metabolism and vascular system of normal man. *Am. J. Physiol.* 95, 71–8.

Esler, M. Jennings, G., Meredith, I., Horne, M., and Eisenhofer, G. (1990). Overflow of catecholamine neurotransmitter to the circulation: source, fate and function. *Physiol. Rev.*, 70, 963–85.

Frayn, K. N. and Macdonald I. A. (1996). Adipose tissue circulation. In *Nervous control of blood vessels*, (ed. T. Bennett and S. M. Gardiner), pp. 505–39. Hardwood Academic Publishers, UK.

Fredholm, B. B. (1985). Nervous control of circulation and metabolism in white adipose tissue. In *New perspectives in adipose tissue: structure, function and development*, (ed. A. Cryer and R. L. R. Van), pp. 45–64. Butterworths, London.

Heller, S. R. and Macdonald, I. A. (1991). Physiological disturbances in hypoglycaemia: effect on subjective awareness. *Clin. Sci.* 81, 1–9.

Hjemdahl, P. and Linde, B. (1983). Influence of circulating NE and Epi on adipose tissue vascular resistance and lipolysis in humans. *Am. J. Physiol.* 245, H447–H452.

Jessen, K., Rabol, A., and Winkles, K. (1990). Total body and splanchnic thermogenesis in curarized man during a short exposure to cold. *Acta Anaesth. Scand.* 24, 339–44.

Kearney, M. T., Cowley, A. J., Evans, A., Stubbs, T. A., and Macdonald, I. A. (1998). Insulin's depressor action on skeletal muscle vasculative: a novel mechanism for postprandial hypotension in the elderly. *J. Am. Coll. Cardiol.* 31, 209–16.

Kjaer, M., Engfred, K., Fernandes, A., Secher, N. H., and Galbo, H. (1993). Regulation of hepatic glucose production during exercise in humans: role of sympathoadrenergic activity. *Am. J. Physiol.* 265, E275–E283.

Kjaer, M., Keiding, S., Engfred, K. *et al.* (1995). Glucose homeostasis during exercise in humans with a liver or kidney transplant. *Am. J. Physiol.* 268, E636–E644.

Landsberg, L. and Young, J. B. (1985). The influence of diet on the sympathetic nervous system. In *Neuroendocrine perspectives*, (ed. E. E. Muller, R. M. McLeod and L. A. Frohman), pp. 191–218. Elsevier, Amsterdam.

Lautt, W. W. (1980). Hepatic nerves. A review of their functions and effects. *Can. J. Physiol. Pharmacol.* 58, 105–23.

Macdonald, I. A., Bennett, T., and Sainsbury, R. (1984). The effect of a 48 h fast on the thermoregulatory responses to graded cooling in man. *Clin. Sci.* 67, 445–52.

Macdonald, I. A., Bennett, T., and Fellows, I. W. (1985). Catecholamines and the control of metabolism in man. *Clin. Sci.* 68, 613–19.

Miles, J. M., Nissen, S. L., Gerich, J. E., and Haymond, M. W. (1984). Effect of epinephrine infusion on leucine and alanine kinetics in humans. *Am. J. Physiol.* 247, E166–E172.

Niijima, A. (1989). Nervous regulation of metabolism. *Prog. Neurobiol.* 33, 135–47.

Peterson, H. R., Rothschild, M., Winberg, C. R., Fell, R. D., McLeish, K. R., and Pfeiffer, M. A. (1988). Body fat and the activity of the autonomic nervous system. *New Engl. J. Med.* 318, 1077–83.

Robinson, A. M., Parkin, H. M., Macdonald, I. A., and Tattersall, R. B. (1995). Antecedent hypoglycaemia in non-diabetic subjects reduces the adrenaline response for 6 days but does not affect the catecholamine response to other stimuli. *Clin. Sci.* 89, 359–66.

Rothwell, N. J. and Stock, M. J. (1981). Regulation of energy balance. *Ann. Rev. Nutr.* 1, 235–56.

Samra, J. S., Clark, M. L., Humphreys, S. M., Macdonald, I. A., Matthews, D. R., and Frayn, K. N. (1996). Effects of morning rise in cortisol concentration on regulation of lipolysis in subcutaneous adipose tissue. *Am. J. Physiol.* 271, E996-E1002.

Schwartz, R. W., Jaeger, L. F., and Veith, R. C. (1988). Effect of clonidine on the thermic effect of feeding in humans. *Am. J. Physiol.* 254, R90–R94.

Scott, A. R., Bennett, T., and Macdonald, I. A. (1988*a*). Effects of hyperinsulinaemia on the cardiovascular responses to graded hypovolaemia in normal and diabetic subjects. *Clin. Sci.* 75, 85–92.

Scott, A. R., Macdonald, I. A., Bennett, T., and Tattersall, R. B. (1988*b*). Abnormal thermoregulation in diabetic autonomic neuropathy. *Diabetes* 37, 961–8.

Webber, J. and Macdonald, I. A. (1993). Metabolic actions of catecholamines in man. *Baillière's Clin. Endocrinol. Metab.* 7, 393–413.

Young, J. B. and Landsberg, L. (1977). Catecholamines and intermediary metabolism. *Clin. Endocrinol. Metab.* 6, 599–631.

18. The kidney and the sympathetic nervous system

Gerald F. DiBona and Christopher S. Wilcox

Introduction

It is the purpose of this chapter to review the physiology and pharmacology of the renal sympathetic nervous system in the regulation of renal function (DiBona and Kopp 1997) and to integrate this information into a clearer understanding of the abnormalities in body fluid regulation which are observed in autonomic failure (AF), a condition thought to be characterized by partial or complete renal sympathetic denervation.

Neural control of renal function: physiology and pharmacology

Control of the renal circulation

Alterations in renal nerve activity

It is generally agreed that under physiological conditions basal efferent renal sympathetic nerve activity (ERSNA) is too low to influence renal haemodynamics. In the conscious state, surgical or pharmacological renal denervation does not affect renal blood flow (RBF) or renal vascular resistance. When ERSNA is elevated above its baseline, its effect on renal haemodynamics can be profound. Studies in anaesthetized rats and conscious dogs have shown a frequency-dependent reduction in RBF in response to graded increases in the frequency of electrical renal nerve stimulation with a threshold frequency of about 1 Hz. Current available evidence supports the concept that renal nerves do not play a role in the mechanisms involved in autoregulation of RBF.

Effector loci of renal nerves

The effector loci for renal nerves within the renal cortical microcirculation have been localized by micropuncture techniques to both the afferent and efferent glomerular arteriole. Renal nerve stimulation decreases single-nephron glomerular filtration rate (SNGFR) and single-nephron plasma flow (SNPF). The decreases are due to the increases in afferent and efferent glomerular arteriolar resistances, with a resultant decrease in the glomerular hydrostatic pressure gradient and a decrease in the glomerular capillary ultrafiltration coefficient (K_f). Renal nerve stimulation at lower intensities produces similar but quantitatively smaller effects. When ERSNA is low, as is the case in euvolaemic rats, the renal nerves play a minimal role in the control of SNGFR. However, acute renal denervation of euvolaemic rats increases urinary sodium excretion in the absence of a change in SNGFR. When ERSNA is elevated, e.g. by sodium depletion, SNGFR is reduced due to a reduction in SNPF and K_f. SNGFR is restored towards control levels by either volume repletion, which lowers ERSNA, or renal denervation via reductions in afferent and efferent glomerular arteriolar resistances and increases in SNPF and K_f. The marked fall in K_f caused by renal nerve stimulation is at least partly related to decreased glomerular capillary surface area since morphological studies show that glomeruli (as well as afferent and efferent glomerular arterioles) from the stimulated kidney are markedly smaller than glomeruli (and arterioles) from the contralateral non-stimulated kidney.

Adrenergic receptors

The renal vasoconstrictor response to renal nerve stimulation is predominantly mediated by renal vascular α_1-adrenoceptors (α_{1A} subtype) with a lesser role being identified for α_2-adrenoceptors under certain conditions in some mammalian species.

Whether the renal circulation can be affected by activation of presynaptic α- and/or β_2-adrenoceptors has been examined. The intrarenal administration of the α_2-adrenoceptor antagonist yohimbine or the β_2-agonist adrenaline enhances the renal venous overflow of noradrenaline and the renal vasoconstrictor response to renal nerve stimulation. Thus it is possible that neurogenic renal vasoconstriction can be enhanced by increased circulating adrenaline concentration, i.e. during stress.

Recent studies comparing the effects of catecholamines on renal haemodynamics in innervated and denervated kidneys show that chronically denervated kidneys (7–10 days) exhibit supersensitivity to noradrenaline. The denervation supersensitivity is not due to a loss of neuronal uptake of noradrenaline and is not restricted to noradrenaline, since denervated kidneys also showed enhanced renal vasoconstrictor responses to vasopressin (ADH), serotonin, and prostaglandin $F_{2\alpha}$.

Although there is considerable evidence for the existence in the kidney of nerves that contain dopamine, and for renal vasodilator effects of exogenous dopamine, the physiological significance of neurally released dopamine is still controversial. Although electrical and reflex renal nerve stimulation result in a small increase in renal venous output of dopamine, there is no functional evidence for the existence of renal vasodilator nerves. While the kidney contains acetylcholinesterase, this is located in the adrenergic nerve terminals and there is no functional evidence for the existence of renal parasympathetic cholinergic innervation. Direct electrical renal nerve stimulation fails to produce a renal vasodilator response in canine kidneys treated with guanethidine or prazosin (α_1-adrenoceptor antagonist).

Control of renal tubular solute and water transport

Renal denervation

Renal denervation results in decreased proximal tubular reabsorption of sodium, chloride, bicarbonate, phosphate, and water in association with an increased urinary excretion of these ions and water. These changes occur in the absence of alterations in single-nephron or whole-kidney GFR or RBF, interstitial or peritubular capillary oncotic or hydrostatic pressure. Renal denervation also decreases water, sodium, and potassium reabsorption in the loop of Henle and decreases water, sodium, and bicarbonate reabsorption in the distal convoluted tubule. Renal denervation decreases proximal tubular Na^+, K^+-ATPase activity and Na^+/H^+ exchange.

The occurrence of denervation diuresis and natriuresis in conscious rats with chronic renal denervation clearly indicate that the renal response to renal denervation is not due to the removal of an artefactually increased level of ERSNA, as is present in anaesthetized, surgically stressed animals. The effects of renal denervation are not transient and have been observed for up to 35 weeks after renal denervation.

In consideration of the effect of renal denervation on urinary water and sodium excretion, the potentially confounding issue of supersensitivity of the vasculature and tubules of the acutely or chronically denervated kidney to circulating noradrenaline is important. There is evidence of both renal vascular and tubular supersensitivity to noradrenaline in the chronically but the not the acutely denervated kidney; however, the plasma noradrenaline concentrations required to demonstrate this are high, producing vasoconstriction with resultant increases in mean arterial pressure and/or decreases in GFR and RBF which could independently influence urinary water and sodium excretion. Thus, it seems unlikely that, at prevailing basal plasma noradrenaline concentrations, supersensitivity of the renal vasculature or tubules of the chronically denervated kidney masks the effect of renal denervation to increase urinary flow rate and sodium excretion. It is known, however, that infusions of noradrenaline that produce physiological increments (<50–100 per cent 'increase) in plasma noradrenaline concentration decrease urinary sodium excretion without affecting mean arterial pressure, GFR, or RBF in both dogs and humans with innervated kidneys.

Direct and reflex activation of the renal nerves (Table 18.1)

Using a frequency of renal nerve stimulation that was subthreshold for renal vasoconstriction, it has been demonstrated in dogs, rabbits, rats, and monkeys that direct low-frequency electrical stimulation of the renal nerves produced a reversible decrease in urinary sodium excretion without a change in renal perfusion pressure, GFR, RBF, or intrarenal distribution of blood flow. Micropuncture techniques localize the increased renal tubular sodium reabsorption to the proximal convoluted tubule, the thick ascending limb of the loop of Henle, and the collecting duct.

Reflex increases in ERSNA produce changes in renal sodium and water handling similar to those seen after direct electrical stimulation of the renal nerves. In both anaesthetized and conscious animals, unloading carotid arterial baroreceptors increases ERSNA and decreases urinary sodium and water excretion without changes in GFR,

Table 18.1. Renal functional responses to graded renal nerve stimulation

Renal nerve stimulation frequency (Hz)	Renin secretion rate	$U_{Na}V$	GFR	RBF
0.25	No effect on basal; modulation of non-neural mechanisms	0	0	0
0.50	Direct neural release from juxtaglomerular granular cells without alterations in stimuli to macula densa receptor or vascular baroreceptor	0	0	0
1.0	Alteration in stimulus to macula densa receptor	↓	0	0
2.5	Alteration in stimulus to vascular baroreceptor	↓	↓	↓

$U_{Na}V$, urinary sodium excretion; GFR, glomerular filtration rate; RBF, renal blood flow.

RBF, or intrarenal distribution of blood flow. The antidiuretic and antinatriuretic responses were shown to be prevented by renal arterial administration of phenoxybenzamine, phentolamine, or guanethidine as well as by renal denervation or carotid sinus nerve section.

Activation of left atrial mechanoreceptors ('cardiopulmonary receptors', 'volume receptors') decreases ERSNA. Distension of the left atrium by inflating a balloon in the left atrium or head-out water immersion produced a reversible decrease in ERSNA which was accompanied by a diuresis and a natriuresis in the absence of changes in renal perfusion pressure, GFR, RBF, or intrarenal distribution of blood flow. The reduction in ERSNA during left atrial receptor stimulation and the accompanying diuresis and natriuresis are mediated by the Paintal-type atrial receptors with myelinated vagal afferent fibres. Left atrial receptor stimulation produces a reflex whose afferent limb is in the vagus nerves (prevented by vagotomy or cardiac denervation) and whose efferent limb for the diuretic response is suppression of ADH release (prevented by hypophysectomy) and for the natriuretic response is suppression of ERSNA (prevented by renal denervation).

Studies in conscious rats, dogs, monkeys, and sheep demonstrate that prior bilateral renal denervation attenuates the diuretic and natriuretic response to acute intravascular volume expansion. These findings indicate that the withdrawal of ERSNA that occurs during the volume expansion is a significant contributor to the diuretic and natriuretic responses observed.

Central nervous system lesions

Although a variety of central nervous system lesions have been associated with alterations in the renal handling of water and solutes, the most extensively characterized lesion is that involving the anteroventral portion of the third ventricle (Johnson 1990). Acutely, there is adipsia, hypernatraemia, and marked extracellular fluid volume depletion. Chronically, there is impaired drinking response to thirst challenges, hypernatraemia, impaired natriuretic response to volume expansion, increased plasma renin activity, and increased blood volume.

Adrenergic receptors

The antinatriuretic response (increased renal tubular sodium reabsorption) is mediated by α_1 (α_{1B} subtype) adrenoceptors located at neuroeffector junctions on the basolateral aspect of the tubule throughout the extent of the nephron. Increased ERSNA (*in vivo*) and noradrenaline (*in vitro*, via α_1-adrenoceptors) increase proximal tubular Na^+, K^+-ATPase activity and Na^+/H^+ exchange.

Non-neuronal dopamine produced locally within the kidney acts as an autocrine or paracrine substance, producing a decrease in renal tubular sodium reabsorption. Aromatic L-amino acid decarboxylase, which converts L-dopa to dopamine, is present in the proximal convoluted tubule and its activity is up-regulated by increased dietary sodium intake. Dopamine, via binding to D_1 receptors, decreases proximal tubular Na^+/H^+ exchange and Na^+, K^+-ATPase activity throughout the nephron, resulting in decreased renal tubular sodium reabsorption and natriuresis.

Role of renal nerves in sodium and water homeostasis

Denervation diuresis and natriuresis is observed in the conscious animal in the absence of anaesthesia and traumatic operative procedures. Chronic renal denervation attenuates the diuretic and natriuretic response to acute intravascular volume expansion in conscious animals. These studies in the conscious state provide compelling evidence for a significant role for ERSNA in the regulation of sodium and water homeostasis under physiological conditions.

As another approach to understanding the role of the renal nerves in sodium homeostasis, investigators have used experimental designs which would test the requirement for intact renal innervation under conditions where there existed a requirement for maximum renal sodium conservation in conscious animals. Severe dietary sodium restriction represents a sufficient challenge to engage maximally all mechanisms required for a normal renal adaptive response in order to avoid a negative Sodium balance. Under such conditions, the absence or malfunction of any one of these redundant mechanisms cannot be made up for by another and a negative sodium balance results. Thus, under these circumstances, renal denervation eliminates an essential mechanism which is revealed by the development of a negative sodium balance. A lesser degree of dietary sodium restriction would not activate maximally this complex multicomponent homeostatic system and elimination of one component (e.g. renal denervation) would not result in a defect in renal sodium conservation. The overall results lend further support to the argument that the dependence of normal renal sodium conservation on intact renal innervation is related to the magnitude of the dietary sodium restriction, with a severe degree of restriction requiring intact renal innervation and lesser degrees of restriction not requiring intact renal innervation. The studies of Gill and Bartter (1966) and Wilcox *et al.* (1977) support the view that intact renal innervation is also essential for the kidney to express its full ability to reabsorb sodium maximally in response to a reduction in dietary sodium intake in humans.

Control of renin secretion

Alterations in renal nerve activity

Renal nerve stimulation at a frequency of 0.3–0.5 Hz results in an increase in renin secretion rate in the absence of changes in renal haemodynamics and urinary sodium excretion; thus the resultant increase in renin secretion rate occurred in the absence of stimulatory input to the vascular baroreceptor and tubular macula densa receptor mechanisms. The increases in renin secretion rate observed with renal nerve stimulation are frequency dependent.

The increase in renal secretion rate that occurs with dietary sodium restriction in human subjects is associated with increased renal noradrenaline spillover as an index of increased ERSNA.

Adrenergic receptors

It is well established that the renin secretion rate response to increases in ERSNA at intensities causing no or minimal changes in renal haemodynamics (low-level renal nerve stimulation) is mediated by activation of renal β_1-adrenoceptors; β_2-adrenoceptors are not involved. There is little doubt that the increase in renin secretion rate produced by renal nerve stimulation at intensities causing marked decreases in urinary sodium excretion and RBF is partly related to activation of vascular and/or tubular α_1 adrenoceptors. The role of α-adrenoceptors in the increase in renin secretion rate produced by renal nerve stimulation at intensities causing minimal renal haemodynamic changes is small. Dopamine increases renin secretion rate by stimulating D_1 receptors located on juxtaglomerular granular cells.

Interaction between neural and non-neural mechanisms

There is an important augmenting interaction between the neural and non-neural mechanisms in the control of renin secretion rate. This is dependent on the level of renal arterial pressure (magnitude of vascular baroreceptor stimulation) and on the intensity of the renal nerve stimulation. At a low magnitude of vascular baroreceptor stimulation (small reduction in renal arterial pressure), a greater intensity of renal nerve stimulation is required for augmentation of renin secretion rate than when the magnitude of vascular baroreceptor stimulation is higher (large reduction in renal arterial pressure). Similarly, studies in humans show that reflex renal nerve stimulation produced by cold pressor stress enhances the increase in renal venous plasma renin activity (PRA) produced by renal arterial pressure reduction.

Body fluid homeostasis and renal function in patients with autonomic failure

This section contains a concise review of studies of body fluid homeostasis, renal function, and relevant hormones in patients with autonomic failure (AF). These studies are of practical interest since they provide a rational basis for management of orthostatic hypertension.

Studies in patients with AF first established the importance of the autonomic nervous system for body fluid homeostasis. In the original description of pure autonomic failure in 1925, the nocturnal polyuria from which these patients often suffer was reported. Thirty years later, abnormal patterns of water and sodium excretion were described which Gill and Bartter (1966) related to failure of the sympathetic nervous system, since they reproduced these defects in normal human subjects by administration of guanethidine. More recently, important differences in key hormones and in body fluid homeostasis have been found between patients whose AF is due to tetraplegia and those with pure AF or multiple system atrophy (MSA).

Body fluid volumes

The median value for plasma volume (PV) derived from a survey of published studies of 53 patients with AF due to pure AF or MSA is 99.2 per cent of normal (Wilcox *et al.* 1984). However, the regulation of PV during changes in sodium intake or posture is clearly abnormal in such patients. When healthy subjects stand or are tilted upright, their blood pressure (BP) does not change substantially, yet PV is reduced by an average of 10 per cent. This orthostatic fall in PV is normally accompanied by a corresponding increase in interstitial volume of the lower limbs due to an increase in the hydraulic pressure in skin and muscle capillaries. In contrast, when patients with AF stand or are tilted upright, there is a sharp fall in BP yet PV is maintained. The absence of a postural decline of PV in patients with AF suggests that the orthostatic fall in BP is sufficient to counter any increase in capillary hydraulic pressure.

During dietary sodium restriction, one study showed that the PV fell by a similar degree in normal subjects and patients with AF, yet the AF patients lost three times as much body weight due to defective renal sodium conservation (see below). Thus, the excessive loss of body fluid derived exclusively from the interstitial (or intracellular) compartment(s). As with head-up tilt, the sharp fall in BP of patients with AF during dietary sodium restriction may have reduced the hydraulic pressure in the capillary bed sufficiently to redistribute interstitial fluid into the intravascular compartment (Wilcox *et al.* 1984).

Preservation of the PV during standing or dietary sodium restriction is a vital last line of defence against catastrophic hypotension. In the absence of effective cardiovascular control mechanisms that normally increase peripheral arterial resistance and reduce venous capacitance, the BP of patients with AF is closely dependent on cardiac output and venous return (Fig. 18.1). Therefore, the initial

fall in BP and cardiac output during standing or sodium depletion may prevent a loss of PV and thereby limit the fall in venous return and progressive hypotension.

Hormonal control of renal function

Renin–angiotensin–aldosterone system

The median value of plasma renin activity (PRA) from a survey of 33 reports in 127 patients with AF due to pure AF, MSA, or diabetes mellitus (DM) is only 53 per cent of normal while the patients are recumbent and only 48 per cent of normal while they are upright. The reduced levels of PRA in patients while upright indicates a profound blunting of renin release since orthostatic hypotension should be a potent stimulus to renin release. Moreover, cardiac output is sharply reduced on standing and this may reduce hepatic blood flow and prolong the circulatory half-life of renin. These blunted renin levels have been ascribed to a defect in renal renin release, probably due to defective ERSNA or subnormal plasma catecholamine concentrations, rather than to a defect in renal renin stores since PRA rises normally in patients with pure AF or MSA during severe hypotension produced by a combination of standing and dietary sodium restriction (Wilcox *et al.* 1977) or in response to infusions of dopamine, isoproterenol (isoprenaline), or furosemide (frusemide).

In striking contrast are the reports of patients with the Riley–Day syndrome or tetraplegia complicating high cervical spinal cord lesions, where the median values for PRA are increased by 688 per cent and 277 per cent, respectively. The reasons for the difference between the elevated values of PRA in these two categories of AF compared to the low values seen in patients with pure AF, MSA, or DM, despite similar degrees of blockade of sympathetic neural reflexes, have not been adequately explained. One theory ascribes the subnormal PRA values in patients with pure AF, MSA, or DM to defective ERSNA. However, an anatomical explanation is unsatisfactory since the dominant lesion in the sympathetic nervous system in patients with MSA is a degenera-

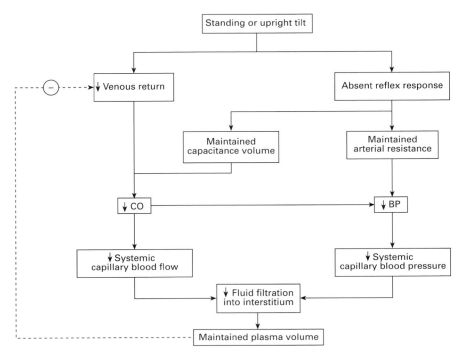

Fig. 18.1. Diagrammatic representation of the cardiovascular responses to orthostasis in patients with autonomic failure. CO, cardiac output; BP, blood pressure.

tion of cells in the intermediolateral column of the cervicolumbar spinal cord, yet their subnormal values of PRA differ radically from the elevated values seen in tetraplegic patients who also have blockade of sympathetic neural reflexes at this site. Tetraplegic patients can have overactive autonomic reflexes which might increase ERSNA and hence renin release. However, Mathias et al. (1980) found that activation of such reflexes in tetraplegics by bladder stimulation, although provoking a rise in BP and plasma noradrenaline levels indicative of widespread spinal sympathetic reflex activation, did not increase PRA. Whereas blockade of β-adrenoceptors with propranolol prevented the rise in PRA that normally occurs during upright tilting in normal subjects, it failed to block the rise in PRA in patients with tetraplegia. Since the PRA of these patients increased normally during infusion of isoproterenol (isoprenaline), indicating that β-adrenoceptor-mediated stimulation of renin release was intact, these authors concluded that the rise in PRA on tilting was not due to residual sympathetic neural reflex activity acting through β-adrenoceptors. They postulated a renal baroreceptor-mediated stimulus to renin release caused by the tilt-induced fall in renal perfusion pressure. However, there remains, first, the problem of explaining the high basal values of PRA in tetraplegic patients while they are recumbent with relatively normal levels of BP and, secondly, the subnormal PRA responses to tilt in patients with pure AF and MSA despite equally impressive orthostatic falls in BP.

As anticipated from the values of PRA, a survey of measurements of the rate of secretion or excretion of aldosterone in 30 patients with pure AF or MSA shows that the median values are only 43 per cent of normal, while plasma aldosterone levels in patients with the Riley–Day syndrome or tetraplegia are normal or raised. The subnormal aldosterone secretion observed in patients with pure AF or amyloidosis was accompanied by a blunted response to short-term stimulation with angiotensin or ACTH. Since more prolonged stimulation provided either by dietary sodium restriction or by prolonged infusions of angiotensin increased aldosterone secretion into the normal range, it was concluded that the low basal values and subnormal short-term responses represented the effects of a prolonged reduction in angiotensin stimulation of the zona glomerulosa of the adrenal gland due to defective renin release.

The regulation of the renin–angiotensin–aldosterone system in patients with DM has attracted considerable interest. PRA is reduced in DM with AF when compared to those with normal autonomic function. However, the interpretation is complicated because patients with advanced DM, but without AF, can have sufficiently low values of PRA and aldosterone to lead to overt hypoaldosteronism with hyperkalaemia and metabolic acidosis (type IV renal tubular acidosis). The suppressed renin–aldosterone axis in these patients with DM has variously been related to hyalinosis of the renin–containing cells in the afferent arteriole, to reduced renin release from prolonged volume expansion, or to a specific defect in renin synthesis. Regardless, it is clear that the cause for hyporeninaemic hypoaldosteronism in DM is usually not AF.

Antidiuretic hormone (ADH)

ADH release is triggered either by a rise in plasma osmolality or by a reduction in blood volume or venous return, leading to reduced stretch of low-pressure receptors in the atria and pulmonary vascular circuit. On standing, there is normally a reduction in central venous pressure and PV which can account for the observed increase in ADH release. Although the osmotic regulation of ADH release appears intact in patients with pure AF or MSA, postural regulation of ADH release is often abnormal. Thus, some patients with MSA cannot dilute their urine normally in response to a water load while standing, which implies an exaggerated postural release of, or response to, ADH (Wilcox et al. 1975). However, other studies have disclosed that patients with MSA can have a blunted postural release of ADH due to abnormal central control via dopaminergic and opiodergic mechanisms in the brainstem (Puritz et al. 1983). Further studies are required to resolve these issues.

Renal haemodynamics

Measurements of RBF and GFR in patients with AF while they are recumbent are usually normal. Moreover, these patients retain normal renal vasoconstrictor responses to infused angiotensin or ADH. During stepwise head-up tilt to progressively reduce the BP, the RBF and GFR are maintained until the lower limits of the autoregulatory response are exceeded at 65–70 mmHg.

Renal sodium conservation

Schalekamp et al. (1985) varied the mean arterial pressure of patients with pure AF by graded tilting. They showed a steep increase in renal sodium and potassium excretion when mean arterial pressure rose above 55–60 mmHg. A concurrent infusion of aldosterone reduced the sodium excretion and increased the potassium excretion. This study illustrates the predominant importance of renal perfusion pressure and mineralocorticosteroids in regulating sodium excretion in patients with pure AF.

Normal subjects given a low dietary sodium intake reduce their renal sodium excretion rapidly over 2–5 days to achieve sodium balance at the lower level of sodium intake. A survey of published reports of 23 patients with pure AF or MSA studied during dietary sodium restriction revealed that renal sodium conservation was impaired in two-thirds; some manifested a remarkable inability to conserve sodium. Wilcox et al. (1977) contrasted renal sodium conservation in a group of five patients with pure AF or MSA with five age-matched controls. As shown in Fig. 18.2, while urinary sodium excretion fell rapidly over 3–5 days in the normal subjects, it was not significantly altered over a week of dietary sodium restriction in those with AF. This excessive sodium loss in the patients with AF was accompanied by a greater loss of body weight, a worsening of orthostatic hypotension, and a deterioration in their clinical state. The worsening orthostatic hypotension was directly related to the fall in PV in these patients. Failure of sodium conservation in patients with AF may be ascribed, in part, to subnormal aldosterone secretion. Administration of a mineralocorticosteroid improves, but does not normalize, sodium homeostasis in these subjects (Wilcox et al. 1977). However, these patients display inappropriately high urinary sodium excretion while they are recumbent even while receiving supramaximal doses of mineralocorticosteroid replacement. This implies additional mineralocorticosteroid-independent defects which may include a reduced action of angiotensin and catecholamines (noradrenaline) to enhance renal tubular sodium and water reabsorption. Interestingly, patients with tetraplegia lack the exaggerated natriuresis of recumbency seen in those with pure AF or MSA, although they do have an exaggerated diuresis. Sutters et al. (1992) have shown also that they can conserve sodium during dietary salt restriction. This difference in sodium concentration was ascribed

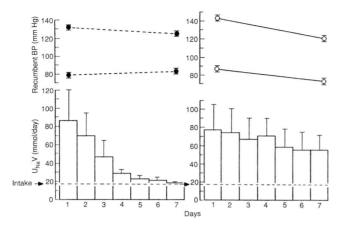

Fig. 18.2. Mean ± SEM values for systolic and diastolic blood pressure (BP) while recumbent and urinary sodium excretion ($U_{Na}V$) in five patients with AF due to pure AF and MSA (right panel, open circles) and five aged-matched control subjects (left panel, closed circles) during 7 days of reduced dietary sodium intake (17 mmol/24 h). Note the failure of the patients with AF to achieve sodium balance and their decrease in BP. (From Wilcox *et al.* (1977), with permission.)

to the higher levels of PRA and aldosterone in tetraplegic subjects. Further studies are required to define the precise role of renal nerves in renal sodium and fluid homeostasis in patients with AF.

Renal sodium wasting in patients with pure AF or MSA provides a rational basis for provision of a liberal sodium intake supplemented, during periods of intercurrent illness or anorexia, with sodium chloride capsules or intravenous sodium chloride solutions. Moreover, subnormal aldosterone levels in these patients can be addressed by administration of a mineralocorticosteroid agent. Indeed, 9-α-fluorocortisone (Fluorinef®) can alleviate orthostatic hypotension due to prolonged bed-rest, DM, pure AF, MSA, and a variety of other categories of AF. Whereas about one-third of patients show a striking benefit, a similar fraction show little or no response and eventually most patients become refractory. Soon after starting treatment with 9-α-fluorocortisone, patients usually retain sodium and fluid; there is an expansion of the PV and the body weight increases by 1–3 kg. However, after some weeks or months of therapy, the PV and body weight return to baseline yet some improvement in orthostatic hypotension persists (Schalekamp *et al.* 1985). This apparent improvement in autonomic control of the circulation has been ascribed to an enhanced vascular responsiveness to noradrenaline, since 9-α-fluorocortisone can increase the pressor sensitivity to infused noradrenaline in patients with pure AF or MSA independent of sodium or fluid retention.

Overzealous treatment with 9-α-fluorocortisone and sodium chloride can lead to excessive sodium and fluid retention, recumbent hypertension, potassium depletion and alkalosis. This requires a temporary discontinuation of therapy which can later be restarted at a reduced dosage.

Effects of posture on sodium and fluid excretion

Some patients with pure AF or MSA are troubled with nocturnal polyuria which can reduce extracellular fluid volume (ECV) in the morning sufficiently to worsen orthostatic hypotension. Patients with

MSA have a normal capacity to eliminate a water load while recumbent, yet a subnormal diuretic response while standing due to an inability to dilute the urine maximally (Wilcox *et al.* 1975). Conversely, during prolonged water deprivation, urine flow and sodium excretion decrease, and urine osmolality increases normally during standing, yet these changes in patients with AF are reversed during recumbency. Two mechanisms have been identified which could account for these striking effects of posture. First, Schalekamp *et al.* (1985) demonstrated a steep relationship between arterial pressure and sodium excretion in patients with pure AF. Therefore, the greater diuresis and natriuresis while recumbent may relate to higher BP. Secondly, patients with AF may have exaggerated postural changes in central blood volume due to excessive pooling of blood in the periphery on standing and excessive return of blood to the central compartment on lying down. These excessive postural changes could generate exaggerated responses by the low pressure volume receptors that would be complemented by exaggerated responses by the high pressure baroreceptors due to the orthostatic decreases in BP. Therefore, any intact volume-sensitive mechanism may generate abnormal signals that could dictate excessive postural changes in renal function. One such mechanism could be the release of atrial natriuretic peptide. A second may be release of ADH which is regulated by low-pressure receptors. Indeed, measurements in one subject with MSA demonstrated excessive postural changes in ADH excretion (Wilcox *et al.* 1975), although this was not confirmed in a later study of plasma ADH concentration during tilting (Puritz *et al.* 1983). Thus, a role for ADH in the abnormal diuresis of recumbency in patients with AF has yet to be defined clearly. As described above, tetrapelgic patients also show an excessive diuresis when recumbent, but, unlike those with pure AF or MSA, they do not have major posture-induced changes in sodium excretion. The neuroendocrine factors that contribute to maintenance of the plasma volume during orthostasis, and major sites of abnormality in patients with AF, are reviewed in Fig. 18.3.

The demonstration of an inappropriate diuresis and natriuresis in patients with pure AF or MSA while recumbent provides a rational basis for postural therapy whereby the patient is kept in the semisitting position at night. Such a change in posture can diminish the recumbency-induced natriuresis and diuresis of patients with pure AF or MSA and thereby prevent the ensuing worsening of orthostatic hypotension during the following morning. Where such postural therapy is effective, patients often gain 1–3 g in weight and have a diminished orthostatic fall in BP. Postural therapy may be combined with 9-α-fluorocortisone. In contrast, the normal or elevated values for renin and aldosterone in tetraplegic patients, together with the absence of a recumbency-induced natriuresis, or clear evidence of sodium wasting in this group of patients, suggest that postural therapy or supplementary 9-α-fluorocortisone may not be of major benefit to them.

Renal consequences of denervation following human cardiac or renal transplantation

The transplantation of a donor heart into a subject with normal kidneys, or the replacement of diseased kidneys with a functioning

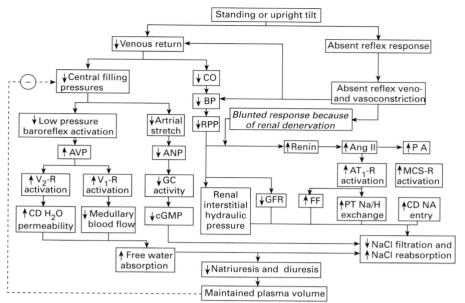

Fig. 18.3. Diagrammatic representation of the neuroendocrine response to orthostasis and factors that protect against plasma volume depletion. CO, cardiac output; BP, blood pressure; RPP, renal perfusion pressure; AVP, arginine vasopressin (antidiuretic hormone, ADH); ANP, atrial natriuretic peptide; V_1-R and V_2-R, vasopressin receptors, types 1 and 2; GC, guanylyl cyclase; CD, collecting duct; cGMP, cyclic guanosine 3′,5′-monophosphate; GFR, glomerular filtration rate; FF, filtration fraction; Ang II, angiotensin II; PA, plasma aldosterone; AT_1-R, angiotensin II type 1 receptor; MCS-R, mineralocorticosteroid receptor; PT, proximal tubule.

renal transplant, provides a unique opportunity to study the role of sympathetic neural control of renal function in man. Unfortunately, interpretation is complicated by the often profound effects of antirejection therapy, notably with cyclosporin A or FK-506 (Sander and Victor 1995). These agents contribute to renal vasoconstriction and hypertension, which is typically low-renin and salt sensitive. Cyclosporin induces preferential pre-renal vasoconstriction. Nevertheless, recent studies by Braith *et al.* (1996, 1998) have dissociated the effects of cyclosporin from those of cardiac denervation by contrasting renal function and fluid volume homeostasis in normal subjects, patients receiving cyclosporin for liver transplant, and patients receiving an equal cyclosporin dose but with cardiac denervation following cardiac transplantation. The results demonstrated a striking failure of patients following cardiac transplantation to respond appropriately to a modest isotonic saline load. Unlike the controls or those receiving cyclosporin for liver transplantation, the cardiac transplant recipients responded to the isotonic saline infusion with paradoxical increases in PRA, plasma angiotensin II, plasma aldosterone, and plasma ADH concentrations and an exaggerated increase in plasma atrial natriuretic peptide concentration. Again, in contrast to the controls, their BP rose linearly with increasing isotonic saline infusion. Despite the increase in BP, they exhibited a blunted natriuretic and diuretic response. These studies demonstrate graphically the role of cardiac afferent nerves in volume-sensing mechanisms and their critical role in co-ordinating neurohumoral and renal excretory responses to isotonic saline volume loading. In the absence of cardiac innervation, the appreciation of a volume load is diminished and the renal excretory response is influenced predominantly by the increases in BP and plasma atrial natriuretic peptide concentration.

Two recent studies have examined renal function following renal transplantation in subjects with good post-transplant GFR. Hansen *et al.* (1994) showed that, in patients transplanted more than 2 years previously, there was a supersensitive renal vasoconstrictor response to infused noradrenaline and a failure to engage reflex renal vasoconstriction during lower-body negative pressure. This study suggested that these human transplanted kidneys were not completely function-

ally reinnervated. A second study by Rabelink *et al.* (1993), of patients between 24 and 56 days following renal transplantation, examined the renal response to an increase in central blood volume induced by head-out water immersion. The patients failed to exhibit the normal increase in RBF and decrease in renal vascular resistance and failed to suppress PRA. However, the patients had elevated levels of plasma atrial natriuretic peptide and exhibited appropriate rates of urinary sodium excretion and urine flow. This study suggests that renal sympathetic nerves are required for precise volume-sensitive regulation of renal haemodynamics and renin release.

Collectively, the studies on cardiac transplantation have shown the quantitative importance of cardiac afferent innervation for volume sensing in man, while those on renal transplantation have shown that renal sympathetic nerves are also required for precise regulation of renal function in response to alterations in body fluid volumes.

Acknowledgements

Work from the laboratory of GFD was supported by National Institutes of Health grants DK 15843 and HL 55006 and by the Veterans Administration. Work from the laboratory of CSW was supported by National Institutes of Health grants DK 36079 and DK 49870 and from the George E. Schreiner Chair of Nephrology.

References

Braith, R. W., Mills, R. M., Wilcox, C. S., Convertino, V. A., Davis, G. L., and Wood, C. E. (1996). Breakdown of blood pressure and body fluid homeostasis in heart transplant recipients. *J. Am. Coll. Cardiol.* **27**, 375–83.

Braith, R. W., Mills, R. M. Jr., Wilcox, C. S., Convertino, V. A., Davis, G. L., and Wood, C. E. (1996). Fluid homeostasis after heart transplantation: the role of cardiac denervation. *J. Heart Lung Transpl.*, **15**, 872–80.

DiBona, G. F. and Kopp, U. C. (1997). Neural control of renal function. *Physiol. Rev.* **77**, 75–197.

Gill, J. R. and Bartter, F. C. (1966). Adrenergic nervous system in sodium metabolism. II. Effects of guanethidine on the renal response to sodium deprivation in normal man. *New Eng. J. Med.* **275**, 1466–71.

Hansen, J. M., Abildgaard, U., Fogh-Andersen, N. *et al.* (1994). The transplanted human kidney does not achieve functional reinnervation. *Clin. Sci.* **87**, 13–20.

Johnson, A. K. (1990). Brain mechanisms in the control of body fluid homeostasis. In *Perspectives in exercise science and sports medicine, vol. 3: fluid homeostasis during exercise*, (ed. C. V. Gisolfi and D. R. Lamb), pp. 347–424. Benchmark, Carmel, Indiana.

Mathias, C. J., Christensen, N. J., Frankel, H. L., and Peart, W. S. (1980). Renin release during head-up tilt occurs independently of sympathetic nervous activity in tetraplegic man. *Clin. Sci.* **59**, 251–6.

Puritz, R., Lightman, S. L., Wilcox, C. S., Forsling, M., and Bannister, R. (1983). Blood pressure and vasopressin in progressive autonomic failure: response to postural stimulation, l-dopa and naloxone. *Brain* **106**, 503–11.

Rabelink, T. J., van Tilborg, K. A., Hené, R. J., and Koomans, H. A. (1993). Natriuretic response to head-out immersion in humans with recent kidney transplants. *Clin. Sci.* **85**, 471–7.

Sander, M. and Victor, R. G. (1995). Hypertension after cardiac transplantation: pathophysiology and management. *Curr. Opin. Nephrol. Hypertens.* **4**, 443–51.

Schalekamp, M. A. D. H., Man in't Veld, A. J., and Wenting, G. J. (1985). The second Sir George Pickering Memorial Lecture: What regulates whole body autoregulation? Clinical observations. *J. Hypertension.* **3**, 97–107.

Sutters, M., Wakefield, C., O'Neil, K. *et al.* (1992). The cardiovascular, endocrine and renal response of tetraplegic and paraplegic subjects to dietary sodium restriction. *J. Physiol.* **457**, 515–23.

Wilcox, C. S., Aminoff, M. J., and Penn, W. (1975). The basis of the nocturnal polyuria in patients with autonomic failure. *J. Neurol. Neurosurg. Psychiat.* **37**, 677–84.

Wilcox, C. S., Aminoff, M. J., and Slater, J. D. H. (1977). Sodium homeostasis in patients with autonomic failure. *Clin. Sci.* **53**, 321–8.

Wilcox, C. S., Puritz, R., Lightman, S. L., Bannister, R., and Aminoff, M. J. (1984). Plasma volume regulation in patients with progressive autonomic failure during changes in salt intake or posture. *J. Lab. Clin. Med.* **104**, 331–9.

19. Neural control of the urinary bladder and sexual organs

William C. de Groat

Introduction

Various functions of the urogenital tract are controlled by extrinsic nervous pathways that involve neurones in the brain, spinal cord, and peripheral ganglia. Many of these functions are complex, requiring the participation of somatic as well as autonomic efferent mechanisms and the integration of neural and endocrine systems. Due to the complexities of the neurohumoral factors regulating the urogenital organs, the activities of these organs are sensitive to a wide variety of injuries, diseases, and chemicals which affect the nervous system. Thus, neurological mechanisms are an important consideration in the diagnosis and treatment of disorders of the urogenital tract.

This chapter will review experimental studies in animals which have provided insights into the anatomical organization and the transmitters involved in the neural control of urogenital function.

Innervation of the lower urinary tract

The storage and periodic elimination of urine is dependent upon the activity of two functional units in the lower urinary tract: (1) a reservoir (the urinary bladder) and (2) an outlet, consisting of bladder neck, urethra, and striated muscles of the urethral sphincter. These structures are, in turn, controlled by three sets of peripheral nerves: sacral parasympathetic (pelvic nerves), thoracolumbar sympathetic (hypogastric nerves and sympathetic chain), and sacral somatic nerves (pudendal nerves) (Fig. 19.l) (de Groat et al. 1993).

Sacral parasympathetic pathways

The sacral parasympathetic outflow provides the major excitatory input to the urinary bladder. Cholinergic preganglionic neurones located in the intermediolateral region of the sacral spinal cord send axons via the pelvic nerves to ganglion cells in the pelvic plexus and in the wall of the bladder. Transmission in bladder ganglia is mediated by a nicotinic cholinergic mechanism, which can be modulated by activation of various receptors including muscarinic, adrenergic, purinergic, and peptidergic (Table 19.1) (de Groat and Booth 1993a). Ganglia in some species (cats and rabbits) also exhibit a prominent frequency-dependent facilitatory mechanism that can amplify parasympathetic activity passing from the spinal cord to the bladder. The ganglion cells in turn excite bladder smooth muscle via the release of cholinergic (acetylcholine) and non-cholinergic, non-adrenergic transmitters. Cholinergic excitatory transmission in the bladder is mediated by muscarinic receptors, which are blocked by

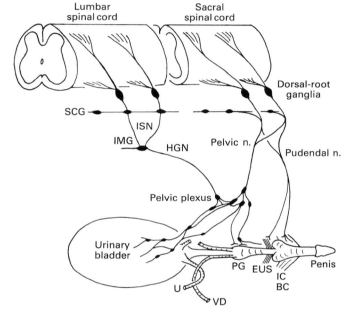

Fig. 19.1. Diagram showing the sympathetic, parasympathetic, and somatic innervation of the urogenital tract of the male cat. Sympathetic preganglionic pathways emerge from the lumbar spinal cord and pass to the sympathetic chain ganglia (SCG) and then via the inferior splanchnic nerves (ISN) to the inferior mesenteric ganglia (IMG). Preganglionic and postganglionic sympathetic axons then travel in the hypogastric nerve (HGN) to the pelvic plexus and the urogenital organs. Parasympathetic preganglionic axons which originate in the sacral spinal cord pass in the pelvic nerve to ganglion cells in the pelvic plexus and to distal ganglia in the organs. Sacral somatic pathways are contained in the pudendal nerve, which provides an innervation to the penis, the ischiocavernosus (IC), bulbocavernosus (BC), and external urethral sphincter (EUS) muscles. The pudendal and pelvic nerves also receive postganglionic axons from the caudal sympathetic chain ganglia. These three sets of nerves contain afferent axons from the lumbosacral dorsal root ganglia. Abbreviations: ureter (U), prostate gland (PG), vas deferens (VD).

atropine, whereas non-cholinergic transmission is mediated by the purinergic transmitter, adenosine triphosphate (ATP), acting on P_{2X} purinergic receptors (Table 19.1). Modulatory receptors are also present prejunctionally on parasympathetic nerve terminals. Activation of these receptors by acetylcholine can enhance (M_1 receptors) or suppress (M_4 receptors) transmitter release, depending upon the intensity of neural firing (Somogyi et al. 1996). Inhibitory input

Table 19.1. Receptors for putative transmitters in the lower urinary tract*

Tissue	Cholinergic	Adrenergic	Other
Bladder body	+ [M_2] + [M_3]	− [β_2] + [α_1]	+ Purinergic [P_{2x}] − VIP + PG + Substance P
Bladder base	+ [M_2] + [M_3]	+ [α_1]	+ Purinergic [P_{2x}] − VIP
Ganglia	+ [N] + [M_1]	+ [α_1] − [α_2] + [β]	− Enkephalinergic [δ] ± Purinergic [P_1, P_{2x}] + Substance P
Urethra	+ [M]	+ [α_1] + [α_2] − [β_2]	− NO ± Purinergic [P_{2x}] − VIP
Parasympathetic terminals	+ [M_1] − [M_4]	+ [α_1] − [α_2]	− NPY + 5HT
Afferent neurones			+ CAPS + PG + Purinergic [P_{2x}]
Sphincter striated muscle	+ [N]		

Letters in parentheses indicate receptor type, e.g. M (muscarinic) and N (nicotinic).

+, excitatory; −, inhibitory. CAPS, capsaicin; PG, prostaglandins; NO, nitric oxide.

See text for other abbreviations.

to the urethral smooth muscle is mediated by nitric oxide released by parasympathetic nerves (Andersson 1993). Postganglionic neurones innervating the bladder also contain neuropeptides, such as vasoactive intestinal polypeptide (VIP), neuropeptide Y (NPY), and enkephalin. These substances are co-released with acetylcholine or ATP and may function as modulators of neuroeffector transmission.

Thoracolumbar sympathetic pathways

Sympathetic pathways to the lower urinary tract originate in the lumbosacral sympathetic chain ganglia as well as in the prevertebral inferior mesenteric ganglia (de Groat *et al.* 1993). Input from the sacral chain ganglia passes to the bladder via the pelvic nerves, whereas fibres from the rostral lumbar and inferior mesenteric ganglia travel in the hypogastric nerves. Sympathetic efferent pathways in the hypogastric and pelvic nerves in the cat elicit similar effects in the bladder, consisting of:

(1) inhibition of detrusor muscle via β-adrenergic receptors;

(2) excitation of the bladder base and urethra via α_1-receptors; and

(3) inhibition and facilitation in bladder parasympathetic ganglia via α_2- and α_1-receptors, respectively (Table 19.1) (de Groat and Booth 1993*a*).

Somatic efferent pathways

The efferent innervation of the urethral striated muscles in various species originates from cells in a circumscribed region of the lateral ventral horn which is termed Onuf's nucleus. Sphincter motoneurones send their axons into the pudendal nerve and excite sphincter muscles via the release of acetylcholine which stimulates postjunctional nicotinic receptors.

Afferent pathways

Afferent axons innervating the urinary tract are present in the three sets of nerves (de Groat *et al.* 1993). The most important afferents for initiating micturition are those passing in the pelvic nerve to the sacral spinal cord. These afferents are small myelinated (Aδ) and unmyelinated (C) fibres, which convey information from receptors in the bladder wall to second-order neurones in the spinal cord. Aδ bladder afferents in the cat respond in a graded manner to passive distension as well as active contraction of the bladder and exhibit pressure thresholds in the range of 5–15 mmHg, which are similar to those pressures at which humans report the first sensation of bladder filling. These fibres also code for noxious stimuli in the bladder. On the other hand, C-fibre bladder afferents in the cat have very high thresholds and commonly do not respond to even high levels of intravesical pressure. However, activity in some of these afferents is unmasked or enhanced by chemical irritation of the bladder mucosa. These findings indicate that C-fibre afferents in the cat have specialized functions, such as the signalling of inflammatory or noxious events in the lower urinary tract. In the rat, A-fibre and C-fibre bladder afferents can not be distinguished on the basis of stimulus modality; thus both types of afferents consist of mechanosensitive and chemosensitive populations. C-fibre afferents are also sensitive to the neurotoxin capsaicin (Maggi 1993). Approximately 70 per cent of bladder afferent neurones in the rat are of the capsaicin-sensitive, C-fibre type.

Reflex control of the lower urinary tract

The neural pathways controlling lower urinary tract function are organized as simple on–off switching circuits (Figs 19.2, 19.3) that maintain a reciprocal relationship between the urinary bladder and urethral outlet. The principal reflex components of these switching circuits are listed in Table 19.2 and illustrated in Figs 19.4 and 19.5. Intravesical pressure measurements during bladder filling in both humans and animals reveal low and relatively constant bladder pressures when bladder volume is below the threshold for inducing voiding (Fig. 19.3a). The accommodation of the bladder to increasing volumes of urine is primarily a passive phenomenon dependent upon the intrinsic properties of the vesical smooth muscle and quiescence of the parasympathetic efferent pathway. In addition, in some species urine storage is also facilitated by sympathetic reflexes which mediate an inhibition of bladder activity, closure of the bladder neck, and contraction of the proximal urethra (Table 19.2, Fig. 19.4). During bladder filling the activity of the sphincter electromyogram (EMG) also increases (Fig. 19.3b), reflecting an increase in efferent firing in the pudendal nerve and an increase in outlet resistance which contributes to the maintenance of urinary continence.

The storage phase of the urinary bladder can be switched to the voiding phase either involuntarily (reflexly) or voluntarily (Fig. 19.3). The former is readily demonstrated in the human infant (Fig. 19.3a).

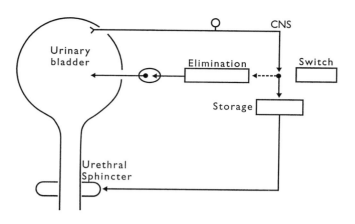

Fig. 19.2. Diagram illustrating the anatomy of the lower urinary tract and the switch-like function of the micturition reflex pathway. During urine storage, a low level of afferent activity activates efferent input to the urethral sphincter. A high level of afferent activity induced by bladder distention activates the switching circuit in the central nervous system (CNS), producing firing in the efferent pathways to the bladder, inhibition of the efferent outflow to the sphincter, and urine elimination.

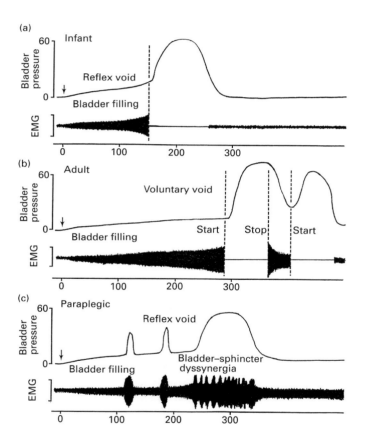

Fig. 19.3. Combined cystometrograms and sphincter electromyograms (EMG) comparing reflex voiding responses in an infant (a) and in a paraplegic patient (c) with a voluntary voiding response in an adult (b). The abscissa in all records represents bladder volume in millilitres and the ordinates represent bladder pressure in cmH$_2$O and electrical activity of the EMG recording. On the left side of each trace the arrows indicate the start of a slow infusion of fluid into the bladder (bladder filling). Vertical dashed lines indicate the start of sphincter relaxation which precedes by a few seconds the bladder contraction in (a) and (b). In part (b) note that a voluntary cessation of voiding (stop) is associated with an initial increase in sphincter EMG followed by a reciprocal relaxation of the bladder. A resumption of voiding is again associated with sphincter relaxation and a delayed increase in bladder pressure. On the other hand, in the paraplegic patient (c) the reciprocal relationship between bladder and sphincter is abolished. During bladder filling, transient uninhibited bladder contractions occur in association with sphincter activity. Further filling leads to more prolonged and simultaneous contractions of the bladder and sphincter (bladder–sphincter dyssynergia). Loss of the reciprocal relationship between bladder and sphincter in paraplegic patients interferes with bladder emptying.

Table 19.2. Reflexes to the lower urinary tract

Afferent pathway	Efferent pathway		Central pathway
Urine storage Low-level vesical afferent activity (pelvic nerve)	1.	External sphincter contraction (somatic nerves)	Spinal reflexes
	2.	Internal sphincter contraction (sympathetic nerves)	
	3.	Detrusor inhibition (sympathetic nerves)	
	4.	Ganglionic inhibition (sympathetic nerves)	
	5.	Sacral parasympathetic outflow inactive	
Micturition High level vesical afferent activity (pelvic nerve)	1.	Inhibition of external sphincter activity	Sphinobulbospinal reflexes
	2.	Inhibition of sympathetic outflow	
	3.	Activation of parasympathetic outflow to the bladder	
	4.	Activation of parasympathetic outflow to the urethra	Spinal reflex

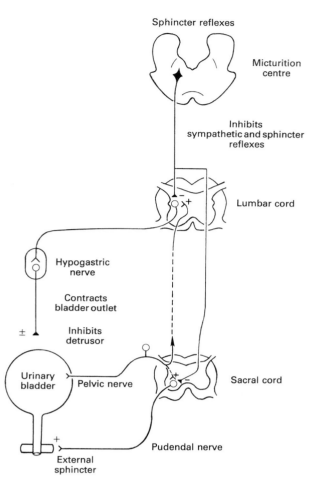

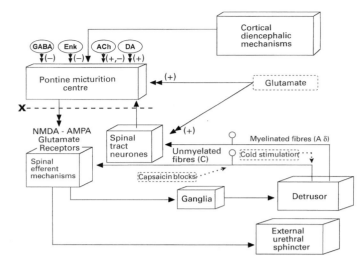

Fig. 19.4. Diagram showing detrusor–sphincter reflexes. During the storage of urine, distention of the bladder produces low-level vesical afferent firing, which in turn stimulates (1) the sympathetic outflow to the bladder outlet (base and urethra) and (2) pudendal outflow to the external urethral sphincter. These responses occur by spinal reflex pathways and represent 'guarding reflexes', which promote continence. Sympathetic firing also inhibits detrusor muscle and transmission in bladder ganglia. At the initiation of micturition, intense vesical afferent activity activates the brainstem micturition centre, which inhibits the spinal guarding reflexes.

Fig. 19.5. Diagram of the central reflex pathways that regulate micturition in the cat. In an animal with an intact neuraxis, micturition is initiated by a supraspinal reflex pathway passing through the pontine micturition centre (PMC) in the brainstem. The pathway is triggered by myelinated afferents (Aδ) connected to tension receptors in the bladder wall (detrusor). Spinal-tract neurones carry information to the brain. During micturition, pathways from the PMC activate the parasympathetic outflow to the bladder and inhibit the somatic outflow to the urethral sphincter. Transmission in the PMC is modulated by cortical–diencephalic mechanisms. In spinal-cord-transected animals, connections between the brainstem and the sacral spinal cord are interrupted and micturition is initially blocked. In chronic spinal animals, a spinal micturition reflex emerges which is triggered by unmyelinated (C-fibre) bladder afferents. The C-fibre reflex pathway is usually weak or undetectable in animals with an intact nervous system. Stimulation of the C-fibre bladder afferents by instillation of ice-water into the bladder (cold stimulation) activates voiding reflexes in patients with spinal-cord injury. Capsaicin (20–30 mg/kg, subcutaneously) blocks the C-fibre reflexes in chronic spinal cats, but does not block micturition reflexes in intact cats. Intravesical capsaicin also suppresses detrusor hyper-reflexia and cold-evoked reflexes in patients with neurogenic bladder dysfunction. Glutamic acid is the principal excitatory transmitter in the ascending and descending limbs of the micturition reflex pathway, as well as in the reflex pathway controlling sphincter function. Glutamate acts on both NMDA and AMPA glutamatergic receptors. Other neurotransmitters that regulate transmission in the micturition reflex pathway include: γ-aminobutyric acid (GABA), enkephalins (Enk), acetylcholine (ACh), and dopamine (DA). ACh has both excitatory and inhibitory effects on the pathway; (+), excitatory and (–), inhibitory synapses.

or in the aneaesthetized animal when the volume of urine exceeds the micturition threshold. At this point, increased afferent firing from tension receptors in the bladder reverses the pattern of efferent outflow, producing firing in the sacral parasympathetic pathways and inhibition of sympathetic and somatic pathways. The expulsion phase consists of an initial relaxation of the urethral sphincter (Fig. 19.3a) followed in a few seconds by a contraction of the bladder, an increase in bladder pressure, and flow of urine. Relaxation of the urethral outlet is mediated by activation of a parasympathetic reflex pathway to the urethra (Table 19.2) that triggers the release of nitric oxide, an inhibitory transmitter (Andersson 1993), as well as by removal of adrenergic and somatic cholinergic excitatory inputs to the urethra. Secondary reflexes elicited by flow of urine through the urethra facilitate bladder emptying (de Groat et al. 1993).

These reflexes require the integrative action of neuronal populations at various levels of the neuraxis (Figs. 19.4 and 19.5). Certain reflexes, for example those mediating the excitatory outflow to the sphincters and the sympathetic inhibitory outflow to the bladder, are organized at the spinal level (Fig. 19.4), whereas the parasympathetic outflow to the detrusor has a more complicated central organization involving spinal and spinobulbospinal pathways (Fig. 19.5).

Anatomy of central nervous pathways controlling the lower urinary tract

The reflex circuitry controlling micturition consists of four basic components: spinal efferent neurones, spinal interneurones, primary afferent neurones and neurones in the brain that modulate spinal reflex pathways. New research methodologies, including transneuronal virus tracing, measurements of gene expression, and patch-clamp recording in spinal cord slice preparations, have recently provided new insights into the morphological and electrophysiological properties of these reflex components (de Groat *et al.* 1993, 1995). Neurotropic viruses, such as pseudorabies virus (PRV), have been particularly useful since they can be injected into a target organ (urinary bladder, urethra, urethral sphincter), from which they move intra-axonally, from the periphery to the central nervous system, where they replicate and then pass retrogradely across synapses to infect second- and third-order neurones in the neural pathways (Nadelhaft and Vera 1995; Vizzard *et al.* 1995). Since PRV can be transported across many synapses, it can sequentially infect all of the neurones that connect directly or indirectly to the lower urinary tract (Fig. 19.6).

Pathways in the spinal cord

The spinal-cord grey matter is divided into three general regions:

(1) the dorsal horn, which contains interneurones that process sensory input;

(2) the ventral horn, which contains motoneurones; and

(3) an intermediate region located between the dorsal and ventral horns which contains interneurones and autonomic preganglionic neurones.

These regions are further subdivided into layers or laminae which are numbered, starting with the superficial layer of the dorsal horn (lamina I) and extending to the ventral horn (lamina IX) and the commissure connecting the two sides of the spinal cord (lamina X) (Fig. 19.7d).

Preganglionic neurones

Parasympathetic preganglionic neurones innervating the lower urinary tract are located in the intermediolateral grey matter (laminae V–VII) in the sacral segments of the spinal cord (Fig. 19.6); whereas sympathetic preganglionic neurones are located in both medial (lamina X) and lateral sites (laminae V–VII) in the rostral lumbar spinal cord. As shown in Fig. 19.8, parasympathetic preganglionic neurones send dendrites to discrete regions of the spinal cord, including:

(1) the lateral and dorsal lateral funiculus;

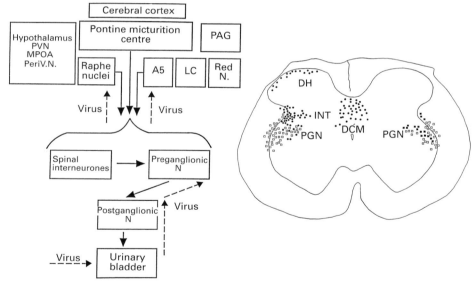

Fig. 19.6. Transneuronal virus tracing of the central pathways controlling the urinary bladder of the rat. Injection of pseudorabies virus into the wall of the urinary bladder leads to retrograde transport of virus (dashed arrows) and sequential infection of postganglionic neurones, preganglionic neurones, and then various central neural circuits synaptically linked to the preganglionic neurones. Normal synaptic connections are indicated by solid arrows. At long survival times virus can be detected with immunocytochemical techniques in neurones at specific sites throughout the spinal cord and brain, extending to the pontine micturition centre in the pons (i.e. Barrington's nucleus) and to the cerebral cortex. Other sites in the brain labelled by virus are: (1) the paraventricular nucleus (PVN), medial preoptic area (MPOA) and periventricular nucleus (Peri V.N.) of the hypothalamus; (2) periaqueductal grey (PAG); (3) locus coeruleus (LC) and subcoeruleus; (4) red nucleus; (5) medullary raphe nuclei; and (6) the noradrenergic cell group designated A5. L6 Spinal-cord section, showing on the left side the distribution of virus-labelled parasympathetic preganglionic neurones (□) and interneurones (●) in the region of the parasympathetic nucleus, the dorsal commissure (DCM), and the superficial laminae of the dorsal horn (DH), 72 h after injection of the virus into the bladder. The right side shows the entire population of preganglionic neurones (PGN) (□) labelled by axonal tracing with the fluorescent dye (fluorogold), injected into the pelvic ganglia and the distribution of virus-labelled bladder PGN (■). Composite diagram of neurones in 12 spinal sections (42 μm). (From de Groat 1995).

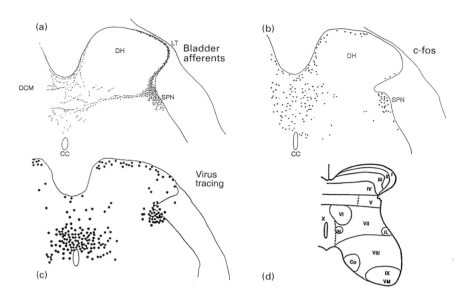

Fig. 19.7. Comparison of the distribution of bladder afferent projections to the L6 spinal cord of the rat (a), with the distribution of c-*fos*-positive cells in the L6 spinal segment following chemical irritation of the lower urinary tract of the rat (b), and the distribution of interneurones in the L6 spinal cord labelled by transneuronal transport of pseudorabies virus injected into the urinary bladder (c). Afferents labelled by WGA-HRP injected into the urinary bladder. C-*fos* immunoreactivity is present in the nuclei of cells. DH, dorsal horn; SPN, sacral parasympathetic nucleus; CC central canal. Calibration represents 500 μm. (Modified from de Groat *et al.* 1993). (d) The laminar organization of the cat spinal cord. (From Rexed, B. 1952). These data show that spinal interneurones involved in the reflex control of the urinary bladder are concentrated in specific regions of the spinal cord that receive afferent input from the lower urinary tract. Some of these interneurones provide excitatory input to the parasympathetic preganglionic neurones and represent an essential component of the spinal micturition reflex pathway.

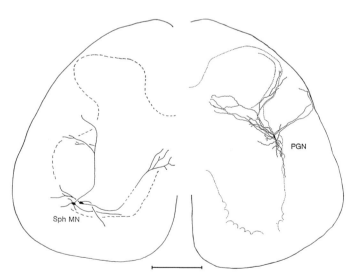

Fig. 19.8. Comparison of the dendritic distributions of external urethral sphincter motoneurones (left side) and a sacral parasympathetic preganglionic neurone (right side) in the cat. The sacral preganglionic neurones which was filled intracellularly with neurobiotin, exhibits dendrites which extend into: (1) the lateral funiculus, (2) lateral lamina I, (3) the dorsal commissure, and (4) within the sacral autonomic nucleus. Dendrites were reconstructed from serial sections extending 500 μm rostral and caudal to the cell body. Two sphincter motoneurones (left side) were labelled by retrograde axonal transport following injections of cholera toxin-HRP into the external urethral sphincter. Although the dendritic distributions are incomplete, they show prominent dendritic projections of one cell to lamina X around the central canal and projections of another cell to the intermediolateral region. Right and left sides are at sightly different rostrocaudal levels. Calibration represents 500 μm. (From de Groat *et al.* 1993). These data, coupled with results shown in Fig. 19.7, show that the dendritic distribution of preganglionic and sphincter efferent neurones coincides with the distribution of bladder interneurones and primary afferent pathways

(2) lamina I on the lateral edge of the dorsal horn;

(3) the dorsal grey commissure (lamina X); and

(4) grey matter and lateral funiculus ventral to the autonomic nucleus.

This dendritic structure very likely indicates the origin of important synaptic inputs to these cells.

Sphincter motoneurones

Retrograde axonal tracing has identified pudendal motoneurones innervating the external urethral sphincter (EUS). In the cat, EUS motoneurones are located in the ventrolateral division of Onuf's nucleus and send dendritic projections into:

(1) the lateral funiculus;

(2) lamina X;

(3) intermediolateral grey matter; and

(4) rostrocaudally within the nucleus (Fig. 19.8).

Thus, the dendritic distribution of sphincter motoneurones is similar to that of sacral preganglionic neurones, indicating that these two populations of neurones may receive synaptic inputs from the same interneuronal and fibre tracts in the spinal cord.

Afferent projections in the spinal cord

Afferent pathways from the lower urinary tract (LUT) project to discrete regions of the dorsal horn that contain interneurones as well as the soma and/or dendrites of efferent neurones innervating the LUT. Pelvic nerve afferent pathways from the urinary bladder of the cat and rat project into Lissauer's tract at the apex of the dorsal horn and then pass rostrocaudally, giving off collaterals that extend laterally and medially through the superficial layer of the dorsal horn (lamina I) into the deeper layers (laminae V–VII and X) at the base of the dorsal horn (Fig. 19.7a). The lateral pathway, which is the most prominent projection, terminates in the region of the sacral parasympathetic nucleus and also sends some axons to the dorsal commissure (Fig. 19.7a). Pudendal afferent pathways from the urethra and urethral sphincter exhibit a similar pattern of termination in the sacral spinal cord (de Groat et al. 1993); whereas pudendal afferent pathways from cutaneous receptors (e.g. penis) have a prominent projection to deeper layers of the dorsal horn and the dorsal commissure. The overlap of bladder and urethral afferents in the lateral dorsal horn and dorsal commissure indicates that these regions are likely to be important sites of viscerosomatic integration and involved in co-ordinating bladder and sphincter activity.

Immunohistochemical studies have shown that a large percentage of bladder afferent neurones contain peptides, including calcitonin-gene-related peptide (CGRP), vasoactive intestinal polypeptide (VIP), substance P, and enkephalins. In the spinal cord, certain peptidergic afferent terminals, e.g. VIP, have a distribution very similar to that of bladder afferents. Nerves containing these peptides are also common in the bladder wall within the subepithelial and submucosal layers and around blood vessels.

Spinal interneurones

As shown in Figs 19.6 and 19.7, interneurones retrogradely labelled by injection of pseudorabies virus into the urinary bladder of the rat are located in regions of the spinal cord receiving afferent input from the bladder (de Groat et al. 1995; Nadelhaft and Vera 1995; Vizzard

et al. 1995). Large populations of interneurones are located just dorsal and medial to the preganglionic neurones as well as in the dorsal commissure and lamina I (Figs 19.6 and 19.7b). A similar distribution of labelled interneurones has been noted following injections of virus into the urethra or the external urethral sphincter, indicating a prominent overlap of the interneuronal pathways controlling the various target organs of the lower urinary tract.

The spinal neurones involved in processing afferent input from the lower urinary tract have been identified by the expression of the immediate early gene, c-fos (Fig. 19.7b). In the rat, noxious or non-noxious stimulation of the bladder and urethra increases the levels of Fos protein primarily in the dorsal commissure, the superficial dorsal horn, and in the area of the sacral parasympathetic nucleus (Fig. 19.7b). Some of these interneurones send long projections to the brain; whereas others make local connections in the spinal cord and participate in segmental spinal reflexes. The former are involved in transmitting sensory input to supraspinal centres for subsequent relay to the cerebral cortex or to micturition reflex circuits in the brainstem. According to traditional concepts, ascending visceral sensory pathways travel in the lateral funiculus. However recent studies indicate that nociceptive signals from the pelvic viscera can also ascend in the dorsal funiculus (Al Chaer et al. 1996). Ascending axons terminate in several areas, including the periaqueductal grey (PAG) (Blok et al. 1995) and the gracile nucleus (Al-Chaer et al. 1996). Anatomical and electrophysiological studies in cats and rats indicate that the projection to the PAG originates from neurones in the lateral dorsal horn. It is believed that neurones in the PAG relay information to the pontine micturition centre and initiate the micturition reflex. Projections to the gracile nucleus seem to arise primarily from neurones in the dorsal commissure and carry nociceptive signals which are eventually routed to the thalamus and cortex (Al-Chaer et al. 1996).

Patch–clamp recordings from parasympathetic preganglionic neurones in the neonatal rat spinal slice preparation have revealed that interneurones located immediately dorsal and medial to the parasympathetic nucleus make direct monosynaptic connections with the preganglionic neurones (Araki and de Groat 1996). Microstimulation of interneurones in both locations elicits glutamatergic, N-methyl-d-aspartare (NMDA), and non-NMDA excitatory postsynaptic currents in preganglionic neurones (Fig. 19.9). Stimulation of a subpopulation of medial interneurones elicits GABAergic and glycinergic inhibitory postsynaptic currents (Fig. 9). Thus local interneurones are likely to play an important role in both excitatory and inhibitory reflex pathways controlling the preganglionic outflow to the lower urinary tract.

Pathways in the brain

The neurones in the brain that control the lower urinary tract have been studied using a variety of anatomical tracing techniques in several species (de Groat et al. 1993, 1995; Nadelhaft and Vera 1995; Vizzard et al. 1995). In the rat, transneuronal virus tracing methods have identified many populations of central neurones that are involved in the control of bladder, urethra, and the urethral sphincter, including Barrington's nucleus (the pontine micturition centre, PMC); medullary raphe nuclei, which contain serotonergic neurones; the locus coeruleus, which contains noradrenergic neurones; periaqueductal grey, and the A5 noradrenergic cell group (Fig. 19.6).

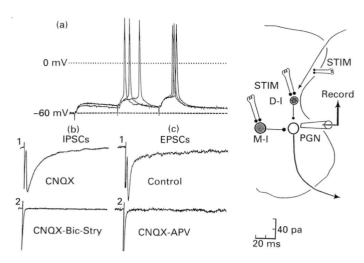

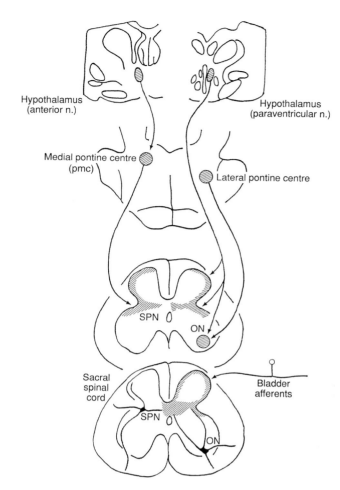

Fig. 19.9. Excitatory glutamatergic (a,c) and inhibitory GABAergic and glycinergic (b) interneuronal inputs to sacral parasympathetic preganglionic neurones (PGN) in the neonatal rat spinal cord slice preparation. (a) Repetitive stimulation of a dorsal interneurone (D-I) (three pulses at 50-ms intervals) induced action potentials in a preganglionic neurone. Recordings were made using whole-cell patch–clamp methods. Note that action potentials were induced by the second and third EPSPs but not by the first EPSP. Dashed horizontal lines: membrane potential. (b1) Inhibitory postsynaptic currents (IPSCs) evoked in a PGN by stimulating a medial interneurone (M-I) in the presence of 5 μM CNQX (6-cyano-7-nitro-quinoxaline-2-3-dione) to block glutamatergic transmission. (b2) Block of IPSCs by 10 μm bicuculline (GABA$_A$ antagonist) and 1 μM strychnine (glycine antagonist). (c1) Fast AMPA (α-amino-3-hydroxy-5-methyl-4-isoxazole propionic acid) and slow NMDA (N-methyl-D-aspartate) excitatory postsynaptic currents (EPSCs) evoked in a PGN by stimulation of a dorsal interneurone (D-I) in Mg^{2+} free solution. (c2) EPSCs were blocked by combined administration of 5 μM CNQX (AMPA glutamatergic receptor antagonist) and 50 μM APV (2-amino-5-phosphonovalerate) (an NMDA antagonist). Holding potentials were –60 mV. Records represent averages of 20–30 individual responses. Diagram shows stimulation and recording methods for the patch slice preparation. Electrical stimulation in the region of primary afferent pathways in the lateral dorsal horn activates dorsal interneurones (D-I).

Fig. 19.10. Neural connections between the brain and the sacral spinal cord that may be involved in the regulation of the lower urinary tract in the cat. Lower section of spinal cord shows the location and morphology of a preganglionic neurone in the sacral parasympathetic nucleus (SPN), a sphincter motoneurone in Onuf's nucleus (ON), and the sites of central termination of afferent projections from the urinary bladder. Upper section of the spinal cord shows the sites of termination of descending pathways arising in the pontine micturition centre (medial), the pontine sphincter or urine storage centre (lateral), and the paraventricular nuclei of the hypothalamus. Section through the pons shows the projection from the anterior hypothalamic nuclei to the pontine micturition centre.

Several regions in the hypothalamus and the cerebral cortex also exhibited virus-infected cells. Neurones in the cortex were located primarily in the medial frontal cortex.

Other anatomical studies in which anterograde tracer substances were injected into brain areas and then identified in terminals in the spinal cord (Fig. 19.10) are consistent with the virus tracing data. Tracer injected into the paraventricular nucleus of the hypothalamus labelled terminals in the sacral parasympathetic nucleus as well as the sphincter motor nucleus. On the other hand, neurones in the anterior hypothalamus project to the pontine micturition centre (PMC). Neurones in the PMC in turn project primarily to the sacral parasympathetic nucleus and the lateral edge of the dorsal horn and the dorsal commissure, areas containing dendritic projections from preganglionic neurones, sphincter motoneurones, and afferent inputs from the bladder. Conversely, projections from neurones in the lateral pons terminate rather selectively in the sphincter motor nucleus

(Fig. 19.10). Thus the sites of termination of descending projections from the pontine micturition centre are optimally located to regulate reflex mechanisms at the spinal level.

Organization of urine storage and voiding reflexes

Sympathetic storage reflex

The integrity of the sympathetic input to the lower urinary tract is not essential for the performance of micturition. However, physiological experiments in animals indicate that during bladder filling the sympathetic system does provide a tonic inhibitory input to the bladder as well as an excitatory input to the urethra. This sympathetic input is physiologically significant since surgical interruption or pharmacological blockade of the sympathetic innervation can reduce urethral outflow resistance, reduce bladder capacity, and increase the frequency and amplitude of bladder contractions recorded under constant volume conditions (de Groat *et al.* 1993).

Sympathetic reflex activity is elicited by a sacrolumbar intersegmental spinal reflex pathway which is triggered by vesical afferent activity in the pelvic nerves (Fig. 19.4). The reflex pathway is inhibited when bladder pressure is raised to the threshold for producing micturition. This inhibitory response is abolished by transection of the spinal cord at the lower thoracic level, indicating that it originates at a supraspinal site, possibly the pontine micturition centre. Thus, the vesicosympathetic reflex represents a negative feedback mechanism whereby an increase in bladder pressure tends to increase inhibitory input to vesical ganglia and smooth muscle, thus allowing the bladder to accommodate large volumes (Fig. 19.4). Increased sympathetic excitatory input to the bladder base and urethra would compliment these mechanisms by increasing outflow resistance. During micturition these reflexes are suppressed by supraspinal controls, thereby facilitating bladder emptying.

Urethral sphincter storage reflex

Motoneurones innervating the striated muscles of the urethral sphincter exhibit a tonic discharge which increases during bladder filling. This activity is mediated in part by low-level afferent input from the bladder (Fig. 19.4). During micturition the firing of sphincter motoneurones is inhibited. This inhibition is dependent in part on supraspinal mechanisms, since it is not prominent in chronic spinal animals. Electrical stimulation of the pontine micturition centre induces sphincter relaxation, suggesting that bulbospinal pathways from the pons may be responsible for maintaining the normal reciprocal relationship between bladder and sphincter.

Voiding reflexes

Spinobulbospinal micturition reflex pathway

Micturition is mediated by activation of the sacral parasympathetic efferent pathway to the bladder and the urethra as well as reciprocal inhibition of the somatic pathway to the urethral sphincter (Table 19.2) (Fig. 19.3b). Studies in cats using brain-lesioning techniques revealed that neurones in the brainstem at the level of the inferior colliculus have an essential role in the control of the parasympathetic component of micturition (Fig. 19.5). Removal of areas of the brain above the inferior colliculus by intercollicular decerebration usually facilitates micturition by elimination of inhibitory inputs from more rostral centres (Fig. 19.5). However, transections at any point below the colliculi abolish micturition. Bilateral lesions in the rostral pons in the region of the locus coeruleus in cats, or Barrington's nucleus in rats, also abolishes micturition; whereas electrical or chemical stimulation at these sites triggers bladder contractions and micturition. These observations led to the concept of a spinobulbospinal micturition reflex pathway that passes through a centre in the rostral brainstem (the pontine micturition centre) (Fig. 19.5). The pathway functions as an 'on–off' switch (Figs 19.2 and 19.5) that is activated

by a critical level of afferent activity arising from tension receptors in the bladder and is, in turn, modulated by inhibitory and excitatory influences from areas of the brain rostral to the pons (e.g. diencephalon and cerebral cortex) (Fig. 19.5).

In contrast to the reflex control of the bladder, the parasympathetic control of the urethra in the rat appears to be dependent on pathways organized in the spinal cord that are modulated by input from the brain. Nitric-oxide-mediated relaxation of the urethra that occurs in response to bladder distension is reduced but not eliminated by transection of the spinal cord. The reflex relaxation of the urethra is also very prominent in chronic spinal-cord-transected rats.

Electrophysiological studies in cats and rats have confirmed that the parasympathetic efferent outflow to the urinary bladder is activated by a long latency supraspinal reflex pathway. In cats, recordings from sacral parasympathetic preganglionic neurones innervating the urinary bladder show that reflex firing occurs with a long latency (65–100 ms) following stimulation of myelinated (Aδ) afferents in the pelvic nerve. Afferent stimulation also evokes negative field potentials in the rostral pons at latencies of 30–40 ms; whereas electrical stimulation in the pons excites sacral preganglionic neurones at latencies of 45–60 ms. The sum of the latencies for the spinobulbar and bulbospinal components of the reflex pathway approximate the latency for the entire reflex.

Pontine micturition centre (PMC)

Physiological and anatomical experiments have provided substantial support for the concept that neuronal circuitry in the PMC functions as a switch in the micturition reflex pathway. The switch seems to regulate bladder capacity and also co-ordinate the activity of the bladder and external urethral sphincter. Electrical or chemical stimulation in the PMC of the rat, cat and dog induces:

(1) a suppression of urethral sphincter EMG;
(2) firing of sacral preganglionic neurones;
(3) bladder contractions and;
(4) release of urine (de Groat *et al.* 1993).

On the other hand, microinjections of putative inhibitory transmitters into the PMC of the cat can increase the volume threshold for inducing micturition and, in high doses, completely block reflex voiding, indicating that synapses in this region are important for regulating the set-point for reflex voiding and also are an essential link in the reflex pathway.

Suprapontine control of micturition

The organization of suprapontine pathways controlling micturition is less well defined, despite the fact that there is large body of literature dealing with the responses of the lower urinary tract to lesions or electrical stimulation of the brain (de Groat *et al.* 1993). In brief, it appears that the voluntary control of micturition in humans is dependent upon:

(1) connections between the frontal cortex and the septal and the preoptic regions of the hypothalamus and;
(2) connections between the paracentral lobule and the brainstem and spinal cord.

Lesions in these cortical areas resulting from tumours, aneurysms, or cerebrovascular disease appear to remove inhibitory control over the anterior hypothalamic region which normally provides an excitatory input to micturition centres in the brainstem.

Electrical stimulation of anterior and lateral hypothalamic regions in animals induces bladder contractions and voiding; whereas stimulation of posterior and medial hypothalamic areas inhibits bladder activity. According to results obtained in cats, the inhibitory and excitatory effects of hypothalamic stimulation are believed to be mediated, respectively, by activation of sympathetic inhibitory pathways and activation of parasympathetic excitatory pathways to the bladder.

Axonal tracing studies in cats have shown that the anterior hypothalamic area sends direct projections through the medial forebrain bundle to the pontine micturition centre (Fig. 19.10). On the other hand, medial and posterior hypothalamic areas, including the paraventricular nucleus, send direct projections to the sacral parasympathetic nucleus, the sphincter motor nucleus (Onuf's nucleus), and to certain sites of bladder afferent termination (laminae I and X) in the sacral spinal cord. Thus the modulatory effect of hypothalamic centres on the reflex pathways to the lower urinary tract are probably mediated by direct inputs to both pontine and sacral micturition centres.

Human PET (position emission tomography) scan studies revealed that two cortical areas (the right dorsolateral prefrontal cortex and the anterior cingulate gyrus) are active (i.e. exhibited increased blood flow) during voiding (Blok *et al.* 1997). The hypothalamus, including the preoptic area as well as the pons and the PAG, also showed activity in concert with voluntary micturition. It is noteworthy that the active areas were predominately on the right side of the brain, which is consistent with reports that urge incontinence is correlated with lesions in the right hemisphere.

Spinal micturition reflex pathway

Spinal-cord injury rostral to the lumbosacral level eliminates voluntary and supraspinal control of voiding, leading initially to an areflexic bladder and complete urinary retention followed by a slow development of automatic micturition and bladder hyperactivity (Fig. 19.3c) mediated by spinal reflex pathways (de Groat 1995). However, voiding is commonly inefficient due to simultaneous contractions of the bladder and urethral sphincter (bladder–sphincter dyssynergia) (Fig. 19.3c).

Electrophysiological studies in rats and cats have shown that the reflex pathways in intact and chronic animals are markedly different (de Groat *et al.* 1993). In both species, the central delay for the micturition reflex in chronic spinal animals is considerably shorter (<5 ms in rats; 15–40 ms in cats) than in intact animals (60–75 ms) . In addition, in chronic spinal cats the afferent limb of the micturition reflex consists of unmyelinated (C-fibre) afferents, whereas in intact cats it consists of myelinated (Aδ) afferents (Fig. 19.5). This was not only demonstrated with electrophysiological recording but also by administering capsaicin, a neurotoxin that is known to disrupt the function of C-fibre afferents. In normal cats, capsaicin injected systemically in large doses did not block reflex contractions of the bladder or the Aδ-fibre-evoked bladder reflex. However in chronic spinal cats (3–6 weeks after spinal transection) capsaicin completely blocked the rhythmic bladder contractions induced by bladder distension and blocked the C-fibre-evoked reflex firing recorded on bladder postganglionic nerves. These data indicate that two distinct central pathways (supraspinal and spinal), utilizing different peripheral afferent limbs (A and C fibre) can mediate detrusor to detrusor reflexes in the cat (Fig. 19.5). The properties of the peripheral C-fibre afferent receptors also appear to be changed in the spinal-injured cat

(de Groat 1995). C-fibre bladder afferents in the cat usually do not respond to bladder distension (i.e. silent C-fibres). However, in chronic spinal cats bladder distension initiates automatic micturition by activating C-fibre afferent neurones. Thus, spinal injury must change the properties of these afferent receptors in the bladder. The mechanisms contributing to the emergence of C-fibre-mediated bladder reflexes have been discussed in several recent papers (de Groat *et al.* 1993; de Groat *et al.* 1995).

Other reflexes that are unmasked following spinal-cord injury also appear to be mediated by C-fibre afferents. For example, it is known that instillation of cold water into the bladder of patients with upper motoneurone lesions induces reflex voiding (the Bors ice-water test) (de Groat 1995; Geirsson *et al.* 1995). This reflex does not occur in normal patients. Recently, it has been shown in the cat that C-fibre bladder afferents are responsible for cold-induced bladder reflexes (Fig. 19.5). Intravesical administration of capsaicin to spinal-cord-injured patients suppresses the Ice Water Reflex indicating that it is mediated by C-fibre afferents in humans as well (Geirsson *et al.* 1995). The ice-water-test is also positive in patients with multiple sclerosis, cerebrovascular disease, Parkinson's disease, and benign prostatic hypertrophy, as well as in normal infants. These observations suggest that cold-evoked bladder reflexes are mediated by a primitive spinal pathway that is present in the immature nervous system and then suppressed during postnatal development as supraspinal mechanisms assume the dominant role in controlling micturition. However, when supraspinal controls are damaged by spinal-cord injury or neurological diseases, such as multiple sclerosis, it appears that the spinal reflexes re-emerge.

It is noteworthy that the cold-induced bladder reflex also has been detected in elderly patients who have uninhibited, overactive bladders and an impaired perception of bladder fullness. Since these patients did not exhibit other neurological problems, it is possible that subtle cerebral dysfunctions that selectively affect micturition pathways eliminate supraspinal input to the spinal cord and allow the emergence of primitive bladder reflexes that can trigger bladder hyperactivity and incontinence.

Other reflexes also emerge after spinal-cord injury. For example, arterial pressor responses induced by bladder distension occur in spinal-injured patients and animals. In normal and spinal-injured rats the increase in blood pressure induced by isometric bladder contractions or distension is suppressed by capsaicin (de Groat *et al.* 1993; Maggi 1993). This suggests that C-fibre afferents mediate bladder–vascular reflexes in this species. Similar capsaicin-sensitive afferents may be responsible for autonomic dysreflexia in quadriplegic patients.

Capsaicin has also been used in a few patients for the treatment of various types of neurogenic disorders of the lower urinary tract. When administered intravesically in concentrations between 100 μM and 2 mM capsaicin decreased voiding frequency and nocturia in patients with hypersensitive bladders (Maggi 1993) and increased bladder capacity and reduced the frequency of incontinence in patients with multiple sclerosis (Fowler *et al.* 1994). The effects of high concentrations of capsaicin in multiple sclerosis patients persist for weeks to months after treatment, presumably due to degeneration of the bladder C-fibre afferents.

In preliminary studies on a small population of spinal-cord-injured patients with detrusor hyper-reflexia and autonomic dysreflexia, intravesical capsaicin treatment increased bladder capacity, depressed the micturition contraction pressure, decreased autonomic dysreflexia, decreased urge incontinence, and suppressed the bladder cooling reflex in some patients (Geirsson *et al.* 1995). These observations suggest that capsaicin-sensitive, C-fibre bladder afferents are involved in several pathological conditions associated with neurogenic bladder hyperactivity.

Neurotransmitters in micturition reflex pathways

Since the sacral parasympathetic reflex pathway to the bladder is essentially a positive feedback circuit, tonic inhibitory modulation of the pathway is necessary to properly store urine and to prevent voiding at low bladder volumes. Damage to central inhibitory mechanisms following disease or injury to the nervous system leads to failure of urine storage, bladder hyperactivity, and incontinence. Animal studies indicate that multiple transmitters may be involved in regulating transmission in the PMC (Fig. 19.5) and in the spinal cord (reviewed in detail by de Groat *et al.* 1993; Yoshimura and de Groat 1997).

Inhibitory neurotransmitters

Several types of inhibitory transmitters, including (1) opioid peptides (enkephalins); (2) inhibitory amino acids (GABA, glycine); (3) 5-hydroxytryptamine (serotonin), (4) acetylcholine; (5) dopamine; and (6) non-opioid peptides (corticotrophin-releasing factor and neuropeptide Y (NPY), can inhibit the micturition reflex when applied to the central nervous system. Experimental evidence in anaesthetized animals indicates that GABA and enkephalins exert a tonic inhibitory control in the PMC and regulate bladder capacity. The inhibitory effects are mediated by $GABA_A$ and μ opioid receptors, respectively. Administration of $GABA_A$ or opioid receptor antagonists into the PMC reduced the micturition volume threshold, indicating that the set-point for reflex voiding is regulated by inhibitory mechanisms in the brain (Fig. 19.5).

GABA and enkephalins also have inhibitory actions in the spinal cord (Fig. 19.9). Baclofen, a $GABA_B$ agonist, which mimicks a part of the inhibitory action of GABA, has been used clinically via intrathecal administration in patients with hyperactive bladders to suppress bladder activity and to promote urine storage (de Groat *et al.* 1993).

Interest in the role of dopamine in the control of bladder function arises from the clinical observation that patients with idiopathic Parkinson's disease often exhibit bladder hyperactivity (Yoshimura and de Groat 1997). Parkinson's disease is a disorder of basal ganglia function caused by degeneration of dopamine-containing neurones. An animal model for Parkinson's disease has been developed in monkeys by administration of a neurotoxin 1-methyl-4-phenyl-1,2,3,6 tetrahydropyridine (MPTP) that destroys dopamine neurones. Animals treated with MPTP show motor symptoms typical of Parkinson's disease and also have hyperactive bladders. Pharmacological studies in MPTP-treated monkeys revealed that the bladder hyperactivity was due to the loss of dopaminergic inhibition mediated by D_1 dopaminergic receptors. On the other hand, D_2 dopaminergic receptors can mediate a facilitation of micturition. The functional significance of the latter receptors is not known.

Excitatory neurotransmitters

Excitatory transmission in the central pathways to the lower urinary tract may depend on several types of transmitters, including (1) glutamic acid, (2) neuropeptides (substance P, vasoactive intestinal polypeptide), (3) noradrenaline; (4) acetylcholine; and (5) nitric oxide.

Pharmacological experiments in rats have revealed that glutamic acid is an essential transmitter in the ascending, pontine, and descending limbs of the spinobulbospinal micturition reflex pathway and in the reflex pathways controlling the external urethral sphincter. NMDA and non-NMDA glutamatergic synaptic mechanisms appear to interact synergistically to mediate transmission in these pathways (Fig. 19.9c). Glutamatergic transmission also contributes to the micturition reflex in chronic spinal rats.

Innervation of sexual organs

In humans the physiological changes initiated by erotic stimuli are divided into four distinct phases (excitement, plateau, orgasm, and resolution) which are designated collectively the sexual response cycle. Although anatomical differences obviously preclude identical responses in male and female during each phase of the cycle it is clear that similar secretory responses (vaginal lubrication, prostatic and bulbourethral gland secretion), vascular responses (penile and clitoral erection), and responses of smooth and striated muscles occur in both sexes (Table 19.3). This section will review experimental studies in animals that examined the neural mechanisms regulating these physiological responses.

The sex organs, like the lower urinary tract, receive an innervation from three sets of nerves: sacral parasympathetic (pelvic), thoracolumbar sympathetic (hypogastric and lumbar sympathetic chain), and somatic (pudendal) nerves (Fig. 19.l).

Parasympathetic pathways

Preganglionic axons arising from neurones in the sacral spinal cord provide an excitatory input to parasympathetic ganglion cells (Fig. 19.11) in the pelvic plexus which in turn innervate:

(1) erectile tissue in the penis and clitoris;

(2) smooth muscle and glandular tissue in the prostate, urethra, seminal vesicles, vagina, uterus and;

(3) blood vessels and possibly secretory epithelia in various structures.

Among the numerous sexual functions controlled by the sacral parasympathetic pathway, the one that has attracted the most research interest and for which there is the most detailed information is penile erection.

Since the initial observation by Eckhard in 1863 that electrical stimulation of the pelvic nerves in the dog produced penile erection, the mechanisms involved in erection have been investigated in various species (de Groat and Booth 1993*b*). It was known for many years that parasympathetic neural activity induces vasodilation in penile blood vessels and increases blood flow to the cavernous tissue. However, the mechanisms underlying the vasodilation and the transmitters mediating the response have only recently been elucidated (Burnett *et al.* 1992; Andersson 1993; Argiolas and Melis 1995). It is clear that parasympathetic postganglionic neurones

Table 19.3. Male sexual reflexes

Response	Afferent nerves	Efferent nerves	Central pathway	Effector organ
Penile erection				
Reflexogenic	Pudendal nerve	Sacral parasympathetic	Sacral spinal reflex	Dilatation of arterial supply to corpus cavernosum and corpus spongiosum
Psychogenic	Auditory, imaginative, visual,	Sacral parasympathetic, lumber sympathetic	Supraspinal origin	
Glandular secretion	Pudendal nerve	Sacral parasympathetic, lumber sympathetic	Sacral spinal reflex	Seminal vesicles and prostate
Seminal emission	Pudendal nerve	Lumbar sympathetic	Intersegmental spinal reflex (sacrolumbar)	Contraction of vas deferens, ampulla, seminal vesicles, prostate, and closure of bladder neck
Ejaculation	Pudendal nerve	Somatic efferents in pudendal nerve	Sacral spinal reflex	Rhythmic contractions of bulbocavernosus and ischiocavernosus muscles

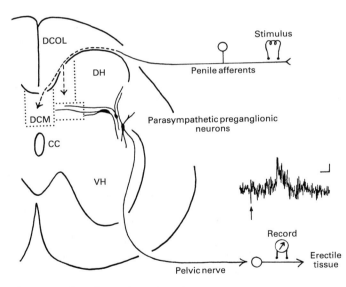

Fig. 19.11. The reflex pathway for inducing penile erection. Horseradish peroxidase axonal tracing studies in the cat have shown the relationship between sacral parasympathetic preganglionic neurones and afferent projections from the penis. Penile afferents in the pudendal nerve project to the medial side of the dorsal horn (DH) and the dorsal commissure (DCM) in the S2 segment of the spinal cord. Preganglionic neurones send dendrites into regions of afferent termination. DCOL, dorsal column; VH, ventral horn; CC, and central canal. In the rat electrical stimulation of penile afferents in the dorsal nerve of the penis elicits reflex firing in efferent pathways to the penis. Inset is an example of a reflex discharge in parasympathetic postganglionic axons in penile nerves. The reflexes, which occur at a long latency (mean 75 ms), are present in normal and chronic spinal rats and are blocked by section of the pelvic nerve. Stimulus marked by arrow. Horizontal calibration 20 ms, vertical calibration 10 μV.

innervating the cavernous tissue can release multiple transmitters, including acetylcholine, vasoactive intestinal polypeptide (VIP), and nitric oxide (Burnett *et al.* 1992; Andersson 1993; de Groat and Booth 1993*a*).

Cholinergic mechanisms

Under certain experimental conditions exogenous acetylcholine (ACh) can act on muscarinic receptors to relax cavernous smooth muscle; however, pharmacological experiments in humans and animals showed convincingly that endogenously released ACh is not the principal mediator of penile erection. Atropine, a muscarinic receptor antagonist, that blocks parasympathetic responses in the bladder, does not block erection. Nevertheless it is possible that ACh contributes to erection by acting prejunctionally or postjunctionally to block adrenergic vasoconstrictor mechanisms or by acting on other targets such as endothelium to release non-cholinergic relaxing factors (Andersson 1993).

Peptidergic mechanisms

The identification of neuropeptides as mediators of non-cholinergic, non-adrenergic transmission at various sites in the mammalian peripheral nervous system focused attention on the possible role of these agents in the vasodilator pathways to the penis. Among the neuropeptides, VIP has been the most interesting transmitter candidate since it is present in penile nerves in many species, including humans. VIP elicits an increase in penile volume after local administration, relaxes *in vitro* preparations of penile smooth muscle, and is present at high levels in the venous effluent of the penis of man and dog during psychogenic, drug, or electrically induced erections (Andersson 1993; de Groat and Booth 1993*b*). However intracavernosal injection of VIP does not elicit full erections in humans, indicating that it is not the major transmitter involved in erection.

Nitric oxidergic mechanisms

Various evidence indicates that nitric oxide (NO) is the principal mediator of penile erection in humans and animals (Burnett *et al.* 1992; Andersson 1993; Argiolas and Melis 1995). Nerves in the cavernous tissue as well as neurones in the pelvic plexus that innervate the penis exhibit neuronal nitric oxide synthase (NOS), the enzyme responsible for the synthesis of NO. Inhibitors of NOS suppress the penile erection induced by penile nerve stimulation; and this effect can be reversed by the administration of the NO precursor L-arginine. In addition, local application or intracavernosal injection of NO-donors elicits penile erection in animals as well as in impotent men. NO acts to induce smooth muscle relaxation by stimulating guanylate cyclase and increasing the concentrations of cyclic GMP, a second messenger that leads to a suppression of contractile mechanisms in the smooth muscle. Although neurally released NO is the major mechanism for eliciting penile erection, gene knock-out experiments indicate that other mechanisms may also be involved. When neuronal NOS was eliminated in transgenic mice, copulation and fertility were not blocked. This observation has led to the suggestion that another form of NOS, such as endothelial NOS, may also be able to mediate erections.

Sympathetic pathways

Sympathetic pathways to the reproductive organs follow three routes:

(1) the hypogastric nerves;

(2) the pelvic nerves, and (3) the pudendal nerves (Fig. 19.1).

The sympathetic nerves provide an input to penile and clitoral erectile tissue as well as to smooth muscle of the ductus deferens, seminal vesicles, prostate, vagina, and uterus.

Sympathetic postganglionic neurones release primarily noradrenaline and adenosine triphosphate (ATP), but some neurones that elicit penile erection presumably release ACh, NO, and neuropeptides (de Groat and Booth 1993*b*). Inputs from the caudal sympathetic chain ganglia which contain noradrenaline and possibly neuropeptide Y produce vasoconstriction of penile blood vessels and detumescence via actions on α-adrenergic and peptidergic receptors. On the other hand, inputs from the hypogastric nerve which pass through ganglionic relay stations in the pelvic plexus can produce vasodilation and penile erection as well as detumescence.

Sympathetic nerves provide excitatory inputs to the ductus deferens, seminal vesicles, prostate, vaginal and uterine smooth muscle. These excitatory responses are mediated by an action of noradrenaline on α-adrenergic receptors. In the ductus deferens and seminal vesicles a second excitatory transmitter, ATP, is co-released with noradrenaline and acts on P_{2X} purinergic receptors.

Somatic pathways

The pudendal nerves arising from the lumbosacral segments of the spinal cord provide efferent excitatory input to the bulbocavernosus and ischiocavernosus muscles (Fig. 19.1). These muscles are responsible for ejaculation in male and contribute to the rhythmic perineal contractions during orgasm in the female. In many species, including cat, monkey, and humans, the motoneurones innervating these muscles are located in Onuf's nucleus, whereas in the rat they are located in a separate nucleus in the medial part of the ventral horn.

Afferent pathways

Afferent pathways to the penis, clitoris, and vagina are present in the pudendal nerves. Afferent pathways to deeper structures such as the uterine cervix and uterine horns are present in the pelvic and hypogastric nerves, respectively. Cervical afferent neurones are located primarily in the sacral dorsal root ganglia; whereas uterine horn afferent neurones are located primarily in the rostral lumbar dorsal root ganglia. Electrophysiological studies have shown that afferents from the penis respond to tactile stimuli; whereas the great majority of afferents from the uterus are of the polymodal type which respond to noxious and non-noxious mechanical and chemical stimuli.

Substance P and CGRP are present in a considerable proportion of the afferent neurones innervating the genital organs. For example, it has been estimated that 45–80 per cent of the lumbosacral dorsal root ganglia cells innervating the female genital tract contain CGRP. VIP is present in a large percentage (70 per cent) of the sacral afferent neurones innervating the uterine cervix of the cat. At many sites the two peptides are colocalized in the same neurone and, therefore, may function as co-transmitters in afferent pathways to the genital organs.

Central reflex mechanisms controlling the sexual organs

Penile erection

Penile erection is primarily an involuntary or reflex phenomenon that can be elicited by a variety of reflexogenic and psychogenic stimuli and by at least two distinct central mechanisms (i.e. spinal and supraspinal) (Table 19.3) which probably act synergistically. The central control of clitoral erection is likely to be mediated by similar mechanisms but has not been studied in detail.

Reflexogenic erections

Reflexogenic penile erections which are elicited by exteroceptive stimulation of the genital regions are mediated by a sacral spinal reflex pathway having an afferent limb in the pudendal nerve and an efferent limb in the sacral parasympathetic nerves (Table 19.3; Fig. 19.11). The central organization of the reflex pathway has been studied in several species of animals. Axonal tracing techniques have revealed that pudendal afferent pathways from the penis of the cat and rat terminate in the medial dorsal horn and dorsal commissure (Fig. 19.11). Interneurones in these regions are activated by tactile stimulation of the penis and presumably are involved in transmitting sensations to the brain in addition to activating parasympathetic preganglionic neurones that induce erection. The preganglionic neurones are located in the intermediolateral nucleus of the sacral spinal cord and send dendritic projections into areas of laminae V–VII and the dorsal commissure which receive afferent input from the penis (Fig. 19.11). Pseudorabies virus tracing in the rat (Marson *et al.* 1993) and cat have revealed sympathetic and parasympathetic preganglionic neurones and interneurones in the thoracolumbar and lumbosacral spinal cord in locations similar to those labelled by virus injected into the urinary bladder and urethra. Similar labelling was also noted in the brain. Injection of PRV into the rat penis labelled neurones in the Barrington's nucleus, A5 noradrenergic cell group, raphe magnus and pallidus, the paraventricular nucleus of the hypothalamus, the parapyramidal reticular formation of the medulla, and the nucleus paragigantocellularis (Marson *et al.* 1993). The PRV labelling in Barrington's nucleus was unexpected since neurones in this area were previously thought to be involved exclusively in lower urinary tract function. However, transneuronal labelling of this nucleus following PRV injection into the penis and the colon raises the possibility that it might have broader functions to control the activity of all the pelvic viscera. Virus labelling in the nucleus paragigantocellularis is particularly significant since neurones in this nucleus have been shown to mediate a tonic inhibition of sexual reflexes. Electrolytic lesions in this area significantly increase copulatory efficiency in male rats and reduce latencies in *ex copula* sexual reflex tests (Marson *et al.* 1993).

In the rat, electrical stimulation of the dorsal nerve of the penis evokes long latency (mean 75 ms) reflex discharges in postganglionic axons passing from the major pelvic ganglion into the penile nerves (Fig. 19.11). Since these reflexes are obtained in both normal and chronic spinal rats and are eliminated by transection of the pelvic nerves, it is clear that they are mediated by a polysynaptic spinal reflex pathway involving efferent neurones in the sacral autonomic outflow.

In the rat, penile afferents also project into the ventral horn and appear to make contacts with the soma and dendrites of motoneurones. These connections could be involved in the somatic reflex mechanisms involved in copulation.

Psychogenic erections

Psychogenic erections are initiated by supraspinal centres in response to auditory, visual, olfactory, and imaginative stimuli. The efferent limb of the reflex pathway traverses both the thoracolumbar and the sacral autonomic outflow (Table 19.3). Studies conducted in monkeys and rats indicate that hypothalamic and limbic pathways play a key role in erection and that the medial preoptic–anterior hypothalamic area is an important integrating centre (de Groat and Booth 1993*b*; Argiolas and Melis 1995). Electrical stimulation at this site produces full erections in anaesthetized and unanaesthetized animals, whereas lesions at the same site generally suppress sexual behaviour.

Efferent pathways from the medial preoptic area enter the medial forebrain bundle and then pass caudally into the midbrain tegmental region near the lateral part of the substantia nigra. Caudal to the midbrain the efferent pathway for erection travels in the ventrolateral pons and medulla and then in the lateral funiculus of the spinal cord. Descending projections from the hypothalamic nuclei terminate in lumbosacral spinal autonomic and somatic centres involved in erection (Fig. 19.10).

Secretion

During the first and second phases of the sexual response cycle, activity in parasympathetic and sympathetic pathways in the male stimulates mucus secretion from the bulbourethral and Littre's glands and secretion from the seminal vesicles and prostate gland (Table 19.3). Acetylcholine has been implicated as an efferent transmitter since cholinomimetic agents mimic neurally evoked secretion from some glands.

Erotic stimuli in the female elicit vaginal lubrication and mucus secretion from Bartholin's glands. Vaginal lubrication is thought to be secondary to increased vaginal blood and changes in capillary permeability, leading to increased formation of plasma transudate which passes through the epithelium to the vaginal surface. An active secretory mechanism is unlikely since the vaginal epithelium is devoid of glands. VIP has been implicated as the efferent transmitter in vaginal lubrication and increased vaginal blood flow.

Emission–Ejaculation

The third phase of the sexual act (orgasm) which is accompanied by emission and ejaculation of semen involves the co-ordination of autonomic and somatic reflex mechanisms at different levels of the lumbosacral spinal cord. During the first step in the process (emission) reflex activity in the thoracolumbar sympathetic outflow elicits rhythmic contractions of the smooth muscle of the seminal vesicles, prostate, ductus deferens, and ampulla, resulting in the ejection of sperm and glandular secretions into the urethra and at the same time closure of the bladder neck to prevent backflow of semen into the bladder. Pharmacological studies have shown that these responses are mediated by the adrenergic transmitter noradrenaline acting on α-adrenergic receptors and by the purinergic transmitter, ATP.

After emission of semen into the proximal urethra, rhythmic contractions of the bulbocavernosus, ischiocavernosus, and periurethral striated muscles results in ejaculation. The afferent and efferent limbs of the ejaculatory reflex are contained in the pudendal nerve. The sensations accompanying ejaculation, or rhythmic vaginal contractions in the female, represent a major component of the orgasmic response.

Neurotransmitters in sexual reflex pathways

Pharmacological studies in animals have implicated many neurotransmitter systems in the central control of sexual function. The literature relevant to this topic is extensive (de Groat and Booth 1993*b*; Argiolas and Melis 1995).

Monoamines

The monoaminergic transmitters (5-hydroxytryptamine, dopamine, and noradrenaline) appear to have varied roles in the central mechanisms underlying sexual behaviour. For example, pharmacological blockade or destruction of the 5-hydroxytryptamine (5-HT)-containing pathways in the brain facilitates sexual activity in male rats and rabbits, whereas the administration of a 5-HT precursor decreases sexual activity. These data indicate that 5-HT pathways in the brain exert a general depressant effect on sexual motivation. However, other studies imply that at the level of the spinal cord 5-HT mechanisms facilitate seminal emission, but have mixed effects on penile erection in the rat. The tonic inhibitory control of spinal penile reflexes by the nucleus paragigantocellularis is mediated by a bulbospinal 5-HT pathway (Marson *et al.* 1993; Argiolas and Melis 1995).

Dopaminergic pathways have a facilitatory effect on male copulatory behavior in the rat. Administration of L-dopa, a precursor of dopamine, or the administration of dopamine receptor agonists increases mounting, intromissions, and ejaculations in male rats. On the other hand, lesions of the dopamine system in rats depress copulatory behaviour. In rhesus monkeys, apomorphine, a dopamine receptor agonist and quinelorane, a D_2 dopamine receptor agonist, facilitate penile erections.

Noradrenergic pathways exert an inhibitory influence on sexual function. Clonidine, a centrally acting α_2-adrenergic receptor agonist, inhibits erections and copulatory activity in rats. The inhibitory effects of clonidine are reversed by yohimbine, an α_2-adrenergic receptor antagonist. The administration of yohimbine alone increases sexual motivation, suggesting that sexual activity is tonically inhibited by a noradrenergic pathway.

Neuropeptides and GABA

Oxytocin, a neuropeptide that is present in efferent pathways from the hypothalamus to spinal autonomic centres, facilitates penile erectile mechanisms in the rat when administered in nanogram quantities into the cerebral ventricles (de Groat and Booth 1993*b*; Argiolas and Melis 1995). Injection of NOS inhibitors into the hypothalamus prevented the penile erection induced by oxytocin as well as dopamine, indicating that NO plays a role centrally as well as peripherally in erectile responses. Opioid peptides and GABA inhibit copulatory behaviour when administered into the brain of male rats, whereas the administration of receptor antagonists for either type of transmitter facilitates copulatory behaviour indicating that sexual function is under tonic inhibitory control via these transmitters.

Thus a broad spectrum of neurotransmitters seems to be involved in the control of sexual behaviour in the rodent. It is uncertain whether these findings are generally applicable to humans. However, the susceptibility of human sexual function to a broad range of drugs suggests that sexual behaviour in humans, as in rodents, depends on a variety of neurochemical mechanisms.

References

Al-Chaer, E. D., Lawand, N. B., Westlund, K. N., and Willis, W. D. (1996). Pelvic visceral input into the nucleus gracilis is largely mediated by the postsynaptic dorsal column pathway. *J. Neurophysiol.* **76**, 2675–90.

Andersson, K.-E. (1993). Pharmacology of lower urinary tract smooth muscles and penile erectile tissues. *Pharmacol. Rev.* **45**, 253–308.

Araki, I. and de Groat, W. C. (1996). Unitary excitatory synaptic currents in preganglionic neurons mediated by two distinct groups of interneurons in neonatal rat sacral parasympathetic nucleus. *J. Neurophysiol.* **76**, 215–26.

Argiolas, A. and Melis, M. R. (1995). Neuromodulation of penile erection: an overview of the role of neurotransmitters and neuropeptides. *Prog. in Neurobiol.* **47**, 235–55.

Blok, B. F. M., DeWeerd, H., and Holstege, G. (1995). Ultrastructure evidence for the paucity of projections from the lumbosacral cord to the M-region in the cat. A new concept for the organization of the micturition reflex with the periaqueductal gray as central relay. *J. Com. Neurol.* **359**, 300–9.

Blok, B. F. M., Willemsen, A. T. M., and Holstege, G. (1997). A PET study on the brain control of micturition in humans. *Brain*, **120**, 111–21.

Burnett, A. L., Lowenstein, C. J., Bredt, D. S., Chang, T. S. K., and Snyder, S. H. (1992). Nitric oxide: A physiologic mediator of penile erection. *Science* **257**, 401–3.

de Groat, W. C. (1995). Mechanisms underlying the recovery of lower urinary tract function following spinal cord injury. *Paraplegia* **33**, 493–505.

de Groat, W. C. and Booth, A. M. (1993*a*). Synaptic transmission in pelvic ganglia. In *The autonomic nervous system.* Vol. 3, *Nervous control of the urogenital system*, (ed. C. A. Maggi), pp. 291–347. Harwood Academic, London.

de Groat, W. C. and Booth, A. M. (1993*b*). Neural control of penile erection. In *The Autonomic nervous system.* Vol. 3, *Nervous control of the urogenital system*, (ed. C. A. Maggi), pp. 467–524. Harwood Academic, London.

de Groat, W. C., Booth, A. M., and Yoshimura, N. (1993). Neurophysiology of micturition and its modification in animal models of human disease. In *The autonomic nervous system.* Vol. 3, *Nervous control of the urogenital system*, (ed. C.A. Maggi), pp. 227–90. Harwood Academic, London.

de Groat, W. C., Vizzard, M. A., Araki, I., and Roppolo, J. R. (1995). Spinal interneurons and preganglionic neurons in sacral autonomic reflex pathways. In *The emotional motor system, progress in brain research*, (ed. G. Holstege, R. Bandler, and C. Saper), pp. 97–111, Vol 107. Elsevier Science Publishers, Amsterdam.

Fowler, C. J., Beck, R. O., Gerard, S., Betts, C. D., and Fowler, C. G. (1994). Intravesical capsaicin for treatment of detrusor hyperreflexia. *J. Neurol., Neurosurg. Psychiat.* **57**, 169–73.

Geirsson, G., Fall, M. and Sullivan, L. (1995). Clinical and urodynamic effects of intravesical capsaicin treatment in patients with chronic traumatic spinal detrusor hyperreflexia. *J. Urol.* **154**, 1825–9.

Maggi, C. A. (1993). The dual, sensory and efferent function of the capsaicin-sensitive primary sensory nerves in the bladder and urethra. In *The autonomic nervous system.* Vol. 3, *Nervous control of the urogenital system*, (ed. C. A. Maggi), pp. 383–422. Harwood Academic, London.

Marson, L., Platt, K. B., and McKenna, K. E. (1993). Central nervous system innervation of the penis as revealed by the transneuronal transport of pseudorabies virus. *Neuroscience* **55**, 263–80.

Nadelhaft, I. and Vera, P. L. (1995). Central nervous system neurons infected by pseudorabies virus injected into the rat urinary bladder following unilateral transection of the pelvic nerve. *J. Comp. Neurol.* **359**, 443–55.

Rexed, B. (1952). The cytoarchitectonic organization of the spinal cord of the cat. *J. Comp. Neurol.* **96**, 415–95.

Somogyi, G. T., Tanowitz, M., Zernova, G., and de Groat, W. C. (1996). M_1 muscarinic receptor facilitation of ACh and noradrenaline release in the rat urinary bladder is mediated by protein kinase C. *J. Physiol.* **496**, 245–54.

Vizzard, M. A., Erickson, V. L., Card, J. P., Roppolo, J. R., and de Groat, W. C. (1995). Transneuronal labeling of neurons in the adult rat brainstem and spinal cord after injection of pseudorabies virus into the urethra. *J. Comp. Neurol.* **355**, 629–40.

Yoshimura, N. and de Groat, W. C. (1997). Neural control of the lower urinary tract. *Int. J. Urol.* **4**, 111–25.

PART III

Clinical Autonomic Testing

20. Investigation of autonomic disorders
Christopher J. Mathias and Roger Bannister

Introduction

In a patient with a suspected autonomic disorder the major aims of investigation are:

(1) to determine whether autonomic function is normal or abnormal;

(2) if the latter, to assess the degree of dysfunction, with an emphasis on the site of the lesion and on the functional deficit;

(3) to ascertain whether the abnormality is of the primary variety, or secondary to recognized disorders, as the prognosis and management may depend on the diagnostic category.

In this chapter an overview of the ways to investigate the autonomic nervous system is provided (Table 20.1). A range of systems is covered, with an emphasis on the cardiovascular system, where there have been more numerous advances, especially in non-invasive measurement and in recognizing the role of compensatory systems, including various hormones. It should be emphasized that assessment of autonomic function depends not only on reflex arcs and on efferent nerve activity but also on end-organ responsiveness, where factors that include the metabolic clearance and disposition of transmitters, postsynaptic receptors, postreceptor translation, and second messenger systems influence the final response. Therefore each test, and the information from it, should be considered in relation to the whole clinical picture, and closely linked with factors in daily life where relevant. The information from investigations is needed not only for diagnosis but also for evaluation of therapy and assessment of its benefits; this is of particular importance in patients with generalized autonomic disorders.

Table 20.1. Outline of investigations in autonomic failure

Cardiovascular	
Physiological	Head-up tilt (45°)*; Standing*; Valsalva manoeuvre*
	Pressor stimuli—isometric exercise*, cutaneous cold*, mental arithmetic*
	Heart rate responses—deep breathing*, hyperventilation*, standing*, head-up tilt*, 30 : 15 ratio
	Liquid meal challenge
	Exercise testing
	Carotid sinus massage
Biochemical	Plasma noradrenaline—supine and head-up tilt or standing; urinary catecholamines; plasma renin activity and aldosterone
Pharmacological	Noradrenaline—α-adrenoceptors—vascular
	Isoprenaline—β-adrenoceptors—vascular and cardiac
	Tyramine—pressor and noradrenaline response
	Edrophonium—noradrenaline response
	Atropine—parasympathetic cardiac blockade
Sudomotor	Central regulation—thermoregulatory sweat test
	Sweat gland response—intradermal acetylcholine, quantitative sudomotor axon reflex test (Q-SART), localized sweat test
	Sympathetic skin response
Gastrointestinal	Barium studies, videocinefluoroscopy, endoscopy, gastric emptying studies
Renal function and urinary tract	Day and night urine volumes and sodium/potassium excretion
	Urodynamic studies, intravenous urography, ultrasound examination, sphincter electromyography
Sexual function	Penile plethysmography
	Intracavernosal papaverine
Respiratory	Laryngoscopy
	Sleep studies to assess apnoea/oxygen desaturation
Eye	Schirmer's test
	Pupil function—pharmacological and physiological

* indicate screening tests used in our units..

In certain autonomic disorders specific 'non-autonomic' investigations may be needed. An example is in Horner's syndrome where further investigation in identifying the cause is of greater importance than the assessment of the autonomic deficit. The tests may include a computed tomography (CT) or magnetic resonance imaging (MRI) scan to exclude midbrain or medullary infarction, a CT scan of the thorax along with bronchoscopy to exclude Pancoast's syndrome (a malignancy in the apex of the lung), or carotid angiography to exclude dissection of the internal carotid artery.

Interpretation of test results

No single test can provide a global assessment of autonomic function. Even if directed towards a single system, testing often involves a variety of procedures. Those used as 'screening' or 'routine' tests in our Autonomic Units in London are listed in Appendix I. These are directed predominantly towards cardiovascular autonomic function and are of value as postural hypotension is often a cardinal feature, especially in patients with a generalized autonomic disorder. The detection and evaluation of postural hypotension is important because it may be an early sign of sympathetic vasoconstrictor failure; many also have impaired heart rate responses to various stimuli because of cardiac parasympathetic failure. If the responses to cardiovascular reflex testing are within expected limits, this information, in conjunction with the rest of the clinical picture, is often helpful in excluding the primary autonomic failure syndromes and indicates that other explanations for the features should be sought. If the responses are abnormal and suggest neurogenic failure, they reinforce the case for further evaluation. The majority of screening tests are directed towards the determination of autonomic underactivity. However, autonomic overactivity is of importance in certain disorders and contributes to morbidity or even mortality. Examples are increased cardiac vagal activity in neurally mediated syncope (see Chapters 44 and 45), and paroxysmal hypertension as part of autonomic dysreflexia in high spinal-cord injuries (see Chapter 51); specific testing is needed if such disorders are suspected.

The need for 'normal' and ideally 'control' values, and their relevance, warrants discussion. Although the principles of autonomic testing, and the interpretation of the results should be universally applied, the precise levels and ranges of responses to various stimuli depend upon a large number of factors. Some of these include the specific laboratory conditions during testing (such as the room temperature), the nature and specification of testing equipment used, the sophistication of the recording equipment and computer facilities, the protocol followed, and equally important the quality of staff, who should be trained to consistently and rigorously follow testing schedules. To obtain normal values, the basic requirements are age, gender, body weight, and control of food intake, including, in certain investigations, the avoidance of laboratory personnel as their responses may reflect the effects of habituation. To obtain true 'control' values many other factors may need to be matched, and some of these include drug therapy (which can affect either autonomic nerve activity or function of the target organ from which measurements often are derived), the level of physical fitness, smoking, alcohol intake, and previous medical disorders (such as a myocardial infarction) that may influence the results. In clinical practice, therefore, information from testing if matched against normal values alone may be of limited value, and may even be misleading if not considered along with the overall clinical picture and in relation to the individual case. However, each laboratory, needs to have a range of 'expected values', preferably within different age bands (Appendix I).

Cardiovascular autonomic tests lend themselves to objective rather than descriptive assessment that may not be applied as readily to the testing of other areas affected in autonomic disorders. An example is the videocinefluoroscopic examination of dysphagia, that may provide a clear indication of dysfunction and the risk of aspiration, but is less easy to quantify precisely and therefore interpret if used in longitudinal studies to assess progression of disease, or to determine the responses to therapy. The natural history of certain autonomic disorders also is important when evaluating the responses to intervention. For instance, pancreatic transplantation in diabetic autonomic neuropathy and hepatic transplantation in familial amyloid polyneuropathy prevent further neurological and autonomic damage, but testing may not show improvement; however, this in itself is a positive response, as relentless progression would occur without such intervention.

Cardiovascular testing

The prime concern of the cardiovascular system is tissue perfusion, with blood pressure and blood flow therefore of critical importance. These are influenced by a number of factors, with beat-to-beat control of blood pressure dependent upon the autonomic nervous system and, in particular, the sympathetic efferent pathways. In addition, a number of secondary mechanisms, involving systemically acting hormones, such as angiotensin II and aldosterone, and locally acting substances, such as the prostaglandins, nitric oxide, and endothelin, play a role. These substances may act directly or indirectly on the heart and vasculature, and may control or influence the intravascular and extravascular fluid compartments, each of which may modify the level of blood pressure and thus tissue perfusion. A schematic diagram of the main neurological pathways involved in the regulation of blood pressure is provided in Fig. 20.1. There are cortical, limbic, anterior and posterior hypothalamic, and medullary centres, where the input from a range of afferents can be integrated. The major cardiovascular afferents are those from the carotid sinus, the aortic arch, and the cardiopulmonary region. A range of other afferents (from skeletal muscle, skin, and viscera) also contribute, as is observed in patients with cervical or high thoracic spinal-cord transection (in whom the spinal and peripheral autonomic pathways are devoid of cerebral control), in whom stimulation of such afferents may induce autonomic dysreflexia (Chapter 51). Normally from the cerebral centres, the output through the vagus and the sympathetic nervous system to the heart and blood vessels is co-ordinated. A variety of investigative approaches in animals (Chapter 6) indicate that the major baroreceptor afferents pass to the nucleus tractus solitarius, that the vagal output is through the nucleus ambiguus, and that the sympathetic output is through the reticular paramedian nucleus.

Lesions resulting in autonomic dysfunction may involve the afferent pathways, the central connections, the efferent pathways, the target organs, or a combination of these, depending upon the disorder. Impairment of cardiovascular reflex activity usually results

Afferent   Efferent

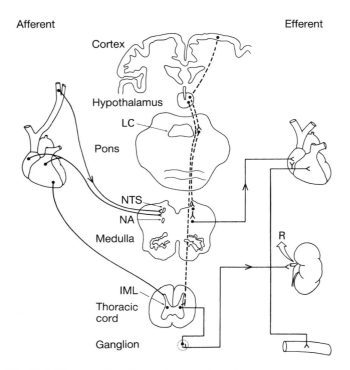

Fig. 20.1. Diagram of cardiovascular control mechanism. LC, locus ceruleus; NA, nucleus ambiguus; NTS, nucleus tractus solitarius; IML, intermediolateral column; R, renin. (Taken with permission from Bannister (1979).)

Table 20.2. Some of the symptoms resulting from postural (orthostatic) hypotension and impaired perfusion of various organs

Cerebral hypoperfusion
  Dizziness
  Visual disturbances
    blurred—tunnel
    scotoma
    greying out—blacking out
    colour defects
  Loss of consciousness
  Impaired cognition

Muscle hypoperfusion
  Paracervical and suboccipital ('coathanger') ache
  Lower back/buttock ache

Cardiac hypoperfusion
  Angina pectoris

Spinal cord hypoperfusion

Renal hypoperfusion
  Oliguria

Non-specific
  Weakness, lethargy, fatigue
  Falls

Adapted from Mathias (1995a).

Head-up postural challenge

Postural (orthostatic) hypotension is a cardinal manifestation of autonomic failure and therefore the cardiovascular responses to head-up postural change are particularly important (Fig. 20.2). Previously we arbitrarily had defined postural hypotension as a fall of more that 20 mmHg systolic blood pressure on standing. This now has been accepted by a Consensus Committee of international experts (Consensus Statement 1996); their definition also includes a fall in diastolic blood pressure of at least 10 mmHg within 3 minutes of standing or head-up tilt (to 60°). Postural hypotension results in a number of symptoms (Table 20.2), characteristically associated with head-up postural change and relieved by sitting or lying flat. In some there may be few symptoms, despite postural hypotension (Fig. 20.3), presumably because of improved cerebral autoregulation. In the presence of relevant symptoms, a fall of less than 20 mmHg systolic blood pressure also may be of importance and will warrant further investigation. The presence of vascular disease may enhance susceptibility to cerebral ischaemia, as in patients with carotid artery stenosis (Fig. 20.4).

In the clinic, brachial artery blood pressure usually is measured non-invasively using a standard mercury or aneroid sphygmomanometer. Semi-automated machines, that utilize the auscultatory or oscillometric method to measure systolic and diastolic blood-pressure in addition to deriving heart rate, are of value in the laboratory. A considerable advance has been the non-invasive technique to measure finger arterial blood pressure, using a sophisticated system (Finapres; Chapter 21) which provides beat-to-beat pressure. This obviates the need for invasive intra-arterial (radial or brachial artery) catheterization, which previously was the only reliable means of obtaining continuous blood pressure measurements. The Finapres provides a reliable measure of change in

in abnormalities of blood pressure control, although hormones that influence blood vessels, intravascular volume and the kidneys may help to buffer these abnormalities. These aspects need to be borne in mind when we consider the range of tests to assess cardiovascular aspects of autonomic function, to determine the site or sites of lesions, and to ascertain hormonal factors which may be contributing to, or may be utilized for, the benefit of the patient.

The responses to postural change (head-up tilt and standing), pressor tests, the Valsalva manoeuvre, deep breathing, and hyperventilation form the core of screening tests in most laboratories, as in our two London Autonomic Units. These are described below, together with the results obtained from subjects without autonomic abnormalities that provide 'expected' results in different age bands (see Appendix I). When non-invasive techniques are used with standard laboratory precautions, these screening tests are safe, as in the experience of our units (starting in 1975 and with now over 1500 investigations per year), and that of other major centres. During certain tests (such as isometric hand grip) cardiac dysrhythmias may be more likely to occur in patients with cardiac disease, as after a myocardial infarction; however an electrocardiograph (ECG) analysis of 925 consecutive patients indicated rhythm disturbances during testing in only nine subjects, in whom these resolved without intervention (Piha and Voipio-Pulkki 1993). Although the risk is minimal, continuous ECG monitoring and resuscitation facilities should be available. Depending upon the questions raised, investigations additional to the screening tests may be needed, such as evaluating the responses to food ingestion, exercise, and carotid sinus massage. The limitations and risks of these investigations are individually listed where relevant.

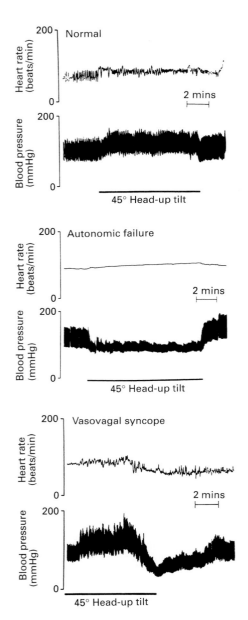

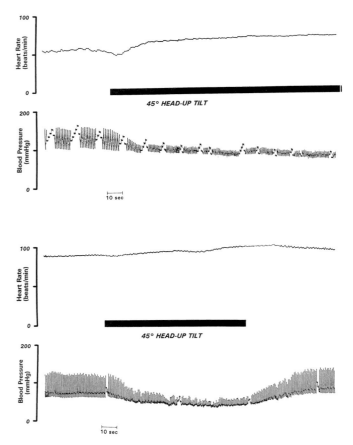

Fig. 20.3. Blood pressure and heart rate, measured by the Finapres, in two patients with autonomic failure. In the patient in the upper panel blood pressure falls to low levels, with the patient maintaining head-up tilt for over 20 min with virtually no symptoms. This patient had autonomic failure for many years and could tolerate such levels of blood pressure, presumably because of the improved cerebrovascular autoregulation. This is in contrast to the patient in the lower panel, who had to be put back to the horizontal after a short period of head-up tilt; she recently had developed severe postural hypotension after surgery. (From Mathias (1996a).)

Fig. 20.2. Blood pressure and heart rate before, during and after head-up tilt in a normal subject (uppermost panel), a patient with pure autonomic failure (middle panel), and a patient with vasovagal syncope (lowermost panel). In the normal subject there is no fall in blood pressure during head-up tilt, unlike the patient with autonomic failure in whom blood pressure falls promptly and remains low with a blood pressure overshoot on return to the horizontal. In the patient with autonomic failure there is only a minimal change in heart rate despite the marked blood pressure fall. In the patient with vasovagal syncope there was initially no fall in blood pressure during head-up tilt; in the latter part of tilt, as indicated in the record, blood pressure initially rose and then markedly fell, to extremely low levels, so that the patient had to be returned to the horizontal. Heart rate also fell. In each case continuous blood pressure and heart rate were recorded with the Portapress II.

blood pressure, especially when there are rapid responses, as during the Valsalva manoeuvre (Fig. 20.5).

Basal measurements need to be performed with the subject lying supine in a quiet room and as comfortable as possible. An adequate number of readings, over at least a 5–10 min interval, may be needed to determine the stability (or lability), of supine blood pressure. Recumbent (supine) hypertension may occur in patients with autonomic failure for reasons that include impaired baroreceptor control, supersensitivity of denervated blood vessels to even small amounts of neurotransmitters or to pressor drug treatment, and fluid shifts from the periphery into the central compartment when changing posture. In our laboratories, blood pressure recordings are performed with the Finapres and also with automated machines using brachial blood pressure measurement. The latter allows comparison with conventional clinic blood pressure recordings and with values

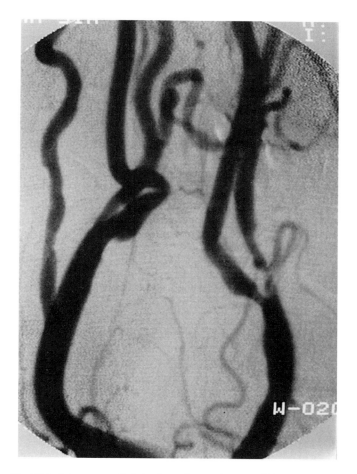

Fig. 20.4. Intravenous digital subtraction angiogram of the cerebral vessels in a patient with hypertension and widespread atherosclerosis, indicating left carotid artery stenosis. She had symptoms that initially were considered to be transient ischaemic attacks resulting from thromboembolism. The history, however, indicated symptoms closely associated with postural change. She had a postural fall in systolic blood pressure of only 10 mmHg, that presumably was sufficient to induce symptoms of cerebral ischaemia because of cerebrovascular disease. A reduction in antihypertensive therapy abolished the small postural fall in blood pressure and also her symptoms. (From Mathias (1998a).)

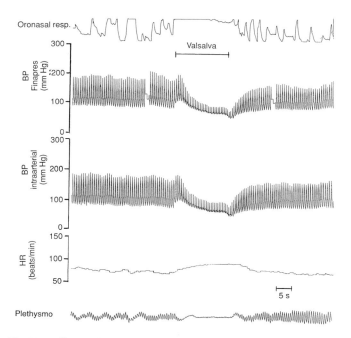

Fig. 20.5. Changes in non-invasive finger blood pressure (BP, Finapres) compared with intra-arterial blood pressure (BP) in a patient with autonomic impairment, before, during, and after a Valsalva manoeuvre. Respiratory rate (oronasal resp.), heart rate (HR), and plethysmograph (Plethysmo) are also continuously recorded; the Finapres recording appears indentical to the intra-arterial trace; the breaks indicate an internal calibration signal. (By courtesy of P. Cortelli and E. Zoni, University of Bologna; from Mathias (1995b).)

obtained from the Finapres, as factors such as cold fingers, especially in those with Raynaud's phenomenon, may impair monitoring. Most intermittent non-invasive blood pressure measurements take around a minute, and as they involve cuff inflation above systolic blood-pressure they should not be repeated too frequently. Postural change can be induced using either a manual or electrically operated tilt table (usually up to 45 or 60°), or by making the subject initially sit and then stand, or stand directly. A tilt table is advantageous, especially in subjects who have neurological disabilities, severe postural hypotension, or both, as it also enables rapid return to the horizontal if symptoms occur. Measurements of brachial blood pressure and heart rate during head-up tilt ideally should be made every $2\frac{1}{2}$ min, preferably for a period of 10 min, as this also enables blood collection for measurements of catecholamines and other vasoactive hormones

released during postural change. It is important with Finapres recordings that the hand is at heart level; this is more reliably and comfortably maintained with an adjustable sling, especially during manoeuvres that cause arm movement.

In normal subjects, head-up tilt or standing results in minimal changes in blood pressure. In autonomic disorders, however, the pressure often falls. The degree and rapidity of fall and extent of recovery can vary considerably even within the same individual. The blood pressure may fall rapidly and progressively in severe autonomic failure (Figs 20.2 and 20.6a); this may not occur in other patients, especially those with partial autonomic failure, as the rate and degree of fall also depends on the ability to recruit non-neurogenic mechanisms that help maintain blood pressure. Thus in patients with high thoracic or cervical spinal-cord transaction, especially those who have been rehabilitated, initially there is a rapid fall in blood pressure because of their inability to activate sympathetic vasoconstrictor pathways in response to postural change; this is followed by partial recovery of blood pressure (see Fig. 20.6b and Chapter 51). The recovery results from activation of spinal sympathetic reflexes or humoral compensatory mechanisms which include the renin– angiotensin–aldosterone system. In patients with autonomic failure who have an immediate and profound fall in blood pressure on postural change it may be difficult, if not impossible, to make accurate measurements using non-invasive techniques other than with the Finapres. Varying the degree of head-up tilt may help.

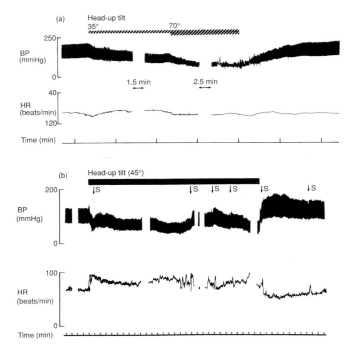

Fig. 20.6. (a) Continuous intra-arterial recording of blood pressure (BP) and heart rate (HR) in a patient with postural hypotension and the Holmes–Adie syndrome. Both systolic and diastolic blood pressure fall progressively during head-up tilt, with no recovery. There are minimal changes in heart rate. There was no change in plasma noradrenaline levels following tilt. Other investigations indicated that the lesions was likely to be on the afferent side of the baroreflex arc. (From Mathias (1987).) (b) Blood pressure (BP) and heart rate (HR) in a tetraplegic patient before, during and after head-up tilt to 45°. Blood pressure falls promptly with partial recovery, which in this case is linked to skeletal muscle spasms (S), inducing spinal sympathetic activity. Some of the later oscillations are probably due to the rise in plasma renin, measured where there are interruptions in the intra-arterial record. In the later phases, muscle spasms occur more frequently and further elevate blood pressure. On return to the horizontal, blood pressure rises rapidly above the previous basal level and slowly returns to supine levels. Heart rate tends to move in the opposite direction. There is a transient increase in heart rate during muscle spasms. (From Mathias and Frankel (1988).)

There is normally a small to moderate rise in heart rate during postural change. In the presence of a substantial fall in blood-pressure, a lack of change in heart rate is indicative of a baroreflex abnormality, as occurs when there is an afferent baroreceptor lesion or when there is both sympathetic and parasympathetic failure, as often occurs in chronic autonomic failure. In tetraplegic patients there is a rise in heart rate in response to the fall in blood pressure, because the vagal and glossopharyngeal afferent and the vagal efferent pathways are intact (Fig. 20.6b). The heart rate, however, does not usually rise above 110 beats/min, which is similar to levels observed after atropine administration and vagal blockade; further elevation of heart rate probably is dependent on adrenomedullary stimulation and elevation of plasma adrenaline levels, which does not occur in such patients. This adrenal component probably accounts for the greater tachycardia observed in subjects with an intact sympathetic nervous system when they have a low blood pressure, as may occur in haemorrhagic shock.

The degree of postural hypotension is dependent upon a large number of factors (Table 20.3). In primary autonomic failure, postural hypotension is often greater in the morning because of nocturnal diuresis, after food ingestion because of splanchnic vasodilatation, after exercise because of skeletal muscle vasodilatation, and in hot weather because of cutaneous vasodilatation. Vasodilatation induced by drugs, including those normally not considered to have significant cardiovascular effects, may cause substantial changes in blood pressure when there is a baroreflex deficit (Fig. 20.7). It is also necessary to consider non-neurogenic causes of postural hypotension (Table 20.2) as these may enhance hypotension considerably in autonomic failure.

A further advance in the assessment of cardiovascular autonomic abnormalities has been the development of 24-hour non-invasive ambulatory blood pressure and heart rate readings, that are of value both in the investigation and also in the evaluation of cardiovascular autonomic abnormalities (Fig. 20.8a,b,c). In normal subjects, blood pressure usually is higher in the day and lower when the subject is asleep at night. This circadian fall usually does not occur in autonomic failure. The technique also allows, with suitable protocols, recordings at different times of the day of responses to stimuli that include postural change, food ingestion, and exercise, each of which can lower blood pressure in autonomic failure. A particular advantage is that the effects of treatment on postural hypotension (Alan et al. 1995), and on hypotension induced by stimuli in daily life, can be assessed in the home situation. These techniques are of value when paroxysmal hypertension also occurs, as in familial dysautonomia (Fig. 20.8c) and tetraplegia (Chapter 51).

There are methods of quantifying the heart rate changes during standing, one of which is the '30–15 ratio'. Normally, on standing the rise in heart rate is greatest by the fifteenth beat, followed by slowing which is maximal at the thirtieth beat. The ratio of the longest P–R interval of the thirtieth to the shortest interval on the fifteenth beat should normally be over one. In the absence of change in heart rate on standing it is 1.0 or less than 1.0. It thus provides a numerical assessment that may be of value in longitudinal or interventional studies; whether it contributes further to assessing or understanding autonomic deficits is debatable. There clearly are difficulties in those who cannot readily stand.

The responses in two groups of patients, who do not have detectable autonomic impairment but are prone to fainting or presyncopal

Table 20.3. Factors influencing postural (orthostatic) hypotension

Speed of positional change
Time of day (worse in the morning)
Prolonged recumbency
Warm environment (hot weather, central heating, hot bath)
Raising intrathoracic pressure—micturition, defaecation or coughing
Food and alcohol ingestion
Physical exertion
Manoeuvres and positions (bending forward, abdominal compression, leg crossing, squatting, activating calf muscle pump)[*]
Drugs with vasoactive properties (including dopaminergic agents)

[*] These manoeuvres usually reduce the postural fall in blood pressure, unlike the others.

Adapted from Mathias (1995).

Table 20.4. Non-neurogenic causes of postural hypotension

Low intravascular volume	
Blood/plasma loss	Haemorrhage, burns, haemodialysis
Fluid/electrolyte	Inadequate intake—anorexia nervosa
	Fluid loss—vomiting, diarrhoea, losses from ileostomy
	Renal/endocrine—salt-losing nepropathy, adrenal insufficiency (Addison's disease), diabetes insipidus, diuretics
Vasodilatation	Drugs—glyceryl trinitrate
	Alcohol
	Heat, pyrexia
	Hyperbradykinism
	Systemic mastocytosis
	Extensive varicose veins
Cardiac impairment	
Myocardial	Myocarditis
Impaired ventricular filling	Atrial myxoma, constrictive pericarditis
Impaired output	Aortic stenosis

symptoms, should be mentioned. The first are those with neurally mediated syncope such as due to vasovagal syncope or emotional fainting (Chapters 44 and 45). There may be a family history of syncope, especially when the onset is below the age of 20 (Mathias *et al.* 1998). In these patients detailed autonomic testing usually reveals no abnormalities, but they may faint during postural change (Fig. 20.2 and 20.9), sometimes when prolonged, or when exposed to a variety of stimuli, including the sight or mere mention of a venepuncture needle. Continuous bloodpressure and heart rate monitoring, as with the Finapres, is of particular value in such cases. Additional physiological and pharmacological stimuli have been used to induce an episode and these include simultaneous lower-body negative pressure and drugs such as isoprenaline and glyceryl trinitrate. It is debatable whether such stimuli provide information of value, especially as they may induce syncope in normal subjects without a previous history of fainting; moreover, some carry a potential risk. In patients with vasovagal syncope the blood pressure often is maintained initially during head-up tilt, but then suddenly falls; this may be preceded by a fall in heart

rate. The responses are consistent with withdrawal of sympathetic nervous activity to blood vessels, in the presence of vagal overactivity to the heart (see Chapter 23). The former appears to be of greater importance, as vagal blockade with atropine, or maintenance of heart rate with a demand pacemaker, usually do not protect against syncope.

The second group of patients with symptoms on postural change are those in whom an autonomic deficit cannot be clearly defined but who have a pronounced tachycardia during postural change, following which there may be a fall in blood pressure. Many have symptoms of postural intolerance despite a lack of postural hypotension. For reasons that are unclear, there is a marked chronotropic cardiac response which presumably results either in inadequate filling of the right side of the heart or activation of cardiac sensory receptors followed later by sympathetic withdrawal, as postulated in some patients with vasovagal syncope. In some, hyperventilation may contribute. The association of postural intolerance with tachycardia is likely to have multiple causes (Khurana 1995).

The Valsalva manoeuvre

The changes in blood pressure and heart rate during the Valsalva manoeuvre, when intrathoracic pressure ideally is raised to 40 mmHg, provide a further assessment of the baroreflex pathways. To perform this the subject blows with an open glottis into a disposable syringe connected to the mercury column of a sphygmomanometer and maintains a forced expiratory pressure of up to 40 mmHg for 10 seconds. This may be difficult in some subjects, in whom levels between 20 and 40 mmHg often suffice to induce the necessary changes. Normally, with the rise in intrathoracic pressure the venous return falls along with blood pressure (Fig. 20.10). On releasing intrathoracic pressure there is a blood pressure overshoot because of persistence of sympathetic activity. Baroreflex activation then results in a secondary fall in heart rate to below basal levels. In sympathetic vasoconstrictor failure, the Valsalva manoeuvre results in a continuous fall in blood pressure with no stabilization; following release there is no blood pressure overshoot and thus there is no compensatory bradycardia. If the afferent and vagal efferent components of the baroreflex pathways are intact, as in tetraplegics and some patients with autonomic failure, heart rate rises while the blood pressure falls. There is also a sympathetic component to this response, because in normal subjects the rise in heart rate is blunted following administration of the

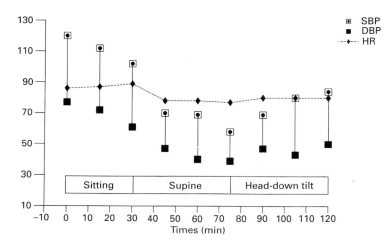

Fig. 20.7. Systolic and diastolic blood pressure in a patient with parkinsonian features before and after a standard laevodopa challenge (250 mg of laevodopa along with 25 mg carbidopa). The patient was initially seated but blood pressure fell and was so low that he needed to be laid supine and horizontal, and then head down. On further investigation, the final diagnosis in this patient was autonomic failure and the parkinsonian form of multiple system atrophy. (From Mathias (1999).)

β-adrenoceptor blocker propranolol. In diabetics with a proliferative retinopathy, some feel that there may be a risk of intraocular haemorrhage, because of the pressure transients.

It often is not possible, without a Finapres, to obtain beat-to-beat blood pressure during the Valsalva manoeuvre; the continuous measurement of heart rate with an electrocardiograph (ECG) often suffices in obtaining relevant information. However, spuriously abnormal responses may occur if the cheek muscles are used to produce an apparent but false rise in intrathoracic pressure. Beat-to-beat blood pressure monitoring, as with the Finapres (Fig. 20.5), is of

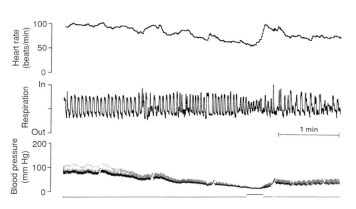

Fig. 20.9. blood pressure changes towards the end of a period of head-up tilt in a patient with recurrent episodes of vasovagal syncope. Blood pressure which was previously maintained begins to fall. There is also a fall in heart rate. Initially there are relatively minor changes in respiratory rate. The patient was about to faint and was put back to the horizontal (indicated by elevated time signal below) and then to 5° head-down tilt. Blood pressure and heart rate recover but still remain lower than previously. This patient had no other autonomic abnormalities on detailed testing. Blood pressure was measured non-invasively by the Finapres.

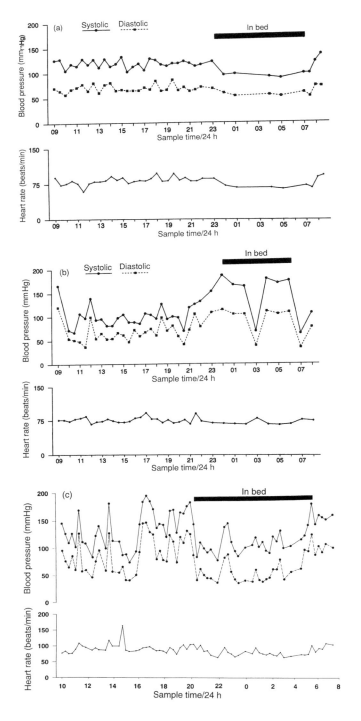

particular value in this situation, as it will identify a lack of fall in blood pressure, indicating that intrathoracic pressure was not elevated adequately.

There are various measurements and derived ratios of heart rate during the different phases of the Valsalva manoeuvre. A commonly used ratio (the Valsalva ratio), relates to the changes in heart rate in response to the variations in blood pressure. Normally, when intrathoracic pressure is elevated (phase II), the blood pressure falls and heart rate risks, while in the first 30 seconds after release of intrathoracic pressure (phase IV), the heart rate should fall in response to the rise in blood pressure. The Valsalva ratio is the derivative of the maximum rise and fall in these two phases (phase II ÷ phase IV) and should normally be over 1. It is 1 or less in the presence of autonomic failure. In our laboratories in London we attempt to obtain a Valsalva in the supine position while maintaining intrathoracic pressure at 40 mmHg, but this

Fig. 20.8. Twenty-four hour non-invasive ambulatory blood pressure profile, showing systolic (●——●) and diastolic (■– – –■) blood pressure and heart rate at intervals through the day and night. (a) The changes in a normal subject with no postural fall in blood pressure; there was a fall in blood pressure at night while asleep, with a rise in blood pressure on wakening. (b) The marked fluctuations in blood pressure in a patient with pure autonomic failure. The marked falls in blood pressure are usually the result of postural changes, either sitting or standing. Supine blood pressure, particularly at night, is elevated. Getting up to micturate causes a marked fall in blood pressure (at 03:00 hours). There is a reversal of the diurnal changes in blood pressure. There are relatively small changes in heart rate, considering the marked changes in blood pressure. (c) The marked variability in the blood pressure even at night in a patient with the Riley–Day syndrome (familial dysautonomia). The profile indicates episodes of profound hypotension, and at times marked hypertension. (From Mathias (1996*b*).)

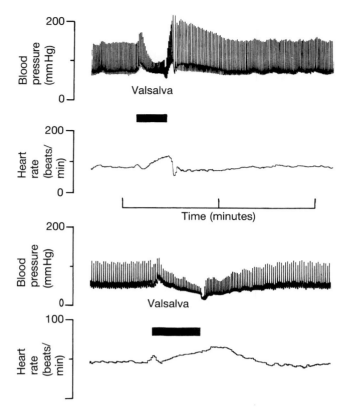

Fig. 20.10. Changes in intra-arterial blood pressure and heart rate before, during, and after the Valsalva manoeuvre, when intrathoracic pressure was raised to 40 mmHg in a normal subject (upper trace) and in a patient (lower trace). In the normal subject release of intrathoracic pressure was accompanied by an increase in blood pressure and a reduction in heart rate below basal levels. In the patient there was a gradual increase in blood pressure implying impairment of sympathetic vasoconstrictor pathways. The heart rate scale varies in the two subjects.

may not be achieved for reasons that include the patient's co-operation and strength, especially if there is impairment of muscles (diaphragm, intercostal, and accessory) involved in respiratory effort. The position of the patient (lying or sitting), and the time of day when the Valsalva manoeuvre is performed, are also factors that may influence the response (see Chapter 21). The responses also need to be considered in relation to factors known to affect heart rate, such as drug therapy and the myocardial state. We record the responses to three wellperformed Valsalva manoeuvres as this verifies an abnormal response, if present. It is debatable if averaging the results from three manoeuvres provides any further information; it may even be misleading in a subject with normal autonomic function who, for a variety of reasons, may be unable to adequately perform the Valsalva repeatedly. It may be that the best 'normal' response should be considered for the ratio in such subjects.

Analysis of the continuous blood pressure and heart rate record during the Valsalva often provides valuable information on the baroreflex. A rise in heart rate in response to the rise in intrathoracic pressure, when the blood pressure falls, suggests that the afferent and vagal efferent pathways are operative. Recovery of the blood pressure while intrathoracic pressure is maintained often occurs in normal

subjects, but not in those with sympathetic vasoconstrictor failure, when blood pressure usually falls inexorably; with release of intrathoracic pressure in such patients there is only a slow return to the baseline without the overshoot, consistent with the lack of sympathetic vasoconstrictor function. These form the characteristic blood pressure features of a 'blocked' Valsalva manoeuvre (Fig. 20.10).

Pressor stimuli

These raise blood pressure by stimulating sympathetic efferent pathways in a variety of ways. With isometric exercise or cutaneous cold there is activation of peripheral receptors, although there is an important cerebral component, especially with the former. Other stimuli, such as sudden noise or mental arithmetic, are dependent predominantly on cerebral stimulation.

Isometric exercise is performed by using either a dynamometer or a partially inflated sphygmomanometer cuff, and sustaining handgrip for 3 min, usually at a third of the maximum voluntary contraction pressure. The cold pressor (cutaneous cold) test consists of immersing the hand for up to 2 min in ice slush, usually just below 4 °C. Cortical arousal is performed by sudden noise, mental arithmetic (subtraction or addition of 7 or 17), or a variety of more complex tasks. These stimuli normally elevate blood pressure and heart rate (Fig. 20.11a, b). In patients with central or efferent sympathetic lesions the response to these stimuli is impaired or absent.

In tetraplegic patients with complete cervical spinal-cord lesions, mental arithmetic and stimuli above the cutaneous level of the lesion (such as with an ice pack) do not raise blood pressure, in contrast to stimuli below the lesion which activate spinal sympathetic reflexes (independently of the brain) and cause a rise in pressure, often accompanied by a fall in heart rate because of a baroreflex induced increase in vagal activity. Stimuli capable of such effects include cutaneous cold or other noxious cutaneous stimuli (including pin-prick), activation of abdominal or pelvic visceral reflexes by urinary bladder or large bowel contraction, and skeletal muscle spasms (Fig. 20.11c) (see Chapter 51). This elevation in blood pressure, along with a range of other cardiovascular changes, is an important component of the syndrome of autonomic dysreflexia and may be mistaken for a hypertensive crisis as in patients with a phaeochromocytoma, when there is excessive secretion of catecholamines from the tumour. Exaggerated pressor responses may occur in patients with partial or complete afferent baroreceptor impairment.

Responses to isometric exercise, cutaneous cold, and mental arithmetic can be obtained within a short period of time, and often provide valuable information in a wide range of disorders. The most useful responses probably are those induced by isometric exercise and cutaneous cold. Factors independent of the autonomic nervous system may affect the responses; thus disordered muscle function may influence the pressor response during isometric exercise and the presence of a sensory deficit may limit the response to cutaneous cold. The sensitivity, specificity, and reproducibility of these tests have been studied. The results obtained during isometric exercise with handgrip compare favourably with tilt-table tests (Khurana and Setty 1996). With the cold pressor test, systolic blood pressure was the more reliable measurement; reproducibility however, was lower when testing was repeated over the same day, or over 3 consecutive days, presumably because of habituation or anticipation (Fasano *et al.* 1996). The responses to mental arithmetic can vary; these may be reduced when

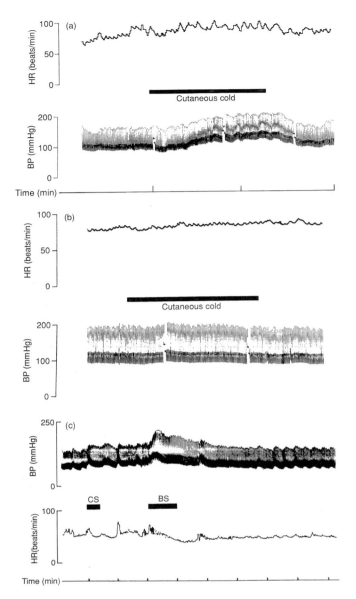

Fig. 20.11. Blood pressure (BP) and heart rate (HR) responses to cutaneous cold (hand up to wrist in ice slush) (a) in a normal subject and (b) in a patient with autonomic failure. The time scale is similar in (a) and (b). In the patient there is no rise in BP. Non-invasive recordings were made with the Finapres. (c) Intra-arterial BP and HR in a chronic tetraplegic before, during and after cutaneous stimulation (CS) and bladder stimulation (BS) 6 months after injury when reflex isolated spinal-cord activity had returned. Cutaneous stimulation is performed by the application of ice over the chest below the level of the lesion, and urinary bladder stimulation is by suprapubic percussion of the anterior abdominal wall. There is a rise in BP with both stimuli, this being greater with bladder stimulation. (From Mathias *et al.* (1979).)

the stimulus is too trivial as in those who are highly numerate, or when they cannot be performed adequately as in those with dementia. There is a variety of mental stress tests, many computerized both for execution and evaluation, that have been used successfully for research purposes (Mounier-Vehier *et al.* 1995). Interpretation of the results of

pressor tests, therefore, should be linked with the clinical characteristics and diagnosis of each patient, and related to the information that needs to be derived from such testing.

Heart rate responses to respiratory change

Changes in respiration result in rapid responses in heart rate and often provide a guide to the activity of the cardiac vagi. These results can be used in conjunction with the heart rate response to head-up tilt, standing, and the Valsalva manoeuvre. Normally with inspiration there is a rise, and with expiration a fall, in heart rate; this is the basis of sinus arrhythmia (Fig. 20.12). A considerable number of variations are available to exploit and standardize this objectively. A single deep breath, a short period of quiet breathing, or a fixed rate of 6 breaths/min has been used; each is claimed to be a better discriminator. Hyperventilation is probably a stronger stimulus to vagal withdrawal and causes a rise in heart rate. However, it may also lower blood-pressure and this could influence heart rate; the precise mechanisms for the fall in pressure with hyperventilation are unclear. Heart rate responses to respiratory manoeuvres are dependent on age, and this is an important factor in interpretation of results (Appendix I).

In autonomic neuropathy complicating diabetes mellitus and alcoholism, cardiac vagal lesions may occur prior to sympathetic impairment, and the heart rate responses to these tests may be abnormal before postural hypotension ensues. Although this provides evidence of an autonomic neuropathy, this should not be equated with a generalized or sympathetic deficit, or both.

Food challenge

Food lowers supine blood pressure in a large number of patients with primary autonomic failure (Chapter 29). In these patients, postprandial hypotension is linked to the release of vasodilatatory gut peptides and splanchnic vasodilatation, which is not accompanied by compensatory changes in cardiac output and skeletal muscle resistance vessels, as occur in normal subjects in whom blood pressure does not

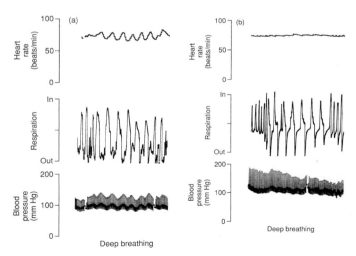

Fig. 20.12. The effect of deep breathing on heart rate and blood pressure in (a) a normal subject and (b) a patient with autonomic failure. There is no sinus arrhythmia in the patient, despite a fall in blood pressure. Respiratory changes are indicated in the middle panel.

fall after food ingestion. In addition to the fall in supine blood pressure, food is now recognized as unmasking or aggravating postural hypotension. The responses to food ingestion are thus of value in the assessment of post prandial hypotension, and in determining whether drugs (such as octreotide) reduce the blood pressure fall. This can be measured objectively by assessing the responses to head-up tilt ideally after an overnight fast, before and 45 min after food ingestion. For practical reasons, ingestion of liquids is preferable. Glucose can be used but the solution provides a caloric load of high osmolality which may be a problem, especially in diabetics. A clinically relevant and probably more physiological alternative is a balanced liquid meal using commercially available Complan (containing various food components) with added glucose, either in a milk or soya-bean base, made up to 300 ml with a caloric load of 330 Kcal (Mathias *et al.* 1991b). This can be prepared easily and ingested readily via a straw while lying flat, so that the effects of food ingestion also can be obtained independently of postural change. A fall of more than 20 mmHg systolic while supine clearly is abnormal; comparison of blood pressure during head-up tilt pre- and postprandially enables determination of whether there is enhancement or unmasking of postural hypotension by food. This can be of importance as there are patients who, when fasted, have modest postural hypotension, which is considerably exaggerated by food ingestion (Fig. 20.13).

Exercise testing

It is recognized increasingly that exercise, even in the supine position, lowers blood pressure in patients with autonomic failure (Smith *et al.* 1995). In these patients the hypotension induced by exercise is accompanied by a rise in cardiac output similar to that in normal subjects, but there is a coincidental marked fall in systemic vascular resistance. The latter is probably the result of vasodilatation in exercising skeletal muscle, without the compensatory responses elsewhere of increased sympathetic nerve traffic and sympathoadrenal activation which occur normally (Puvi-Rajasingham *et al.* 1997). Separating the responses of exercise from posture and gravity is important, and a technique has been devised so that increasing workloads (from 25 to 75 watts) on a bicycle ergometer can be performed while horizontal (Fig. 20.14). The responses to supine exercise therefore can be assessed, in addition to responses to either head-up tilt or standing, before and after exercise. In normal subjects exercise raises blood pressure; in autonomic failure usually there is a fall during the period of exercise. In some, however, the pressure does not fall (or rise) during exercise, but falls immediately on ceasing exercise; this is presumably due to peripheral vasodilatation and pooling not opposed by the calf muscle pump (Fig. 20.15). In autonomic failure, there is often an aggravation of postural hypotension post-exercise (Fig. 20.16), which is likely to be of importance in daily life. In patients who also have suspected ischaemic heart disease it may be best to limit or avoid even the mild degree of exercise that these patients are subjected to during this test.

The responses to exercise vary in the different autonomic disorders, with a greater fall in blood pressure in PAF than in MSA (Smith *et al.* 1995). Furthermore, differences may occur even with the various forms of MSA; in the parkinsonian form there is a smaller fall in blood pressure while supine when compared to the cerebellar form, although the enhancement of postural hypotension post-exercise is similar in the two groups (Smith and Mathias 1996). The

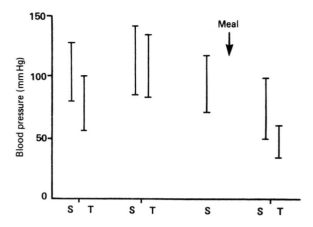

Fig. 20.13 Systolic and diastolic blood pressure in a patient with multiple system atrophy, while supine (S) and after 45° head-up tilt (T) on three occasions. On the first, food intake was not controlled and the patient had eaten earlier. On the second the patient had not eaten and the postural blood pressure fall was negligible. The patient then had a liquid meal. Following food challenge supine blood pressure fell and on the third occasion of tilt there was a considerably greater fall in blood pressure. These observations emphasize the importance of food intake on postural hypotension. (From Mathias (1991b).)

reasons are unclear. It may be that there is more extensive autonomic impairment in the cerebellar form as the lesions are more caudal, and in closer proximity and more likely to impair central autonomic mechanisms. In patients with an isolated peripheral autonomic disorder (dopamine β-hydroxylase deficiency), there is neither a rise nor a fall in blood pressure during exercise while supine, but there is a considerable worsening of postural hypotension post-exercise (Fig. 20.16). The reasons for the lack of blood pressure fall while supine are probably similar to those that prevent supine postprandial hypotension in these patients (see Chapter 29).

Carotid sinus massage

This should be performed if the history suggests that syncope is caused by movements of the neck or pressure over the carotid sinus by a collar or tie, especially in the presence of apparently normal cardiovascular autonomic function. Carotid sinus hypersensitivity is recognized increasingly in the elderly as a potential cause of unexplained falls (McIntosh *et al.* 1993), and it needs to be sought actively in this group. Carotid sinus massage may provoke asystole and cardiac dysrhythmias, so it is essential that adequate resuscitation measures are available readily in the event of cardiovascular collapse. Continuous monitoring of heart rate, the ECG (on an oscilloscope, preferably with a printing facility), and blood pressure, ideally with a noninvasive beat-to-beat machine such as the Finapres, is needed. Only one carotid sinus should be stimulated each time, using gentle pressure that compresses the carotid bulb against the transverse processes of the upper cervical vertebrae. There are normally minor changes in heart rate and blood pressure. In carotid sinus hypersensitivity, severe bradycardia and hypotension may occur (Fig. 20.17). The former may precede the hypotension, and in the cardioinhibitory form may be prevented by atropine or a demand cardiac pacemaker. There is a less common vasodepressor form,

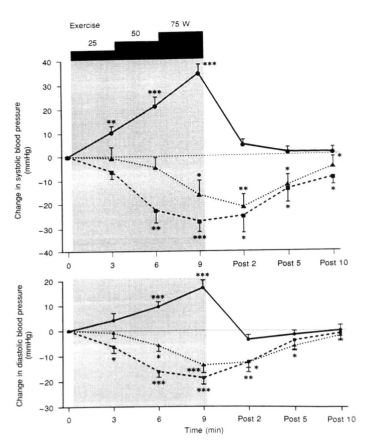

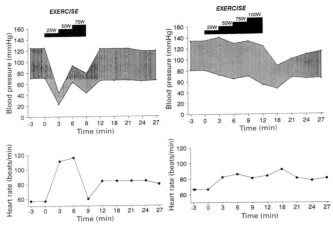

Fig. 20.15. Systolic and diastolic blood pressure (top) and heart rate (lower panel) in two patients with autonomic failure, before, during, and after bicycle exercise performed with the patients in the supine position at different workloads, ranging from 25 to 100 watts. In the patient on the left there is a marked fall in blood pressure on initiating exercise; she had to crawl upstairs because of severe exercise-induced hypotension. In the patient on the right, there are minor changes in blood pressure during exercise, but a marked decrease soon after stopping exercise. This patient was usually asymptomatic while walking, but developed postural symptoms when he stopped walking and stood still. It is likely that the decrease in blood pressure post-exercise was due to vasodilatation in exercising skeletal muscle, not opposed by the calf muscle pump. (From Mathias and Williams (1994).)

Fig. 20.14. Change in systolic (upper panel) and diastolic (lower panel) blood pressure during 9 minutes of incremental supine exercise on a bicycle at 25, 50, and 75 watts, with supine measurements continued post exercise at 2, 5, and 10 minutes. Blood pressure rises in normal subjects (●—●), and rapidly falls back towards normal on cessation of exercise. In patients with multiple system atrophy (MSA; ▲---▲) and pure autonomic failure (PAF; ■---■), there is a work-related fall in blood pressure that is at its lowest towards the end of the exercise period; post-exercise, blood pressure slowly recovers and even 10 minutes later has not entirely returned to normal (From Smith *et al.* (1995).)

where hypotension occurs without bradycardia (Fig 20.18); this appears to be due to withdrawal of sympathetic nerve activity (Chapter 23). Many fall into the mixed form, with a fall in both heart rate and blood pressure. Therapeutic approaches in the vasodepressor and mixed forms include unilateral or bilateral carotid sinus denervation. Predicting the outcome can be difficult and testing may need to be repeated after intravenous atropine (Fig. 20.19) and occasionally after local anaesthetic infiltrated around the carotid sinus.

Other measures of assessing baroreceptor reflex function

A variety of techniques ranging from lower-body suction to stimulation of carotid sinus afferents by a neck chamber have been utilized. Negative pressure to the lower half of the body can be exerted by having the subject in a box or capsule extending up to the midthoracic region, with an airtight seal allowing suction, usually by a vacuum cleaner, which unloads and thus stimulates cardiopulmonary

baroreceptor afferents. In normal subjects this should increase sympathetic neural activity, with constriction of resistance vessels, a rise in heart rate, and maintenance of blood pressure. This does not occur in sympathetic vasoconstrictor failure, when blood pressure rapidly falls (Fig. 20.20). In neurally mediated syncope the combination of lower-body negative pressure along with head-up tilt has been used to provoke syncope (El-Badawi *et al.* 1994).

A specially designed cervical collar enables assessment of carotid sinus afferents, which may be either inhibited or stimulated by localized elevation or lowering of pressure. The relationship between heart rate and blood pressure helps to construct indices of baroreflex sensitivity. Pharmacological approaches using pressor agents (phenylephrine) or vasodilators (glyceryl trinitrate), given either as a bolus injection or sublingually to transiently raise or lower blood pressure respectively, have also been used. The use of physiological and pharmacological approaches have particular value in the research setting and provide considerable information when combined with haemodynamic measurements in different regions.

Cardiac and regional haemodynamic measurements

Non-invasive techniques are now used widely to measure cardiac and regional haemodynamics. Their main value has been in clinical research laboratories, although the information derived in various disorders increasingly has been utilized in diagnosis and management. The measurements include various aspects of cardiac function (such as stroke volume and cardiac output), and blood flow to skin, skeletal muscle, the splanchnic region, and the brain. Some

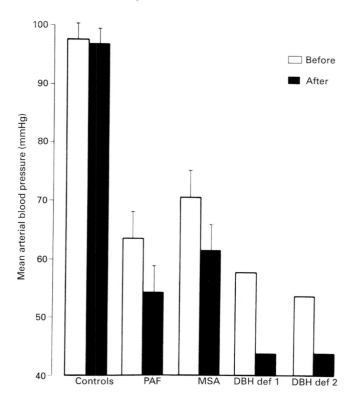

Fig. 20.16. Mean arterial blood pressure during head-up tilt before (open histograms) and 10 minutes after supine exercise (filled histograms) in normal subjects (controls), patients with pure autonomic failure (PAF), multiple system atrophy (MSA), and in two siblings (a brother and sister) with dopamine β-hydroxylase (DBH) deficiency. Blood pressure on standing does not change in the controls, either before or after exercise, unlike the autonomic failure groups in whom standing blood pressure after exercise is considerably lower in PAF and MSA, with a substantial accentuation of postural hypotension in the two patients with DBH deficiency. (From Smith and Mathias (1995).)

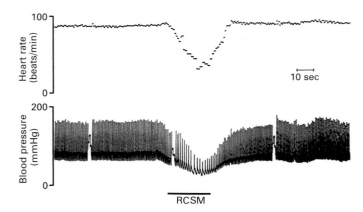

Fig. 20.17. Heart rate and blood pressure before, during, and after right carotid sinus massage (RCSM) in a patient with syncopal episodes. There is a fall in both heart rate and blood pressure during carotid sinus massage, typical of the mixed (cardioinhibitory and vasodepressor) form of this disorder. The breaks in the record indicate interval calibration by the Finapres machine. (From Mathias (1999).)

Spectral analytical techniques to study short- and long-term cardiovascular changes

These are being utilized increasingly, although largely in a research setting (details in Chapter 22). The use of such techniques to study heart rate changes as a measure of cardiac autonomic function during sleep has been of value, especially in certain neuropsychiatric disorders (Ferini-Strambi and Smirne 1997); in narcolepsy there are changes related to impairment of the sleep–awake cycle while in panic disorders sympathetic overactivity occurs only in the day and not at night, thus excluding an intrinsic defect in autonomic regulation.

Electrophysiological assessment of sympathetic activity

Intraneural recordings of sympathetic activity

Skin and muscle sympathetic nerve activity can be recorded using tungsten microelectrodes inserted into a cutaneous nerve in the arm or leg (Chapter 23). Skin sympathetic activity is affected by thermal stimuli (activity increases with cold and decreases with heat), in contrast to muscle sympathetic activity which responds to maneouvres activating baroreceptors and is time-locked to blood pressure changes within the cardiac cycle.

Microneurographic techniques have confirmed and advanced our understanding of a considerable number of physiological and pathophysiological processes. However, there are limitations and disadvantages to this technique. Measurements can only be made in a restricted region and although there is a surprisingly good correlation with plasma noradrenaline levels, it may not provide specific answers when stimuli cause differential regional sympathetic responses. More importantly, the procedure is dependent upon considerable skill and, although safe, is an invasive one. It is likely to be unreliable or of no value when sympathoneuronal activity is low or absent, as in autonomic failure.

techniques, such as those for cardiac function and skeletal muscle blood flow, are widely available (Smith *et al.* 1995). Technological advances have contributed substantially to measurements in other regions. In the splanchnic region, measurement of superior mesenteric artery blood flow can be measured accurately and reproducibly and has enhanced our understanding of the role of the splanchnic circulation in various disorders (Chaudhuri *et al.* 1991) (see Chapter 29). Cutaneous blood flow can be measured continuously using laser Doppler flowmetry that has been used in various disease states (Abbott 1993; Faes *et al.* 1993). Blood flow in the middle cerebral artery can be measured using Doppler sonography, which has provided useful information in patients with autonomic failure (Brooks *et al.* 1989; Lagi *et al.* 1994) and in neurally mediated syncope (Diehl *et al.* 1996) (Fig. 20.21). Near infrared spectroscopy (Elwell *et al.* 1994), positron emission tomography scanning (Dolan *et al.* 1997), and functional magnetic resonance imaging are providing further information on cerebral blood flow changes, especially in localized regions of the brain (Fig. 20.22).

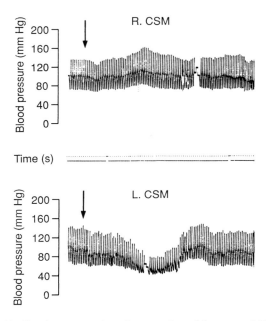

Fig. 20.18. Continuous non-invasive recording of finger arterial blood pressure (Finapres) before, during, and after carotid sinus massage on the right (R. CSM) and left (L. CSM). The fine dots indicate the time marker in seconds. The arrow indicates when stimulation began. Stimulation on the right for 10 sec did not lower blood pressure and heart rate. On the left, carotid sinus massage caused a substantial fall in both systolic and diastolic blood pressure, during which the patient felt light-headed and had greying-out of vision. There was only a modest fall in heart rate. The syncopal attacks were abolished by left carotid sinus denervation. The breaks in the record indicate internal calibration by the Finapres machine. (From Mathias et al. (1991a).)

Sympathetic skin response

Electrical potentials can be recorded from electrodes on the foot and hand using standard electromyographic equipment, before and after stimuli which increase sympathetic cholinergic activity to sweat glands. A variety of these stimuli activate sweat glands, cause -production of sweat, and change skin resistance, hence the use of the terms sympathetic skin response (SSR), electrodermal activity, and galvanic skin response (Fig. 20.23a). The SSR can be induced by stimuli that are physiological (inspiratory gasp, loud noise, or touch) or electrical (median nerve stimulation). The response is usually absent in axonal neuropathies, but is present in demyelinating disorders (Shahani et al. 1984); this was the original basis of the test which was later adapted as a means of determining sympathetic cholinergic function.

There have been numerous reports on the SSR in a variety of disorders (Arunodaya and Taly 1995), but there have been limited observations on influencing factors and few studies in adequate numbers of clearly defined autonomic disorders. This is compounded by the variability of responses when latency and amplitude are incorporated into calculations. This results in poor sensitivity and specificity, as has been observed previously with polygraph recordings used as a 'lie detector', when the response was measured along with blood pressure, heart rate, and respiration rate (Brett et al. 1986). This problem may be avoided by using responses that are either consistently present or absent. When this approach is

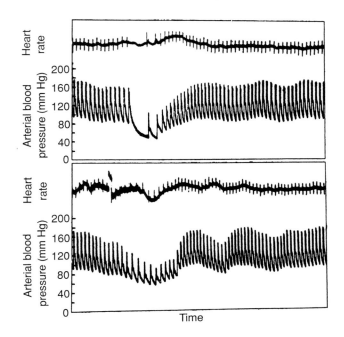

Fig. 20.19. The effect of carotid sinus massage on heart rate and blood pressure in a patient with carotid sinus hypersensitivity before (upper panel) and after (lower panel) 1 mg of atropine intravenously. The bradycardia is prevented by atropine but the blood pressure falls on repeat stimulation, indicating that vasodilatation, probably due to sympathetic withdrawal, is also contributory in the mixed forms of carotid sinus hypersensitivity. (From Hutchinson and Stock (1960).)

used the SSR has been reproducibly elicited in normal subjects and patients with dopamine β-hydroxylase deficiency (with preserved cholinergic function) and is absent in patients with pure autonomic failure and pure cholinergic dysautonomia (Fig. 20.23a, b) (Magnifico et al. 1998). Thus, the SSR may be helpful in patients with peripheral autonomic lesions.

The SSR has the advantage of being a non-invasive test that can be applied readily in most laboratories. However, its value needs further assessment, especially in patients with different types of central autonomic disorders. In MSA with confirmed sympathetic adrenergic failure, up to a third with either the parkinsonian or cerebellar forms had a definite SSR (Fig. 20.24), making it unlikely that it would be a valuable discriminatory test in separating MSA from idiopathic Parkinson's disease (without autonomic failure), especially in the early stages (Magnifico et al. 1997). The precise basis for the response also needs clarification, as the skin electric potential may reflect not only sweat-gland activity, but also changes in the property of surrounding skin. This is of relevance to recent observations where the SSR was present, although with a diminished amplitude, in patients who were treated successfully for palmar hyperhidrosis by endoscopic thoracic sympathectomy (Magnifico et al. 1996).

Biochemical and hormonal
Catecholamines and their metabolites

Noradrenaline is the major neurotransmitter at sympathetic nerve endings, while adrenaline and noradrenaline are both released from the

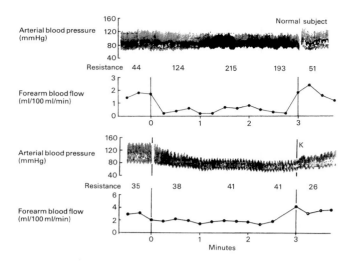

Fig. 20.20. The effect of lower-body negative suction on arterial blood pressure, forearm vascular resistance, and forearm blood flow in a normal subject (upper panel, and in a patient with autonomic failure (lower panel). This rise in forearm vascular resistance in the normal subject during suction is not seen in the patient, in whom there is a substantial fall in blood pressure. (From Bannister *et al.* (1967).)

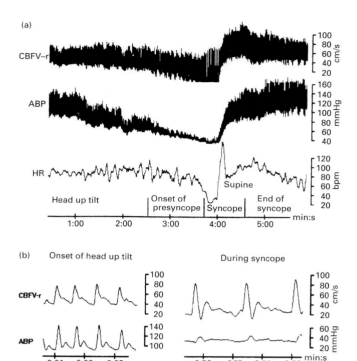

Fig. 20.21. Continuous measurements of right middle cerebral blood flow velocity (CBFV-r), arterial blood pressure (ABP) and heart rate (HR) in a patient before, during, and after tilt-induced neurally mediated (vasovagal) syncope (a). There is a marked fall in ABP that precedes the fall in HR. (b) In the left panel, cerebral blood flow velocity during head-up tilt before the fall in blood pressure shows a relatively low pulsatility, unlike the arterial blood pressure wave, while this is interchanged during syncope. The findings favour cerebral vasoconstriction during neurally mediated syncope with milder proximal and stronger peripheral vasoconstriction in the cerebral vessels. (From Diehl *et al.* (1996).)

adrenal medulla. Stimuli such as head-up tilt, that result in sympathoneural activation, elevate levels of noradrenaline in plasma. In sympathetic failure there is no rise in plasma noradrenaline levels and thus the combination of measurement of basal levels along with the response to head-up tilt or standing is necessary (Fig. 20.25). The concentration of noradrenaline in plasma, however, is the net result of a number of processes, involving secretion, neuronal uptake, intraneuronal and extraneuronal metabolism, and clearance. As arterial measurements usually are not made, changes in a venous bed may reflect regional characteristics which may not be applicable globally.

The basal supine plasma level itself may help in pointing to the possible diagnosis. In PAF, levels are often low because these patients are likely to have more complete distal lesions, while in MSA, with more central lesions, levels are often within the normal range (Fig. 20.25). It should be noted that basal levels in tetraplegics with a definite preganglionic lesion are about 35 per cent of normal (see Chapter 51). Extremely low or virtually undetectable levels of plasma noradrenaline and adrenaline occur in patients with deficiency of the enzyme dopamine β-hydroxylase (Chapter 40). The characteristic difference from other groups with low levels, such as PAF, is that plasma dopamine levels uniquely are elevated (Fig. 20.25). The diagnosis can be confirmed by the absence of dopamine β-hydroxylase in both plasma and tissue. Levels of plasma adrenaline normally often are just at the detection limit of most assays, and basal levels alone do not usually provide useful information. In normal subjects, hypoglycaemia and exercise predominantly raise plasma adrenaline levels; this does not occur in autonomic failure. An excess of plasma noradrenaline and adrenaline may suggest a phaeochromocytoma; such patients characteristically have paroxysms of hypertension, headache and sweating but also may suffer from postural hypotension, because of a low plasma volume and subsensitivity of α-adrenoceptors.

Measurements of catecholamines and their metabolites in urine have certain advantages, as they provide a measure of secretion over a longer period, which may be of value in phaeochromocytoma where

there may be intermittent secretion. They also may help in the diagnosis of rarer forms of autonomic failure and the monitoring of their treatment. In dopamine β-hydroxylase deficiency, urinary dopamine metabolites are normal or elevated, while those of noradrenaline and adrenaline are almost undetectable; with adequate treatment with DL- or L-threo-dihydroxyphenylserine, noradrenaline metabolites increase (Chapter 40). A number of other urinary metabolites provide indices of central or peripheral catecholamine metabolism (Chapter 24).

Techniques such as total-body and regional noradrenaline spillover have provided valuable information on sympathetic activation in the body, heart, and vascular regions (such as the splanchnic and renal circulations), and in the brain (Esler *et al.* 1993; Lambert *et al.* 1997). The use of radioactive substances and cannulation of arteries and major veins, however, restrict their use to highly specialized research laboratories. There also are non-invasive approaches to assess regional sympathetic innervation and function, using [123I]meta-iodobenzyl guanidine (MIBG) that is taken up into sympathetic nerve terminals and can be measured by single photon emission computed tomography (SPECT). This technique successfully images adrenal and extra-adrenal phaeochromocytoma and has been used to image the heart in autonomic disorders, such as diabetic autonomic neuropathy (Claus

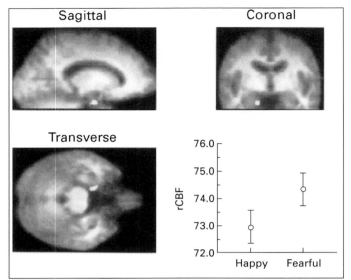

Fig. 20.22. Views of the brain showing activation of the left amygdala using positron emission tomography scanning with $H_2^{15}O$ superimposed on structural magnetic resonance images, and the construction of a statistical parametric map. This was in response to visual stimuli using photographs showing happy and fearful facial expressions. Regional cerebral blood flow (rCBF) is indicated on the right. Faces with fearful expressions caused a greater change in the blood flow to the amygdala than happy faces. (From Morris *et al.* (1996).)

et al. 1994). It is unclear whether the technique currently has the sensitivity of the invasive methods; in normal subjects there is no relationship with age when global values are considered, although there is a relationship with specific cardiac regions (Tsuchimochi *et al.* 1995). A recent approach has been positron emission tomographic (PET) scanning, (Goldstein *et al.* 1997a) using 6-[¹⁸F]fluorodopamine to visualize sympathetic innervation of cardiac tissue in various forms of autonomic failure (Goldstein *et al.* 1997b).

Renin–angiotensin–aldosterone system

This system has a major influence on blood pressure. Renin is released from the juxtaglomerular cells of the renal afferent arterioles and, by a series of steps, results in the formation of the active pressor agent, angiotensin II, which has multiple actions on blood vessels, sympathetic nerves, the brain, and also on the adrenal cortex (to cause secretion of aldosterone). In adrenocortical deficiency (such as Addison's disease), postural hypotension may occur, and there is a compensatory and marked elevation in renin and angiotensin II levels while plasma aldosterone levels are extremely low. In such patients plasma cortisol levels do not rise after administration of adrenocorticotrophic hormone.

In autonomic disorders, the renin response to head-up tilt or standing may be of relevance to the use of head-up tilt at night to reduce postural hypotension (Chapter 36). In some patients with primary autonomic failure the renin response is impaired, especially when related to their marked hypotension during head-up tilt (Bannister *et al.* 1979). In others, however, there may be an exaggerated rise (Mathias *et al.* 1977), as is also observed in tetraplegic patients (Chapter 51). If renin measurements are made,

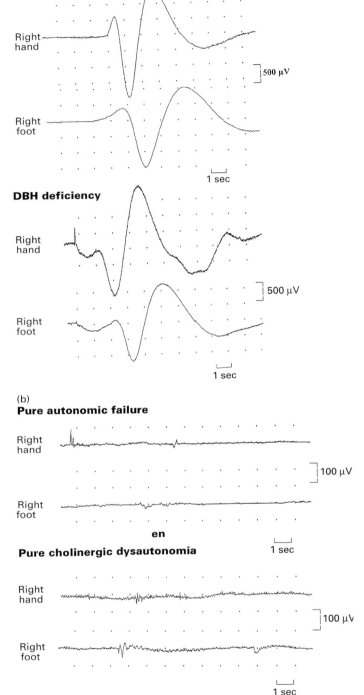

Fig. 20.23. (a) The sympathetic skin response (in microvolts) from the right hand and right foot of a normal subject (control) and a patient with dopamine β-hydroxylase (DBH) deficiency. (b) The sympathetic skin response could not be recorded in two patients, one with pure autonomic failure (PAF) and the other with pure cholinergic dysautonomia. (From Magnifico *et al.* (1998).)

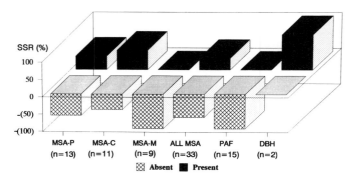

Fig. 20.24. Presence or absence of the sympathetic skin response (SSR) in 33 patients with MSA, 15 patients with pure autonomic failure (PAF), and two siblings with dopamine β-hydroxylase (DBH) deficiency. The SSR (as occurs in normal subjects) was present in the two DBH-deficiency patients who had adrenergic failure but preserved cholinergic function; it was absent in all PAF patients with a peripheral sympathetic lesion. A proportion of patients (up to 30 per cent) with the parkinsonian (MSA-P) and cerebellar (MSA-C) forms had preservation of the SSR, despite postural hypotension and definite sympathetic adrenergic failure. (data from Magnifico *et al.* (1997).)

care should be taken to obtain an adequate basal level, keeping in mind the long half-life of renin. A 10 min period of tilt may suffice to demonstrate an exaggerated response (Fig. 20.26), although a longer period is preferable, especially if plasma aldosterone is also being measured. A variety of influences, including salt intake and drugs such as fludrocortisone, can modify renin release.

Antidiuretic hormone (vasopressin)

In normal subjects, there is a rise in plasma vasopressin levels with head-up tilt and with hyperosmotic stimuli (see Chapter 24). Vasopressin levels have been used to assess the integrity of the afferent and central autonomic pathways. In afferent lesions vasopressin levels do not rise with head-up tilt, unlike patients with central lesions of the baroreceptor pathways, in whom there is no response; in both however, there is a preserved response to an osmotic stimulus, confirming integrity of the relevant hypothalamic nuclei and their posterior pituitary connections. In PAF, vasopressin levels rise with head-up tilt, unlike in MSA (Kaufmann *et al.* 1992). In patients with cervical spinal-cord injuries there is an exaggerated rise in vasopressin levels with head-up tilt (see Chapter 51).

Pharmacological

Information on the integrity of autonomic pathways, the number and sensitivity of receptors on target organs, and on functional components of the autonomic nervous system may be obtained by using drugs that are either agonists or antagonists. When combined with relevant hormonal responses they provide further information on central and peripheral autonomic pathways and on autonomic receptors. It is important, especially in patients with suspected autonomic disorders who may have abnormal responses, that drugs to reverse their effects are available along with resuscitation facilities.

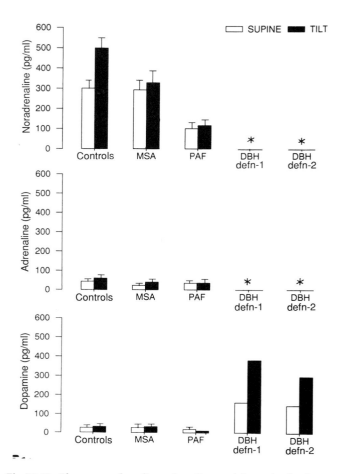

Fig. 20.25. Plasma noradrenaline, adrenaline, and dopamine levels (measured by high pressure liquid chromatography) in normal subjects (controls), patients with multiple system atrophy (MSA), pure autonomic failure (PAF), and two individual patients with dopamine β-hydroxylase deficiency (DBH def) while supine and after head-up tilt to 45° for 10 min. The asterisk indicates levels below the detection limits for the assay, which are less than 5 pg/ml for noradrenaline and adrenaline and less than 20 pg/ml for dopamine. Bars indicate ± SEM.

Drugs acting on the sympathetic nervous system

Noradrenaline

Noradrenaline is the major neurotransmitter at sympathetic nerve endings and predominantly stimulates α-adrenoceptors, with some effects on β-adrenoceptors. Pressor sensitivity to noradrenaline can be tested by intravenous infusion, beginning with a low dose (in case of supersensitivity) followed by increments every 5–10 min, with careful monitoring of blood pressure, heart rate, and the ECG. Construction of a dose–response curve will indicate whether there is an enhanced pressor response, when compared to normal responses. In more distal sympathetic lesions, as in PAF, the dose–response curve is shifted considerably to the left, and there is also a greater slope, indicating that these patients have a greater degree of pressor supersensitivity than MSA patients (Fig. 20.27) see (Chapter 24). The mechanisms responsible for pressor supersensitivity appear to be

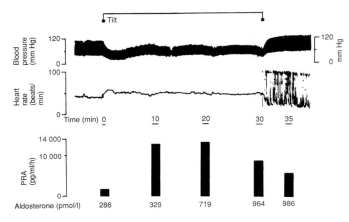

Fig. 20.26. Blood pressure (BP), heart rate, plasma renin activity (PRA), and plasma aldosterone levels in a patient with autonomic failure before, during and after head-up tilt to 45° for 30 min. There was an immediate fall in both systolic and diastolic BP which gradually recovered. There was a small elevation in BP over previous basal levels on return to the horizontal. Heart rate rose when BP fell, but the response was modest. Following return to the horizontal, bigeminal rhythm occurred, accounting for the abnormal trace. Levels of plasma renin activity rose markedly during head-up tilt, reaching the levels often seen in severely hypertensive patients with renal artery stenosis. Plasma aldosterone levels rose later. (From Bannister *et al.* (1986).)

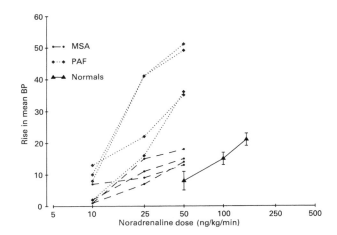

Fig. 20.27. Rise in mean blood pressure (BP) in four patients with pure autonomic failure (PAF), four patients with multiple system atrophy (MSA), and normal subjects (± SEM) during graded intravenous infusions of noradrenaline. Both groups of patients with autonomic failure had increased sensitivity to infused noradrenaline. In the PAF patients there appears to be a considerably greater response.

multiple. Indirect evidence from studies of α_2-adrenoceptors on platelets suggest that there is up-regulation of adrenoceptors, probably because of the low levels of plasma noradrenaline. This may account for the difference in slope. The shift to the left that occurs in both PAF and MSA suggests that impairment of the baroreceptor reflex and the inability to compensate in different vascular beds (as also occurs in tetraplegic patients), may be major factors. Finally, clearance of noradrenaline is likely to be affected, depending upon both the site and the degree of sympathetic nerve impairment. The reverse, an impaired pressor response to noradrenaline and other vasopressor agents, may occur in systemic amyloidosis because of infiltration of blood vessels by amyloid tissue.

Assessment of sensitivity to noradrenaline or other adrenoceptor agonists (such as phenylephrine), is of value in providing evidence of sensitivity of blood vessels and the possible response to sympathomimetic treatment. As with other pharmacological tests, these should be performed in laboratories familiar with the techniques. Because of pressor supersensitivity, testing in patients with suspected autonomic disorders should begin cautiously, using doses of a fifth or less than usual. Supine hypertension may occur in patients with autonomic failure and the clinical investigator will need to decide which level of blood pressure can be reached safely in individual patients. One should be on guard for cardiac dysrhythmias. The ready availability of suitable drugs and resuscitation measures in an emergency is a necessity. Rapid relief of severe hypertension may be obtained by placing patients in the head-up position.

Tyramine

Tyramine releases noradrenaline from both the granules and the cytosol within the sympathetic nerve terminal. A lack of rise in blood pressure and in plasma noradrenaline levels is indicative of absent noradrenaline stores and is characteristic of widespread postganglionic denervation or noradrenaline depletion, as in dopamine β-hydroxylase deficiency (Chapter 40). In incomplete lesions, however, release of even subnormal amounts of noradrenaline may cause a substantial pressor response because of supersensitivity; this impairs interpretation of tyramine-induced responses.

Isoprenaline

Isoprenaline is a β-adrenoceptor agonist which acts on both the β_1 and β_2 subtypes. The β_1 subtype is concerned predominantly with raising heart rate, and the β_2 subtype with vasodilatation and bronchodilatation. Isoprenaline can be given either as a bolus or as an intravenous infusion and its effects on heart rate and blood-pressure provide an indication of β-adrenoceptor responsiveness. In patients with autonomic failure and in tetraplegics, bolus intravenous injections cause an exaggerated but transient fall in both systolic and diastolic blood pressure (Fig. 20.28).

Similar changes occur with intravenous infusion of isoprenaline (Fig. 20.29). This may result from β_2-adrenoceptor supersensitivity, and from unopposed β_2-adrenoceptor-induced vasodilatation because of the baroreceptor deficit. Chronotropic supersensitivity to isoprenaline does not occur in autonomic failure with vagal denervation (Fig. 20.30), despite indirect *in vitro* evidence from lymphocyte studies that suggest an increase in β-adrenoceptor numbers. In tetraplegics the fall in blood pressure in the presence of the preserved afferent baroreceptor and efferent vagal pathways may result in a greater rise in heart rate, that is not necessarily attributable to β-adrenoceptor supersensitivity.

Clonidine

Clonidine is an α-adrenoceptor agonist which has a number of effects, including a predominant cerebral action in reducing sympathetic neural activity and thus lowering blood pressure. In normal subjects after clonidine, plasma noradrenaline levels fall and serum growth hormone levels rise. The latter is dependent upon intact central autonomic pathways. Clonidine can be given intravenously (2 μg/kg body weight over 10 min to avoid a transient pressor effect), with observations for a period of 75–90 min after administration. Its side-effects include dryness of mouth and sedation. After an hour following intravenous infusion most subjects are awake, although drowsy.

The uses of clonidine include:

1. Determining residual sympathetic nervous activity and its contribution to the maintenance of blood pressure. In PAF patients there is usually a rise in blood pressure (because of supersensitivity) with a small fall or no further reduction in the low levels of plasma noradrenaline, unlike normal subjects in whom both blood-pressure and plasma noradrenaline levels fall (Thomaides *et al.* 1992). In patients with MSA or with incomplete autonomic lesions, there is usually a fall in supine blood pressure and plasma noradrenaline levels. Similar changes to those in PAF are observed in dopamine β-hydroxylase deficiency (Chapter 40). In tetraplegics there is a transient pressor response with intravenous clonidine; after oral clonidine, blood pressure is unchanged (Chapter 51).

2. Distinguishing phaeochromocytoma patients with autonomous noradrenaline secretion from patients with essential hypertension and labile hypertension who have elevated basal noradrenaline levels. In phaeochromocytoma, plasma noradrenaline levels remain elevated, unlike normal subjects or essential hypertensive patients in whom levels fall after clonidine (Fig. 20.31).

3. Measuring the growth hormone response as a neuroendocrine marker of integrity of the central adrenergic system. In normal subjects, serum growth hormone levels rise substantially within

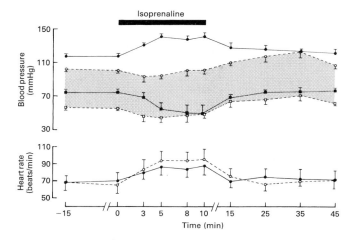

Fig. 20.29. Blood pressure and heart rate in five tetraplegic patients (open circles and squares and broken line) and five control subjects (full circles and squares and continuous line) before, during, and after intravenous infusion of isoprenaline (0.01 μg/min/kg). The shaded area indicates blood pressure in the tetraplegics; bars indicate ± SEM. In the tetraplegics there is a fall in both systolic and diastolic blood pressure. (From Mathias *et al.* (1981).)

15 min after clonidine. There is a similar rise in growth hormone levels in patients with PAF in whom the lesions are peripheral, unlike those with MSA in whom there is no rise (Thomaides *et al.* 1992). These results have been confirmed in larger numbers of PAF and MSA patients, and include MSA with either the parkinsonian or cerebellar form (Fig. 20.32a) (Kimber *et al.* 1997). More important, in patients with idiopathic Parkinson's disease, there is a rise in serum growth hormone levels after clonidine (Fig. 20.32b), indicating that in addition to being a useful means of distiguishing central from peripheral autonomic failure, the clonidine–growth hormone test may distinguish MSA from Parkinson's disease. In MSA patients who have an absent or impaired growth hormone response to clonidine, the oral administration of the growth hormone secretagogue, L-dopa, raises levels of plasma growth hormone releasing factor (GHRF) and growth hormone, thus indicating the integrity of hypothalamic GHRF-secreting neurones and confirming responsiveness of the anterior pituitary cells. Furthermore, this favours a specific α_2-adrenoceptor–hypothalamic deficit in MSA. The clonidine– growth hormone test therefore, may help further in the evaluation of central neurotransmitter abnormalities, in addition to its potential diagnostic capabilities.

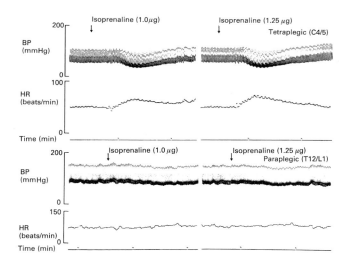

Fig. 20.28. Blood pressure (BP) and heart rate (HR) in a tetraplegic patient (upper panel) and a paraplegic patient with an almost intact sympathetic nervous system (lower panel) in response to bolus injections of isoprenaline. In the tetraplegic there is a clear fall in blood pressure after isoprenaline. This probably results from β_2-adrenoceptor-mediated vasodilatation. There is a rise in heart rate before the blood pressure falls and this is likely to be β_1-adrenoceptor-mediated effect which is then enhanced by the fall in blood pressure. In the paraplegic patient there are considerably smaller changes. (From Mathias and Frankel (1986).)

Drugs acting on the cholinergic system

Edrophonium

This is a short-acting cholinesterase inhibitor which may help differentiate pre- from postganglionic sympathetic lesions by stimulating nicotinic receptors within paravertebral ganglia (Gemmill *et al.* 1988). In PAF with distal lesions edrophonium has no effects, and there is no change in plasma noradrenaline levels. In MSA, where it is presumed there is an intact postganglionic system, there is a rise in noradrenaline levels. The limitations and value of edrophonium testing in different autonomic disorders remain to be evaluated.

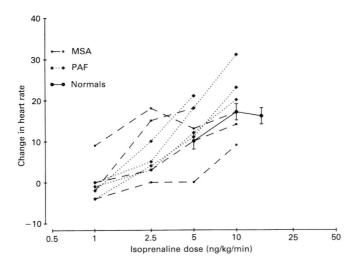

Fig. 20.30. Change in heart rate in response to incremental infusion of isoprenaline in four patients with pure autonomic failure (PAF) and in four patients with multiple system atrophy (MSA). The response in normal subjects (± SEM) is indicated. Despite a fall in blood pressure in the majority of patients with autonomic failure, only a few had a greater increase in sensitivity. Chronotropic β-adrenergic supersensitivity does not therefore appear to be as marked as pressor sensitivity in autonomic failure patients.

Atropine

Postsynaptic parasympathetic and sympathetic cholinergic receptors are of the muscarinic subtype and are effectively blocked by atropine sulphate. It can be used to determine the degree of cardiac vagal (cholinergic) involvement. In normal subjects bolus intravenous doses of 5 μg/kg body weight at 2 min intervals raise heart rate. Doses up to a total of 1800 μg are usually sufficient to assess responsiveness and construct a dose–response curve (Fig. 20.38). Further atropine should not be given if the heart rate rises above about 110 beats/min, or if there is evidence of an abnormal cardiac rhythm. After atropine, side-effects are usually mild, but may be troublesome. Dilatation of the pupils and blurring of vision, because of its cycloplegic effects, may occur. It may impair detrusor muscle activity and the urinary bladder should be emptied before the test. A dry mouth is common and may last for an hour. Subjects should be cautioned not to drink fluids in excess.

In the majority of patients with PAF and MSA, there is vagal impairment with a flat dose–response curve. This is consistent with neuropathological observations on the vagus that indicate lesions either in the dorsal vagal nuclei within the brainstem or more peripherally.

Thermoregulatory and sweat testing

The regulation of body temperature is dependent upon a number of factors that influence heat generation and disposal. Heat disposal depends upon the sudomotor system and the ability of the cutaneous circulation to respond appropriately. Thermoregulatory sweating is tested by raising the core temperature by 1 °C, using hot-water

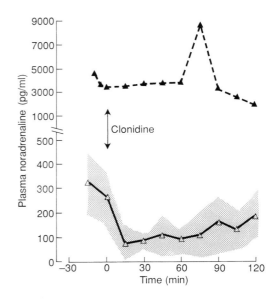

Fig. 20.31. Plasma noradrenaline levels in a patient with a phaeochromocytoma (▲– –▲) and in a group of patients with essential hypertension (△——△) before and after intravenous clonidine, indicated by an arrow (2 μg/kg over 10 min). Plasma noradrenaline levels fall rapidly in the essential hypertensives after clonidine and remain low over the period of observation. The stippled area indicates the ± SEM. Plasma noradrenaline levels are considerably higher in the phaeochromocytoma patient and are not affected by clonidine.

bottles and a space blanket. Normally, sweating occurs through stimulation of eccrine sweat glands which are widely distributed over the body. This can be aided by pretreatment with a diaphoretic, paracetamol (0.5 or 1 g orally). The detection of sweat production can be enhanced by using indicator dyes such as quinizarine red or ponso red; when sprinkled on the skin they turn from pale pink to bright red on exposure to moisture. In patients with PAF and MSA thermoregulatory sweating is often impaired. In dopamine β-hydroxylase deficiency, however, sweating is preserved and provides an important clue to the diagnosis (Chapter 40). Other tests of sweat gland function are described in Chapter 27.

The indicator dyes can be used to determine local abnormalities of sudomotor function as in the patchy denervation caused by leprosy (Karat *et al.* 1969). When applied over the skin and covered by a transparent tape, especially with the subject in a warm room, a colour change occurs in normal but not denervated areas; this may provide a rapid and semi-quantitative assessment applicable to multiple sites if needed, as has been demonstrated in PAF and MSA patients (Riedel and Mathias 1997). Other approaches include the acetylcholine sweatspot test (Ryder *et al.* 1988). Local disorders of sweating may need special methods of study. In gustatory sweating (Frey's syndrome), severe and socially embarrassing sweating may occur after ingestion of spicy or acidic foods and those containing tyramine. Challenge with food, together with the use of the indicator dye over the head, neck, and trunk, helps determine the area of distribution.

In patients who cannot control their cutaneous circulation, hypothermia may occur in temperate or cold climates, especially in tetraplegics who are unable to shiver (Chapter 51). The reverse,

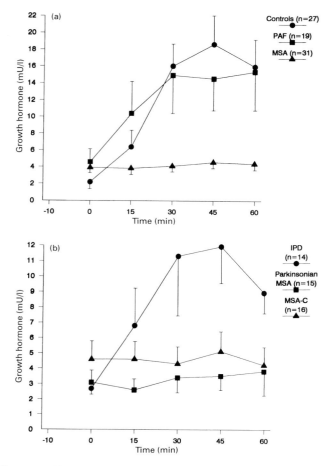

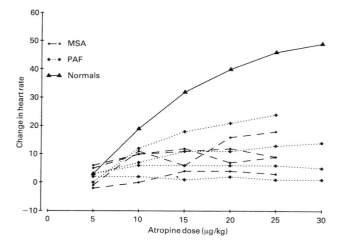

Fig. 20.33. Change in heart rate in four patients with pure autonomic failure (PAF) and four patients with multiple system atrophy (MSA) in response to atropine. In the majority of patients there is minimal change in heart rate unlike the change expected in normal subjects. Cardiac vagal impairment seems to occur equally in both groups of patients.

Fig. 20.32. (a) Serum growth hormone (GH) concentrations before (0) and at 15-minute intervals for 60 minutes after clonidine (2 μg/kg/min) in normal subjects (controls) and in patients with pure autonomic failure (PAF) and multiple system atrophy (MSA). GH concentrations rise in controls and in patients with PAF with a peripheral lesion; there is no rise in patients with MSA with a central lesion. (From Kimber *et al.* (1997).) (b) Indicates lack of serum GH response to clonidine in MSA (the cerebellar form; MSA-C and the parkinsonian form) in contrast to patients with idiopathic Parkinson's disease with no autonomic deficit IPD), in whom there is a significant rise in GH levels. (From Kimber *et al.* (1997).)

Gastrointestinal system

The gastrointestinal system is often involved in autonomic disorders. Investigations will depend upon the specific problem.

Oropharyngeal dysphagia may occur, especially in the later states of MSA. Although often asymptomatic, it is of clinical importance as it may result in tracheal aspiration, especially in the presence of laryngeal abductor cord paresis. Videocinefluoroscopic examination is a valuable means of assessing swallowing disturbances (Fig. 20.34) (Mathias 1996). The upper gastrointestinal tract may be assessed using a barium swallow and follow-through. In localized oesophageal involvement (as in Chagas' disease) a barium swallow alone may help. Studies of pressure changes, especially in the oesophago-gastric sphincter region may be of value. If gastroscopy is utilized, an advantage is biopsy of tissue, thus enabling diagnosis of conditions such as systemic amyloidosis. Assessment of gastric motility may be of importance (Chapter 29). In some disorders rapid gastric emptying is a problem, while in others, such as diabetes, gastroparesis may be particularly troublesome (Chapter 39).

Constipation is a common complaint in autonomic failure. Occasionally other coincidental disorders, such as neoplasia in the elderly, need to be considered. A barium enema or colonoscopy may be helpful. A rectal biopsy and staining with Congo red may provide a definitive diagnosis in amyloidosis.

Renal and urinary bladder function

Nocturnal polyuria is common in autonomic disorders, and in autonomic failure may result in overnight weight loss of over a kilogram with a reduction in extracellular fluid volume; this appears to aggravate postural hypotension in the morning. This can be assessed by 12-hourly evaluations (day and night) of urine volume and, if possible, of sodium and potassium secretion (Mathias *et al.* 1986). If there is urinary bladder or sphincter involvement, nocturnal polyuria

hyperpyrexia, may occur in extremely hot weather, especially when sweating is also impaired. In such patients it is important that core temperature (for example, using a rectal thermometer) is measured. If hypothermia is suspected, a low-reading thermometer should be used. In patients with MSA and PAF there is a lack of circadian variation in body temperature, which either does not fall at night, or only minimally in MSA with autonomic failure, unlike in normal subjects (Pierangeli *et al.* 1997). Details of thermoregulation and its investigation are in Chapter 12.

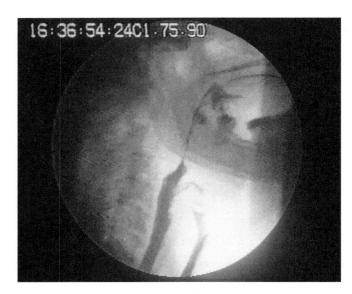

Fig. 20.34. Stills from a videocinefluoroscopic examination in a subject with oropharyngeal dysphagia, showing penetration of the larynx, with the potential to lead to tracheal aspiration. (From Mathias (1996c).)

may cause even greater difficulties because of the frequency of micturition, and at times incontinence. The assessments are helpful in predicting the value of the antidiuretic agent, desmopressin, which may be used intranasally or in an oral form at night to reduce nocturnal polyuria (Chapter 36).

Urodynamic measurements provide information on the nature of bladder dysfunction, such as detrusor areflexia or hyper-reflexia. Urethral sphincter electromyography shows a distinct pattern in patients with MSA, and may help distinguish them from those with idiopathic Parkinson's disease (Chapter 30). Urinary infections and calculi may complicate bladder dysfunction and suitable investigations, including intravenous urography and ultrasound examination, may be needed.

Sexual function

Impotence in the male is common in autonomic failure. Organic erectile failure can be difficult to distinguish from psychogenic impotence, though nocturnal erections do not occur in the former. Penile plethysmography may help. Intracorporeal injection of papavarine causes an erection in both groups and therefore is not a means of differentiating between the two (Chapter 30). In situations such as diabetes mellitus, vascular factors also may contribute. In dopamine β-hydroxylase deficiency erection is preserved but there is delayed ejaculation, which can be corrected by the drug dihydroxy-phenylserine (DOPS), which replenishes noradrenaline levels (Chapter 40).

Respiratory system

Stridor, particularly at night, may occur in the later stages in MSA because of paralysis of abductor muscles of the vocal cord

(Chapter 26). This can be detected by laryngoscopy. Brainstem dysfunction causing periods of apnoea may further contribute to hypoxia and complicate the problem. Blood gas monitoring during sleep may be necessary to determine whether significant oxygen desaturation occurs. These investigations are of relevance to management, including the decision on proceeding to a tracheostomy (Harcourt et al. 1996).

The eye

Lacrimal secretion may be diminished as a result of direct involvement of the gland, as in Sjögren's syndrome. Lacrimal secretion can be tested by using a special absorbent paper, which forms the basis of Schirmer's test. Diminished secretion or alacrima may result in corneal abrasions which may need to be assessed using either fluorescein or Bengal red dyes, and a slit lamp.

Intraocular pressure may be reduced in sympathetic lesions, as in Horner's syndrome, but has minimal clinical significance when compared with the elevation of intraocular pressure that may occur with anticholinergic drugs, especially in patients who are prone to glaucoma. Intraocular pressure may be dependent on systemic blood pressure, as has been demonstrated recently in patients with PAF and MSA (Dumskyj et al. 1997). In these patients, intraocular pressure was lower when blood pressure was reduced during head-up tilt and rose when blood pressure was elevated by returning them to the horizontal and during head-down tilt. This may have implications in the consideration and assessment of glaucoma in such patients.

The pupil is involved in a number of autonomic disorders and can be assessed using either pharmacological approaches (sympathomimetics and cholinomimetics and testing for supersensitivity) or specialized physiological function tests (Chapter 25).

Miscellaneous investigations

In this section a range of investigations which may be of value in the assessment of patients with autonomic disorders are described briefly. Some of these investigations are concerned directly with diagnosis, others with elimination of disorders that may mimic autonomic failure, and in addition there are those that provide valuable information in understanding the pathophysiological basis of certain autonomic disorders.

Neurophysiological tests

Electroencephalography may be needed as the distinction between syncope (due to autonomic impairment) and epilepsy can be difficult (Lempert 1996). Occasionally, epileptic seizures may be induced because of an extremely low cerebral perfusion pressure. A variety of motor abnormalities have been recorded in normal subjects in whom syncope was induced (Lempert et al. 1994).

Auditory evoked responses are of value in separating patients with cerebral lesions as in MSA, from those with more distal lesions as in PAF (Chapter 31). A variety of peripheral electrophysiological studies are of value to determine the specific type of neuropathy, or its absence. Thermal threshold testing is a sensitive means of determining unmyelinated fibre involvement. The absence of the

'H' reflex is characteristic of patients with the Holmes–Adie syndrome, where there is a myotonic pupil and absent tendon reflexes.

Neuro-otological studies

Dizziness is a common symptom in both neuro-otological and autonomic disorders. In the majority the history and clinical examination separates one from the other, although in some this may not be so. Neuro-otological investigations are of particular value in excluding or confirming primary or coincidental vestibular dysfunction when suspected.

Cardiac investigations

There are a number of cardiac causes of syncope, the most dramatic probably being Stokes–Adams attacks (Chapter 46). In the young the long Q–T syndrome needs to be excluded, while in the elderly cardiac dysrhythmias are common and the use of a 24-hour tape with computerized analysis of cardiac rhythm may be necessary. In rare cases, postural hypotension may be the result of an atrial myxoma and two-dimensional echocardiography is the ideal non-invasive means of making or excluding this diagnosis.

Biopsies

Tissue can be subjected to light microscopy, electron microscopy, and a range of immunohistochemical studies. In amyloidosis, biopsy of the kidney or a sural nerve may provide the diagnosis when tissues are stained with Congo red. Sural nerve biopsies provide valuable information on the nerve fibres and on both degenerative and regenerative peripheral neural processes (Chapter 38). Muscle biopsies in autonomic failure are described in Chapter 35. Skin biopsies have proved to be of value in patients with dopamine β-hydroxylase deficiency, as they have confirmed the integrity of perivascular sympathetic nerves and demonstrated the normal distribution of a range of neuropeptides, some associated with sympathetic nerves (such as neuropeptide Y) and others with parasympathetic nerves (such as vasoactive intestinal polypeptide) (Chapter 40). In these patients, there is lack of immunoreactivity to dopamine β-hydroxylase in skin tissue containing sympathetic nerves that further confirms the diagnosis. Immunoreactivity to dopamine β-hydroxylase, tyrosine hydroxylase, and the sensory neuropeptides, substance P and CGRP, could not be detected in a skin biopsy in a patient with autonomic and sensory neuropeptide deficiency resulting from a presumed nerve growth factor deficiency (see Chapter 40).

Intradermal histamine test

The use of the intradermal histamine test to assess the Lewis response may be of value in certain disorders, especially if correlation with the composition of skin tissue is possible. An abnormal skin histamine response is a characteristic feature of patients with familial dysautonomia (Riley–Day syndrome; Chapter 41); in a patient with diminished sensory neuropeptides (see Chapter 40), there was a diminished histamine response consistent with low or absent sensory neuropeptide levels in skin.

Neuroimaging

A range of non-invasive technological advances now enables assessment of cerebral and spinal morphology. A CT scan is often of value but there are considerable advantages in performing an MRI scan (Schrag et al. 1998), especially when determining abnormalities within the basal ganglia, brainstem, and spinal cord. In addition, positron emission tomography (PET) scans can provide details of the formation, distribution, and receptor configuration of neurotransmitters within the central nervous system. The value of PET scans in separating MSA from PAF, and in the evaluation of neurochemical abnormalities, is discussed in Chapters 31 and 32.

Concluding remarks

The autonomic nervous system innervates every organ and in the generalized autonomic disorders there may be impaired function of virtually every organ in the body. As indicated in this chapter, there is a wide range of investigative approaches and, depending upon the clinical questions raised, specific tests will need to be performed. Further details of certain tests can be found in relevant chapters.

The rapid advances in investigation and diagnosis of various autonomic disorders, and recognition of their complications in various diseases, have resulted in autonomic laboratories now fulfilling an important clinical service role, as distinct from the past where these activities were incorporated, sometimes loosely, into research units. A basic requirement of such laboratories should be the provision of screening autonomic function tests, the capacity to perform additional investigations (such as carotid sinus massage and sudomotor/thermoregulatory tests), and in conjunction with other units if needed, the ability to advise on, and direct, the evaluation and management of suspected autonomic disorders. Such activities are probably best incorporated into a regional neuroscience or cardiovascular unit or, as in our case, national referral units. The setting up of an autonomic laboratory will depend upon the acquisition of appropriate equipment, which is likely to vary because of dependence on a large number of factors ranging from finance to access for servicing and maintenance of equipment. A crucial factor however, is the training of the physicians directing the unit, and the technical staff performing the investigations. The increasing complexity of autonomic testing, and more importantly its interpretation, now demands that a trainee spends an adequate period in an established autonomic unit which ideally deals with an extensive range of disorders and has wide expertise on many fronts. The formalized training of technical staff also may need to be considered. This would be similar to medical and paramedical training programmes in neurophysiological, cardiovascular, and cardiology laboratories. A recognized period of training, with accreditation when completed, may become a necessary requirement as autonomic investigation increasingly becomes an integral part of clinical practice in the diagnosis and management of a wide variety of neurological and other medical disorders. Furthermore, interpretation of autonomic testing may be of crucial importance in litigation, especially involving the effects of drugs and toxins.

It is re-emphasized that results obtained from the investigation of autonomic disorders need to be interpreted in conjunction with the clinical state and confounding variables that relate not only to the autonomic nervous system but also to organs they supply, as the majority of tests are dependent upon target organ function. The complexities in many of the systems involved also make it more appropriate that responses to testing are described individually, so as to have a measure of both the defect and the associated dysfunction, rather than having them incorporated as part of a scoring system. Some of these scoring systems (Low 1993) combine the results of adrenergic, cardiovagal, and sudomotor testing, and although they provide a numerical figure, this often does not aid understanding of the specific attendant abnormalities, or recognition of functional deficits. However, in certain situations as in a research setting, they may be of value.

Finally, it cannot be stressed too strongly that autonomic investigation has to be determined selectively, ideally by a clinician, and preferably by one with a background in integrative physiology, who will take account of various factors, which should also include time, patient tolerance, and cost. This is because after the initial screening tests, subsequent investigations are often not routine and must be designed to answer specific questions. It is intended that this chapter, by providing an overview of the investigation of those autonomic abnormalities that cause morbidity and contribute to mortality, will help in early diagnosis and comprehensive assessment, each of which is important for prognosis and for appropriate management.

References

Abbott, N. G., Beck, J. S. Wilson, S. B., and Khan, F. (1993). Vasomotor reflexes in the fingertip skin of patients with Type 1 diabetes mellitus and leprosy. *Clin. Auton. Res.* **3**, 189–93.

Alam, M., Smith, G. D. P., Bleasdale-Barr, K., Pavitt, D. V., and Mathias, C. J. (1995). Effects of the peptide release inhibitor, Octreotide, on daytime hypotension and on nocturnal hypertension in primary autonomic failure. *J. Hypertension* **13**, 1664–9.

Arunodaya, G. R. and Taly, A. B. (1995). Sympathetic skin response: a decade later. *J. Neurol. Sci.* **129**, 81–9.

Bannister, R. (1979). Chronic autonomic failure with postural hypotension. *Lancet* **ii**, 404–6.

Bannister, R., Ardill, L., and Fentem, P. (1967). Defective autonomic control of blood vessels in idiopathic orthostatic hypotension. *Brain* **90**, 725–46.

Bannister, R., Davies, I. B., Holly, E., Rosenthal, T., and Sever, P. S. (1979). Defective cardiovascular reflexes and supersensitivity to sympathomimetic drugs in autonomic failure. *Brain* **102**, 163–76.

Bannister, R., da Costa, D. F., Hendry, W. G., Jacobs, J., and Mathias, C. J. (1986). Atrial demand pacing to protect against vagal overactivity in sympathetic autonomic neuropathy. *Brain* **109**, 345–56.

Brett, A. S., Phillips, M., and Beary, J. F. (1986). Predictive power of the polygraph: Can the "lie detector" really detect liars? *Lancet* **i**, 544–7.

Brooks, D. J., Redmond, S., Mathias, C. J., Bannister, R., and Symon, L. (1989). The effect of orthostatic hypotension on cerebral blood flow and middle cerebral artery velocity in autonomic failure, with observations on the action of ephedrine. *J. Neurol. Neurosurg. Psychiat.* **52**, 962–6.

Chaudhuri, K. R., Thomaides, T., Hernandez, P., Alam, M., and Mathias, C. J. (1991). Non-invasive quantification of superior mesenteric artery blood flow during sympathoneural activation in normal subjects. *Clin. Auton. Res.* **1**, 37–42.

Claus, D., Feistel, H., Brunholzl, C., Platsch, G., Neundorfer, B., and Wolf, F. (1994). Investigation of parasympathetic and sympathetic cardiac innervation in diabetic neuropathy: heart rate variation versus meta-iodobenzylguanidine measured by single photon emission computed tomography. *Clin. Auton. Res.* **4**, 117–23.

Consensus statement (1996). Consensus statement on the definition of orthostatic hypotension, pure autonomic failure and multiple system atrophy. *Clin. Auton. Res.* **6**, 125–6.

Diehl, R. R., Linden, D., Chalkiadaki, A., Ringelstein, E. B., and Berlit, P. (1996). Transcranial doppler during neurocardiogenic syncope. *Clin. Auto. Res.* **6**, 71–4.

Dolan, R. J., Fink, G. R., Rolls, E. *et al.* (1997). How the brain learns to see objects and faces in an impoverished context. *Nature* **389**, 596–9.

Dumskyj, M. J., Mathias, C. J., Dore, C. J., Bleasdale-Barr, K., and Kohner, E. M. (1998). Intraocular pressure, blood pressure and body position in normal human subjects and patients with autonomic failure. *Clin. Auton. Res.* **8**, 9.

El-Badawi, K. M. and Hainsworth, R. (1994). Combined head-up tilt and lower body suction: a test of orthostatic tolerance. *Clin. Auton. Res.* **4**, 41–7.

Elwell, C. E., Cope, M., Edwards, A. D., Wyatt, J. S., Delpy, D. T., and Reynolds, E. O. (1994). Quantification of adult cerebral hemodynamics by near-infrared spectroscopy. *J. Appl. Physiol.* **77**, 2753–60.

Esler, M. (1993). Clinical application of noradrenaline spillover methodology: delineation of regional human sympathetic nervous responses. *Pharmacol. Toxicol.* **75**, 243–53.

Faes, T. J. C., Wagemans, M. F. M., Cillekens, J. M., Scheffer, G.- J., Karemaker, J. M., and Bertelsmann, F. W. (1993). The validity and reproducibility of the skin vasomotor test – studies in normal subjects, after spinal anaesthesia, and in diabetes mellitus. *Clin. Auton. Res.* **3**, 319–24.

Fasano, M. L., Sand, T., Brubakk, A. O., Kurszewski, P., Bordini, C., and Sjaastad, O. (1996). Reproducibility of the cold pressor test: studies in normal subjects. *Clin. Auton. Res.* **6**, 249–53.

Ferini-Strambi, L. and Smirne, S. (1997). Cardiac autonomic function during sleep in several neuropsychiatric disorders. *J. Neurol.* **244**, S29–S36.

Gemmill, J. D., Venables, G. S., and Ewing, D. J. (1988). Noradrenaline response to edrophonium in primary autonomic failure: distinction between central and peripheral damage. *Lancet* **i**, 1018–21.

Goldstein, D. S., Holmes, C., Stuhlmuller, J. E., Lenders, J. W. M., and Kopin I. J. (1997*a*). 6-[^{18}F] Fluorodopamine positron emission tomographic scanning in the assessment of cardiac sympathoneural function – studies in normal humans. *Clin. Auton. Res.* **7**, 17–29.

Goldstein, D. S., Holmes, C., Cannon, R. O. III, Eisenhofer, G., and Kopin, I. J. (1997*b*). Sympathetic cardioneuropathy in dysautonomias. *New Engl. J. Med.* **336**, 696–702

Harcourt, J., Spraggs, P., Mathias, C. J., and Brookes, G. (1996). Sleep-related breathing disorders in the Shy-Drager syndrome. Observations on investigation and management. *Eur. J. Neurol.* **3**, 186–90

Hutchinson, E. C. and Stock, J. P. P. (1960). Carotid sinus syndrome. *Lancet* **ii**, 445–9.

Karat, A. B. A., Karat, S., and Pallis, C. (1969). Sweating under cellulose tape. A test of autonomic function. *Lancet* **i**, 651–2

Kaufmann, H., Oribe, E., Miller, M., Knott, P., Wiltshire-Clement, M., and Yahr, M. (1992). Hypotension induced vasopressin release distinguishes between PAF and MSA with autonomic failure. *Neurology* **42**, 590–3.

Khurana, R. K. (1995). Orthostatic intolerance and orthostatic tachycardia: a heterogeneous disorder. *Clin. Auton. Res.* **5**, 12–18.

Khurana, R. K. and Setty, A. (1996). The value of the isometric hand-grip test – studies in various autonomic disorders. *Clin. Auton. Res.* **6**, 211–18.

Kimber, J. R., Watson, .L, and Mathias, C. J. (1997). Distinction of idiopathic Parkinson's disease from multiple system atrophy by stimulation of growth hormone release with clonidine. *Lancet* **349**, 1877–81.

Lagi, A., Bacalli, S., Cencetti, S., Paggetti, C., and Colzi, L. (1994). Cerebral autoregulation in orthostatic hypotension: a transcranial doppler study. *Stroke* **25**, 1771–75.

Lambert, G. W., Thompson, J. M., Turner, A. G. *et al.* (1997). Cerebral noradrenaline spillover and its relation to muscle sympathetic nervous activity in healthy human subjects. *J. Autonom. Nerv. Syst.* **64**, 57–64.

Lempert, T. (1996). Recognizing syncope: pitfalls and surprises. *J. R. Soc. Med.* **89**, 372–5.

Lempert, T., Bauer, M., and Schmidt, D. (1994). Syncope: a videometric analysis of 56 episodes of transient cerebral hypoxia. *Ann. Neurol.* **36**, 233–7.

Low, P. A. (1993). Composite autonomic scoring scale for laboratory quantification of generalized autonomic failure. *Mayo Clin. Proc.* **68**, 748–52.

McIntosh, S. J, Lawson, J., and Kenny, R. A. (1993). Clinical characteristics of vasodepressor, cardioinhibitory and mixed carotid sinus syndrome in the elderly. *Am. J. Med.* **95**, 203–8.

Magnifico, F., Misra, V. P., Murray, N. M. F., and Mathias. C. J. (1996). The sympathetic skin response following successful upper limb sympathectomy in primary hyperhidrosis. *Clin. Auton. Res.* **6**, 289.

Magnifico, F., Misra, V. P., Murray, N. M. F., and Mathias. C. J. (1997). The laboratory detection of autonomic dysfunction in multiple system atrophy – the role of the sympathetic skin response. *Neurology* **48** (suppl), A190.

Magnifico, F., Misra, V. P., Murray, N. M. F., and Mathias, C. J. (1998). The sympathetic skin response in peripheral autonomic failure – evaluation in pure autonomic failure, pure cholinergic dysautonomia and dopamine beta-hydroxylase deficiency. *Clin. Auton. Res.*, **8**, 133–8.

Mathias, C. J. (1987). Autonomic dysfunction. *Br. J. Hosp. Med.* **38**, 238–43.

Mathias, C. J. (1995a). Orthostatic hypotension – causes, mechanisms and influencing factors. *Neurology* **45**, (Suppl. 5), s6–s11.

Mathias, C. J. (1995b). Assessment of autonomic function. In *Clinical Neurophysiology*, (ed. J. Osseslton with C. Binnie, R. Looper, C. Fowler, F. Maguire and P. Prior). Heinemann, Butterworth, London. pp. 218–32.

Mathias, C.J. (1996a). Disorders affecting autonomic function in Parkinsonian patients. In *Parkinson's disease*, (ed. L. Battistin, G. Scarlato, T. Caraceni, and S. Ruggieri), Advances in Neurology, **69**, pp. 383–91. Lippincott-Raven Press, New York.

Mathias, C. J. (1996b). Disorders of the autonomic nervous system in childhood. In *Principles of child neurology*, (ed. B. Berg), pp. 413–36. McGraw-Hill, New York.

Mathias, C. J. (1996c). Gastrointestinal dysfunction in multiple system atrophy. *Semin. Neurol.* **16**, 251–5.

Mathias, C. J. (1997). Pharmacological manipulation of human gastrointestinal blood flow. *Fund. Clin. Pharmacol.* **11**, 29–34.

Mathias, C. J. (1998). Autonomic disorders. In *Textbook of neurology*, (ed. J. Bogousslavsky and M. Fisher). Chap. 35, pp. 519–45. Butterworth Heinemann, Massachusetts.

Mathias, C. J. (1999). Autonomic dysfunction and the elderly. In *Oxford textbook of geriatric medicine*, (2nd edn), (ed. J. Grimley-Evans). Oxford University Press, Oxford, in press.

Mathias, C. J. and Frankel, H. L. (1986). The neurological and hormonal control of blood vessels and heart in spinal man. *J. autonom. nerv. Syst.* (suppl.), 457–64.

Mathias, C. J. and Frankel, H. L. (1988). Cardiovascular control in spinal man. *Ann. Rev. Physiol.* **50**, 577–92.

Mathias, C. J. and Williams, A. C. (1994). The Shy Drager syndrome (and multiple system atrophy). In *Neurodegenerative diseases*, (1st edn), (ed. Donald B. Calne), Chap. 43, pp. 743–68. WB Saunders, Philadelphia, Pennsylvania, USA.

Mathias, C. J., Matthews, W. B., and Spalding, J. M. K. S. (1977). Postural changes in plasma renin activity and responses to vasoactive drugs in a case of Shy–Drager syndrome. *J. Neurol. Neurosurg. Psychiat.* **40**, 138–43.

Mathias, C. J., Christensen, N. J., Frankel, H. L., and Spalding, J. M. K. (1979). Cardiovascular control in recently injured tetraplegics in spinal shock. *Q. J. Med. New Series* **48**, 273–87.

Mathias, C. J., Frankel, H. L., Davies, I. B., James, V. H. T., and Peart, W. S. (1981). Renin and aldosterone release during sympathetic stimulation in tetraplegia. *Clin. Sci.* **60**, 399–604.

Mathias, C. J., Fosbraey, P., da Costa, D. F., Thornley, A., and Bannister, R. (1986). Desmopressin reduces nocturnal polyuria, reverses overnight weight loss and improves morning postural hypotension in autonomic failure. *BMJ* **293**, 353–4.

Mathias, C. J., Armstrong, E., Browse, N., Chaudhuri, K. R., Enevoldson, P., and Ross-Russell, R. W. (1991a). Value of non-invasive continuous blood pressure monitoring in the detection of carotid sinus hypersensitivity. *Clin. Auton. Res.* **1**, 157–9.

Mathias, C. J., Holly, E. R., Armstrong, E., Shareef, M., and Bannister, R. (1991b). The influence of food and postural hypotension in three groups of chronic autonomic failure; clinical and therapeutic implications. *J. Neurol. Neurosurg. Psychiat.* **54**, 726–30.

Mathias, C. J., Deguchi, K., Bleasdale-Barr, K., and Kimber, J. (1998). Frequency of family history in vasovagal syncope. *Lancet* **352**, 33–4.

Morris, J. S., Frith, C. D., Perrett, D. I. *et al.* (1996). A differential neural response in the human amygdala to fearful and happy facial expressions. *Nature* **383**, 812–15.

Mounier-Vehier, C., Girard, A., Consoli, S., Laude, D., Vacheron, A., and Elghozi, J. L. (1995). Cardiovascular reactivity to a new mental stress test: the maze test. *Clin. Auton. Res.* **5**, 145–50.

Pierangeli, G., Cortelli, P., Provini, F., Plazzi, G., and Lugaresi, E. (1997). Circadian rhythm of body core temperature in neurodegenerative diseases. In *Somatic and autonomic regulation in sleep: physiological and clinical aspects*, pp. 55–71, (ed. E. Lugaresi and P. L. Parmeggiani). Springer-Verlag, Italia, Milano.

Piha, S. J. and Voipio-Pullki, L. M. (1993). Cardiac dysrhythmias during cardiovascular autonomic reflex tests. *Clin. Auton. Res.* **3**, 183–7.

Puvi-Rajasingham, S., Smith, G. D. P., Akinola, A., and Mathias, C. J. (1997). Abnormal regional blood flow responses during and after exercise in human sympathetic denervation. *J. Physiol.* **505**, 481–9.

Puvi-Rajasingham, S., Smith, G. D. P., Akinola, A., and Mathias, C. J. (1998). Hypotensive and regional haemodynamic effects of exercise, fasted and after food, in human sympathetic denervation. *Clin. Sci.* **94**, 49–55.

Riedel, A. and Mathias, C. J. (1997). A rapid response sweat test with potential clinical applications – studies in normal subjects, pure autonomic failure and multiple system atrophy. *Clin. Auton. Res.* **7**, 208.

Ryder, R. E. J., Johnson, K., Owens, D. R., Marshall, R., Ryder, A. P. P., and Hayes, T. M. (1988). Acetylcholine sweatspot test for autonomic denervation. *Lancet* **ii**, 1303–5.

Schrag, A., Kingsley, D., Phatouros, C. *et al.* (1998). Clinical usefulness of magnetic resonance imaging in multiple system atrophy. *J. Neuroc. Neurosurg. Psychiat.*. **65**, 65–71.

Shahani, B. T., Halpern, J. J., Boulu, P., and Cohen, J. (1984). Sympathetic skin response-a method of assessing unmyelinated axon dysfunction in peripheral neuropathies. *J. Neurol. Neurosurg. Psychiat.* **47**, 536–42.

Smith, G. D. P. and Mathias, C. J. (1995). Postural hypotension enhanced by exercise in patients with chronic autonomic failure. *Q. J. Med.* **88**, 251–6.

Smith, G. D. P. and Mathias, C. J. (1996). Differences in the cardiovascular responses to supine exercise and to standing post-exercise in two clinical subgroups of the Shy–Drager syndrome (multiple system atrophy). *J. Neurol. Neurosurg. Psychiat.* **61**, 297–303.

Smith, G. D. P., Watson, L. P., Pavitt, D. V., and Mathias, C.J. (1995). Abnormal cardiovascular and catecholamine responses to supine exercise in human subjects with sympathetic dysfunction. *J. Physiol. (London)* **485**, 255–65.

Thomaides, T., Chaudhuri, K. R., Maule, S., Watson, L., Marsden, C.D., and Mathias, C. J. (1992). The growth hormone response to clonidine in central and peripheral primary autonomic failure. *Lancet* **340**, 263–6.

Tsuchimochi, S., Tamaki, N., Tadamura, E. *et al.* (1995). Age and gender differences in normal myocardial adrenergic neuronal function evaluated by iodine-123 MIBG imaging. *J. Nucl. Med.* **36**, 969–74.

Appendix I

Data from standard autonomic function tests in 122 subjects who are grouped in different age bands. None of the subjects had autonomic failure or were on drugs that could have interfered with the responses. All measurements were made with an automated sphygmomanometer. Mean change in systolic or diastolic blood pressure (SBP and DBP respectively) or in heart rate (HR), with the standard error of the mean are provided. The figures below these are the 95 per cent confidence intervals, with both lower and upper values.

Age groups (years)	20–29	30–39	40–49	50–59	60–69	≥70
Standing						
2 minutes						
Δ SBP	3 ± 2	–1 ± 3	–2 ± 2	2 ± 3	2 ± 3	7 ± 3
	(–1 to 7)	(–7 to 6)	(–6 to 3)	(–1 to 5)	(–1 to 5)	(4 to 10)
Δ DBP	6 ± 3	5 ± 3	6 ± 2	5 ± 3	3 ± 1	5 ± 2
	(0 to 12)	(–1 to 11)	(1 to 11)	(–1 to 11)	(0 to 6)	(1 to 9)
Δ HR	15 ± 3	10 ± 3	11 ± 2	8 ± 2	8 ± 2	7 ± 1
	(9 to 21)	(4 to 16)	(8 to 15)	(4 to 12)	(4 to 12)	(5 to 9)
5 minutes						
Δ SBP	1 ± 3	0 ± 2	–1 ± 2	1 ± 2	4 ± 2	5 ± 3
	(–4 to 6)	(–3 to 4)	(–5 to 3)	(–1 to 3)	(2 to 6)	(2 to 8)
Δ DBP	4 ± 3	4 ± 2	5 ± 2	5 ± 2	6 ± 1	4 ± 2
	(–2 to 10)	(0 to 8)	(1 to 9)	(1 to 9)	(4 to 8)	(0 to 8)
Δ HR	14 ± 3	11 ± 2	11 ± 2	8 ± 2	9 ± 1	9 ± 1
	(8 to 20)	(7 to 15)	(7 to 14)	(4 to 12)	(7 to 11)	(7 to 11)
Head-up tilt						
2 minutes						
Δ SBP	–1 ± 3	3 ± 3	–3 ± 2	–2 ± 4	–8 ± 2	–7 ± 2
	(–7 to 9)	(0 to 9)	(–7 to 1)	(–10 to 2)	(–12 to –4)	(–11 to –3)
Δ DBP	4 ± 3	7 ± 2	2 ± 1	0 ± 2	3 ± 1	2 ± 3
	(–2 to 10)	(3 to 11)	(0 to 4)	(–4 to 4)	(0 to 6)	(–4 to 8)
Δ HR	8 ± 3	8 ± 3	7 ± 2	3 ± 5	2 ± 2	1 ± 2
	(2 to 14)	(2 to 14)	(3 to 11)	(–7 to 13)	(–2 to 6)	(–3 to 5)
5 minutes						
Δ SBP	–4 ± 3	7 ± 2	–2 ± 2	0 ± 4	–5 ± 3	3 ± 4
	(–10 to 2)	(3 to 11)	(–6 to 2)	(–8 to 8)	(–11 to 1)	(–5 to 11)
Δ DBP	0 ± 4	5 ± 2	3 ± 1	3 ± 2	1 ± 2	1 ± 2
	(–8 to 8)	(1 to 9)	(1 to 5)	(–1 to 7)	(–3 to 5)	(–3 to 5)
Δ HR	10 ± 4	7 ± 2	5 ± 1	4 ± 3	3 ± 1	4 ± 2
	(2 to 18)	(3 to 11)	(3 to 7)	(–2 to 10)	(1 to 5)	(0 to 8)
Isometric exercise						
Δ SBP	15 ± 3	13 ± 2	15 ± 3	19 ± 3	17 ± 3	22 ± 4
	(9 to 21)	(9 to 17)	(9 to 21)	(13 to 25)	(11 to 23)	(14 to 30)
Δ DBP	13 ± 2	11 ± 2	12 ± 2	11 ± 3	11 ± 2	11 ± 1
	(9 to 17)	(7 to 15)	(8 to 14)	(5 to 17)	(7 to 15)	(9 to 13)
Δ HR	7 ± 1	7 ± 2	9 ± 2	7 ± 2	4 ± 1	6 ± 1
	(5 to 9)	(3 to 11)	(5 to 13)	(3 to 11)	(2 to 6)	(4 to 8)
Cutaneous cold						
Δ SBP	9 ± 1	9 ± 2	12 ± 3	16 ± 3	15 ± 2	21 ± 3
	(7 to 11)	(5 to 13)	(6 to 18)	(10 to 22)	(11 to 19)	(15 to 27)
Δ DBP	10 ± 2	12 ± 3	10 ± 2	8 ± 4	10 ± 2	12 ± 4
	(6 to 13)	(7 to 17)	(6 to 14)	(5 to 12)	(7 to 13)	(5 to 19)
Δ HR	0 ± 1	3 ± 2	3 ± 2	3 ± 2	1 ± 1	5 ± 1
	(–2 to 2)	(–1 to 7)	(–1 to 7)	(–1 to 7)	(–2 to 3)	(3 to 7)
Mental arithmetic						
Δ SBP	17 ± 4	10 ± 2	12 ± 3	19 ± 3	13 ± 3	13 ± 4
	(10 to 24)	(5 to 15)	(7 to 17)	(16 to 21)	(7 to 19)	(6 to 20)
Δ DBP	12 ± 2	5 ± 3	8 ± 2	6 ± 2	9 ± 2	8 ± 2
	(9 to 15)	(0 to 11)	(5 to 11)	(2 to 10)	(5 to 13)	(3 to 13)
Δ HR	7 ± 3	5 ± 2	8 ± 2	8 ± 2	8 ± 2	5 ± 1
	(2 to 12)	(1 to 9)	(5 to 11)	(6 to 10)	(5 to 11)	(3 to 7)

Appendix I. (*continued*)

Age groups (years)	20–29	30–39	40–49	50–59	60–69	≥70
Valsalva ratio	1.84 ± 0.12	1.81 ± 0.1	1.76 ± 0.06	1.72 ± 0.11	1.62 ± 0.06	1.33 ± 0.06
	(1.6 to 2.08)	(1.6 to 2.02)	(1.67 to 1.92)	(1.50 to 1.94)	(1.50 to 1.74)	(1.21 to 1.45)
Deep breathing						
Δ HR	20 ± 2	19 ± 3	15 ± 2	17 ± 2	12 ± 1	9 ± 1
	16 to 24	13 to 24	11 to 19	15 to 19	11 to 13	(8 to 10)
Hyperventilation						
Δ HR	21 ± 3	21 ± 3	16 ± 2	18 ± 3	11 ± 1	7 ± 1
	(15 to 27)	(15 to 26)	(12 to 21)	(15 to 21)	(10 to 12)	(6 to 8)

There is no age relationship of BP responses to standing and head-up tilt. With isometric exercise and cutaneous cold, with increasing age there is a rise in SBP but not DBP and heart rate. The responses to mental arithmetic are not age related. The heart rate responses to the Valsalva manoeuvre (as the Valsalva ratio), and to deep breathing and hyperventilation, show an age dependency.

These values are not a definitive source of normal data, for reasons outlined in the text. The data were collected from our two London Autonomic Units (at the National and St Mary's Hospitals), and compiled by A. Akinola, K. Bleasdale-Barr, L. Everall and C. J. Mathias.

21. Measurement of heart rate and blood pressure to evaluate disturbances in neurocardiovascular control

Wouter Wieling and John M. Karemaker

Introduction

The basis of testing any control system is to induce a disturbance and observe the response of the system. In the case of the cardiovascular system rapid correction of the disturbance is dependent on reflexes, of which the arterial baroreflex is the most important one. This autonomic reflex acts in response to blood pressure changes by changing heart rate, cardiac performance, and vasoconstrictor tone. To evaluate correctly the control system's performance, therefore, the physician requires measurement techniques for blood pressure and heart rate to a degree of precision that is adapted to the characteristics of the response under investigation. This implies that for some clinical measurements arm-cuff readings combined with pulse counting may be sufficient, for other measurements one needs a continuous beat-by-beat account of blood pressure and heart rate.

In this chapter the use of non-invasive continuous (finger) blood pressure by the Finapres technique will be described initially. This will be followed by a short account of the role of the arterial baroreflex in the complex of cardiovascular control mechanisms and the difficulties inherent in quantification of its function. The remainder of the chapter is devoted to a systematic account of cardiovascular reflex tests that are commonly used to evaluate specific aspects of baroreflex function. Moreover, a number of reflex tests that bypass the baroreflex system while still exciting its efferents are discussed. Such tests are useful to ascertain the integrity of these pathways when the baroreflex afferents are involved in a disease process.

Non-invasive monitoring of arterial pressure—the Finapres

Counting the pulse and carefully measuring blood pressure with a sphygmomanometer suffices for the routine clinical assessment of patients in the office or at the bedside. Multiple blood pressure readings supine and after standing provide a fair assessment of the typical blood pressure response for an individual. For the evaluation of a patient with disturbances in cardiovascular control mechanisms conventional sphygmomanometry has a major disadvantage: the investigator is not aware of the beat-to-beat fluctuations in arterial pressure (Benditt *et al.* 1996; Low 1996).

Sphygmomanometry, therefore, is not suitable for evaluation of conditions with sudden transient changes in the circulation.

Intra-arterial measurements are not used routinely in cardiovascular laboratories in view of the potential complications. In addition, intravascular instrumentation has the inherent disadvantage of affecting autonomic tone. In this context, the Finapres or volume clamp method, with its ability to measure the arterial pressure in the finger non-invasively and continuously, is an important step forward in the evaluation of autonomic cardiovascular control (Low 1996). The principle of the measurement of finger arterial pressure has been described in detail previously (Imholz *et al.* 1998).

Measurement of finger arterial pressure is almost always possible. Conditions that provoke severe peripheral arterial contraction and, consequently, low arterial flow to the hand are the major limitations. Warming of the hand will improve measurements. When using the Finapres, it is essential that a proper size cuff is snugly applied to the middle or ring finger and, to avoid hydrostatic pressure effects, that the finger cuff is kept at heart level. A skin electrode is placed as a reference point in the mid-axillary line at heart level (the fourth intercostal space at the sternum) and the subject holds the cuffed finger at this place at all times (Fig. 21.1), the hand is further supported by a sling.

Finapres recordings are similar in appearance to intra-arterial blood pressure recordings (Fig. 21.2), but the measurements are not identical. It has long been known that propagation of the pressure wave towards the periphery changes the pulse wave form, and consequently finger blood pressure values differ from values obtained more proximally. The physiological brachial-to-finger pressure gradient causes mean and diastolic pressures to be lower in the finger compared to brachial pressure; amplification of the pulse wave, especially in young subjects, may result in higher finger systolic pressure values (reviewed by Imholz *et al.* 1998).

When results are averaged for a group of subjects, the differences between intra-arterial and finger pressures are small, for systolic and diastolic pressure usually less than 5 mmHg (Fig. 21.3). However, the standard deviation of these differences is not small and Finapres readings, therefore, do not guarantee a reliable estimate of actual intrabrachial pressure levels in the individual patient. We still recommend a sphygmomanometric reading for this.

In practice, the clinician must interpret a blood pressure response in an individual patient; a reliable estimate of the *changes* in blood pressure is therefore of crucial importance. The Finapres is an excellent device in this respect; changes in mean and diastolic pressure during steady-state conditions and during manoeuvres such as Valsalva's and hypotensive orthostatic stress are measured reliably

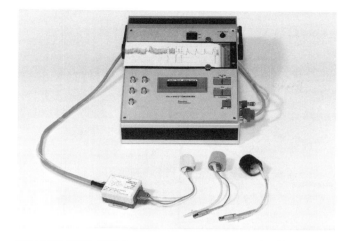

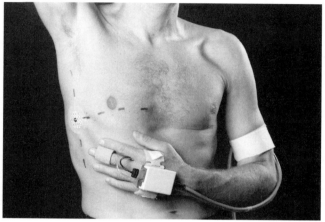

Fig. 21.1. Above, basic components of TNO model 5. A small, inflatable cuff is connected to a small box (front end), which is connected via a 5 m long cable to the main unit. Below, to avoid hydrostatic pressure effects, the finger is held at heart level.

(Imholz *et al.* 1990a; Petersen *et al.* 1995; Jellema *et al.* 1996). The finger-to-brachial differences within one subject are relatively stable; the 95 per cent individual limits of agreement of the standard deviation are between 0 and 4 mmHg. Finger systolic pressures are more variable, but on the whole the performance of Finapres allows it to be used to evaluate autonomic cardiovascular control even in patients over 70 years of age.

Recently, solutions to the drawbacks of peripheral finger blood pressure measurements have been described. Reconstruction of brachial artery pressure waves from finger measurements by correction for pulse wave distortion and individual pressure gradients has been found to be feasible and reliable (Bos *et al.* 1996; Gizdulich *et al.* 1997). The availability of optimally corrected finger pressure measurements will be especially helpful during experiments that require continuous knowledge of the exact blood pressure level and in circumstances where finger pressure measurements have been shown to represent brachial artery pressure with reduced accuracy. These include measurements in subjects with severe cardiovascular disease and measurements during infusion of phenylephrine and strenuous dynamic exercise (Imholz *et al.* 1998).

Monitoring of finger arterial pressure enables one to study the dynamics of circulatory responses in detail. As explained further

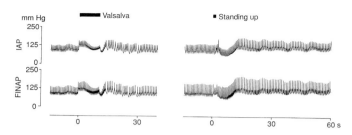

Fig. 21.2. Original recordings of intrabrachial (IAP) and finger (FINAP) arterial blood-pressure responses induced by Valsalva's manoeuvre (left panel) and standing up (right panel). Duration of Valsalva strain and time needed to stand up are indicated. Note similarity between the IAP and FINAP tracings.

below, components of blood pressure and heart rate variability can be studied by techniques such as spectral analysis and sequence analysis, which attempt to assess baroreflex function dynamically (De Boer *et al.* 1987; Omboni *et al.* 1993, 1996). The ambulatory version of Finapres, the TNO Portapres device, enables one to study circulatory responses during 24 hours under everyday circumstances (Imholz *et al.* 1993; Omboni *et al.* 1995). Finapres and Portapres have even made it into space as key instruments in complex experimental human physiology settings (Karemaker 1995).

A recent derivation is the calculation of beat-to-beat changes in stroke volume from the arterial pulse wave (Stok *et al.* 1993; Wesseling *et al.* 1993). Mathematical pulse-wave analysis enables the clinician to evaluate the haemodynamics underlying changes in blood pressure in terms of cardiac output and total peripheral resistance. This has opened new avenues of investigation both in the laboratory and under ambulatory conditions (Wieling *et al.* 1992; De Jong *et al.* 1995, 1997a; Veerman *et al.* 1995).

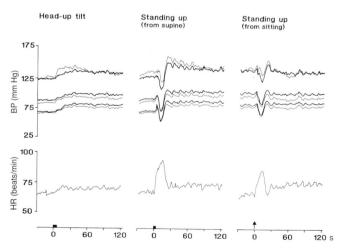

Fig. 21.3. Average intrabrachial (IAP) and finger (FINAP) arterial blood-pressure (BP) and heart-rate (HR) responses in 11 healthy adult subjects aged 22–40 years to three orthostatic manoeuvres. Bold trace, IAP; thin trace, FINAP. (Taken with permission from Imholz *et al.* (1990*a*).)

Cardiovascular control and the arterial baroreflex

The control mechanisms involved in circulatory homeostasis include the following major subsets of pressure buffering systems (in acting order): the neurocardiovascular or neural system, the humorocardiovascular or humoral system, the capillary-fluid-shift system and the renal-body-fluid control system. The renal-body-fluid system acts as a slow, long-term blood pressure integral controller, with the humoral and, especially, the neural control systems serving as fast, fine-tuning feed back mechanisms to match the needs of the body more closely. Among the many reflexes that act upon the cardiovascular system, the arterial baroreceptor reflex is the most relevant reflex in autonomic function testing; it is the key regulatory mechanism for short-term control of systemic blood pressure (Eckberg and Sleight 1992; Wieling and Wesseling 1993). We will restrict the following discussion to the arterial baroreflex for the sake of brevity, although we are aware that this neglects other neural mechanisms impinging on the cardiovascular system.

Arterial baroreceptors are stretch receptors located in the blood vessel walls of the carotid sinuses and aortic arch, which mainly react to increases in arterial pressure at each arterial pulse wave. The afferents from the carotid sinus areas form, together with the chemoreceptor afferents from the carotid bodies, the (bilateral) carotid sinus nerves, which join the glossopharyngeal nerves on their way to the brainstem. Afferents from the aortic baroreceptors join the vagus nerves inside the thorax. The baroreceptor afferents, both from the carotid sinuses and the aortic arch, have their first synapse in the nucleus tractus solitarii in the brainstem. After this synapse the central 'wiring diagram' very quickly becomes obscure, since even the most simple cardiovascular reflexes are known to have a large degree of central integration.

To regulate beat-to-beat blood pressure the autonomic nervous system has three levers to operate: the heart (heart rate, inotropy), venous supply, and systemic vascular resistance. The efferent limbs of the autonomic nervous system consist of sympathetic and parasympathetic fibres to the heart as well as sympathetic fibres to the smooth muscles in the peripheral blood vessels (Fig. 21.4).

The arterial baroreceptors excite the cardiac vagal centres and, at the same time, inhibit sympathetic vasomotor centres in the brainstem. A decrease in arterial pressure and thereby in vascular stretch diminishes vagal excitation and sympathetic inhibition with a resultant decrease in vagal outflow to the heart and increase in sympathetic outflow, causing increases in heart rate, cardiac contractility, and vasomotor tone, all geared towards blood pressure restoration. Conversely, augmented arterial pressure increases baroreceptor discharge and results in neural reflex adjustments that oppose the blood pressure rise. These adjustments act rapidly. Modulation of vagus nerve activity allows changes in heart rate within one or two beats after a changed pulse pressure. Sympathetically mediated changes in heart rate, cardiac contractility, and arteriolar vasomotor tone take 2–3 seconds before they begin.

Quantification of baroreflex function

Theoretically, direct evaluation of baroreflex effectiveness in the intact human is not possible. In order to do so, one would have to isolate vascularly the baroreceptor afferent areas and impose stable

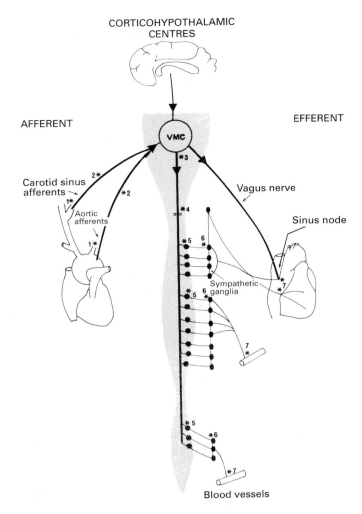

Fig. 21.4. Schematic drawing of the baroreceptor afferent and autonomic efferent pathways of the baroreflex arc. VMC indicates vasomotor centres in brainstem. Possible mechanisms of failure of cardiovascular control are indicated 1, lesion of carotid sinus/aortic baroreceptors; 2, lesion in afferent carotid and/or aortic afferents; 3, lower brainstem lesion; 4, spinal cord transsection; 5, lesion in intermediolateral columns; 6, preganglionic/ganglionic lesion; 7, postganglionic lesion.

blood pressure to them while observing the induced level of blood pressure and heart rate in the remaining part of the vascular tree. Such experiments have been performed in acute animal studies under general anaesthesia, resulting in 'Koch's blood pressure characteristic curves' (Koch 1931), which relate blood pressure in the isolated receptor areas to effective blood pressure or heart rate. In the intact organism we are in the 'closed-loop situation': when blood pressure changes, activation of the baroreflex will tend to annihilate this change. Therefore, input to the arterial baroreflex system, the blood pressure change, cannot be quantified separately from the output of the same system, the new level of blood pressure.

One way around this predicament is to impose a very fast blood pressure change and observe the ensuing vagal change in heart rate. Since the vagal effects are much faster than the sympathetically induced effects on heart and vessels, we may consider the relation between the change in blood pressure and heart rate, with some restrictions, without having to take the closed loop into account. This way of measuring baroreflex sensitivity (BRS) is exploited in a common test known as the phenylephrine test. Here a bolus injection of the vasoactive drug induces a rapid blood pressure rise, which provokes a vagally mediated heart rate drop via the baroreflex. BRS is commonly quantified as the quotient of induced change in pulse interval over the causing change in (systolic) blood pressure, thus yielding a measure in ms/mmHg. Normal values for baroreflex sensitivity range from 15 to 50 ms/mmHg for young adult subjects (Eckberg and Sleight 1992).

We must be aware that this measure of baroreflex quality is restricted to the blood pressure to heart rate arm of the reflex. Important though this may be, it is not essential for blood pressure control in normal daily life: heart transplant patients do not have this reflex, since their hearts are essentially denervated, but they still maintain a normal blood pressure, even when standing up quickly (Wieling and Wesseling 1993). Obviously, a good control of vascular resistance is much more important for the cardiovascular system, but this cannot be quantified as easily as the vagal arm by BRS due to the closed-loop problem.

Direct information on activity of sympathetic nerves in humans can be obtained by transcutaneous microneurographic recordings of superficial peripheral nerves in the limbs. By careful positioning of the electrode and selection of nerve fascicles, the experienced microneurographer can select activity of postganglionic fibres to skeletal muscle or to the skin. The former is mostly related to blood pressure control, the latter to emotion and thermoregulation. The measurement of muscle sympathetic nerve activity (MSNA) has taught us a considerable amount about the nature of baroreflex-modulated sympathetic outflow. The nerves are active in bursts, each burst probably needs a sufficiently low level of baroreceptor activity to start, i.e. in the diastolic portion of the blood pressure pulse. This burst increases in intensity until it is shut off by the baroreceptor afferent burst induced by the next pulse wave. Sympathetic bursts do not occur in all heart beats; the average number of bursts per 100 beats is an accepted measure to quantify the activity. This may be increased by bloodpressure-lowering interventions such as lower-body negative pressure (LBNP) or nitroprusside infusion, or decreased by drugs that increase blood pressure such as infusions of phenylephrine (Pagani et al. 1997). Strangely enough, there is no clear-cut relation between the prevalence of high or low blood pressure and MSNA activity. The number of bursts per 100 beats seems to be some individually determined parameter, which is highly reproducible even over periods of years (Fagius and Wallin 1993; Chapter 23).

A more global measure of sympathetic activity may be obtained by measuring the amount of noradrenaline that appears in the bloodstream as a result of neurotransmitter spillover. Each organ has a specific rate of extraction of noradrenaline from the arterial blood and another rate of excretion to the venous blood due to its own sympathetic activity. Therefore, one should either obtain arterial samples (where the lung will have exerted its own process of extraction and excretion on the mixed venous blood that enters the heart), or measure organ-specific rates by radiotracer methodology involving elaborate catheterization and infusion schemes (Eslen 1993).

Alternatives to the baroreflex sensitivity measurement are offered by computer-oriented techniques applied to continuous recordings of arterial blood pressure and heart rate (see Chapter 22).

Physiological interpretation of the outcome requires some background knowledge of signal analysis techniques and the inherent assumptions and limitations. The most used techniques at present are derived in one way or the other from Fourier analysis. This is a mathematical tool to decompose any signal into a spectrum of sinusoids that, when added together, will reconstitute the original signal. This implies that irregularities in the signal (for example due to extrasystoles) will result in many spectral components, which do not make very much sense, physiologically speaking, but they will tend to obscure the actual spectrum one is trying to obtain.

The spectrum of variations in a resting heart rate recording can be represented as in Fig. 21.5. This shows that the variations can be broadly ascribed to three peaks. One at low frequencies (below 0.05 Hz or one period per 20 s), one around 0.1 Hz (1/10 s) and one around the respiratory rate (mostly 1/4 s). Of these three spectral peaks we know that the respiratory peak is due to vagus nerve activity, since it completely disappears under atropine. The 0.1 Hz peak is due to underlying oscillations in blood pressure at the same frequency, which are probably due to the slowness of the sympathetic system in correcting blood pressure perturbations. The concomitant peak in heart rate oscillations is due to combined vagal and sympathetic activity impinging on the sinus node (De Boer et al. 1987). The still slower variations are due to various regulatory mechanisms, such as chemoreception, temperature regulation, and probably many more. These mechanisms may influence heart rate directly (chemoreflexes) or via the baroreflex.

From the known physiology underlying spontaneous variations in heart rate, various ways to extract information on the baroreflex have

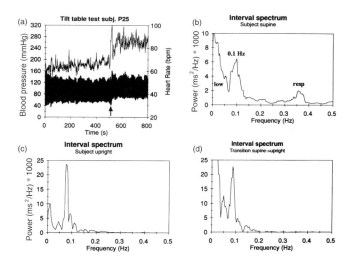

Fig. 21.5. Tilt experiment in a healthy 21-year-old male subject (a) Recording of BP and HR; at the arrow the subject is tilted from supine to 70° head up. (b) Fourier spectrum of heart interval variability for the supine period. Low frequency variability (< 0.05 Hz), 0.1 Hz, and respiratory variability are all present. (c) Spectrum for the standing period. Mainly 0.1 Hz variability is present, respiratory variability has vanished. (Note the adapted scale.) (d) Result when the transition from supine to upright is taken into the analysis: spurious pronounced low-frequency variability dominates the spectrum. This demonstrates the requirement of steady-state conditions for proper application of Fourier analysis to a data set. (Data from Baisch et al. (1992).)

been devised. The most simple being the 'sequences' method, where a recording is scanned for sequences of three or more heart beats where both systolic pressures and the accompanying heart periods go up, or when both are going down together. Such sequences are supposed to be baroreflex mediated and the regression coefficient of the sequences should give an indication of the sensitivity of the reflex (Omboni *et al.* 1993). Alternatively, one can study the coherence between spectral peaks in blood pressure and heart period. If there is sufficient coherence between say, the variations around 0.1 Hz in both parameters, one can assume that the transfer from blood pressure to heart period is made via the baroreflex. Once again, a number for its sensitivity can be obtained in ms heart-period change per mmHg BP change (De Boer *et al.* 1986; Robbe *et al.* 1987). Moreover, as we have seen above, the peak in heart-period variations around the respiratory frequency is uniquely vagally mediated. This makes it a good object of study in the case of suspected loss of vagal control, as may occur in developing neuropathy in a diabetic patient (Lishner *et al.* 1987; Freeman *et al.* 1991; Weston *et al.* 1996).

The computer-oriented techniques have not yet made it from the clinical physiology laboratory to routine clinical use. This may be due both to lack of sufficiently established computational techniques and a reference database of normal (age-related) values with which to compare clinical results. Uncertain reproducibility and sensitivity to erroneous outcome due to measurement difficulty (e.g. by extrasystoles) are further stumbling blocks to the use of this technique (Camm *et al.* 1996; Omboni *et al.* 1996; Wieling *et al.* 1997). Finally, the interpretation of computer findings is by no means undisputed in current literature (Karemaker 1997). The following paragraphs will detail a set of more-or-less classical non-invasive methods of arterial baroreflex pathways testing based on analysing blood pressure and heart rate responses to a variety of physiological stresses. These stresses are easy to apply and provide valuable information about the presence or absence of functional disturbances in baroreflex control of systemic pressure. For these tests more-or-less well-established lower limits of normal values per age group are known. In as far as heart rate responses are important for the test outcome, the reflex tests suffer much less from cardiac irregularities than do spectral analysis techniques. On the other hand, most tests require some form of patient co-operation, which may be difficult to obtain in elderly, physically or mentally disabled patients. In the latter, spectral measures, where patient compliance is much less an issue, can have certain advantages.

Cardiovascular reflex tests

Procedures and analysis data

In earlier studies we used the combination of continuous heart rate monitoring and conventional sphygmomanometry, to define normal and abnormal circulatory responses. Presently, in our laboratory continuous blood pressure recording by Finapres is used instead of sphygmomanometry. In the following both methods will be discussed.

Standardization is a key factor in the assessment of cardiovascular reflex control. Ambient conditions such as time of day and room temperature, breathing pattern, and body posture during the test and the preceding period of supine rest should all be considered. In our laboratory, studies are performed in the morning in a quiet room at a pleasant ambient temperature (21–23 °C) at least 1hour after breakfast. Subjects abstain from coffee and cigarettes from the previous evening.

Medications known to influence the cardiovascular system are not allowed from 48 h prior to testing. Subjects are informed about the procedures involved and are instructed to empty their bladder prior to the start of testing. The actual protocol is begun after a test run to train the subject to perform the test manoeuvres correctly.

Our common order of tests is a forced breathing test in supine position, followed by a standing-up test from supine and a Valsalva manoeuvre in sitting position (Table 21.1). This 'classical series' may be followed by long-duration orthostatic stress testing using a tilt table. The latter is only performed on special indication after previous testing. We want to have the classical tests performed first, since long-duration tilt (in particular if it leads to fainting) may have prolonged effects on cardiovascular control due to neuro-hormonal changes. Compared to the test times in the classical battery (Table 21.1) longer supine resting periods (at least 20 min) are advised for the assessment of disturbances in humoral control. This issue will not be elaborated further in this chapter.

To keep track of the procedure a strip chart recorder at low speed (50 mm/min) is used. Beat-by-beat heart rate is monitored with a cardiotachometer or is obtained from the Finapres arterial pulse pressure interval. Arm-cuff blood pressure is measured supine and in the upright position with the arm relaxed at the side when sphygmomanometry is used. When using Finapres the cuffed finger is kept at heart level, to avoid hydrostatic pressure influences. Just prior to the procedure Finapres' Physiocal- or Servo-selfadjust-option is switched off to ascertain a continuous recording during the transient phases of the manoeuvres.

Calculations are made from the original tracings. Control values for heart rate are obtained by averaging a 10 s period prior to the manoeuvres. In case of marked fluctuations in heart rate a 10–30 s period prior to the manoeuvres should be used. Changes in heart rate from control values induced by forced breathing, standing, and Valsalva's manoeuvre are computed. Control sphygmomanometer blood pressure values are obtained by averaging three measurements. Control values for finger arterial pressure are computed by averaging a 10–30 s period prior to the manoeuvres. Changes in blood pressure from control values induced by the three test manoeuvres are computed.

Overall baroreflex integrity

Overall integrity of the baroreflex arc can be assessed by analysing continuous heart rate and blood pressure responses to orthostasis and Valsalva straining. These manoeuvres impede venous return and reduce cardiac output, thus taxing arterial baroreflex regulatory mechanisms aimed at the stabilization of systemic blood pressure.

Table 21.1. Order of observations in standard cardiovascular reflex testing

- Supine instrumentation
- Instruction of manoeuvres
- 5 min supine rest
- 1 min forced breathing test
- 2–3 min supine rest
- Standing up
- 5 min free standing
- 2–3 min sitting
- Valsalva's manoeuvre (sitting)

Orthostatic stress testing using standing

It is useful to divide the short-term circulatory response to the upright posture into an initial phase (first 30 s) with marked changes in heart rate and blood pressure and an early phase of stabilization (after 1–2 min standing) (Fig. 21.6a). Prolonged standing is defined as at least 5 min upright.

Initial heart rate and blood pressure responses to standing

After a total of 5–10 min of preceding rest, subjects are instructed to move from supine to standing in about 3 s, if necessary with assistance (cf. Table 21.1). They stand for at least 2 min without support. Standing up in healthy adult subjects induces characteristic changes in heart rate (Fig. 21.6a). The heart rate increases abruptly towards a primary peak around 3 s, increases further to a secondary peak around 12 s, declines to a relative bradycardia around 20 s, and then gradually rises again. The primary hear-rate peak is vagally mediated and may be attributed to an exercise reflex that operates when voluntary muscle contractions are performed. The more gradual secondary heart rate rise, starting around 5 s after standing up, is mainly due to further reflex inhibition of cardiac vagal tone and increased sympathetic outflow to the sinus node, and can be attributed to diminished activation of arterial baroreceptors by the fall in arterial pressure. The subsequent decrease in heart rate is associated with the recovery of arterial pressure and is again mediated through the arterial baroreflex by an increase in vagal outflow to the sinus node (Fig. 21.6a).

In quantifying the initial heart rate response to standing, the secondary heart rate peak is generally used. The highest heart rate in the first 15 s from the onset of standing is determined and expressed as the increase from baseline (ΔHR_{max}, 1 in Fig. 21.6a). This approach also allows a quantification of the response in patients with a more gradual heart rate increase, but without a relative bradycardia and consequently without a clear secondary peak. Ewing expressed the relative bradycardia originally as the ratio between the thirtieth and fifteenth R–R interval after the onset of standing. Indeed, on average, the maximal heart rate increase is reached at around the fifteenth beat and the relative bradycardia at around beat 30. However, since there are considerable interindividual differences, measurement of the 30/15 ratio at exactly beats 15 and 30 may underestimate the true RR_{max}/RR_{min} ratio. It is now generally recommended to use the highest and lowest heart rate in the first 30 s from the onset of standing (1 and 2 in Fig. 21.6a) to quantify the relative bradycardia (HR_{max}/HR_{min} ratio) (Ewing 1991; Wieling et al. 1997). The magnitude of ΔHR_{max} and the HR_{max}/HR_{min} ratio decrease with age. Another factor that has a large influence on the initial circulatory response is the duration of the period of supine rest prior to standing (Ten Harkel et al. 1990). The magnitude of ΔHR_{max} after 20 min rest exceeds the value after 1 min rest by about 30 per cent. Our reference values (Table 21.2) are, therefore, only valid for resting periods

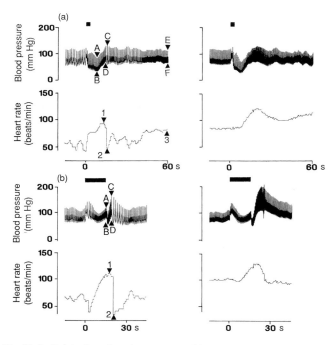

Fig. 21.6. Original tracings in a 33-year-old male subject of blood pressure and heart rate responses induced by (a) standing and (b) Valsalva's manoeuvre. Pharmacological blockade with atropine abolished the large vagally mediated transient heart rate changes, a sluggish, sympathetically mediated heart rate increase remains (right panels). The arrows indicate the timing of characteristic response extremes of interest. For standing: A, systolic pressure and B, diastolic pressure trough; C, systolic pressure and D, diastolic pressure overshoot; E, systolic and F, diastolic pressure level after 1 min standing; 1, initial peak heart rate increase (HR_{max}); 2 relative bradycardia (HR_{min}; 3, heart rate after 1 min standing. For Valsalva's manoeuvre: A, systolic and B, diastolic pressure at the end of straining; C, systolic and D, diastolic pressure overshoot; 1, initial peak heart rate increase (HR_{max}); 2, bradycardia (HR_{min}).

Table 21.2. Assessment of initial heart rate response following 5–10 min resting period and assessment of early steady-state heart rate response

| Age (years) | Initial heart rate response | | Early steady state |
	ΔHR_{max}* (beats/min)	HR_{max}/HR_{min}[†]	$\Delta HR_{2\,minutes}$[‡] (beats/min)
10–14	<20	<1.20	>35
15–19	19	1.18	>34
20–24	19	1.17	>33
25–29	18	1.15	>32
30–34	17	1.13	>31
35–39	16	1.11	>30
40–44	16	1.09	>29
45–49	15	1.08	>28
50–54	14	1.06	>27
55–59	13	1.04	>26
60–64	13	1.02	>25
65–69	12	1.01	>24
70–74	12	1.00	>23
75–80	11	—	>22

*Abnormally low scores for ΔHR_{max} are defined as scores below $P_{0.025}$ (see Fig. 21.9).

[†]Abnormally low values for relative bradycardia are numerically expressed as HR_{max}/HR_{min} ratio.

[‡]Heart rate increases above $P_{0.975}$ of early steady-state values (after 2 min standing) are defined as excessive increase in heart rate.

between 5 and 10 min. The influence of the level of resting heart rate on the magnitude of test scores is small compared to the effect of age and supine rest both in healthy subjects and in patients.

The test range for ΔHR_{max} is sufficient also in the elderly and its long-term within-subject repeatability is high. Thus ΔHR_{max} is a good test to assess instantaneous heart rate control. In contrast, the test range for the HR_{max}/HR_{min} ratio does not allow the distinction to be made between normal and abnormal heart rate control in subjects older than 65 years (Table 21.2) (Piha 1993).

Using the Finapres, the magnitude of the initial blood pressure response can be quantified by determining the systolic and diastolic blood pressure trough (A and B in Fig. 21.6a) and the subsequent systolic and diastolic blood pressure overshoot (C and D in Fig. 21.6a). In patients in whom a recovery of blood pressure is not observed, the value at 10 s after the onset of standing up is taken to indicate the trough and the value at 20 s to indicate the (absence of an) overshoot. The ratio of the change in pulse interval to mean arterial pressure (ms/mmHg) at the moment of the blood pressure trough (1 and A,B in Fig. 21.6a) has been used to compute an estimate of the sensitivity of the arterial baroreflex. This estimate decreases linearly with age (Goedhard *et al.* 1985).

Reference values for the magnitude of the initial blood pressure trough have not yet been established. Based on preliminary experience we consider an initial fall of more than 40 mmHg in systolic pressure and/or more than 25 mmHg in diastolic pressure as abnormally large (Wieling *et al.* 1992; Tanaka *et al.* 1994). The initial fall in blood pressure does not increase with age (Fig. 21.7). An initial overshoot of systolic and/or diastolic pressure is generally observed in healthy adult subjects. Its absence has been suggested as an indicator of sympathetic vasomotor dysfunction (Lindqvist *et al.* 1997).

Heart rate and blood pressure adjustments in the early phase of stabilization (1–2 min standing) and during prolonged standing (5–10 min standing)

The circulatory response in the early phase of stabilization is commonly used in the evaluation of neural circulatory control. This can be established by sphygmomanometer blood pressure readings or by averaging 10 s periods of heart rate and finger blood pressure centred at 1 (3 and E, F in Fig. 21.6a) and 2 min after the change of posture. When there are marked fluctuations in heart rate and blood pressure a 30 s period of the Finapres recording should be averaged. Sphygmomanometric readings are erratic under these conditions. To quantify the circulatory response during prolonged standing, heart rate and blood pressure are taken at 5 and 10 min after the onset of standing.

The normal adjustments in the early phase of stabilization are an increase in diastolic pressure by about 10 mmHg, with little or no change in systolic pressure and an increase in heart rate of about 10 beats/min. During prolonged standing only minor further changes are observed in healthy adult subjects and in the vast majority of patients with abnormal orthostatic responses. Nevertheless, measurements should be continued for 10 minutes when there is a strong clinical suspicion of orthostatic hypotension without the earlier finding of a drop in blood pressure (Streeten and Anderson 1992).

The heart rate increase after 1–2 min standing depends predominantly on increased activity of the sympathetic nervous system; an excessive increase (postural tachycardia) indicates functionally intact neurocardiovascular control and a strong adrenergic drive to the sinus node (Low *et al.* 1995). The orthostatic rise in heart rate

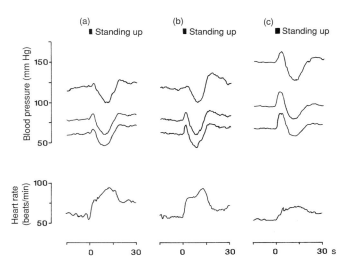

Fig. 21.7. Average systolic, mean and diastolic blood pressure and heart rate responses upon standing in (a) ten 10–14-year-old boys; (b) ten 20–40-year-old adult subjects; and (c) twenty over-70-year-old male subjects. (Data kindly provided by Ten Harkel *et al.* (1990), Imholz *et al.* (1990*b*), and Dambrink *et al.* (1991*a*).)

decreases with age (Table 21.2). A decrease in arterial pressure in the upright position can involve both systolic and diastolic pressures at the same time or be restricted to systolic pressure only. A fall of systolic pressure only is most likely caused by a non-neurogenic disturbance such as central hypovolaemia. Orthostatic hypotension due to autonomic failure involves both systolic and diastolic pressures. Ageing *per se* has little effect on sympathetic-circulatory regulation of arterial pressure during orthostasis; in upright, well-hydrated, normotensive elderly subjects arterial pressure is maintained just as well as in young adult subjects (Taylor *et al.* 1992). A persistent fall of more than 20 mmHg in systolic pressure after 1–2 min standing and/or in diastolic pressure of more than 5–10 mmHg is considered abnormal irrespective of age. The larger systolic blood pressure fall is easier to account for than the diastolic fall. Patients with a high supine systolic pressure tend to have a larger fall in pressure. If supine systolic blood pressure is over 160 mmHg or under 120 mmHg these effects should be taken into account (Van Dijk *et al.* 1994).

Orthostatic stress testing using head-up tilting

The initial circulatory response upon a passive change of posture distinctly differs from the response on standing. A 70° head-up tilt results in a gradual rise in diastolic pressure, little change in systolic pressure, and a gradual initial heart rate rise with little or no overshoot (Fig. 21.3). The different initial responses can be attributed to the effects of contraction of leg and abdominal muscles on the circulation during standing up; the underlying mechanisms have been addressed elsewhere (Sprangers *et al.* 1991; Wieling *et al.* 1996). A 70° angle of tilt may be considered to induce an almost identical hydrostatic effect as a 90° head-up tilt since sin 70° = 0.94 and sin 90° = 1.00. Even with tilt times of between 2 and 5 s, the speed of the manoeuvre has little or no influence on the initial orthostatic response to upright tilting.

The initial heart rate response induced by a 70° head-up tilt does not differentiate between patients with mild vagal impairment and those with normal heart rate control; this is in contrast to the response induced by active standing up. Active standing is, therefore, more suitable to assess orthostatic neural control in the initial phase. The circulatory adjustments during quiet standing and passive head-up tilting in the early phase of stabilization (after 1–2 min upright) and during prolonged orthostatic stress (5–10 min upright) are similar. Both procedures seem appropriate in the clinical evaluation of neural circulatory control in these phases. In subjects with neurological disabilities and for long-duration orthostatic stress testing (20–45 min upright) head-up tilting is preferred since it gives the experimenter better control and allows rapid return to the supine posture in case of impending syncope in the head-up posture (Benditt *et al.* 1996).

Valsalva manoeuvre

Valsalva manoeuvre as used in the cardiovascular laboratory is an abrupt voluntary elevation of intrathoracic and intra-abdominal pressure by straining. It is provoked by blowing through a mouthpiece in a closed system where pressure is measured (e.g. a blood pressure meter). The patient maintains a prescribed airway pressure and to force an open connection between mouth and airways a small leak in the tubing (e.g. via a fine-bore hypodermic needle) is advised. After a brief period of increased peripheral arterial pressure, the blood pumped out is not adequately replenished due to the pressure-induced hindrance of inflow of blood to the trunk; this results in a temporary fall in blood volume in the central vessels. A serious fall in arterial pressure is prevented by reflex vasoconstriction (Sandroni *et al.* 1991; Smith *et al.* 1996). Typical responses are shown in Fig. 21.6b). Preferably, Valsalva manoeuvre is performed while sitting, because the circulatory effects are larger in that position compared to the changes observed in the supine position (Fig. 21.8) (Ten Harkel *et al.* 1990).

An expiratory pressure of 40 mmHg is maintained for 15 s. Care is taken to prevent deep breathing prior to and directly following release of the strain, since this influences test scores considerably. If straining produces marked falls in blood pressures, the manoeuvre should be performed supine. In our experience, some elderly patients, especially those with neurological disorders, and the majority of very young subjects, cannot carry out the procedure adequately (De Jong *et al.* 1997b). Valsalva straining should be avoided in patients with proliferative retinopathy.

Valsalva manoeuvre elicits typical changes in heart rate in young adult subjects (Fig. 21.6b). An immediate heart rate decrease during the rise in systolic and diastolic pressure at the onset of straining is usually observed. It is followed by an increase in heart rate during and directly after release of intrathoracic pressure and a subsequent bradycardia.

The heart rate increase during and directly after release of the strain (peak 1 in Fig. 21.6b) is mediated by withdrawal of vagal tone and increased sympathetic outflow to the sinus node due to the fall in blood pressure. The bradycardia (2 in Fig. 21.6b) is the result of a vagal reflex, which depends on a blood pressure overshoot relative to control blood pressure. The magnitude of the heart rate responses induced by Valsalva manoeuvre again decreases with age (Table 21.3).

In quantifying the heart rate increase induced by Valsalva manoeuvre the maximum heart rate is determined and expressed as the difference from baseline (ΔHR_{max}, peak 1 in Fig. 21.6b). The ratio

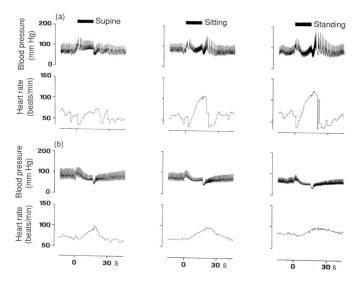

Fig. 21.8. Influence of posture on Valsalva manoeuvre in (a) a healthy 33-year-old subject and (b) a 43-year-old patient with autonomic failure. Note marked influences of posture on the blood pressure responses in both subjects. The square-wave response observed in the healthy adult subject in supine position is a normal finding. (Taken with permission from Ten Harkel *et al.* (1990).)

between highest and lowest heart rate directly after release of the strain (1 and 2 in Fig. 21.6b) is generally used to quantify the relative bradycardia (HR_{max}/HR_{min} ratio or Valsalva ratio). The test range for the Valsalva ratio does not allow one to distinguish between normal and abnormal heart rate control in subjects older than 65 years (Table 21.3) (Piha 1993). Long-term reproducibility of the Valsalva ratio in adult subjects is high.

Table 21.3. Assessment of heart rate responses induced by forced breathing and the Valsalva manoeuvre

Age (years)	I–E difference* (beats/min)	Valsalva ratio[†]
10–14	<17	<1.53
15–19	<16	<1.48
20–24	<15	<1.43
25–29	<14	<1.38
30–34	<13	<1.33
35–39	<12	<1.28
40–44	<11	<1.24
45–49	<11	<1.20
50–55	<10	<1.16
55–60	<9	<1.12
60–65	<9	<1.08
65–70	<8	<1.04
70–75	<7	<1.00
75–80	<7	—

*Abnormally low scores for I⁻–E difference are defined as scores below $P_{0.025}$ (see Fig. 21.6).

[†]Abnormally low values for heart rate changes induced by the Valsalva manoeuvre are expressed as the Valsalva ratio.

Using the Finapres, the magnitude of the blood pressure response can be quantified by determining the systolic and diastolic blood pressure at the end of straining (A and B in Fig. 21.6b) and the subsequent systolic and diastolic blood pressure overshoot after release of Valsalva straining (C and D in Fig. 21.6b) relative to control levels of blood pressure. An overshoot of systolic and/or diastolic pressure is generally observed in healthy adult subjects. These pressure elevations provide acceptable estimates of preceding sympathetic nerve responses and the integrity of arterial baroreceptor sympathetic vasomotor control mechanisms (Smith *et al.* 1996). In patients without a blood pressure overshoot the highest blood pressure in the first 15 s after release of the strain is taken.

It has been suggested that the absence of a partial recovery of arterial pressure during straining is an index of impairment of sympathetic vasomotor function that occurs earlier than the lack of overshoot of arterial pressure above baseline values (Sandroni *et al.* 1991). For older subjects, no data are available on this topic. Baroreflex sensitivity on heart rate can be estimated by measuring the change in interbeat interval per unit change in systolic blood pressure (ms/mmHg) during the overshoot of blood pressure after the straining (Palmero *et al.* 1981). This estimate, again, decreases with age.

Afferent arterial baroreflex pathways

If failure of the baroreflex arc is demonstrated by orthostatic stress or Valsalva straining, the question is whether the lesion on the arterial baroreflex arc is on the afferent, central, or efferent side. Afferent and central lesions cannot be assessed directly in patients. The common approach is to evaluate efferent sympathetic and parasympathetic pathways. If these are normal, the lesion is supposed to be on the afferent or central site of the arterial baroreflex arc.

Efferent sympathetic pathways

Placing one hand in ice water (*cold pressor test*), mental stress, and isometric exercise such as sustained handgrip, result in increased systemic blood pressure. The afferent pathways involved in these stresses (pain, central command, muscle receptors) are distinct from the afferent pathways of the arterial baroreflex. In subjects with evidence of disturbances in control of systemic blood pressure during orthostatic stress or Valsalva straining, a rise in blood pressure in response to these stresses suggests that efferent sympathetic pathways are functioning. The influence of age on the blood pressure responses to such acute stresses is not agreed upon; hyper- and hyporeactivity have been reported. Recent evidence suggests that application of the above-mentioned stressors evokes similar absolute increases in sympathetic neural activity and arterial pressure in healthy young and elderly subjects (Ng *et al.* 1994).

The arterial blood pressure response to the cold pressor test is, in our experience, a useful index of sympathetic outflow to systemic blood vessels. Sustained handgrip has been found consistently to be of limited sensitivity and specificity in the assessment of efferent sympathetic activity (Ziegler *et al.* 1992) (Piha 1993). The cold pressor test is easily applied even in older subjects. The test is performed in the semi-recumbent position. Responses are measured before and during immersion of one hand in ice water for 2 min. The changes in blood pressure during the last 10 s of the test are compared to baseline values. A blood pressure rise of 10–15 mmHg in systolic pressure and of 10 mmHg in diastolic is considered to be a normal response, and an

increase of more than 20 mmHg in systolic pressure *and* 15 mmHg in diastolic pressure as excessive. Hyper-reactivity has been a frequent finding in hypertensive subjects. Little or no increase in arterial pressure is supposed to indicate failure of efferent sympathetic vasomotor pathways, but some normal subjects may also have little or no response.

Efferent cardiac vagal control

The instantaneous heart rate responses elicited by changes in arterial pressure induced by standing up and Valsalva straining (Fig. 21.6a, b) are used as measures of the arterial baroreflex effectiveness on heart rate, as discussed above. For a selective evaluation of efferent cardiac vagal pathways it is useful to apply manoeuvres that elicit non-baroreflex-mediated changes in vagal outflow to the heart. Stimulation of vagal outflow can be evoked by apnoeic face immersion (diving reflex), the cold face test or eyeball pressure (oculovagal reflex). An instantaneous heart rate decrease induced by these manoeuvres indicates intact efferent cardiac vagal pathways. Decreased heart rate responsiveness at older age during these manoeuvres does not allow us to distinguish between normal and diminished efferent cardiac vagal control in the elderly.

Cardiac vagal stimulation and inhibition can be tested by the forced breathing manoeuvre. The afferent pathways and central mechanisms underlying the heart response to this test are complex and the mechanisms involved remain uncertain. There is, however, general agreement that the efferent path is predominantly the parasympathetic supply to the heart by the vagus nerve and it is assumed that the magnitude of the oscillations in heart rate provide the best estimate of efferent neural traffic of the vagus nerve to the heart in man. Compliance to the test is easy, the test range is sufficient (also in the elderly, cf. Table 21.3), and long-term reproducibility is good.

The forced breathing test is performed supine, since vagal effects are then most pronounced. After 5 min rest the subject is instructed to perform six consecutive maximal inspiration and expiration cycles at a rate of 6 breaths/min. To quantify the test score the difference between maximal and minimal heart rate for each of the six cycles is determined and averaged to obtain the inspiratory–expiratory (I–E) difference in beats/min. The magnitude of the I–E difference is age-related (Fig. 21.9) (Wieling *et al.* 1982).

The influence of the level of resting heart rate on the I–E difference is small compared to the effect of age. Thus, a correction for resting heart rate is not important in the measurement of the I–E difference. However, to observe vagally mediated changes in heart rate, some vagal tone should be present. This test, therefore, cannot be interpreted when the resting heart rate is high (>100 beats/min). This principle applies to all tests aiming to assess cardiac vagal tone.

Test battery: clinical interpretation of one or more abnormal test results

We are in favour of using a combination of tests in the evaluation of patients suspected of suffering from autonomic disturbances. We feel that a (patho) physiological interpretation of test results is more important than simply to add test scores as was done in the now almost classical 'Ewing protocol'. Here outcomes of various tests were scored as normal, borderline, or pathological; points were awarded

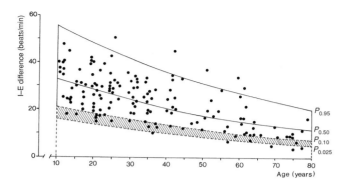

Fig. 21.9. Magnitude of the I-E difference in relation to age. The regression line ($P_{0.50}$) and confidence limits were calculated from log-transformed values. The hatched area indicates values between the lower 2.5th and 10th percentile, which we have defined as borderline. The values below this range are considered abnormally small, values above it are considered normal. (Data from Wieling *et al.* (1982) and Dambrink *et al.* (1991*a*).)

per score; and all scores added to find a final label (Ewing 1992). This 'battery approach' masks the basic pathophysiological abnormalities in cardiovagal or adrenergic control.

The clinical relevance of the search for highly sensitive estimates of alterations in short-term cardiovascular control, be it cardiovagal (Weston *et al.* 1996) or adrenergic (Low *et al.* 1996; Lindqvist 1997), needs to be reconsidered. A sensitive test to screen patients for an abnormality is only indicated if efficacious treatments for the primary disease and/or efficacious preventive manoeuvres for its sequelae exist. Early detection of subclinical autonomic dysfunction has been suggested to be important for risk stratification and subsequent management in patients with cardiovascular disease. However, at this moment there is neither efficacious treatment for autonomic dysfunction nor for the associated increase in sudden death. Large-scale screening for impairment of short-term cardiovascular control is, therefore, not yet indicated, except maybe for research purposes (Wieling *et al.* 1997). In addition, it is important to realize that cardiovascular reflex tests are more difficult to interpret than, for example, nerve conduction measurements, since both autonomic nerve function and cardiovascular haemodynamics are involved.

Moreover, medication and unstable clinical conditions can influence test scores greatly. In daily practice, therefore, it is of far more importance to work towards a definite (patho) physiological diagnosis than to aim for detection of subtle abnormalities.

We use the I–E difference induced by forced breathing as a sensitive measure to assess vagal heart rate control. We have found the combination of abnormally low test scores for both the I–E difference and for ΔHR_{max} upon standing to be eminently suited to identify definite cardiac vagal neuropathy in individual patients (Wieling *et al.* 1982). HR_{max}/HR_{min} ratios induced by standing and the Valsalva heart rate ratios are, in our experience also abnormally low in these conditions.

In earlier studies we used the circulatory response to standing, evaluated by continuous heart rate monitoring and conventional sphygmomanometry, to define a spectrum of normal and abnormal circulatory responses. Using the Finapres we have continued to use this approach (Wieling *et al.* 1991). Our reasons for doing so are:

1. In patients with disturbances in autonomic circulatory control, orthostatic dizziness and fainting are the main clinical problems.
2. Orthostatic stress testing can be applied and interpreted both with and without sophisticated equipment.
3. Orthostatic stress testing can be used not only to evaluate instantaneous, but also prolonged orthostatic circulatory responses.

The Valsalva manoeuvre provides, in our experience, mainly confirmatory information (see next section).

Spectrum of normal and abnormal orthostatic responses

Five main types of responses are clinically important in the evaluation of complaints of orthostatic dizziness (Table 21.4). The first three are common and transient and are found in subjects with intact circulatory reflexes. The last two are rare and characterized by a significant and persistent fall in blood pressure in the upright position due to autonomic failure.

A careful evaluation of the patient's history and the conventional measurement of blood pressure by a sphygmomanometer and heart rate by pulse-counting, supine and after 1–2 min standing, are simple procedures to evaluate complaints of orthostatic dizziness in general

Table 21.4. Classification of patients according to their response to standing

Response	Early steady-state blood pressure		Initial heart rate response	Early steady-state heart rate response
Normal	Systolic	=	Biphasic	↑
	Diastolic	↑		
Hyperadrenergic	Systolic	↓	Large ΔHR_{max}	↑↑
	Diastolic	↑↑	– little or no relative bradycardia	
Vasovagal	Systolic	↓	Normal or hyperadrenergic	↓
	Diastolic	↓		
Hypoadrenergic (vagus intact)	Systolic	↓	Large ΔHR_{max}	↑↑
	Diastolic	↓	– no relative bradycardia	
Hypoadrenergic (with cardiac denervation)	Systolic	↓	Absent	=
	Diastolic	↓		

practice. Based on the heart rate and blood pressure responses in the early phase of stabilization a distinction can be made into:

(1) normal orthostatic heart rate and blood pressure control;
(2) normal orthostatic blood pressure control in combination with a postural tachycardia; and
(3) orthostatic hypotension with or without postural tachycardia (Table 21.4).

Below we will show that, although continuous measurement of arterial blood pressure is no prerequisite for a classification of patients, analysis of both heart rate and blood pressure changes contributes to a more fundamental understanding of the pathophysiological mechanisms involved.

Initial orthostatic dizziness on standing in healthy subjects

A normal initial heart rate response, including an immediate heart rate increase, a large secondary heart rate peak, and a marked subsequent bradycardia (1 and 2 in Fig. 21.6a) is an important clinical finding. It indicates, for reasons explained above, that intact afferent, central, and efferent cardiac vagal and efferent sympathetic vasomotor pathways are present. Nevertheless, it should be realized that subjects with intact autonomic cardiovascular control can still have complaints of dizziness shortly after standing up. In fact most people have experience with a brief feeling of dizziness 5–10 s after the onset of standing up rapidly, especially after prolonged supine rest. Such common spells of dizziness are characterized by their time of onset and short duration and appear to be more common in young subjects.

In teenagers with severe complaints of orthostatic dizziness immediately on standing up, an extraordinary large initial blood pressure drop and sluggish recovery has been observed (Fig. 21.10a) (Dambrink et al. 1991b; Tanaka et al. 1994). This impairment of postural blood pressure adjustment is associated with postural tachycardia and vasovagal attacks during prolonged standing (see below). The observation that a similar impaired initial blood pressure response can be found after clonidine administration (Coupland et al. 1995) supports the view that blunted sympathetic activation of the resistance vessels is involved. Nevertheless, the circulatory response to Valsalva's manoeuvre in these subjects is, in our experience, qualitatively normal (Fig. 21.10a). An abnormally large initial blood pressure fall and sluggish recovery upon active standing can also be found in patients with bilateral denervation of the carotid baroreceptors (operation for carotid body tumours) (Wieling and Wesseling 1993). This abnormality is to be expected since the carotid baroreceptors are of key importance for adjustments to rapid changes in arterial pressure.

Hyperadrenergic orthostatic response

An excessive heart rate increment (cf. Table 21.2) after 1–2 min of standing can be considered as a compensatory response to a variety of conditions; an abnormal degree of central hypovolaemia and a strong adrenergic drive in the upright posture are common to these conditions (Low et al. 1995). Classically, such a response consists of an immediate heart rate increase and a large secondary peak with little or no subsequent relative bradycardia, resulting in an excessive increase in heart rate in the upright position (Fig. 21.10b), together with a fall in systolic pressure and a marked increase in diastolic

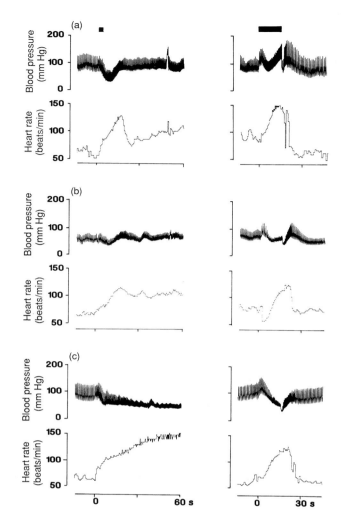

Fig. 21.10. Blood pressure and heart rate responses induced by standing (■) and Valsalva manoeuvre (▬). (a) A 17-year-old female patient with complaints of orthostatic dizziness almost immediately upon standing and a large initial fall in blood pressure. (b) A 32-year-old female patient with a postural tachycardia. (c) Orthostatic hypotension (hypoadrenergic) with intact heart rate control in a 23-year-old female patient.

pressure. A marked increase in both systolic and diastolic pressure has also been described. The normal circulatory response to Valsalva's manoeuvre in these conditions confirms functionally intact arterial baroreflex pathways.

Vasovagal orthostatic response

Typical for a vasovagal response is a temporary phase of tachycardia in the upright position, which changes into a decrease in heart rate and a fall in blood pressure due to reflex vagal facilitation and adrenergic inhibition, respectively (Fig. 21.11; Van Lieshout et al. 1991a).

Using pulse contour analysis the variability of haemodynamic responses leading up to a vasovagal faint can be analysed (Fig. 21.12) (De Jong et al. 1997a). An impaired ability to generate or to maintain vasomotor tone seems to be the key factor in vasovagal fainting both

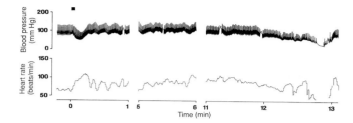

Fig. 21.11. Vasovagal fainting in a healthy 22-year-old male subject. Note normal initial heart rate and blood pressure response and marked increase in heart rate after 6 min standing. After 11–12 min standing, blood pressure and heart rate start to decrease to very low values during the actual faint; the heart rate tracing in the faint is interrupted in a period of asystole of 7 s. On lying down, heart rate and blood pressure recover almost immediately. (Taken with permission from Van Lieshout *et al.* (1991*a*).)

in young and in adult subjects (Ten Harkel *et al.* 1993; De Jong *et al.* 1995; Novak *et al.* 1996; Tanaka *et al.* 1997). In our experience the circulatory response to Valsalva's manoeuvre is normal in subjects with a vasovagal orthostatic response.

Hypoadrenergic orthostatic response with intact heart rate control

In patients with sympathetic vasomotor lesions but intact vagal heart rate control, an immediate large heart rate increase without a relative bradycardia and consequently a persistent and marked heart rate rise is observed (Van Lieshout *et al.* 1989). This is accompanied by a progressive fall of both systolic and diastolic blood pressures (Fig. 21.10c). This response can be attributed to correct baroreceptor sensing of an absence of recovery of blood pressure due to the defective vasoconstrictor mechanisms (compare Fig. 21.6a with Fig. 21.10c). Hypoadrenergic orthostatic hypotension, combined with a marked postural tachycardia, can be found in some patients with dysautonomia, in tetraplegic patients, and after extensive sympathectomy.

The blood pressure response induced by Valsalva's manoeuvre in these patients indicates loss of sympathetic vasomotor control. If the heart rate response is considered without the simultaneous blood pressure recording, the result can be misleading, since a reflex brady-cardia and high Valsalva ratios can be observed in some of these patients (Fig. 21.10c) The rare combination of hypoadrenergic orthostatic response with intact vagal heart rate control (Fig. 21.10c) may be interpreted as the mirror image of the common pattern of autonomic circulatory denervation, where impaired vagal heart rate control precedes overt sympathetic damage, i.e. orthostatic hypotension (Fig. 21.13a).

Hypoadrenergic orthostatic response with impairment of vagal and sympathetic innervation of the heart

In subjects with a normal resting heart rate, a delayed and sluggish primary heart rate response upon standing indicates that vagal heart rate control is absent (compare Fig. 21.6a right and left panels with Fig. 21.13b left panel). The heart rate increase in these patients

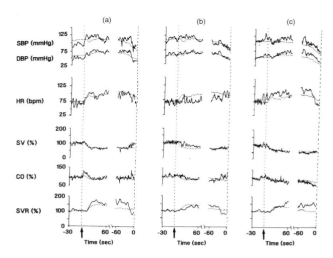

Fig. 21.12. Typical individual of examples vasovagal response (a); a vasodepressor response (b); and a vagal response (c). The dotted lines represent the group averages of 29 6–16 year old near-fainting subjects. Supine control, the first 60s of the head-up tilt and the last 60s before tilt-back are presented. The arrow indicate the moment of tilt-up. SBP, systolic blood pressure; DBP, diastolic blood pressure; HR, heart rate; SV, stroke volume; CO, cardiac output; SVR, systemic vascular resistance. (Taken with permission from De Jong *et al.* (1997*a*).)

represents the remaining sympathetic response mentioned before. Thus, a delayed onset of cardioacceleration and a substantial heart rate increase afterwards suggest cardiac vagal denervation with intact sympathetic heart rate control. A small heart rate increase after prolonged standing in patients with orthostatic hypotension should be interpreted as a sign of impaired sympathetic heart rate control. Valsalva's manoeuvre will confirm the abnormality (compare Fig. 21.6b right and left panels, with Fig. 21.13b right panel.

Complete denervation of the heart can be found in patients with a cardiac transplant. The blood pressure adjustment to orthostatic stress shows that when vasomotor innervation is intact, orthostatic blood pressure control remains undisturbed in spite of complete cardiac denervation (Fig. 21.13c) (Wieling and Wesseling 1993). A square-wave response is induced by Valsalva's manoeuvre. Obviously, the marked blood pressure changes induced by standing and Valsalva's manoeuvre will not be noticed in this patient if continuous monitoring is not available.

Square-wave response during Valsalva straining

A square-wave response during Valsalva straining occurs in subjects with congestive heart failure, but also during a supine Valsalva's manoeuvre in some normal subjects (Ten Harkel *et al.* 1990). In the latter the square-wave response changes to 'normal' in the sitting and the standing position (Fig. 21.8). These observations suggest that the blood pressure responses during Valsalva straining can be used to monitor changes in central blood volume. The diurnal and postural effects on blood pressure during Valsalva straining in a patient with autonomic failure are another example of this concept (Fig. 21.14; Van Lieshout *et al.* 1991*b*).

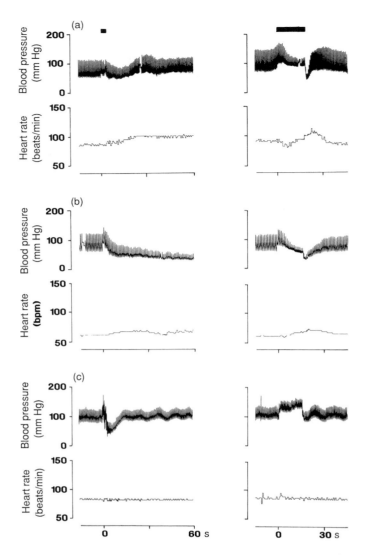

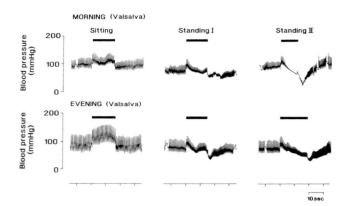

Fig. 21.14. Diurnal and postural effects on the blood pressure response to Valsalva manoeuvre. The manoeuvre was performed in the sitting position, after 10 min of standing upright (Standing I) and was repeated after a further 2 min in the upright position (Standing II). Bars indicate the duration of the straining period. Note the higher sitting and standing mean blood pressure in the evening and the square-wave response during Valsalva's manoeuvre in the sitting position in the evening. (Taken with permission from Van Lieshout et al. (1991b).

Fig. 21.13. Blood pressure and heart rate responses induced by standing (■) and Valsalva manoeuvre (▬▬). (a) A 64-year-old male patient with polyneuropathy and impairment of cardiac vagal control, but normal blood pressure responses. (b) A 69-year-old male patient with orthostatic hypotension (hypoadrenergic) with impairment of vagal and sympathetic cardiac control (Valsalva's manoeuvre is performed supine). (c) Total cardiac denervation with intact vasomotor control in a 38-year-old fit patient with a cardiac transplant.

Concluding remarks

An active standing test provides much insight about human neuro-cardiovascular control as both instantaneous and sustained orthostatic circulatory responses can be assessed. ΔHR_{max} is a good test to assess instantaneous heart rate control in the elderly, but the HR_{max}/HR_{min} ratio is *probably* not. The combination of sphygmomanometric blood pressure readings in the supine position and after 1–2 min standing and monitoring of the instantaneous heart rate response on standing provides sufficient information for a classification of normal and abnormal orthostatic circulatory responses. However, for a full physiological evaluation of an abnormal heart rate response it is necessary

to monitor the concomitant blood pressure responses continuously using the Finapres.

In contrast to the orthostatic stress test, Valsalva's manoeuvre only assesses instantaneous circulatory responses. The advantage of Valsalva's manoeuvre is that both the capacities for cardioacceleration and cardiodeceleration are tested. Lack of reference values for blood pressure indices of the manoeuvre in elderly subjects and problems in the correct execution make the procedure less suitable for the assessment of cardiovascular control than orthostatic stress testing.

Reference

Baisch, F., Beck, L., Karemaker, J. M., Arbeille, P., Gaffney, F. A., and Blomqvist, C. G. (1992). Head-down tilt bedrest. HDT'88—an international collaborative effort in integrated systems physiology. *Acta Physiol. Scand. Suppl.* **604**, 1–12.

Benditt, D. G., Ferguson, D .W., Grubb, B. P. et al. (1996). Tilt table testing for assessing syncope. ACC expert consensus documents. *J. Am. Coll. Cardiol.* **28**, 263–75.

Bos, W. J., Van Goudoever, J., Van Montfrans, G. A., Van den Meiracker, A. J., and Wesseling, K. H. (1996). Reconstruction of brachial artery pressure from non-invasive finger pressure measurements. *Circulation* **94**, 1870–5.

Camm, A. J., Malik, M., Bigger, J. T. et al. (1996) Heart rate variability—standards of measurement, physiological interpretation, and clinical use. *Circulation* **93**, 1043–65.

Coupland, N. J., Bailey, J. E., Wilson, S. J., Horvath, R., and Nutt, D. (1995). The effects of clonidine on cardiovascular responses to standing in healthy volunteers. *Clin. Auton. Res.* **5**, 171–7.

Dambrink, J. H. A., Imholz, B. P. M., Karemaker, J. M., and Wieling, W. (1991a). Circulatory adaptation to orthostatic stress in healthy 10–14 year old children. *Clin. Sci.* **81**, 51–8.

Dambrink, J. H. A., Imholz, B. P. M., Karemaker, J. M. and Wieling, W. (1991b). Postural and transient hypotension in two healthy teenagers. *Clin. Auton. Res.* **1**, 281–7.

De Boer, R. W., Karemaker, J. M., and Strackee, J. (1986). Determination of baroreflex sensitivity by spectral analysis of spontaneous blood pressure and heart rate fluctuations in man. In *Neural mechanisms and cardiovascular disease.* (ed. B. Lown, A. Malliani, and M. Prosdocimi), pp. 303–15. Liviana Press, Padova.

De Boer, R. W., Karemaker, J. M. and Strackee, J. (1987). Hemodynamic fluctuations and baroreflex sensitivity in humans: a beat-to-beat model. *Am. J. Physiol.* 253, H680–H689.

De Jong-de Vos van Steenwijk, C. C. E., Wieling, W., Johannes, J. M., Harms, M. P. M., Kuis, W., and Wesseling, K. H. (1995). Incidence and hemodynamics of near-fainting in healthy 6–16 old subjects. *J. Am Coll. Cardiol.* 25, 1615–21.

De Jong-de Vos van Steenwijk, C. C. E., Wieling, W., Harms, M. P. M., and Wesseling, K. H. (1997a). Variability of near-fainting responses in healthy 6–16 year old subjects. *Clin. Sci.* 93, 205–11.

De Jong-de Vos van Steenwijk, C. C. E., Imholz, B. P. M., Wesseling, K. H., and Wieling, W. (1997b). The Valsalva manoeuvre as a cardiovascular reflex test in healthy children and teenagers. *Clin. Auton. Res.* 7, 167–71.

Eckberg, D. L. and Sleight, P. (1992). *Human baroreflexes in health and disease.* Oxford University Press, Oxford.

Esler, M. (1993). Clinical application of noradrenaline spillover methodology: delineation of regional human sympathetic nervous responses. *Pharmacol. Toxicol.* 73, 243–53.

Ewing, D. J. (1992). Analysis of heart rate variability and other non-invasive tests with special reference to diabetic mellitus. In *Autonomic failure. A textbook of clinical disorders of the autonomic nervous system,* (ed. R. Bannister and C. J. Mathias), pp. 312–33. Oxford University Press, Oxford.

Fagius, J. and Wallin, B. G. (1993). Long-term variability and reproducibility of resting human muscle nerve sympathetic activity at rest, as reassessed after a decade. *Clin. Auton. Res.* 3, 201–5.

Freeman, R., Saul, J. P., Roberts, M. S., Berger, R. D., Broadbridge, C., and Cohen, R. J. (1991). Spectral analysis of heart rate in diabetic autonomic neuropathy. *Arch. Neurol.* 48, 185–90.

Gizdulich, P., Prentza, A., and Wesseling, K. H. (1997). Models of brachial to finger pulse wave distorsion and pressure decrement. *Cardiovasc. Res.* 33, 698–705.

Goedhard, W. J. A., Wesseling, K. H., and Settels, J. J. (1985). Baroreflex pressure control responding to orthostasis changes with age. In *Psychophysiology of cardiovascular control.* (ed. J. F. Orlebeke, G. Mulder, and L. P. J. Van Doornen), pp. 191–202. Plenum, New York.

Imholz, B. P. M., Settels, J. J., Van den Meiracker, A. H., Wesseling, K. H., and Wieling, W. (1990a). Noninvasive beat-to-beat finger blood pressure measurement during orthostatic stress compared to intra-arterial pressure. *Cardiovasc. Res.* 24, 214–21.

Imholz, B. P. M., Dambrink, J. H. A., Karemaker, J. M., and Wieling, W. (1990b). Orthostatic circulatory control in the elderly evaluated by non-invasive continuous blood pressure measurement. *Clin. Sci.* 79, 73–9.

Imholz, B. P. M., Langewouters, G. J., Van Montfrans, G. A. et al. (1993). Feasibility of ambulatory, continuous 24-hour finger arterial pressure recording. *Hypertension* 21, 65–73.

Imholz, B. P. M., Wieling, W., Van Montfrans, G. A., and Wesseling, K. H. (1998). Fifteen years experience with finger arterial pressure monitoring: assessment of the technology. *Cardiovascular. Res.* 38, 605–16.

Jellema, W. T., Imholz, B. P. M., Van Goedoever, J., Wesseling, K. H., and Van Lieshout, J. J. (1996). Finger arterial versus intrabrachial pressure and continuous cardiac output during head-up tilt testing in healthy subjects. *Clin. Sci.,* 91, 193–200.

Karemaker, J. M. (1995). Blood pressure measurement under extreme circumstances: Finapres in actual and simulated weightlessness. *Homeostasis* 36, 275–80.

Karemaker, J. M. (1997). Heart rate variability: why do spectral analysis? *Heart* 77, 99–101.

Koch, E. (1931). *Die reflektorische Selbststeuerung des Kreislaufes.* Steinkopff Verlag, Dresden.

Lindqvist, A., Torffvit, O., Rittner, R., Agardh, C. D., and Pahlm, O. (1997). Artery blood pressure oscillation after active standing up: an indicator of sympathetic function in diabetic patients. *Clin. Physiol.* 17, 159–69.

Lishner, M. S., Akselrod, S., Avi, V. M., Oz, O., Divon, M., and Ravid, M. (1987). Spectral analysis of heart rate fluctuations. A non-invasive, sensitive method for the early diagnosis of autonomic neuropathy in diabetes mellitus. *J. Auton. Nerv. Syst.* 19, 119–25.

Low, P. A. (1996). Clinical autonomic testing report of the therapeutics and technology assessment subcommittee of the American Academy of Neurology. *Neurology* 46, 873–80.

Low, P. A., Opfer-Gehrking, T. L., Textor, S. C. et al. (1995). Postural tachycardia syndrome. *Neurology* 45, S19–25.

Ng, A. V., Callister, R., Johnson, D. G., and Seals, D. R. (1994). Sympathetic neural reactivity to stress does not increase with age in healthy humans. *Am. J. Physiol.* 267, H344–353.

Novak, V., Honos, G., and Schondorf, R. (1996). Is the heart empty at syncope? *J. Auton. Nerv. Syst.* 60, 83–92.

Omboni, S., Parati, G., Frattola, A. et al. (1993). Spectral and sequence analysis of finger blood pressure variability. Comparison with analysis of intra-arterial recordings. *Hypertension* 22, 26–33.

Omboni, S., Smit, A. A. J., and Wieling, W. (1995). Twenty-four hour non-invasive finger pressure monitoring: a novel approach to the evaluation of therapy in patients with autonomic failure. *Br. Heart J.* 73, 290–2.

Omboni, S., Parati, G., Di Rienzo, M., Wieling, W., and Mancia, G. (1996). Blood pressure and heart rate variability in autonomic disorders: a critical review. *Clin. Auton. Res.* 6, 171–82.

Pagani, M., Montano, N., Porta, A., et al. (1997). Relationship between spectral components of cardiovascular variabilities and direct measures of muscle sympathetic nerve activity in humans. *Circulation* 95, 1441–8.

Palmero, H. A., Caeiro, T. F., Iosa, D. J., and Bas, J. (1981). Baroreceptor reflex sensitivity index derived from Phase 4 of the Valsalva maneuver. *Hypertension* 3, II-134-7.

Petersen, M. E. V., Williams, T. R., and Sutton, R. (1995). A comparison of non-invasive continuous finger blood pressure measurement (Finapres) with intra-arterial pressure during head-up tilt. *Eur. Heart J.* 16, 1647–54.

Piha, S. J. (1993). Age-related diminution of the cardiovascular autonomic responses: diagnostic problems in the elderly. *Clin. Physiol.* 13, 507–17.

Robbe, H. W., Mulder, L. J., Ruddel, H., Langewitz, W. A., Veldman, J. B., and Mulder, G. (1987). Assessment of baroreceptor reflex sensitivity by means of spectral analysis. *Hypertension* 10, 538–43.

Sandroni, P., Benarroch, E. E., and Low, P. A. (1991). Pharmacologic dissection of components of the Valsalva maneuver in adrenergic failure. *J. Appl. Physiol.* 71, 1563–7.

Smith, M. L., Beightol, L. A., Fritsch-Yelle, J. M., Ellenbogen, K. A., Porter, T. R., and Eckberg, D. L. (1996). Valsalva's maneuver revisited—A quantitative method yielding insights into human autonomic control. *Am. J. Physiol.* 271, 1240–9.

Sprangers, R. L. H., Wesseling, K. H., Imholz, A. L. T., Imholz, B. P. M., and Wieling, W. (1991). The initial blood pressure fall upon stand up and onset to exercise explained by changes in total peripheral resistance. *J. Appl. Physiol.* 70, 523–30.

Stok, W. J., Baisch, F., Hillebrecht, A., Schulz, H., Meyer, M., and Karemaker, J. M. (1993). Noninvasive cardiac output measurement by arterial pulse analysis compared with inert gas rebreathing. *J. Appl. Physiol.* 74, 2687–93.

Streeten, D. H. P. and Anderson, G. H. (1992). Delayed orthostatic intolerance. *Arch. Int. Med.* 152, 1066–72.

Tanaka, H., Thulesius, O., Yamaguchi, H., and Mino, M. (1994). Circulatory responses in children with unexplained syncope evaluated by continuous non-invasive finger blood pressure monitoring. *Acta Paediatr.* 83, 754–61.

Tanaka, H., Yamaguchi, H., Tamai, H., Mino, M., Konishi, K., and Thulesius, O. (1997). Haemodynamic changes during vasodepressor syncope in children and autonomic function. *Clin. Physiol.* 17, 121–33.

Taylor, J. A., Hand, G. A., Johnson, D. G., and Seals, D. R. (1992). Sympathoadrenal-circulatory regulation of arterial pressure during orthostatic stress in young and older men. *Am. J. Physiol.* 263, R1147–1155.

Ten Harkel, A. D. J., Van Lieshout, J. J., Van Lieshout, E. J., and Wieling, W. (1990). Assessment of cardiovascular reflexes: influence of posture and period of preceding rest. *J. Appl. Physiol.* **68**, 147–53.

Ten Harkel, A. D., van Lieshout, J. J., Karemaker, J. M., and Wieling, W. (1993). Differences in circulatory control in normal subjects who faint and who do not faint during orthostatic stress. *Clin. Auton. Res.* **3**, 117–24.

Van Dijk, J. G., Tjon-A-Tsien, A. M.., Kamzoul, B. A., Kramer, C. G., and Lemkes, H. H. (1994). Effects of supine blood pressure on interpretation of standing up test in 500 patients with diabetes mellitus. *J. Autonom. Nerv. Syst.* **47**, 23–31.

Van Lieshout, J. J., Wieling, W., Wesseling, K., and Karemaker, J. M. (1989). Pitfalls in the assessment of cardiovascular reflexes in patients with sympathetic failure but intact vagal control. *Clin. Sci.* **76**, 523–8.

Van Lieshout, J. J., Wieling, W., Karemaker, J. M., and Eckberg, D. L. (1991a). The vasovagal response. *Clin. Sci.* **81**, 575–86.

Van Lieshout, J. J., Ten Harkel, A. D., van Leeuwen, A. M., and Wieling, W. (1991b). Contrasting effects of acute and chronic volume expansion on orthostatic blood pressure control in a patient with autonomic circulatory failure. *Neth. J. Med.* **39**, 72–83.

Veerman, D. P., Imholz, B. P. M., Wieling., Wesseling, K. H., and Van Montfrans, G. A. (1995). Circadian profile of systemic hemodynamics. *Hypertension* **26**, 55–9.

Wesseling, K. H., Jansen, J. R. C., Settels, J. J., and Schreuder, J. J. (1993). Computation of aortic flow from pressure in humans using a nonlinear, three-element model. *J. Appl. Physiol.* **74**, 2566–73.

Weston, P. J., James, M. A., Panerai, R. *et al.* (1996). Abnormal baroreceptor-cardiac reflex sensitivity is not detected by conventional tests of autonomic function in patients with insulin-dependent diabetes mellitus. *Clin. Sci.* **91**, 59–64.

Wieling, W. and Wesseling, K. H. (1993). Importance of reflexes in the circulatory adjustments to postural change. In *Cardiovascular reflex control in health and disease*, (ed. R. Hainsworth and A. L. Mark), pp. 35–65. W.B. Saunders, London.

Wieling, W., Van Brederode, J. F. M., De Rijk, L. G., Borst, C., and Dunning, A. J. (1982). Reflex control of heart rate in normal subjects in relation to age; a data base for cardiac vagal neuropathy. *Diabetologia* **22**, 163–6.

Wieling, W., Ten Harkel, A. D. J., and Van Lieshout, J. J. (1991). Spectrum of orthostatic disorders: classification based on an analysis of the short-term circulatory response upon standing. *Clin. Sci.* **81**, 241–8.

Wieling, W., Veerman, D. P., Dambrink, J. H. A., and Imholz, B. P. M. (1992). Disparities in circulatory adjustment to standing between young and elderly subjects explained by pulse contour analysis. *Clin. Sci.* **83**, 149–55.

Wieling, W., Harms, M. P. M., Ten Harkel, A. D. J., Van Lieshout, J. J., Wesseling, K. H., and Sprangers, R. L. H. (1996). Circulatory response at the onset of dynamic leg exercise in humans. *J. Physiol.* **494**, 601–11.

Wieling, W., Smit, A. A. J., and Karemaker, J. M. (1997). Autonomic dysfunction in diabetic patients. *Neurosci. Res. Comm.* **21**, 67–74.

Ziegler, D., Laux, G., Dannehl, K. *et al.* (1992). Assessment of cardiovascular autonomic function: age-related normal ranges and reproducibility of spectral analysis, vector analysis, and standard tests of heart rate variation and blood pressure responses. *Diabet. Med.* **9**, 166–75.

22. Computer analysis of blood pressure and heart rate variability in subjects with normal and abnormal autonomic cardiovascular control

G. Parati, M. Di Rienzo, S. Omboni, and G. Mancia

Introduction

Autonomic cardiovascular regulation in humans is usually investigated by measurement of blood pressure and/or heart rate responses to laboratory stimuli which interfere in different ways with the central and reflex control of circulation. Although providing important information on autonomic cardiovascular control in health and disease, this approach is affected by several limitations. Some of these can be overcome by analysis of spontaneous fluctuations in cardiovascular signals which appear to offer, in several instances, a deeper insight into normal and deranged mechanisms of autonomic cardiovascular control. The aim of this chapter is to describe basic features of spontaneous blood pressure and heart rate variability, and to discuss the possible diagnostic value of the data obtained in patients with autonomic dysfunction.

Laboratory methods for the assessment of autonomic cardiovascular regulation

Typical examples of laboratory methods used to investigate autonomic cardiovascular control are:

(1) the assessment of the reflex changes in R–R interval induced by blood pressure changes that follow intravenous injection or infusion of vasopressor and vasodepressor drugs and thus the increase and decrease in the activity of arterial baroreceptors, respectively (Mancia and Mark 1983);

(2) the reflex blood pressure and heart rate responses to changes in carotid baroreceptor activity obtained through the application of either positive or negative pneumatic pressures within a neck-chamber device (Ludbrook *et al.* 1977);

(3) the cardiovascular responses to mental or physical stressors (Parati *et al.* 1988*a*);

(4) the reflex cardiovascular changes that accompany application of negative pneumatic pressure within a lower-body chamber and thus the unloading of volume cardiac receptors (Mancia *et al.* 1988); and

(5) the cardiovascular responses to changes in respiratory activity or posture (see Chapters 20 and 21).

This has allowed important knowledge on autonomic cardiovascular regulation to be obtained, together with assessment of whether this

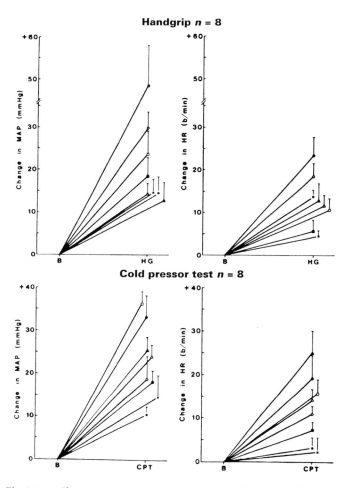

Fig. 22.1. Changes in mean arterial pressure (MAP), measured by an intra-arterial catheter, and heart rate (HR) induced by handgrip exercise (upper panels) and cold pressor test (lower panels) in 8 subjects. Different symbols refer to individual subjects. Each symbol indicates the average response of a given subject to six identical performances of either test. Vertical bars are the standard deviations of the individual average response, and reflect within-subject response variability. (From Parati *et al.* (1985), with permission.)

egulation is altered in a number of diseases, including primary and secondary autonomic failure. There are limitations with this approach, however, because: some of the stimuli delivered to the cardiovascular system may interfere with the autonomic mechanisms under evaluation; the assessment of neural cardiovascular control is usually in a stressful laboratory environment; the reproducibility of the haemodynamic responses is low (Parati *et al.* 1985) (Fig. 22.1); and, finally, responses are usually measured as average stimulus-induced stepwise changes, thus disregarding information on the dynamic features of neural cardiovascular modulation.

Blood pressure and heart rate variability: historical and methodological aspects

Blood pressure, although continuously perturbed by external stimuli, invariably displays a tendency to return to a reference level. This suggests that attention has to be paid not only to the average blood pressure value but also to the fluctuations of blood pressure around its average level. These fluctuations appear therefore to be not an undesirable noise but phenomena which need to be fully understood in order

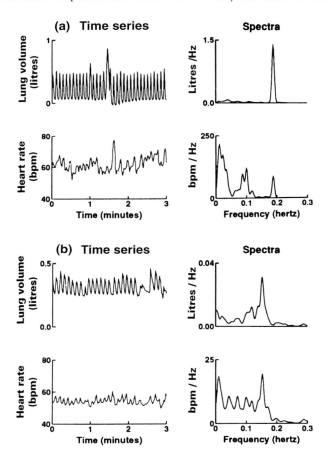

Fig. 22.2. Plots show respiratory activity and heart rate time series (left panels) and their spectra (right panels). Data from one subject with 'peaky' heart rate spectra (a) and from another subject with 'broadband' heart rate spectra (b), are shown separately. (From Parati *et al.* (1995*a*), with permission.)

to determine how cardiovascular regulation normally operates and whether a derangement has occurred (Parati *et al.* 1995*a*).

Important findings in this direction, were obtained in the 1960s with the introduction of a technique for continuous intra-arterial blood pressure monitoring in ambulant individuals, which provided unequivocal evidence that blood pressure fluctuates continuously and markedly in normal individuals (Mancia *et al.* 1983, 1997*a*), that heart rate behaves in a similar fashion, and that the degree of these fluctuations vary in different clinical conditions. For example, when blood pressure variability was quantified by the standard deviation of its average 24 h value, blood pressure fluctuations were greater in hypertensive as compared to normotensive subjects, and in elderly as compared to young individuals. Conversely, when similarly quantified as the standard deviation of their average value, heart rate fluctuations were reduced in diseases such as diabetes mellitus, congestive heart failure, myocardial infarction, and autonomic failure.

The standard deviation, although providing a comprehensive description of the signal dispersion around the mean, offers no information on the patterns that characterize the variability of the signal under study over a period of time (De Boer *et al.* 1987; Mancia *et al.* 1997*a*). This has led to the development of other methods for quantification of cardiovascular signal variability, among which spectral analysis has been used widely. This approach allows the overall variance of a signal to be split into its various frequency components (Fig. 22.2), making use of either the fast Fourier transform (FFT) or the autoregressive modelling (AR) method (Parati *et al.* 1995*a*). The FFT spectrum is derived from all data present in the recorded signal, regardless of whether their various frequency components appear as spectral peaks (reflecting regular oscillations) or as more irregular fluctuations, which do not result in clearly identifiable peaks in the spectrum (see below) (Fig. 22.2). In contrast, with the AR approach the raw data are used to identify the best-fitting model from which the final spectrum, consisting of the direct current (d.c.) component and a variable number of peaks, is derived (Parati *et al.* 1995*a*).

It should be emphasized that these methods yield similar results when FFT is used with some degree of signal smoothing and the AR method is applied with a sufficiently high model order (Fig. 22.3; Parati *et al.* 1995*a*). Yet, current use of the FFT and AR approach has led investigators to proceed in different directions. With the AR method, attention has been largely focused on the spectral peaks that correspond to regular oscillations having a frequency greater than 0.025 Hz (i.e. relatively fast oscillations with a period shorter than 30 s), which appear to reflect sympathetic and parasympathetic modulation of the heart and vascular tone. This offers a method for quantifying the autonomic cardiovascular modulation either under controlled laboratory conditions, when a stationary signal is employed, or as a change over time in daily life, when the amplitude and frequency modulations of the above peaks are quantified by time-varying spectral analysis techniques (Fig. 22.4; Parati *et al.* 1990). With the FFT method, attention has also been directed to the slower components of blood pressure and heart rate variability and the ability of this method to include the whole blood pressure or heart rate recording in a single spectrum has allowed spectral components to be assessed over a broad range of frequency from the lowest to the highest (Fig. 22.5; Di Rienzo *et al.* 1992). This broad-band approach indicates that 24 h blood pressure and heart rate spectra are characterized by a $1/f$ trend, i.e. that the amplitude of both fluctuations increases progressively with the reduction in their frequency, which implies that total 24 h blood pressure and heart rate spectral powers depend more

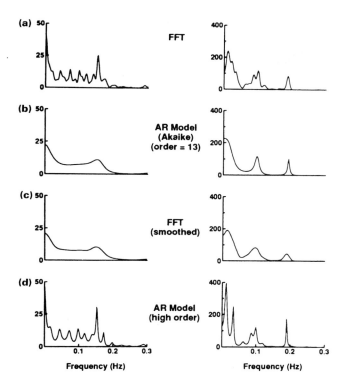

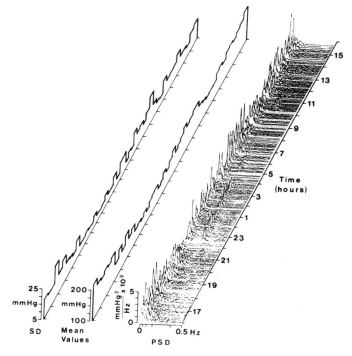

Fig. 22.3. Plots show the same heart rate spectra as Fig. 22.2a (right panels) and Fig. 22.2b (left panels), obtained by means of different analysis methods. (a) data are obtained using an unsmoothed fast Fourier transform (FFT) algorithm. (b) Data are obtained with an autoregressive (AR) model, the order of which (13) was determined by Akaike criteria. (c) Data are obtained with an FFT algorithm smoothed with a Gaussian window, and appear like those obtained with the AR model having an order of 13(a). (d) Data are obtained with an AR model with a high order (=30), and appear like those obtained with the unsmoothed FFT algorithm (a). (From Parati *et al.* (1995a), with permission.)

Fig. 22.4. Sequential power spectrum densities (PSD) of low-frequency (0.025–0.07 Hz), mid-frequency (0.07–0.14 Hz), and high-frequency (0.14–0.35 Hz) systolic blood pressure (SBP) oscillations computed over consecutive segments of 256 beats throughout a 24 hour period in a representative subject. SBP mean values and standard deviations (SD) for each half-hour of the recording are also shown. Data are derived from a 24-hour intra-arterial ambulatory BP recording. Dotted lines in the right panel refer to segments in which PSD could not be estimated because the recorded signal, was not stationary. (From Parati et al. (1990), with permission.)

on lower- than on higher-frequency components. The $1/f$ trend of blood pressure and heart rate spectra also undergoes marked changes following surgical or pharmacological intervention interfering with autonomic cardiovascular influences (Fig. 22.6; Castiglioni *et al.* 1993) and varies in different diseases and conditions, thus offering an additional means by which to assess normal and deranged autonomic mechanisms (Fig. 22.7; Parati *et al.* 1997).

Regardless of the method, there are concerns about the specificity and the reproducibility of the information provided by spectral analysis techniques. The specificity of the low-frequency (LF, around 0.1 Hz) and high-frequency (HF, the respiratory frequency) powers of heart rate as markers of sympathetic and vagal cardiac tone, respectively, is highly debated, particularly when signal variability is reduced (Daffonchio *et al.* 1991; Kingwell *et al.* 1995); this also applies for the LF spectral powers of blood pressure as markers of sympathetic vasomotor tone. Discordant evidence also exist as to the reproducibility of these and other spectral indices (Freed *et al.* 1994; Parati *et al.* 1995a). Autonomic cardiovascular modulation is characterized by a high degree of non-linearity in the relationship between external inputs and cardiovascular response; this may impair the use of spectral analysis to assess autonomic cardiovascular control. This important issue, which is exemplified for baroreflex

control of RR interval in Fig. 22.8 (Parati *et al.* 1995a), is largely ignored as the generally accepted, but incorrect, assumption is that cardiovascular responses are approximately linear. Additional methodological problems are that the signal recorded needs to be stationary in order to allow blood pressure and heart rate spectra to be interpreted correctly; that there has to be an appropriate degree of spontaneous fluctuation in the signal under evaluation, in order to avoid the risk of having no input data in the frequency range of interest; and that frequency domain techniques may better quantify changes in autonomic cardiovascular modulation than mean neural autonomic activity. As an example, Fig. 22.9 (Parati *et al.* 1995a) shows how a marked increase in parasympathetic cardiac drive was associated with a reduction, rather than with an increase, in heart rate variability.

In the attempt to address some of these issues, other methods have been proposed. These include the analysis of non-linear dynamics in cardiovascular signals, such as the calculation of the slope of $1/f$ trends, the Fractal dimension, Lyiapunov exponents, and Poincaré plots (Elbert *et al.* 1994). They also include methods that aim at coupling the information obtained from the biological signal with the information derived from physiological or mathematical models. Examples are the approaches that consider the relationship between two or more cardiovascular signals physiologically related to

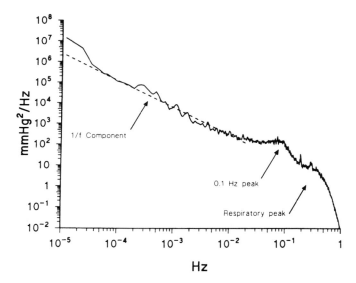

Fig. 22.5. Representative example of a broad-band spectrum of systolic blood pressure obtained from the analysis of a 24 hour ambulatory intra-arterial blood pressure recording performed in a normotensive volunteer. Spectral components with frequencies ranging from 1 to approximately 0.000023 Hz (i.e. with periods ranging from 1 s to 12 h) are considered. The continuous line refers to the actual spectral powers; the discontinuous line is the $1/f$ line modelling the spectrum in the frequency region where the $1/f$ model is suitably applicable. (From Di Rienzo et al. (1992), with permission.)

each other. Some of these multivariate models are based on the evaluation of the gain and phase relationship between respiration and either blood pressure or heart rate changes by transfer function analysis (Saul et al. 1991), the relationship between specific components of blood pressure and pulse interval fluctuations in the time (sequence technique) (Fig. 22.10) or frequency domain (Fig. 22.11) (Parati et al. 1995b) to obtain a dynamic assessment of 'spontaneous' baroreflex sensitivity (see below), and the relationship between blood pressure and pulse interval in a closed-loop fashion by either autoregressive moving average techniques (ARMA models) (Patton et al. 1996) or, more simply, through Fourier-based transfer function techniques (Parati et al. 1995b). In a number of instances these approaches have also been employed in the analysis of longer-term blood pressure or heart rate recordings in ambulant subjects, which has allowed study of autonomic cardiovascular influences out of an artificial laboratory setting and under the conditions of daily life.

Insights into neural cardiovascular regulation from blood pressure and heart rate variability analysis

Between-subject differences in blood pressure or heart rate variability can be related to differences in the neural influences responsible for cardiovascular regulation. These factors include both central and reflex influences, with the arterial baroreflex playing a fundamental role (Mancia et al. 1997a). Examples of central influences are hypotension and bradycardia due to the transition from wakefulness to sleep (Mancia et al. 1983, 1997a), the pressor and tachycardic responses to physical exercise, to unusual emotional stresses (such as

gambling or a medical visit), or even to common situations (such as talking) (Parati et al. 1992a). These cannot, however, be used easily to quantify whether autonomic cardiovascular influences are normal, reduced, or enhanced because the behavioural challenges are difficult to standardize between individuals.

Different conclusions can be reached for the arterial baroreflex, however. Evidence is available that this reflex exerts an important buffering action on spontaneous blood pressure variability in conscious animals (Cowley et al. 1973; Ramirez et al. 1985; Di Rienzo et al. 1991), with its inactivation by section of the carotid sinus and aortic nerves, followed by a striking increase in the magnitude of the blood pressure fluctuations. Increased variability in blood pressure following anaesthesia or section of the carotid sinus nerves occurs in human subjects undergoing neck surgery (Mancia et al. 1997a). The buffering effect of the arterial baroreflex on blood pressure variability in humans undergoing 24 h intra-arterial blood pressure monitoring, is also demonstrated by the finding that baroreflex sensitivity is inversely related to the 24 h blood pressure standard deviation (Mancia et al. 1986).

Baroreflex sensitivity also enhances heart rate variability. Sinoaortic denervated animals display a reduced degree of heart rate fluctuations compared to intact animals (Ramirez et al. 1985). Between-subject differences in heart rate variability are related to differences in their baroreflex sensitivity as assessed by traditional methods (Mancia et al. 1986). Also, in an individual subject, changes in baroreflex sensitivity over 24 h are inversely related to changes in blood pressure variability but directly related to changes in heart rate variability. Thus the stabilizing effect of the baroreflex on blood pressure may be exerted through the ability of baroreceptors to modulate neural cardiac drive in a way that compensates, through changes in cardiac output, for the blood pressure changes. This is further supported by studies in the rat where an atropine-induced reduction in heart rate variability is accompanied by an increase in blood pressure variability (Mancia et al. 1997a). However, in other

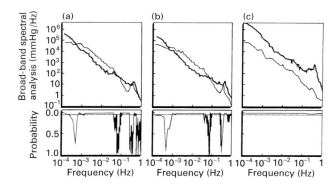

Fig. 22.6. Broad-band spectra of systolic blood pressure (a), diastolic blood pressure (b), and pulse interval, the reciprocal of heart rate (c), derived from 3 h intra-arterial recordings obtained both in the intact condition (thick line) and 7 days after surgical baroreceptor deafferentation through sinoaortic denervation (thin line) in a group of eight conscious cats. The lower traces are the probabilities of the null hypothesis for the differences in the average spectral powers between intact and sinoaortic denervated conditions. The level of statistical significance ($p = 0.05$) is represented by the dotted horizontal line, and power differences are statistically significant if the corresponding p values fall into the zone above the dotted line. (From Castiglioni et al. (1993), with permission.)

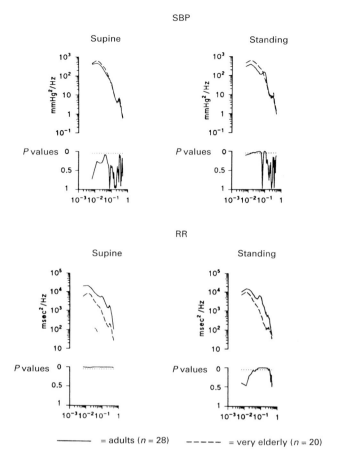

Fig. 22.7. Broad-band spectra of systolic blood pressure (SBP, upper panels) and RR interval (bottom panels) are computed separately for the supine (left) and the standing (right) positions. Data are shown as averages for a group of 28 adult individuals (_____) and a group of 20 very elderly individuals (age >75 years, ----). Spectral powers are expressed in absolute units after logarithmic transformation. The lower portion of each panel illustrates the level of statistical significance of the differences between the broad-band spectra of adult and very elderly individuals assessed for each spectral line. For other explanations see Fig. 22.6. (From Parati et al. (1997), with permission).

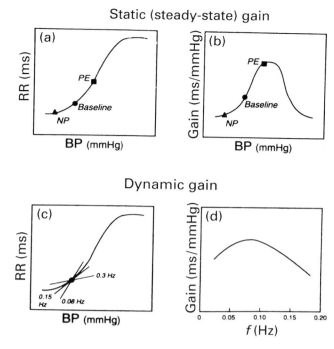

Fig. 22.8. Schematic drawing illustrating several features of baroreflex heart rate control. (a) Sigmoid curve describing the relationship between changes in the input (blood pressure, BP) and reflex changes in the output (RR interval). As BP increases, RR interval increases, approximating a sigmoidal relationship with threshold and saturation values at either end of the curve. The gain of the heart rate baroflex is defined as the slope at any given point on the response curve. Administration of vasoactive agents (nitroprusside (NP) or phenylephrine (PE)) induces changes in mean arterial pressure, moving the normal baroreflex operating point (baseline) into a different operating range. This may lead potentially to different gains. (b) Plot of the baroreceptor heart rate gain as a function of BP. As the baroreflex stimulus-response curve is sigmoidal, maximal gain is observed in the linear portion of the curve, occurring at intermediate BP levels. At more extreme BP values, steady-state gain is diminished. (c) Dynamic or beat-to-beat baroreflex gain as measured by the autoregressive moving average (ARMA), the spectral and the sequence techniques at the mean operating point in a may be higher or lower than the 'steady-state' gain, depending on the characteristics of the BP signal. (d) In particular, the dynamic gain may depend on the frequency content of the input signal. In this example the maximal gain is found to occur around 0.10 Hz, with a decreased gain at both ends of the frequency range, suggesting band-pass characteristics. (From Parati et al. (1995a), with permission.)

animals and in humans this is certainly not the only stabilizing blood pressure mechanism, because blood pressure variability is not increased by reducing heart rate variability through atropine (Fig. 22.12; Parati et al. 1987) or by abolishing heart rate variations through cardiac pacing (Mancia et al. 1997a), indicating that the stabilizing effect on blood pressure also is accounted for by vascular influences of the baroreflex.

Studies in animals and in humans (Saul et al. 1991; Parati et al. 1995a; Mancia et al. 1997a) have allowed the following additional conclusions to be reached. Heart rate fluctuations at frequencies above 0.15 Hz (i.e. in the HF or respiratory band) are due primarily to modulation of sinus node activity by changing vagal cardiac influences, associated with the respiratory cycle, although mechanical modulation of sinus rate by atrial stretch also seems to be involved to some degree (Bernardi et al. 1989). These fluctuations, therefore, can be considered as a relatively satisfactory parasympathetic marker. On the other hand, HF blood pressure fluctuations are caused by the mechanical effects of

respiration and no direct vagal modulation of vasomotor tone is involved (Mancia et al. 1997a). Heart rate fluctuations at frequencies above 0.025 but below 0.15 Hz (variably defined as LF or mid-frequency, MF, when using methods that split this frequency band into two components) are mediated by both sympathetic and parasympathetic influences and, to a minor degree, also by non-neural influences; thus, they cannot be regarded invariably as purely sympathetic markers (Mancia et al. 1997a). The specificity of these fluctuations as indices of sympathetic cardiac modulation can be enhanced, however, in conditions where the sympathetic system is activated (Saul et al. 1990). When blood pressure is considered, spectral powers below 0.15 Hz predominantly reflect fluctuations in vasomotor

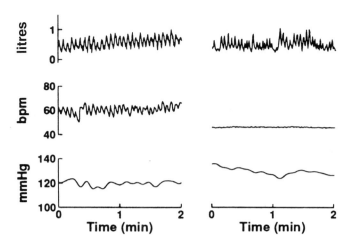

Fig. 22.9. Time series of respiratory activity (respiratory volume, top), heart rate (middle), and mean blood pressure (bottom) in one subject. Data were obtained under control conditions (left) and during intravenous infusion of phenylephrine (right), which determined an increase in blood pressure and a reflex bradycardia. Note that at the time of maximal reflex cardiac vagal stimulation under phenylephrine infusion, respiratory sinus arrhythmia disappeared. (From Parati *et al.* (1995*a*), with permission).

tone and systemic vascular resistance. At frequencies between 0.04 and 0.025 Hz, this vascular modulation may be dependent on the renin–angiotensin system, endothelial factors, and local influences related to thermoregulation (Mancia *et al.* 1997*a*), although conclusive evidence is not available. In contrast, at frequencies between 0.04 and 0.15 Hz blood pressure fluctuations have repeatedly been interpreted as a marker of sympathetic vasomotor tone (Malliani *et al.* 1991; Mancia *et al.* 1993, 1997*a*) although this is not invariably so in both animals and man when correlated with other measures of sympathetic activity (Parati *et al.* 1995*a*); furthermore, they persist even after substantial removal of sympathetic vascular influences by surgical and/or pharmacological sympathectomy (Mancia *et al.* 1993).

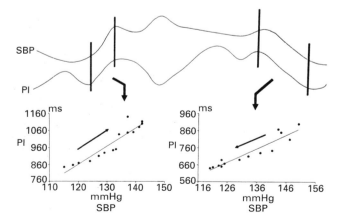

Fig. 22.10. Schematic drawing that illustrates how spontaneous baroreflex sensitivity is assessed through the sequence technique. An example of hypertension/bradycardia sequence is shown on the left, while an example of hypotension/tachycardia sequence is shown on the right. SBP, systolic blood pressure; PI, pulse interval. (From Parati *et al.* (1995*b*), with permission.)

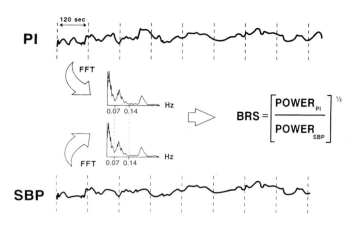

Fig. 22.11. Schematic drawing that illustrates how spontaneous baroreflex sensitivity can be assessed in the frequency domain by computing the 'alpha' coefficient, i.e. the squared ratio of the spectral powers of PI and SBP in the frequency regions where these powers are coherent. BRS, baroreflex sensitivity; FFT, fast Fourier transform. For other explanations see Fig. 22.10. (From Parati *et al.* (1995*b*), with permission.)

In conclusion, while spectral analysis of blood pressure and heart rate variability provides substantial information, the interpretation of the blood pressure and heart rate spectra as quantitative markers of autonomic cardiovascular influences is still controversial, particularly when signals are recorded in the absence of standardized conditions and without simultaneous recording of respiratory activity (Bernandi *et al.* 1989; Saul *et al.* 1991; Mancia *et al.* 1993).

Measurement of slower blood pressure and heart rate fluctuations (i.e. fluctuations <0.025 Hz) provided by broad-band spectral analysis has recently raised interest because it may offer further insights into cardiovascular control mechanisms. An example is the alteration of these fluctuations in conscious cats after baroreceptor denervation by sinoaortic nerve section (SAD) (Cerutti *et al.* 1991; Parati *et al.* 1995*b*; Di Rienzo *et al.* 1996). As shown in Fig. 22.6, baroreceptor denervation changes all the spectral components of systolic blood pressure and pulse interval (the reciprocal of heart rate), indicating that the baroreflex was responsible for the genesis of faster (frequencies >0.025 Hz) and also slower components variability (with periods up to 1.5 h). After SAD, pulse interval powers were reduced at all frequencies while blood pressure powers showed more complex changes. This included a reduction in the power of spectral components from 0.2 to 0.007 Hz and below 0.0003 Hz; an increase in the power of spectral components from 0.05 to 0.0005 Hz; almost no change in the power of spectral components at the respiratory frequency (around 0.3 Hz) and a change in the slope of the $1/f$ trend of the blood pressure spectrum, thus supporting the concept that the baroreflex is involved in this phenomenon.

The arterial baroreflex thus plays different roles depending on the frequency of blood pressure fluctuations; it has a negligible effect on respiratory blood pressure fluctuations; it buffers blood pressure fluctuations between 0.05 and 0.0005 Hz, and it exerts a pro-oscillatory role on fluctuations around 0.1 Hz and at very low frequencies. This paradoxical pro-oscillatory role of the baroreflex is in agreement with the hypothesis of Wesseling *et al.* (1985) that the spectral peak observed at 0.1 Hz is at least in part due to resonance in the baroreflex loop.

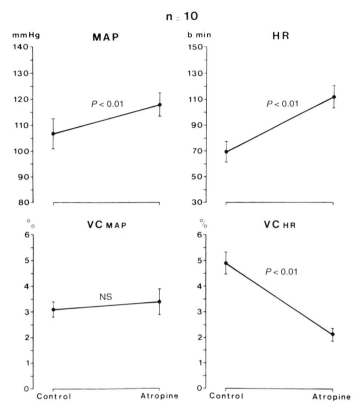

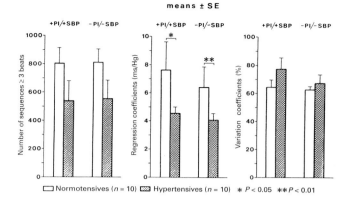

Fig. 22.13. Histograms illustrating the number of sequences characterized by a progressive increase (+PI/+SBP) or by a progressive reduction (−PI/−SBP) in pulse interval and systolic blood pressure during 24 hours (left panel), their mean 24-hour slopes or regression coefficients (middle panel), and the 24-hour variation coefficients of these slopes (right panel). Sequences of different duration are pooled. Data are shown separately as means ± SE for 10 normotensive and 10 hypertensive subjects. (From Parati *et al.* (1988*b*), with permission.)

Fig. 22.12. The changes in the average values of mean arterial pressure (MAP) and heart rate (HR) and in their coefficient of variations (VC, i.e. (SD/average value) × 100) from a control condition induced by intravenous bolus injection of atropine (0.04 mg/kg in two refracted doses) in 10 subjects under intra-arterial ambulatory blood pressure monitoring. The BP and HR recordings obtained before and under atropine administration were both carried out over 1 h (Oxford recorder).

Dynamic assessment of baroreflex sensitivity through analysis of blood pressure and heart rate variability

Because the arterial baroreflex is involved in a major way in the modulation of both spontaneous blood pressure and heart rate variability, joint analysis of these phenomena has been proposed to obtain information on baroreflex function in daily life (Parati *et al.* 1992*b*). This can be achieved both in the time and in the frequency domain. By computer analysis of continuous blood pressure and heart rate recordings it is possible to identify sequences of contiguous heart beats characterized by progressive and linearly related increases in systolic blood pressure and pulse interval (hypertension/bradycardia sequences, +PI/+SBP) or by progressive and linearly related reductions in systolic blood pressure and pulse interval (hypotension/tachycardia sequences, −PI/−SBP) (Fig. 22.10). As with the laboratory technique based on injection of vasoactive drugs, the slope of the regression line between changes in systolic

blood pressure and subsequent changes in pulse interval can be taken as an index of the sensitivity of baroreflex control of the heart (Bertinieri *et al.* 1988; Parati *et al.* 1988*b*, 1995*b*) and has led to various conclusions. In cats, these sequences almost completely disappear following surgical baroreceptor denervation, demonstrating their dependence on the arterial baroreflex (Bertinieri *et al.* 1988; Parati *et al.* 1995*b*). In normotensive subjects undergoing ambulatory intraarterial blood pressure recordings the slope of the hundreds of sequences seen over 24 h changes continuously over time (Fig. 22.13) and displays a marked day–night difference, with a marked increase in slope (i.e. in baroreflex sensitivity) from wakefulness to sleep (Fig. 22.14; Parati *et al.* 1988*b*). In essential hypertensive patients, the number of 24 h sequences is markedly reduced. Furthermore, the sequence slope is substantially lower than in normotensive individuals (Fig. 22.13), with an alteration of day–night modulation (Fig. 22.14; Parati *et al.* 1988*b*, 1994). Finally, similar alterations in baroreflex sensitivity have been observed in the elderly (Fig. 22.15; Parati *et al.* 1995*c*).

Spontaneous baroreflex sensitivity can be assessed in the frequency domain by computing the modulus of the cross-spectrum (Robbe *et al.* 1987) or the squared ratio (Pagani *et al.* 1988; Parati *et al.* 1992*b*, 1995*b*) between blood pressure and heart rate powers in the frequency regions where these powers are coherent (Fig. 22.11), e.g. around 0.1 Hz. As in the case for the sequence slope, this spectral index of baroreflex sensitivity (termed the alpha coefficient), displays a clear 24 h modulation in normotensive individuals, with a marked increase during night sleep, its magnitude and day–night modulation being markedly reduced in hypertensives and in the elderly (Parati *et al.* 1992*b*, 1995*b*, *c*) with patterns similar to those seen with the time-domain method (Fig. 22.16). Blood pressure and heart rate powers are usually also coherent around 0.25 Hz, but at variance from the 0.1 Hz coherence; this 'high-frequency' coherence partially survives sinoaortic denervation (Parati *et al.* 1992*b*; 1995*b*; Di Rienzo *et al.* 1996). Thus, in the high-frequency region this coherence is accounted for substantially by non-baroreceptor mechanisms, which makes use of the HF alpha coefficient in order to quantify the baroreflex sensitivity questionable.

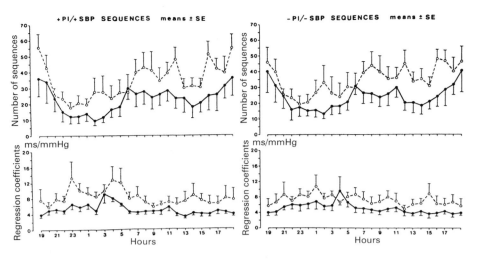

Fig. 22.14. Number and mean regression coefficients (or slopes) of +PI/+SBP and –PI/–SBP sequences during each hour of a 24-hour intra-arterial ambulatory blood pressure recording. Data are shown as means ± SE for 10 normotensive (○) and 10 hypertensive (●) subjects. Sequences of different duration are pooled. (From Parati *et al.* (1988*b*), modified, with permission.)

Analysis of spontaneous baroreflex sensitivity by time-domain and frequency-domain methods has recently been shown to be able to identify early autonomic abnormalities. In diabetic patients with normal autonomic function, based on deep breathing and heart rate and blood pressure changes from lying to standing, the sequence method and the spectral approach showed clear evidence of reduced baroreflex modulation of the heart (Fig. 22.17; Frattola *et al.* 1997). This evidence was also obtained in smokers, where these methods identified a baroreflex impairment (Fig. 22.18) which escaped recognition when traditional baroreflex evaluation by laboratory stimuli (such as the neck chamber) was employed (Mancia *et al.* 1997*b*).

These different observations support the conclusion that joint computer analysis of blood pressure and pulse interval variability (either in the time or in the frequency domain) may provide an innovative and sensitive method of quantifying the efficiency of the baroreceptor–heart rate reflex and to obtain such measurement also in conditions of daily life. There are advantages with this approach, because it avoids the limited number of measurements, the artificial external stimuli, and the abnormal environmental conditions typical of laboratory methods, that may influence neural control of the circulation.

Intra-arterial and non-invasive finger blood pressure monitoring in the assesssment of autonomic cardiovascular regulation in daily life

Computer analysis of blood pressure variability requires beat-to-beat blood pressure signals of good quality, that previously have been possible only by intra-arterial recordings. The recent development of

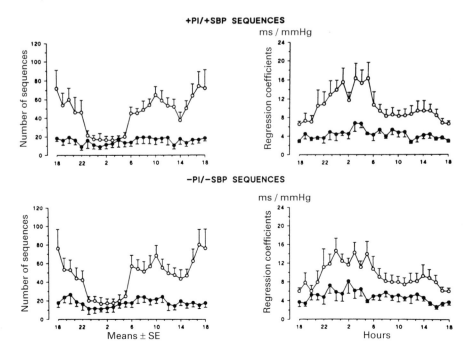

Fig. 22.15. Number and regression coefficients of +PI/+SBP and –PI/–SBP sequences in a group of eight young and eight elderly (○) subjects. Data are shown as average values ±SE for each hour of a 24-hour ambulatory intra-arterial blood pressure recording. (From Parati *et al.* (1995*c*), with permission.)

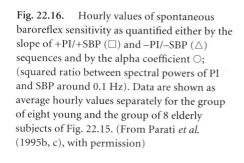

Fig. 22.16. Hourly values of spontaneous baroreflex sensitivity as quantified either by the slope of +PI/+SBP (□) and −PI/−SBP (△) sequences and by the alpha coefficient ○; (squared ratio between spectral powers of PI and SBP around 0.1 Hz). Data are shown as average hourly values separately for the group of eight young and the group of 8 elderly subjects of Fig. 22.15. (From Parati *et al.* (1995b, c), with permission)

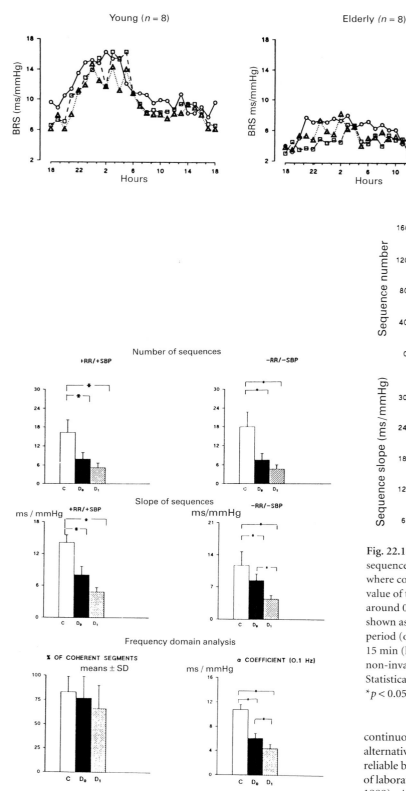

Fig. 22.17. Time- and frequency-domain estimates of the spontaneous baroreceptor–heart rate reflex in control subjects (C) and in diabetic patients with no or with autonomic dysfunction at classical laboratory tests (D_0 and D_1, respectively), *$P < 0.05$. (From Frattola *et al.* (1997), with permission).

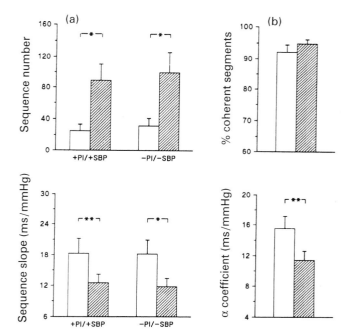

Fig. 22.18. (a) Number and slope of +PI/+SBP and −PI/−SBP sequences. (b) Percentage of signal segments (each including 256 beats) where coherence between PI and SBP around 0.1 Hz was > 0.5, and value of the alpha coefficient (squared ratio between PI and SBP powers around 0.1 Hz) was computed. Data from group of 10 subjects are shown as average values ± SE from a 1-hour non-smoking control period (open bars) period during which one cigarette was smoked every 15 min (hatched bars). Blood pressure was continuously recorded in a non-invasive fashion by a Finapres (Finapres, Ohmeda) device. Statistical significance of differences between control and smoking: *$p < 0.05$; **$p < 0.01$. (From Mancia *et al.* (1997b), with permission.)

continuous finger blood pressure recorders has offered a non-invasive alternative to the intra-arterial approach (see Chapter 21). It provides reliable blood pressure values not only at rest but also during a number of laboratory tests inducing pressor or depressor responses (Parati *et al.* 1989). Analysis of finger pressure recordings also offers a reliable quantification of the standard deviation of mean arterial pressure (although less so for systolic blood pressure), thereby also being suitable for an estimate of overall blood pressure variability. Recent studies have focused on whether this approach is adequate for more complex time- and frequency-domain analysis of blood pressure variability. In

14 untreated mild or moderate essential hypertensive patients, spectral analysis by FFT was performed on finger (Finapres, TNO) and intra-arterial blood pressure recordings simultaneously obtained for 30 min at rest while supine. Spectral powers of blood pressure and pulse interval were integrated over three frequency bands, defined as low frequency (LF, 0.025–0.07 Hz), mid frequency (MF, 0.07–0.14 Hz), and high frequency (HF, 0.14–0.35 Hz). The standard deviations of the average blood pressures of the whole recording period were slightly higher when assessed by finger than by intra-arterial recordings, the difference being statistically significant for systolic blood pressure only. The spectral powers of pulse interval were similar for finger and intra-arterial recordings at all frequencies; this being the case also for spectral powers of mean and diastolic blood pressure. However, the spectral powers of systolic blood pressure located in the lower portion of the spectrum (MF and LF powers, and powers of lower frequencies down to 0.001 Hz) were overestimated by analysis of finger blood pressure (Fig. 22.19; Omboni *et al.* 1993). Despite this, the coherence (i.e. a measure of linear relationship between two signals in the frequency domain) between intra-arterial and finger blood pressure or pulse interval powers was greater than 0.5 at all frequencies, and was highest at approximately 0.1 Hz (Omboni *et al.* 1993). Based on these data, analysis of finger blood pressure recordings should, in general, be accepted in estimating blood pressure variability, even on the background of the reported overestimation of systolic blood pressure powers. This is because such an overestimation represents a nearly constant offset, which can be accounted for by use of correction factors, and the occurrence of a high coherence between finger blood pressure and intra-arterial powers in the frequency regions where the analysis of BP variability is of clinical interest. When finger blood pressure

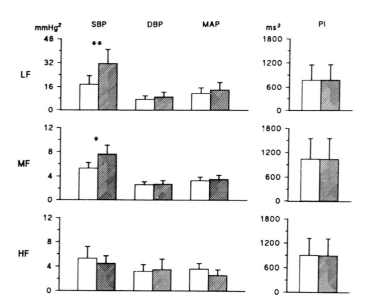

Fig. 22.19. Low-frequency (LF, upper panels), mid-frequency (MF, mid panels) and high-frequency (HF, lower panels) power spectral densities of systolic blood pressure (SBP), diastolic blood pressure (DBP), mean arterial pressure (MAP), and pulse interval (PI) obtained intra-arterially (open bars) and by Finapres (striped bars). Data are shown as average values ± SE for 14 subjects. Asterisks refer to statistical significance of the between-method differences **, p < 0.01; *, p < 0.05. For further details, see text. (From Omboni *et al.* (1993), with permission.)

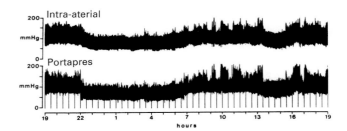

Fig. 22.20. Original tracing of a 24-hour intra-arterial blood pressure recording (Oxford technique, upper panel) and a beat-to-beat finger blood pressure recording (Portapres, lower panel) obtained simultaneously in an ambulant subjects. Vertical lines refer to between-finger shift of Portapres measurement every 30 minutes.

recordings are used to assess spontaneous baroreflex sensitivity non-invasively through the sequence technique, the number of sequences and their slope can be superimposed onto the data derived from analysis of intra-arterial recordings (Omboni *et al.* 1993)

Similar analyses were carried out on non-invasive and intra-arterial 24 h ambulatory blood pressure recordings obtained simultaneously through a Portapres (the portable version of the Finapres device) (Langewouters *et al.* 1990) and an Oxford recorder. The Portapres device is equipped with two finger cuffs, and shifts automatically from one to the other at pre-set time intervals, with a hydrostatic height correction system, that previously was shown to reproduce simultaneous ambulatory intra-arterial blood pressure recordings satisfactorily (Imholz *et al.* 1993) (Fig. 22.20). The results obtained in 20 subjects by quantifying non-invasive and intra-arterial 24 h blood pressure variability have largely confirmed the data obtained in resting conditions, i.e. that pulse interval, diastolic and mean blood pressure powers are similar when derived from finger and intra-arterial signals, while systolic blood pressure powers, in particular very low frequency (with periods up to a few hours) and LF powers, are overestimated by finger blood pressure recordings. The overestimation appears to be relatively constant with time and does not seem to prevent reliable tracking of changes in blood-pressure variability in different clinical and experimental conditions (Omboni *et al.* 1998).

Data from patients with autonomic failure

In patients with orthostatic hypotension due to primary or secondary autonomic failure (Omboni *et al.* 1995) the combined use of beat-to-beat finger blood pressure monitoring (Parati *et al.* 1989; Omboni *et al.* 1993) and computerized assessment of baroreflex sensitivity (Robbe *et al.* 1987; Bertinieri *et al.* 1988; Pagani *et al.* 1988; Parati *et al.* 1988b, 1992b, 1994, 1995b, c) also helps in the determination of the autonomic dysfunction. This can be done in the laboratory, during controlled conditions and standardized activities, and over 24 h, during the dynamic conditions of daily-life, using the Portapres device (Langewouters *et al.* 1990; Imholz *et al.* 1993; Omboni *et al.* 1995) (see Chapter 21).

An example of the usefulness of finger blood pressure monitoring in evaluating autonomic failure is provided in Fig. 22.21, which shows beat-to-beat finger blood pressure and heart rate in a young normal subject and in a patient with orthostatic hypotension. The patient had a marked fall in blood pressure, with presyncopal symptoms, and a small heart rate change during standing, in contrast with the young subject who maintained his blood pressure with a normal heart rate increase during standing. Autonomic tests (Valsalva manoeuvre, forced respiratory sinus arrhythmia, and handgrip exercise) confirmed that the patient had cardiac vagal and sympathetic vasomotor denervation. Use of spectral analysis and sequence analysis indicated minimal baroreflex sensitivity in the patient as compared to the normal subject not only during supine rest (1 ms/mmHg versus 15 ms/mmHg) but also during active standing (1 ms/mmHg versus 14 ms/mmHg). The percentage of coherent segments between blood pressure and heart rate powers was similarly reduced in a striking fashion, i.e. it was 7 per cent in the supine and 4 per cent in the standing position in the patient, as compared to 86 per cent in the supine and 79 per cent in the standing position in the normal subject. The sequence analysis showed very few sequences in the dysautonomic patient (none in the supine position and two during standing) as compared to the normal subject (three in the supine position and 19 during standing). Thus, although an alteration of neural cardiovascular control was evident using traditional tests, this was complemented by the computerized assessment of baroreflex sensitivity that was able to quantify the striking impairment of 'spontaneous' reflex cardiac control.

The usefulness of computer analysis of blood pressure and heart rate variability in assessing autonomic dysfunction is further emphasized by the data obtained in 10 patients with orthostatic hypotension due to pure autonomic failure, in whom 24 h beat-to-beat finger blood pressure recordings were performed by Portapres. As previously observed by intra-arterial recordings (Tulen *et al.* 1991), their 24 h blood pressure variability is greater, while pulse interval variability is less, when compared to normal subjects (Omboni *et al.* 1996). Night sleep was associated either with a small blood pressure reduction, no blood pressure reduction, or in some instances even a reversal of the circadian blood pressure profile. In patients with autonomic failure, the sensitivity of the baroreflex, as assessed by the sequence slope and the alpha coefficient, was strikingly lower than in control subjects throughout the 24 h, with a loss of its day–night modulation. The percentage of segments with a high coherence was

smaller in patients with autonomic failure than in control subjects, indicating a reduced ability of the baroreflex to couple pulse interval with systolic blood pressure changes. An example of these alterations in a representative patient as compared to a healthy control, is provided (Fig. 22.22).

Concluding remarks

The data reviewed suggest that analysis of blood pressure and heart rate variability provides insight into cardiovascular regulation that cannot be obtained by traditional analysis of stepwise changes in mean blood pressure and heart rate, when induced by external stimuli. Furthermore, these approaches can be used in daily life and with techniques that allow non-invasive beat-to-beat blood pressure recordings. However, cautious interpretation of result is needed, especially for clinical application, and particularly when dealing with fluctuations in a single cardiovascular signal obtained in uncontrolled conditions, when no information on respiratory activity is available. Multivariate analysis techniques, such as the joint quantification of blood pressure and heart rate fluctuations, may provide more reliable information. Studies in autonomic failure suggest that these methods

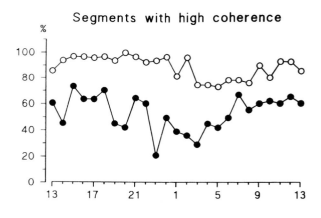

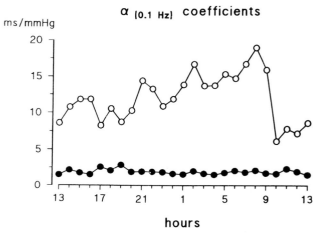

Fig. 22.22. Frequency of segments with high coherence (top panel) and their corresponding alpha coefficient values (bottom panel) in one young healthy subject (○) and in one patient with pure autonomic failure (●). Data are shown as hourly average values. (From Omboni *et al.* (1996), permission.)

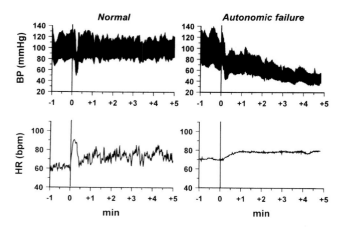

Fig. 22.21. Original beat-to-beat finger blood pressure (upper panels) and heart rate (lower panels) tracing obtained by Finapres in a young normal subject (left panels) and in a patient with autonomic failure (right panels) during supine rest and active standing.

may be complementary to, and sometimes even more sensitive and specific than, traditional laboratory tests. However, the clinical impact of these methods in the diagnostic and prognostic evaluation of patients with autonomic failure needs to be tested in longitudinal controlled studies.

References

Bernardi, L. F., Keller, M., Sanders, M., Reddy, P. S., Meno F., and Pinsky, M. R. (1989). Respiratory sinus arrhythmia in the denervated human heart. *J. Appl. Physiol.* **67**, 1447–55.

Bertinieri, G., Di Rienzo, G., Cavallazzi, A., Ferrari, A. U., Pedotti, A., and Mancia, G. (1988). Evaluation of baroreceptor reflex by blood pressure monitoring in unanesthetized cats. *Am. J. Physiol.* **254**, H377–H383.

Castiglioni, P., Daffonchio, A., Ferrari, A. U., Mancia, G., Pedotti, A., and Di Rienzo, M. (1993). Blood pressure and heart rate variability in conscious rats before and after autonomic blockade: evaluation by wide band spectral analysis. *Proc. Computers in Cardiology 1993*, pp. 487–90. IEEE Computer Society Press, Los Alamitos.

Cerutti, C., Gustin, M. P., Paultre, C. Z. *et al.* (1991). Autonomic nervous system and cardiovascular variability in rats: a spectral analysis approach. *Am. J. Physiol.* **261**, H1292–H1299.

Cowley, A. W., Liard, L. F., and Guyton, A. C. (1973). Role of the baroreceptor reflex in daily control of arterial blood pressure and other variables in dogs. *Circ. Res.* **32**, 564–76.

Daffonchio, A., Franzelli, C., Di Rienzo, M. *et al.* (1991). Effects of sympathectomy on blood pressure variability in the conscious rat. *J. Hypertension* **9** (Suppl. 6), S70–S71.

De Boer, R. W., Karemaker, J. M., and Strackee, J. (1987). Haemodynamic fluctuation baroreflex sensitivity in humans: a beat-to-beat model. *Am. J. Physiol.* **253**, (*Heart Circ. Physiol.* **22**), H680–H689.

Di Rienzo, M., Parati, G., Castiglioni, P. *et al.* (1991). Role of sinoaortic afferents in modulating BP and pulse interval spectral analysis in unanesthetized cats. *Am. J. Physiol.* **261**, H1811–H1818.

Di Rienzo, M., Castiglioni, P., Ramirez, A. J., Mancia, G., and Pedotti, A. (1992). Sequential spectral analysis of blood pressure and heart rate in humans and animals. In *Blood pressure and heart rate variability*, (ed. M. Di Rienzo, G. Mancia, G. Parati, A. Pedotti, and A. Zanchetti), pp. 24–38. IOS, Amsterdam.

Di Rienzo, M., Castiglioni, P., Parati, G., Mancia, G., and Pedorri, A. (1996). Effects of sino-aortic denervation on spectral characteristic of blood pressure and pulse interval variability: a wide-band approach. *Med. Biol. Eng. Comput.* **34**, 133–41.

Elbert, T., Ray, W. J., Kowalik, Z. J., Skinner, J. E., Graf, K. E., and Birbaumer, N. (1994). Chaos and physiology: deterministic chaos in excitable cell assemblies. *Physiol. Rev.* **74**, 1–40.

Frattola, A., Parati, G., Gamba, P. *et al.* (1997). Time and frequency domain estimates of spontaneous baroreflex sensitivity provide early detection of autonomic dysfunction in diabetes mellitus. *Diabetologia* **40**, 1470–5.

Freed, L. A., Stein, K. M., Gordon, M., Urban, M., and Kligfield, P. (1994). Reproducibility of power spectral measures of heart rate variability obtained from short-term sampling periods. *Am. J. Cardiol.* **74**, 972–3.

Imholz, B. P. M., Langewouters, G. J., and Van Montfrans, G. A. *et al.* (1993) Feasibility of ambulatory, 24-hour-continuous, finger arterial recording. *Hypertension* **21**, 65–73.

Kingwell, B. A., Thompson, J. M., McPerson, G. A., Kaye, D., Jennings, G. L., and Esler, M. D. (1995). Comparison of heart rate spectral analysis with cardiac noradrenaline spillover and muscle sympathetic nerve activity in human subjects. In *Computer analysis of cardiovascular signals*, (ed. M. Di Rienzo, G. Mancia, G. Parati, A. Pedotti, and A. Zanchetti), pp. 167–76. IOS Press, Amsterdam.

Langewouters, G. J., De Witt, B., Van Der Hoeven, G. M. A. *et al.* (1990). Feasibility of continuous non invasive 24 h ambulatory measurements of finger arterial blood pressure with Portapres. *J. Hypertension* **8** (Suppl. 3), S88.

Ludbrook, J., Mancia, G., Ferrari, A., and Zanchetti, A. (1977). The variable neck chamber method for studying the carotid baroreflex in man. *Clin. Sci. Mol. Med.* **53**, 165–71.

Malliani, A., Pagani, M., Lombardi, F., and Cerutti, S. (1991). Cardiovascular neural regulation explored in the frequency domain. *Circulation*, **84**, 482–92.

Mancia, G. and Mark, A. L. (1983). Arterial baroreflexes in humans. In Shepherd J. T., Abboud F. M. (Eds), *Handbook of physiology*, Sect 2, *The cardiovascular system IV*, Vol 3. *Peripheral circulation and organ blood flow*, (ed. J. T. Shepherd and F. M. Abboud), Part 2, pp. 755–94. American Physiological Society, Bethesda, MD.

Mancia, G., Ferrari, A., Gregorini, L., *et al.* (1983). Blood pressure and heart rate variabilities in normotensive and hypertensive human beings. Circ. Res. **53**, 96–104.

Mancia, G., Parati, G., Pomidossi, G., Casadei, R., Di Rienzo, M., and Zanchetti, A. (1986). Arterial baroreflex and blood pressure and heart rate variabilities in humans. *Hypertension* **8**, 147–53.

Mancia, G., Grassi, G., and Giannattasio, C. (1988). Cardiopulmonary receptor reflex in hypertension. *Am. J. Hypertens.* **1**, 249–55.

Mancia, G., Grassi, G., Parati, G., and Daffonchio, A. (1993). Evaluating sympathetic activity in human hypertension. *J. Hypertension* **11**, (Suppl. 5), S13–S19.

Mancia, G., Parati, G., Di Rienzo, M., and Zanchetti, A. (1997*a*). Blood pressure variability. In *Handbook of hypertension*, (ed. A. Zanchetti and G. Mancia) Vol. 17, pp. 117–69. Elsevier Science.

Mancia, G., Groppelli, A., Di Rienzo, M., Castiglioni, P., and Parati, G. (1997*b*). Smoking impairs baroreflex sensitivity in humans. *Am. J. Physiol.* **273**, (Heart Circ Physiol. **42**), H1555–H1560.

Omboni, S., Parati, G., Frattola, A. *et al.* (1993). Spectral and sequence analysis of finger blood pressure variability: Comparison with analysis of intra-arterial recordings. *Hypertension* **22**, 22–6.

Omboni, S., Smit, A. A. J., and Wieling, W. (1995). Twenty four hour continuous non-invasive finger blood pressure monitoring: a novel approach to the evaluation of treatment in patients with autonomic failure. *Br. Heart J.* **73**, 290–2.

Omboni, S., Parati, G., Di Rienzo, M., Wieling, W., and Mancia G. (1996). Blood pressure and heart rate variability in autonomic disorders: a critical review. *Clin. Auton. Res.* **6**, 171–82.

Omboni, S., Parati, G., Castiglioni, P., and Di Rienzo, M. *et al.* (1998). Estimation of blood pressure variability from 24 hour ambulatory finger blood pressure. *Hypertension* **32**, 52–8.

Pagani, M., Somers, V., Furlan, R. *et al.* (1988). Changes in autonomic regulation induced by physical training in mild hypertension. *Hypertension* **12**, 600–10.

Parati, G., Pomidossi, G., Ramirez, A. J., Cesana, B., and Mancia, G. (1985). Variability of the haemodynamic responses to laboratory test employed in assessment of neural cardiovascular regulation in man. *Clin. Sci.* **69**, 533–40.

Parati, G., Pomidossi, G., Casadei, R. *et al.* (1987). Role of heart rate variability in the production of blood pressure variability in man. *J. Hypertension* **5**, 557–60.

Parati, G., Pomidossi, G., Casadei, R., *et al.* (1988*a*). Comparison of the cardiovascular effects of different laboratory stressors in their relationship with blood pressure variability. *J. Hypertension* **6**, 481–8.

Parati, G., Di Rienzo, M., Bertinieri, G. *et al.* (1988*b*). Evaluation of the baroreceptor-heart rate reflex by 24-hour intra-arterial blood pressure monitoring in humans. *Hypertension* 12, 214–22.

Parati, G., Casadei, R., Groppelli, A., Di Rienzo, M., and Mancia, G. (1989). Comparison of finger and intra-arterial blood pressure monitoring at rest and during laboratory testing. *Hypertension* 13, 647–655.

Parati, G., Castiglioni, P., Di Rienzo, M., Omboni, S., Pedotti, A., and Mancia, G. (1990) Sequential spectral analysis of 24-hour blood pressure and pulse interval in humans. *Hypertension* 16, 414–21.

Parati, G., Mutti, E., Omboni, S., and Mancia, G. (1992*a*). How to deal with blood pressure variability. In *Ambulatory blood pressure recording*, (ed. H. Brunner and B. Waeber), pp. 71–99. Raven Press, New York.

Parati, G., Omboni, S., Frattola, A., Di Rienzo, M., Zanchetti, A., and Mancia, G. (1992*b*). Dynamic evaluation of the baroreflex in ambulant subjects. In *Blood Pressure and Heart rate Variability*, (ed. M. Di Rienzo, G. Mancia, G. Parati, A. Pedotti, and A. Zanchetti), pp. 123–37. IOS Press, Amsterdam.

Parati, G., Mutti, E., Frattola, A., Castiglioni, P., Di Rienzo, M., and Mancia, G. (1994). Beta-adrenergic blocking treatment and 24-hour baroreflex sensitivity in essential hypertensive patients. *Hypertension* 23, 992–6.

Parati, G., Saul, J. P., Di Rienzo, M., and Mancia, G. (1995*a*). Spectral analysis of blood pressure and heart rate variability in evaluating cardiovascular regulation. A critical appraisal. *Hypertension* 25, 1276–86.

Parati, G., Di Rienzo, M., Castiglioni, P. *et al.* (1995*b*). Daily life baroreflex modulation: new perspectives from computer analysis of cardiovascular signals. In *Computer analysis of cardiovascular signals*, (ed. M. Di Rienzo, G. Mancia, G. Parati, A. Pedotti, and A. Zanchetti), pp. 209–18. IOS Press, Amsterdam.

Parati, G., Frattola, A., Di Rienzo, M., Castiglioni, P., Pedotti, A., and Mancia, G. (1995*c*). Effects of aging on 24 h dynamic baroreceptor control of heart rate in ambulant subjects. *Am. J. Physiol.* 268, H1606–H1612.

Parati, G., Frattola, A., Di Rienzo, M., Castiglioni, P., and Mancia, G. (1997). Broad band spectral analysis of blood pressure and heart rate variability in very elderly subjects. *Hypertension* 30, 803–8.

Patton, D. J., Triedman, J. K., Perrott, M., Vidian, A. A., and Saul, P. (1996*b*). Baroreflex gain: characterization using autoregressive moving average analysis. *Am. J. Physiol.* 270, (Heart Circ. Physiol. 39), H1240–H1249.

Ramirez, A. J., Bertinieri, G., Belli, L. *et al.* (1985). Reflex control of blood pressure and heart rate by arterial baroreceptors and by cardiopulmonary receptors in the unanesthetized rat. *J. Hypertension* 3, 327–35.

Robbe, H. W. J., Mulder, L. J. M., Ruddel, H., Langewitz, W. A., Veldman, J. B. P., and Mulder, G. (1987). Assessment of baroreceptor reflex sensitivity by means of spectral analysis. *Hypertension* 10, 538–43.

Saul, J. P., Rea, R. F., Eckberg, D. L., Berger, R. D., and Cohen, R. J. (1990). Heart rate and muscle sympathetic nerve variability during reflex changes of autonomic activity. *Am. J. Physiol.* 258, H713–H721.

Saul, J. P., Berger, R. D., Albrecht, P., Stein, S. P., Chen, M. H., and Cohen, R. J. (1991). Transfer function analysis of the circulation: unique insight into cardiovasscular regulation. *Am. J. Physiol.* 261, H1231–H1245.

Tulen, J. H. M., Man in 't Veld, A. J., van Steenis, H. G., and Mechelse, K. (1991). Sleep patterns and blood pressure variability in patients with pure autonomic failure. *Clin. Auton. Res.* 1, 309–5.

Wesseling, K. H. and Settels, J. J. (1985) Baromodulation explains short-term blood pressure variability. In *Psychophysiology of cardiovascular control. Models, methods and data.* (ed. T. F. Orlebeke, G. Mulder, and J. J. P. van Doochen), pp. 69–97. Plenum, New York.

23. Intraneural recordings of normal and abnormal sympathetic activity in humans

B. Gunnar Wallin

Introduction

Sympathetic neural activity is difficult to evaluate in humans. Clinically, the common method is to record sympathetic effector activities, such as heart rate, blood flow, or sweat production, and use the results to draw conclusions about the neural drive. This approach has the drawback that data are difficult to interpret because effector organs react slowly to variations in sympathetic neural drive and because they may respond also to hormonal, local chemical, and mechanical stimuli. In addition, resting sympathetic activity cannot be evaluated. By using percutaneous microelectrodes to record action potentials from postganglionic sympathetic axons in human peripheral nerves (microneurography), many of these difficulties can be circumvented. This method provides direct information about sympathetic impulse traffic to skin and muscle, both at rest and during various manoeuvres (visceral sympathetic activity and parasympathetic activity are still inaccessible). The technique is not used for routine diagnostic work (see below) but is well suited for the study of sympathetic physiology and pathophysiology. This chapter will summarize the characteristics of normal sympathetic activity to skin and muscle and abnormalities found in certain diseases. A number of drug studies have also been reported (such as the effects of general anaesthetics, e.g. Ebert and Muzi 1994) but will not be dealt with here. Specific references will be given mostly to recent work and pathophysiological findings. Other references can be found in Mano (1990) and Wallin (1994).

Methods

Most microneurographic recordings are made with monopolar tungsten microelectrodes with tip diameters of a few micrometres, but a concentric electrode type has also been described. The recording electrode is inserted manually through the skin into an underlying nerve and a reference electrode is placed subcutaneously 1–2 cm away. In most cases multi-unit activity is obtained, but single units may be recorded. Most recordings are made in the large median, radial, peroneal, or tibial nerves, but sometimes small cutaneous nerves in arm, leg, or face have been used. Human peripheral nerves contain a varying number of fascicles, each of which is surrounded by a barrier of connective tissue. Action potentials can be recorded only with the tip inside a fascicle and there is no cross-talk from neighbouring fascicles. Mixed nerves are impaled as far distally as possible in order to obtain recordings from relatively 'pure' muscle or skin nerve fascicles. During the search for a sympathetic recording site, subjects

may experience minor discomfort, but they feel nothing during the recording. In most cases there are no after-effects, but around 10 per cent of the subjects may feel skin paraesthesia or mild muscle tenderness for a few days after the recording.

For analysis, multi-unit bursts of sympathetic impulses are detected either visually or by computer. In a given electrode site the strength of activity is usually expressed as the number of bursts multiplied by their mean voltage amplitude or area. Since burst amplitude/area depends on the electrode site, only the number of bursts can be used for interindividual comparisons. For detailed descriptions of techniques and evidence for the sympathetic nature of the recorded impulses see Vallbo *et al.* (1979), Gandevia and Hales (1997).

The microelectrode can also be used for evoking action potentials by intraneural electrical stimulation. Stimulation-induced cutaneous sympathetic effector responses can be detected by monitoring blood flow, skin resistance, and/or water evaporation. Local anaesthetic blocks of the nerve proximal or distal to the stimulation site will reveal whether the effector responses are caused by reflexes or evoked directly by centrifugally conducted impulses.

Normal sympathetic activity

Functional organization of sympathetic outflow

Sympathetic impulses in human skin and muscle nerves occur spontaneously and are grouped in synchronized bursts separated by more or less complete neural silence. The average firing frequency in single sympathetic fibres is around 0.5 Hz at rest but the irregularity of firing leads to instantaneous firing rates that occasionally exceed 50 Hz. The bursting pattern has functional implications in that transmitter release may be more efficient with irregular than with regular frequencies.

At one time sympathetic reactions were thought to occur in parallel in nerves to different tissues. This view of a diffusely acting system led to the term 'sympathetic tone' to describe the strength of a presumed global level of sympathetic activity. This concept is no longer tenable: both in experimental animals and humans there are clear differences in nerve traffic between different sympathetic subdivisions, indicating that sympathetic outflows to different tissues are controlled separately. However, there is a remarkable parallelism between two neurograms when resting sympathetic activity is recorded simultaneously in different muscle nerves (or in different skin nerves innervating hands and feet). These findings suggest that there are different populations of sympathetic neurones, each of which is subjected to its own homogeneous supraspinal drive which differs from that of other populations. With some maneouvres there is still a high degree of parallelism between muscle sympathetic nerve activity (MSNA) in the arm and leg, whereas quantitative differences are induced by other stimuli. Differences have also been found between skin sympathetic nerve activity (SSNA) in the hand and forearm. Thus, the sympathetic system can be regarded as consisting of a number of subdivisions that can be activated in varying combinations and to different degrees depending on the functional demand.

Skin nerve sympathetic activity

Resting activity

Skin blood vessels and sweat glands are innervated by separate sympathetic fibres (vasomotor and sudomotor) which are intermingled and can be recorded from in the same intrafascicular site. At rest at normal room temperature, SSNA in nerves to hand and foot is dominated by irregular bursts of vasoconstrictor impulses. Sudomotor discharges may be present if the subject is tense or stressed. The conduction velocity is approximately 1.3 m/s in sudomotor and 0.8 m/s in vasoconstrictor fibres and this difference contributes to the shorter duration of sudomotor bursts. There is also evidence from microneurographic recordings suggesting that a subset of vasomotor fibres induces active vasodilatation. Since the different types of impulses cannot be separated in the neurogram, meaningful quantitation of SSNA is difficult to achieve.

Arterial baroreceptor modulation of skin vasoconstrictor impulses is weak or absent: impulse bursts are not pulse synchronous, they show no systematic correlation to spontaneous blood pressure fluctuations, they are not affected in a reproducible way by electrical stimulation of the carotid sinus nerves or temporary baroreceptor deafferentation. Surprisingly, however, both single- and multi-unit recordings show that sudomotor activity displays weak cardiac rhythmicity, presumably related to reflex influence from cardiopulmonary receptors (see below). The bursts show a respiratory rhythmicity, and a deep breath usually evokes a strong discharge containing a mixture of vasoconstrictor and sudomotor impulses. During non-REM sleep both decreased and unchanged SSNA have been reported,whereas clear increases occur in association with K-complexes and during REM sleep.

Effects of manoeuvres

The skin is important for thermoregulation and SSNA is sensitive to thermal stimuli. Body cooling selectively increases outflow of vasoconstrictor impulses, and moderate warming decreases the strength of this activity to a minimum. When body warming leads to sweating, SSNA increases due to activation of sudomotor impulses. Thus, changes of environmental temperature may activate selectively either the vasoconstrictor or the sudomotor neural system with suppression of activity in the other system. So far convincing microneurographic evidence of activation of vasodilator impulses has not been obtained during body heating.

Stimuli with emotional effects activate both vasoconstrictor and sudomotor impulses (cold sweat). Any arousal stimulus regularly evokes a single burst, whereas mental stress leads to a more long-lasting increase of activity. Arousal discharges occur after a latency of 0.5–1.0 s, depending on the recording site and the subject's height. The latency differences are related to differences in conduction time in postganglionic C fibres, and the reflex latency can be used as an indirect measure of sympathetic conduction velocity. Arousal-induced changes of electrodermal activity (skin resistance or potential) have been used as an indirect measure of the strength of SSNA. However, such data have to be interpreted with great caution, since there is no simple quantitative relationship between the number of sudomotor impulses and the size of the electrodermal response (Kunimoto et al. 1992).

There are interactions between thermoregulatory and other cutaneous vasomotor reflex effects. In the extremities of thermoneutral or warm subjects arousal, a deep breath, or mental stress causes transient activation of vasoconstrictor fibres. After cooling the same stimuli induce vasodilatation. For a deep breath it was recently found that the vasodilatation in cold subjects is due to a transient reduction of vasoconstrictor activity following the initial respiration-induced discharge (Wallin et al., 1998). The transition from vasoconstrictor to vasodilator responses occurs at a skin temperature around 28 °C in the hand and 33 °C in the foot. Thus, to avoid ambigous results in skin blood-flow studies, subjects should probably be either warm or cold rather than thermoneutral.

As mentioned above, sudomotor traffic displays weak cardiac rhythmicity. This may be due to reflex influences from low pressure- rather than arterial baroreceptors: sudomotor activity is not influenced by blood pressure changes whereas reduction of blood volume in the chest by lower body negative pressure (LBNP) at 5 or 10 mmHg (or head-up tilt) leads to a reduction of sudomotor nerve traffic (Dodt et al. 1995). Presumably, the low-pressure-receptor reflex may serve as protection against excessive loss of blood volume during profuse sweating. Conversely, low-level LBNP seems to have little effect on skin vasoconstrictor activity

Isometric handgrip has been found to increase SSNA in nerves to the forearm and the sole of the foot. The increase of activity seems to be dominated by sudomotor impulses and occurs with short latency. It is probably influenced more by central command and the thermal state of the subject than by intramuscular chemoreceptors.

Metabolic–hormonal effects: studies on the coupling between glucose metabolism and sympathetic outflow have shown that intravenous infusion of insulin or 2-deoxy-D-glucose increases sudomotor and inhibits vasoconstrictor outflow to the skin, probably due to CNS glucopenia. Oral intake of D-glucose does not change SSNA.

Muscle nerve sympathetic activity

Resting activity

Sympathetic activity in muscle nerve fascicles (MSNA) consists of bursts of vasoconstrictor impulses. The temporal pattern of activity differs from that found in skin nerves in that most bursts have similar duration and display strong cardiac rhythmicity. There is also a relationship to respiration, and bursts occur most frequently during late expiration and early inspiration. The level of activity is reduced during non-REM sleep and increases during REM sleep. In an awake individual the strength of activity at rest (expressed as bursts/100 heart beats or bursts/min) is similar in arm and leg nerves and remarkably constant in repeated recordings at intervals of 10 years or more (Fig. 23.1). There are, however, wide interindividual differences. The burst incidence increases with age, body mass index,

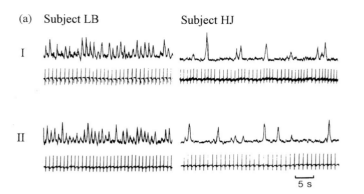

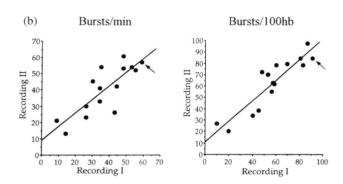

Fig. 23.1. Similarity of MSNA in repeated recordings in the same subjects. (a) Peroneal mean voltage neurograms and ECG from two subjects; interval between recordings 2 months (LB) and 3 weeks (HJ), respectively. (b) Correlation between repeated recordings of MSNA expressed as bursts/min (left, $r = 0.81$, $P < 0.001$) and bursts/100 heart beats ($r = 0.90$, $P < 0.001$) in 15 healthy subjects. Mean interval between recordings, 12 years. Arrow indicates subject LB. (a) taken with permission from Sundlöf and Wallin (1997) and (b) from Fagins and Wallin (1993).

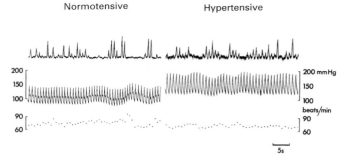

Fig. 23.2. Relationship between blood pressure and MSNA at rest in one normotensive subject and one subject with essential hypertension. Upper traces, mean voltage neurograms of MSNA; second traces, intra-arterial blood pressure; third traces, heart rate. Note inhibition of sympathetic bursts (peaks in the neurograms) with transient blood pressure and similar number of sympathetic bursts in spite of large difference in mean blood pressure levels. (Taken with permission from Wallin and Sundlöf (1979).)

and waist-to-thigh ratio, and males have higher levels than females. Genetic factors may be important for the interindividual differences since the differences in level of activity were much less for homozygotic twins than for age-matched pairs of subjects who were unrelated (Wallin *et al.* 1993).

Relationship to blood pressure: the occurrence of sympathetic bursts in muscle nerves shows an intimate relationship to spontaneous blood pressure variations. Bursts are more frequent during reductions of blood pressure and disappear when blood pressure rises (Fig. 23.2). This, and the findings that electrical stimulation of the carotid sinus nerves inhibits MSNA and that cardiac rhythmicity is eliminated by temporary baroreceptor deafferentation, show that the activity is influenced by arterial baroreflexes. This implies that bursts correspond to diastolic pressure reductions and pauses between successive bursts to systolic inhibitions. In agreement with this, a sudden fall of diastolic blood pressure in a single heart beat is regularly followed by an unusually strong sympathetic burst. In the peroneal nerve the (baroreflex) latency between pressure fall and burst is approximately 1.3 s. The delay varies depending on the strength of the burst (Wallin *et al.* 1994) but mean latency at rest is related to the subject's height and serves as an indirect measure of sympathetic conduction velocity. Variations of MSNA are related primarily to fluctuations of diastolic blood pressure

and cardiac interval, whereas other blood pressure parameters seem to be of little importance.

Although variations of MSNA are intimately coupled to *variations* of blood pressure, there is no corresponding close relationship between mean levels of MSNA and blood pressure: individual subjects may have high or low blood pressure regardless of MSNA level (Fig. 23.2). Several explanations are possible:

(1) strong vasoconstrictor activity in nerves to one vascular bed may be coupled to weak activity in nerves to other beds (sympathetic differentiation);

(2) a high total peripheral vascular resistance induced by strong nerve traffic may be balanced by a low cardiac output; and

(3) the vasoconstrictor effect of strong nerve traffic may be counteracted by a low transmitter release/impulse, by a low number/ sensitivity of vascular adrenergic receptors, or by a high level of a circulating dilating factor.

The recent finding of a positive correlation between resting MSNA and the plasma concentration of nitrate in young males (Skarphedinsson *et al.*, 1997) may indicate a coupling between sympathetic nerve traffic and the release of the endogenous vasodilator nitric oxide, which could contribute to the poor relationship between resting levels of MSNA and blood pressure.

Reflex effects on MSNA

1. *Arterial baroreceptors* have complex effects on MSNA. Dynamic stimulation of carotid baroreceptors is effective in influencing the activity, whereas static stimuli only have minor effects. In contrast, aortic baroreceptors seem to have more static effects on MSNA. This suggests that changes of MSNA evoked by changes of posture (which alters carotid but presumably not aortic arterial baroreceptor firing) are evoked to a lesser degree from arterial baroreceptors. In addition, there is evidence that the left carotid baroreceptors have a greater influence on MSNA than those on the right side (Williamson *et al.* 1996). This agrees with previous evidence of asymmetry of arterial baroreflex effects on the human heart.

2. *Cardiopulmonary baroreceptors,* which are volume receptors in the heart and the great vessels entering the heart, are stimulated by increases of central blood volume. Reduction of central blood volume increases the level of MSNA to a similar degree in arm and leg nerves. Conversely, head-out water immersion, which increases central blood volume, leads to a sustained decrease of MSNA. These findings agree with the notion that postural changes of MSNA are evoked to a large extent from cardiopulmonary baroreceptors. However, this is difficult to reconcile with the finding that a reduction of central blood volume in hearttransplanted patients still evokes a marked increase of MSNA.

3. *Systemic chemoreceptors.* Both hypoxia and hypercapnia increase MSNA, which probably contributes to the increase of MSNA seen during voluntary apnoea. The sympathoexcitatory effects of chemoreceptor stimulation are blunted, presumably from pulmonary stretch receptors, if there are simultaneous increases of ventilation. The respiratory rhythmicity of MSNA is probably a consequence of a primary central respiratory rhythm but pulmonary stretch receptors may also contribute.

4. *Intramuscular chemoreceptors.* During isometric muscle contraction MSNA recorded in a peroneal nerve (i.e. supplying non-contracting muscles) is unchanged during the first minute but increases thereafter. The effect increases with increasing muscle mass and the increase can be maintained for minutes after the end of contraction if circulation to the contracting muscles is arrested. Presumably, the response is evoked from chemoreceptors in the contracting muscles and there is a coupling between changes of intramuscular pH and increases of MSNA. In agreement with this, the increase of MSNA during handgrip contraction is reduced after endurance training of forearm muscles. Central command does not contribute significantly to the increase of MSNA until near maximal efforts. For a review on sympathetic activation during exercise see Mitchell and Victor (1996).

5. *Miscellaneous receptors.* Immersion of a hand in cold water ('cold pressor test') leads to increases of MSNA, heart rate, and blood pressure, presumably evoked from cutaneous cold and/or pain receptors. Face immersion in cold water also increases MSNA. Although evoked in part from cutaneous receptors in the face, this 'diving reflex' is more complex and differs functionally from the reflex evoked by the cold pressor test. Mechanical stimulation of receptors in the pharynx and larynx in paralysed patients under general anaesthesia causes pronounced and long-lasting sympathetic excitation, both in muscle and skin nerves. Accumulation of urine in the bladder increases MSNA, an effect which may be induced from stretch receptors in the bladder wall. Pain induced by electrical stimulation of skin nerves has little or no effect on MSNA, but pain induced by mechanical pressure of a hard object against a finger or toe nail or against bone evokes marked increases of nerve traffic (Nordin and Fagius 1995).

Mental stress

Stimuli that cause mental stress evoke complex sympathetic reactions. MSNA does not change significantly with arousal or short-lasting mental arithmetic, but with stress of longer duration MSNA increases in the peroneal nerve but remains unchanged in the radial nerve. Presumably, the arm–leg difference is of central origin. The increase of MSNA is influenced by task difficulty and the subject's emotional state. When stress was induced by delayed auditory feedback, tibial MSNA increased already during the first minute. If plasma adrenaline concentrations increase during the stress, this may also contribute to an increase of MSNA (see below).

Hormonal influence

Several hormones influence MSNA. Insulin-induced hypoglycaemia increases the activity as does infusion of 2-deoxy-D-glucose. The underlying mechanisms are complex, but central nervous effects may be important (Munzel *et al.* 1995). This is underlined by the finding that the MSNA increase induced by euglycaemic hyperinsulinaemic clamp is abolished by pretreatment with dexamethasone. Food intake (carbohydrate, protein, or fat) causes an increase of MSNA, which lasts more than 90 min (Fagius and Berne 1993). The underlying mechanism is unclear (insulin probably contributes only to a minor degree). Lack of this response may explain postprandial hypotension in autonomic failure.

MSNA increases moderately during, and markedly after, infusion of high concentrations of adrenaline; the increase after the infusion may be related to a reduced central venous pressure. A central nervous mechanism has been implied for the transient increase of MSNA following subcutaneous injections of thyrotrophin-releasing hormone. MSNA correlates negatively with serum levels of free triiodothyronine and thyroxine, and positively with thyroid-stimulating hormone. Taken together, the findings suggest an inverse relationship between thyroid function and sympathetic nerve activity.

Relationship between MSNA and transmitter release

Noradrenaline is the principal postganglionic sympathetic transmitter, and there is a positive linear correlation between the sympathetic burst incidence of MSNA at rest and the plasma concentration of noradrenaline in, and spillover to, forearm venous plasma in normotensive subjects. Also, the plasma concentration of neuropeptide Y (NPY) increases but primarily at very high levels of MSNA. Correlations between MSNA and plasma concentrations of noradrenaline have also been found in hypertensive subjects, in patients with cardiac failure, and in patients with liver cirrhosis with ascites. Several factors probably contribute to the relationships:

(1) skeletal muscle is a large tissue, responsible for 10–20 per cent of the total spillover to blood;

(2) the contribution of noradrenaline from muscle is disproportionately high in forearm venous blood;

(3) at rest, the strength of MSNA is also correlated with noradrenaline spillover in the heart and the kidney (Wallin *et al.* 1996).

On a group basis, several manoeuvres that increase MSNA, are followed by increases of forearm venous plasma noradrenaline concentration, but individual increases of MSNA and plasma concentration often show a poor correlation. Furthermore, the increase of MSNA occurring with systemic hypoxia is not associated with increased plasma noradrenaline levels. Since plasma noradrenaline concentrations are also influenced by factors other than noradrenaline spillover (e.g. plasma clearance, blood flow) the finding is not surprising.

Abnormal sympathetic activity

Theoretically, nervous lesions may result in pathological sympathetic activity which could be detected in microneurographic recordings. Unfortunately, however, there are several limitations for the diagnostic use of the method in individual patients. Obviously, the technique is inappropriate for abnormalities in peripheral fibres distal to the recording site, or in the neuroeffector junction. It is also difficult to diagnose *quantitative* abnormalities, for two main reasons. First, in normal subjects there are large interindividual differences in the strength of activity and this makes it difficult to define meaningful normal values. Secondly, since it is sometimes impossible in normal subjects to find a recording site with acceptable signal-to-noise ratio, failure to find a sympathetic site in an individual patient has no diagnostic significance. The consequence of these limitations is that microneurography is useful mainly for comparing groups of subjects but not as a diagnostic tool in individual patients. However, the technique may be used for detecting *qualitative* abnormalities in exceptional individual patients, i.e. when reflex effects are evoked from a stimulus which normally is ineffective, or if a normally excitatory response is turned into an inhibitory one, or vice versa. The following section gives examples of different types of abnormalities rather than a complete coverage of all diseases studied by microneurography.

Peripheral efferent lesions: polyneuropathy

Many cases of polyneuropathy have symptoms suggestive of autonomic involvement. In myelinated nerve fibres the conduction velocity is usually lowered, but in polyneuropathy of different aetiology sympathetic conduction velocities are normal, even if patients have autonomic symptoms (Fig. 23.3). However, failure to find sympathetic activity is increased, especially in diabetic polyneuropathy. The findings suggest that, in polyneuropathy, sympathetic conduction velocity is normal as long as the fibres conduct. With sympathetic involvement in the disease successive loss of functioning fibres causes clinical symptoms and finally disappearance of

detectable activity. If fibres on the afferent side of different reflex arcs also become affected by the disease, symptoms due to failure of conduction in postganglionic sympathetic fibres may be mixed with symptoms due to the afferent lesion.

Peripheral afferent lesions

If nerve fibres on the afferent side of a sympathetic reflex arc are damaged, different effects will arise depending on whether the reflex is excitatory or inhibitory. The following diseases involve defects in arterial and/or cardiopulmonary baroreflexes which have inhibitory effects on MSNA.

Decreased afferent activity

If afferent nerve traffic from arterial and cardiopulmonary baroreceptors should decrease, one would expect increases of sympathetic activity, heart rate, and blood pressure. This may occur in the Guillain-Barré syndrome. In three such patients MSNA still displayed cardiac rhythmicity but all patients had higher activity during the acute phase than after recovery. When recordings were repeated after clinical recovery, the incidence of sympathetic bursts was normal (Fig. 23.4). The abnormality can be explained by reduced inhibition of brainstem vasomotor centres caused by involvement of afferent baroreceptor fibres in the disease. Since cardiac rhythmicity was maintained, it is likely that mainly fibres from cardiopulmonary receptors were affected.

Paroxysmal attacks of hypertension have been described in a patient with a history of neck and mediastinal radiation who had loss of cardiac rhythmicity in MSNA but preserved MSNA responses to lower-body negative pressure. In this case selective loss of arterial baroreceptor function may explain the findings.

Increased afferent activity: syncope

Increased afferent nerve traffic from baroreceptors should be expected to inhibit sympathetic activity, decrease heart rate, and

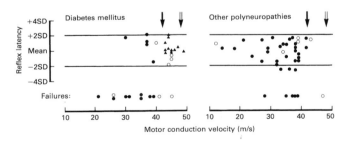

Fig. 23.3. Sympathetic reflex latencies (proportional to conduction velocity in postganglionic sympathetic fibres) expressed as standard deviations from normal and related to motor conduction velocity of the nerve recorded from in patients with polyneuropathy. The reflexes used were the arterial baroreflex (for MSNA) and an arousal reflex (for SSNA). (o and ●) patients with polyneuropathy (peroneal and median nerve, respectively) and (▲) diabetic patients without polyneuropathy, peroneal nerve. Failures, motor conduction velocity of the nerves in which no sympathetic activity could be found. The lower normal limit for motor conduction velocity in the peroneal and median nerve is indicated by filled and open arrows, respectively. SD, standard deviation. (Taken with permission from Fagius (1982).)

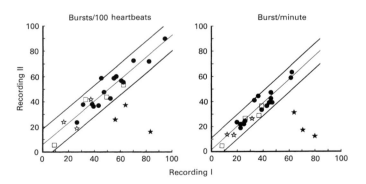

Fig. 23.4. Quantity of sympathetic bursts at two consecutive recordings of MSNA plotted against each other. ★, Guillain–Barré syndrome with tachycardia and hypertension; acute and first follow-up recording. ☆, Guillain–Barré syndrome with tachycardia and hypertension; both recordings after recovery. □, Guillain–Barré syndrome without autonomic involvement. o, Healthy subjects. Thick lines indicate 2 standard deviations (SD) from the regression line. $r = 0.94$ for both graphs. Note clear aberration of the three Guillain–Barré syndrome patients with hypertension and tachycardia at the recording during their acute illness. (Taken with permission from Fagius and Wallin (1983).)

lower blood pressure. Physiologically, this occurs as part of normal homeostatic blood pressure regulation whenever a transient blood pressure increase is buffered by baroreceptor mechanisms. If buffering reactions become exaggerated, they will cause more pronounced blood pressure falls and ultimately syncope. A syncopal reaction can probably be induced by increased activity both from arterial and cardiopulmonary receptors, and it has been suggested that activation of sympathetic vasodilator fibres also forms part of the syncopal reaction. MSNA has been recorded both during typical vasovagal syncope and in atypical long-lasting vasodepressive attacks. In all patients, sympathetic activity suddenly disappeared when syncope occurred. This does not exclude activation of vasodilator fibres but it does show that withdrawal of vasoconstrictor activity contributes importantly to muscle vasodilatation during syncope. The sympathetic withdrawal may be a reflex effect evoked by increased activity from cardiac ventricular receptors. However, since syncope with cessation of MSNA may also occur in patients without innervated ventricular receptors (after heart transplantation), vasovagal syncope is not always dependent on ventricular baroreceptor activation.

In patients with carotid sinus hypersensitivity carotid massage has been found to inhibit MSNA and reduce heart rate and blood pressure (e.g. Luck *et al.* 1996). Presumably, syncope in these patients occurs because the carotid baroreceptors are abnormally sensitive to mechanical stimuli.

In a case of glossopharyngeal neuralgia with syncope, each syncope episode was associated with cessation of MSNA. In glossopharyngeal neuralgia the patient gets short-lasting severe pain attacks in the throat evoked by chewing, swallowing, coughing, etc. Afferent sensory fibres from the throat and from carotid baroreceptors both run in the glossopharyngeal nerve. In the rare cases when syncope occurs during neuralgia there may be a pathological 'synapse' (an ephapse) in the glossopharyngeal nerve at which pain impulses are misdirected and jump over to baroreceptor fibres. Presumably, when this afferent barrage reaches brainstem vasomotor centres there is profound inhibition and fainting occurs.

Central nervous disorders

In patients with traumatic spinal-cord injury spontaneous sympathetic activity was virtually absent and, when it occurred in muscle nerve fascicles, there was no cardiac rhythmicity. Furthermore, sympathetic reflex discharges were weak and difficult to evoke; nevertheless, long-lasting pronounced blood pressure increases occurred. Thus, attacks of high blood pressure in these patients are probably not due to sympathetic hyperactivity. Pressure over the bladder and arousal-like skin stimuli (e.g. skin pinching) below the lesion gave rise to excitatory responses both in skin and muscle nerve fascicles (Fig. 23.5). Normally, such responses occur only in skin nerves; thus, the finding represents a qualitative abnormality similar to that observed after experimental baroreceptor deafferentation. A possible explanation is that normal afferent baroreceptor activity, in addition to being involved in blood pressure regulation, also serves as a powerful brake on reflex effects in MSNA from other afferent inputs; therefore, when baroreceptor inhibition is eliminated such reflexes are unmasked. This hypothesis agrees with other examples of central nervous lesions revealing patterns which normally are concealed due to inhibitory regulation, e.g. the Babinski sign and reflex grasping.

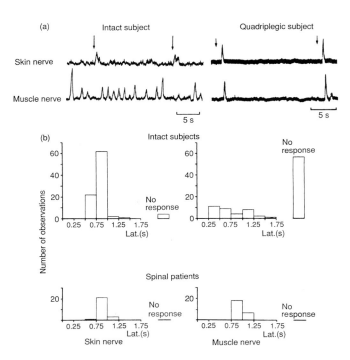

Fig. 23.5. (a) Mean voltage neurograms from simultaneous recordings in peroneal nerve fascicle to skin in the right leg and to muscle in the left leg in an intact subject (left) and a patient with complete cervical spinal-cord lesion (right). Arrows indicate electrical stimulations to the left upper thigh, inducing synchronous neural responses in skin and muscle nerve fascicles in the quadriplegic patient but responses only in the skin fascicle in the intact subject. (b) Relationship between electrical skin stimuli applied to the upper part of the thigh and sympathetic discharges in nerves to skin and muscle in five intact subjects (upper) and two patients with spinal-cord lesion (lower). Sympathetic discharges recorded simultaneously from the two peroneal nerves. In skin nerves of intact subjects, bursts were usually (85 cases, 93 per cent) recorded 0.5–1.0 s after stimuli and only in four cases (4 per cent) were there no bursts within 0.25–1.75 s after stimuli. In muscle nerves bursts were often lacking (56 cases, 61 per cent) and the bursts recorded showed no systematic relationship to the stimuli. In patients with spinal-cord lesions all stimuli evoked bursts in both skin and muscle nerves. (Data from Stjernberg *et al.* (1986).)

In a case of the Shy-Drager syndrome, oral administration of L-threo-dops markedly enhanced both a weak resting activity and the response to tilting, suggesting that in some patients with this disease a biochemical defect may contribute to the symptoms. Dopamine ß-hydroxylase deficiency provides an example of a biochemical defect causing autonomic failure in spite of normal MSNA (Rea *et al.* 1990).

In amyotrophic lateral sclerosis increased resting MSNA has been reported but the significance is unclear.

Miscellaneous conditions

Pathological sympathetic activity has been found in several cardiovascular and other diseases but the reason for the abnormality is often unknown. For some of the conditions mentioned below only a brief summary of microneurographic results are given—details are provided in special chapters.

Hypertension

To compare the strength of MSNA at rest between groups is complicated by the large interindividual variability and confounding factors such as age, sex, and body weight. With such factors taken into account, both normal (e.g. Gudbjörnsdottir *et al.* 1996) and increased (e.g. Yamada *et al.* 1989) MSNA has been found in established essential hypertension. Recent studies indicate increased MSNA in borderline hypertension, renovascular hypertension, and primary aldosteronism. Patients with accelerated hypertension were found to have higher nerve traffic than patients with benign hypertension.

Reflex abnormalities have also been demonstrated in borderline and/or essential hypertension during mental stress, apnoea during hypoxia, the cold pressor test, and lower-body negative pressure, but not with isometric handgrip. Recently, offspring of hypertensive patients and normotensive controls were found to have similar resting levels of activity but the hypertensive offspring had higher MSNA-responses to mental stress than the control group (Noll *et al.* 1996). For details on hypertension see Chapter 48.

Heart failure

Several studies have shown that moderate–severe heart failure is associated with a marked increase of MSNA (Ferguson 1993). The increase of MSNA may be preceded by an increased sympathetic outflow to the heart: cardiac noradrenaline spillover was increased in patients with mild failure who had normal MSNA and total-body noradrenaline spillover. The mechanisms underlying the increased nerve traffic are unknown but impaired baroreflex function may contribute. Cardiac glycosides reduce MSNA in heart failure (but not

in healthy subjects) and this effect may be mediated in part by arterial and/or low pressure baroreflexes. Chemoreflex activation does not seem to be involved. After cardiac transplantation an early study found that MSNA remained increased, whereas in subsequent studies this was not confirmed. In fact, in one study (Rundqvist *et al.* 1997), MSNA returned almost to normal within 1 month after transplantation (Fig. 23.6).

Others

Patients with sleep apnoea have increased resting MSNA in the awake state and marked surges of activity during apnoeic episodes during sleep. The sympatho-excitation is reduced by therapy with continous positive airway pressure. In cirrhosis of the liver MSNA was reported to be increased only if the patients had *ascites*. Also pre-eclampsia has been found to have increased MSNA which returned to normal after delivery (Schobel *et al.* 1996).

Acknowledgement

Supported by the Swedish Medical Research Council, Grant No 3546.

References

Dodt, C., Gunnarsson, T., Elam, M., Karlsson, T., and Wallin, B. G. (1995). Central blood volume influences sympathetic sudomotor nerve traffic in warm humans. *Acta Physiol. Scand.* **155**, 41–51.

Ebert, T.J. and Muzi, M. (1994). Propofol and autonomic reflex function in humans. *Anesth. Analg.* **78**, 369–75.

Fagius, J. (1982). Microneurographic findings in diabetic polyneuropathy with special reference to sympathetic activity. *Diabetologia* **23**, 415–20.

Fagius, J. and Berne, C. (1993). Increase in muscle nerve sympathetic activity in humans after food intake. *Clin. Sci.* **86**, 159–67.

Fagius, J. and Wallin, B. G. (1983). Microneurographic evidence of excessive sympathetic outflow in the Guillain–Barré syndrome. *Brain* **106**, 589–600.

Fagius, J. and Wallin, B. G. (1993). Long-term variability and reproducibility of resting human muscle nerve sympathetic activity at rest, as reassessed after a decade. *Clin. Auton. Res.* **3**, 201–5.

Ferguson, D. W. (1993). Sympathetic mechanisms in heart failure. Pathophysiological and pharmacological implications. *Circulation* **87**, (Suppl. VII), VII68–VII75.

Gandevia, S. C. and Hales, J. P. (1997). The methodology and scope of human microneurography. *J. Neurosci. Methods* **74**, 123–36.

Gudbjörnsdottir, S., Lönnroth, P., Sverrisdottir, Y. B., Wallin, B. G., and Elam, M. (1996). Sympathetic nerve activity and insulin in obese normotensive and hypertensive men. *Hypertension* **27**, 276–80.

Kunimoto, M., Kirnö, K., Elam, M., Karlsson, T., and Wallin, B. G. (1992). Non-linearity of skin resistance response to intraneural electrical stimulation of sudomotor nerves. *Acta Physiol. Scand.* **146**, 385–92.

Luck, J. C., Hoover, R. J., Biederman, R. W., Ettinger, S. M., Sinoway, L. I., and Leuenberger, U. A. (1996). Observations on carotid sinus hypersensitivity from direct intraneural recordings of sympathetic nerve traffic. *Am. J. Cardiol.* **77**, 1362–5.

Mano, T. (1990). Sympathetic nerve mechanisms of human adaptation to environment—findings obtained by recent microneurographic studies. *Environ. Med.* **34**, 1–35.

Mitchell, J. H. and Victor, R. G. (1996). Neural control of the cardiovascular system: insights from muscle sympathetic nerve recordings in humans. *Med. Sci. Sports Exerc.* **28**, S60–S69.

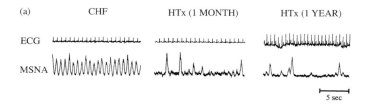

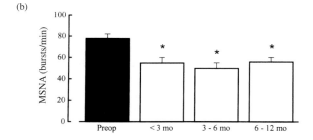

Fig. 23.6. Results of recordings of MSNA in patients with cardiac failure obtained before and at different times after heart transplantation. (a) Integrated neurograms of MSNA and heart rate from one patient recorded before (left) and 1 and 12 months after transplantation. (b) Group data on MSNA (expressed as bursts/min) in heart-failure patients pre-transplantation ($n = 21$) and at <3 ($n = 21$), 3–6 ($n = 18$), and 6–12 ($n = 13$) months post-transplantation. * indicates $p < 0.05$ versus values pre-transplantation. (Data from Rundqvist *et al.* (1997).)

Munzel, M. S., Anderson, E. A., Johnson, A. K., and Mark, A. L. (1995). Mechanisms of insulin action of sympathetic nerve activity. *Clin. Exp. Hypertens.* 17, (1 and 2), 39–50.

Noll, G., Wenzel, R. R., Schneider, M. *et al.* (1996). Increased activation of sympathetic nervous system and endothelin by mental stress in normotensive offspring of hypertensive parents. *Circulation* 93, 866–9.

Nordin, M. and Fagius, J. (1995). Effect of noxious stimulation on sympathetic vasoconstrictor outflow to human muscles. *J. Physiol. (Lond.)* 423, 241–55.

Rea, R. F., Biaggioni, I., Robertson, R. M., Haile, V., and Robertson, D. (1990). Reflex control of sympathetic nerve activity in dopamine β-hydroxylase deficiency. *Hypertension* 15, 107–12.

Rundqvist, B., Casale, R., Sverrisdottir, Y., Friberg, P., Mortara, A., and Elam, M. (1997). Rapid fall in sympathetic nerve hyperactivity in patients with cardiac failure after cardiac transplantation. *J. Cardiac Failure* 3, 21–6.

Schobel, H. P., Fischer, T., Heuszer, K., Geiger, H., and Schmieder, R. E. (1996). Preeclampsia—a state of sympathetic overactivity. *New Engl. J. Med.* 335, 1480–5.

Skarphedinsson, J. O., Elam, M., Jungersten, L., and Wallin, B. G. (1997). Sympathetic nerve traffic correlates to release of nitric oxide in humans: implications for blood pressure control. *J. Physiol. (Lond.)* 501, 671–5.

Stjernberg, L., Blumberg, H., and Wallin, B. G. (1986). Sympathetic activity in man after spinal cord injury. Outflow to muscle below the lesion. *Brain* 109, 695–715.

Sundlöf, G. and Wallin, B. G. (1977). The variability of muscle nerve sympathetic activity in resting recumbent man. *J. Physiol (Lond.)* 272, 383–97.

Vallbo, Å. B., Hagbarth, K.-E., Torebjörk, H. E., and Wallin, B. G. (1979). Somatosensory, proprioceptive and sympathetic activity in human peripheral nerves. *Physiol. Rev.* 59, 919–57.

Wallin, B. G. (1994). Assement of sympathetic mechanisms from recordings of postganglionic efferent nerve traffic. In Cardiovascular reflex control in health and disease, (ed. R. Hainsworth and A. L. Mark), pp. 65–93 Saunders, London.

Wallin, B. G. and Sundlöf, G. (1979). A quantitative study of muscle nerve sympathetic activity in resting normotensive and hypertensive subjects. *Hypertension* 1, 67–77.

Wallin, B. G., Kunimoto, M., and Sellgren, J. (1993). Possible genetic influence on the strength of human muscle nerve sympathetic activity at rest. *Hypertension* 22, 282–4.

Wallin, B. G., Burke, D., and Gandevia, S. (1994). Coupling between variations in strength and baroflex latency of sympathetic discharges in human mucle nerves. *J. Physiol. (Lond.)* 474, 331–8.

Wallin, B. G., Thompson, J. M., Jennings, G. L., and Esler, M. D. (1996). Renal noradrenaline spillover correlates with muscle sympathetic activity in humans. *J. Physiol. (Lond.)* 491, 881–7.

Wallin, B. G., Båtelsson, K., Kienbaum, P., Karlsson, T., Gazelius, B., and Elam, M. (1998). Two neural mechanisms for respiration-induced cutaneous vasodilatation in humans. *J. Physiol. (Lond.)* In press.

Williamson, J. W., Muzi, M., and Ebert, T. J. (1996). Unilateral carotid sinus stimulation and muscle sympathetic nerve activity in man. *Med. Sci. Sports Exerc.* 28, 815–21.

Yamada, Y., Miyajima, E., Tochikubo, O., Matsukawa, T., and Ishii, M. (1989). Age-related changes in muscle sympathetic nerve activity in essential hypertension. *Hypertension* 13, 870–7.

24. Neuropharmacological investigation of autonomic failure

Ronald J. Polinsky

Introduction

Autonomic nervous system testing has evolved over the past 25 years in conjunction with advances in analytical capability in the laboratory. Development of sensitive specific assays for measuring neurotransmitters and neuropeptides in various biological fluids has fostered a new era in clinical neuroscience. It is now feasible to carry out investigations in man that parallel studies in experimental animals. Neuropharmacological assessment of autonomic function has a distinct advantage over the physiological approach. Although both strategies yield useful information that help to localize lesions, the pharmacological characteristics of the disorder often provide a rational foundation for treatment.

The contrast between two distinct disorders, pure autonomic failure (PAF) and multiple system atrophy (MSA), illustrates the value of a neuropharmacological approach. Despite similar clinical manifestations of autonomic failure the underlying lesions have different characteristics in these two syndromes. Application of the various tests listed in Table 24.1 has substantially increased our

understanding of PAF and MSA. Abnormal functioning of the nervous system and related control mechanisms contributes to the pathophysiology in these disorders.

Much work in this area has been directed towards postural hypotension, the most disabling aspect of autonomic failure. Consequently, postganglionic noradrenergic neuronal function is a major focus of research efforts since this unit is the primary link between the nervous system and blood pressure control. Several neurological and neuroendocrine mechanisms participate in the regulation of other vital functions under automatic control. This chapter summarizes the neuropharmacological approach to evaluating the autonomic nervous system. A discussion of neurotransmitter and neuropeptide function in patients with autonomic failure emphasizes the distinction between peripheral and central disorders.

Peripheral mechanisms

Relatively simple, non-invasive access to the appropriate biological compartments facilitates evaluation of the peripheral components of autonomic control. In addition, the peripheral origins of neurotransmitters and their metabolites in plasma and urine have been more clearly defined in comparison with central nervous system contributions.

Sympathetic noradrenergic neuronal function

Noradrenaline is the primary neurotransmitter released from most postganglionic sympathetic neurones. Several aspects of sympathetic neuronal function provide the basis for characterizing abnormalities in autonomic failure: synthesis, storage, release, uptake, and metabolism. The general approach for evaluating these functional characteristics involves measurement of noradrenaline and metabolite levels in plasma and urine under baseline conditions and after application of various physiological and pharmacological stimuli.

Plasma noradrenaline

Following release of noradrenaline into the synaptic cleft in response to nerve impulses, a small amount (approximately 10 per cent) reaches the plasma. This 'spillover' of noradrenaline provides a biochemical window to view sympathetic nerve activity. Great care must be observed in obtaining and handling blood samples for plasma noradrenaline measurement. The levels in blood change very rapidly and are extremely responsive to external and internal stimuli. The age

Table 24.1. Neuropharmacological approaches for investigating autonomic failure

Target	Strategy
Postganglionic sympathetic neurone	Plasma NA at rest and in response to stimuli
	NA metabolites in plasma, urine Clearance of NA Pressor responsivity
Peripheral parasympathetic function	Pancreatic polypeptide response to hypoglycaemia Basal gastrin levels
Adrenal medullary activity	Plasma A responses to hypoglycaemia, cholinergic stimulation
Sympathetic ganglia	Plasma NA responses to acetylcholine
CNS pathways	Cardiovascular responses to various drugs PET scanning Neurotransmitters, metabolites, enzymes, peptides in CSF Plasma and/or urinary levels of hormones, peptides, metabolites following activation

NA, noradrenaline; A, adrenaline.

of the subject and site of sampling also affect plasma noradrenaline. Despite these limitations, the neurotransmitter levels in plasma can be used as an index of sympathetic function as long as the experimental protocol and methods for analysis are rigorously controlled and standardized. Plasma noradrenaline levels correlate with electrophysiological measurements of muscle sympathetic nerve activity in man (Wallin *et al.* 1981).

Plasma noradrenaline levels in PAF and MSA reflect distinct pathophysiological consequences of autonomic failure in the two disorders. MSA patients generally have normal (150–300 pg/ml) or slightly elevated supine plasma noradrenaline levels. Occasional patients manifest low levels (less than 100 pg/ml), suggestive of peripheral involvement. Although direct recording of sympathetic nerve activity in a single patient with MSA reveals evidence of preganglionic dysfunction (Dotson *et al.* 1990), electromyographic studies have demonstrated denervation changes in selected muscle groups. Cohen *et al.* (1987) identified somatic neuropathy in approximately 20 per cent of their MSA patients. In contrast to MSA, the basal supine plasma noradrenaline levels in PAF are lower than normal. The only group of PAF patients reported to have nearly normal noradrenaline levels also manifested significantly decreased clearance which could elevate the plasma level (Esler *et al.* 1980). This aspect of sympathetic neuronal function will be discussed later in the chapter.

Most studies confirm the above difference in supine plasma noradrenaline levels; however, the diagnostic value of this neurochemical measure is limited by substantial overlap among normal, MSA, and PAF groups. In the author's experience, only 4 per cent of patients with MSA have a plasma level less than 100 pg/ml. In contrast, approximately 20 per cent of PAF patients manifest levels greater than 100 pg/ml. Thus, a normal plasma noradrenaline level supports the clinical diagnosis of MSA. However, a low value has much greater significance in establishing the diagnosis of PAF, especially if observed early in the course of the disease.

It must be emphasized that this index of sympathetic activity should be used in conjunction with the results of other investigative procedures. A single value for plasma noradrenaline is analogous to an individual frame of a moving picture. Although it bears a relationship to the preceding and subsequent frames, an isolated shot contributes little to understanding the entire sequence. Consider the example of measuring plasma noradrenaline after a venepuncture: the level rises dramatically following needle insertion and then gradually declines to basal levels in approximately 15–20 min. Without knowledge of the basal level and time from the stimulus, measurement of noradrenaline levels could lead to different conclusions about clinical status. Postural change is a standardized stimulus that elicits an increase in sympathetic nerve activity; at least 5 min should elapse before samples are taken to assess the plasma noradrenaline response. This protocol is based on the relatively short half-life of noradrenaline in plasma; interpretation is facilitated by sampling after a steady state has been achieved. Plasma noradrenaline levels double when normal subjects stand. This increment reflects the increased sympathetic nerve activity required to maintain blood pressure despite gravity-induced pooling of blood in the lower extremities. Neither patients with MSA nor PAF manifest an adequate increase in plasma noradrenaline on standing. The implication of these observations is that both groups have lesions that prevent normal operation of the baroreflex arc. Low basal supine noradrenaline levels in PAF suggest primary

involvement of postganglionic sympathetic neurones, whereas the normal or slightly elevated levels in MSA are consistent with a more central lesion that causes failure to activate relatively intact peripheral noradrenergic neurones.

Neuronal uptake of noradrenaline

As mentioned above, plasma noradrenaline levels are affected by a variety of factors, including the processes involved with its disposition following release at the nerve ending. The neuronal uptake mechanism can be evaluated qualitatively by measuring the physiological and biochemical effects of an indirectly acting sympathomimetic drug. Such agents require: (1) an intact uptake mechanism to enter the nerve ending; and (2) adequate neuronal stores of noradrenaline. Their pharmacological effects are exerted through release of endogenous neurotransmitter. This approach is more relevant to the distinction between denervation and decentralization which will be discussed in a subsequent section. An alternative strategy, though not practical at most institutions, consists of measuring the kinetic disposition of radiolabelled catecholamines. In theory it is necessary to achieve steady-state conditions so that the various processes that determine the plasma noradrenaline concentration are at equilibrium. From a practical standpoint, tracer infusion should be maintained for at least 3 half-lives of the substance under investigation. The advantage of this method lies in the quantitative values that can be derived from equations for calculating the clearance of noradrenaline and its endogenous secretion rate into plasma. Since neuronal uptake is the primary mechanism for terminating the effects of released noradrenaline, assessment of clearance provides a useful index of sympathetic function.

Despite the importance of evaluating neuronal uptake, there have been only two studies of noradrenaline kinetics in autonomic failure (Esler *et al.* 1980; Polinsky *et al.* 1985). Although both groups found reduced noradrenaline clearance in PAF, the patients studied by Esler *et al.* (1980) had normal basal levels of the catecholamine. Uptake may have been affected out of proportion to synthesis and release so that the slower removal of noradrenaline resulted in an increase of the plasma level into the normal range. These findings highlight the need to investigate clearance. Delayed clearance could also explain the prolonged pressor effect observed following injection of sympathomimetic amines in some patients with autonomic failure. Polinsky *et al.* (1985) demonstrated a striking deficit of neuronal uptake in PAF by comparing the disappearance rates of radiolabelled noradrenaline and isoprenaline. The latter compound is only cleared through extraneuronal mechanisms; hence, its disappearance from plasma is normally much slower than that of noradrenaline. In patients with PAF, noradrenaline and isoprenaline are removed from plasma at similar rates. The very low plasma levels and clearance in these patients reflect severe involvement of postganglionic sympathetic neurones. Normal noradrenaline clearance in MSA indicates that these neurones remain functionally intact.

Noradrenaline metabolism

Another approach to evaluating sympathetic function is based on the dissociation in metabolic fate between noradrenaline taken up into sympathetic neurones and that which escapes into plasma. Intraneuronal metabolism results in the formation of deaminated metabolites following the action of monoamine oxidase on cytoplasmic noradrenaline. Neuronal uptake and leakage of vesicular noradrenaline contribute to the cytoplasmic pool of neurotransmitter. Dihydroxyphenylglycol (DHPG) results from intraneuronal noradrenaline metabolism; subsequent enzymatic reactions yield vanillylmandelic acid (VMA) and 3-methoxy,4-hydroxyphenylglycol (MHPG). Through the action of extraneuronal catechol-O-methyltransferase, normetanephrine is formed from released noradrenaline that is not taken up into sympathetic nerve endings. Conjugation protects a small portion of normetanephrine from de-amination; this conjugated normetanephrine is excreted by the kidney.

In MSA there is a disproportionate reduction in the urinary excretion of normetanephrine; total metabolites are normal or slightly decreased (Kopin *et al.* 1983*b*). This metabolite pattern is consistent with failure to activate functionally intact noradrenergic neurones since the selective decrease in normetanephrine reflects a reduction in noradrenaline release. All noradrenaline metabolites are decreased in PAF, consistent with an overall reduction in noradrenergic neurones. These results have been confirmed and extended through measurement of plasma catecholamine patterns (Fig. 24.1). The rate-limiting step in catecholamine synthesis involves tyrosine hydroxylase; thus, plasma levels of dihydroxyphenylalanine (dopa) may serve as an index of noradrenaline synthesis. Although plasma dopa levels are normal, noradrenaline and DHPG are low in PAF, as anticipated (Goldstein *et al.* 1989). A preganglionic dysfunction in MSA is supported by the observation of normal catechol levels in plasma; basal levels of dopa, noradrenaline, and DHPG confirm normal operation of synthetic and degradative pathways in sympathetic neurones. Although the number of patients is small, Goldstein *et al.* (1989) suggest that peripheral involvement may occur in MSA. The relationship between DHPG and noradrenaline in MSA patients differs from that in normal subjects; less noradrenaline may be released through exocytosis relative to the amount of noradrenaline synthesized. In one subgroup, low noradrenaline attended

by normal dopa and DHPG levels reflects a greater discrepancy between synthesis and release. Another pattern in MSA consists of normal noradrenaline and low dopa and DHPG; this is consistent with a reduction in synthesis accompanied by a compensatory increase in exocytotic release of noradrenaline.

In PAF the DHPG/noradrenaline ratio is much higher than in control subjects. Since newly synthesized noradrenaline preferentially leaks into the cytoplasm, DHPG formation continues in the absence of noradrenaline release. Two subgroups of PAF patients were identified: (1) low noradrenaline and normal dopa and DHPG; and (2) low noradrenaline and DHPG and substantially reduced dopa. The former group may have increased noradrenaline synthesis in remaining neurones as a compensatory mechanism but the high DHPG/noradrenaline ratio suggests either decreased postganglionic sympathetic activity or defective exocytotic release. In the latter group vesicular uptake might be affected. Of special importance are the findings in patients with dopamine β-hydroxylase deficiency which causes a selective disturbance in noradrenaline production (see Chapter 40). As predicted, noradrenaline and DHPG are virtually absent from plasma. However, high dopa levels suggest an attempt to increase synthesis, consistent with the increase in sympathetic nerve activity identified by microneurography. These results demonstrate the value of examining noradrenaline metabolism, which may not only facilitate the distinction between central and peripheral lesions but may elucidate intraneuronal abnormalities as well.

Noradrenergic cardiovascular responses

Pharmacological assessment of sympathetic nervous system function is based on the descriptions of supersensitivity that appeared in the literature more than a century ago. This important facet depends indirectly on the function of noradrenergic neurones since postsynaptic end-organ changes may be secondary to noradrenaline output. The ability of the baroreflex to modulate changes in cardiovascular parameters is also critical. Drugs with selective mechanisms of action test various components of the system. A non-adrenergic pressor drug, e.g. angiotensin, may be used to assess the endorgan response (vasoconstriction). Noradrenaline and isoprenaline affect cardiovascular changes through stimulation of α- and β-adrenoceptors, respectively. Tyramine causes a pressor effect through release of endogenous noradrenaline stores.

The neuropharmacological consequences of lesioning experiments in animals provide a basis for interpreting the results of pressor infusion studies in patients with autonomic failure. A postganglionic lesion (denervation) enhances the response to noradrenaline; there is also a loss of sympathetic neuronal noradrenaline stores. A more modest increase in pressor responsivity follows a preganglionic lesion; however, this change is non-specific and is not attended by a reduction in the response to indirectly acting sympathomimetics. Both types of lesions interrupt the sympathetic nervous system component of the baroreflex arc. Several principles regarding interpretation of pharmacological dose–response curves are relevant to understanding clinical investigations. Although these relationships have a sigmoidal shape when appropriately plotted on a semi-logarithmic scale, it is the linear portion that has clinical importance. Two characteristics, threshold and gain, are crucial to the distinction between denervation and decentralization. Gain is the slope of the dose–response curve and threshold is the dose at which the response begins. With respect

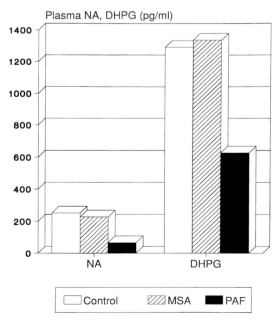

Fig. 24.1. Plasma noradrenaline (NA) and dihydroxyphenylglycol (DHPG) levels in control subjects and patients with autonomic failure.

to blood pressure–log dose relationships, gain and threshold, respectively, reflect baroreflex modulation and adrenoceptor sensitivity. Discussion of the results obtained using the pharmacological approach in patients with autonomic failure will illustrate this type of analysis.

Exaggerated cardiovascular responses to a variety of drugs have been reported in MSA and PAF. These include noradrenaline, angiotensin, isoprenaline, dopamine, tyramine, methoxamine, vasopressin, and somatostatin (and its analogues). The wide array of pharmacological agents reflects the non-specific nature of this hyperresponsivity. An increase in gain of the blood pressure–dose response curves to noradrenaline and angiotensin is manifested in patients with PAF and MSA (Fig. 24.2). The increased slope of the pressor response is consistent with a lesion in the baroreflex arc preventing normal modulation of blood pressure (Polinsky *et al.* 1981*a*). Bannister *et al.* (1979) found that the magnitude of the pressor response to noradrenaline appeared to correlate with the degree of baroreflex impairment. They also observed the greatest sensitivity to noradrenaline in a PAF patient who had a prolonged pressor effect following a bolus injection, suggesting that the mechanism of hyperresponsivity in PAF might differ from that in MSA. In contrast to MSA, the blood pressure response to intravenous noradrenaline in PAF is characterized by a shift to the left (Fig. 24.2). This leftward shift is a manifestation of true adrenoceptor supersensivity, presumably the result of a postganglionic lesion (Polinsky *et al.* 1981*a*). Chronotropic and vasodepressor responses to isoprenaline in PAF are characterized by similar evidence of β-adrenergic supersensitivity (Baser *et al.* 1991). These results further confirm the pharmacological distinction between PAF and MSA observed by Kontos *et al.* (1976). In their study, both groups decreased forearm blood flow in response to intra-arterial administration of noradrenaline, but only those with MSA responded to tyramine. Polinsky *et al.* (1981*a*) found that patients with PAF manifested a significantly smaller increment in plasma noradrenaline following intravenous bolus injections of tyramine compared to normal subjects or patients with MSA. The reduced response to an indirectly acting sympathomimetic in PAF gives additional support for the presence of a postganglionic lesion in this disorder.

In summary, pressor responsivity is increased in both PAF and MSA, but the mechanism underlying this change differs in the two disorders. Low resting plasma noradrenaline and metabolites, decreased neuronal uptake, leftward shift of the cardiovascular dose–response curves to adrenergic agonist drugs, and diminished

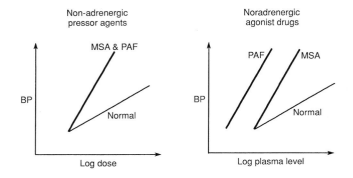

Fig. 24.2. Schematic representation of pressor responses to different drug classes in autonomic failure.

responses to tyramine provide clear evidence for postganglionic noradrenergic dysfunction in PAF. Normal indices of peripheral noradrenergic function together with a non-specific increase in pressor responsivity point to a primary involvement of the central nervous system in MSA. Thus, pharmacological investigations can be used to localize lesions within the nervous system pathways that control cardiovascular function. In addition, assessment of plasma catechol patterns shows promise for further defining abnormalities of the sympathetic nervous system.

Peripheral parasympathetic function

Neurochemical research on autonomic failure has focused on the noradrenergic nervous system because biochemical indices are available for evaluating sympathetic neuronal function. Acetylcholine, the neurotransmitter of parasympathetic neurones in the periphery, is extremely labile in plasma and attempts to measure and use it as a meaningful index, analogous to noradrenaline, have been unsuccessful. Another approach, which overcomes these limitations, is the assessment of hormonal mechanisms controlled by the parasympathetic nervous system; pancreatic polypeptide and gastrin are two examples that illustrate this strategy. Unlike true circulating hormones, these peptides are released locally through nerve stimulation and produce functional changes in nearby structures. Their levels in plasma may have little to do with physiological parameters (e.g. blood pressure, heart rate) but may serve as an index of parasympathetic activity.

Although the physiological importance of pancreatic polypeptide is unclear, it is one of several gut peptides released during insulin hypoglycaemia. Release of pancreatic polypeptide appears to be mediated through a vagal, cholinergic mechanism (see Polinsky *et al.* 1982 for references). The increase in plasma levels of pancreatic polypeptide induced by insulin is blocked by muscarinic anticholinergic drugs and truncal vagotomy. Since hypoglycaemia also elicits elevation of plasma catecholamines, insulin administration can be used to assess sympathetic and parasympathetic function simultaneously. In normal subjects hypoglycaemia is attended by a precipitous rise in plasma levels of pancreatic polypeptide. This response is virtually absent in PAF and in most patients with MSA (Fig. 24.3). Polinsky *et al.* (1982) found no correlation between catecholamine and peptide responses, consistent with their independent neural control. In the few MSA patients who manifested an increment in pancreatic polypeptide, subsequent testing revealed a loss of this response as the illness progressed. Deficient or absent pancreatic polypeptide responses provide biochemical evidence for parasympathetic involvement in PAF and MSA. Unfortunately, this test has no localizing value since the response to hypoglycaemia depends on the functional integrity of central and peripheral pathways.

Control of gastrin release is more complicated. Although vagal stimulation increases gastrin release, basal levels are increased following vagotomy. The physiological consequences of vagotomy, i.e. gastric distension and increased stomach pH, predominate in this situation. Hypoglycaemia continues to elicit a gastrin response even after highly selective vagotomy. An adrenergic mechanism appears to be involved in mediating the response during hypoglycaemia. Infusion of adrenaline releases gastrin through β-adrenergic stimulation; there is also a correlation between the gastrin increment and the plasma adrenaline response during hypoglycaemia. The pattern of

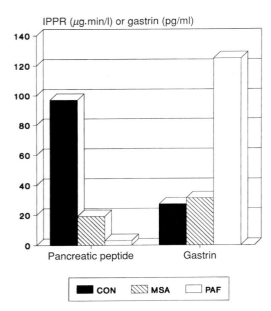

Fig. 24.3. Integrated pancreatic polypeptide response (IPPR) to hypoglycaemia and basal gastrin levels in normal controls (CON) and patients with MSA or PAF.

basal and stimulated gastrin levels differs in PAF and MSA (Polinsky *et al.* 1988*b*). High basal levels in PAF reflect peripheral parasympathetic involvement (Fig. 24.3); in fact, gastrin levels in some patients are similar to those observed in achlorhydric subjects. Gastrin responses during hypoglycaemia are respectively lower and higher than normal in MSA and PAF. As discussed earlier in this chapter, only patients with PAF have adrenoceptor supersensitivity. Thus, although both groups have deficient catecholamine responses, the effects on gastrin release differ since β-adrenergic sensitivity is normal in MSA. Infusion studies with isoprenaline confirm this pathophysiological distinction. Only patients with PAF manifest a greater than normal increase in plasma gastrin levels during isoprenaline administration. Hence, measurement of basal and isoprenaline-induced gastrin levels permits assessment of peripheral vagal and β-adrenoceptor function. The response to hypoglycaemia may give an indirect indication of the latter.

Adrenal medullary activity

In accord with its teleological function, the adrenal gland secretes adrenaline and a small amount of noradrenaline into the bloodstream in response to stressful stimuli. Although adrenaline plays a critical role during catastrophic circulatory compromise, adrenal medullary activity is more directly related to metabolic control (see Chapter 17). Catecholamines can effect an increase in various metabolic mechanisms to counter the consequences of hypoglycaemia. In this manner, adrenaline functions more like a hormone than a neurotransmitter. The primary function of this protective response is highlighted by the order in which glucose counter-regulatory hormones are secreted: adrenaline, noradrenaline, glucagon, growth hormone, and cortisol. Studies of insulin-induced hypoglycaemia as a stimulus for evaluating adrenal medullary activity began in the early part of this century. Despite the importance of this specialized ganglion, few additional

studies have been conducted since Luft and von Euler (1953) reported a lack of catecholamine excretion in response to insulin-induced hypoglycaemia in two patients with postural hypotension.

Investigation of catecholamines during insulin-induced hypoglycaemia has yielded valuable insight into the normal physiological response (Polinsky *et al.* 1980). The glucose recovery curve following the nadir of hypoglycaemia is characterized by two phases in normal subjects: an initial rapid rise precedes a slower return towards euglycaemia. The fall in blood glucose is attended by a dramatic rise in plasma adrenaline which peaks within minutes of the lowest blood sugar. This striking adrenaline response is analogous to an intravenous injection of the neurotransmitter. Its importance is exemplified by the absence of the initial rapid phase of glucose recovery in patients who lack catecholamine responses during hypoglycaemia. Fortunately, other counter-regulatory mechanisms, including glucagon, growth hormone, and cortisol, function normally in these patients (Polinsky *et al.* 1981*b*). Most patients with MSA or PAF manifest deficient catecholamine responses to hypoglycaemia because a lesion at any point in the pathway from central glucose receptors to the adrenal medulla would block the reflex. Thus, assessment of the adrenal medullary response has important clinical and therapeutic implications but cannot be used to identify the site of lesions in autonomic failure. It is possible, however, to employ a pharmacological strategy to further characterize an abnormal adrenaline response. Arecoline, a cholinergic agonist, stimulates muscarinic and nicotinic receptors. Following pretreatment with a muscarinic blocking drug, only patients with MSA increase their plasma adrenaline levels, consistent with a central lesion preventing the response to hypoglycaemia (Polinsky *et al.* 1991*a*). Primary involvement of adrenal medullary innervation probably occurs in PAF since these patients do not respond to arecoline or hypoglycaemia (Fig. 24.4).

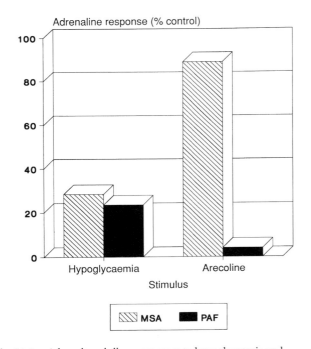

Fig. 24.4. Adrenal medullary responses to hypoglycaemia and intravenous arecoline in patients with autonomic failure.

Counter-regulatory mechanisms can be examined in the absence of catecholamine responses in patients with adrenergic insufficiency. As indicated above, their glucose recovery curves demonstrate that adrenaline is responsible for the initial rapid phase of glucose elevation in man. This is consistent with the view that adrenaline release protects against severely stressful insults until other more slowly responsive mechanisms come into play. Furthermore, these patients are able to recover from severe hypoglycaemia, indicating that adrenaline is not essential for restoring euglycaemia or eliciting other glucose counter-regulatory hormones. The noradrenaline response during hypoglycaemia may be a compensatory mechanism to counter the hypotensive effect of insulin.

Central mechanisms

Although sympathetic ganglia are anatomically located in the periphery, their synaptic function is primarily governed by cholinergic neurones whose cell bodies are in the intermediolateral cell column of the spinal cord. Thus, evaluation of ganglion function provides a natural transition from peripheral to central mechanisms.

Sympathetic ganglia

As discussed earlier in this chapter, tests of peripheral noradrenergic function in MSA reveal findings characteristic of decentralization. Furthermore, the number of intermediolateral column neurones is reduced in MSA. In order to investigate ganglionic function, Polinsky et al. (1991c) measured plasma noradrenaline responses to intravenously administered acetylcholine in patients with autonomic failure. Peripheral muscarinic effects were blocked in order to study ganglionic (nicotinic) effects of the drug. Normal subjects increase their plasma noradrenaline levels in proportion to the acetylcholine infusion rate. Lack of a noradrenaline increase in PAF is consistent with postganglionic sympathetic involvement, previously demonstrated by a variety of neurochemical and pharmacological methods. However, two distinct response patterns were evident in the MSA patients. One group did not increase their plasma noradrenaline levels while the other MSA patients manifested an exaggerated response at low doses followed by a decrease to normal levels as the infusion rate was increased. The biphasic response in the latter group suggests cholinergic supersensitivity with depolarization blockade at higher doses. Although the lack of response in the former group might indicate peripheral involvement as in PAF, extreme supersensitivity could produce blockade at even the lowest acetylcholine doses. Pharmacological demonstration of ganglionic supersensitivity further distinguishes peripheral and central lesions of the sympathetic nervous system. Although somewhat speculative, lesions more central than the intermediolateral column might not result in cholinergic ganglionic supersensitivity.

Central nervous system neurotransmitter pathways

Three general approaches have been utilized to overcome the inherent difficulties in studying central nervous system (CNS) neurotransmitter function in man: (1) neuroimaging; (2) neurochemical; and (3) neuro-endocrine. Each strategy has limitations which differ according to practical and theoretical issues. Functional neuroimaging studies are very expensive and depend critically upon access to a cyclotron, required to produce neurotransmitter precursors and ligands labelled with positron-emitting isotopes. From a theoretical standpoint it is important to verify the behaviour of these compounds. The primary advantage of this positron emission tomography (PET) application is that technological advances permit direct visualization and quantitation of regional brain function. Although less direct than the previous approach, measurement of neurotransmitter-related substances in the cerebrospinal fluid (CSF) provides an opportunity to study multiple systems simultaneously with little risk or inconvenience to the patient. However, standardized methods for collection and storage are imperative. In addition, the use of particular substances as indices of specific neuronal systems requires a thorough knowledge of their origin in CSF and the various factors that affect interpretation of the findings. The most indirect method involves the application of neuroendocrine paradigms. In some instances, it is possible to measure the levels of substances in plasma or urine. Otherwise, drugs with specific mechanisms of action must be employed to elicit hormonal/peptide responses. In this approach peripheral effects should be blocked to facilitate interpretation.

Neuroimaging studies

This strategy will only be discussed briefly since neuroimaging studies are covered in Chapter 32. Cerebral glucose metabolism is decreased in those areas primarily involved with the degenerative process in MSA; patients with PAF do not exhibit abnormal metabolism (Fulham et al. 1991). Hypometabolism within specific brain regions in MSA correlates with clinical severity: (1) reductions in the caudate/putamen with parkinsonism; (2) hypometabolism in cerebellum with cerebellar signs; and (3) decreased metabolism in thalamus, frontal, and temporal regions with autonomic dysfunction (Perani et al. 1995). Various subtypes of MSA have also been studied using the ^{18}F-2-flouro-2-deoxy-D-glucose (^{18}F-FDG) method. A comparison of the pattern of cerebral glucose metabolism among sporadic olivopontocerebellar atrophy (OPCA), dominant OPCA, and MSA suggests that sporadic OPCA may progress to MSA (Gilman et al. 1994). There appears to be a relative sparing of the brainstem and cerebellum in the striatonigral degeneration (SND; parkinsonian, MSA-P) form (Otsuka et al. 1996). Local cerebral flow measured by PET after administration of ^{15}O-H$_2$O was found to be a useful predictor of diagnosis in patients with sporadic OPCA (Gilman et al. 1995b). Unfortunately, only indirect inferences about neurotransmitter systems can be made from these results.

Although cerebral glucose metabolism has been investigated extensively over the past 15 years in various neurological disorders, PET studies of neurotransmitter systems have only been possible more recently. Bhatt et al. (1990) observed a reduction of ^{18}F-fluorodopa uptake in two patients with MSA; another patient with normal uptake manifested mild parkinsonism which had been present for only a short time. Brooks et al. (1990) applied this approach to patients with PAF and MSA. In addition to ^{18}F-fluorodopa, they used S-^{11}C-nomifensine, which binds to thalamic dopamine sites. A reduction in putaminal ^{18}F-fluorodopa uptake correlated with locomotor disability in MSA; caudate uptake was also impaired. Normal caudate function in Parkinson's disease differentiated the two disorders. It appears that the striatal abnormality was attended by a loss of nigrostriatal nerve terminals, as indicated by the reduction in nomifensine binding. A decrease in D_2 dopamine receptors in MSA has also been demonstrated using single photon emission computed tomography with ^{123}I-iodobenzamide (IBZM) (van Royen *et al.* 1993). Patients with PAF generally have normal striatonigral function. Thus, this approach not only distinguishes among patients with MSA, PAF, and Parkinson's disease but points to regional localization of lesions involving specific CNS neurotransmitters.

More recently, other PET ligands have been applied to study various neurotransmitter systems in patients with MSA. For example, Gilman *et al.* (1996) used ^{11}C-dihydrotetrabenazine, a ligand for type 2 vesicular monoamine transporter, to demonstrate decreased binding in the striatum of patients with MSA; smaller reductions in sporadic OPCA suggests that these patients also have nigrostriatal involvement. In the OPCA (cerebellar, MSA-C) variant of MSA, there is decreased opioid binding in the putamen attended by reduced uptake of ^{18}F-fluorodopa (Rinne *et al.* 1995). These results provide further evidence for subclinical nigrostriatal dysfunction in the OPCA subtype of MSA. Benzodiazepine receptor binding is preserved in the various forms of MSA (Gilman *et al.* 1995*a*).

Another imaging modality, proton magnetic resonance spectroscopy (MRS), has also been used recently to investigate brain metabolism in neurological disorders. Davie *et al.* (1995) observed a reduction in the *N*-acetyl aspartate (NAA): creatine ratio within the lentiform nucleus in the various types of MSA. This neurochemical change likely results from neuronal loss, predominantly in the putamen. In contrast, this ratio is normal in patients with Parkinson's disease. Further development and evaluation of this approach will be required to assess the full potential for its application in the investigation of degenerative disorders of the brain.

Neurochemical measurements in CSF

Despite limitations that hamper application of this approach, the levels of neurotransmitters, metabolites, and neuronal enzymes have been used to examine the functional integrity of CNS pathways. Since access is generally limited to lumbar CSF, it is important not to over-interpret the significance of abnormalities. This strategy has been most extensively employed in the investigation of monoamine systems; however, the development of sensitive, specific radio-immunoassay methods permits measurement of peptides in CSF as well.

Noradrenaline plays an important role as a central neurotransmitter in addition to its role in the periphery. Noradrenergic neurones in the locus ceruleus, one of the nuclei consistently affected by the degenerative process in MSA, innervate the hypothalamus; other fibres project to the cerebellum, hippocampus, cerebral cortex, and hypothalamus. Another pathway originates from diffuse brainstem areas to innervate the hypothalamus, limbic system, and other brainstem centres. Descending bulbospinal fibres project to preganglionic sympathetic neurones and anterior horn cells.

In man, MHPG is the predominant metabolite of noradrenaline in the central nervous system. Approximately one-third of the total MHPG in plasma is unconjugated; most of the metabolite in CSF is in the free form. Although there is a significant correlation between CSF and plasma MHPG, the levels in CSF are consistently higher than in plasma (Kopin *et al.* 1983*a*). This is true even in patients with phaeochromocytoma, a rare tumour of the adrenal medulla that secretes large amounts of catecholamines and is not under nervous system control. Since free MHPG readily crosses the blood–brain barrier, it appears that a component of CSF MHPG is derived from peripheral sources. In order to use CSF levels of MHPG as an index of central noradrenaline metabolism, a correction for the contribution from free plasma MHPG must be made. A method for estimating the central component of CSF MHPG has been derived from a kinetic model in which the plasma and CSF are considered as a two-compartment system with similar rate constants for entry into and exit from the CSF. The slope of the line relating CSF to plasma MHPG in normal subjects and patients with phaeochromocytoma gives the proportion of plasma MHPG which must be subtracted from the total CSF level since the elevation of CSF MHPG in the latter group results solely from diffusion of free MHPG from plasma into CSF. The empirically determined value for the slope, 0.9, fits well with theoretical predictions since it represents the ratio of entry and exit constants for MHPG. The constant for exit of MHPG from CSF should be slightly greater than the entry constant due to bulk flow of CSF.

Application of this strategy to patients with autonomic failure illustrates the importance of understanding the various factors required to interpret CSF neurotransmitter metabolite levels. Patients with MSA and PAF have low total CSF MHPG levels (Polinsky *et al.* 1984). As expected on the basis of their low plasma noradrenaline, patients with PAF have low levels of plasma MHPG. In contrast, plasma MHPG is normal in MSA. Thus, when the low total CSF MHPG levels are corrected for the respective plasma contributions in these two disorders, only those with MSA manifest a decrease in the component due to central nervous system noradrenaline metabolism (Fig. 24.5). Low total CSF MHPG in PAF results from the small contribution of peripheral noradrenaline metabolism. The findings in MSA are in accord with the neuropathology; several brain areas innervated by noradrenergic pathways are involved. Furthermore, Spokes *et al.* (1979) found reduced noradrenaline content in the

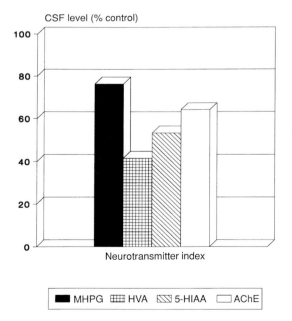

Fig. 24.5. Reduced levels of CSF neurotransmitter indices in multiple system atrophy.

locus ceruleus, hypothalamus, and septal nuclei in MSA. Although corrected CSF levels of MHPG provide clinical evidence of central noradrenergic lesions in MSA, this approach cannot be used at present to further localize the lesions. Normal central nervous system metabolism in PAF is consistent with primary postganglionic involvement demonstrated through investigations of peripheral mechanisms.

Two other brain monoamine systems have also been investigated in patients with MSA and PAF. Dopaminergic involvement is the likely cause of parkinsonism in MSA. The importance of the serotonergic system is highlighted by its regional distribution in the CNS; high concentrations parallel the pathways responsible for wakefulness and vegetative control. Brainstem serotonergic neurones with spinal cord projections make this system a likely neurochemical target for the degenerative process. The primary brain metabolites in man of dopamine and serotonin are, respectively, homovanillic acid (HVA) and 5-hydroxyindoleacetic acid (5-HIAA); both acid metabolites are removed from CSF through the same mechanism. Interpretation of their measurements in CSF is less complicated than for MHPG since there does not appear to be a contribution from the periphery. However, the collection method must be standardized because of the rostral–caudal concentration gradient. Both metabolites are reduced to approximately 50 per cent of control values in patients with MSA (Fig. 24.5; Polinsky et al. 1988a). A deficit in turnover rather than transport is supported by the observation that probenecid elevates both metabolites in MSA. Bromocriptine lowers CSF HVA in patients with MSA (Williams et al. 1979), consistent with the functional integrity of dopaminergic receptors. The increase in CSF HVA following treatment with Sinemet® suggests that some synthesis, release, and metabolism of dopamine may continue despite degeneration in the areas of dopaminergic projections (Polinsky et al. 1988a). This latter observation may explain the modest therapeutic benefit from antiparkinsonian drugs during the early and middle stages of the illness.

Polinsky et al. (1988a) noted some interesting clinical correlations among the patients with MSA in their study. Patients were subdivided according to the presence and severity of parkinsonian features. All subgroups, including those without clinical signs of parkinsonism, manifested low CSF levels of HVA. The MSA subgroup with OPCA (MSA-C) may not have exhibited clinical evidence of dopaminergic deficiency because the degree of involvement may not have reached the 80 per cent threshold estimated for appearance of symptoms in idiopathic Parkinson's disease. In addition, other brain dopamine systems unrelated to motor control might be affected since there are widespread neuropathological lesions in olivopontocerebellar atrophy. As anticipated, MSA patients with the most severe parkinsonism had the lowest CSF HVA levels. The reductions in CSF HVA in MSA are consistent with neuronal loss and decreased dopamine content in the striatum and substantia nigra. Although low CSF 5-HIAA in MSA probably reflects decreased serotonin turnover, the significance of this finding is unclear. Neurochemical studies of post-mortem brain tissue have not revealed consistent changes in serotonin content in MSA. Reductions in various brain regions have been observed, however, in Parkinson's disease. Since the rostral–caudal gradient is less than for HVA, the spinal cord may make a larger contribution to the CSF level (perhaps as much as one-third of the total). Thus, low CSF 5-HIAA in MSA may result from the well-documented neuropathological involvement in spinal

cord pathways. Similar levels of the serotonin metabolite in the various MSA subgroups adds further support to the notion that this deficit is not related to the abnormality in motor control. Normal levels of HVA and 5-HIAA in patients with PAF provide further evidence that this disorder is limited to peripheral autonomic involvement. In addition, these neurochemical results do not support an association between PAF and Parkinson's disease. The changes in MSA confirm central nervous system dysfunction in dopaminergic and serotonergic systems but this strategy does not allow a more precise definition or characterization of the areas responsible for these functional deficits.

Cholinergic function is important for the normal operation of several brain regions including the cerebral cortex, basal ganglia, hypothalamus, and brainstem nuclei. Involvement of this neurotransmitter system in MSA has been demonstrated by measuring decreases in the regional concentration of choline acetyltransferase, a marker of cholinergic neuronal integrity. Assessment of the cholinergic system in man presents a greater challenge in comparison with the monoamine systems discussed above, as there is no comparable index of central acetylcholine turnover. This neurotransmitter is extremely labile in biological fluids due to the ubiquitous presence of degradative enzymes. Efforts to measure CSF levels of choline acetyltransferase have been unsuccessful. However, acetylcholinesterase (AChE) is present in CSF and appears to be derived from a neuronal source. The enzyme may be a marker of cholinergic innervation since its activity in frontal cortex parallels that of choline acetyltransferase. Various drugs and electrical stimulation cause secretion of AChE into the spinal fluid. The rates of recovery for various molecular forms of the enzyme following irreversible inhibition support a brain-tissue source for AChE. It is important to separate AChE activity from butyrylcholinesterase although there is little activity of the latter enzyme in CSF. Polinsky et al. (1989a) found low levels of CSF AChE in patients with MSA (Fig. 24.5) but not PAF. This observation is consistent with central cholinergic involvement in MSA; since the low enzyme levels did not correlate with reduced monoamine metabolites it appears that these neurotransmitter systems are independently affected by the degenerative disorder. Dopaminergic dysfunction could contribute to the low CSF AChE in MSA since nigral neurones appear to release the enzyme. Specific localization of the lesions responsible for the decrease in CSF AChE activity would be speculative. Patients with Parkinson's disease do not have low levels of the enzyme. Thus, it would appear that extrapyramidal lesions do not contribute to the abnormality; furthermore, reduced cholinergic turnover in the basal ganglia would yield the opposite clinical effects in MSA since anticholinergic drugs improve the parkinsonian features. Cholinergic dysfunction may involve cortical, hypothalamic, brainstem, or spinal cord pathways.

Peptides may function as neurotransmitters or neuromodulators throughout the nervous system. Many gut peptides are present in the brain. In addition, pituitary peptides appear to act in other non-hormonal capacities. Autonomic pathways in the spinal cord also contain a variety of neuropeptides. Substance P was perhaps the first peptide proposed as a neurotransmitter. Its importance in the control of blood pressure is underscored by its potential role as a neurotransmitter in the baroreflex arc. It also appears to be released by unmyelinated sensory fibres in the skin. Despite their role in mediating a variety of actions, relatively few studies of CSF peptides have been conducted in patients with autonomic failure. The levels in

CSF of substance P (Nutt *et al.* 1980), somatostatin (Polinsky *et al.* 1989*b*), and corticotrophin-releasing factor (CRF) (Polinsky *et al.* 1991*b*) are low only in patients with MSA. Low levels of substance P and somatostatin are consistent with the reductions in their spinal cord concentration. However, Kwak (1985) also demonstrated markedly decreased levels of substance P in the basal ganglia. In view of the postulated role for substance P in producing the skin flare, it is interesting that histamine-induced flares are normal in patients with MSA (Anand *et al.* 1988). The CSF levels of somatostatin and CRF in MSA do not correlate with dysfunction in the other neurotransmitter systems described earlier in this section. Although Polinsky *et al.* (1989*b*) found a significant negative correlation between CSF somatostatin and a clinical rating of parkinsonism, low levels in those patients without parkinsonian features suggest that the relationship may be a reflection of disease progression. The levels of CRF are not related to clinical ratings of parkinsonism, depression, or dementia. Normal CSF peptide levels in PAF are consistent with the known pathophysiology in this disorder and indicate that autonomic dysfunction does not affect the levels of these peptides in CSF.

Recently, nitric oxide (NO) has been proposed as an important brain neurotransmitter in addition to its roles as a mediator of vasodilation and macrophage cytotoxicity. NO synthase forms NO from a pathway in which L-arginine is oxidized to citrulline. The NO degradation products nitrite and nitrate are detectable in CSF. Patients with MSA and Parkinson's disease have only decreased levels of nitrate in CSF (Kuiper *et al.* 1994), consistent with decreased production of NO in the central nervous system. This may allow more oxygen radicals to be formed, contributing to the neurodegeneration in these disorders.

Neuroendocrine strategies

The release of endocrine substances into the plasma from specific brain regions justifies their measurement to investigate pathways that mediate these responses. Various physiological and pharmacological stimuli comprise strategies to probe these central nervous system mechanisms. Several hormonal/peptide substances have been studied in patients with autonomic failure.

Although the function of melatonin in man is not known, its diurnal pattern of secretion by the pineal gland permits an indirect assessment of the central mechanisms and peripheral pathways that mediate its release. The rhythmic pattern is controlled by an endogenous circadian oscillator (perhaps the 'biological clock') located in the suprachiasmatic nucleus. Light plays a major role in modulating the diurnal cycle; the effects of environmental illumination are transmitted via retinohypothalamic pathways. A projection from the suprachiasmatic nucleus terminates in the hypothalamus. The central pathways that provide pineal innervation arise from the medial forebrain bundle and midbrain reticular formation, terminating on the cells of the intermediolateral column in the thoracic spinal cord. Preganglionic fibres innervate the superior cervical ganglion which sends ascending sympathetic nerve fibres to the pineal gland. These postganglionic neurones release increased amounts of noradrenaline at night; pineal noradrenergic receptors respond to β-adrenergic stimulation by increasing melatonin synthesis and release. Plasma melatonin is rapidly metabolized to 6-hydroxymelatonin and subsequently excreted as a conjugate through the kidney. Urinary levels of the metabolite can be used to assess pineal activity.

Normal subjects excrete most of their melatonin during the night with relatively little during the day. Distinct differences between MSA and PAF reflect the underlying pathophysiology in these disorders (Tetsuo *et al.* 1981). Although the total daily amount of 6-hydroxymelatonin is low in PAF, the diurnal pattern appears to be preserved; this finding suggests that pineal innervation may be affected. Presumably, reduced synthesis and release results from a decrease in nocturnal stimulation since postganglionic activity would be diminished in PAF. In contrast, the daytime excretion in many MSA patients was equal to or in excess of the nocturnal amount. This alteration in the pattern is consistent with disruption in central pathways which control the timing of synthesis and release. Decentralization of the pineal is further supported by the findings in patients with cord transection; a complete cervical but not a lumbar lesion alters the normal day–night pattern of melatonin excretion. Thus, investigation of this β-adrenergic sympathetically controlled substance biochemically distinguishes central and peripheral autonomic nervous system disorders.

The pituitary peptides, β-endorphin and adrenocorticotrophic hormone (ACTH), are among the many central and peripheral hormonal responses activated during hypoglycaemia. Insulin only releases these peptides if hypoglycaemia occurs. Although hypothalamic releasing factors primarily control anterior pituitary hormones, neurotransmitters also modulate their release. Arecoline, a cholinergic agonist, increases β-endorphin even after peripheral effects of the drug are blocked; atropine prevents the rise in β-endorphin during insulin hypoglycaemia. Thus, it appears that a central cholinergic pathway mediates the β-endorphin and ACTH responses to hypoglycaemia. Polinsky *et al.* (1987) found that patients with MSA but not PAF had essentially absent β-endorphin and ACTH responses to insulin-induced hypoglycaemia. This observation suggests CNS involvement, probably at the level of the hypothalamus. Normal responses in PAF would be expected on the basis of a peripheral disorder.

The abnormality in β-endorphin and ACTH indicates that at least one central cholinergic pathway is affected in MSA. In order to further examine this possibility, Polinsky *et al.* (1991*a*) administered arecoline to patients with autonomic failure. Patients with MSA and PAF failed to increase plasma ACTH in response to the drug (Fig. 24.6). This paradoxical result emphasizes the importance of considering interactions among various neurotransmitter and peptide control systems. As mentioned in the discussion of adrenal medullary function, patients with MSA but not PAF manifested an increase in plasma adrenaline following administration of arecoline. Peripheral administration of isoprenaline releases ACTH in intact rats and in those who have either pituitary stalk sectioning or lesioning of the median eminence. The effects of insulin hypoglycaemia or isoprenaline on ACTH release can be blocked by propranolol. Since adrenaline crosses the blood–brain barrier in the region of the hypothalamus, it appears that peripheral adrenergic activity may be required for cholinergic-mediated release of ACTH. Thus, PAF patients do not increase their plasma ACTH levels following arecoline because they lack the adrenaline increment. In MSA, the response is absent due to the degenerative process that is known to affect several areas with dense, cholinergic innervation including the hypothalamus. Choline acetyltransferase activity is reduced in the brains of MSA patients. Surprisingly, no evidence of central cholinergic supersensitivity was observed in relation to the

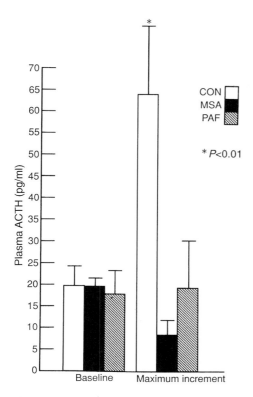

Fig. 24.6. Plasma ACTH responses to arecoline in normal subjects (CON) and patients with autonomic failure.

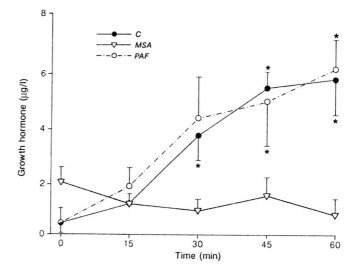

Fig. 24.7. Mean serum growth hormone concentrations before (0) and 15, 30, 45 and 60 minutes after clonidine (1.5 g/kg) in normal subjects (controls, C) and in subjects with multiple system atrophy (MSA) and pure autonomic failure (PAF). The error bars indicate ± SEM. (From Thomaides, T. *et al.* (1992)).

ACTH responses to arecoline. Degeneration may have also affected postsynaptic elements.

Growth hormone is produced by acidophil cells of the anterior pituitary and is released by stimulation of the hypothalamo-pituitary axis. Variable plasma growth hormone responses to insulin-induced hypoglycaemia in MSA have been reported. This inconsistency limits the localizing value of this approach. Normal growth hormone responses in PAF patients with adrenergic insufficiency suggest that peripheral catecholamines are not required to mediate the response to hypoglycaemia (Polinsky *et al.* 1981*b*). A pharmacological challenge with intravenous clonidine, an α_2-adrenoceptor agonist, was carried out by Thomaides *et al.* (1992) (Fig. 24.7) in patients with PAF and MSA. Plasma growth hormone increased normally in response to clonidine only in patients with PAF. Lack of a response in MSA is presumably the result of central lesions affecting the neural pathways involved with control of growth hormone release. These observations provide the basis for a useful neuroendocrine approach for differentiating patients with central and peripheral disorders of the autonomic nervous system.

Recent work indicates that administration of the growth hormone secretagogue, laevodopa, to MSA patients (with an absent growth hormone response to clonidine), causes a rise in growth hormone releasing hormone and also growth hormone (Fig. 24.8) (Kimber *et al.* 1997). This indicates that in MSA hypothalamic GHRH neurones are functional, and it confirms the ability of anterior pituitary cells to secrete growth hormone. These studies, therefore, favour a selective α_2-adrenoceptor hypothalamic deficit in MSA. Kimber *et al.* also studied the rise in growth hormone response to

clonidine in patients with idiopathic Parkinson's disease; their response differed markedly from the response of those with parkinsonian and cerebellar forms of MSA. This suggests that the clonidine–growth hormone stimulation test might be a useful means of differentiating disorders with similar neurological features (but without central autonomic failure), such as Parkinson's disease, progressive supranuclear palsy, and cerebellar degeneration, from the different forms of MSA. Whether this will enable differentiation at an early stage, remains to be determined.

Vasopressin, named for its potent vasoconstrictor actions, is released by the posterior pituitary in response to water deprivation or extracellular fluid volume depletion. Although the peptide also serves as a central neurotransmitter, plasma levels reflect its hormonal function. Its localizing value is diminished by the spectrum of general and local stimuli that affect its release: primary stimuli include serum osmolality and activation of thoracic stretch receptors. A brisk rise in plasma vasopressin occurs when normal subjects are tilted head-up, with a greater rise in tetraplegics, in whom the blood pressure falls (Poole *et al.* 1987). The postural increment is blunted in patients with autonomic failure (Zerbe *et al.* 1983; Williams *et al.* 1985). Williams *et al.* (1985) suggested an afferent lesion since the response to infusion of normal saline was preserved. Central lesions in MSA presumably prevent the suppression of vasopressin by laevodopa or naloxone. Normal vasopressin responses to osmotic stimuli in tetraplegic patients provide additional support for localizing the deficit. Unfortunately, this information only points out the areas that are not functionally involved.

Summary

Neurochemical and pharmacological strategies clearly distinguish pathophysiological differences between central and peripheral disorders of the autonomic nervous system. In addition, underlying

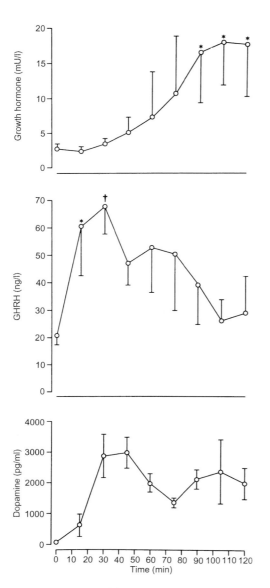

Fig. 24.8. Mean serum growth hormone; plasma growth hormone releasing hormone (GHRH) and plasma dopamine concentrations before and after 250 mg of oral L-dopa and 25 mg of a dopa decarboxylase inhibitor in combination (Sinemet®) in nine multiple system atrophy subjects with parkinsonian features, each of whom had no GH response to clonidine. *, $P < 0.05$ versus basal (time 0). (From Kimber, J.R., Watson, L., and Mathias, C.J., (1997))

Table 24.2. Neurochemical and pharmacological differences between PAF and MSA

	PAF	MSA
Peripheral		
Supine plasma NA	Low	Normal
Neuronal uptake	Decreased	Normal
Neuronal NA stores	Low	Normal
Urinary NA metabolites		
Total	Decreased	Normal
NM/Total	Normal	Decreased
Plasma NA metabolites	Low	Normal
NA receptor sensitivity	Increased	Normal
Gastrin		
Basal level	Increased	Normal
Response to hypoglycaemia	Increased	Decreased
Response to isoprenaline	Increased	Normal
Adrenaline response to arecoline	Absent	Normal
Central		
Plasma NA response to acetylcholine	Absent	Increased
Neuroimaging		
Glucose metabolism	Normal	Decreased
Dopamine uptake	Normal	Deceased
CSF studies		
MHPG	Normal	Low
HVA	Normal	Low
5-HIAA	Normal	Low
AChE	Normal	Low
Substance P	?	Low
Somatostatin	Normal	Low
CRF	Normal	Low
Neuroendocrine mechanisms		
Melatonin		
Total	Low	Normal
Diurnal pattern	Normal	Reversed
β-endorphin/ACTH	Normal	Decreased
Growth hormone response to clonidine	Normal	Absent

NA, noradrenaline; NM, normetanephrine; all other abbreviations defined in text.

deficits in circulatory and metabolic homeostasis have been elucidated. Investigation of patients with autonomic failure provides an opportunity to study lesions involving various neurotransmitter and neuropeptide pathways in man. Their results have often enlightened our understanding of normal function and metabolism and allowed us to validate hypotheses otherwise tested only in experimental animal preparations. Table 24.2 summarizes the results of applying these methods to patients with MSA and PAF. Some of the results clarify functional abnormalities while others contribute to the development of rational therapeutic approaches. Unfortunately, progress in our understanding and management of these patients has not been attended by comparable advances in improving the prognosis, particularly in MSA. Sustained efforts to further define the cause and consequences of these disorders will undoubtedly focus our attempts to succeed in that regard.

References

Anand, P., Bannister, R., McGregor, G. P., Ghatei, M. A., Mulderry, P. K., and **Bloom, S. R.** (1988). Marked depletion of dorsal spinal cord substance P and calcitonin gene-related peptide with intact skin flare responses in multiple system atrophy. *J. Neurol. Neurosurg. Psychiat.* 51, 192–6.

Bannister, R., Crowe, R., Eames, R., Rosenthal, T., and Sever, P. (1979). Defective cardiovascular reflexes and supersensitivity to sympathomimetic drugs in autonomic failure. *Brain* 102, 163–76.

Baser, S. M., Brown, R. T., Curras, M. T., Baucom, C. E., Hooper, D. H., and Polinsky, R. J. (1991). Beta-receptor sensitivity in autonomic failure. *Neurology* 41, 1107–12.

Bhatt, M. H., Snow, B. J., Martin, W. R. W., Cooper, S., and Calne, D. B. (1990). Positron emission tomography in Shy–Drager syndrome. *Ann. Neurol.* 28, 101–3.

Brooks, D. J., Salmon, E. P., Mathias, C. J. *et al.* (1990). The relationship between locomotor disability, autonomic dysfunction, and the integrity of the striatal dopaminergic system in patients with multiple system atrophy, pure autonomic failure, and Parkinson's disease, studied with PET. *Brain* 113, 1539–52.

Cohen, J., Low, P., Fealey, R., Sheps, S., and Jiang, N.-S. (1987). Somatic and autonomic function in progressive autonomic failure and multiple system atrophy.

Davie, C. A., Wenning, G. K., Barker, G. J. *et al.* (1995). Differentiation of multiple system atrophy from idiopathic Parkinson's disease using proton magnetic resonance spectroscopy. *Ann. Neurol.* 37, 204–10.

Dotson, R., Ochoa, J., Marchettini, P., and Cline, M. (1990). Sympathetic neural outflow directly recorded in patients with primary autonomic failure: clinical observations, microneurography, and histopathology. *Neurology* 40, 1079–85.

Esler, M., Jackman, G., Kelleher, D. *et al.* (1980). Norepinephrine kinetics in patients with idiopathic autonomic insufficiently. *Circ. Res.* 46, (Suppl. 1), 47–8.

Fulham, M. J., Dubinsky, R. M., Polinsky, R. J. *et al.* (1991). Computerized tomography, magnetic resonance imaging and positron emission tomography with [^{18}F] flurodeoxyglucose in the assessment of multiple system atrophy and pure autonomic failure. *Clin. Auton. Res.* 1, 27–36.

Gilman, S., Koeppe, R. A., Junck, L., Kluin, K. J., Lohman, M., and St. Laurent, R. T. (1994). Patterns of cerebral glucose metabolism detected with positron emission tomography differ in multiple system atrophy and olivopontocerebellar atrophy. *Ann. Neurol.* 36, 166–75.

Gilman, S., Koeppe, R. A., Junck, L., Kluin, K. J., Lohman, M., and St. Laurent, R. T. (1995a). Benzodiazepine receptor binding in cerebellar degenerations studied with positron emission tomography. *Ann. Neurol.* 38, 176–85.

Gilman, S., St. Laurent, R. T., Koeppe, R. A., Junck, L., Kluin, K. J., and Lohman, M. (1995b). A comparison of cerebral blood flow and glucose metabolism in olivopontocerebellar atrophy using PET. *Neurology* 45, 1345–52.

Gilman, S., Frey, K. A., Koeppe, R. A. *et al.* (1996). Decreased striatal monoaminergic terminals in olivopontocerebellar atrophy and multiple system atrophy demonstrated with positron emission tomography. *Ann. Neurol.* 40, 885–92.

Goldstein, D. S., Polinsky, R. J., Garty, M. *et al.* (1989). Patterns of plasma levels of catechols in neurogenic orthostatic hypotension. *Ann. Neurol.* 26, 558–63.

Kimber, J. R., Watson, L., and Mathias, C. J. (1997). Distinction of idiopathic Parkinson's disease from multiple system atrophy by stimulation of grown hormone release with clonidine. *Lancet* 349, 1877–81.

Kontos, H. A., Richardson, D. W., and Norvell, J. E. (1976) Mechanisms of circulatory dysfunction in orthostatic hypotension. *Trans. Am. Clin. Climatol. Ass.* 87, 26–33.

Kopin, I. J., Gordon, E. K., Jimerson, D. C., and Polinsky, R. J. (1983a). Relationship between plasma and cerebrospinal fluid levels of 3-methoxy-4-hydroxyphenylglycol. *Science* 219, 73–5.

Kopin, I. J., Polinsky, R. J., Oliver, J. A., Oddershede, I. R., and Ebert, M. H. (1983b). Urinary catecholamine metabolites distinguish different types of sympathetic neuronal dysfunction in patients with orthostatic hypotension. *J. Clin. Endocrinol. Metab.* 47, 632–7.

Kuiper, M. A., Visser, J. J., Bergmans, P. L. M., Scheltens, P., and Wolters, E. C. (1994). Decreased cerebrospinal fluid nitrate levels in Parkinson's disease, Alzheimer's disease and multiple system atrophy patients. *J. Neurol. Sci.* 121, 46–9.

Kwak, S. (1985). Biochemical analysis of transmitters in the brains of multiple system atrophy. *No Shinkei* 37, 691–4.

Luft, F. and von Euler, U. (1953). Two cases of postural hypotension showing a deficiency in release of norepinephrine and epinephrine. *J. Clin. Invest.* 32, 1065–9.

Nutt, J. G., Mroz, E. A., Leeman, S. E., Williams, A. C., Engel, W. K., and Chase, T. N. (1980). Substance P in human cerebrospinal fluid: reductions in peripheral neuropathy and autonomic dysfunction. *Neurology* 30, 1280–5.

Otsuka, M., Ichiya, Y., Kuwabara, Y. *et al.* (1996). Glucose metabolism in the cortical and subcortical brain structures in multiple system atrophy and Parkinson's disease: a positron emission tomographic study. *J. Neurol. Sci.* 144, 77–83.

Perani, D., Bressi, S., Testa, D. *et al.* (1995). Clinical/metabolic correlations in multiple system atrophy: a fluorodeoxyglucose F^{18} positron emission tomographic study. *Arch. Neurol.* 52, 179–85.

Polinsky, R. J., Kopin, I. J., Ebert, M. H., and Weise, V. (1980). The adrenal medullary response to hypoglycaemia in patients with orthostatic hypotension. *J. Clin. Endocrinol. Metab.* 51, 1401–6.

Polinsky, R. J., Kopin, I. J., Ebert, M. H., and Weise, V. (1981a). Pharmacologic distinction of different orthostatic hypotension syndromes. *Neurology* 31, 1–7.

Polinsky, R. J., Kopin, I. J., Ebert, M. H., Weise, V., and Recant, L. (1981b). Hormonal responses to hypoglycaemia in orthostatic hypotension patients with adrenergic insufficiency. *Life Sci.* 29, 417–25.

Polinsky, R. J., Taylor, I. L., Chew, P., Weise, V., and Kopin, I. J. (1982). Pancreatic polypeptide responses to hypoglycaemia in chronic autonomic failure. *J. Clin. Endocrinol. Metab.* 54, 48–52.

Polinsky, R. J., Jimerson, D. C., and Kopin, I. J. (1984). Chronic autonomic failure: CSF and plasma 3-methoxy-4-hydroxyphenylglycol. *Neurology* 34, 979–83.

Polinsky, R. J., Goldstein, D. S., Brown, R. T., Keiser, H. R., and Kopin, I. J. (1985). Decreased sympathetic neuronal uptake in idiopathic orthostatic hypotension. *Ann. Neurol.* 18, 48–53.

Polinsky, R. J., Brown, R. T., Lee, G. K. *et al.* (1987). Beta-endorphin, ACTH, and catecholamine responses in chronic autonomic failure. *Ann. Neurol.* 21, 573–7.

Polinsky, R. J., Brown, R. T., Burns, R. S., Harvey-White, J., and Kopin, I. J. (1988a). Low lumbar CSF levels of homovanillic acid and 5-hydroxyin-doleacetic acid in multiple system atrophy with autonomic failure. *J. Neurol. Neurosurg. Psychiat.* 51, 914–19.

Polinsky, R. J., Taylor, I. L., Weise, V., and Kopin, I. J. (1988b). Gastrin responses in patients with adrenergic insufficiency *J. Neurol. Neurosurg. Psychiat.* 51, 67–71.

Polinsky, R. J., Holmes, K. V., Brown, R. T., and Weise, V. (1989a). CSF acetylcholinesterase levels are reduced in multiple system atrophy with autonomic failure. *Neurology* 39, 40–4.

Polinsky, R. J., Hooper, D., and Baser, S. M. (1989b). Reduced CSF somatostatin in multiple system atrophy with autonomic failure. *Neurology* 39, (Suppl. 1), 142.

Polinsky, R. J., Brown, R. T., Curras, M. T. *et al.* (1991a). Central and peripheral effects of arecoline in patients with autonomic failure. *J. Neurol. Neurosurg. Psychiat.* 54, 807–12.

Polinsky, R. J., Hooper, D., Nee, L., Marini, A., and Scott, J. (1991b). CSF corticotropin releasing factor in patients with autonomic failure. *Neurology* 41, (Suppl. 1), 283.

Polinsky, R. J., Baser, S. M., Brown, R. T., Marini, A. M., and Baucom, C. E. (1991c). Ganglionic responsivity in patients with autonomic failure. *Clin. Autonom. Res.* 1, 83.

Poole, C.J.M., Williams, T.D.M., Lightman, S.L., and Frankel, H.L. (1987). Neuroendocrine control of vasopressin secretion and its effect on blood pressure in subjects with spinal cord transection. *Brain.* 110, 727–35.

Rinne, J. O., Burn, D. J., Mathias, C. J., Quinn, N. P., Marsden, C. D., and Brooks, D. J. (1995). Positron emission tomography studies on the dopaminergic system and striatal opioid binding in the olivopontocerebellar atrophy variant of multiple system atrophy. *Ann. Neurol.* **37**, 568–73.

Spokes, E. G. S., Bannister, R., and Oppenheimer, D. R. (1979). Multiple system atrophy with autonomic failure: clinical, histological and neurochemical observations on four cases. *J. Neurol. Sci.* **43**, 59–82.

Tetsuo, M., Polinsky, R. J., Markey, S. P., and Kopin, I. J. (1981). Urinary 6-hydroxymelatonin excretion in patients with orthostatic hypotension. *J. Clin. Endocrinol. Metab.* **53**, 607–10.

Thomaides, T. N., Chaudhuri, K. R., Maule, S., Watson, L., Marsden, C. D., and Mathias, C. J. (1992). Growth hormone response to clonidine in central and peripheral autonomic failure. *Lancet* **340**, 263–6.

van Royen, E., Verhoeff, N. F. L. G., Speelman, J. D., Wolters, E. C., Kuiper, M. A., and Janssen, A. G. M. (1993). Multiple system atrophy and progressive supranuclear palsy: diminished striatal D_2 dopamine receptor activity demonstrated by ^{123}I-IBZM single photon emission computed tomography. *Arch. Neurol.* **50**, 513–6.

Wallin, B. G., Sundlof, G., Eriksson, B.-M., Dominiak, P., Grobecker, H., and Lindblad, L.-E. (1981). Plasma noradrenaline correlates to sympathetic muscle nerve activity in normotensive man. *Acta Physiol. Scand.* **111**, 69–73.

Williams, A. C., Nutt, J., Lake, C. R. *et al.* (1979). Actions of bromocriptine in the Shy–Drager and Steele–Richardson–Olszewski syndromes. In *Dopaminergic ergots and motor control*, (ed. K. Fuxe and D. B. Calne), pp. 271–83. Pergamon Press, New York.

Williams, T. D. M., Lightman, S. L., and Bannister, R. (1985). Vasopressin secretion in progressive autonomic failure: evidence for defective afferent cardiovascular pathways. *J. Neurol. Neurosurg. Psychiat.* **48**, 225–8.

Zerbe, R. L., Henry, D. P., and Robertson, G. L. (1983). Vasopressin response to orthostatic hypotension: etiologic and clinical implications. *Am. J. Med.* **74**, 265–71.

25. Pupil function: tests and disorders

Shirley A. Smith and S. E. Smith

Introduction

This chapter describes how to assess pupil function and its involvement in a number of autonomic disorders. Ocular parasympathetic deficits are seen most commonly in Adie's syndrome. Increased parasympathetic activity resulting from central disinhibition occurs in Argyll Robertson pupils and narcolepsy. Sympathetic deficits result in the classical ptosis and miosis of Horner's syndrome, whereas sympathetic overactivity causes large pupils in oculosympathetic spasm. Pupils are involved in the generalized disorders of pure autonomic failure and diabetic autonomic neuropathy. First, the anatomy and physiology that underlies normal pupil function is described.

Pupillary constriction

Contraction of the circular smooth muscle fibres of the sphincter pupillae constricts the pupil during the reflex responses to light and near vision. Both reflexes involve activation of parasympathetic preganglionic neurones whose cell bodies lie in the Edinger–Westphal nuclei, a pair of slim columns of small cells situated dorsorostrally to the main mass of the oculomotor nuclear complex in the anterior midbrain. These preganglionic neurones pass uncrossed in the superficial part of the third cranial nerve to synapse in the ciliary ganglion which lies about 10 mm in front of the superior orbital fissure in the loose fatty tissue at the orbital apex. This ganglion contains cell bodies of the postganglionic parasympathetic fibres whose axons travel forward to the ciliary muscle and iris sphincter via the short ciliary nerves that penetrate the eyeball at its posterior pole. Fibres subserving pupillary constriction comprise only 3 per cent of the parasympathetic outflow from the ciliary ganglion; the majority subserve accommodation, in accordance with the relatively greater bulk of the ciliary compared with the sphincter muscle.

The course of the light reflex pathway from the retina to the sphincter is illustrated in Fig. 25.1. Afferent impulses for visual perception and pupillary constriction diverge in the posterior (central) third of the optic tracts. The visual fibres relay in the lateral geniculate bodies, whereas the pupillary fibres leave the optic tracts and synapse in the pretectal nuclei in the midbrain. Fibres from these nuclei carry the pupillomotor impulses to Edinger–Westphal nuclei of both sides. In man this crossing, together with the preceding one at the optic chiasm, is essentially symmetrical. Thus, illumination of only one eye produces reflex constriction of both pupils of approximately equal magnitude.

During fixation on a near object, the pupil constricts in association with accommodation produced by ciliary muscle contraction and convergence elicited by contraction of the medial rectus muscles. The light and near pupillary reflexes share a common neuronal path only from

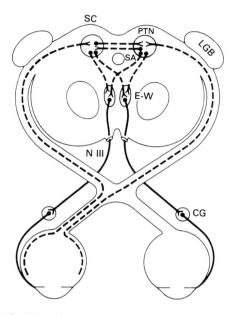

Fig. 25.1. The light reflex pathway from the retina to the iris sphincter. SC, superior colliculus; PTN, pretectal nucleus; LGB, lateral geniculate body; SA, Sylvian aqueduct; E–W, Edinger–Westphal nucleus; N III, oculomotor (third) nerve; CG, ciliary ganglion. (Taken with permission from Alexandridis (1985).)

the Edinger–Westphal nucleus onward. Prior to that, the near reflex pathway descends from the occipital cortex, bypassing the pretectal nucleus on its way to the Edinger–Westphal nucleus. As the fibres approach the nucleus they are probably situated more ventrolaterally than the light reflex fibres because they are often spared in patients in whom pineal or collicular tumours have abolished the light reflex by pressure from the dorsal side (Lowenstein and Loewenfeld 1969).

The postganglionic nerves release acetylcholine to activate muscarinic receptors on the sphincter pupillae. Some muscarinic receptors are present on the dilator which may relax the radial smooth muscle fibres during pupil constriction.

Pupillary dilatation

Dilatation of the pupil in darkness and during arousal is elicited by two mechanisms: central inhibition of the Edinger–Westphal nucleus and activation of the peripheral sympathetic innervation of the radial smooth muscle fibres of the dilator pupillae. The central inhibition is said to be via sympathetic fibres from the posterior hypothalamus to the oculomotor nucleus (Lowenstein and Loewenfeld 1950).

The peripheral sympathetic pathway comprises three parts (Fig. 25.2). The first neurone arises in the hypothalamus where connections from higher centres, including the cortex, influence sympathetic control of the pupil. From the hypothalamus the fibres descend uncrossed through the brainstem to the ciliospinal centre of Budge in the intermediolateral columns at the level of the last cervical and the first two thoracic segments. This centre contains the cell bodies of the preganglionic neurones which form the second stage of the pathway. Their axons leave the cord by the ventral roots of the first two thoracic segments and enter the cervical sympathetic trunk. They traverse the inferior and middle cervical ganglia before reaching the superior cervical ganglion near the bifurcation of the internal and external carotid arteries. Since these preganglionic axons pass close to the apex of the lung, the sympathetic pathway to the pupil may be interrupted by malignancy in this area arising from pulmonary or breast tissue. Within the superior cervical ganglion they synapse with the cell bodies of the postganglionic nerves which form the third stage of the pathway. Fibres which subserve pupillary dilatation, movement of the eyelids via Müller's (smooth) muscle, and local vasomotor function leave the ganglion and follow the course of the internal carotid arteries into the cranium. The pupillary fibres join the fifth (trigeminal) nerve and approach the orbit in its ophthalmic branch, entering via the superior orbital fissure. They continue in its nasociliary division and enter the eye in the long ciliary nerves. In man, some of the sympathetic fibres to the pupil may traverse, but do not synapse in, the ciliary ganglion.

The postganglionic nerves release noradrenaline on to α-adrenoceptors on the dilator pupillae. A small number of β-adrenoceptors are present on the sphincter which relax these circular fibres during pupillary dilatation. As with the cholinergic reciprocal innervation, there is no indication that these are of physiological significance and they do not mediate a change of pupil size during glaucoma treatment with β-adrenoceptor blocking drugs.

Pupillometric methods

There is a wide range of techniques available. Television systems, though expensive, enable dynamic parameters to be measured. Photographic methods are useful for accurate measurement of static pupil size. For all types of pupillometry, the subjects should fix on a distant target to avoid accommodative effort and the room should be quiet with stable, reproducible, and preferably variable background lighting.

Television pupillometry

These systems can be monocular or binocular. The eyes are illuminated with infrared light so that pupils can be measured in darkness. The infrared-sensitive television cameras scan the front of the eye and the image is analysed to provide a measure of either vertical pupil diameter or pupil area. Light stimulation is provided from a bright source to one or both eyes at a length, frequency, and brightness all of which can be varied over a wide range. Light reflexes are usually elicited with open-loop stimulation, i.e. the stimulus light is too small to be reduced in size by a constricting pupil. The pupillometric output can be both analogue for chart display and digital for direct computer analysis.

Photographic methods

Any camera that can provide a clear magnified image of the front of the eye will suffice. Infrared illumination will allow the eye to be viewed in darkness, and infrared-sensitive film can be used for darkness diameter measurement. However, light reflex latencies are in excess of 0.2 s, so that conventional flash-light photographs can be taken even in darkness before the pupil starts to constrict. Close-up Polaroid photography gives instant results that are convenient clinically. Monocular photography allows for greater magnification and thus accuracy, but for measuring drug effects on pupil size it is better to photograph both pupils together.

Physiological pupil function tests

Darkness diameter

The size of the healthy pupil at rest in darkness is determined by the amount of central inhibition of the parasympathetic outflow and the level of peripheral sympathetic drive. It is age-dependent, being small in infancy but gradually increasing to a peak diameter in adolescence (Miller 1985). Thereafter, it decreases linearly at about 0.4 mm per decade. Presumably, changing levels of supranuclear inhibition and decreasing sympathetic tone contribute to this decline in adults.

An age-related normal range must be used to identify abnormality in darkness pupil size, such as that in Table 25.1 which was constructed from a healthy population of 163 subjects aged 16–92 years (Smith and Dewhirst 1986). A convenient way of expressing pupil size is the pupil diameter per cent (PD%: Table 25.1). This represents the amount of iris taken up by the dilated pupil and is calculated as the ratio of the pupil to the iris diameter. It is dependent only on age, which accounts for 48 per cent of the total variance, and is independent of the image magnification.

Measuring pupil size in darkness allows for universal applicability of such a normal range as darkness, unlike a light environment, can be reproduced consistently. The range shown was obtained using monocular Polaroid photography, and the results agreed well with those from television pupillometry (Smith and Smith 1983a) and infrared photography in a larger population (Miller 1985). Darkness

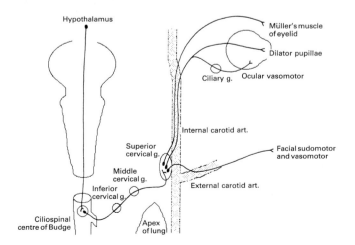

Fig. 25.2.   The sympathetic pathway subserving pupillary dilatation.

Table 25.1. Age-related normal range for pupil diameter in darkness expressed as the absolute measure and as a percentage of iris diameter (PD%). Values shown are the 2.5, 50, and 97.5 percentiles which define the lower, mean, and upper limits of normal

Age range (year)	Mean (year)	Pupil diameter (mm)			PD%		
		Lower	Expected	Upper	Lower	Expected	Upper
15–19	17	6.0	7.4	8.8	52.0	63.3	74.6
20–24	22	5.8	7.2	8.6	50.5	61.8	73.1
25–29	27	5.6	7.0	8.4	49.0	60.3	71.5
30–34	32	5.4	6.8	8.2	47.5	58.8	70.0
35–39	37	5.2	6.6	8.0	46.0	57.3	68.5
40–44	42	5.0	6.4	7.8	44.5	55.8	67.0
45–49	47	4.8	6.2	7.6	43.0	54.3	65.5
50–54	52	4.6	6.0	7.4	41.5	52.7	64.0
55–59	57	4.4	5.8	7.2	40.0	51.2	62.5
60–64	62	4.2	5.6	7.0	38.5	49.7	61.0
65–69	67	4.0	5.4	6.8	37.0	48.2	59.5
70–74	72	3.8	5.2	6.6	35.4	46.7	58.0

pupil diameter is a highly reproducible measure with coefficients of variation averaging 3 per cent.

Near reflex

When a subject changes fixation from far to near there is a miosis which accompanies the accommodation and convergence. The three functions are associated but are not dependent on each other, and focal electrical stimulation in the oculomotor nucleus and the third nerve have been shown in animal studies to elicit each function independently. The time course and amplitude of the pupillary near reflex can be measured with television pupillometry. The amplitude of the miosis increases with the amount of accommodative effort. It is a less useful test of parasympathetic integrity than the light reflex, because the stimulus is subjective. An absent near reflex indicates either parasympathetic dysfunction or a lack of accommodative effort by the subject. However, it is a useful sign when found to be greater than the light reflex, as such 'light-near dissociation' is an important diagnostic sign in some autonomic neuropathies.

Light reflex amplitude and dynamics

Normal reflex responses to light depend on intact parasympathetic innervation and sensitivity to light. Thus, light reflexes are reduced if retinal pathology or optic nerve lesions have reduced visual perception. However, a patient blind from a lesion to the lateral geniculate nucleus or beyond will retain intact light reflexes. If the efferent side of the light reflex is to be tested independently, visual perception threshold should be measured first so that any afferent defects can be quantified and light intensity adjusted accordingly.

Measurement of static pupil size in the light can be made photographically to indicate parasympathetic integrity. More comprehensive information is obtained from continuous measurement of response to short-duration light stimuli in background darkness. Smooth light reflex profiles can be obtained by standard averaging techniques, as illustrated in Fig. 25.3. The amplitude of the reflex from its starting darkness diameter to its peak is a measure of the

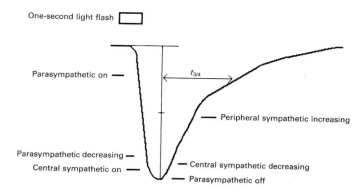

Fig. 25.3. Diagram of a pupillographic tracing of a light reflex to show the $t_{3/4}$ measure of redilatation time. The presumed activity of the autonomic system in shaping the reflex is indicated.

parasympathetic response. This is attenuated first by central inhibition of the Edinger–Westphal nuclei via probable adrenergic inputs from the hypothalamus, then by peripheral sympathetic activation of the iris dilator.

Reflex amplitude is not affected by age directly, but it is reduced in pupils which are small in darkness due to age or sympathetic neuropathy. This is a mechanical restriction, whereby a small pupil has limited scope for further constriction (Smith and Smith 1983b).

Analysis of the averaged reflex provides data on latency, time to peak constriction, and the maximum velocities of constriction and dilatation. All these kinetic parameters are strongly dependent on amplitude, so that small reflexes have prolonged latencies, reduced times to peak, and slower maximum velocities of constriction and dilatation. These dynamic variables thus also reflect parasympathetic events, and are generally less reproducible than amplitude as pupillary measures.

Hippus

When pupils from healthy subjects are stimulated with continuous bright light they constrict initially, then redilate partially as the eye adapts to the stimulus. Pupil size oscillates slowly as the redilatation ensues, a phenomenon known as hippus (Lowenstein and Loewenfeld 1969). This pupillary unrest is always synchronous in the two eyes and is therefore likely to be central in origin. The oscillations can be measured by Fourier frequency analysis, which separates them into their component sinusoidal wavelengths. Hippus comprises mostly low-frequency waves of less than 0.2 Hz.

Redilatation time

The recovery from a light reflex is shown in Fig. 25.3. Initially, the pupil dilates rapidly as the parasympathetic drive finishes and it is during this phase that the pupil reaches its maximum dilatation velocity. Thereafter, the peripheral sympathetic widens the pupil more slowly, and studies with adrenoceptor antagonists have shown that the time to three-quarter dilatation ($t_{3/4}$) accurately reflects this sympathetic activity (Smith and Smith 1990). A healthy population was studied to define a normal range for $t_{3/4}$ using television pupillometry. Bright lights elicited large reflexes in the dark-adapted state. Starting diameter and age had little influence, but $t_{3/4}$ time increased proportionally with amplitude (Table 25.2). Times that exceed the

Table 25.2. Normal range for the $t_{3/4}$ redilatation time. Values shown are the 2.5, 50, and 97.5 percentiles which define the lower, mean, and upper limits of normal

Reflex amplitude (mm)	$t_{3/4}$(s)		
	Lower	Expected	Upper
1.0	0.00	1.46	3.07
1.2	0.04	1.62	3.20
1.4	0.23	1.79	3.34
1.6	0.42	1.95	3.49
1.8	0.60	2.12	3.63
2.0	0.78	2.28	3.79
2.2	0.95	2.45	3.94
2.4	1.12	2.61	4.11
2.6	1.29	2.78	4.27
2.8	1.44	2.94	4.45
3.0	1.60	3.11	4.62
3.2	1.74	3.28	4.81
3.4	1.89	3.44	4.99
3.6	2.03	3.61	5.18

97.5 percentile indicate a significant redilatation lag. This is a sensitive indicator of peripheral sympathetic dysfunction if reflex averaging is used to improve reproducibility.

A photographic method can be used to identify dilatation lag in patients with unilateral Horner's syndrome, where there is a normal pupil available for comparison (Thompson 1977b). Binocular photographs are taken at 5 and at 15 s after turning the room lights out. If there is more anisocoria in the 5-s photograph than in the 15-s one, the subject has a relative dilatation lag. The 5-s photograph corresponds approximately to the $t_{3/4}$ time.

Psychosensory dilatation

When a subject is aroused, alarmed, or afraid, the pupils dilate. Central inhibition of the parasympathetic outflow, peripheral sympathetic drive, and circulating adrenaline may all contribute. The binocular dilatation can be measured with television pupillometry in background light to a stimulus such as a loud noise. This test has limited reproducibility.

Pupil cycle time

Another method of testing pupillary parasympathetic function is the pupil cycle time (Martyn and Ewing 1986). The test was first described as a means of quantifying afferent pupillary defects in optic neuritis. Regular oscillations of the pupil are induced by focusing a narrow beam of light on the pupil margin using a slit lamp. The constricting pupil interrupts the light beam, removing the stimulus and thereby dilating the pupil, enabling the light to restimulate the retina ('closed-loop stimulation'). The mean time is calculated from 100 cycles with a stop watch. It has been found to increase with increasing age. The pupil cycle time is lengthened by para-sympathetic, but not sympathetic, drug blockade. It does not differentiate between afferent and efferent pupillary defects, and pupils in a proportion of patients cannot be made to cycle.

Pharmacological pupil function tests

These are a useful supplement to clinical and physiological signs. However, pupillary responses to drugs show wide inter- and intra-individual variability. There is poor bioavailability from eyedrops because of low and variable corneal penetration. Dark eyes are more resistant to drug effects, due to a thicker iris stroma reducing access to the smooth muscle. Many drugs are absorbed by melanin pigment, which will reduce bioavailability in dark eyes more than in light eyes which have less melanin.

Sources of variability should be minimized where possible. Binocular measurement can eliminate arousal effects, which affect the pupils equally. The effects of drugs on the pupil are often long-lasting, and at least 48 h should elapse between repeated drug tests. Systemic drugs with pupillary effects should be discontinued temporarily if possible. Ideally, dilutions of drugs should be made up freshly in a buffered diluent at room temperature to avoid lacrimation from stinging drops. Two drops should be given at 1 min apart to ensure effective dosing. Experiments with miotics are best performed in darkness, whereas mydriatics need stable background light to increase the available range of pupillary movement. Pupils should be measured several times post-instillation so that peak responses can be identified. Between-subject variation should be defined in healthy controls so that normal ranges can be constructed (Smith and Smith 1983a; Cremer et al. 1990a).

Denervation supersensitivity

An important principle utilized in drug tests is that of denervation supersensitivity. An organ deprived of its innervation becomes more sensitive to the transmitter normally released from those nerves. This 'up-regulation' is thought to be mediated by an increase in the number and activity of the receptors on the end organ. The increased sensitivity extends to other agonists active at those receptors. It is a general principle applying to denervated voluntary muscle, glands, postsynaptic nerve cell bodies, and smooth muscle. It occurs not only with complete lesions to the postganglionic nerve, but also to a lesser degree with partial lesions, lesions more proximal in the nerve pathway, and even with functional, not anatomical, deficits. It is now understood to be one end of a regulatory spectrum, the other end of which is the decreased sensitivity or 'down-regulation' that follows excessive excitation as, for example, after treatment with high doses of miotic drugs.

Cholinergic tests

A large pupil with poor light and near reflexes may be caused by a parasympathetic deficit, local iris sphincter trauma, or cholinolytic mydriatic treatment. The former can be usefully differentiated from the latter two with a muscarinic agonist. The denervated pupil will show a supersensitive miosis, whereas the damaged or atropinized pupil will not constrict. If only one pupil is large, binocular responses to a weak concentration of the agonist should be measured to establish a relative supersensitivity. If both pupils are large, one eye should be treated and the drug effect taken as the difference in anisocoria before and after miosis. The response can then only be judged as super-sensitive if data are available from matched healthy controls.

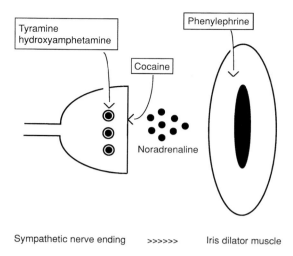

Sympathetic nerve ending   >>>>>>   Iris dilator muscle

Fig. 25.4. Diagram to show the site of action of drugs used in the diagnosis of sympathetic dysfunction. Phenylephrine excites receptors on the dilator muscle, cocaine blocks the uptake of noradrenaline into the terminal, and tyramine and hydroxyamphetamine release noradrenaline from the terminal.

Table 25.3. Age-related normal ranges for 2 per cent phenylephrine and 0.5 per cent hydroxyamphetamine drug tests. Values shown are the 2.5, 50, and 97.5 percentiles which define the lower, mean and upper limits of normal

Age range (year)	Mean (year)	Phenylephrine mydriasis (mm)			Hydroxyamphetamine mydriasis (mm)		
		Lower	Expected	Upper	Lower	Expected	Upper
15–19	17	—	0.2	1.6	0.25	1.6	2.9
20–24	22	—	0.4	1.8	0.3	1.7	3.0
25–29	27	—	0.6	2.0	0.4	1.7	3.05
30–34	32	—	0.85	2.2	0.5	1.8	3.1
35–39	37	—	1.1	2.4	0.55	1.9	3.2
40–44	42	—	1.3	2.6	0.6	1.9	3.2
45–49	47	0.2	1.5	2.8	0.7	2.0	3.3
50–54	52	0.4	1.7	3.0	0.75	2.05	3.4
55–59	57	0.6	1.9	3.25	0.8	2.1	3.4
60–64	62	0.8	2.1	3.5	0.9	2.2	3.5
65–69	67	1.0	2.4	3.7	0.9	2.25	3.6
70–74	72	1.2	2.6	3.9	1.0	2.3	3.6

Pilocarpine, an alkaloid with good corneal penetration that is resistant to cholinesterase destruction, is often used to test for sphincter supersensitivity. Thompson (1977*a*) recommends pilocarpine 0.125 per cent, which usually gives a small miosis in a healthy pupil. He studied patients with Adie's pupils having unilateral postganglionic parasympathetic denervation and found that 80 per cent of affected pupils constricted 0.2 mm more than the fellow eyes. Peak effects occur at approximately 1 h after instillation.

A supersensitive response indicates dysfunction anywhere from the midbrain to the nerve endings in the iris sphincter (Ponsford *et al.* 1982; Jacobson, 1990). The response to pilocarpine is age-dependent and control studies in healthy pupils should be included when investigating binocular parasympathetic neuropathies.

Sympathetic tests

There is a wider range of drug tests for sympathetic deficits (Fig. 25.4). Phenylephrine and cocaine are used to establish whether a small pupil is caused by sympathetic dysfunction, and hydroxyamphetamine, pholedrine, or tyramine can help to locate the lesion.

Phenylephrine is an α-adrenoceptor agonist which is used to test for supersensitivity caused by a lesion anywhere along the three stages of the peripheral sympathetic pathway. Phenylephrine 2 per cent causes a small mydriasis in young adults, which increases markedly with age (Table 25.3). It is thus again important to use age-matched controls when testing binocular conditions which do not have a normal pupil available for comparison.

Cocaine (4–10 per cent) dilates the normal pupil by blocking reuptake of noradrenaline, which then accumulates at the adrenoceptors. A lesion anywhere in the pathway will reduce the mydriasis, since there is less transmitter being released. Cocaine thus gives the same information as phenylephrine, the former showing a reduction and the latter an increase in mydriatic response in pupillary sympathetic dysfunction.

Hydroxyamphetamine (0.5 or 1 per cent), pholedrine (0.5 per cent), and tyramine (2–5 per cent) are indirect-acting sympathomimetics which dilate the pupil by displacing noradrenaline from its storage sites in sympathetic nerve endings. None of them has significant direct action on the receptors. If the postganglionic sympathetic nerve is damaged, these agents cause less mydriasis than normal as there is less transmitter available to release. If the lesion is preganglionic or central in origin, these agents give a normal or somewhat enhanced mydriasis as decentralized nerves have normal transmitter stores which after release act on supersensitive receptors. Such agents can therefore be used to determine whether a lesion is pre- or postganglionic. The response to hydroxyamphetamine 0.5 per cent is weakly age-dependent (Table 25.3).

Most experience with indirect-acting sympathomimetics in the localization of lesions in Horner's syndrome has been gained with hydroxyamphetamine (Cremer *et al.* 1990*b*). Pholedrine appears to have exactly similar actions (Bates *et al.* 1995). Unfortunately, at the time of writing neither agent is freely available for clinical use.

Pupillary disorders

Tonic pupils

Lesions to the postganglionic parasympathetic innervation give 'tonic' pupils, i.e. the constrictions to light and near are slow and inextensive. Acutely, there may be complete internal ophthalmoplegia but reinnervation often restores some function. A variety of inflammatory, infective, malignant, or traumatic conditions can cause tonic pupils by damaging the ciliary ganglion or the short ciliary nerves. They are, however, seen most commonly in Adie's syndrome.

Adie's syndrome

This is a benign condition in which the idiopathic ciliary ganglion pathology is associated with loss of deep tendon reflexes. Usually, a patient with Adie's syndrome of recent onset presents with accommodative paresis and has one large pupil with poor or absent light reflexes. Further examination shows segmental iris sphincter palsy, denervation supersensitivity to topical pilocarpine, and deep tendon areflexia of the upper and lower extremities. Corneal sensation may be reduced from involvement of sensory nerves, some of which pass through the ciliary ganglion to join the ophthalmic division of the trigeminal nerve.

Many cases of Adie's pupils are investigated in the clinic some time after the initial onset of symptoms when the affected pupil is in fact smaller than the normal one. An Adie's pupil only remains larger than its fellow for about 2–6 months (Thompson 1977a). Thereafter, aberrant regeneration of fibres subserving accommodation, which are far in excess of those subserving pupil constriction, causes innervation of the affected sections of the sphincter pupillae (Loewenfeld and Thompson 1981). The neuronal drive associated with ciliary muscle function then constricts the pupil via its aberrant nerves to give a small pupil. This also results in a 'light–near dissociation' with pupillary constriction to near exceeding that to light, though both reflexes are abnormally slow. The initial accommodative difficulties resolve as the ciliary muscle reinnervates. The pupils at this stage may be difficult to distinguish from spastic miotic pupils (Argyll Robertson pupils, see next section) caused by midbrain lesions anterior to the oculomotor nucleus. The differential diagnosis may be made on the presence of segmental sphincter palsy and denervation supersensitivity (as in Adie's pupils) and the nature of the pupillary near reflex response which is slow in Adie's but brisk in Argyll Robertson's syndrome.

Adie's syndrome is a progressive condition with loss of the light reaction in further segments of the sphincter, further loss of the deep tendon reflexes, and eventual second eye involvement. This has led to the suggestion that a slow virus may be the cause of Adie's syndrome, although immunological studies have, as yet, proved inconclusive.

There is clear histological evidence of loss of ganglion cells from the ciliary ganglia which explains the ocular signs. The cause of the progressive areflexia is less clear. However, post-mortem evidence has indicated that there is degeneration in the dorsal columns of the spinal cord, notably in the fasciculus gracilis and the fasciculus cuneatus.

There is recent evidence from patients with longstanding Adie's syndrome that sweating deficits are much more common than previously supposed (Bacon and Smith 1993). Thus the separately classified Ross's syndrome, defined as Adie's syndrome with segmental hypohidrosis, may be part of the same disorder. These and other workers (Hope-Ross et al. 1990) have also reported that some Adie's patients have impaired cold pressor responses and reduced Valsalva responses, although the vasomotor sympathetic deficit was not enough to cause postural hypotension. One can speculate that the spinal cord pathology cited above could involve the efferent sympathetic pathway. Thus, although the symptoms of Adie's that trouble the patient are exclusively ocular, it appears that there is often a much wider neurological involvement.

Argyll Robertson pupils

Pupillary dysfunction occurs in some conditions from disinhibition of the Edinger–Westphal nuclei which results in spastically miotic pupils. Such is the case in Argyll Robertson pupils of neurosyphilis, now a clinical rarity but still of considerable theoretical interest.

In the Argyll Robertson syndrome the pupils are small and light reflexes are reduced or absent, whereas the pupillary constriction to near is well preserved. The pupil signs are usually bilateral and may be associated with tabes dorsalis and general paresis although vision is not impaired. The pupillary abnormalities are thought to be due to pathology close to and slightly anterior to the oculomotor nucleus in the midbrain (Lowenstein and Loewenfeld 1969). Such a lesion would destroy the terminal branches of both the crossed and the uncrossed pretectal fibres subserving the light reflex, but would spare the more ventrally situated supranuclear pathways for the near vision reaction. Other inhibitory inputs from higher brain centres would also be interrupted, thereby disinhibiting the parasympathetic motor nuclei. Marked, diffuse damage around the Sylvian aqueduct and the posterior portion of the third ventricle has been found post-mortem, which could explain the pupillary signs. The pupils are often irregular and tonic, which is thought to be due to postganglionic parasympathetic function in addition to the central pathology.

Narcolepsy

Other situations in which there is a small pupil due to central disinhibition are fatigue, sleep (Physiological or drug-induced), and narcolepsy. This is a condition of chronic hypersomnia for which pupillography can be a valuable diagnostic tool (Yoss et al. 1969). Responses to light and near are normal, but measurement in darkness reveals abnormally small pupils which show large spontaneous oscillations in diameter reflecting the sleepiness that characterizes this condition. These 'fatigue waves' are of much larger amplitude and slower frequency than hippus. Treatment with amphetamines, which usually give an excellent clinical response, reverses these pupillary abnormalities which represent one end of the spectrum of arousal effects on pupil size.

Narcotic dependence

Small pupils are a characteristic sign of dependence on opioid narcotics. A central parasympathetic disinhibition is accompanied by a smaller local miotic action, probably involving inhibition of transmitter release from sympathetic terminals in the iris dilator muscle. In this condition there is a resulting mydriatic response to naloxone eyedrops (Ghodse et al. 1986).

Alzheimer's disease

Supersensitivity to dilute tropicamide eyedrops has been reported in dementia of the Alzheimer type (Scinto et al. 1994) as in people with Down's syndrome (Sacks and Smith 1989). However, subsequent observations (Loupe et al. 1996) suggest that the test is unreliable for diagnostic purposes.

Horner's syndrome

In this condition, sympathetic dysfunction leads to small pupils which have normal reflex constriction to light and near. This miosis is usually accompanied by ptosis and, in cases of preganglionic lesions, by sweating deficits of the face and neck. There is sometimes an apparent, not a real, enophthalmos due to the narrowing of the palpebral fissure caused by denervation of Müller's smooth muscles of the eyelids. Horner's syndrome results from partial or complete interruption of the sympathetic pathway in any of its three parts. Patients with damage to the first neurone may have had a medullary infarction or have cervical cord disease. Second-neurone lesions can occur when a lung or breast malignancy has spread to the thoracic outlet, or when surgery or trauma to the neck has involved the sympathetic nerves. Causes of postganglionic lesions include vascular headache syndromes, intraoral or retroparotid trauma, internal carotid artery pathology, and tumours of the middle cranial fossa or the cavernous sinus.

The pupillary behaviour in Horner's syndrome is illustrated in Fig. 25.5. This pupillographic record from a 62 year-old patient with cluster headaches shows a left-sided Horner's pupil. Compared with the normal right pupil, the affected one has a small darkness diameter, normal constriction to light, and a redilatation lag. The $t_{3/4}$ time in the affected pupil was 6.4 s, considerably prolonged in comparison with the 3.1 s measured in the fellow eye. Drug tests in postganglionic Horner's pupils show reduced mydriasis to cocaine and tyramine, and an enhanced response to phenylephrine.

A painful Horner's syndrome characterized by unilateral headache or facial pain in the distribution of the first division of the trigeminal nerve is termed Raeder's syndrome (Grimson and Thompson 1980). Some patients with Raeder's syndrome have multiple cranial nerve involvement and require thorough investigation for possible tumours or aneurysms involving the internal carotid artery. Other patients with Raeder's syndrome without multiple cranial nerve involvement have a benign condition such as cluster headache.

In cluster headache the unilateral pain is very severe, lasts up to 2 h, and may occur several times daily during the cluster period which lasts for several weeks or months. Patients with cluster headache may show signs of sympathetic hyperactivity during attacks on the side affected by pain which include lacrimation, nasal stuffiness, conjunctival hyperaemia, and hyperhidrosis. Between attacks, there is some-

times reduced forehead sweating on heating and a relative miosis with drug tests suggestive of a partial Horner's syndrome (Salvesen *et al.* 1987). Grimson and Thompson (1980) state that 5–22 per cent of patients with cluster headache have clinically evident Horner's syndrome. Presumably the position of the postganglionic fibres in the plexus surrounding the internal carotid artery renders them susceptible to irritation during attacks and ultimately to permanent damage. The occurrence of pupillary abnormalities due to sympathetic dysfunction in various idiopathic headache syndromes has been the subject of a recent review (De Marinis 1994).

Congenital Horner's syndrome, which is rarer than the acquired syndrome, is accompanied by heterochromia iridis since an intact noradrenaline synthetic pathway is required for melanin synthesis. Loss of pigment in acquired Horner's syndrome occurs rarely.

Oculosympathetic spasm

Irritation of sympathetic nerves anywhere from the brainstem to the iris dilator can cause intermittent ipsilateral mydriasis, the 'springing pupil', sometimes associated with hyperhidrosis. Clinically it is not difficult to distinguish from parasympathetic dysfunction as light and near reflexes are intact. This irritation can be associated with Horner's syndrome, as in cluster headache described above. Other causes are cervical cord disease, lung malignancy, and carotid artery trauma.

One type of oculosympathetic spasm dilates just a section of the pupil to give peaked or 'tadpole' pupils. Episodes last about a minute, may occur several times a day, are unilateral and benign, and resolve with no neurological or systemic sequelae apart from mild Horner's syndrome in some cases.

Pupil abnormalities in generalized autonomic neuropathies and autonomic failure

In our experience (Smith and Smith, unpublished observations) the pupil is frequently involved in conditions characterized by widespread autonomic dysfunction. Patients with pure autonomic failure (PAF) usually have bilateral Horner's syndrome, as do many patients with diabetic autonomic neuropathy (see below). The autonomic neuropathy of generalized systemic amyloidosis is associated in some cases with bilateral Horner's syndrome, in others with bilateral tonic pupils, depending presumably on the location of the amyloid deposits. By contrast, in the autonomic neuropathy of AIDS the pupil is usually normal, even in the presence of abnormal cardiovascular autonomic function (Shahmanesh *et al.* 1991).

In multiple system atrophy (MSA) the pupils are often remarkably normal, even when there is evidence of severe autonomic damage affecting the cardiovascular system and the urinary tract. In some patients the resting pupil may be larger than normal in the dark, but its reflex responses to light and near are usually preserved. The reasons for this are not known and are hard to determine, particularly because many of these cases are under treatment with dopaminergic and anticholinergic drugs which can themselves influence the pupil. In patients free of drug effects, the unique preservation of the pupillary reflexes presumably indicates that the midbrain centres involved are unaffected by the disease process, unlike those concerned with cardiovascular and genitourinary regulation. More detailed studies of the relevant pathology are needed to resolve this apparent enigma.

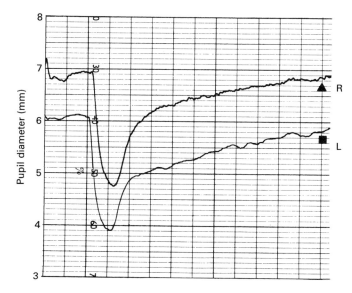

Fig. 25.5. Pupillograph from a patient with a left-sided Horner's syndrome obtained with infrared television pupillometry. The right (R) and (L) traces are separated on the time axis (1 vertical bar = 1 s) for convenience.

Diabetic autonomic neuropathy

Small pupils for age are a characteristic sign in this condition (Smith *et al.* 1978; Hreidarsson 1982). There is evidence that sympathetic dysfunction is partly responsible. However, the size is sometimes smaller than that seen in Horner's syndrome in non-diabetics and it usually affects both pupils equally, implying that central control mechanisms may be damaged. There is also evidence for parasympathetic dysfunction but, as small pupils with normal light reflexes are found to be much more common than large pupils with reduced reflexes, it appears that the sympathetic pupillary innervation is the more susceptible in diabetes. Histological studies of irides from diabetic patients removed during cataract surgery have confirmed that loss of nerve terminals occurs mostly from the dilator pupillae (Ishikawa *et al.* 1985).

Significant associations between small pupils and a wide range of diabetic complications have been recorded: cardiovascular autonomic dysfunction (Smith and Smith 1983*a*), peripheral sensory loss (Smith *et al.* 1978; Hreidarsson 1982), retinopathy (Hayashi and Ishikawa 1979), and nephropathy (Hreidarsson 1982). Patients are more likely to have small pupils if their hyperglycaemia has been of a marked degree and duration (Hreidarsson 1982; Smith and Smith 1983*a*).

Redilatation lag occurs in diabetic miosis. Figure 25.6 shows redilatation in two healthy non-diabetic subjects and one diabetic with autonomic neuropathy. The diabetic patient has small pupils in darkness which constrict well to light but are slow to redilate. The $t_{3/4}$ times are 6 and 6.5 s in the right and left eyes, respectively, which are significantly prolonged for this 1.4 mm reflex size (Table 25.2).

The mydriatic response to directly acting sympathomimetic agents is exaggerated in patients with diabetic autonomic neuropathy, suggesting that there is denervation supersensitivity as in Horner's syndrome (Hayashi and Ishikawa 1979; Smith and Smith 1983*a*). However, the response to hydroxyamphetamine does not differ significantly from normal, from which one can conclude that post-ganglionic nerve function is essentially normal. It would be surprising if a multifactorial disorder such as diabetes caused dysfunction at one specific point in the pathway. More probably the sympathetic deficit results from a composite of mildly reduced function throughout.

The finding that small diabetic pupils dilate well to sympathomimetics shows that damage to the muscle itself is not responsible for the limited movement in darkness. In severe diabetic eye disease rubeosis iridis and glaucoma will eventually limit pupillary movements but the evidence available shows that muscle function in most patients is remarkably well preserved.

Diabetics with neuropathy show reduced hippus (Fig. 25.6), which indicates that central pupillary control may be affected.

Light reflex amplitude is reduced in diabetic autonomic neuropathy (Smith and Smith 1983*b*; Hreidarsson and Gundersen 1985). This reduction is usually only seen in pupils which are already small from sympathetic dysfunction. Figure 25.7 shows a pupil recording from a patient with severe autonomic neuropathy. Pupil size remained almost the same despite a change in illumination from darkness to bright flash stimulation. Myopathy was not responsible for the limited mobility since drugs were effective in changing pupil size, nor was an afferent defect reducing reflex response since visual perception was intact. Presumably the iris was essentially denervated in both autonomic branches.

It is difficult to establish genuine reductions in reflex amplitude in pupils that start small due to sympathetic dysfunction. However Smith and Smith (1983*b*) found that light reflexes in diabetic miosis were significantly smaller than in non-diabetic senile miosis. It is likely that the additional reduction in diabetics is due to parasympathetic dysfunction. The supersensitive response to cholinomimetic drugs (Hayashi and Ishikawa 1979) supports this hypothesis.

Reversal of chronic hyperglycaemia does not appear to improve autonomic function. the St Thomas's Diabetic Study Group (1986) reported a prospective trial of a 2-year improvement in glycaemic control in 20 insulin-treated diabetic patients with established autonomic dysfunction. There was no reversal of the neuropathy and, in fact, two pupillary and three cardiovascular tests indicated a significant deterioration which exceeded that explicable by ageing.

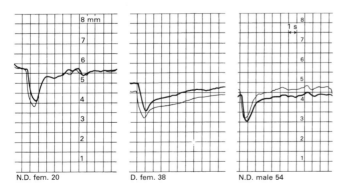

Fig. 25.6. Pupillographs from a non-diabetic (N.D.) 20-year-old female, a diabetic (D.) 38-year-old female with autonomic neuropathy, and a non-diabetic 54-year-old male subject. The bolder line indicates the right pupil, and the responses from the two pupils are separated on the time axis (1 vertical bar = 1 s) for convenience. For each subject, measurements were made in darkness interrupted by a single 1-s light flash. The diameter scale in mm is shown on the left graph. Note the bilateral redilatation lag and absent hippus in the diabetic patient.

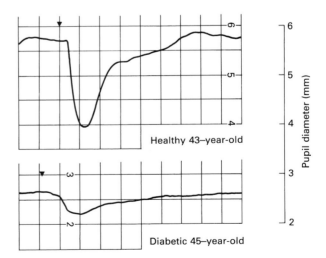

Fig. 25.7. Pupillographic record from a diabetic patient with marked autonomic neuropathy (lower trace). A normal light reflex from an age-matched healthy subject (upper trace) is shown for comparison. The pupil of the diabetic patient failed to dilate in the dark, and constricted poorly to a bright 1-s light flash (▼).

Drug effects on the pupil

Many drugs, given locally or systemically, affect pupil size and may thus complicate the diagnosis of neurological disease. Glaucoma may be treated with eyedrops that constrict the pupil, as with pilocarpine, or dilate the pupil, as with adrenaline. Certain mydriatic agents, such as cyclopentolate, used to enable fundal inspection can dilate the pupil for several days after a single application. Many insecticides contain powerful anticholinesterase agents which may give pinpoint pupils if the eyes have been contaminated.

Patients taking tricyclic antidepressant drugs will have large pupils as these drugs are muscarinic antagonists. Drugs used to treat Parkinson's disease, particularly the anticholinergic agents such as procyclidine, may cause mydriasis. Arteriolar vasodilator agents used to treat hypertension will constrict the pupil by α-adrenoceptor blockade. Patients using or abusing opiates will have small pupils. Many sedative drugs constrict the pupils in association with the sleepiness they induce.

References

Alexandridis, E. (1985). *The pupil.* Springer-Verlag, New York.

Bacon, P. J. and Smith, S. E. (1993). Cardiovascular and sweating dysfunction in patients with Holmes–Adie Syndrome *J. Neurol. Neurosurg. Psychiat.* 56, 1096–102.

Bates, A., Chamberlain, S., Champion, M. *et al.* (1995). Pholedrine: a substitute for hydroxyamphetamine as diagnostic eyedrop test in Horner's syndrome. *J. Neurol. Neurosurg. Psychiat.* 58, 215–17.

Cremer, S. A., Thompson, H. S., Digre, K. B., and Kardon, R. H. (1990a). Hydroxyamphetamine mydriasis in normal subjects. *Am. J. Ophthalmol.* 110, 66–70.

Cremer, S. A., Thompson, H. S., Digre, K. B., and Kardon, R. H. (1990b). Hydroxyamphetamine mydriasis in Horner's syndrome. *Am. J. Ophthalmol.* 110, 71–6.

De Marinis, M. (1994). Pupillary abnormalities due to sympathetic dysfunction in different forms of idiopathic headache. *Clin. Auton. Res.* 4, 331–8.

Ghodse, A. H., Bewley, T. H., Kearney, M. K., and Smith, S. E. (1986). Mydriatic response to topical naloxone in opiate abusers. *Br. J. Psychiat.* 148, 44–6.

Grimson, B. S. and Thompson, H. S. (1980). Raeder's syndrome. A clinical review. *Survey Ophthalmol.* 24, 199–210.

Hayashi, M. and Ishikawa, S. (1979). Pharmacology of pupillary responses in diabetics–correlative study of the responses and grade of retinopathy. *Jap. J. Ophthalmol.* 23, 65–72.

Hope-Ross, H., Buchanan T. A. S., Archer, D. B., and Allen, J. A. (1990). Autonomic function in Holmes–Adie syndrome. *Eye* 4, 607–12.

Hreidarsson, A. B. (1982). Pupil size in insulin-dependent diabetes. *Diabetes* 31, 442–8.

Hreidarsson, A. B. and Gundersen, H. J. G. (1985). The pupillary response to light in Type I (insulin-dependent) diabetes. *Diabetologia* 28, 815–21.

Ishikawa, S., Bensaoula, T., Uga, S., and Mukono, K. (1985) Electron microscopic study of iris nerves and muscles in diabetes. *Ophthalmologica* 191, 172–83.

Jacobson, D. M. (1990). Pupillary responses to dilute pilocarpine in preganglionic 3rd nerve disorders. *Neurology* 40, 804–8.

Loewenfeld, I. E. and Thompson, H. S. (1981). Mechanism of tonic pupil. *Ann. Neurol.* 10, 275–6.

Loupe, D. N., Newman, N. J., Green, R. C., and Lynn, M. J. (1996). Pupillary response to tropicamide in patients with Alzheimer's disease. *Ophthalmology* 103, 495–503.

Lowenstein, O. and Loewenfeld, I. E. (1950). Mutual role of sympathetic and parasympathetic in shaping of the pupillary reflex to light. Pupillographic studies. *Arch. Neurol. Psychiatry* 64, 341–77.

Lowenstein, O. and Loewenfeld, I. E. (1969). The pupil. In *The eye*, Vol. 3, (ed. H. Davson), pp. 255–337. Academic Press, New York.

Martyn, C. N. and Ewing, D. J. (1986). Pupil cycle time: a simple way of measuring an autonomic reflex. *J. Neurol. Neurosurg. Psychiat.* 49, 771–4

Miller, N. R. (1985). The autonomic nervous system: pupillary function, accommodation and lacrimation. In *Walsh and Hoyt's clinical neuro-ophthalmology*, (4th edn), Vol. 2, (ed. N. R. Miller), pp. 385–556. Williams & Wilkins, Baltimore.

Ponsford, J. R., Bannister, R., and Paul E. A. (1982). Methacholine pupillary responses in third nerve palsy and Adie's syndrome. *Brain* 105, 583–97.

Sacks, B. and Smith, S. E. (1989). People with Down's syndrome can be distinguished on the basis of cholinergic dysfunction. *J. Neurol. Neurosurg. Psychiat.* 52, 1294- 5.

Salvesen, R., Bogucki, A., Wysocka-Bakowska, M. M., Antonaci, F., Fredricksen, T. A., and Sjaastad, O. (1987). Cluster headache pathogenesis: a pupillometric study. *Cephalalgia* 7, 273–84.

Scinto, L. F. M., Daffner, K. R., Dressler, D. *et al.* (1994). A potential noninvasive neurobiological test for Alzheimer's disease. *Science* 266, 1051–3.

Shahmanesh, M., Bradbeer, C. S., Edwards, A. E., and Smith, S. E. (1991). Autonomic dysfunction in patients with human immunodeficiency virus infection. *Int. J. STD. AIDS* 2 419–23.

Smith, S. A. and Dewhirst, R. R. (1986). A simple diagnostic test for pupillary abnormality in diabetic autonomic neuropathy. *Diabetic Med.* 3, 38–41.

Smith, S. A. and Smith, S. E. (1983a). Evidence for a neuropathic aetiology in the small pupil of diabetes mellitus. *Br. J. Ophthalmol.* 67, 89–93.

Smith, S. A. and Smith, S. E. (1983b). Reduced pupillary light reflexes in diabetic autonomic neuropathy. *Diabetologia* 24, 330–2.

Smith, S. A. and Smith, S. E. (1990). The quantitative estimation of pupillary dilatation in Horner's syndrome. In *Sympathicus und Auge*, (ed. A. Huber), pp. 152–65. Enke, Stuttgart.

Smith, S. E., Smith, S. A., Brown, P. M., Fox C., and Sonksen, P. H. (1978). Pupillary signs in diabetic autonomic neuropathy. *BMJ* 2, 924–7.

St Thomas's Diabetic Study Group (1986). Failure of improved glycaemic control to reverse diabetic autonomic neuropathy. *Diabetic Med.* 3, 330–4.

Thompson, H. S. (1977a). Adie's syndrome: some new observations. *Trans. Am. Ophthalmol. Soc.* 75, 587–626.

Thompson, H. S. (1977b). Diagnosing Horner's syndrome. *Trans. Am. Acad. Ophthalmol. Otolaryngol.* 83, 840–2.

Yoss, R. E., Moyer, N. J., and Ogle, K. N. (1969). The pupillogram and narcolepsy. *Neurology* 19, 921–8.

26. The assessment of sleep disturbances in autonomic failure

Sudhansu Chokroverty

Introduction

The autonomic nervous system (ANS) is involved intimately in the control of sleep and breathing. The nucleus of the tractus solitarius (NTS) in the medulla orchestrates the central autonomic network by its ascending and descending projections. The NTS also contains the lower brainstem hypnogenic and central respiratory neurones. Dysfunction of the ANS may therefore have serious impact on human sleep and respiration during sleep. Furthermore, sleep has a profound effect on the functions of the ANS. It is, therefore, logical to expect sleep disorder and respiratory dysfunction during sleep in patients with autonomic failure. Sleep and breathing disturbances in conditions associated with autonomic failure should be easy to understand when one also remembers that the peripheral respiratory receptors and central respiratory and lower brainstem hypnogenic neurones are linked intimately by the ANS. This chapter is concerned with an assessment of sleep and respiratory disturbances in autonomic failure, including the influence of the ANS on cardiac rhythm during sleep. A basic familiarity with the stages of sleep, the control of breathing, and the inter-relationship between the central autonomic network and the neuronal network controlling breathing and sleep–wake states is a prerequisite to an understanding of sleep and breathing dysfunction in autonomic failure.

Central autonomic network

Over the past 20 years, a central circuitry of the autonomic network has been identified (Loewy and Spyer 1990). The NTS in the medulla is the single most important structure of the autonomic network in the brainstem. It receives afferents from the cardiovascular and the respiratory systems for autonomic control of cardiac rhythm, circulation, and respiration. Lower brainstem hypnogenic neurones are also located in the NTS. The NTS has ascending projections to the supramedullary structures including the hypothalamic and limbic regions and descending projections to ventral medulla which also sends efferents to intermediolateral neurones of the spinal cord (Loewy and Spyer 1990). Many of the ascending and descending projections (Figs 26.1 and 26.2) are reciprocal in nature. Through its connections in the dorsal and ventral medulla, the NTS influences directly the inputs to the vagal (the dorsal nucleus of the vagus and the nucleus ambiguus) and sympathetic preganglionic neurones in the spinal cord. The NTS, thus, orchestrates the central autonomic network for autonomic control of the vital cardiorespiratory functions during sleep.

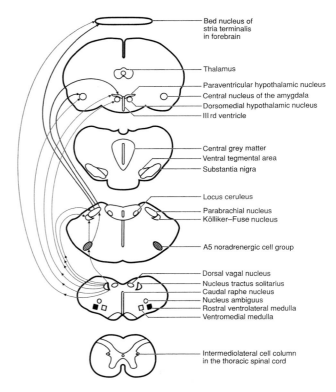

Fig. 26.1. Central autonomic network: ascending projections (schematic). (Modified from Loewy and Spyer (1990); reproduced with permission from Chokroverty (1991) and the American Academy of Neurology.)

An overview of sleep

Based on electroencephalographic (EEG), behavioural, and physiological observations, two types of sleep have been recognized (Chokroverty 1999): non-REM sleep, comprising 75–80 per cent, and REM or paradoxical sleep, comprising 20–25 per cent of sleep time in adults. EEG criteria establish four stages of non-REM sleep: stages I–IV. In normal individuals the REM sleep begins 60–90 min after sleep onset and recurs in a cyclic manner every 90 min throughout the night. REM sleep is divided into tonic and phasic stages based on EEG, electromyographic (EMG), and eye movements criteria.

Based on the ablation and stimulation experiments, single-unit recordings, and pathological findings, it is believed that non-REM or synchronized sleep results from a combination of two factors

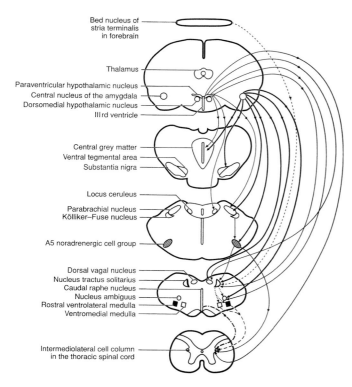

Fig. 26.2. Central autonomic network: descending projections (schematic). (Modified from Loewy and Spyer (1990); reproduced with permission from Chokroverty (1991) and the American Academy of Neurology.)

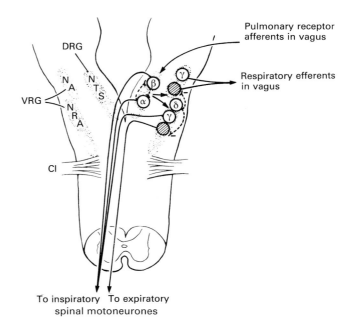

Fig. 26.3. Medullary respiratory neurones, cell types, and inter-connections are shown schematically. DRG, Dorsal respiratory group; VRG, ventral respiratory group; NTS, nucleus tractus solitarius; NA, nucleus ambiguus; NRA, nucleus retroambigualis; CI, first cervical dorsal root; subscripts α, β, γ, δ, inspiratory cell subtype designations. The DRG located in the ventrolateral NTS is the site where vagal sensory information is first incorporated into a respiratory motor response. The DRG drives the VRG and some spinal inspiratory motoneurones. The VRG is composed of NA and NRA. Vagal respiratory motoneurones arise from NA. Axons from NRA project to some spinal inspiratory and probably all spinal expiratory motoneurones. Inspiratory cells are indicated by open circles, and expiratory by hatched circles. Dashed lines indicate some of the hypothesized intramedullary neural inter-connections. (Taken with permission from Berger *et al.* (1977).)

(Chokroverty 1999): inhibition of the ascending reticular activating system and activation of the hypnogenic neurones in the anterior hypothalamus and the preoptic region as well as the NTS in the dorsomedial medulla. The original concept of a reciprocal inter-active model for REM sleep generation has recently been revised (Chokroverty 1999). The recent theory suggests that there are anatomically distributed and neurochemically interpenetrated REM 'on' and REM 'off' cells in the brainstem. The interaction and oscillation between the cholinergic REM-promoting and aminergic REM-inhibiting neurones generate the REM–non-REM cycle.

Control of breathing during sleep and wakefulness

The anatomical relationship suggests a close functional interdepend-ence between the central autonomic network, the respiratory and hypnognic neurones. Two separate and independent controlling systems are responsible for breathing (Chokroverty 1999): the metabolic or automatic system and a voluntary or behavioural system. Both voluntary and metabolic systems operate during wake-fulness but respiration during sleep depends upon the inherent rhythmicity of the automatic respiratory control system located in the medulla. These two controlling systems are complimented by a third system, the reticular arousal system exerting a tonic influence on the brainstem respiratory neurones (McNicholas *et al.* 1983).

Upper brainstem respiratory neurones located in the rostral pons in the region of parabrachial and Kölliker–Fuse nuclei (pneumotaxic centre), and in the dorsolateral region of the lower pons (apneustic centre) influence the automatic respiratory neurones. The medullary (automatic) respiratory neurones consist of two principal groups (Berger *et al.* 1977): the dorsal respiratory group located in the NTS responsible predominantly, but not exclusively, for inspiration, and the ventral respiratory group located in the region of the nucleus ambiguus and retroambigualis, responsible for both inspiration and expiration (Fig. 26.3). These respiratory premotor neurones send axons which decussate below the obex and descend in the reticulospinal tracts in the ventrolateral spinal cord to synapse with spinal respiratory motor neurones innervating the various respiratory muscles. Respiratory rhythmogenesis depends upon tonic inputs from the peripheral and central structures converging on the medullary neurones. Figure 26.4 shows schematically the effects of various brainstem and vagal transections on the ventilatory patterns.

The voluntary breathing system originating in the cerebral cortex (forebrain and limbic system) controls respiration during wakeful-ness in addition to participating in non-respiratory functions. The system descends partly to the automatic medullary controlling system

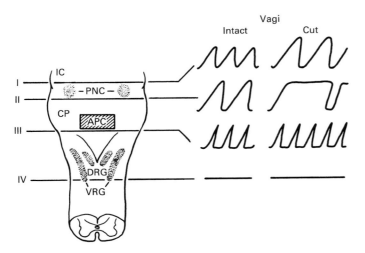

Fig. 26.4. Schematic representation of effects of various brainstem and vagal transections on the ventilatory pattern of the anaesthetized animal. IC, Inferior colliculus; PNC, pneumotaxic centre; CP, cerebellar peduncle; APC, apneustic centre; DRG, dorsal respiratory group; VRG, ventral respiratory group. On the left is a representation of the dorsal surface of the lower brainstem and, on the right, a representation of tidal volume with inspiration upwards. Transection I, just rostral to the PNC, does not affect normal breathing, but, in combination with vagotomy, slow deep breathing results. Transection II, isolating the PNC from the lower brainstem, causes slow deep breathing with the vagi intact, and either apneusis (sustained inspiration) or apneustic breathing (rhythmic respiration with marked increase in inspiratory time) when the vagi are cut. Transection III, isolating structures rostral to the medulla, results in most cases in a regular gasping breathing that is generally not affected by vagotomy. Transection IV, at the medullospinal junction, results in respiratory arrest. (Taken with permission from Berger *et al.* (1977).)

and integrates in part there but mostly descends with the cortico-bulbar and corticospinal tracts to the spinal respiratory motor neurones where the fibres finally integrate with the reticulospinal fibres originating from the automatic medullary respiratory neurones.

The control of respiration during non-REM sleep in normal individuals is entirely dependent upon the automatic control system. The ventilation, tidal volume, and respiratory rate decrease in non-REM sleep. Ventilatory responses to hypercapnia and hypoxia are attenuated during non-REM sleep in normal individuals. These findings suggest decreased sensitivity of the central chemoreceptors subserving medullary respiratory neurones. In REM sleep respiration is rapid and erratic; tonic and phasic activities in the intercostal and upper airway muscles decrease while phasic activity is maintained in the diaphragm but the tonic activity in the diaphragm is reduced. There is some uncertainty about the ventilatory responses to CO_2 and hypoxia in REM sleep. Compared with the responses during non-REM sleep the hypercapnic and hypoxic ventilatory responses in the adult human are reduced during REM sleep. The voluntary respiratory control system may be active during some part of REM sleep. Thus, in normal individuals, respiration is vulnerable during sleep; mild respiratory irregularities and pauses may occur in normals, but in disease states these may assume a pathological significance.

Sleep and respiratory disturbances in autonomic failure

Autonomic failure (AF) may be classified into primary and secondary AF. Primary AF (without known cause) includes pure AF without any somatic neurological deficits and multiple system atrophy (MSA or the Shy–Drager syndrome) (see Chapter on Introduction and Classification of autonomic disorders). The best-known condition with AF in which sleep and respiratory disturbances have been reported and well described is MSA or the Shy–Drager syndrome. Familial dysautonomia, a recessively inherited disease with autonomic failure, is also known to be associated with disturbances of breathing and sleep. A large number of neurological and general medical disorders are associated with prominent secondary autonomic failure. In many patients with diabetic autonomic neuropathies, amyloidotic neuropathy, and Guillain–Barré syndrome, sleep and sleep-related respiratory disturbances have been noted. In a large number of neurological conditions, sleep and respiratory disturbances are secondary to the structural lesions involving the central hypnogenic or respiratory neurones.

In this section an assessment of sleep and respiratory disturbances in multiple system atrophy and familial dysautonomia will be given. In addition, a brief account will also be presented of the following conditions in which sleep disturbances or sleep-related breathing disorders may be the prominent features: diabetic autonomic neuropathy, Parkinson's disease with autonomic failure, and fatal familial insomnia, a recently described rare prion disease with severe sleep disturbances and dysautonomia.

Primary autonomic failure

Multiple system atrophy (Shy–Drager syndrome)

Since the original description by Shy and Drager (1960) of a neurodegenerative disorder characterized by autonomic failure and multiple system atrophy, there have been numerous reports (Chokroverty *et al.* 1969; Bannister and Oppenheimer 1972; Bannister *et al.* 1981; Chokroverty 1999) of the condition that has generally come to be known as multiple system atrophy (MSA). Patients with this syndrome frequently manifest sleep and respiratory disturbances, particularly in the later stage of the illness. Further clinical details are given in Chapter 31.

Some patients may complain of insomnia and many patients may manifest REM behaviour disorder which may occasionally be the presenting feature. However, sleep-related respiratory dysrhythmias associated with repeated arousals and hypoxaemia are the most common sleep disorders in MSA. The clinical manifestations resulting from respiratory dysfunction may consist of daytime hypersomnolence, resulting from severe nocturnal sleep disruption, early morning headache, daytime fatigue, intellectual deterioration, pulmonary hypertension, cor pulmonale, congestive cardiac failure, and cardiac arrhythmias. Sudden nocturnal death in some patients with MSA may be due to respiratory arrest or cardiac arrhythmia. Polysomnographic study may show the following: a reduction of total sleep time, decreased sleep efficiency, increased number of awakenings during sleep, a reduction of slow-wave and REM sleep, absence of muscle atonia in REM sleep in those with REM behaviour disorder, and a variety of respiratory dysrhythmias, as described below.

The spectrum of respiratory dysrhythmias in MSA may be summarized as follows (Chokroverty 1994):

(1) central, upper-airway obstructive, and mixed apnoeas associated with oxygen desaturation during non-REM stages I and II and REM sleep;

(2) irregular rate, rhythm, and amplitude of respiration, with and without oxygen desaturation becoming worse in sleep (dysrhythmic breathing);

(3) transient occlusion of the upper airway or transient uncoupling of the intercostal and diaphragmatic muscle activities;

(4) prolonged periods of central apnoea accompanied by mild oxygen desaturation in relaxed wakefulness;

(5) Cheyne–Stokes pattern and Cheyne–Stokes variant (hypopnoea substitutes apnoea) pattern of breathing becoming worse in sleep;

(6) periodic breathing in the erect posture accompanied by postural fall of blood pressure;

(7) inspiratory gasps and apnoeustic-like breathing;

(8) nocturnal stridor; and

(9) transient sudden respiratory arrest.

Figure 26.5 shows schematically the various breathing patterns.

The most common respiratory dysrhythmias in MSA include central, upper airway obstructive, or mixed (Fig. 26.6) apnoeas–hypopnoeas (Chokroverty *et al.* 1978, 1984; Guilleminault *et al.* 1981; Munschauer et al. 1990; Chokroverty 1999), dysrhythmic breathing (McNicholas *et al.* 1983; Chokroverty 1999), and laryngeal stridor due to laryngeal abductor paralysis (Bannister *et al.* 1981; Munschauer *et al.* 1990; Sadaoka *et al.* 1996). The nocturnal stridor can be inspiratory, expiratory or both and cause excessive snoring and upper airway obstruction during sleep. Stridor may give rise to a striking noise which may be likened to a 'donkey braying'. Less commonly, apnoeustic breathing, inspiratory gasping, or Cheyne–Stokes breathing may occur.

Impaired hypoxic or hypercapnic ventilatory responses and mouth occlusion pressure response in some patients suggested impairment of the metabolic respiratory system (McNicholas *et al.* 1983; Chokroverty 1999) while normal hypercapnic and hypoxic

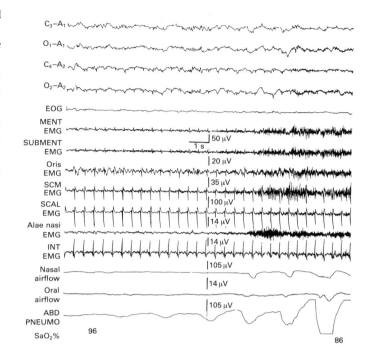

Fig. 26.6. Polygraphic recordings in a patient with MSA showing EEG (top four channels), vertical electro-oculogram (EOG), EMG of mentalis (MENT), submental, oris, sternocleidomastoideus (SCM), scalenus anticus (SCAL), alae nasi and intercostal (INT) muscles, nasal and oral airflow, abdominal pneumogram (ABD PNEUMO), and oxygen saturation (SaO$_2$%). The patient has mixed apnoea (only a portion of the episode is shown) associated with oxygen desaturation during stage II non-REM sleep

ventilatory responses in some patients in the presence of an abnormal respiratory pattern indicated that the chemoreceptor control and respiratory pattern generator are probably subserved by different population of neurones with selective vulnerability of these neurones in MSA (Lockwood 1976; Chokroverty 1999).

Post-mortem findings of marked loss of neurones in the pontine tegmentum and medullary reticular formation including neurones around the nucleus tractus solitarius in those MSA patients with sleep-related respiratory dysrhythmias confirmed involvement of the respiratory neurones in the brainstem (Chokroverty *et al.* 1978; Munschauer *et al.* 1990).

The suggested pathogenetic mechanisms for respiratory dysrhythmia in MSA include:

(1) direct involvement of the medullary respiratory neurones;

(2) involvement of the arousal system (ascending reticular activating system) and severe compromise of the wakefulness stimulus;

(3) involvement of the respiratory and non-respiratory motor neurones in the brainstem, e.g. the nucleus ambiguus and hypoglossal nuclei causing laryngeal abductor paresis, and pharyngeal and genioglossal weakness causing upper airway obstructive apnoea;

(4) involvement of the respiratory motor neurones (anterior horn cells) in the cervical and thoracic spinal cord, thereby reducing impulse traffic along the phrenic and intercostal nerves to the diaphragm and intercostal muscles. If there is differential affec-

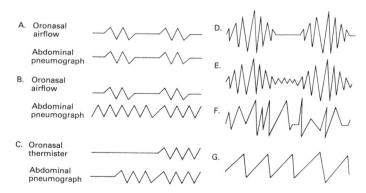

Fig. 26.5. Different respiratory patterns in MSA are shown schematically. A, central apnoea; B, upper-airway obstructive apnoea; C, mixed apnoea; D, Cheyne-Stokes breathing; E, Cheyne–Stokes variant pattern; F, dysrhythmic breathing; G, apneustic breathing.

tion between the upper airway motor neurones and spinal respiratory motor neurones, there may be obstructive and mixed apnoeas;

(5) interference with the forebrain, midbrain, and pontine inputs to the medullar respiratory neurones causing dysrhythmic and apnoeustic breathing;

(6) involvement of the direct projections from the hypothalamus and central nucleus of amygdala to the respiratory neurons in the NTS and nucleus ambiguus;

(7) involvement of the vagal afferents from the lower and upper airway receptors may reduce the input to the central respiratory neurones, causing respiratory dysrhythmia;

(8) sympathetic denervation of the nasal mucosa causing increased nasal resistance may promote upper airway obstructive apnoea; and

(9) finally, discrete neurochemical alterations in MSA may interfere with normal regulation of breathing.

Familial dysautonomia

This condition is a recessively inherited disorder confined to the Jewish population and presenting in childhood. The clinical manifestations comprise autonomic, neuromuscular, cardiovascular, skeletal, renal, and respiratory abnormalities. Patients show a characteristic absence of the fungiform papillae of the tongue. Other features include defective lacrimation and sweating, vasomotor instability, fluctuation of blood pressure (postural hypotension and paroxysmal hypertension), relative insensitivity to pain, and absent muscle stretch reflexes. Most patients have a mild respiratory and sleep disorder associated with both central and obstructive sleep apnoeas (Gadoth et al. 1983). The sleep abnormalities include increased arousals and awakenings; prolonged sleep onset; prolonged REM sleep onset but reduced total REM sleep time; and apnoeas during sleep. The patients with familial dysautonomia often show severe breath-holding spells due to defective responses of central respiratory neurones to changes in $PaCO_2$. Guilleminault et al. (1981) and McNicholas et al. (1983) found an irregular pattern of breathing in patients with familial dysautonomia similar to that noted in Shy–Drager syndrome. Oesophageal reflux during sleep causing frequent awakenings was noted in one patient by Guilleminault et al. (1981).

Secondary autonomic failure (those associated with other medical and neurological disorders)

Diabetic autonomic neuropathy

Autonomic neuropathies have been described in many neurological and medical disorders. However, the sleep and respiratory functions have not been studied well in most of these conditions. In diabetic polyneuropathies, however, there have been reports of disturbances of sleep and respiration. Similar disturbances have been described in some patients with autonomic failure associated with amyloidosis and Guillain–Barré syndrome.

Central or upper airway obstructive apnoeas have been described in several patients with diabetes mellitus and autonomic neuropathy (Guilleminault et al. 1981; Rees et al. 1981). However, controversy about the association of diabetes mellitus and symptomatic sleep apnoea remains (Strohl 1996).

Parkinson's disease with autonomic failure

Sleep disturbances and sleep-related respiratory dysrhythmias are common in patients with Parkinson's disease (PD), especially those with evidence of autonomic failure (Chokroverty 1996). Distinguishing dopa-responsive idiopathic PD with autonomic failure from dopa non-responsive MSA with predominant parkinsonism and dysautonomia may be difficult but important for prognosis and treatment. Sleep complaints in PD include insomnia, hypersomnia, parasomnia, and circadian rhythm sleep disorders. Isolated reports of pulmonary dysfunction and respiratory abnormalities have been reported in PD. It is of note that Parkinson himself in his original description alluded to respiratory problems in his patients and stated that some 'fetched their breath rather hard'. Most of the respiratory problems are the results of direct effects of PD, particularly those with autonomic dysfunction. However, some are levodopa-treatment-related. Obstructive, central and mixed apnoeas have been described in PD patients, though not all authors have observed them. Some investigators have speculated that respiration-related sleep disorders in PD may be responsible for early morning mortality in some of these patients.

The spectrum of sleep-related respiratory dysrhythmias in PD includes sleep apnoea–hypopnoea, hypoventilation, Cheyne–Stokes and Cheyne–Stokes variant pattern of breathing, dysrhythmic breathing, and nocturnal stridor. The mechanisms of sleep-related respiratory dysrhythmias in PD include an impairment of the central control of breathing; an upper airway obstructive ventilatory defect related to frequent involvement of the upper airway muscles in PD; stridor or laryngeal spasms associated with off-states or dystonic episodes and diaphragmatic dyskinesias as well as end-of-the-dose and peak-dose levodopa-related dysrhythmias.

Another important sleep disturbance in PD is emergence of REM behaviour disorder (RBD). Many patients with idiopathic RBD (Schenck and Mahowald. 1996) after many years developed PD, and many PD patients also had manifestations of RBD as diagnosed by history and video-polysomnographic study.

Fatal familial insomnia

Fatal familial insomnia (FFI) is a rare autosomal dominant prion disease akin to Creutzfeldt–Jakob disease (Medori et al. 1992) with onset in adults. The term 'prion' refers to a proteinacous infectious particle resistant to inactivation by most standard procedures. The major clinical findings include progressive insomnia, motor abnormalities in the form of spontaneous and reflex myoclonus, ataxia, dysarthria, and hyper-reflexia, neuroendocrine abnormalities, and dysautonomia. Insomnia is progressive with worsening within a few months. The autonomic dysfunction is manifested by sympathetic hyper-reflexia as evidenced by hypertension, tachycardia, tachypnoea, hyperhidrosis as well as urinary dysfunction and impotence. Tests for parasympathetic function are normal. Neuroendocrine dysfunction is characterized by elevated plasma cortisol and catecholamines, reduced circadian oscillations of cortisol and failure of rise of melatonin during darkness, and absence of a tight relationship between slow-wave sleep and rise of growth hormone and prolactin. There is no evidence of dementia but neuropsychological tests may show frontal lobe type dysfunction. The most prominent finding in the polysomnographic recording is progressive decrement of non-REM and REM sleep to only brief non-REM sleep. EEG shows diffuse background slowing and periodically recurring spikes in some cases in the later stage. Cerebral evoked potentials, brain CT and MRI are normal. PET scan shows glucose hypometabolism in the thalamus.

The course of the illness is relentlessly progressive, lasting for 1 to 4 years. In the final stage, the patients display random myoclonus and dream-like hallucinatory behaviour in wakefulness. In the final terminal months, sleeplessness gives way to stupor and coma.

Neuropathological findings consist of degneration and loss of neurones in the dorsomedial and anterior thalamic nuclei with normal hypothalamus and brainstem reticular formation. Frontal and temporal cortex shows mild to moderate gliosis. DNA analysis shows that FFI results from a point mutation at codon 178 and a polymorphism on codon 129 on the prion gene on chromosome 20.

Autonomic nervous system and sleep

There are several changes in the autonomic functions during sleep affecting particularly the cardiovascular and the respiratory systems (Loewy and Spyer 1990). The neural regulation of the heart predominantly involves the sympathetic and parasympathetic divisions of the ANS but to an extent involves the whole CNS axis. The limbic–hypothalamic region, by controlling the central autonomic network (Loewy and Spyer 1990), affects cardiac rhythm. Sympathetic preganglionic neurones in the intermediolateral column of the spinal cord and the parasympathetic preganglionic neurones in the nucleus ambiguus and dorsal motor nucleus of the vagus, along with the extensive connections with the central autonomic network and the peripheral afferent inputs to the central autonomic network, control the cardiovascular regulation in wakefulness and sleep (Loewy and Spyer 1990). Based on animal experiments and human studies, it is known that heart rate slows during non-REM sleep due to tonic increase in parasympathetic activity. There is further slowing of the heart rate during REM sleep due to combination of two factors: persistence of parasympathetic predominance and an additional decrease of sympathetic activity. Similarly, the blood pressure falls during non-REM with further fall during REM sleep due to the same mechanism. Blood pressure and heart rate are unstable during phasic REM due to phasic inhibition of the vagus and phasic activation of sympathetic tone, resulting from changes in the brainstem neural activity. The reduction in cardiovascular haemodynamic activities in normal sleep, involving the heart rate, peripheral vascular resistance, blood pressure, blood flow, and cardiac output, becomes critical in patients with cardiopulmonary diseases (e.g. ischaemic heart disease, congestive cardiac failure, pulmonary emphysema, and chronic obstructive pulmonary disease).

Sleep and cardiac arrhythmias

Several studies have been obtained in normal individuals using Holter monitoring to understand the effect of sleep on cardiac rhythm (Parish and Shepard 1990). The most frequent nocturnal dysrhythmia is sinus arrhythmia which is noted in 50 per cent of young individuals (see Parish and Shepard 1990). One-third of

them had sinus pauses lasting from 1.8 to 2 seconds and in another 6 per cent there were episodes of atrioventricular block. In young healthy adults sinus arrest has been noted lasting up to 9 seconds during REM sleep without associated apnoeas or significant oxygen desaturation (see Parish and Shepard 1990).

Although human studies revealed contradictory results about the effect of sleep on ventricular arrhythmia, the majority (Verrier and Kirby 1988) showed an antiarrhythmic effect of sleep on ventricular premature beats. This seems to be due to enhanced parasympathetic tone during sleep conferring protection against ventricular arrhythmia and sudden cardiac death.

There are also several reports of ventricular arrhythmias occurring during arousal from sleep. A classic example was a 14-year-old girl who was awakened from sleep by a loud auditory stimulation with ventricular tachyarrhythmia (see Verrier and Kirby 1988). This was thought to be due to an increase of sympathetic activity as the episodes could be prevented by propranolol, a β-blocker.

In patients with ischaemic heart disease, 24 h Holter monitoring may reveal several different electrocardiographic changes during sleep: ST segment depression and T-wave inversion. Nocturnal cardiac ischaemia associated with ST segment depression or elevation has been noted in some middle-aged men and also in postmenopausal women during sleep.

Sleep and sudden cardiac death

Muller et al. (1987) analysed the time of sudden cardiac death in 2203 individuals dying out of hospital in 1983. There was low incidence during the night and high incidence from 7 to 11 a.m. This pattern is similar to the incidence of non-fatal myocardial infarction and episodes of myocardial ischaemia which are more likely to occur in the morning. One suggestion is that the sudden cardiac death may result from a primary arrhythmic event. It is known that in the morning there is increased sympathetic activity which may increase myocardial electrical instability giving rise to fatal arrhythmia. Besides myocardial infarction as a risk factor for sudden cardiac death, another clinical entity, known as the congenital long QT syndrome (CLQTS), may cause syncope or sudden death. In CLQTS, ECG shows a prolonged QT interval with abnormal T and U waves, and torsade de pointes (polymorphic ventricular tachycardia).

Cardiac arrhythmias, autonomic deficits, and obstructive sleep apnoea syndrome (OSAS)

Several varieties of cardiac dysrhythmias are noted in patients with obstructive sleep apnoea syndrome (Parish and Shepard 1990). These arrhythmias are determined by the changes in autonomic nervous system. The most common is bradytachyarrhythmia alternating during apnea and immediately after termination of apnoea. The other dysrhythmias consist of the following: sinus bradycardia with less than 30 beats per minute; sinus pauses lasting for 2–13 seconds; second-degree heart block; and ventricular ectopic beats including complex and mutifocal ectopic beats, and ventricular tachycardia. There is a clear relationship between the level of oxygen saturation (SaO_2) and premature ventricular complex, and sleep apnoea syndrome. Patients with SaO_2 below 60 per cent are the most vulnerable. Hoffstein and Mateika (1994), using nocturnal polysomnography, prospectively studied 458 patients with OSAS. They found a high prevalence (58 per cent) of cardiac arrhythmias in these patients and those with arrhythmias had more severe apnoea and nocturnal hypoxaemia than those without arrhythmias.

Micieli *et al.* (1995) found evidence of mild hypofunction of both sympathetic and parasympathetic divisions of the autonomic nervous system in 5 of 13 cases with OSAS. Most reports emphasize hyperactivity of the sympathetic nervous system, causing increased plasma noradrenaline levels and urinary catecholamine secretions which are attributed to hypoxaemia associated with apnoeic episodes. Waravdekar *et al.* (1996) recorded muscle sympathetic nerve activity (MSNA) during wakefulness by using peroneal microneurography in seven patients with OSAS before and 1 month after nasal CPAP (continuous positive airway pressure) therapy. These authors found a direct linear relationship between the decrease in MSNA and treatment with CPAP. The mechanism of sympathetic overactivity and its reduction by CPAP treatment remains undetermined.

Laboratory diagnosis of sleep and respiratory dysfunction in autonomic failure

The diagnosis of primary and secondary autonomic failure is based on a combination of clinical manifestations, documentation of autonomic dysfunction, and exclusion of other causes of dysautonomia and somatic neurological diseases. Computed tomography (CT), magnetic resonance imaging, positron emission tomography using fluorodopa, electromyographic (EMG) and nerve conduction study, cerebrospinal fluid examination, and routine EEG in addition to special autonomic function studies may be necessary to establish the diagnosis. EMG of the external urethral or anal sphincter muscles may be helpful in the diagnosis of some suspected cases of MSA by showing evidence of denervation and reinnervation. Once the diagnosis of MSA or other secondary autonomic failure is made, further studies are necessary in patients suspected of sleep and respiratory dysrhythmia to diagnose and treat the specific disturbance. A thorough history and physical examination including orolaryngological examination to detect laryngeal and oropharyngeal muscle weakness should precede the special studies described.

Polysomnographic study

For the assessment of sleep and respiratory dysfunction in autonomic failure, it is important to obtain a complete polysomnographic study. To assess the severity of the sleep and respiratory disturbances, and to fully understand the structure of sleep, all-night recordings should be obtained. The study should include simultaneous recordings of multiple channels of EEG, EMG of orofacial and tibialis anterior muscles, electrocardiogram, electro-oculogram, respiratory recordings, and continuous oxygen saturation by an oximeter. Respiration can be monitored by oronasal thermistors to detect airflow and by use of an abdominal pneumograph or inductive plethysmograph (Respitrace) to detect respiratory effort. Inclusion of video polysomnographic study may be needed in some patients to diagnosis REM behaviour disorder which may occur in patients with MSA and PD.

The importance of studying the sleep architecture is that sleep may accentuate respiratory abnormalities, and respiratory dys-

function may affect sleep structure adversely; both these factors may alter the long-term course of the illness. One may also obtain 24 h ambulatory recording of sleep and breathing to assess their circadian variation.

Multiple sleep latency test

This is an objective test for assessment of daytime pathological sleepiness. This test may help in assessing the severity of daytime hypersomnolence and for monitoring the effect of treatment. In this recording, 4 or 5 daytime tests at 2-h intervals, each time lasting for 20 min, are obtained. The patients are encouraged to remain awake in between the recordings and the recording must follow a standardized protocol to validate the results of the tests adequately. Sleep onset latency and sleep onset REM are noted. Sleep onset latency of less than 5 min is indicative of pathological sleepiness.

Pulmonary function tests

In order to exclude intrinsic bronchopulmonary disease contributing to respiratory dysfunction in autonomic failure, one should obtain measurements of spirometry, lung volumes, pulmonary diffusing capacity, and blood gases. One should also measure the maximum static inspiratory and expiratory pressures. These are more important than the dynamic measurements in detecting respiratory muscle weakness. To measure the chemical control of breathing, hypercapnic or hypoxic ventilatory and mouth occlusion pressure ($Po.1$) responses, with or without load, should be studied. Mouth occlusion pressure reflects central respiratory drive and inspiratory muscle strength independent of pulmonary mechanical factors. These measurements may be impaired in patients with dysfunction of the metabolic respiratory control system.

EMG of respiratory muscles

Electrical activity of the respiratory and upper airway including genioglossus and laryngeal muscles may be obtained to assess ventilatory activity and upper airway muscle tone. Laryngeal EMG is important in patients suspected of laryngeal paresis.

Electrocardiogram (ECG)

ECG recording is essential in patients with suspected cardiac dysrhythmia or in those at high risk for developing such arrhythmias. Continuous monitoring of ECG by Holter monitoring for one or more days is required in some patients. This will give an indication about the circadian variation of the heart rate as well as the circadian influence on the cardiac dysrhythmias.

Treatment of sleep-related respiratory dysfunction

In the absence of an adequate understanding of the pathogenesis and a lack of a definite aetiological agent causing MSA and other neurodegenerative diseases, treatment remains unsatisfactory and consists of symptomatic measures only. Similarly, the pathogenesis of sleep-related respiratory dysfunction in MSA and other disorders with autonomic failure is not clearly understood; therefore, the treatment remains difficult. Repeated hypoxaemias during sleep are potentially harmful, not only to the immediate health of the patient but also to the long-term course of the illness. It is, therefore, important to diagnose and assess the type of respiratory dysrhythmia and take appropriate measures to ameliorate the disability. Improvement of the quality of life and prevention of life-threatening cardiac arrhythmias, pulmonary hypertension, and congestive heart failure should be the aim of treatment.

General measures

Reduction or elimination of the risk factors that may enhance the sleep-related respiratory dysrhythmias constitute the fundamental general principles. The patient must avoid alcohol and sedative–hypnotic drugs which may further depress the respiratory centre. The role of alcohol and sedative–hypnotic drugs in disrupting the sleep architecture and in increasing the frequency and duration of sleep apnoeas is well established but the mechanism is not known. These agents may depress genioglossal muscle activity, thus selectively promoting upper airway obstructive apnoea.

Pharmacological treatment

Ideally, this should be directed towards agents that will change the respiratory centre motor output selectively to stimulate the upper airway muscles to overcome the hypotonia of the genioglossal and other upper airway muscles, and so prevent central and obstructive apnoea. By correcting apnoea these agents might then improve the sleep architecture. However, no such selective and ideal agents have yet been found. Protriptyline, a non-sedating tricyclic antidepressant, and medroxyprogesterone acetate have been used with some success in patients with mild-to-moderate obstructive sleep apnoea. Acetazolamide has been used to treat central apnoea in MSA. However, one must be cautious because of the danger of increasing orthostatic hypotension resulting from diuresis and natriuresis. Unfortunately, these pharmacological agents have not been very helpful in patients with MSA because the natural history of the illness shows relentless progression despite treatment.

Continuous positive airway pressure (CPAP)

CPAP treatment delivered through the nose has been the most significant recent development in the treatment of patients with obstructive sleep apnoea syndrome. This treatment may be tried in patients with MSA showing predominantly obstructive or mixed sleep apnoea. One should use the lowest pressure that will be effective in decreasing the number and duration of apnoeic events. Some patients may need bilevel positive airway pressure (BiPAP) where the inspiratory and the expiratory pressure can be altered independently. CPAP uses same pressure during inspiration/expiration but in BiPAP, the expiratory pressure can be lowered and this is more comfortable in some patients who cannot tolerate CPAP. If nasal CPAP or BiPAP shows a good response during polysomnographic study in the laboratory, then this treatment may be considered in patients with moderate to severe obstructive or mixed sleep apnoea. There are several types of home CPAP or BiPAP units available for this purpose. In patients with obstructive sleep apnoea, following CPAP or BiPAP treatment there is dramatic improvement in apnoea–hypopnoea index along with amelioration of daytime hypersomnolence and correction of oxygen desaturation. However, it should be noted that the polysomnographic study will show REM rebound with increased REM density and reduction of REM latency along with marked increase of slow-wave sleep. The long-term effect of CPAP or BiPAP treatment in the usual patients of obstructive sleep apnoea syndrome is probably beneficial but cannot be stated definitely without prolonged follow-up, and the mechanism of its action is not definitely known. Patients with MSA showing obstructive sleep apnoea syndrome may show temporary improvement following the nasal CPAP or BiPAP treatment but, as stated above, the natural history of the disease is one of relentless progression and, therefore, the benefit appears to be transient.

Tracheostomy

This remains the only effective treatment, used as an emergency measure in patients with severe respiratory dysfunction accompanied by marked hypoxaemia and cyanosis, and in patients with sudden respiratory arrest after resuscitation by intubation. Tracheostomy is also the only form of treatment used successfully in patients with severe laryngeal stridor due to laryngeal abductor paralysis. An attempt should be made to wean a patient from a tracheostomy but the weaning procedure may be difficult in patients with MSA because of the progressive course of the illness.

Despite considerable advances in our understanding of MSA and the sleep and respiratory disturbances observed in this illness an effective therapy for the respiratory dysrhythmias continues to elude us. In autonomic failure other than MSA causing sleep and respiratory disturbances similar lines of treatment may be tried.

Acknowledgement

I wish to thank Errika Thompson for typing the manuscript.

References

Bannister, R. and Oppenheimer, D. R. (1972). Degenerative disease of the nervous system associated with autonomic failure. *Brain* **95**, 457–74.

Bannister, R., Gibson, W., Michaels, L., and Oppenheimer, D. R. (1981). Laryngeal abductor paralysis in multiple system atrophy. *Brain* **104**, 351–68.

Berger, A. J., Mitchel, R. A., and Severinghaus, J. N. (1977). Regulation of respiration. *New Engl. J. Med.* **297**, 138–43.

Chokroverty, S. (1991). Functional anatomy of the autonomic nervous system: autonomic dysfunction and disorders of the CNS. In Correlative nevroanatomy and nevropathology for the clinical neurologist. American Academy of Nevrology Course No. 144. American Academy of Nevrology, Minneapolis.

Chokroverty, S. (1999). Sleep, breathing and neurological disorders. In *Sleep disorders medicine: basic science, technical considerations and clinical aspects*, 2nd edition, (ed. S. Chokroverty), Butterworth–Heinemann, Boston.

Chokroverty, S. (1996). Sleep and degenerative neurologic disorders. In *Sleep disorders II*, (ed. M. S. Aldrich), pp. 807–26. W. B. Saunders, Philadelphia.

Chokroverty, S., Barron, K. D., Katz, F. M., Del Greco, F., and Sharp, J. T. (1969). The syndrome of primary orthostatic hypotension. *Brain* 92, 743–68.

Chokroverty, S., Sharp, J. T., and Barron, K. D. (1978). Periodic respiration in erect posture in Shy–Drager syndrome. *J. Neurol. Neurosurg. Psychiat.* 41, 980–6.

Chokroverty, S., Sachdeo, R., and Masdeu, J. (1984). Autonomic dysfunction and sleep apnea in olivopontocerebellar degeneration. *Arch. Neurol.* 41, 926–31.

Gadoth, N., Solol, J., and Lavie, P. (1983). Sleep structure and nocturnal disordered breathing in familial dysautonomia. *J. Neurol. Sci.* 60, 117–25.

Guilleminault, C., Briskin, J. G., Greenfield, M. S., and Silvestri, R. (1981). The impact of autonomic nervous system dysfunction on breathing during sleep. Sleep 4, 263–78.

Hoffstein, V. and Mateika, S. (1994). Cardiac arrhythmias, snoring and sleep apnea. *Chest* 106, 466–71.

Lockwood, A. H. (1976). Shy–Drager syndrome with abnormal respirations and antidiuretic hormone release. *Arch. Neurol.* 33, 292–5.

Loewy, A. D. and Spyer, K. M. (1990). *Central regulation of autonomic functions.* Oxford University Press, Oxford.

McNicholas, W. T., Rutherford, R., Grossman, R., Moldofsky, H., Zamel, N., and Phillipson, E. A. (1983). Abnormal respiratory pattern generation during sleep in patients with autonomic dysfunction. *Am. Rev. Respir. Dis.* 128, 429–33.

Medori, R., Tritchler, H. J., LeBlanca, A. *et al.* (1992). Fatal familial insomnia is a prion disease with a mutation at codon 178 of the prion diseases. *New Engl. J. Med.* 326, 444–9.

Micieli, G., Manni, R., Tassorelli, C. *et al.* (1995). Sleep-apnea and autonomic dysfunction: a cardiopressor and pupillometric study. *Acta Neurol. Scand.* 91, 382–8.

Muller, J. E., Ludmer, P. L., Willich, S. N. *et al.* (1987). Circadian variation in the frequency of sudden cardiac death. *Circulation* 75, 131–8

Munschauer, F. E., Loh, L., Bannister, R., and Newsom-Davis, J. (1990). Abnormal respiration and sudden death during sleep in multiple system atrophy with autonomic failure. *Neurology* 40, 677–9.

Parish, J. M. and Shepard, J. W., Jr (1990). Cardiovascular effects of sleep disorders. *Chest* 97, 1220–6.

Rees, P. J., Cochrane, G. M., Prior, J. G., and Clark, T. J. H. (1981). Sleep apnea in diabetic patients with autonomic neuropathy. *J. R. Soc. Med.* 74, 192–5.

Sadaoka T., Kakitsuba, N., Fujiwara, Y. *et al.* (1996). Sleep-related breathing disorders in patients with multiple system atrophy and vocal fold palsy. *Sleep* 19, 479–84.

Schenck, C. H. and Mahowald, M. W. (1996). Delayed emergence of a parkinsonian disorder in 38% of 29 older males initially diagnosed with idiopathic REM sleep behavior disorder. *Neurology* 46; 388–93.

Shy, G. M. and Drager, G. A. (1960). A neurological syndrome associated with orthostatic hypotension. *Arch. Neurol., Chicago* 2, 511–27.

Strohl, K. P. (1996). Diabetes and sleep apnea. *Sleep* 19, s225–s228.

Verrier, R. L. and Kirby, D. A. (1988). Sleep and cardiac arrhythmias. *Ann. New York Acad. Sci.* 533, 238–51.

Waravdekar, N. V., Sinoway, L. I., Zwillich, C. W. *et al.* (1996). Influence of treatment on muscle sympathetic nerve activity in sleep apnea. *Am. J. Respir. Crit. Care Med.* 153, 1333–8.

27. Evaluation of sudomotor function

Phillip A. Low and Robert D. Fealey

Introduction

Anatomy and physiology of sweating

Thermoreceptors are present in the preoptic-anterior hypothalamus area, in skin, in viscera and in spinal cord. In addition to the spino-thalamic tract afferent pathways ascend as multisynaptic fibres diffusely in lateral spinal cord, to reticular formation of brainstem and finally to hypothalamus and thalamus. These signals are integrated in the posterior hypothalamus where a set-point is established.

Efferent pathways as crossed and uncrossed fibres from the hypo-thalamus travel via the tegmentum of the pons and the lateral reticular substance of the medulla to the intermediolateral column. Recent studies indicate that many fiber connections are polysynaptic.

The intermediolateral column neurones, are cholinergic and synapse with paravertebral sympathetic ganglia from whence post-ganglionic sympathetic cholinergic sudomotor axons supply eccrine sweat glands. There are about 5000 preganglionic neurones per segment of thoracic cord in humans and there is an attrition rate of 5–7 per cent per decade (Low *et al.* 1977).

There are less precise sudomotor than sensory dermatomes since a single ganglion receives fibres from 5–6 preganglionic levels and skin is multi-innervated. Approximate sudomotor dermatomes are: T1–2, ipsilateral face; T2–6, upper limb; T5–12, trunk; T10–L3, lower limb. As a rule, concordance of sudomotor dermatomes is good once post-ganglionic fibres enter the nerve trunk but poor proximal to that.

There are two types of sweat glands, eccrine and apocrine (Ogawa and Low 1993). The eccrine sweat glands are simple, tubular glands that extend down from the epidermis to the lower dermis. The lower portion is a tightly coiled secretory apparatus consisting of two types of cells. One is a dark basophilic cell that secretes mucous material and the other a light acidophilic cell that is responsible for the passage of water and electrolytes. Surrounding the secretory cells are myo-epithelial cells, which are thought to aid the expulsion of sweat by contraction. These glands receive a rich supply of blood vessels and sympathetic nerve fibres, but are unusual in that sympathetic innervation is cholinergic. The full complement of eccrine glands develops in the embryonic state (Kuno 1956). No new glands develop after birth.

The postganglionic sweat response fails progressively with increasing age (Low 1997*b*). We evaluated 357 normal subjects aged 10–83 years, evenly distributed by age and gender. There is a proximo-distal gradient of severity. All lower-extremity sites, measured by the quantative sudomoter axon reflex rest (QSART), underwent a significant reduction with age ($P < 0.001$) with a slope of 0.02 $\mu l/cm^2/year$ for proximal leg and foot and 0.03 $\mu l/cm^2$

for the distal leg. The sweat loss is associated with a loss of cholinergic unmyelinated fibre stained with the panaxonal marker PGP9.5 & AChE (Abdel-Rahman *et al.* 1992).

The distribution of eccrine glands shows area differences (Kuno 1956), with the greatest density in the palms and soles. They vary in density from 400/mm² on the palm to about 80/cm² on the thighs and upper arm and least in the back. The total numbers are approximately 2–5 million (Kuno 1956). They weigh is about 30–40 μg each (Sato and Sato 1983).

The physiology of the human sweat response is known from the detailed *in vitro* studies of Sato *et al.* (1993). Acetylcholine secretion results in the production of an ultrafiltrate (isotonic) by the secretory coil. Directly collected sweat has identical Na$^+$ and K$^+$ values to plasma. Reabsorption of sodium ions by the eccrine sweat duct results in hypotonic sweat. Directly collected sweat from the proximal duct is hypotonic (Na$^+$, 20–80 mM; K$^+$, 5–25 mM) (Sato and Sato 1983). Extracellular Ca^{2+} is important since removal of periglandular Ca^{2+} with [ethylene-bis(oxy-ethylenenitrilo)] tetraacaic acid (EGTA) completely inhibits sweat secretion, while the calcium ionophore A23187 strongly and persistently stimulates sweating (Sato and Sato 1983). Magnesium ions appear to be unimportant.

Sato and Sato (1983) made additional key observations on isolated human eccrine sweat gland regulation. The regulation of sweating is cholinergic and muscarinic since it is completely inhibited by atropine. Sudomotor function is metabolically active. It is inhibited by cold (4 °C) and involves active transport, being inhibited by ouabain and by the metabolic inhibitors, cyanide or dinitrophenol (DNP). The prostaglandin, PGE$_1$, has sudorific effect *in vitro* comparable to acetylcholine (ACh) and was thought to act via cyclic AMP (cAMP). Microtubules may be important since vinblastine strongly but reversibly inhibits sweating. Endogenous cAMP appears to be the second messenger, since theophylline, by inhibiting phosphodiesterase, markedly increases the sweat response.

The major function of the sweat gland in humans is thermo-regulatory. With repeated episodes of profuse sweating, the salt content of the sweat declines progressively. In the individual acclimatized to a hot climate the salt content is reduced, probably reflecting an increase of mineralocorticoids in response to thermal stress (Kuno 1956).

The long efferent course of autonomic sudomotor fibres can be interrupted by autonomic disorders, both central and peripheral, and results in an impairment of the sweat response. This impairment can be evaluated using the thermoregulatory sweat test (TST). The post-ganglionic fibres can be evaluated using the quantitative sudomotor axon reflex (QSART) and related tests.

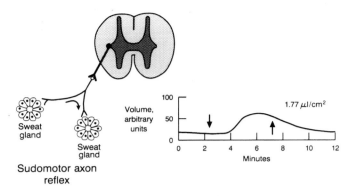

Fig. 27.1. Left: The neural substrate for the axon-reflex sweat response. Right: A representative axon-reflex sweat response. (From Low *et al.* (1992).)

Tests of sudomotor function

Quantitative sudomotor axon reflex test (QSART)

The principle of the test can be gathered from Fig. 27.1. When post-ganglionic sympathetic terminals are stimulated, an antidromic impulse occurs, reaches a branch-point, then travels orthodromically to release acetylcholine from a nerve terminal. Acetylcholine traverses the neuroglandular junction and binds to M_3 muscarinic receptors on eccrine sweat glands (Torres *et al.* 1991) to evoke the sweat response. Acetylcholinesterase in subcutaneous tissue cleaves acetylcholine to acetate and choline, resulting in its inactivation and cessation of the sweat response. Other neurotransmitters, such as calcitonin-gene-related polypeptide (CGRP) play an important subsidiary role. To avoid direct stimulation of the sweat gland, the stimulus and recording compartments are anatomically separated within a multicompartmental sweat cell, with the recording compartment in the centre,

surrounded by the stimulus compartment, separated by an air-gap (Fig. 27.2). The stimulus is iontophoresed acetylcholine and a constant current of 2 mA for 5 mins is delivered. The sweat response is measured by a sudorometer which determines the sweat volume.

The tests are sensitive and reproducible in controls (Low 1997*a*) and in patients with diabetic neuropathy (Low *et al.* 1986; Low 1997*a*). Tests repeated on two different days regress with a high coefficient of regression. Tests repeated daily to the identical site may evoke local skin alterations, possibly to the sweat duct after about the third or fourth repetition but this 'tolerance' is highly variable. The coefficient of variation is 20 per cent or less (Low 1997*a*).

The recordings are symmetrical so that in normal individuals, the left side is not significantly different to the right. We routinely record from the left but will study the right side when clinically warranted, e.g. following left sural nerve biopsy, or with unilateral symptoms. Four standard recording sites are the medial forearm, the proximal leg, distal leg, and the proximal foot (on a flat surface over the extensor digitorum brevis muscle). The innervation of the forearm, proximal leg, distal leg and proximal foot are by ulnar, peroneal, saphenous, and sural (mainly) nerves, respectively.

The most common abnormality is a loss of sweat volume. A length-dependent neuropathy is typically associated with a loss of sweat volume that is maximal distally (Fig. 27.3). Acute preganglionic nerve lesions result in anhidrosis on the thermoregulatory sweat test, with normal QSART. With long-standing preganglionic denervation, QSART volumes are also reduced. For instance, postganglionic sudomotor failure occurred at the forearm in 50 per cent each of PAF (postganglionic) and MSA (preganglionic) patients and at the foot in 69 per cent and 66 per cent of PAF and MSA patients, respectively (Cohen *et al.* 1987).

Since QSART volumes vary with age and gender (Low 1997*b*), we developed a composite autonomic scoring scale (CASS) that corrects for the confounding effects of age and gender (Low 1993). The sudomotor subset is scored for 0 (no deficit) to 3 (maximal deficit).

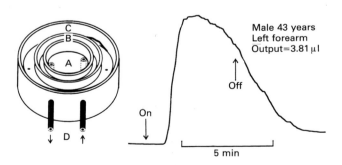

Fig. 27.2. Multicompartmental sweat cell (left) and evoked sweat response (right). The capsule is strapped on to skin, and acetylcholine (compartment C) is iontophoresed using a constant current generator with the anode connected to compartment C. Axon reflex evoked sweat response in compartment A is evaporated off by a stream of nitrogen at a controlled flow rate and quantitated dynamically by a sudorometer. Compartment B and associated ridges prevent diffusion and leakage of acetylcholine. (From Low, (1986) with permission).

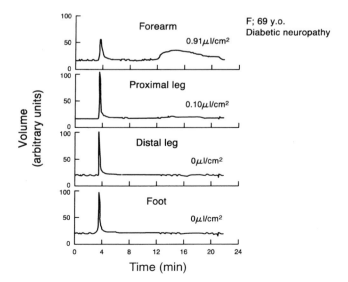

Fig. 27.3 Quantitative sudomotor axon reflex test volumes are normal over forearm and reduced over the entire lower extremity in a patient with diabetic neuropathy. (From Low (1996) with permission).

Disorders of sweating

QSART recordings have been performed in many disorders, including diabetic neuropathy (Low *et al.* 1986), Sjogren's syndrome, Lambert– Eaton myasthenic syndrome, distal small fibre neuropathy (Stewart *et al.* 1992), atopic dermatitis, ageing, idiopathic autonomic neuropathy (Suarez *et al.* 1994) and distal small fibre neuropathy (Stewart *et al.* 1992), acute panautonomic neuroathy (Suarez *et al.* 1994) and Parkinson's disease and related extra-pyramidal and cerebellar disorders (Sandroni *et al.* 1991), a gamut of neuropathies (Low and McLeod 1997), in MSA and PAF (Cohen *et al.* 1987), chronic idiopathic anhidrosis (Low *et al.* 1985), and in studying the pharmacology of sweating (Low *et al.* 1992).

We have reported data based on 26 patients with PAF, 60 patients with PD, 70 patients with mild MSA (MSA-I), 100 patients with classic MSA (MSA-II), and 51 patients with PD with associated autonomic failure (PD-AF). All cases have been evaluated by a neurologist, and quantitative tests of autonomic function to evaluate the severity and distribution of sudomotor, cardiovagal, and adrenergic function were undertaken, and a composite autonomic scoring scale (CASS) was derived, which corrects for the confounding effects of age and gender. In an initial study, confined to MSA and PAF patients (Cohen *et al.* 1987), there was no difference in percentage anhidrosis on thermoregulatory sweat test (TST; >70 per cent anhidrosis). QSART indicated postganglionic sudomotor impairment in the lower extremity in more than 65 per cent of both MSA and PAF patients. In a study on the sensitivity and specificity of CASS in the diagnosis of autonomic failure, we compared MSA (*n*=18), autonomic neuropathy, PD (*n*=20), and common neuropathy (without clinical autonomic failure), CASS for MSA, autonomic neuropathy, and PD were 8.5 ± 1.3, 8.6 ± 1.2, and 1.5 ± 1.1, respectively. All patients with MSA had scores greater than 4 and all patients with PD, less than 4; with 89 per cent of MSA patients having scores above 7.

However, in a review of a larger group of patients referred to the autonomic laboratory (Sandroni *et al.* 1991), comprising PD (*N* = 35), PD-AF (*N* = 54), MSA-I (*N* = 73), and MSA-II (*N* = 75), a range of autonomic failure was found. Clinical autonomic failure was 11 per cent, 83 per cent, 89 per cent, and 100 per cent for PD, PD-AF, MSA-I, and MSA-II, respectively. QSART was reduced in the lower extremity in 40 per cent, 55 per cent, 66 per cent and 70 per cent, respectively. Corresponding values for percentage anhidrosis on TST were 39 per cent, 63 per cent, 72 per cent and 85 per cent, respectively. A similar gradation in cardiovagal and adrenergic function was also found. This gradation seems to translate into outcome. Time in years to evolve from onset to Hoehn–Yahr stage IV was 9.5, 5.1, 4.8, and 3.4 years, respectively. The conclusion was that MSA and PAF are definable, but that it is important to recognize gradations, and that autonomic function tests are helpful in defining these intermediate types.

The nicotinic (indirect or axon-reflex) versus the muscarinic (direct) response in normal subjects and patients with diabetic neuropathy has been compared (Kihara *et al.* 1993). Using a specially designed multicompartmental sweat cell and dual sudorometers, we were able to record the evoked the direct and indirect responses simultaneously. In control subjects, sudorometric direct recordings were consistently larger than axon-reflex mediated responses. There was no difference in sweat droplet density by sex, but the size of droplets was larger in males. In diabetic patients 3 of 23 had absent axon-reflex but preserved direct reponses. Patients with mild neuropathy had an overrepresentation of large-diameter droplets in the silastic imprints, while patients with severe neuropathy had a markedly reduced density and small-diameter droplets.

Thermoregulatory sweat test (TST)

TST provides a sweat stimulus via raised blood and mean skin temperature. The efferent sympathetic response is mediated by pre-ganglionic centres including the hypothalamus, bulbospinal pathways, the intermediolateral cell columns, and white rami; postganglionic paths include the sympathetic chain and postganglionic sudomotor nerves to sweat glands.

The TST conducted in the Mayo Thermoregulatory Laboratory is a modification of Guttmann's quinizarin sweat test (Guttmann 1947). Unclothed subjects lie supine on a cart and the exposed body surface (exclusive of eyes, nose, mouth, and genitalia) is covered with an indicator powder mixture (alizarin red, sodium carbonate, and cornstarch; Fealey *et al.* 1989; Fealey 1996). Subjects are totally enclosed in the sweat cabinet for 45–65 mins (air temperature 44–50 °C, relative humidity 35–45 per cent) and skin temperature is carefully maintained between 39 and 40 °C via overhead infrared heaters. This skin temperature range is critical to recruiting a maximal central response yet is not so high as to cause skin injury, direct sweat gland activation, or somatosympathetic reflex sweating below the level of the lesion (i.e. in complete cervical cord transection). The humidity is regulated to be moderate and the heating time no greater than 70 min, in order to avoid hydromeiosis (Fealey 1996). The oral temperature is monitored continuously and must rise to at least 38.0 °C or by 1.0 °C above baseline temperature, whichever yields the higher value. For normal subjects the mean temperature rise during the TST is 1.2 °C and the average heating time 45 mins. All normal individuals show relatively uniform sweating over the entire body surface, with characteristic areas of heavier or lighter sweating (Fealey 1996).

The sweat distribution is documented by digital photography of the body surface and colour digital pictures are made on standard anatomical drawings for use in report generation. The digital images are also processed by a colour pixel counter to derive an accumulative value for the area of anhidrosis and the percentage of anhidrosis (TST per cent). Alternatively a planimeter (LASICO, model 1252M, resolution = 0.005 cm^2) can be used, with measurement of areas directly from the anatomical drawing. TST per cent is the measured area of anhidrosis divided by the area of the anatomic figure, multiplied by 100. Normal sweat distributions and TST per cent have been published (Fealey *et al.* 1989; Fealey 1996).

Disorders of sweating

Widespread anhidrosis is characteristic of MSA and PAF (see Chapter 31). Cohen *et al.* (1987) found median values of body surface anhidrosis (TST%) of 97 and 91 per cent, respectively. Representative sweat distributions are shown in Fig. 27.4.

We have shown that the severity of clinical autonomic failure in patients with extrapyramidal and cerebellar system disorders regressed significantly with TST per cent (Sandroni *et al.* 1991). The orthostatic blood pressure decrement and TST per cent were found to have a near identical rank order of severity by disease category, being milder for Parkinson's disease and progressive supranuclear palsy and severe for MSA.

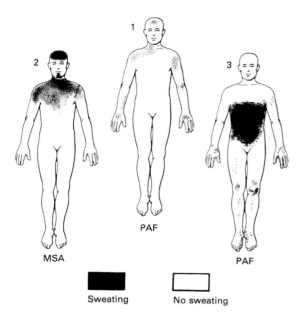

Thermoregulatory sweating abnormalities
in pure autonomic failure (PAF) and multiple system atrophy with autonomic failure (MSA; Shy–Drager syndrome)

Sweating   No sweating

Fig. 27.4. Thermoregulatory sweat test results showing characteristic anhidrosis in MSA and PAF. (From Cohen *et al.* (1987).)

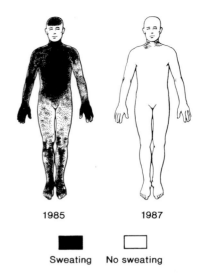

1985   1987

Sweating   No sweating

Fig. 27.5. Progressive sweat test in a patient with an L-dopa responsive, extrapyramidal disorder and mild orthostatic hypotension in 1985 and severe MSA unresponsive to L-dopa with disabling autonomic failure by 1987.

In recent years (1993–97) referrals of patients with 'rule out early MSA' for autonomic testing has increased. Many of these patients are originally diagnosed as having Parkinson's disease but over several years they begin to develop orthostatic hypotension, decreased response to L-dopa, and sleep disturbances. Mild cerebellar and pyramidal findings are often present on their initial exam. Analysis of the extent of anhidrosis in these cases (*n* = 98) reveals mean values of only 67 per cent for the TST per cent. The mean age of these subjects is 67 years and the average temperature rise during the sweat test is 1.9 °C over 48 mins. Progression of sweat loss (Fig. 27.5) has been noted in some of these subjects on serial studies. Initial sweat distributions that portend the occurrence of generalized autonomic failure include regional anhidrosis of the lower legs or of the lower abdomen and legs. Many have some sweating of the distal feet and relatively preserved postganglionic sweat responses (QSART) in areas of TST anhidrosis (the combination of which suggests a preganglionic lesion). Patients who are clinically pure Parkinson's disease, on the other hand, usually have mild distal impairment of sweating on both TST and QSART.

As pathological studies have indicated different anatomical sites of autonomic neuronal degeneration in MSA versus PD versus PAF, at least early on, and prognosis and treatment responses vary with the diagnosis, combined TST/QSART determinations may help to identify early cases of each category, allowing for better predictability of prognosis and response to current and future treatment strategies.

Sympathetic skin response

Skin potential recordings can be used to detect sympathetic sudomotor deficit in the peripheral neuropathies and central autonomic disorders (Shahani *et al.* 1984; Schondorf 1997). The recording electrodes are commonly electrode pairs 1 cm in diameter applied to the dorsal and ventral surfaces of the foot, the hand, or the thighs. The stimulus might be an inspiratory gasp, a cough, a loud noise, or an electric shock. The sources of the skin potential are the sweat gland and the epidermis (Edelberg 1967). It is important to recognize that sudomotor function and skin potential evaluate similar but not identical functions. Human studies have been limited to pharmacological dissection in very few subjects. A reasonable interpretation of studies in mammals, including humans, are that a component of the skin potential (early fast changes) is related to sweating, but that the later changes are due to skin potential changes. The latter can occur in patients who have congenital absence of sweat glands (Lloyd 1961; Shaver *et al.* 1962).

The major advantage of the method is its simplicity so that it can be used in any neurophysiology laboratory. The disadvantages are its enormous variability and the tendency of the responses to habituate although claims for low coefficient of variation have appeared (Levy *et al.* 1992). The responses vary with the recording system, composition of the electrolyte paste, stimulus frequency, age, temperature, stress, status of central structures, and the effects of hormones and drugs (Low 1984).

Following peripheral nerve section, skin potentials are no longer obtainable in the affected dermatome on direct and reflex stimulation. There was usually associated hypothermia and anhidrosis. Following sympathectomy, skin potentials are also lost, but only temporarily, returning in 4–6 months (Sourek 1965).

There is general agreement that a loss of SSR is abnormal. There is some controversy as to whether a reduction of skin potential or a reductions in latency are reliable abnormalities. There is some evidence that unmyelinated fibres conduct without slowing or not at all (Tzeng *et al.* 1993). The test has been reported to correlate well with QSART (Maselli *et al.* 1989), but in our experience it is often present when QSART is clearly impaired. Potentials are reported to become reduced with ageing (Drory and Korczyn 1993).

Disorders of sweating

SSR has been utilized in the evaluation of the peripheral neuropathies, especially diabetic neuropathy (Knezevic and Bajada 1985). The SSR deficit in amplitude and volume is reported to worsen with increasing duration of diabetes and correlates with sweatspot values (Levy et al. 1992) and clinical neuropathy (Braune and Horter 1996). Both amplitude reduction and latency prolongation were seen and abnormalities may precede clinical neuropathy (Braune and Horter 1996). SSR in the foot is abnormal or absent in the majority of patients with well-established neuropathy (Niakan and Harati 1988). For instance, in a study of 72 diabetic patients with electrophysiologically confirmed sensorimotor peripheral neuropathy, SSR was absent in 83 per cent. A statistically significant correlation was found between the Valsalva test abnormality, the degree of peripheral neuropathy, and the SSR (Niakan and Harati 1988). Its sensitivity and specificity to detect early abnormalities or to detect improvement in clinical trials, have not been established.

SSR are reported to be asymmetrical in amplitude or latency in patients with peripheral complex regional pain syndrome (CARP I), previously known as reflex sympathetic dystrophy (Drory and Korczyn 1995). These reports documented either an increase or reduction in amplitude, and suggested that the changes supported the involvement of sympathetic dysfunction in CARP I. Asymmetry should be interpreted with caution in patients who have central nervous system involvement, since lesions of the central pathways are known to cause asymmetry (Korpelainen et al. 1993).

SSR in patients with Parkinson's disease and multiple system atrophy (MSA) have been compared. The frequency of abnormalities in Parkinson's disease is relatively modest, occurring in 8–38 per cent of patients (Wang et al. 1993). These changes are dramatically more marked in patients with MSA or pure autonomic failure (PAF) (Baser et al. 1991) where abnormalities are present in at least two-thirds of patients.

Sweat imprint

Kennedy and colleagues have systematically measured the number and size of sweat droplets activated in response to direct chemical stimulation (Kennedy et al. 1984a,b). The workers used a silastic imprint material that hardens over 1 or 2 minutes, the hardening time varying with the composition of the silastic. They stimulated sweating by a number of methods in the experimental animal and in humans. The most reliable method was the iontophoresis of pilocarpine (Kennedy et al. 1984a,b). They recorded from the same population of sweat glands. The method appears to detect sweat gland failure reliably in diabetic neuropathy.

Disorders of sweating

In a study of 81 diabetic and 30 control subjects, these workers found that many diabetic patients had a reduced number of excitable sweat glands and a low volume of sweat per square centimetre of skin. The results of the sweat tests correlated best with the clinically determined perception of pain from pin-prick. The similar degree of involvement of sudomotor axons and pain-conveying axons may be related to the known similarity in size and reinnervation patterns. There was poor correlation of the sweating deficiency with α motor conduction velocity and with denervation of foot muscles, as determined by the evoked muscle action potential. In another report, where both the silastic sweat imprint and an evaporimeter weres used (Kennedy and Navarro 1989) in 357 type I diabetic patients, the number of active sweat glands was below normal in the hands of 24 per cent of patients and in the feet of 56 per cent, in the foot, while the sweat evaporation rate was low in 17 per cent and 40 per cent of patients, respectively. Computerized analysis of the moulds, which allowed automatic sweat gland counts and estimations of the secretion volume of each sweat gland, detected abnormalities in 36 per cent and 60 per cent of patients. The silastic imprint technique was found to be a sensitive test for detection of sympathetic nerve involvement, even in asymptomatic patients with normal clinical and nerve conduction examinations. Its sensitivity and accuracy has been enhanced by the computerized analysis of the moulds.

Anhidrosis

There are many neurological and some non-neurological causes of anhidrosis and hyperhidrosis. Table 27.1 summarizes the causes, with examples, sites of the lesion and proposed mechanisms of the major causes of anhidrosis. Some characteristic patterns are seen (Fealey 1997). Distal anhidrosis is commonly seen in the peripheral neuropathies and is almost invariably due to postganglionic denervation. When more widespread anhidrosis occurs, e.g. in some cases of amyloid and in diabetic neuropathy, there could be a component of preganglionic anhidrosis.

Global anhidrosis may be central (as in Shy–Drager, idiopathic orthostatic hypotension) or peripheral (as in acute panautonomic neuropathy and Tangier disease). Global anhidrosis with sparing of hands and feet is usually central and may occur not infrequently in PAF and multiple system atrophy.

Lesions of peripheral nerves (root, plexus, trunk or twigs) usually result in sweat impairment of dermatomal distribution. The anhidrosis resulting from sympathectomy has been well described (Fealey 1997). A complete interruption of sympathetic efferent pathways from the hypothalamus to the intermediolateral column of the spinal cord results in hemi-anhidrosis. However, most lesions of brainstem or spinal cord (such as syringomyelia or neoplasms) result in incomplete hemi-anhidrosis since sympathetic efferent bundles are not well compacted.

Skin lesions of various types may damage sweat glands or plug sweat ducts resulting in anhidrosis sometimes with associated compensatory hyperhidrosis of remaining sweat glands.

Hyperhidrosis

Hyperhidrosis may result from lesions of the brain, spinal cord, or peripheral nerves. It can also occur in non-neurological disorders (Table 27.2). Examples of the latter include phaeochromocytoma, thyrotoxicosis, or with lymphomas and certain chronic infectious illnesses, where the neural pathways are intact but the central drive is increased or there is overactivity of certain humoral factors, such as thyroxine, catecholamines, cytokines, or vasoactive intestinal polypeptide.

Damaged peripheral nerves, especially small-diameter fibres, are prone to fire spontaneously. Factors enhancing spontaneous activity

Table 27.1.   Causes and pattern of anhidrosis with examples and proposed mechanisms

Causes	Examples	Pattern	Mechanism
Primary AF	Multiple system atrophy Pure autonomic failure	Global ± acral sparing	Preganglionic denervation Postganglionic denervation
CNS disease	Brain tumour Strokes Traumatic SC injury	Segmental, global or regional	Preganglionic denervation
PNS disease	Distal small fibre neuropathy Diabetic neuropathy Panautonomic neuropathy Chronic idiopathic anhidrosis	Distal Variable Global Global or regional	Postganglionic denervation Postganglionic denervation Postganglionic denervation Postganglionic denervation
Iatrogenic	Anticholinergic medications Sympathectomy	Global Regional typically	Sweat gland postganglionic
Skin lesions	Leprosy Radiation injury	Multifocal Focal	Nerve terminals Sweat gland injury

AF, autonomic failure; CNS, central nervous system; PNS, peripheral nervous system; SC, spinal cord.

include increased sympathetic drive, α-adrenergic activation, mechanostimulation, and nerve microenvironmental perturbations, such as hyperkalaemia. The peripheral neuropathies, especially the toxic and certain metabolic ones (e.g. thallium, arsenic, acrylamide poisoning, and painful diabetic neuropathy), usually have a phase of distal hyperhidrosis, coldness, and pain. Nerve root or plexus irritation may result in a phase of hyperhidrosis followed by an anhidrotic lesion with surrounding hyperhidrosis. A less-pronounced perilesional hyperhidrosis may occur with spinal cord lesion at the edge of the sensory loss, suggesting that central mechanisms may also be involved.

Gustatory sweating following a partial nerve lesion may occur in diabetic neuropathy. The sweating is thought to result from fibre damage with misdirected regeneration, so that a taste stimulus results in excessive sweating. A cardinal feature of reflex sympathetic dystrophy is increased sympathetic traffic with hyperhidrosis.

When a large portion of eccrine sweat glands are denervated, peripherally or centrally, the remaining glands undergo increased sweat secretion and compensatory hyperhidrosis results. This phenomenon may occur with central structural lesions as in cerebral infarction, brain tumours, or following head trauma. Peripheral denervation following

extensive sympathectomy also may result in compensatory hyperhidrosis. Extensive sweat gland disease also may impose an increased secretory burden on remaining sweat glands.

Essential or primary hyperhidrosis is a distressing condition, characterized by excessive sweating of eccrine sweat glands. The sites affected are mainly the hands, axillae, and feet. Onset is early, especially pronounced by the teens, and becomes less by the fourth or fifth decade. The volume of sweat output can be extremely high and can exceed 30 ml/h. Clinically, the sites are confined to those mentioned above, but quantitatively there is generalized hyperhidrosis. Some cases are clinically generalized. The pathophysiology appears to be an exaggerated response to emotional sweating. There is increased sympathetic drive and possibly hypertrophied sweat glands. Patients are typically introverted and anxious. The constant dripping causes social distress. Maceration of skin is not uncommon. A positive family history is present in one-quarter to one-half of the patients (Khurana 1997). It likely has an autosomal dominant inheritance with incomplete penetrance.

Treatment is unsatisfactory, consisting of local treatments, medications, and surgical procedures. Local treatment with iontophoresis of tap water halves the sweat secretion. However, it

Table 27.2.   Causes of hyperhidrosis

Cause	Examples	Pattern	Mechanism
Primary	Primary hyperhidrosis	Acral and axillary	Unknown, ? central
Systemic or neoplastic	Thyroxicosis Lymphoma Phaeochromocytoma	unknown	unknown
CNS disease	Shapiro's syndrome Idiopathic paroxysmal hyperhidrosis	unknown	unknown
PNS disease	Painful peripheral neuropathies Perilesional hyperhidrosis Compensatory hyperhidrosis Gustatory sweating	unknown	unknown
Iatrogenic	Medications and drugs	unknown	unknown

does so by the plugging up of sweat pores. The local application of 20 per cent aluminum chloride hexahydrate in 95 per cent ethyl alcohol yields comparable results. Botulinum toxin will block the autonomic transmission in sympathetic cholinergic fibres to sweat glands. Other local topical therapy has included aluminum chloride, formalin, glutaraldehyde, and topical propantheline bromide. Talc, starch, and other powders have been suggested to absorb excessive sweat. Scopolamine patches have also been used successfully in some patients.

Drug treatment of hyperhidrosis is unsatisfactory but can provide partial improvement for a few hours. Drugs that have been used include anticholinergics such as propantheline and α-adrenergic blocking agents such as phenoxybenzamine. Other drugs have included methantheline bromide, alone or in combination with ergoloid mesylates, mecamylamine, atropine, and propoxyphenel. Other agents that have been used include dibenamine, piperoxan, and phentolamine.

A number of approaches to surgical sympathectomy are in use. All modern approaches lesion the sympathetic outflow below T1. Surgical approaches include the bilateral suction-assisted lipolysis technique, bilateral upper dorsal sympathectomy via the supraclavicular approach, thoracoscopic sympathicolysis, and percutaneous radiofrequency upper thoracic sympathectomy. Sympathetic ganglion blockade has been suggested as an alternative. Compensatory and gustatory sweating were the most frequently stated reasons for dissatisfaction.

References

Abdel-Rahman, T. A., Collins, K. J., Cowen, T., and Rustin, M. (1992). Immunohistochemical, morphological and functional changes in the peripheral sudomotor neuro-effector system in elderly people. *J. autonom. nerv. Syst.* 37, 187–197.

Baser, S. M., Meer, J., Polinsky, R. J., and Hallett, M. (1991). Sudomotor function in autonomic failure. *Neurology* 41, 1564–66.

Braune, H. J. and Horter, C. (1996). Sympathetic skin response in diabetic neuropathy: a prospective clinical and neurophysiological trial on 100 patients. *J. Neurol. Sci.* 138, 120–4.

Cohen, J., Low, P., Fealey, R., Sheps, S., and Jiang, N.-S. (1987). Somatic and autonomic function in progressive autonomic failure and multiple system atrophy. *Ann. Neurol.* 22, 692–9.

Drory, V. E. and Korczyn, A. D. (1993). Sympathetic skin response: age effect. *Neurology* 43, 1818–20.

Drory, V. E. and Korczyn, A. D. (1995). The sympathetic skin response in reflex sympathetic dystrophy. *J. Neurol. Sci.* 128, 92–5.

Edelberg, R. (1967). Electrical properties of the skin. In *Methods in Psychophysiology*, (ed. C. C. Brown), pp. 1–52. Williams and Wilkins, Baltimore.

Fealey, R. D. (1996). Thermoregulatory sweat test. In *Clinical neurophysiology* (ed. J. R. Daube), pp. 396–402. F. A. Davis Co, Philadelphia.

Fealey, R. D. (1997). Thermoregulatory sweat test. In *Clinical autonomic disorders: evaluation and management* (ed. P. A. Low), (2nd edn), pp. 245–57. Lippincott-Raven, New York.

Fealey, R. D., Low, P. A., and Thomas, J. E. (1989). Thermoregulatory sweating abnormalities in diabetes mellitus. *Mayo Clin. Proc.* 64, 617–28.

Guttmann, L. (1947). The management of the quinizarin sweat test (QST). *Postgrad. Med. J.* 23, 353–66.

Kennedy, W. R. and Navarro, X. (1989). Sympathetic sudomotor function in diabetic neuropathy. *Arch. Neurol.* 46, 1182–6.

Kennedy, W. R., Sakuta, M., Sutherland, D., and Goetz, F. C. (1984a). Quantitation of the sweating deficit in diabetes mellitus. *Ann. Neurol.* 15, 482–8.

Kennedy, W. R., Sakuta, M., Sutherland, D., and Goetz, F. C. (1984b). The sweating deficiency in diabetes mellitus: methods of quantitation and clinical correlation. *Neurology* 34, 758–63.

Khurana, R. (1997). Acral sympathetic dysfunction and hyperhidrosis. In *Clinical autonomic disorders: evaluation and management* (ed. P. A. Low), (2nd edn), pp. 809–18. Lippincott-Raven, New York.

Kihara, M., Opfer-Gehrking, T. L., and Low, P. A. (1993). Comparison of directly stimulated with axon reflex-mediated sudomotor responses in human subjects and in patients with diabetes. *Muscle Nerve* 16, 655–60.

Knezevic, W. and Bajada, S. (1985). Peripheral autonomic surface potential. A quantitative technique for recording sympathetic conduction in man. *J. Neurol. Sci.* 67, 239–51.

Korpelainen, J. T., Tolonen, U., Sotaniemi, K. A., and Myllyla, V. V. (1993). Suppressed sympathetic skin response in brain infarction. *Stroke* 24, 1389–92.

Kuno, Y. (1956). *Human perspiration.* Charles C. Thomas, Springfield, IL.

Levy, D. M., Reid, G., Rowley, D. A., and Abraham, R. R. (1992). Quantitative measures of sympathetic skin response in diabetes: relation to sudomotor and neurological function. *J. Neurol. Neurosurg. Psychiat.* 55, 902–8.

Lloyd, D. (1961). Action potential and secretory potential of sweat glands. *Proc. Nat. Acad. Sci. USA* 47, 351–62.

Low, P. A. (1984). Quantitation of autonomic responses. In *Peripheral neuropathy*, (ed P. J. Dyck, P. K. Thomas, E. H. Lambert, and R. Bunge), pp. 1139–65. W. B. Saunders, Philadelphia.

Low, P. A. (1986). Sudomotor function and dysfunction. In *Diseases of the Nervous System* (ed. A. K. Asbury. G. M. McKhann and W. I. McDonald), pp. 596–605. W. B. Saunders, Philadelphia.

Low, P. A. (1993). Composite autonomic scoring scale for laboratory quantification of generalized autonomic failure. *Mayo Clin. Proc.* 68, 748–52.

Low, P. A. (1996). Diabetic autonomic neuropathy. *Semin. Neurol.* 16, 143–51.

Low, P. A. (1997a). Laboratory evaluation of autonomic function. In *Clinical Autonomic disorders: evaluation and management* (ed. P. A. Low), (2nd edn), pp. 179–208. Lippincott-Raven, New York.

Low, P. A. (1997b). The effect of ageing on the autonomic nervous system. In *clinical autonomic disorders: evaluation and management* (ed. P. A. Low), (2nd edn), pp. 161–75. Lippincott-Raven, New York.

Low, P. A., and McLeod, J. G. (1997). Autonomic neuropathies. In: *Clinical autonomic disorders: evaluation and management* (ed. P. A. Low), (2nd edn), pp. 463–86. Lippincott-Raven, New York.

Low, P. A., Okazaki, H., and Dyck, P. J. (1977). Splanchnic preganglionic neurons in man. I. Morphometry of preganglionic cytons. *Acta Neuropath.* 40, 55–61.

Low, P. A., Fealey, R. D., Sheps, S. G., Su, W. P., Trautmann, J. C., and Kuntz, N. L. (1985). Chronic idiopathic anhidrosis. *Ann. Neurol.* 18, 344–8.

Low, P. A., Zimmerman, B. R., and Dyck, P. J. (1986). Comparison of distal sympathetic with vagal function in diabetic neuropathy. *Muscle Nerve* 9, 592–6.

Low, P. A., Opfer-Gehrking, T. L., and Kihara, M. (1992). *In vivo* studies on receptor pharmacology of the human eccrine sweat gland. *Clin. Auton. Res.* 2, 29–34.

Maselli, R. A., Jaspan, J. B., Soliven, B. C., Green, A. J., Spire, J.-P. and Arnason, B. G. W. (1989). Comparison of sympathetic skin response with quantitative sudomotor axon reflex test in diabetic neuropathy. *Muscle Nerve* 12, 420–3.

Niakan, E. and Harati, Y. (1988). Sympathetic skin response in diabetic peripheral neuropathy. *Muscle Nerve* 11, 261–4.

Ogawa, T. and Low, P. A. (1993). Autonomic regulation of temperature and sweating. In *Clinical autonomic disorders: evaluation and management* (ed. P. A. Low), pp. 79–91. Little, Brown and Company, Boston.

Sandroni, P., Ahlskog, J. E., Fealey, R. D., and Low, P. A. (1991). Autonomic involvement in extrapyramidal and cerebellar disorders. *Clin. Auton. Res.* 1, 147–55.

Sato, K. and Sato, F. (1983). Individual variations in structure and function of human eccrine sweat gland. *Am. J. Physiol.* **245**, R203-R208.

Sato, K., Ohtsuyama, M., and Sato, F. (1993). Normal and abnormal eccrine sweat gland function. In *Clinical autonomic disorders: evaluation and management* (ed. P. A. Low), pp. 93–104. Little, Brown and Company, Boston.

Schondorf, R. (1997). Skin potentials: normal and abnormal. In: *Clinical autonomic disorders: evaluation and management* (ed. P. A. Low), (2nd edn), pp. 221–232. Lippincott-Raven, New York.

Shahani, B. T., Halperin, J. J., Boulu, P., and Cohen, J. (1984). Sympathetic skin response—a method of assessing unmyelinated axon dysfunction in peripheral neuropathies. *J. Neurol. Neurosurg. Psychiat.* **47**, 536–42.

Shaver, B. A., Brusilow, S. W., and Cooke, R. E. (1962). Origin of the galvanic skin response. *Proc. Soc. Exp. Biol. Med.* **110**, 559–64.

Sourek, K. (1965). *The nervous control of skin potentials in man.* Rozpravy Ceskoslovenske Akademie Ved Roenik 75-Sesit 1, Prague.

Stewart, J. D., Low, P. A., and Fealey, R. D. (1992). Distal small fibre neuropathy: results of tests of sweating and autonomic cardiovascular reflexes. *Muscle Nerve* **15**, 661–5.

Suarez, G. A., Fealey, R. D., Camilleri, M., and Low, P. A. (1994). Idiopathic autonomic neuropathy: Clinical, neurophysiologic, and follow-up studies on 27 patients. *Neurology* **44**, 1675–82.

Torres, N. E., Zollman, P. J., and Low, P. A. (1991). Characterization of muscarinic receptor subtype of rat eccrine sweat gland by autoradiography. *Brain Res.* **550**, 129–32.

Tzeng, S. S., Wu, Z. A., and Chu, F. L. (1993). The latencies of sympathetic skin responses. *Eu. Neurol.* **33**, 65–8.

Wang, S. J., Fuh, J. L., Shan, D. E. *et al.* (1993). Sympathetic skin response and r-r interval variation in parkinson's disease. *Movement Disorders* **8**, 151–7.

28. Autonomic function and dysfunction in the gastrointestinal tract

David L. Wingate

Historical

In 1901, Langley stated that there were four divisions of the autonomic nervous system: 'sympathetic, cranial, sacral, and enteric'. It is the enteric division that has been the focus of intense interest in the closing decades of the 20th century, after many years of relative neglect. Meissner established the existence of the submucous plexus in 1857 and Auerbach identified the myenteric plexus in 1964. Controversy over whether these were networks of nerves continued for more than a century, but attempts to define their function met with little success. In 1899, Bayliss and Starling demonstrated that the peristaltic reflex is mediated by the intrinsic innervation of the gut wall, but this was a phenomenological observation that could not, at that time, or for many years later, be related to neuroanatomy, neurophysiology, or neurochemistry. Obstacles to progress included the belief that the autonomic nervous system relied upon only two transmitters, acetylcholine and adrenaline, defining neural pathways according to the concept of 'one nerve, one transmitter' proposed by Henry Dale. The ganglia were viewed as, at best, interruptions in the sympathetic and parasympathetic pathways that allowed neurones to be labeled as 'pre-ganglionic' or 'post-ganglionic'; the post-ganglionic fibres were still considered to be sympathetic or parasympathetic components.

The impetus for the advances of recent decades came from several directions:

(1) When, in 1921, Walter Alvarez demonstrated the inherent electrical rhythmicity of gastrointestinal smooth muscle, it became clear that the timing of contractile events in the gut wall is dictated by electrical pacemaking activity in the smooth muscle. The oesophagus has no pacemaking property; when the act of swallowing places a bolus of food at the orad end of the oesophagus, a peristaltic contraction is initiated which propels the bolus along the length of the oesophageal tube in a matter of seconds. Beyond the oesophagus, peristalsis may occur several times a minute. But chyme takes some hours to traverse the stomach and small bowel, and even longer to pass through the colon. Thus, while pacemakers mark moments when peristalsis *may* occur, peristalsis is not the automatic response to a pacemaking wave, and this implies an additional level of control. In the 1960s, Code and others (Bass 1965; Szurszewski *et al.* 1970) used enteric electromyography in conscious animals to document stereotupic patterns of enteric motor activity.

(2) The complexity of enteric neurotransmission became apparent, starting with the pharmacological discovery of the NANC (non-adrenergic, non-cholinergic) transmitter, postulated by Burnstock to be ATP (Burnstock *et al.* 1970). Serotonin, identified in the myenteric plexus by Gershon (Goodrich *et al.* 1980), was a rival candidate. These advances were overtaken by the tidal wave of neuropeptide research, from which emerged the realization that there are many neuropeptides within the enteric nervous system, and that these neuropeptides are identical with those found in the central nervous system.

(3) Costa, Furness, Wood, and others defined the morphology, electrophysiology, and neurochemistry of the guinea pig myenteric plexus (Wood, 1984). The choice of the guinea pig plexus is more accessible in this species than in others, but there has been sufficient comparative physiological study to confirm that it is an appropriate generic model for the mammalian—including human—myenteric plexus.

Thus, more than a century of limited and laborious progress in understanding the innervation of the gut has been followed by three decades of rapid growth. The major obstacle to progress is the difficulty of physiological study of the digestive tract. Even such an apparently simple function as propulsion is highly complex; the transit speed of material through the digestive tract ranges between a few seconds in the oesophagus and many hours in the colon. Moreover, the content of the digestive tube is transformed in its passage through the bowel by the processes of exocrine secretion, mechanical and chemical digestion, and absorption (Fig. 28.1).

Why motility?

In the sections that follow, there is an emphasis on neural control of the motor activity (or motility) of the gut, and *pari passu*, an apparent neglect of other physiological functions such as secretion, absorption, and blood flow. This reflects the fact it has proved possible to study *in vivo* transient changes in propulsive activity that reflect neural control, but not in other aspects of gut physiology. The same is true of the pathophysiology; so far, only the motor consequences of autonomic dysfunction have been identified in clinical practice. There is, however, another aspect, which is that there is little reserve in the propulsive activity of the gut; it is precisely adapted to the dynamics of digestion and absorption, and even relatively small deviations can cause clinical problems. In contrast, there are considerable reserves of secretory and absorptive capacity in the gut; losses of more than 50 per cent of the total capacity are rapidly compensated by adaptation of the remaining tissue, and therefore do not impose any permanent functional deficit. Furthermore, propulsion is totally dependent upon innervation, whereas mucosal mechanisms

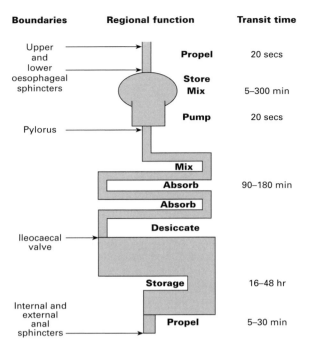

Fig. 28.1. Schematic summary of the anatomy and physiology of the digestive tract, and the time taken for material to pass through the different regions of the gut.

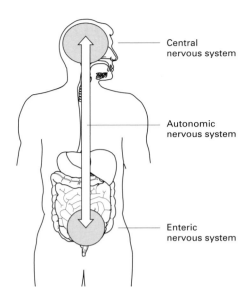

Fig. 28.2. Functional components of gut neural control: (a) block diagram of relationship between neural networks (b) details of parasympathetic and sympathetic innervation of the enteric nervous system.

are regulated largely by physicochemical and biochemical factors. It is thus possible that significant mucosal dysfunction does not occur in gut autonomic failure.

The innervation of the digestive tract

The innervation of the gut can only be understood when it is appreciated that the *intrinsic* innervation—now better known as the enteric nervous system (ENS)—is semi-autonomous (Grundy *et al.* 1996). It functions effectively as a brain that regulates the digestive tract without the need for intervention by the central nervous system (CNS). The overall demands of the organism require co-ordination between the digestive tract and the other systems of the body, and this is achieved by communication between the ENS and CNS along the *extrinsic* parasympathetic and sympathetic neurones that link the two neural networks (Fig. 28.2).

Intrinsic innervation: the enteric nervous system (ENS)

Morphology and chemistry

The enteric nervous system consists of a network of neurones within the gut wall. These are arranged in two principal plexuses, the myenteric plexus of Auerbach, and the submucosal plexus of Meissner. The latter, located between the circular smooth muscle and the submucosa, is probably the main network responsible for regulating the absorptive and secretory activity of the mucosa, the neural modulation of the gut immune system, and local blood flow to

the mucosa. Neural modulation of these functions is not easily studied *in vivo* and consequently knowledge remains fragmentary. More is known about the myenteric plexus, situated between the longitudinal and circular smooth muscle coats, as this plexus is concerned with the regulation of the motor function of the gut. As with skeletal muscle, electrical transients can be recorded that correspond to muscle activity, and it has proved possible to describe patterns of motor activity correspond to neural activation and inhibition.

The structure of the plexuses is relatively simple. Cell bodies are grouped in ganglia, linked by axon bundles. The neuronal population is composed of primary sensory afferents from the gut wall and the mucosal surface, primary efferent motor fibres that regulate effector cells, and interneurones. It is the density and diversity of the interneurones that confer the properties of a neural network on the ENS, with the capacity for implementing programmes of integrated function in response to changes in sensory input. Numerous regulatory peptides have been identified in the ENS, as in the CNS; most neurones appear to contain combinations of several peptides. In addition to the peptide families, other important neurotransmitters include serotonin (5-HT), acetylcholine, and nitric oxide (Burnstock *et al.* 1979).

The ganglia of the ENS are also the location for synaptic communication with the long neurones of the sympathetic and parasympathetic divisions of the autonomic nervous system. In this respect, the classical nomenclature of 'pre-ganglionic' and 'post-ganglionic' for gut autonomic nerves was technically correct; the classification was inadequate because it did not indicate that these two groups were components of different nervous systems.

Basic physiology: peristalsis

The concept of 'The Law of the Intestine' proposed by Bayliss and Starling in 1899 was correct but in some ways misleading. They studied the effect of placing a bolus of material in the lumen of the *in vivo* canine intestine, and showed that it stimulated a wave of contraction that propelled it along the bowel. From this, they concluded that the effect of stimulating the bowel by the arrival of a bolus of material was the production of muscular contraction behind the bolus, and relaxation in front, propelling the bolus onwards. They deduced, correctly, that the nerves responsible for this peristalsis movement are in the gut wall. The misleading implication of their work was the idea that peristalsis is an obligatory response to the presence of material in the gut lumen. In fact, the oesophagus is the only location where this happens, and this is reflected in the rapid transit rate through this region (Fig. 28.1).

It is now clear that the circuitry for peristalsis resides within the intrinsic intramural plexuses. The digestive tube is functionally composed of a series of overlapping segments, each containing the primary afferents, efferents, and interneurones required for peristalsis. These neuronal networks are connected by 'forward feed' neurones to the adjacent functional segment, so that a bolus can be passed, as in the oesophagus, from segment to segment.

The timing of peristaltic contractions is dictated, in the oesophagus, by the act of swallowing, which is a CNS programme. As the bolus enters, it initiates peristalsis, which is propagated along the length of the oesophagus. Beyond the oesophagus, however, the timing of peristalsis is dictated by the electrical rhythmicity of the smooth muscle layers; the frequency of excitation varies from region to region (Fig. 28.3). It was originally believed that the regular electrical oscillation of depolarization and repolarization in the muscle layer reflected the biological properties of the smooth muscle cells themselves, but it is now clear that this oscillation is provided by the interstitial cells of Cajal, which act as an interface between the motor nerves and the smooth muscle cells. It is this basic electrical rhythm, which was first described by Alvarez and Mahoney in 1921, that determines when a smooth muscle contraction may occur.

In the proximal human small bowel, the electrical slow wave allows all opportunities for contraction every minute. If this happened, peristaltic waves would sweep through the entire bowel in a couple of minutes. As this does not happen, it can be deduced that the motor neural input into the smooth muscle is largely *inhibitory*. Discrete motor programmes that have specific functions in delaying transit, and mixing luminal content to allow digestion, absorption, and storage to take place confer this inhibition. To understand this, it is useful to consider the analogy of a child playing a piano. At first, the child will respond to a metronome by hitting a key with all ten fingers and thumbs; a rhythm emerges, but no tune. Teaching the child to play music is essentially teaching them to inhibit most of the fingers on every beat, so that only those notes that form a tune are played. The integrated programmes resident within the central nervous system are the analogue of music; the inhibition is selective and purposeful.

Integrated physiology: methodology

The study of the integrated physiology of the enteric nervous system has, hitherto, focused on the measurement of pressure transients within the gut lumen; these provide a real time indication of neurally controlled motor events. Hence the emphasis in this chapter, and in the published literature, on 'motility'. It must be stressed that the enteric efferents also modulate the function of the mucosal layer, mucosal blood flow, and the mucosal immune system. So far, however, technologies for studying the real time kinetics of these functions *in vivo* have not been developed.

The real time recording of pressure transients with intraluminal sensors is an established clinical technique in the oesophagus and small bowel. In these regions, contractions of the gut wall occlude the lumen, and are easily detected by perfused open tip tubes connected to external pressure transducers, or by miniature strain gauges placed within the lumen. Digital electronic technology permits continuous recording from multiple sensors for 24 hours or more, and miniature data loggers enable data capture in ambulant subjects (Lindberg *et al.* 1990). This has enabled the documentation of periodic activity and circadian variations in the integrated motor patterns of the gut (Kumar *et al.* 1986).

Integrated physiology: the migrating motor complex

V. N. Boldyreff, who was one of Pavlov's research students, was the first to describe the 'periodic' nature of motor activity in the fasting gut at the beginning of the 20th century (Wingate 1981). His work was largely forgotten within a couple of decades, and further progress was not made until the 1960s, when the technique of serosal electromyography in conscious animals was developed in the laboratory of C. F. Code at the Mayo Clinic. In 1969, from that laboratory, J. H. Szurszewski described a regular period variation of motor activity in the canine small bowel that migrated slowly along the length of the bowel (Szurszewski 1969). The concept was further refined in the next few years, and the periodic sequence was divided into three successive phases (Code and Marlett 1975). In Phase I, there is no contractile activity. In phase II, contractile activity is sporadic. Phase III is the most easily identified by pressure manometry; it consists of a sequence of contractions, each one linked to successive electrical slow waves, that lasts for 3–8 minutes. In terms of

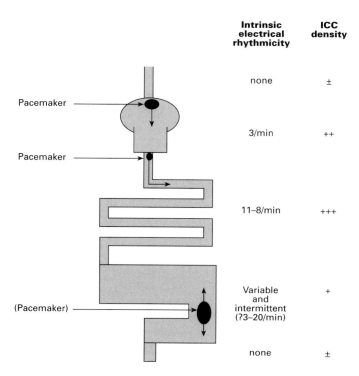

	Intrinsic electrical rhythmicity	ICC density
Pacemaker	none	±
Pacemaker	3/min	++
	11–8/min	+++
(Pacemaker)	Variable and intermittent (?3–20/min)	+
	none	±

Fig. 28.3. Electrical rhythmicity of different regions of the gut, and the associated density of distribution of interstitial cells of Cajal (ICC).

neural input into the smooth muscle, Phase I represents a period of maximal inhibition, while Phase III represents the complete removal of inhibition. Collectively, the three phases are known as the migrating motor complex (MMC), and if the activity of the gut is recorded from sensors along the length of the intestine, the MMC appears to migrate (Fig. 28.4). The period of each MMC cycle is about 90 minutes, although this is extremely variable (Thompson *et al.* 1980), and the migration velocity, again variable, is in the order of 5 centimetres per minute.

The biological significance of periodic motor activity is two-fold. First, it appears to be a property of the *in vivo* digestive tract of virtually all vertebrate species that have been so far studied, but it only occurs in the *in situ* system, and can not be demonstrated in isolated organs. Secondly, the MMC is the only clearly defined integrated motor programme that is attributable to the enteric nervous system. The evidence for this can be summarized briefly, as follows:

(1) MMC activity is invariably **present** in the undamaged *in vivo* gut (Fig. 28.5a)

(2) Phase III is **abnormal** in the enteric neuropathy of Chagas' Disease (Fig. 28.5b)

(3) MMC activity is **absent** in the rare condition of visceral aganglionosis. It can be **abolished** in experimental animals by the topical application of benzalkonium chloride to the mesenteric surface of the gut.

(4) MMC activity is **preserved** in small bowel transplantation, now a treatment option for propulsive failure of the gut (Wallin *et al.* 1992).

The functional significance of the MMC remains a matter of speculation. It seems likely that, in man, it may be important in preventing

the retrograde spread of colonic bacteria (Vantrappen *et al.* 1977); Kellow *et al.* 1990). This is not the case in ruminants, but in herbivorous species, the powerful propulsive force of Phase III may be essential in the propulsion of bulky fibrous material. In clinical terms, however, it is the only indicator that we have to date for evaluating the integrity of the enteric nervous system. Clinically, it is most reliably detected by pressure manometry of the proximal small bowel during diurnal fasting or, preferably, during nocturnal sleep.

Intrinsic innervation: the prevertebral ganglia

Since the three prevertebral ganglia–coeliac, superior mesenteric, and inferior mesenteric (Fig. 28.6)—are anatomically distanced

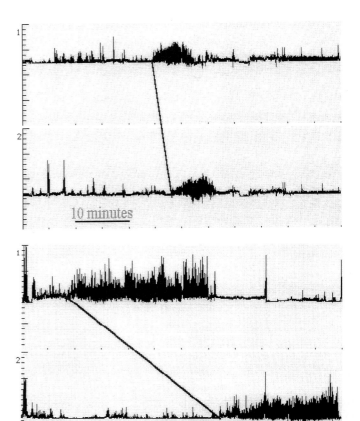

Fig. 28.5. (a) The characteristic cluster of regular contractions marking Phase III of the MMC recorded in a healthy adult at two sites 15 cm apart in the proximal small bowel. The diagonal line illustrates the aboral migration along the bowel. At each recording site, Phase III is preceded by the irregular contractions of Phase II. The motor quiescence of Phase I that follows Phase III is readily apparent in this recording in an ambulant subject, but the deflections that follow Phase III are identical, indicating that these are due to changes in intra-abdominal pressure caused by body movements. (b) A similar recording in a patient suffering from Chagas' disease. Note the prolongation of the clustered contractions. The decreased slope of the diagonal line illustrates the reduced velocity of aboral migration.

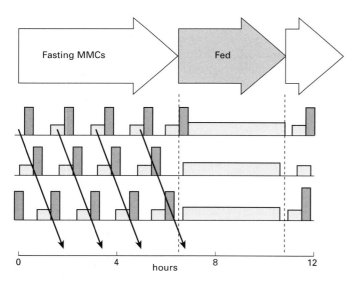

Fig. 28.4. Summary of the intensity of physiological small bowel motor activity at three different sites over 12 hours that include one meal. Low shaded areas represent the irregular activity of Phase II, and vertical bars the regular contractile activity of Phase III. This illustrates the periodic repetition of fasting activity as a motor complex, and the apparent migration down the bowel. Regular periodicity of the MMC, as depicted here, is commonly seen in laboratory animals under controlled conditions, but in man, the periodicity of the MMC is very variable between and within subjects (cf. Figs 28.11 and 28.13).

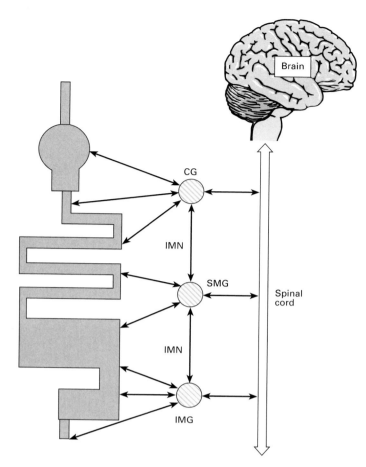

Fig. 28.6. Schematic representation of the prevertebral ganglia (CG—coeliac ganglion; SMG—superior mesenteric ganglion; IMG—inferior mesenteric ganglion) and the intermesenteric nerves (IMN). This illustrates the not only the path of spinal autonomic nerves, but also the route through the intermesenteric nerves that enables the rapid transmission of information between remote areas of the bowel.

from the gut, it may seem illogical to ascribe to them the status of *intrinsic* innervation. They can, after all, be considered merely as relay stations for sympathetic fibres running between gut and spinal cord. Functionally, however, they probably have an equally important function as relay stations in pathways for the rapid transmission of information between remote areas of the gut, mediating intestino-intestinal reflexes. The existence of such reflexes has been well established for many years, but it was always unlikely that the intramural plexuses were the pathway for these reflexes, because of the numerous synapses that would be required for transmission over many centimetres. Studies of *ex vivo* guinea pig colon, with the two mesenteric ganglia and the intermesenteric nerve attached, demonstrated an intact colo-colonic inhibitory reflex even when the proximal and distal ends of the colon were isolated (Kreulen and Szurszewski 1979).

Intestino-intestinal reflexes are probably mostly inhibitory, but excitatory reflexes may also exist. Among the former are the inhibitory reflexes that inhibit the motor activity of the proximal gut when more distal segments are distended (Da Cunha Melo et al. 1981). Human proximal small bowel motor activity can be inhibited

by moderate rectal distension (Kellow et al. 1987); such reflexes may account for the slow bowel transit that occurs in constipated patients who maintain a loaded rectum. The 'gastro-colonic response'—the increased colonic motor activity induced by the ingestion of a meal is likely to be an intestino-intestinal excitatory reflex.

Extrinsic innervation: the gut–brain–gut axis

The conventional view of the extrinsic parasympathetic and sympathetic innervation is that it is largely comprised of efferent neurones, and is therefore mainly a motor system. Recent studies have shown that this is erroneous (Aziz and Thompson 1998). The majority of fibres are afferent, and it is now clear that the extrinsic innervation continually transmits information to the CNS on the functional status of the digestive tract. The extrinsic innervation therefore forms a functional 'gut–brain–gut axis' (Fig. 28.7).

Afferent innervation: gut to brain

The sensory extrinsic innervation of the gut is in two divisions that are anatomically and functionally distinct.

The *parasympathetic* innervation conveys physiological information to the CNS from mucosal receptors that are touch and chemo-sensitive, and smooth muscle nerve endings that encode tension, presumably as a result of deformation. The vagal component of parasympathetic innervation has been the subject of most study, because of its accessibility, and because there are no synapses in vagal fibres between the gut wall and the dorsal vagal complex in the brain stem. Various studies in different animal species have shown that there is continuous afferent traffic in the vagus, and that the pattern of firing encodes physiological change within the gut. It has also been shown that healthy humans do not consciously perceive the types of stimuli that alter vagal input to the brain stem in these animal studies. The logical inference is that while parasympathetic afferent information may modulate function in both gut and brain, the input does not—at least in health—reach the cerebral cortex (Fig. 28.8)

Spinal sympathetic afferents mediate noxious stimuli. The nerve endings are located on the mesenteric surface of the bowel, and respond to distension of the gut. They also respond to direct stimula-

The autonomic nervous system: The gut–brain–gut axis

Parasympathetic		Sympathetic	
Vagus nerves Pelvic nerves		Spinal cord	
Afferent	Efferent	Afferent	Efferent
Physiological stimuli	Excitatory	Noxious stimuli	Inhibitory
● Mucosal touch	to motor and exocrine function	● Excess distention	to motor and exocrine function
● Muscle tension		● Ischaemia	
● Luminal content		● Mucosal damage	

Fig. 28.7. Summary of the parasympathetic and sympathetic systems that link the central and enteric nervous systems.

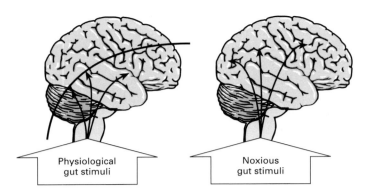

Fig. 28.8. Normally, information relayed from the gut reaches the brain stem, hind brain, and mid brain, but not the cerebral cortex (left). Noxious stimuli are relayed to the cortex (right). In some 'functional disorders', there is evidence from PET scanning that normal physiological stimuli reach the cortex and are relayed into consciousness.

tion, and are almost certainly responsible for the ileus that follows manipulation of the bowel during abdominal surgery. These are pain fibres, and there is evidence from animal studies that they do not respond to the levels of distension that occur during normal movements of the gut, which are picked up by vagal afferents. These afferent fibres mediate pain arising in the gut, and, unlike vagal traffic, this information is relayed to the cerebral cortex; positron emission tomography has been used in man to demonstrate cortical activation by painful distension of the gut (Silverman *et al.* 1997). It is likely that in painful functional disorders of the gut, the threshold of these afferents is lowered so that they respond to distension levels that are within the physiological range (Aziz *et al.* 1995).

Efferent innervation: brain to gut

The classical concept of the extrinsic innervation was that it controlled the motor activity of the gut, with the two divisions, parasympathetic and sympathetic, being respectively excitatory and inhibitory, with acetylcholine and noradrenaline as the respective neurotransmitters. The experiments on which this view was based antedated the identification of the ENS as an autonomous neural network, and the discovery of the numerous neurotransmitters and neuromodulators that we now know to be involved in the neural regulation of the digestive tract. In effect, the two systems were viewed as acting in a manner similar to the accelerator and the brake of a car, with the driver representing the CNS. The analogy is not totally inappropriate, provided it is accepted that the engine now has a mind of its own!

The effect of CNS arousal on the motor and secretory activity of the gut is consistent with the concept of efferent parasympathetic stimulation, but it has not proved possible so far to assess the physiological contribution of extrinsic efferent autonomic activity on the physiological activity of the gut. To describe the innervation as 'motor' or 'sensory' is probably unhelpful; the extrinsic innervation provides pathways for the exchange of information between neural networks. This contemporary approach to the neural control of the gut is exemplified by one aspect of vagal activity that has emerged from relatively recent research. This is the role of the vagus nerve in transforming the motor activity of the stomach and small bowel from the

fasting MMC pattern to the postprandial pattern. Although the ENS has primary afferent neurones, the sensors that detect the arrival of food in the gut are chemosensitive vagal receptors that have no direct input into the ENS. The arrival of food in the gut is signaled to the ENS by information that is relayed by afferent fibres to the dorsal vagal complex (Ewart and Wingate 1984) and thence by vagal efferent fibres to the ENS (Fig. 28.9). Following a meal, acute cooling of the cervical vagus nerves in conscious dogs causes a reversion from the postprandial motor pattern to the fasting MMC pattern, and this effect is reversed when the vagal blockade is removed (Chung and Diamant 1987). This experimental observation explains the postprandial dysfunction that commonly afflicted patients who were submitted to truncal vagotomy for the relief of duodenal ulcer disease. The attenuation of the postprandial response may also account for the meal-stimulated diarrhoea seen in a minority (Thompson *et al.* 1982).

The deficit caused by the interruption of neural circuitry can be used to demonstrate the contribution of the intact system to normal function. Surgical truncal vagotomy is an imperfect example of this type of ablation because the vagal section is incomplete. Even so, if it is taken to provide some kind of indication, then it has to be said that the intact vagus is not an essential condition for normal digestive function. Although some patients do have symptomatic functional deficits, the majority do not. The extant literature on the contribution of extrinsic autonomic innervation to normal gut function is largely based on experimental surgical procedures in animals, and may have little bearing on normal human physiology.

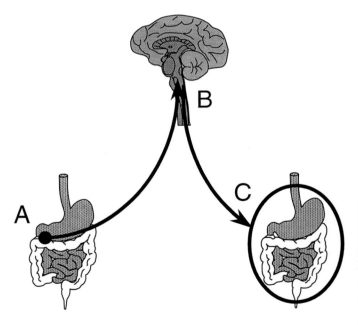

Fig. 28.9. The dependence of the motor response to a meal on the vago-vagal transmission of information. The arrival of a meal in the foregut is detected by gastric and duodenal sensory nerve terminals (A) that respond to volume and chemical stimulation, and this information is transmitted to the dorsal vagal complex (B). From there it passes through the efferent vagus to the effector organs of the gut (C) initiating not only altered motor activity (Fig. 28.4), but also increased bile flow, and exocrine pancreatic secretion.

Brain-gut interaction

The division of control over the operations of the digestive tract is shared between CNS and ENS (Fig. 28.10). The CNS has a major influence on gut-related behaviour, such as eating and defaecation, which requires synchronization with complex body movements. The conscious urge to defaecate is prompted by a cue from rectal receptors that respond to rectal filling. The decision to defaecate is dependent on the conscious perception of a suitable opportunity, and body movements leading to a squatting posture. The actual expulsion of stool requires the synergy of pelvic musculature and sphincters with both CNS and ENS input.

The CNS can modulate enteric function that is within the domain of the ENS. A number of human and animal studies have shown that the motor function of the stomach, small bowel and colon is altered under conditions of psychological stress. In this paradigm, the participation of the CNS is essential for the perception of stressors even if, as appears to be the case in the rat, the stress signal to the bowel is via a humoral messenger (CRF—corticotrophin releasing factor) rather than by information transmission along autonomic pathways. Such influences are bi-directional; satiety signals that terminate eating appear to originate in the gut.

An important advance in the understanding of gut function in recent years has been the development of systems for prolonged monitoring. Until recently, methods for observing the activity of the digestive system, shown in Fig. 28.1, and the time frame of motor events in the gut ranges between a matter of seconds in the oesophagus to many hours in the colon. Until recently periods of observation using invasive sensors were limited by the inability of subjects to tolerate intubation and immobility for more than a few hours. Micro-miniature strain gauges, digital logging, and computer analysis of large volumes of data are now incorporated into systems that permit continuous observation of different regions of the gut for 24 hours or longer. These studies have revealed a circadian modulation of gut function that is evident in both the small intestine (Fig. 28.11) and the colon. From these studies it can be inferred that it is brain-gut interaction that is being modulated in this way, and that the major influence is CNS arousal (Kumar et al. 1990). During sleep, the small bowel is mostly quiescent, but the MMC, represented by the regular contractions of Phase III is omnipresent (Kumar et al. 1989). The colon appears to be virtually inert during sleep, but activity returns on waking (Narducci et al. 1987).

Autonomic dysfunction and failure

In the context of gastrointestinal pathology in most of the world, overt autonomic failure of the gut is exceedingly uncommon. Suspected autonomic dysfunction is more common, but the incidence is sporadic, the aetiology is diverse, and there is no agreed taxonomy. To further obfuscate the situation, histopathological evidence usually is lacking. This summarizes the situation as viewed by most gastroenterologists and neurologists, but this is based on widespread ignorance of the advances in the understanding of the neural control of the gut that have been described above. A simple litmus test of comprehension is done by inviting a clinician to identify the nature and role of the enteric nervous system; most still remain ignorant of its very existence.

The clinical landscape of gut autonomic failure is extensive, but obscured by limited vision. The classification of such disorders into one of the twin categories of 'neuropathy' and 'myopathy' is clearly not only simplistic, but also wrong. Manometric studies that appear to show an inert bowel have been attributed to 'myopathy' (Summers et al. 1983), but may only reflect a dilated bowel, where contractions

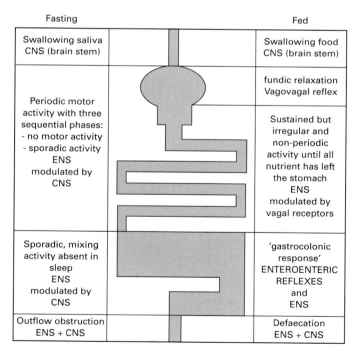

Fig. 28.10. Summary of the regional motor activity, and the relative control exerted by the central nervous system (CNS) and the enteric nervous system (ENS).

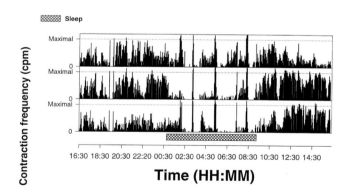

Fig. 28.11. Histogram of the minute by minute incidence of contractions over 24 hours of continuous ambulant manometry at three sites of the proximal small bowel in a healthy adult. In this computer-generated histogram, each line contain 1440 data points. The recording sites were 15 cm proximal to the ligament of Treitz (above), at the ligament of Treitz (centre) and 15 cm distal to it (below). The transient peaks, mostly during sleep, at the maximal contractile frequency (10/min) mark phase III of the MMC. Close inspection reveals the progressive delay of Phase III at successive aboral recording sites, illustrating the migration of Phase III.

do not occlude the lumen and are not detected by intraluminal sensors. The identification of disease-specific pathophysiology is, at present, rarely possible. There is, nonetheless, a common factor to such disorders. As pointed out above, the neural input to the smooth muscle in the pacemaker-driven regions of the gut is largely inhibitory. Neuropathies are marked by an *increase* in contractile activity (Stanghellini *et al.* 1987). This must not be confused with 'increased motility' which implies improved propulsion, as this increased activity is often obstructive rather propulsive, which explains the otherwise paradoxical observation that pseudo-obstruction, or propulsive failure, of the gut is often marked by an excess of motor activity. Clinically, the excess motor activity is most easily detected during sleep, when the bowel is normally relatively quiescent. The excess motor activity is not disease-specific; it is a general property of the neurally-impaired gut.

Clinical presentation

The major functional deficit in autonomic dysfunction is the condition known as pseudo-obstruction (Stanghellini *et al.* 1987). This can be localized, as in achalasia of the cardia and Hirschprung's disease, or generalized. When the colon, or the entire bowel is involved, the clinical picture closely resembles that of mechanical obstruction, with distension, abdominal pain, cessation of the passage of faeces and flatus, nausea, and vomiting. Commonly an exploratory laparotomy is needed to establish the diagnosis with certainty, and to eliminate the possibility of mechanical obstruction by malignant or inflammatory masses, or by fibrous peritoneal adhesions

Usually, the pseudo-obstruction is chronic, and patients may remain in a stable condition. When the problem is chronic, however, there is a common major consequence, which is bacterial overgrowth of the small intestine. In man, the normal migrating motor complex appears to be essential in the prevention of the orad migration of colonic bacterial flora. When motor patterns are abnormal, this protective mechanism fails, and the small bowel is colonised by bacteria (Vantrappen *et al.* 1977). This leads to two clinical problems. Food consumed by the patient is consumed by bacteria, and therefore not absorbed; and the consequence is malnutrition. Secondly, bacterial metabolism of complex crystalloid molecules in the bowel lumen raises intraluminal osmotic pressure and leads to diarrhoea; paradoxically it is thus possible for a patient to have delayed gut transit together with diarrhoea.

Disorders of intrinsic innervation

Regional disorders

Achalasia of the cardia is a neuropathy of the smooth muscle portion of the oesophagus, including the lower oesophageal sphincter. It commonly occurs in adult life, but can occur in childhood. The incidence is said to be about 1 per 100 000 of the population; the true incidence is unknown but certainly higher, as many cases, particularly if the neuropathy is incomplete, remain undiagnosed, or are wrongly diagnosed as either oesophagitis due to gastro-oesophageal reflux or 'non-specific motility disorder of the oesophagus'. The classical presentation is dysphagia due to failure of relaxation of the lower oesophageal sphincter. As the condition advances, the oesophagus becomes chronically dilated and filled with meal residues; this happens because the smooth muscle portion of the oesophagus becomes aperistaltic. A significant proportion of cases present,

however, with disordered motility of the oesophageal body, but with a sphincter that it is still capable of relaxation. Very infrequently, achalasia may be the prodrome of generalized enteric neuropathy, suggesting that it is possibly an autoimmune disorder that enters spontaneous remission. The only available treatment for achalasia is the induction of sphincter incompetence, either by surgical myotomy, or circumferential partial rupture by pneumatic dilatation.

Hirschprung's disease is due to an aganglionic segment of the colon (Rogawski *et al.* 1978) producing a functional obstruction to defaecation, and consequent dilatation of the colon proximal to the aperistaltic segment. It is normally found in children, but it can occur in adults. Treatment is by resection of the affected area.

Generalized disorders

The commonest disease of the enteric nervous system is *Chagas' disease*, also known as South American trypanosomiasis. Dr Carlos Chagas in Brazil first described it, but it is widespread in a number of South American countries, including Chile, Argentina, Paraguay, and Uruguay. The work of Carlos Chagas was largely forgotten after his death, but interest in the disease was revived by the work of F. Koberle, an Austrian pathologist who emigrated to the city of Ribeirao Preto in the Sao Paulo province of Brazil (Koberle 1968). At the present time, there are an estimated 10 million patients suffering from the disease. Sporadic cases have been found in the USA, due to migrant workers who have recently been infected donating their blood to earn money (in South America, but not the USA, donor blood is screened). The pathogen that is implicated is *Trypanosoma cruzii*, but it is, in fact, an autoimmune disease. The vector is an induvid beetle that normally lives in the unplastered walls of peasant shacks, where the inhabitants sleep on mud floors. When the beetle stings a victim, it defaecates on the lesion, expelling the parasite. The victim then rubs the lesion, which ensures the introduction of the trypanosome into the blood stream. There is an infective stage with mild non-specific malaise and malaise and low-grade fever; during this phase, the victim's blood is infective.

The neuropathic stage of the disease starts with the production of anti-trypanosomal antibodies. These antibodies cross-react with a surface antigen on autonomic neuronal cell bodies (Ribeiro dos Santos *et al.* 1979). It is this antibody-antigen fusion that induces the neuropathy. The neuropathy affects the digestive system and the heart. Some patients have only cardiac involvement, others only gastrointestinal involvement, while a minority have involvement of both systems. The clinical manifestations are mega-oesophagus and mega-colon. The presentation of mega-oesophagus is identical to the presentation of achalasia of the cardia, with dysphagia, oesophageal dilatation, and eventually the aspiration of retained food. Mega-colon presents with distension and constipation. Clinical small bowel involvement, when present, is marked by distension and, usually, diarrhoea due to bacterial overgrowth (Aprile *et al.* 1995), but although this is uncommon, histopathology has shown that there is always damage to the myenteric plexus in the small bowel (Costa and Alcantara 1966). Curiously, the stomach does not seem to be greatly damaged in Chagas' disease; no important abnormality of gastric emptying has been demonstrated, although some changes can be found (Troncon and Iazigi 1992).

The biomedical significance of Chagas' disease is that it is the only enteric neuropathy that is sufficiently prevalent to allow the cohorts of patients to be studied in the knowledge that, as confirmed by serology, they have the same disease. The typical functional lesion of the ENS is abnormality of Phase III of the MMC; it is prolonged in duration from about 6 minutes to as much as 20 minutes, and the velocity with which it appears to migrate along the bowel is about 25 per cent of the normal velocity (Fig). Small bowel manometry in Chagas' disease has shown that it is usually abnormal despite the absence of overt small bowel dilatation or pseudo-obstruction (Oliveira *et al.* 1983).

In the Northern hemisphere, *idiopathic enteric neuropathy* is not only very uncommon but also its manifestations are diverse. The commonest age of presentation is in infancy or childhood; paediatric gastroenterologists consequently have more experience of this condition than other clinicians (Hyman *et al.* 1988; Fell *et al.* 1996). Familial cases occur (Camilleri *et al.* 1991), but most appear to be isolated. In adults, neuropathies have been reported in association with small cell bronchial carcinoma (Chinn and Schuffler 1988; Sodhi *et al.* 1989). The presentation of these cases is normally as pseudo-obstruction. Some cases appear to be autoimmune, and are associated with circulating anti-Hu antibodies (Smith *et al.* 1997). Pathological confirmation of the diagnosis is rare, but this position may change with the advent of laparoscopic full-thickness small bowel biopsy. Antroduodenal (Hyman *et al.* 1988) or, preferably, prolonged small bowel manometry (Quigley *et al.* 1997) is usually diagnostic. The point of interest over the manometric findings is the discovery of the features of Chagas' disease in UK patients with pseudo-obstruction. In a series of more than 100 patients with suspected pseudo-obstruction who had prolonged manometry at the Royal London Hospital, 50 per cent of those who had abnormal motility patterns had the Phase III abnormalities found in Chagas' disease (Fig. 28.12) These patients did not, of course, have Chagas' disease, nor did the clinical presentation include mega-oesophagus and mega-colon. The findings do, however, support the hypothesis that there is a stereotypic disruption of the small bowel fasting motility programme in enteric neuropathy.

Management of patients with enteric neuropathy is difficult. Where stasis and distension are severe, limited resection of non-functioning bowel may help, but should only be undertaken with caution and after much thought; when propulsion is abnormal or absent, the consequences of reconstructing the bowel may be difficult to predict. Malnutrition is a frequent problem; treatment of bacterial overgrowth with repeated courses of antibiotics may be helpful, but enteral or parenteral nutritional support may be required. Pain is a frequent problem, probably due to sensory neuropathy rather than 'spasm', and opiate analgesia may be required. 'Prokinetic' drugs, such as substituted benzamides are usually of little help. Finally, small bowel transplantation is now a treatment option, but only as a last resort. In adults, it is only indicated at present when parenteral nutrition is, for whatever reason, unsuccessful. It is more realistic option in children, but the mortality, approximately 30 per cent in the first year, remains high.

Constipation is a problem in *Parkinson's disease*. This was originally attributed to the side-effects of medication, but it now seems that the disease directly affects the enteric nervous system. Loewy bodies have been identified in the myenteric plexus of the oesophagus and colon, and it was recently reported that immunohistochemistry had shown diminished or absent dopamine staining in the colon. There is, however, no other useful information on this topic.

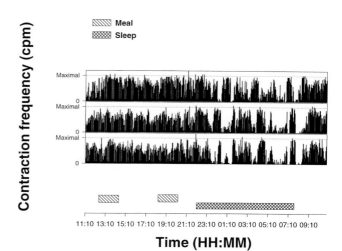

Fig. 28.12. Histogram of small bowel motor activity in a 28-year old woman suffering from a familial enteric neuropathy. Compared with a healthy individual (see Fig. 28.11), there is an overall increase in the incidence of contractions, while the nocturnal Phase III peaks of maximal activity are prolonged in duration, and migrate more slowly. The motor abnormalities in this patient are identical with those found in Chagas' Disease (see Fig. 28.5b).

Disorders of extrinsic innervation

There is little doubt that propulsive activity in the gastrointestinal tract is disturbed in dysautonomia syndromes, but there is, with one major exception, an absence of data. The exception is diabetes mellitus. In Type 1 diabetes, gastroparesis–diminished gastric motor activity with consequent stasis—is common (Ewing and Clarke 1986). It is one of the earliest manifestations of diabetic autonomic neuropathy and may occur in diabetic children (Reid *et al.* 1992), but is often asymptomatic and only detected by gamma scintigraphy. The incidence is such that it is safe to assume that it is present in any Type 1 diabetic who complains of chronic early satiety, epigastric fullness, nausea, and vomiting. The major deficit is in the emptying of solids (Dooley *et al.* 1988); this is partly due to diminished motor activity in the gastric antrum, and partly due to the absence of MMC activity in the stomach. Gastric MMCs are required to empty solid residues; in diabetic gastroparesis, these accumulate and this can lead to the formation of bezoars. The slow emptying of food from the stomach makes diabetic control more difficult, and there is evidence that hyperglycaemia itself exacerbates gastroparesis. Pharmacotherapy can be helpful (Annese *et al.* 1997), in particular with the macrolide antibiotic erythromycin (Tack *et al.* 1992), which attaches to motilin receptors in the stomach and duodenum and stimulates the genesis of MMC activity. The benefit is usually short-lived, due to tachyphylaxis, but it does provide a window of opportunity to improve diabetic control and this may help to minimize gastroparesis. The 'diabetic bowel' is a well-known phenomenon, marked by chronic diarrhoea and evidence of bacterial overgrowth (Rosa *et al.* 1996). The nature of the bowel neuropathy, that is likely to be the cause of the problem remains uncertain (Yoshida *et al.* 1988).

In the primary autonomic failure syndromes, such as multiple system atrophy, there is involvement of the gut (Camilleri and Fealey

1990) that is manifested in various symptoms (see Chapter 00), although precise data, especially on motility, are few (Suarez *et al.* 1994).

Mixed disorders

This is, again, relatively unexplored territory. The only reasonably convincing candidate, largely on the basis of animal studies (Poulakos *et al.* 1990; Summers *et al.* 1992), for a disorder of both intrinsic and extrinsic innervation is post-radiation enteritis (Perino *et al.* 1986; Husebye *et al.* 1994). Fortunately, with better techniques of radiotherapy, it is now a rare occurrence.

Some of the maladies of unknown nature that are now classified as 'functional disorders' may, prove to be neuropathic. Of particular interest in this respect, not least because of its worldwide prevalence, is irritable bowel syndrome. About one quarter of all cases are the sequel of an acute gastroenteritis (McKendrick and Read 1994), often traveller's diarrhoea. There is accumulating evidence that this may be a mild sensory neuropathy. The primary lesion seems to be a lowered sensory threshold of visceral afferents (Prior and Read 1993); the response to this increased sensory input is inappropriate motor responses from the enteric nervous system, and exaggerated visceral perception in the central nervous system (Mertz *et al.* 1995). The motor response has been confirmed by studies of motor activity in the small bowel (Fig. 28.13) and colon (Kumar and Wingate 1985; Kellow *et al.* 1988; Narducci *et al.* 1985), and several groups have demonstrated altered sensory thresholds in the bowel with increased cortical representation (Silverman *et al.* 1997). Progress in this field has been hampered by the absence of an objective marker for the syndrome; the diagnosis at present depends upon the clinician's judgment of whether a combination of symptoms falls within the diagnostic category.

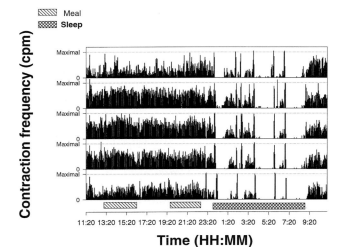

Fig. 28.13 Histogram of small bowel motor activity in a 42-year old woman suffering from irritable bowel syndrome. Note the excess motor activity during the day and the normal activity during sleep. (In this recording five recording sensors were used over the 30 cm of proximal small bowel)

Conclusion

Recently acquired knowledge has transformed our concepts of the physiology of the neural control of the gut; this applies in particular to a clearer understanding of the autonomy of the enteric nervous system. The data suggest that there may be specific types of dysfunction according to the neuronal population affected by autonomic failure in different types of dysautonomia, but, with the exception of Chagas' disease, there is still little information. It is hoped that access to biopsy material will lead to a classification of dysautonomias of the gut, and the development of both diagnostic strategies and clear management protocols.

References

Annese, V., Lombardi, G., Frusciante, V., Germani, U., Andriulli, A., and Bassotti (1997). Cisapride and erythromycin prokinetic effects in gastroparesis due to type 1 (insulin-dependent) diabetes mellitus. *Aliment. Pharmacol. Ther.* 11, 599–603.

Aprile, L. R., Troncon, L. E., Meneghelli, U. G., and de Oliveira, R. B. (1995). [Small bowel bacterial overgrowth syndrome in chagasic megajejunum: report of 2 cases (see comments)]. [Portuguese]. *Arquivos de Gastroenterologia* 32, 71–8.

Aziz, Q., Furlong, P. L., Barlow, J., Hobson, A., Alani, S., Bancewicz, J., Ribbands, M., Harding, G. F., and Thompson, D. G. (1995). Topographic mapping of cortical potentials evoked by distension of the human proximal and distal oesophagus. *Electroencephalography & Clinical Neurophysiology* 96, 219–28.

Aziz, Q. and Thompson, D. G. (1998). Brain-gut axis in health and disease. [Review] [155 refs]. *Gastroenterology* 114, 559–78.

Bass, P. (1965). Electric activity of smooth muscle of the gastrointestinal tract. *Gastroenterology* 49, 391–4.

Burnstock, G., Campbell, G., Satchell, D., and Smythe, A. (1970). Evidence that adenosine triphosphate or a related nucleotide is the transmitter substance released by non-adrenergic inhibitory nerves in the gut. *Br. J. Pharmacol.* 40, 668–88.

Burnstock, G., Hokfelt, T., Gershon, M. D., Iversen, L. L., Kosterlitz, H. W., and Szurszewski, J. H. (1979). Non-adrenergic, non-cholinergic autonomic neurotransmission mechanisms. *Neurosci. Res. Program. Bull.* 17, 377–519.

Camilleri, M., Carbone, L. D., and Schuffler, M. D. (1991). Familial enteric neuropathy with pseudoobstruction. *Dig. Dis. Sci.* 36, 1168–71.

Camilleri, M. and Fealey, R. D. (1990). Idiopathic autonomic denervation in eight patients presenting with functional gastrointestinal disease. A causal association? *Dig. Dis. Sci.* 35, 609–16.

Chinn, J. S. and Schuffler, M. D. (1988). Paraneoplastic visceral neuropathy as a cause of severe gastrointestinal motor dysfunction. *Gastroenterology* 95, 1279–86.

Chung, S. A. and Diamant, N. E. (1987). Small intestinal motility in fasted and postprandial states: effect of transient vagosympathetic blockade. *Am. J. Physiol.* 252, G301–G308

Code, C. F. and Marlett, J. A. (1975). The interdigestive myo-electric complex of the stomach and small bowel of dogs. *J. Physiol. (Lond.)* 246, 289–309.

Costa, R. D. and Alcantara, F. G. de. (1966). [Submucous and myenteric plexuses of the human ileum in Chagas' disease]. [Portuguese]. *Revista Brasileira de Medicina* 23, 399–400.

Da Cunha Melo, J., Summers, R. W., Thompson, H. H., Wingate, D. L. and Yanda, R. (1981). Effects of intestinal secretagogues and distension on small bowel myoelectric activity in fasted and fed conscious dogs. *J. Physiol. (Lond.)* 321, 483–94.

Dooley, C. P., el Newihi, H. M., Zeidler, A., and Valenzuela, J. E. (1988). Abnormalities of the migrating motor complex in diabetics with autonomic neuropathy and diarrhea. *Scand. J. Gastroenterol.* 23, 217–23.

Ewart, W. R. and Wingate, D. L. (1984). Central representation of arrival of nutrient in the duodenum. *Am. J. Physiol.* 246, G750–6.

Ewing, D. J. and Clarke, B. F. (1986). Autonomic neuropathy: its diagnosis and prognosis. [Review] [168 refs]. *Clin. Endocrinol. Metab.* 15, 855–88.

Fell, J. M., Smith, V. V., and Milla, P. J. (1996). Infantile chronic idiopathic intestinal pseudo-obstruction: the role of small intestinal manometry as a diagnostic tool and prognostic indicator. *Gut* 39, 306–11.

Goodrich, J. T., Bernd, P., Sherman, D., and Gershon, M. D. (1980). Phylogeny of enteric serotonergic neurons. *J. Comp. Neurol.* 190, 15–28.

Grundy, D., Enck, P., and Wood, J. D. (1996). Little brain—big brain. IV: Munich, 30 October to 3 November 1995. *Neugastroenterol. Motil.* 8, 153–5.

Husebye, E., Hauer-Jensen, M., Kjorstad, K., and Skar, V. (1994). Severe late radiation enteropathy is characterized by impaired motility of proximal small intestine. *Dig. Dis. Sci.* 39, 2341–9.

Hyman, P. E., McDiarmid, S. V., Napolitano, J., Abrams, C. E., and Tomomasa, T. (1988). Antroduodenal motility in children with chronic intestinal pseudo-obstruction. *J. Pediatr.* 112, 899–905.

Kellow, J. E., Gill, R. C., and Wingate, D. L. (1987). Modulation of human upper gastrointestinal motility by rectal distension. *Gut* 28, 864–8.

Kellow, J. E., Gill, R. C., Wingate, D. L., and Calam, J. E. (1990). Small bowel motor activity and bacterial overgrowth. *J. Gast. Mot.* 2, 180–3.

Kellow, J. E., Phillips, S. F., Miller, L. J., and Zinsmeister, A. R. (1988). Dysmotility of the small intestine in irritable bowel syndrome. *Gut* 29, 1236–43.

Koberle, F. (1968). Chagas' disease and Chagas' syndromes: the pathology of American trypanosomiasis. [Review]. *Adv. Parasit.* 6, 63–116.

Kreulen, D. L. and Szurszewski, J. H. (1979). Reflex pathways in the abdominal prevertebral ganglia: evidence for a colo-colonic inhibitory reflex. *J. Physiol. (Lond.)* 295, 21–32.

Kumar, D., Soffer, E. E., Wingate, D. L., Britto, J., Das-Gupta, A., and Mridha, K. (1989). Modulation of the duration of human postprandial motor activity by sleep *Am. J. Physiol.* 256, G851–5.

Kumar, D., Thompson, P. D., and Wingate, D. L. (1990). Absence of synchrony between human small intestinal migrating motor complex and rectalmotor complex. *Am. J. Physiol.* 258, G171–2.

Kumar, D., Wingate, D., and Ruckebusch, Y. (1986). Circadian variation in the propagation velocity of the migrating motor complex. *Gastroenterology* 91, 926–30.

Kumar, D. and Wingate, D. L. (1985). The irritable bowel syndrome: a paroxysmal motor disorder. *Lancet* 2, 973–7.

Lindberg, G., Iwarzon, M., Stal, P., and Seensalu, R. (1990). Digital ambulatory monitoring of small-bowel motility. *Scand. J. Gastroenterol.* 25, 216–24.

McKendrick, M. W. and Read, N. W. (1994). Irritable bowel syndrome—post salmonella infection. *J. Infect.* 29, 1–3.

Mertz, H., Naliboff, B., Munakata, J., Niazi, N., and Mayer, E. A. (1995). Altered rectal perception is a biological marker of patients with irritable bowel syndrome [published erratum appears in *Gastroenterology* (1997) 113,1054. *Gastroenterology* 109, 40–52.

Narducci, F., Bassotti, G., Gaburri, M., and Morelli, A. (1987). Twenty four hour manometric recording of colonic motor activity in healthy man. *Gut* 28, 17–25.

Narducci, F., Snape, W. J. J., Battle, W. M., London, R. L., and Cohen, S. (1985). Increased colonic motility during exposure to a stressful situation. *Dig. Dis. Sci.* 30,40–4.

Oliveira, R. B., Meneghelli, U. G., de Godoy, R. A., Dantas, R. O., and Padovan, W. (1983). Abnormalities of interdigestive motility of the small intestine in patients with Chagas' disease. *Dig. Dis. Sci.* 28, 294–9.

Perino, L. E., Schuffler, M. D., Mehta, S. J., and Everson, G. T. (1986). Radiation-induced intestinal pseudoobstruction. *Gastroenterology* 91, 994–8.

Poulakos, L., Elwell, J. H., Osborne, J. W., Urdaneta, L. F., Hauer-Jensen, M., Vigliotti, A. P., Hussey, D. H., and Summers, R. W. (1990). The prevalence and severity of late effects in normal rat duodenum following intraoperative irradiation. *Int. J. Rad. Onc., Biol., Phys.* 18, 841–8.

Prior, A. and Read, N. W. (1993). Reduction of rectal sensitivity and post-prandial motility by granisetron, a 5 HT3-receptor antagonist, in patients with irritable bowel syndrome. *Aliment. Pharmacol. Ther.* 7, 175–80.

Quigley, E. M., Deprez, P. H., Hellstrom, P., Husebye, E., Soffer, E. E., Stanghellini, V., Summers, R. W., Wilmer, A., and Wingate, D. L. (1997). Ambulatory intestinal manometry: a consensus report on its clinical role. *Dig. Dis. Sci.* 42,2395–400.

Reid, B., DiLorenzo, C., Travis, L., Flores, A. F., Grill, B. B., and Hyman, P. E. (1992). Diabetic gastroparesis due to postprandial antral hypomotility in childhood. *Pediatrics* 90, 43–46.

Ribeiro dos Santos, R., Marquez, J. O., Von Gal Furtado, C. C., Ramos de Oliveira, J. C., Martins, A. R., and Koberle, F. (1979). Antibodies against neurons in chronic Chagas' disease. *Tropenmedizin und Parasitologie* 30, 19–23.

Rogawski, M. A., Goodrich, J. T., Gershon, M. D., and Touloukian, R. J. (1978). Hirschsprung's disease: absence of serotonergic neurons in the aganglionic colon. *J. Pediatr. Surg.* 13, 608–15.

Rosa, Troncon, L. E. Oliveira, R. B., Foss, M. C., Braga, F. J., Gallo and Junior, L. (1996). Rapid distal small bowel transit associated with sympathetic denervation in type I diabetes mellitus. *Gut* 39, 748–56.

Silverman, D. H., Munakata, J. A., Ennes, H., Mandelkern, M. A., Hoh, C. K., and Mayer, E. A. (1997). Regional cerebral activity in normal and pathological perception of visceral pain. *Gastroenterology* 112, 64–72.

Smith, V. V., Gregson, N., Foggensteiner, L., Neale, G., and Milla, P. J. (1997). Acquired intestinal aganglionosis and circulating autoantibodies without neoplasia or other neural involvement. *Gastroenterology* 112, 1366–71.

Sodhi, N., Camilleri, M., Camoriano, J. K., Low, P. A., Fealey, R. D., and Perry, M. C. (1989). Autonomic function and motility in intestinal pseudoobstruction caused by paraneoplastic syndrome. *Dig. Dis. Sci.* 34, 1937–42.

Stanghellini, V., Camilleri, M., and Malagelada, J. R. (1987). Chronic idiopathic intestinal pseudo-obstruction: clinical and intestinal manometric findings. *Gut* 28, 5–12.

Suarez, G. A., Fealey, R. D., Camilleri, M., and Low, P. A. (1994). Idiopathic autonomic neuropathy: clinical, neurophysiologic, and follow-up studies on 27 patients. *Neurology* 44, 1675–82.

Summers, R. W., Anuras, S., and Green, J. (1983). Jejunal manometry patterns in health, partial intestinal obstruction, and pseudoobstruction. *Gastroenterology* 85, 1290–1300.

Summers, R. W., Glenn, C. E., Flatt, A. J., and Elahmady, A. (1992). Does irradiation produce irreversible changes in canine jejunal myoelectric activity? *Dig. Dis. Sci.* 37, 716–22.

Szurszewski, J. H. (1969). A migrating electric complex of canine small intestine. *Am. J. Physiol.* 217, 1757–63.

Szurszewski, J. H., Elveback, L. R., and Code, C. F. (1970). Configuration and frequency gradient of electric slow wave over canine small bowel. *Am. J. Physiol.* 218, 1468–73.

Tack, J., Janssens, J., Vantrappen, G., Peeters, T., Annese, V., Depoortere I., and Bouillon, R. (1992). Effect of erythromycin on gastric motility in controls and in diabetic gastroparesis. *Gastroenterology* 103, 72–9.

Thompson, D. G., Ritchie, H. D., and Wingate, D. L. (1982). Patterns of small intestinal motility in duodenal ulcer patients before and after vagotomy. *Gut* 23, 517–23.

Thompson, D. G., Wingate, D. L., Archer, L., Benson, M. J., Green, W. J., and Hardy, R. J. (1980). Normal patterns of human upper small bowel motor activity recorded by prolonged radiotelemetry. *Gut* 21, 500–6.

Troncon, L. E. and Iazigi, N. (1992). Scintigraphic study of the gastrointestinal transit of a liquid meal in patients with chronic Chagas' disease. *Braz. J. Med. Biol. Res.* 25, 145–8.

Vantrappen, G., Janssens, J., Hellemans, J., and Ghoos, Y. (1977). The interdigestive motor complex of normal subjects and patients with bacterial overgrowth of the small intestine. *J. Clin. Invest.* 59, 1158–66.

Wallin, C., Engqvist, A., Lindberg, G., Veress, B., and Reichard, H. (1992). [Transplantation of the small intestine can be suitable in patients with pseudoobstruction]. [Swedish]. *Lakartidningen* **89**, 309–10.

Wingate, D. L. (1981). Backwards and forwards with the migrating complex. *Dig. Dis. Sci.* **26**, 641–66.

Wood, J. D. (1984). Enteric neurophysiology. *Am. J. Physiol.* **247**, G585–G598.

Yoshida, M. M., Schuffler, M. D., and Sumi, S. M. (1988). There are no morphologic abnormalities of the gastric wall or abdominal vagus in patients with diabetic gastroparesis. *Gastroenterology* **94**, 907–14.

29. Postprandial hypotension in autonomic disorders

Christopher J. Mathias and Roger Bannister

Introduction

In normal subjects, food ingestion results in a number of hormonal, neural, and regional haemodynamic changes. A variety of pancreatic and gastrointestinal peptides are released. Some of these may affect the cardiovascular system either directly, or indirectly through modulation of autonomic nervous activity. There is a marked increase in splanchnic blood flow, but systemic blood pressure remains virtually unchanged in normal subjects, presumably because activation of the sympathetic nervous system, together with release of vasoactive hormones, results in appropriate readjustment.

In patients with disturbances of autonomic function, ingestion of food may substantially lower blood pressure. Postcibal hypotension as a clinical problem, was first reported by Seyer-Hansen (1977) in a 65-year-old man with autonomic failure and parkinsonism, who suffered from severe dizziness and visual disturbance during almost every meal and in whom hypotension could be provoked by oral glucose. A group of patients with autonomic dysfunction were studied by Robertson et al. (1981) who confirmed a profound fall in both systolic and diastolic blood pressure after food ingestion. In these studies, the patients were seated and it was unclear to what degree the upright posture contributed to the hypotension. Our own interest in postprandial hypotension was triggered in 1982, when a patient complained of considerable worsening of posturally induced dizziness after breakfast, which lowered her pressure to levels of 80/50 mmHg even in the supine position for 3 h (see Fig. 29.1).

Postprandial hypotension can be a major clinical problem in some patients with autonomic failure. In this chapter the pathophysiological mechanisms responsible, with an emphasis on the neural, haemodynamic, and biochemical basis of postprandial hypotension, will be discussed, along with the role of specific components of the meal. The relationship to interventional and therapeutic processes will follow. We shall concentrate on subjects with primary chronic autonomic failure (pure autonomic failure, PAF; and multiple system atrophy, MSA). Studies emphasizing differences between them also will be mentioned. Brief descriptions will be provided of responses to food in other patients with autonomic dysfunction and others who, despite not having an autonomic disorder, may be at risk from the effects of food ingestion.

Haemodynamic changes to food ingestion

In normal subjects, food ingestion in either the seated or the supine position usually causes minimal or no change in blood pressure. In

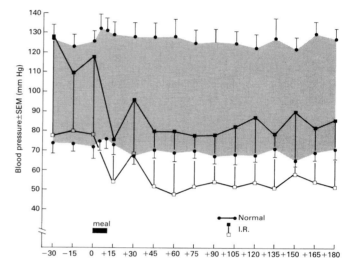

Fig. 29.1. Supine systolic and diastolic blood pressure before and after a standard meal in a group of normal subjects (stippled area, with ± SEM bars) and in a patient with autonomic failure (I.R.). Blood pressure does not change in the normal subjects after a meal. In the patient, there is a rapid fall in blood pressure to levels around 80/50 mmHg which remain low in the supine position over the 3-h observation period.

normal subjects given a standard meal (450 kcal, containing carbohydrate, protein, and fat) in the supine position, there is a rise in heart rate together with an elevation in stroke volume and cardiac output (Mathias et al. 1989a). Forearm muscle blood flow falls with an elevation in forearm vascular resistance. There are no changes in the cutaneous circulation. There is a fall in calculated peripheral vascular resistance (Fig. 29.2a), presumably because of a large increase in splanchnic blood flow, as has been demonstrated by non-invasive measurements of a major splanchnic vessel, the superior mesenteric artery (Fig. 29.2b). Plasma noradrenaline levels rise, suggesting an overall increase in sympathetic nervous activity. There are no changes in plasma adrenaline levels. Plasma renin activity levels double. There is an increase in muscle sympathetic nerve activity measured by microneurographic techniques after ingestion of a nutrient such as glucose (Berne et al. 1989; Fig. 29.3). Studies using noradrenaline spillover techniques indicate that skeletal muscle and the kidneys are major sites of sympathetic activation postprandially, while cardiac spillover is unaltered (Cox et al. 1995; Fig. 29.4). It appears that the nervous and

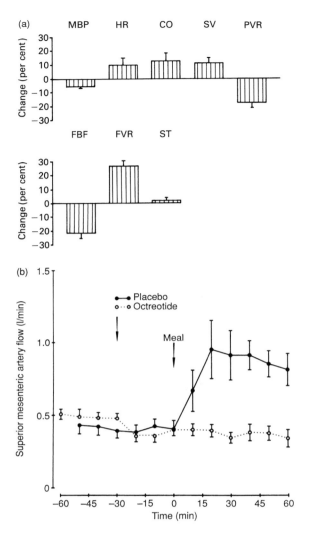

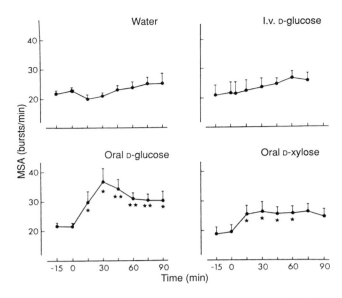

Fig. 29.3. Muscle nerve sympathetic activity (MSA) expressed as the number of bursts per minute in normal subjects after ingestion of either 300 ml of water orally, D-glucose (0.35 g/kg body weight i.v.), 100 g of D-glucose and 75.6 g of D-xylose orally, *, $P < 0.05$; **, $P < 0.01$. (Modified from Berne *et al.* (1989).)

Fig. 29.2. (a) Maximum percentage change in mean blood pressure (MBP), heart rate (HR), cardiac output (CO), stroke volume (SV), calculated peripheral vascular resistance (PVR), forearm muscle blood flow (FBF), calculated forearm vascular resistance (FVR), and skin temperature to the index finger (ST) in six normal subjects in the first hour after food ingestion. Vertical bars indicate ± SEM. (b) Superior mesenteric artery blood flow in normal subjects before and after a balanced liquid meal, when given either saline placebo (continuous line, filled circles) or 50 μg of octreotide (dotted line, open circles), both subcutaneously. (From Kooner *et al.* (1989).)

endocrine systems, among others, exert multiple adjustments that result in the maintenance of blood pressure in normal individuals.

In patients with autonomic failure, even in the supine position, there is a substantial fall in blood pressure which occurs within 10–15 min of ingestion and reaches its nadir within 60 min (Fig. 29.5). There are often modest or no changes in heart rate, particularly if there is associated cardiac parasympathetic denervation. Superior mesenteric artery blood flow rises to an extent similar to that in normal subjects, but there are no changes in blood flow to the skin and forearm vasculature, and no increase in cardiac output,

indicating that appropriate haemodynamic adjustments are not being exerted to counteract splanchnic vasodilatation (Mathias *et al.* 1989*a*; Kooner *et al.* 1990). Plasma noradrenaline and adrenaline levels remain unchanged, consistent with the inability of these patients to activate the sympathetic nervous system. Postural change after food ingestion often results in a fall in blood pressure to even lower levels and has the potential to enhance symptoms of impaired cerebral perfusion markedly (Mathias *et al.* 1991).

Postprandial hypotension appears greater in PAF than in MSA (Mathias *et al.* 1991; Fig. 29.6). Whether this reflects differences in the lesion (peripheral in PAF and central in MSA, see Chapter 24), the ability to release vasodilatatory and vasoconstrictor substances, or supersensitivity of target organs to vasoactive substances, is unclear. The severity of the autonomic lesion may be of importance; thus in MSA, where the disorder is progressive, the autonomic nervous system may not be as impaired as later in the course of the disease and may account for the difference from PAF; longitudinal studies as the disease in MSA progresses have not been described. There also appear to be differential responses to food ingestion within the MSA groups; the cerebellar form has a greater degree of supine postprandial hypotension than the parkinsonian form (Fig. 29.7; von der Thusen *et al.* 1996); this may be related to differences in the central autonomic areas affected in these groups. In the cerebellar form of MSA, where the lesions are more rostral, in addition to neurones affecting motor control, centres influencing cardiovascular autonomic regulation are more likely to be impaired than in the parkinsonian form. Similar differences between the cerebellar and parkinsonian forms of MSA have been reported with exercise-induced hypotension (Smith and Mathias. 1996). These recent observations indicate the importance of clear identification of the autonomic disorder, and especially in MSA even the subgroup, when pathophysiological studies are reported.

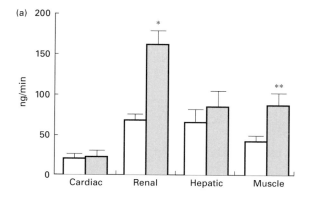

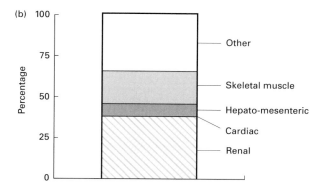

Fig. 29.4 (a) Pre- and postprandial regional plasma noradrenaline spillover, indicating sympathetic nervous system activation in normal subjects. The open histograms indicate the values while fasting, and the filled histograms postprandially, in different vascular beds. The percentage changes are indicated in (b). There is greater activation in the renal and skeletal muscle vasculature than in cardiac or hepatic regions. (From Vaz *et al.* 1995).

Gastrointestinal motility

The gut is richly innervated by autonomic nerves and patients with autonomic failure are likely to have disordered gastrointestinal motility, affecting various segments of the tract (Mathias 1996). The possibility of 'dumping' has been considered, as in many there is evidence of cardiac vagal denervation, favouring vagal impairment of the upper gut. In the classical 'dumping syndrome', which is known to occur after gastric drainage procedures and truncal vagotomy, patients suffer from weakness, sweating, tachycardia, palpitations, and occasionally a modest fall in blood pressure soon after food ingestion, especially if this contains a high carbohydrate load. In this 'early' dumping syndrome, there is rapid entry of a hyperosmotic (often carbohydrate) load into the jejunum, causing fluid absorption within the gut, thus reducing plasma volume and raising the haematocrit. Normally, this would be opposed by an increase in sympathetic activity, thus accounting for some of the symptoms. In autonomic failure there are no changes in plasma osmolality or the haematocrit after food, making it less likely that fluid translocation into the gut, either as a result of osmotic changes or for other reasons, results in a contraction in plasma volume as in the early dumping syndrome (Mathias *et al.* 1989a).

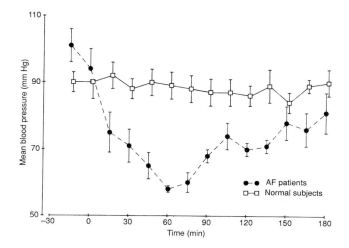

Fig. 29.5. Percentage change in mean blood pressure in a group of patients with chronic autonomic failure (dashed line, filled circles) and in normal subjects (continuous line, open squares) before and after food ingestion at time 0. The bars indicate means ± SEM. (From Mathias *et al.* (1989a).)

To determine whether increased gastric emptying is related to postprandial hypotension, studies have been performed using a technetium-labelled meal with quantification of gastric emptying by γ scintillation scanning in the sitting position. In the majority of patients with autonomic failure there was an increase in gastric emptying (Fig. 29.8), along with postprandial hypotension. In some, however, the rate of emptying was normal, while in others (including one with systemic amyloidosis) gastric emptying was delayed, but they all still developed marked postprandial hypotension. It seems

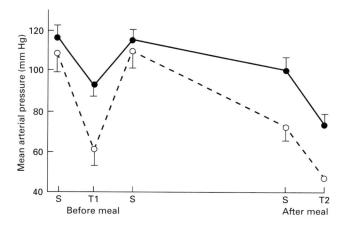

Fig. 29.6. Average levels of mean arterial blood pressure (with standard error of mean) in patients with multiple system atrophy (MSA, ●—●) and pure autonomic failure (PAF, ○---○) before a meal while supine (S) and during head-up tilt to 45° (T1), while supine for 45 minutes postprandially, and before and during retilting (T2 on right, after meal). There is a greater postprandial fall in blood pressure while supine in PAF. After the meal the blood pressure falls to lower levels in both MSA and PAF. The lower pressure, and presumed reduction in cerebral perfusion, is likely to account for the increase in postural symptoms after a meal. (From Mathias *et al.* (1991).)

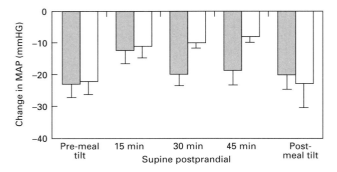

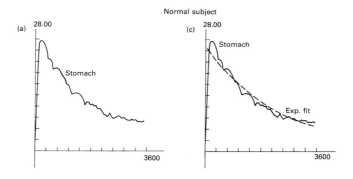

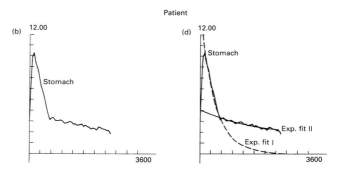

Fig. 29.7. Changes in mean arterial pressure (MAP) ± SEM on head-up tilt and after standard liquid meal ingestion in two subgroups with multiple system atrophy, the cerebellar (MSA-C) (filled histograms) and the parkinsonian (MSA-P) (open histograms). The difference between the groups while supine postprandially was significant at 30 and 45 min. Although there is less supine postprandial hypotension in MSA-P, the postural fall was similar in both groups pre and post-meal. (From von der Thusen *et al.* (1996).)

unlikely, therefore, that increased gastric emptying alone is a major factor accounting for postprandial hypotension.

Food components

Ingestion of a largely solid balanced meal causes a similar fall in blood pressure when compared with the effects of an isocaloric, balanced liquid meal in autonomic failure. A series of further studies using different food components, which were isocaloric, isovolumic, and wherever possible isotonic, indicates major differences between the hypotensive effects of different food components (Fig. 29.9). After glucose, the hypotension is similar to that observed after a balanced meal. Lipid, however, has slower, smaller, and less sustained hypotensive effects while an elemental protein meal causes virtually no change in blood pressure.

The hypotensive effects of oral glucose are not related to its hyperosmolality, as in the same patients an isocaloric, isosmotic, and isovolumic solution of the inert carbohydrate, xylose, causes much smaller falls in blood pressure (Fig. 29.10). However, intravenous administration of hypertonic glucose (25–50 ml of 50 per cent solution) lowers blood pressure rapidly but transiently in patients with tetraplegia and autonomic failure (Mathias *et al.* 1987) (Fig. 29.11). The effects of glucose are not related to its increasing plasma concentration, as intravenous infusions of glucose, despite resulting in higher plasma levels, do not lower blood pressure to the same extent as after oral glucose (Fig. 29.12).

Pancreatic/gut hormones and their effects

Food ingestion causes release of pancreatic and gastrointestinal hormones, some of which are released into the circulation to exert distant effects, while others may act locally. A number were measured in both normal subjects and in autonomic failure patients before and after food ingestion. Changes in plasma levels of gastrin, vasoactive intestinal polypeptide, somatostatin, and cholecystokinin-8 are similar in both groups (Mathias *et al.* 1989a). Enteroglucagon, pancreatic polypeptide, and neurotensin levels rise to a greater extent in patients with autonomic failure (Fig. 29.13); the first two do not

Fig. 29.8. Gastric emptying curves: (a) and (c) in a normal subject and (b) and (d) in a patient with chronic autonomic failure. Integrated counts are indicated on the vertical axis and time in seconds on the horizontal axis. A computer exponential (Exp) fit is indicated on the right. In the autonomic failure patient there is rapid emptying initially (Exp. fit I) with a later slower phase (Exp. fit II).

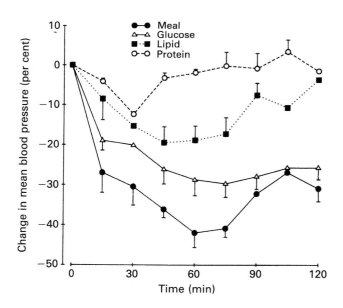

Fig. 29.9. Percentage change in mean blood pressure in six patients with chronic autonomic failure given either a standard meal or an isocaloric and isovolumic solution of carbohydrate (glucose, 1 g/kg body weight), lipid (prosperol 0.95 mg/kg), or protein (maxipro, 1 g/kg) alone, orally. Vertical bars indicate ± SEM.

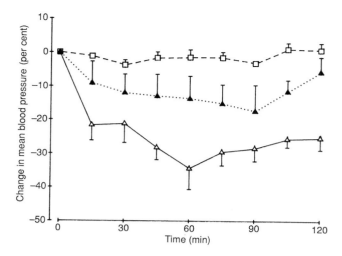

Fig. 29.10 Percentage change in mean blood pressure in eight normal subjects after oral glucose (dashed line, open squares) and in six chronic autonomic failure patients after glucose (continuous line, open triangles) and xylose (dotted line, filled triangles). Results are means ± SEM as vertical bars. The difference between the fall in blood pressure after glucose and xylose in the autonomic failure patients, calculated as the area under the curve, is highly significant (P < 0.01). (From Mathias *et al.* (1989b).)

have vasodilatatory or negative cardiac inotropic effects and are unlikely to contribute to the hypotension. Neurotensin has potential vasodilatatory effects; however, the haemodynamic studies indicated that it was unlikely that postprandial hypotension resulted from its systemic effects. The studies utilizing peripheral venous measurements described above have limitations, as release of peptides and related substances from enteric regions may exert significant autonomic and vascular effects locally without changes reflected in the periphery. An example is recent human studies indicating that feeding almost doubles neuropeptide Y (NPY) overflow in the hepato-mesenteric region independently of noradrenaline spillover,

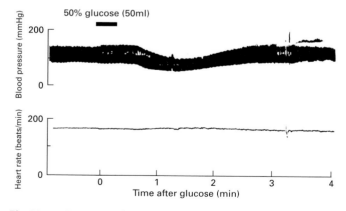

Fig. 29.11 Intra-arterial record showing blood pressure and heart rate in a patient with amyloidosis and severe autonomic failure before, during and after 50% glucose intravenously. There is a rapid but transient fall in blood pressure with no change in heart rate. An equivalent amount of isotonic saline over a similar period (not shown in figure) caused no change in blood pressure. (From Mathias *et al.* 1987).)

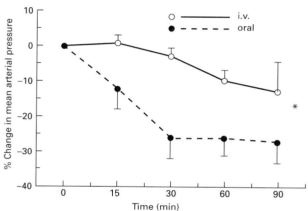

Fig. 29.12. (a) Venous plasma glucose levels in subjects with autonomic failure before (0) and after oral (interrupted lines) and intravenous (continuous lines) glucose. The dose infusion of the latter was calculated to mimic the levels produced by oral glucose, when studied in the same subjects on another occasion. However, the levels with intravenous glucose were higher. Despite this, blood pressure levels (b) were lower after oral glucose. (From data of Mathias, Puvi-Rajasingham, Alam, Raimbach & Cortelli.)

but without similar changes in NPY concentration in peripheral blood (Morris *et al.* 1997).

Of the various peptides, the cardiovascular autonomic effects of insulin have been studied in detail. In normal subjects, exogenous insulin does not lower blood pressure, but increases sympathetic nerve activity and elevates plasma noradrenaline levels (Fagius *et al.* 1986); these changes occur even in adrenalectomized patients, excluding a role for the adrenal medulla. Whether these effects of insulin are through an action on the brain (as suggested by animal studies; Muntzel *et al.* 1994) or directly through causing vasodilatation, is not entirely clear. Vasodilatatory effects of insulin may occur in various vascular regions. In normal subjects, given a high fat meal without an insulin infusion, or in combination with an insulin infusion to raise insulin levels to those observed after a high carbohydrate meal (Kearney *et al.* 1996a; Fig. 29.14), changes were observed in both the skeletal musculature and splanchnic circulation. Vasodilatation in calf muscle did not occur after the

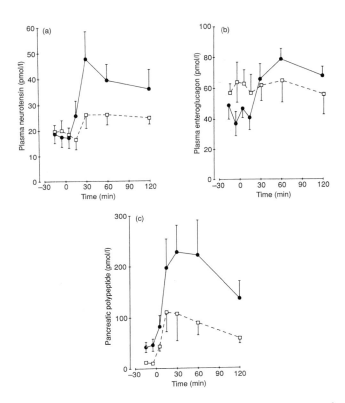

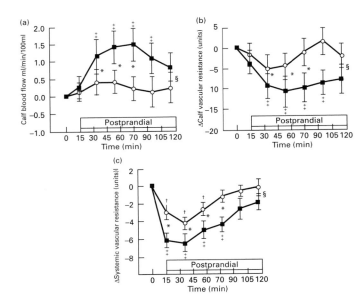

Fig. 29.13. Levels of (a) plasma neurotensin, (b) enteroglucagon, and (c) pancreatic polypeptide in patients with chronic autonomic failure (continuous line, filled circles) and in normal subjects (dashed line, open squares) before and after food ingestion at time 0. The vertical bars are ± SEM. (From Mathias *et al.* (1989*b*).)

Fig. 29.14. Changes in calf blood flow (a), calf vascular resistance (b), and systemic vascular resistance (c) after a high fat meal alone (open circles) and in combination with an insulin infusion to mimic levels after a high carbohydrate meal (filled squares). There were differences over the 120-min. postprandial period. With the high fat meal alone there was no change in calf blood flow which increased when accompanied by insulin. Calf vasculature resistance fell further with insulin infusion. Systemic vascular resistance fell rapidly in both states, with a greater fall after the high fat meal and insulin. §, significant difference in response between meals; †, significant change from baseline after high fat meal; ‡, significant change from baseline after high fat meal with insulin; *, significant difference between individual time points. (From Kearney *et al.* (1996*a*).)

meal alone, but when combined with insulin; there were similar changes in calf muscle vascular resistance. Superior mesenteric artery blood flow responses were similar, with dilatation (consistent with the observations when exogenous insulin was administered without a meal), but vascular resistance was greater when insulin was infused. This suggests that the vasodilatation induced by insulin occurs in both the skeletal muscle and splanchnic vasculature in normal man.

In patients with autonomic failure, exogenous insulin lowers blood pressure substantially, even in the absence of changes in blood glucose (Mathias *et al.* 1987; Brown *et al.* 1989). Bolus intravenous insulin (0.15 units/kg) causes hypotension (Fig. 29.15) but without dilatation in forearm muscle or cutaneous vascular beds. When administered with an euglycaemic clamp, blood pressure falls independently of changes in blood glucose and without changes in cardiac output and forearm muscle or skin blood flow, thus favouring an effect on a large vascular bed such as the splanchnic circulation. In autonomic failure it is likely that insulin causes splanchnic vasodilatation and lowers blood pressure, with no compensatory increase in sympathetic nerve activity as normally seen. This is consistent with the ability of insulin to lower blood pressure in diabetics with autonomic neuropathy (see Chapter 39). Patients with PAF often have a greater degree of postprandial hypotension than those with MSA (Mathias *et al.* 1991); plasma glucose and insulin levels before a meal are similar in both groups

(Fig. 29.16). After a meal, however, glucose levels are similar, but there is a greater rise in post-meal insulin levels in PAF that may account for the greater degree of postprandial hypotension in PAF (Armstrong and Mathias 1991).

In normal subjects the somatostatin analogue, octreotide, is effective in preventing the release of pancreatic and gut hormones in response to various stimuli, including food and alcohol ingestion (Fig. 29.17). Octreotide has to be administered subcutaneously and causes an initial but transient elevation in blood pressure which occurs only in autonomic failure patients and not in normal subjects; the reasons for this are not clear and include pressor supersensitivity, possibly to the venoconstrictor effects of octreotide. Octreotide is effective in preventing both glucose and food-induced hypotension in autonomic failure (Fig. 29.18) (Hoeldtke *et al.* 1986; Raimbach *et al.* 1989). It prevents the rise in insulin, neurotensin, and a range of other hormones in response to food (Fig. 29.19), but it has no effect on cardiac output, muscle or skin blood flow, suggesting that it prevents postprandial hypotension largely by its effects on the splanchnic vasculature. This has been confirmed by non-invasive measurement of superior mesenteric artery blood flow, which rises markedly after a liquid meal but is unchanged after pre-treatment with octreotide (Kooner *et al.* 1990). This emphasizes the role of the splanchnic circulation and of vasodilatatory gut hormones in postprandial hypotension.

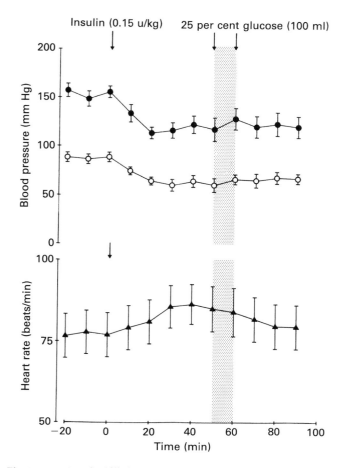

Fig. 29.15. Systolic (filled circles) and diastolic (open circles) blood pressure and heart rate in five patients with chronic autonomic failure before and after intravenous insulin. Both systolic and diastolic blood pressure fall within 10 min. Hypoglycaemia occurred at around 30 minutes and did not result in a further fall in blood pressure. Blood pressure remained low even after reversal of hypoglycaemia with 25 per cent glucose infused over 10 min. (From Mathias *et al.* (1987).)

Investigation of postprandial hypotension

This has been described in Chapter 20.

Management of postprandial hypotension

A better understanding of the pathophysiological mechanisms have increased therapeutic possibilities to limit the problems caused by postprandial hypotension (Mathias, 1997) (Table 29.1). The patient should be made aware of food-induced hypotension and provided with appropriate information concerning the composition, size, and frequency of meals. Carbohydrate increases vulnerability to postural hypotension, especially if refined carbohydrate is used, and dietetic advice about different foods and their composition is needed. The benefit of taking the same caloric intake, but spread as smaller meals

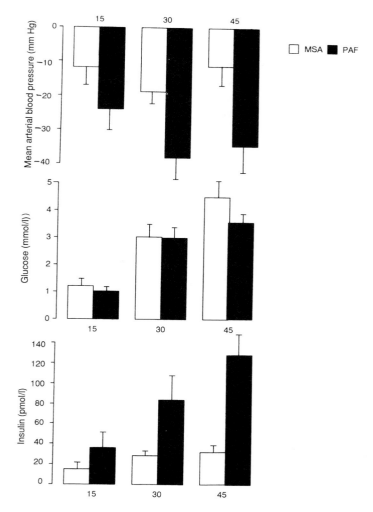

Fig. 29.16. Fall in mean blood pressure in patients with multiple system atrophy (open histograms, MSA) and patients with pure autonomic failure (filled histograms, PAF) at intervals of 15, 30, and 45 min after a balanced liquid meal ingested in the supine position. The middle panel indicates the changes in plasma glucose, and the lower panel in plasma insulin, at similar time points. In PAF there is a greater fall in blood pressure than in MSA. The rise in plasma glucose levels appear similar while the rise in plasma insulin levels are considerably greater in PAF.

given more frequently, had been noted previously by patients and has now been documented as being helpful (Puvi-Rajasingham and Mathias 1996). Food ingestion enhances postural hypotension (Fig. 29.6) and, especially after large meals, it is necessary that patients do not stand or walk. Many are aware that their tolerance to even small amounts of alcohol is low. Alcohol lowers blood pressure and enhances postural hypotension, probably through its vasodilatatory effects, including those on the splanchnic vasculature (Ray Chaudhuri *et al.* 1994; Fig. 29.17).

Various drugs have been used. In the initial studies of Robertson *et al.* (1981), single doses of propranolol, diphenhydramine, cimetidine, and indomethacin were evaluated. Propranolol (40 mg orally) had no beneficial effect and may even have worsened postprandial hypotension. The H₁ antihistaminic, diphenhydramine, and

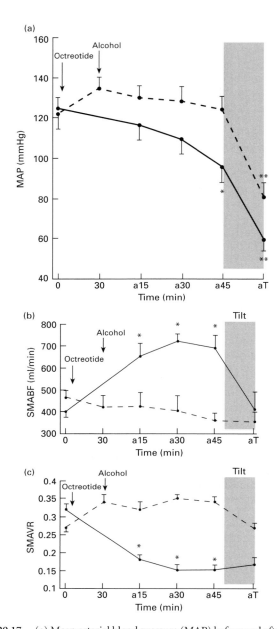

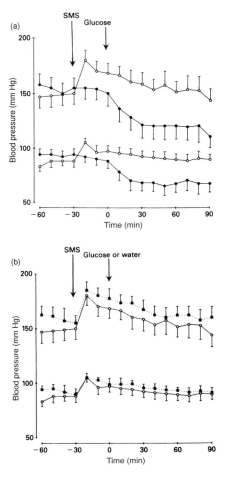

Fig. 29.17. (a) Mean arterial blood pressure (MAP) before and after alcohol ingestion alone without octreotide (continuous line) and after pre-treatment with octreotide (interrupted line), 15, 30, and 45 min (a15, a30, a45) after alcohol ingestion. Blood pressure falls after alcohol alone while supine, and to lower levels during tilt (aT), unlike when ingested after pre-treatment with octreotide. (b) Superior mesenteric artery blood flow (SMABF), and (c) superior mesenteric artery vascular resistance (SMAVR), before and after alcohol ingestion alone (continuous line) and after pre-treatment with octreotide (interrupted line). The fall in SMABF after tilt is greater after alcohol alone (aT). The rise in SMABF is prevented by octreotide. *, $p < 0.05$; **, $p < 0.001$. (From Ray Chaudhuri et al. (1995).)

Fig. 29.18. (a) Systolic and diastolic blood pressure and heart rate in patients with chronic autonomic failure on two occasions when given oral glucose at time 0 with pre-treatment at -30 min with either octreotide (SMS 201–995) 50 μg (open circles) or saline placebo (filled circles) both subcutaneously. (b) Systolic and diastolic blood pressure in patients with chronic autonomic failure given octreotide (SMS 201–995) 50 μg subcutaneously at -30 min followed at 0 min by either oral glucose (open circles) or an equivalent amount of water (filled squares) (From Raimbach et al. (1989).)

the H$_2$ blocker, cimetidine, had no effect, making it unlikely that histamine played a role in the responses. The hypotensive response to food was attenuated by indomethacin (50 mg orally), suggesting that vasodilatatory prostaglandins or arachidonic acid metabolites may be responsible. Long-term studies in postprandial hypotension have not been reported with indomethacin; however, it has the potential to induce gastrointestinal erosions and bleeding.

Caffeine raises blood pressure in normal subjects by stimulating the sympathetic or renin–angiotensin system. It was reported to be highly effective in preventing postprandial hypotension in autonomic failure (Onrot et al. 1985). This occurred independently of stimulation of the sympathetic and renin–angiotensin systems, and a postulated mechanism was blockade of vasodilatatory adenosine receptors. Our experience with caffeine in severe autonomic failure, however, has not been favourable. When administered to PAF and MSA in single doses of 250 and 500 mg, and also on a regular basis, there was neither objective nor subjective evidence of benefit (Armstrong et al. 1990). Similar experiences have been reported in the elderly (Lipsitz et al. 1994). Whether patients with incomplete autonomic lesions (in whom the residual sympathetic or

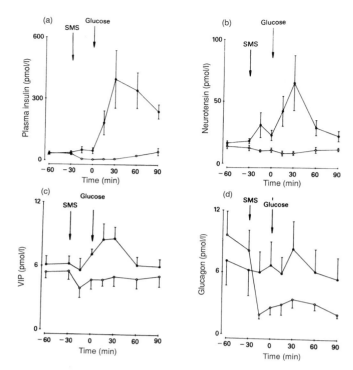

Fig. 29.19. Changes in plasma levels of (a) insulin, (b) neurotensin, (c) vasoactive intestinal polypeptide (VIP), and (d) glucagon in patients with chronic autonomic failure after placebo (filled circles) or octreotide (SMS 201–995) (open circles), given at –30 min followed by oral glucose at 0 min. Results are means ± SEM. (From Raimbach *et al.* (1989).)

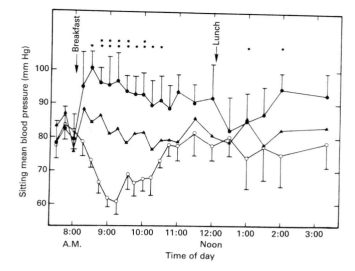

Fig. 29.20. Sitting mean blood pressure after breakfast and lunch in six patients with autonomic failure of different aetiology, when given placebo (open circle) or two different doses of the somatostatin analogue SMS 201–995 (octreotide, filled circles, 0.4 μg/kg and filled triangles, 0.2 μg/kg). For comparisons of drug and placebo, single asterisks signify $P < 0.05$ and double asterisks $P < 0.001$. SEM for low doses of drug are omitted for clarity. (From Hoeldtke *et al.* (1986).)

renin–angiotensin systems may be stimulated) are likely to benefit, remains to be elucidated.

An effective drug in preventing postprandial hypotension is the somatostatin analogue, octreotide (Fig. 29.20). This was first used by Hoeldtke *et al.* (1986) and is a synthetic, long-acting peptide-release inhibitor. It is effective in autonomic failure in reducing glucose- and alcohol-induced hypotension (Raimbach *et al.* 1989; Ray Chaudhuri *et al.* 1995) probably by reducing aplanchnic vasodilatation. Octreotide can be given in small doses, ranging from 25 to 50 μg two or three times daily, ideally about half an hour before meal ingestion. Its disadvantages include its subcutaneous administration and local discomfort because of its low pH; it also may induce nausea, abdomi-

Table 29.1. Some of the approaches used to prevent or reduce postprandial hypotension

Advice

Have smaller meals, more frequently
Reduce refined carbohydrate
Avoid alcohol
Do not stand or walk after meals

Drugs

Indomethacin
Caffeine
Octreotide
Denopamine and midodrine
L-Dihydroxyphenylserine

nal colic, and diarrhoea, the last especially after a fatty meal. Its longer-term side-effects (such as cholelithiasis), although well charted in various endocrine conditions where larger doses usually are used, are less clear in autonomic failure. In one of our patients with pure autonomic failure hyperglycaemia occurred, necessitating oral hypoglycaemics, while in two others intermittent hypoglycaemia was a possibility; the precise cause and relationship was unclear. Beneficial effects of octreotide have been demonstrated on hypotension induced by postural change and even by exercise (Armstrong and Mathias 1991; Smith *et al.* 1995), although these effects may be modest. A further question concerns whether it might enhance nocturnal hypertension in autonomic failure. This has been addressed using 24-hour ambulatory blood pressure profiling, and indicates a favourable effect, with a reduction in nocturnal hypertension (Alam *et al.* 1995). The availability of oral analogues of octreotide should help further.

The splanchnic circulation may be targeted in other ways (Mathias 1997), such as through the known effects of vasopressin on the portal circulation. This provides another possible approach in postprandial hypotension, as demonstrated in five patients with MSA in whom infusion of vasopressin prevented glucose-induced hypotension (Hakusui *et al.* 1991). Analogues such as glypressin (see Chapter 36) may also be of value.

There are increasing data on the value of sympathomimetics in postcibal hypotension. A combination of the α-adrenoceptor agonist midodrine, and the β-adrenoceptor agonist, denopamine, successfully reduced glucose-induced hypotension in eight patients with autonomic failure (Hirayama *et al.* 1993). When given alone, neither drug had a beneficial effect. The combination resulted in an increase in peripheral vascular resistance (presumably through midodrine) and an elevation of cardiac output (probably through denopamine), thus correcting the two major haemodynamic abnormalities contributing to postprandial hypotension. These patients were also placed on long-term treatment, with continuing benefits and no adverse effects.

The prodrug dihydroxyphenylserine (DOPS; in the racaemic, DL form), has recently been shown to reduce postprandial hypotension in both PAF and MSA patients; there was probably a greater response in PAF (Freeman *et al.* 1996). The mechanisms by which DOPS reduces hypotension are discussed in Chapters 36 and 40.

Effects of food in other groups of patients, some with autonomic dysfunction

Patients on ganglionic blockers and following splanchnic denervation

The hypotensive effect of food appears to have been first recorded by Smirk (1953) in hypertensive patients after the ganglionic blocker, pentolinium, was used. He observed a fall in pressure in the lying, sitting, and standing position after lunch. Whether postprandial hypotension occurs after other antihypertensive sympatholytic drugs known to cause postural hypotension, such as reserpine, debrisoquine, guanethidine, and bethanidine, is not clearly documented.

Insulin lowers blood pressure when given to normal subjects after a ganglionic blocker (hexamethonium) (di Salvo *et al.* 1956). Insulin-induced hypotension has been recorded in patients after splanchnic denervation from T7 to L3 inclusive, performed for the relief of severe hypertension (French and Kilpatrick 1955). It is likely in both groups that splanchnic vasodilatation not accompanied by appropriate compensatory sympathetic nervous activity was responsible for the fall in blood pressure.

Diabetes mellitus

Insulin lowers blood pressure in diabetics with autonomic neuropathy and baroreceptor abnormalities and can provoke or enhance postural hypotension (Miles and Hayter 1968) (see Chapter 39). In postprandial hypotension in diabetics with autonomic neuropathy, it has been difficult to separate the effects of food itself from that of insulin. The former is likely to have hypotensive effects, in keeping with the suggestion that factors in addition to insulin are also important in causing hypotension. This is consistent with the observations of Hoeldtke *et al.* (1986) who successfully used octreotide to reduce postprandial hypotension in diabetic autonomic neuropathy; the beneficial effects were not reversed by insulin administration.

The elderly

Postprandial hypotension is now recognized as occurring in a significant number of the elderly, especially in patients over the age of 80 (see Chapter 55). Food predominantly lowers systolic blood pressure but there are additional falls in diastolic pressure. It is unclear whether this is related to autonomic failure associated with the elderly, or to a combination of other factors that include impairment of hormonal responses, baroreceptor activity, and cardiac function. A range of studies indicates that some of the mechanisms responsible for postprandial hypotension in autonomic failure are

similar in the elderly; so also are some of the therapeutic approaches, including the administration of octreotide.

Neurodegenerative disorders

The hypotensive effects of food ingestion in a group of patients with Parkinson's disease were described by Micieli *et al.* (1987); the patients also had postural hypotension, raising the possibility that some had MSA. In a further study in Parkinson's disease without postural hypotension, and with normal autonomic function (Thomaides *et al.* 1993), postprandial hypotension also was observed. When comparisons were made with PAF and MSA, however, the degree of supine hypotension was less, and furthermore food did not induce or accentuate post-meal postural hypotension. Whether postprandial hypotension occurs in other parkinsonian syndromes (such as progressive supranuclear palsy) has not been studied systematically. In Alzheimer's disease, 7 out of 10 patients had hypotension between 20 and 120 mins after food ingestion; none had postural hypotension, making it unlikely that they had underlying autonomic failure (Idiaquez *et al.* 1997).

Tabes dorsalis with an afferent lesion

We have studied one patient with tabes dorsalis who, on detailed autonomic testing, had evidence of an afferent baroreceptor lesion without impairment of central and peripheral sympathetic pathways. He had pronounced hypotension after food, suggesting that the lesion, which probably also involved afferents from the gut, blocked the normal activation of corrective reflexes and thus contributed to the fall in blood pressure after food.

Tetraplegia

Patients with complete cervical spinal-cord transection cannot activate sympathetic activity in response to agents with vasodilatatory properties (see Chapter 51). Exogenous insulin lowers blood pressure

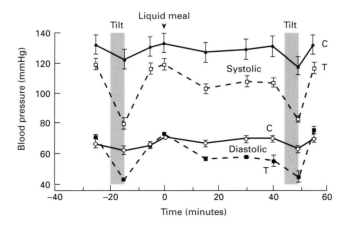

Fig. 29.21.   Blood pressure before and after liquid meal ingestion (at time 0) in tetraplegic (T) and control (C; paraplegic below T12) subjects. There was no significant post-meal fall in supine systolic (upper traces) and diastolic (lower traces) blood pressures (± SEM, bars) in either tetraplegics or in controls. There was no difference in the pre- and post-meal level to which blood pressure fell during postural change in the tetraplegics. (From Baliga *et al.* (1997*a*).)

in tetraplegics (Mathias *et al.* 1979); the fall appears to be smaller than in autonomic failure patients, although no direct comparison has been performed. In tetraplegics, using a similar protocol to those with autonomic failure, ingestion of food causes only modest falls in systolic and diastolic blood pressure, with a rise in heart rate in the supine position (Baliga *et al.* 1997*a*; Fig. 29.21). The reason for the difference from PAF and MSA patients is unclear, and could include the ability of the intact vagus to increase heart rate and cardiac output and thus partially buffer the fall in blood pressure. In these tetraplegics forearm venous plasma noradrenaline did not change after food. However, this does not exclude localized activation of spinal reflexes induced by stimulation of intestinal afferents, as changes in peripheral levels of noradrenaline may not occur because the liver is a major extractor of noradrenaline (Eisenhofer *et al.* 1995). In the tetraplegics postural hypotension post-meal was not enhanced, unlike that observed in PAF and MSA.

Dopamine β-hydroxylase deficiency

Patients with dopamine β-hydroxylase (DBH) deficiency are unable to synthesize either noradrenaline or adrenaline and have severe postural hypotension with selective sympathetic adrenergic failure (see Chapter 40). Food ingestion does not lower their blood pressure (Mathias *et al.* 1990), unlike patients with PAF and MSA. The DBH deficiency patients differ from PAF and MSA in their ability to release dopamine, and presumably other vasoactive chemicals, from otherwise intact sympathetic nerve endings. Whether their ability to release dopamine (which could affect the heart and vasculature) and other vasoconstrictors (such as neuropeptide Y and adenosine triphosphate) from nerve terminals accounts for their resistance to postprandial hypotension, remains to be resolved.

Cerebrovascular and coronary artery disease

These patients do not necessarily have an autonomic deficit, but when on vasoactive drugs they may be prone, because of their regional vascular deficits, to potentially deleterious effects induced by food ingestion. In the presence of carotid artery stenosis an even modest fall in blood pressure may critically impair cerebral perfusion, resulting in a transient ischaemic attack or a stroke; the former has been reported in a single case report (Kamata *et al.* 1994). Recent studies indicate that in patients with haemodynamically significant unilateral and bilateral carotid artery stenosis (with over 80 per cent luminal occlusion), the autonomic control of the circulation is impaired, with postural hypotension occurring in over 50 per cent (Akinola *et al.* 1997). Whether food-induced hypotension further compromises cardiovascular control in such patients remains to be determined.

In patients with coronary artery disease, the increased cardiac workload following food ingestion may contribute to angina pectoris and possibly to myocardial infarction. In his original description in 1772, Heberden noted that angina was exacerbated by exercise, particularly after food. In such patients the composition of food is of importance, as carbohydrate is more likely to induce myocardial ischaemia and reduce exercise capacity than a fat or protein meal (Baliga *et al.* 1997*b*; Fig. 29.22). This may be related to variations in sympathetic activation and an interaction with peptides released by different components in food. Whether there are differences in the efficacy of anti-anginal drugs in preventing

postprandial exacerbations of angina is unclear; α- and/or β-adrenergic blockers may be effective if they prevent sympathetically mediated cardiac work. However, if non-adrenergic vasoconstrictor substances play an important intracoronary role, vasodilatation induced by calcium channel agonists, such as nifedipine, may counteract food-induced myocardial ischaemia; alternatively, preventing peptide release may be beneficial as has been demonstrated with octreotide (Baliga *et al.* 1996).

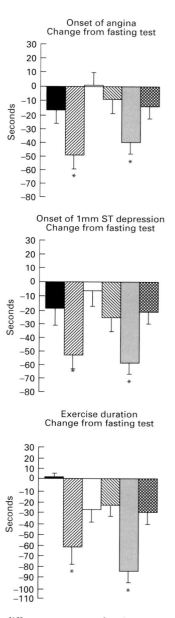

Fig. 29.22. Time differences to onset of angina, 1 mm ST segment depression, and exercise duration after water (black bars), carbohydrate (slashed upwards), fat (white bars), protein (slashed downwards), balanced meal (fine stippled bars), and xylose (boxed bars) compared with corresponding values during exercise in the fasting state in patients with postprandial angina. *, $P = 0.05$. Carbohydrate, either alone or in a mixed balanced meal, was more likely to provoke or worsen angina than other food components. (From Baliga *et al.* (1997*b*).)

Cardiac transplantation

In cardiac transplantees there may be partial or complete cardiac autonomic denervation. In these patients the heart rate and cardiac output response to a high carbohydrate meal is preserved, while the cardiac response appears to be attenuated if a high fat meal has been administered (Kearney *et al.* 1996*b*). The reasons for the rise in heart rate with both meals warrants explanation. In normal subjects there is no rise in noradrenaline spillover post-meal excluding an increase in cardiac sympathetic activation (Cox *et al.* 1995), and suggesting that heart rate changes may be mediated through parasympathetic (vagal) withdrawal. However, the cardiac transplantees were vagally denervated, excluding this possibility. This therefore favours humoral factors, either adrenergic or non-adrenergic, especially if their effects were enhanced in the presence of denervation supersensitivity, as has been demonstrated with isoprenaline (Yusuf *et al.* 1987). Postprandial hypotension did not occur in the transplantees with either meal. With both meals there was an attenuation of the expected postprandial dilatation in the superior mesenteric artery for reasons that are unclear. The studies suggest that neurogenic dysfunction in one region may be compensated for in various ways, in other regions.

References

Akinola A. B., Mathias, C. J., Mansfield, A. *et al.* (1997). Altered neural control of the cardiovascular system in unilateral and bilateral carotid artery stenosis. *Clin. Auton. Res.* 7, 105–6.

Alam, M., Smith, G. D. P., Bleasdale-Barr, K., Pavitt, D. V., and Mathias, C. J. (1995). Effects of the peptide release inhibitor, Octreotide, on daytime hypotension and on nocturnal hypertension in primary autonomic failure. *J. Hypertension* 13, 1664–9.

Armstrong, E. and Mathias, C .J. (1991). The effects of the somatostatin analogue, Octreotide, on postural hypotension, before and after food ingestion, in primary autonomic failure. *Clin. Auton. Res.* 1, 135–40.

Armstrong, E., Watson, L., Hardman, T. C., Bannister, R., and Mathias, C. J. (1990). Effect of oral caffeine on post-prandial and postural hypotension, before and after food ingestion, in primary autonomic failure. *J. autonom. nerv. Syst.* 31, 174–5.

Baliga, R. R., Burden, L., and Kooner, J. S. (1996). Octreotide prevents post-prandial angina pectoris and improves exercise capacity after food ingestion. *Circulation* 94, 8.

Baliga, R. R., Catz, A. B., Watson, L. P., Short, D. J., Frankel, H. L., and Mathias, C. J. (1997*a*). Cardiovascular and hormonal responses to food ingestion in humans with spinal cord transection. *Clin. Auton. Res.* 7, 137–41.

Baliga, R. R., Burden, L., Mandeep, S. K., Rampling, M. W., and Kooner, J. S. (1997*b*). Effects of components of meals (carbohydrate, fat, protein) in causing postprandial exertional angina pectoris. *Am. J. Cardiol.* 79, 1397–400.

Berne, C., Fagius, J., and Niklasson, F. (1989). Sympathetic response to oral carbohydrate administration. Evidence from micro-electrode recordings. *J. Clin. Invest.* 84, 1403–9.

Brown, R. T., Polinsky, R. J., and Bancom, C. E. (1989). Euglycemic insulin-induced hypotension in autonomic failure. *Clin. Neuropharmacol.* 12, 227–31.

Cox, H. S., Kaye, D. M., Thompson, J. M. *et al.* (1995). Regional sympathetic nervous activation after a large meal in humans. *Clin. Sci.* 89, 145–54.

di Salvo, R. J., Bloom, W. L., Brost, A. A., Ferguson, W. F., and Ferris, E. B. (1956). A comparison of the metabolic and circulatory effects of epinephrine, norepinephrine and insulin hypoglycaemia with observations on the influence of autonomic blocking agents. *J. Clin. Invest.* 35, 568–77.

Eisenhofer, G., Aneman, A., Hooper, D., Holmes, C., Goldstein, D., and Friberg, P. (1995). Production and metabolism of dopamine and norepinephrine in mesenteric organs and liver of swine. *Am. J. Physiol.* 268, G641–G649.

Fagius, J., Niklasson, F., and Berne, C. (1986). Sympathetic outflow in human muscle nerves increases during hypoglycaemia. *Diabetes* 35, 1124–9.

Freeman, R., Young, J., Landsberg, L., and Lipsitz, L. (1996). The treatment of postprandial hypotension in autonomic failure with 3,4-DL-threo-dihydroxyphenylserine. *Neurology* 47, 1414–20.

French, E. B. and Kilpatrick, R. (1955). The role of adrenaline in hypoglycemic reactions in man. *Clin. Sci.* 14, 639–51.

Hakusui, S., Sugiyama, Y., Iwase, S. *et al.* (1991). Postprandial hypotension: microneurographic analysis and treatment with vasopressin. *Neurology* 41, 712–15.

Heberden, W. (1772). Some account of a disorder of the breast. *Medical Transactions* (published by the College of Physicians in London) 2, 59–67.

Hirayama, M., Watanabe, H., Koike, Y. *et al.* (1993). Treatment of postprandial hypotension with selective α_1 and β_1 adrenergic agonists. *J. autonom. nerv. Syst.* 45, 149–54.

Hoeldtke, R. D., O'Dorisio, T. M., and Boden, G. (1986). Treatment of autonomic neuropathy with a somatostatin analogue, SMS 201-995. *Lancet* ii, 602–5.

Idiaquez, J., Rios, L., and Sandoval, E. (1997). Post-prandial hypotension in Alzheimer's disease. *Clin. Auton. Res.* 7, 119–20.

Kamata, T., Yokota, T., Furukawa, T., and Tsukagoshi, H. (1994). Cerebral ischaemic attack caused by post-prandial hypotension. *Stroke* 25, 511–13.

Kearney, M. T., Cowley, A. J., Stubbs, T. A., and Macdonald, I. A. (1996*a*). Effect of a physiological insulin infusion on the cardiovascular responses to a high fat meal: evidence supporting a role for insulin in modulating postprandial cardiovascular homoestasis in man. *Clin. Sci.* 91, 415–23.

Kearney, M. T., Cowley, A. J., Stubbs, T. A., Perry, A. J., and Macdonald, I. A. (1996*b*). Central and peripheral haemodynamic responses to high carbohydrate and high fat meals in human cardiac transplant recipients. *Clin. Sci.* 90, 473–83.

Kooner, J. S., Peart, W. S., and Mathias, C. J. (1989). The peptide release inhibitor Octreotide (SMS 201-995), prevents the haemodynamic changes following food ingestion in normal human subjects. *Q. J. Exp. Physiol.* 74, 569–72.

Kooner, J. S., Armstrong, E., Bannister, R., Peart, W. S., and Mathias, C. J. (1990). Octreotide (SMS 201-995) prevents superior mesenteric artery vasodilatation and post-prandial hypotension in human autonomic failure. *Br. J. Clin. Pharmacol.* 29, 154P.

Lipsitz, L. A., Jansen, R. W. M. M., Connelly, C. M., Kelley-Gagnon, M. M., and Parker, A. J. (1994). Haemodynamic and neurohumoral effects of caffeine in elderly patients with symptomatic postprandial hypotension: a double-blind, randomized, placebo-controlled study. *Clin. Sci.* 87, 259–67.

Mathias, C. J. (1996). Gastrointestinal dysfunction in multiple system atrophy. *Semin. Neurol.* 16, 251–5.

Mathias, C. J. (1997) Pharmacological manipulation of human gastrointestinal blood flow. *Fund. Clin. Pharmacol.* 11, 29–34.

Mathias, C. J, Frankel, H. S, Turner, R. C., and Christensen, N. J. (1979). Physiological responses to insulin hypoglycaemia in spinal man. *Paraplegia* 17, 319–26.

Mathias, C. J., Da Costa, D. F., Fosbraey, P., Christensen, N. J., and Bannister, R. (1987). Hypotensive and sedative effects of insulin in autonomic failure. *BMJ.* 295, 161–3.

Mathias, C. J., Da Costa, D. F., Fosbraey, P., *et al.* (1989*a*). Cardiovascular, biochemical and hormonal changes during food induced hypotension in chronic autonomic failure. *J. Neurol. Sci.* 94, 255–69.

Mathias, C. J., Da Costa, D. F., McIntosh, C. M. *et al.* (1989*b*) Differential blood pressure and hormonal effects after glucose and xylose ingestion in chronic autonomic failure. *Clin. Sci.* **77**, 85–92.

Mathias, C. J., Bannister, R., Cortelli, P. *et al.* (1990). Clinical, autonomic and therapeutic observations in two siblings with postural hypotension and sympathetic failure due to an inability to synthesize noradrenaline from dopamine because of a deficency of dopamine β hydroxylase. *Q. J. Med.,* **278**, 617–33

Mathias, C. J., Holly, E., Armstrong, E., Shareef, M., and Bannister, R. (1991). The influence of food on postural hypotension in three groups with chronic autonomic failure—clinical and therapeutic implications. *J. Neurol. Neurosurg. Psychiat.* **54**, 726–30.

Micieli, G., Martignoni, E., Cavallini, A., Sandrini, G., and Nappi, G. (1987). Postprandial and orthostatic hypotension in Parkinson's disease. *Neurology* **37**, 386–93.

Miles, D. W. and Hayter, C. J. (1968). The effects of intravenous insulin on the circulatory responses to tilting in normal and diabetic subjects with special reference to baroreceptor reflex block and atypical hypoglycaemic reactions. *Clin. Sci.* **34**, 419–30.

Morris, M. J., Cox, H. S., Lambert, G. W., *et al.* (1997). Region-specific neuropeptide Y overflows at rest and during sympathetic activation in humans. *Hypertension.* **29**, 137–43.

Muntzel, M., Morgan, D. A., Mark, A. L., and Johnson, A. K. (1994). Intracerebroventricular insulin produces non-uniform increases in sympathetic nerve activity. *Am. J. Physiol.* **267**, R1350–5.

Onrot, J., Goldberg, M. R., Biaggioni, I., Hollister, A. S., Kincaid, D., and Robertson, D. (1985). Haemodynamic and humoral effects of caffeine in autonomic failure. Therapeutic implications for post-prandial hypotension. *New Engl. J. Med.* **313**, 549–54.

Puvi-Rajasingham, S., and Mathias, C. J. (1996). Effect of meal size on the blood pressure before and after postural change in primary autonomic failure. *Clin. Auton. Res.* **6**, 1–6

Raimbach, S. J., Cortelli, P., Kooner, J. S., Bannister, R., Bloom, S. R., and Mathias, C. J. (1989). Prevention of glucose-induced hypotension by the somatostatin analogue Octreotide (SMS 201-995) in chronic autonomic failure haemodynamic and hormonal changes. *Clin. Sci.* **77**, 623–8.

Ray Chaudhuri, K., Maule, S., Thomaides, T., Pavitt, D., and Mathias, C. J. (1994). Alcohol ingestion lowers supine blood pressure, causes splanchnic vasodilatation and worsens postural hypotension in primary autonomic failure. *J. Neurol.* **241**, 145–52.

Ray Chaudhuri, K., Thomaides, T., Watson, L., and Mathias, C. J. (1995). Octreotide reduces alcohol-induced hypotension and orthostatic symptoms in primary autonomic failure. *Q. J. Med.* **88**, 719–25.

Robertson, D., Wade, D., and Robertson, R. M. (1981). Post-prandial alterations in cardiovascular haemodynamics in autonomic dysfunction states. *Am. J. Cardiol.* **48**, 1048–52.

Seyer-Hansen, K. (1977). Post-prandial hypotension. *BMJ* **2**, 1262.

Smirk, F. M. (1953). Action of a new methonium compound in arterial hypotension, M & B 205A. *Lancet* **i**, 457.

Smith, G. D. P., and Mathias, C. J. (1996). Differences in the cardiovascular responses to supine exercise and to standing post-exercise in two clinical subgroups of the Shy–Drager syndrome (multiple system atrophy). *J. Neurol. Neurosurg. Psychiat.* **61**, 297–303

Smith, G. D. P., Alam, M., Watson, L. P., and Mathias, C. J. (1995). Effects of the somatostatin analogue, octreotide, on exercise induced hypotension in human subjects with chronic sympathetic failure. *Clin. Sci.* **89**, 367–73.

Thomaides, T., Bleasdale-Barr, K. Chaudhuri, K. R., Pavitt, D. V., Marsden, C. D., and Mathias, C. J. (1993). Cardiovascular and hormonal responses to liquid food challenge in idiopathic Parkinsons disease, multiple system atrophy and pure autonomic failure. *Neurology* **43**, 900–4.

Vaz, M., Cox, H. S., Kaye, D. M., Turner, A. G., Jennings, G. L., and Esler, M. D. (1995). Fallibility of plasma noradrenaline measurements in studying postprandial sympathetic nervous responses. *J. Autonom. Nerv. Syst.* **56**, 97–104.

von der Thusen, J. H., Smith, G. D. P., Bleasdale-Barr, K., and Mathias, C. J. (1996). Differences in postprandial hypotension in two subtypes with human central autonomic failure (Shy–Drager syndrome/multiple system atrophy). *J. Physiol.* **495**, 129P.

Yusuf, S., Theodropoulos, S., Mathias, C. J. *et al.* (1987). Increased sensitivity of the denervated transplanted human heart to isoprenaline both before and after beta-adrenergic blockade. *Circulation* **75**, 696–704.

30. Investigation and treatment of bladder and sexual dysfunction in diseases affecting the autonomic nervous system

Clare J. Fowler

Introduction

The lower urinary tract and genitalia are largely innervated by autonomic fibres and consequently disturbances of bladder and sexual function are common in patients with diseases of the autonomic nervous system. Poor bladder emptying, failure of bladder storage, and impaired sexual responses, usually erectile failure, can be either presenting symptoms of autonomic nervous system failure or occur as troublesome problems in patients with established disease. Investigation of such complaints using urodynamic or neurophysiological methods may be carried out for the purpose of establishing a neurological diagnosis, particularly if some local structural disorder could produce similar symptoms or with a view to introducing treatment. The management of urinary and sexual dysfunction arising from autonomic failure is mostly symptomatic and many of the treatments now available are highly effective.

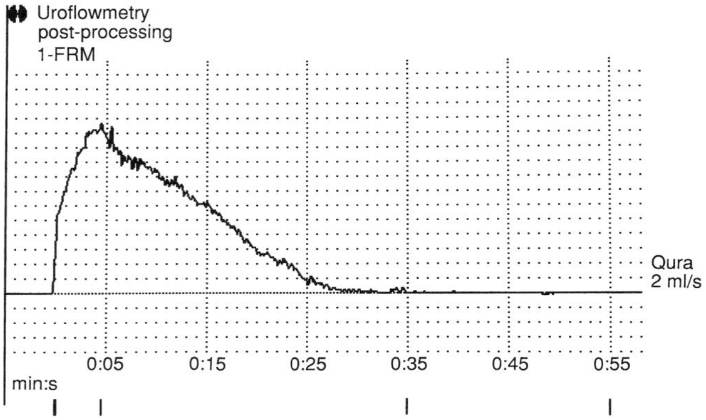

Uroflowmetry
post-processing
1-FRM

Qura
2 ml/s

min:s   0:05   0:15   0:25   0:35   0:45   0:55

Fig. 30.1. Normal uroflowmetry. Qura is the urinary flow rate. The maximum flow rate is 22 ml/s and the trace is smooth, indicating an uninterrupted urine flow.

Methods of investigation

Urodynamic studies

Urodynamic studies include various tests devised to investigate the storage and emptying functions of the lower urinary tract. Although of value in providing descriptive information about the pathophysiological behaviour of the bladder, such tests cannot be expected to provide a diagnosis in neurological terms. Furthermore, very similar findings may occur in urological and neurological disease.

Tests range from simple charting of voided volumes over a 24 h period to complex studies involving the simultaneous recording of the intravesical pressure, intra-abdominal pressure, urinary flow, and sphincter electromyography.

Uroflowmetry and post micturition studies

Measurement of the urinary flow rate and the postmicturition urinary volume are useful initial screening tests. Small and inexpensive flow meters are now available which provide a graphic trace of urinary flow (Fig. 30.1). Most devices are able to give values for maximum flow rate, voided volume and the time taken to complete micturition. Urinary flow rates can only properly be assessed if the patient voids at least 150 ml, when nomograms adjusted for age, sex, and voided volume can be used to interpret the results. After voiding, the residual

urine can be measured either by passing a urethral catheter into the bladder or by ultrasound (Fig. 30.2). If the patient voids with a normal flow rate and has a residual of less than 50 ml, a significant abnormality of the innervation of the bladder is unlikely.

Cystometry—filling and voiding

Cystometry involves monitoring the detrusor pressure while the bladder is filled and during voiding. Intravesical pressure is measured using a fine catheter (1 mm diameter) passed into the bladder alongside a larger Nelaton catheter (3 mm diameter) which is used to fill the bladder at a controlled rate. Rectal pressure provides a measure of intra-abdominal pressure and is recorded by means of another fine catheter inserted into the rectum. The urodynamic machine calculates the detrusor pressure by subtraction of the rectal pressure from the total intravesical pressure. The filling phase of cystometry is most useful in the investigation of patients with symptoms of urgency and frequency and incontinence. Normally during filling there is only a small rise in the detrusor pressure which occurs when the bladder is nearly full (Fig. 30.3). Abnormal detrusor contractions may be recorded during filling (Fig. 30.4) and if they occur in a patient with known neurological disease the patient is said to have 'detrusor hyper-reflexia'. Detrusor hyper-reflexia occurs very commonly in patients with spinal-cord disease but may also occur in patients with

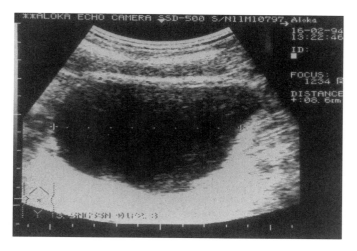

Fig. 30.2. Ultrasound image of bladder. Cursors are placed on the image and, after measurement in three planes, the volume of urine is estimated assuming the bladder to be nearly spherical.

sphincter can then be seen on the video during attempts to void and EMG recordings are unnecessary.

Neurophysiological investigation of the urogenital tract

Electromyography (EMG) of the urethral sphincter can be carried out as part of a urodynamic study as described above or can be performed as a separate neurophysiological study. A concentric needle electrode can be used to examine for changes of denervation and chronic reinnervation in either the urethral or anal sphincter and this has proved to be of value in recognizing multiple system atrophy (MSA) (Eardley *et al.* 1989; Beck *et al.* 1994; Palace *et al.* 1997). (Figure 30.3)

The other neurophysiological investigations that have been used to examine the innervation of the pelvic floor and lower urinary tracts suffer mostly from the defect that they test only the somatic innervation of the region. It is possible to record sacral reflex latencies electrophysiologically, i.e. recordings made from striated muscle structures in the pelvic floor in response to stimulation of the

parkinsonism or other forms of cerebral disease. However, exactly the same appearance may be seen in patients who do not have neurological disease and then the activity is called 'detrusor instability'. Thus the cause of bladder overactivity can not be deduced from urodynamic studies and its correct classification depends on the clinician recognizing that the patient has an underlying neurological disease. The urinary symptoms reported by patients with detrusor hyper-reflexia or instability include frequency, urgency, and urge incontinence.

Pressure-flow studies during micturition are useful in the investigation of patients with difficulty in voiding and incomplete emptying. Analysis of the urinary flow and the detrusor pressure sustained during voiding may show that a low urine flow rate is due either to a failure of detrusor contraction or obstructed outflow. An abnormality of the parasympathetic innervation of the bladder will result in weak, poorly sustained detrusor contractions during attempts to void, a low urinary flow rate, and possibly a raised postmicturition residual volume. By contrast, a local urological abnormality such as prostatic hypertrophy may cause poor urine flow but with a high detrusor pressure. The literature on the cystometric findings in urological and neuro-urological disease is extensive and reference to recent textbooks is recommended for further reading (Mundy *et al.* 1994; Chancellor and Blavias, 1996).

Any interruption of the neural connections between the pons and the sacral cord causes a loss of the co-ordinated activity of the bladder and sphincter so that instead of the sphincter relaxing with the initiation of micturition, the bladder may contract spontaneously due to detrusor hyper-reflexia and the sphincter contract at the same time. This disorder is known as 'detrusor-sphincter dyssynergia' and may be demonstrated by simultaneous recordings of sphincter EMG activity and urine flow rate. For some while sphincter EMG was recommended as part of cystometry and many urodynamics machines have a channel for EMG recordings. However, now most centres with a particular interest in the urological problems of patients following spinal-cord injury use fluoroscopy during cystometry to visualize the upper renal tracts and to detect the potentially serious problem of ureteric reflux. Abnormal contractions of the

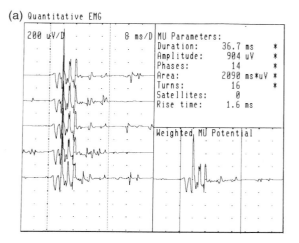

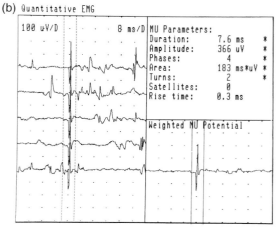

Fig. 30.3. (a) An abnormally prolonged motor unit recorded from the anal sphincter of a patient with MSA using a trigger and delay line. The unit is shown on the left in a falling leaf display and the inset shows the 'weighed motor potential'. The cursors have been set to show its duration of 36.7 ms. (b) A normal duration motor unit, recorded and displayed in the same way as Figure 30.5.

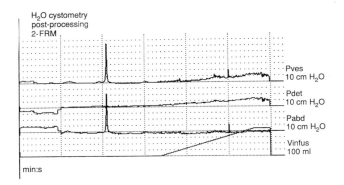

Fig. 30.4. A 'stable' bladder on cystometry. Vinfus, filling rate; Pabd, intra-abdominal pressure; Pves, intravesical pressure; Pdet, the detrusor pressure, is derived by subtracting Pabd from Pves. This trace shows the detrusor pressure rising to less than 10 cm of water on filling to 450 ml. The sudden increase in Pves, which also occurs in Pabd occurred when the subject was asked to cough.

dorsal nerve of the penis/clitoris, and although the latency of responses may be abnormal in a patient with a cauda equina lesion or peripheral neuropathy, the test only examines conduction in the large myelinated fibres innervating the region, not the unmyelinated fibre autonomic innervation. Likewise, the pudendal evoked potential can be delayed in patients with spinal-cord disease and urogenital dysfunction but there is usually other clinical evidence of such a problem, and the test is very rarely diagnostic (Delodovici and Fowler 1995). A similar criticism can be made of measurement of the latency of pelvic floor muscle contraction in response to cortical magnetic stimulation.

Sympathetic skin responses recorded from the genital region do, however, give information about local sympathetic innervation. Using the same technique as is used to record the responses from the hands or the feet, surface electrodes can be attached to the perineum or genitalia and record either spontaneous ongoing activity or the response to stimulation of a distant nerve (Ertekin et al. 1995). Unfortunately no significance can be attached to a low amplitude response and only an absent response can only be considered definitely abnormal. The question as to whether the

activity, which has been called 'SPACE' (single potential analysis of cavernosus electrical activity) (Stief et al. 1991), is significantly different from sympathetically generated electrodermal activity is not yet resolved.

Investigation of sexual dysfunction

Investigation of sexual dysfunction is predominantly treatment orientated and the main complaint for which there is effective management is male erectile dysfunction. Although female sexual dysfunction may occur in autonomic nervous system disease, there are no specific treatments and it is a problem which has been very little researched.

The introduction of intracorporeal injections of vasoactive substances for treatment of male erectile dysfunction transformed management such that the need to distinguish between neurogenic and psychogenic erectile dysfunction became mainly of academic interest. Nocturnal penile tumescence studies are no longer regarded as being of diagnostic value in demonstrating organic erectile dysfunction, although they may still have some place in the assessment of a diabetic man complaining of impotence.

An adequate response to prostaglandin E, indicates that the problem must be either neurogenic or psychogenic, whereas repeated failure to develop an erection suggests a vascular pathology such as inadequate arterial inflow or abnormal venous outflow.

Neurophysiological studies are mostly non-contributory although absence of a sympathetic skin response from the genital region or failure to record SPACE (see above) may confirm the presence of a local autonomic neuropathy (Fowler 1998).

Treatments
Treatment of neurogenic bladder disorders

When a patient with neurological disease complains of urinary urgency and frequency it is reasonable to assume the pathophysiological basis of the symptoms is detrusor hyper-reflexia and prescribe anticholinergic medication. However, this course of action however overlooks the possible contribution that incomplete bladder emptying might be making to the problem. In several of the neurological disorders that affect the innervation of the bladder, both detrusor hyper-reflexia and incomplete bladder emptying occur, although symptoms of the existence of the latter may be relatively minor. A constant residual urine volume in the bladder is likely to act as a stimulus for detrusor hyper-reflexia so that urgency and frequency will persist as long as the bladder is not emptied. For this reason it has been proposed that measurement of the postmicturition residual volume be made in all patients with neurogenic incontinence (Fowler 1996). If this is in excess of 100 ml, it will be necessary for the patient to achieve better bladder emptying before anticholinergics can be effective, particularly since drugs with anticholinergic action may exacerbate poor bladder emptying. An algorithm for bladder management is outlined in Fig. 30.6 which requires minimal investigation and offers the best possibility for effective therapy of patients with neurogenic incontinence. If the patient fails to report sustained improvement after starting anticholinergic medication, the postmicturition residual volume should be re-measured.

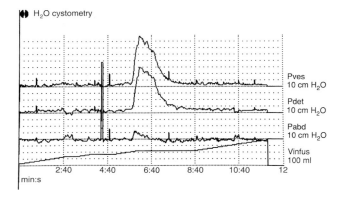

Fig. 30.5. Detrusor hyper-reflexia. At about 5 min into the study with the bladder filled to 200 ml, there is an abrupt rise in detrusor pressure (60 cm water) which the patient was unable to suppress.

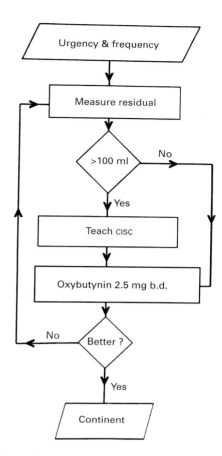

Fig. 30.6. Algorithm for management of neurogenic incontinence (Fowler, 1996). In a patient with known neurological disease with urinary symptoms of urgency and frequency, detrusor hyper-reflexia requiring treatment with an anticholinergic can reasonably be assumed to be the underlying cause. An essential measurement is the postmicturition residual urine volume since if this is raised urine in the bladder will act as a constant stimulus, causing continued bladder contractions. Clean intermittent self-catheterization (CISC) can be highly effective in emptying the bladder and thus reducing symptoms.

Treatment of incomplete bladder emptying

Incomplete bladder emptying may result from a disturbance of the parasympathetic innervation of the detrusor or poorly co-ordinated detrusor–sphincter activity and is best managed by intermittent catheterization. Introduced for the treatment of urinary dysfunction in patients with spinal injuries, the technique has since greatly improved the management of patients with urinary dysfunction resulting from many different neurological causes. In general the greatest symptomatic improvement can be expected in those patients with large residual volumes and good storage function.

A specialist nurse is the most suitable person to instruct the patient, or if necessary his or her carer in the technique. In general, female patients find the procedure more difficult initially and usually require a mirror to help locate the urethral orifice. Most patients performing clean intermittent self-catheterization will void a variable amount before passing the catheter but after commencing anticholinergic medication, effective voiding may be so reduced that the

patient relies more on intermittent self-catheterization. Frequency of catheterization will best be determined by the patients but initially they should be advised to perform the procedure three or four times a day, ensuring that the residuals are kept lower than 500 ml. Asymptomatic bacteriuria is not an uncommon finding in those using intermittent self-catheterization but serious urinary tract infections are, fortunately, less common.

Recently the use of a vibrating stimulus applied to the suprapubic region has been found to improve bladder emptying in some patients with detrusor hyper-reflexia and incomplete bladder emptying (Dasgupta *et al.* 1997).

Anticholinergic medication

Detrusor hyper-reflexia is best treated by drugs with anticholinergic properties. Oxybutynin (2.5 mg two or three times a day) is often highly effective if the patient has detrusor hyper-reflexia. It has a smooth muscle relaxant effect in addition to anticholinergic action. Propantheline (15–30 mg four times a day) can be used as an alternative but the side-effects of this and other non-selective anticholinergics include a dry mouth, impaired accommodation, and constipation. New anticholinergic preparation selective for the M_3 muscarinic receptor to terodine has recently been introduced.

Capsaicin

An alternative approach to lessening detrusor hyper-reflexia if patients have spinal-cord disease has been the use of intravesical capsaicin. Following a spinal-cord lesion that disconnects the sacral cord from the pontine micturition centre, a new segmental reflex emerges at the sacral level of the cord, the afferents of which are unmyelinated C fibres. Although the fibres and the receptors they subserve are present in the neurologically intact, they are usually quiescent unless activated by irritations such as bacterial infection. A strong solution of capsaicin (100 ml of 2 mM) instilled into the bladder for 30 min was found to have the effect of lessening of detrusor hyper-reflexia for some months (Fowler *et al.* 1994). It is thought that the mechanism of action of capsaicin is to deafferent the bladder by its selectively C-fibre neurotoxic effect. Alternative drugs that selectively block the afferent limb of the reflex that causes detrusor hyper-reflexia are currently under development.

DDAVP

The synthetic antidiuretic hormone DDAVP® (Desmospray®) was initially introduced for the treatment of diabetes insipidus but in recent years it has become widely accepted for the treatment for nocturnal enuresis in children. Desmospray® has also been used to treat patients with muitiple sclerosis who are troubled by night-time frequency and some of these patients have taken to using it during the day if they particularly require a 4–6 hour period free from urinary urgency. This is safe provided that the patient understands the importance of only using the medication once in 24 h. Patients with autonomic failure are often troubled by night-time frequency, possibly as a result of progressive daytime hypotension causing poor renal profusion. Desmospray® may lessen nocturnal frequency in these patients and seems to have an added beneficial effect in the management of postural hypotension. DDAVP is now available in a tablet form. Whereas a metered dose of 10 μg is administered from the nasal spray, the tablets contain either 0.1 or 0.2 mg of desmopressin, the higher dosage being necessary because of enzymatic degradation when the substance is taken orally.

Treatment of male erectile dysfunction (MED)

Patients should be counselled before commencing treatment and many benefit from an explanation of their sexual difficulties in relation to their illness. If appropriate the situation should also be explained to the patient's partner.

The advent of an oral drug for MED has transformed the treatment of this disorder as there were considerable disadvantages to the management options previously available.

Sildenafil (Viagra)

Release of nitric oxide nerves supplying the arterioles of the corpora cavernosa results in smooth muscle relaxation and penile erection. Nitric acid increases intracellular levels of cyclic GMP (guanosine monophosphate) which acts on vascular smooth muscle and the effect of cGMP is terminated by the enzyme phosphodiesterase. Slidenafil is an orally active selective phosphodiesterase inhibitor and it prolongs the effect of cGMP on erectile tissue. Because of its mode of action Sildenafil would only be expected to cause erection following sexual stimulation.

Sildenafil is rapidly absorbed from the stomach so that it reaches effective blood levels within one hour and has a half life of 3–5 hours. The selective nature of its phosphodiesterase inhibitory action (PDI type 5 found mostly in the cavernosal tissue with small amounts present also in the retina) means that there are few side effects. Its clearance is reduced in patients with renal and hepatic impairment.

Initial clinical trials showed it was effective in producing erection following visual sexual stimulation (Boolell *et al.* 1996) and a large scale, double-blind placebo controlled study in men with a wide range of causes of MED demonstrated effectiveness as judged by a self-administered questionnaire (Goldstein *et al.* 1998). Studies published in abstract form only to date have demonstrated Sildenafil to be effective in treating MED in diabetics and men with spinal cord injury.

Intracorporeal pharmacotherapy

Prior to the advent of Sildenafil there were various methods of treatment available, intracorporeal injection therapy being the most reliable. The use of Papaverine was first described by Virag, a vascular surgeon in 1982 and the use of Phentolamine for the same purpose was reported by Brindley in 1983. Papaverine has a direct relaxant effect on smooth muscle and for some years was the preferred agent, but bruising and local discomfort were not uncommon and corporal fibrosis sometimes occurred. Patients with neurogenic impotence were particularly prone to develop episodes of prolonged erection which if they lasted for more than 4 hours required reversal by aspiration of the corpora or possibly intracorporeal injections of alpha-adrenergic agents such as metaraminol or adrenaline. Prostaglandin E1, (alprostadil) was then approved world-wide for self-injection therapy (Porst, 1996) and this rapidly replaced the use of papaverine. Prostaglandin E1 is an endogenous substance which is rapidly metabolised so that priaprism was very uncommon, as was local fibrosis. The substance has almost no systemic side effects and was highly effective—the only frequent problem being of penile pain

and the need to self-inject. The same active agent was then developed as a pellet which was inserted into the urethra as MUSE (medicated urethral system for erection) and although this obviated the need for injection there appear to be a number of problems with the therapy (Fulgham *et al.* 1998).

Vacuum pumps

These devices consist of a cylinder which is placed over the penis and by pumping air out of the tube and creating a vacuum the penis enlarges within it. The increased blood is maintained in the penis by placing a tourniquet around the base and although the resulting erection is less stiff and the base remains flaccid, good success rates for uses of these devices are reported in motivated patients.

Prosthesis

If all non-surgical treatments fail or are unsuitable, some patients may consider having implantation of a penile prosthesis. There are malleable or inflatable types available (Kirby *et al.* 1991). The former are reliable but since the penis remains semi-rigid, concealment can be a problem. The inflatable types have the advantage of being only rigid at the time of intercourse but are considerably more expensive. The corporeal structures are removed at the time of the implant so that if this approach fails no further forms of therapy are available. Implanting these devices is a highly specialized surgical procedure and there is a risk of infection.

Ejaculatory disturbance

Little is known about the neurophysiology of ejaculation in man but it is thought to be under sympathetic control. Sympathetic fibres control the emission of semen from the seminal vesicles and the closure of the bladder neck at the time of ejaculation. Yohimbine is a drug that is claimed to improve ejaculatory function and orgasm. Its action is through an α sympathetic agonist effect and it has been recommended that 5–10 mg should be taken 1–2 h before intercourse is attempted.

Semen can be obtained by electroejaculation, but this technique is used only for purposes of fertilization and has no role in improving sexual performance.

Bladder and sexual dysfunction resulting from specific conditions

Spinal cord pathology

Spinal cord pathology resulting form traumatic injury, demyelination, or neoplastic changes causes a severe disruption of bladder function. This is because the efferent and afferent spinal pathways that pass between the pontine micturition centre and sacral spinal cord are interrupted. In health these pathways are important in maintaining the bladder as a low-pressure, compliant organ during filling and co-ordinating the relaxation of the striated muscle of the urethral sphincter preceding a detrusor contraction during voiding. With loss of this modulating activity the bladder becomes hyper-reflexic and emptying can also be affected both by poorly sustained detrusor contractions and detrusor sphincter dyssynergia. In patients following spinal cord injury, upper-tract disease can ensue, leading to renal failure unless effective preventive measures are taken. However, in patients with progressive neurological disease upper-tract involvement is, for unknown reasons, uncommon and effective management of incontinence for most patients, particularly those less severely disabled, can be achieved by following the algorithm shown in Fig. 30.5.

Multiple system atrophy (MSA)

Urinary and sexual symptoms are a pronounced feature of patients with MSA and erectile dysfunction is frequently the first symptom of the disease in men. In a retrospective review of symptoms in 64 patients with definite multiple system atrophy, 14 of 24 male patients recalled impotence as being the first symptom (Beck et al. 1994). Early urinary symptoms include urgency and frequency of micturition and patients may also complain of a reduced urinary stream. These symptoms are also typical of the much more common condition of prostatic hypertrophy and men with MSA not infrequently undergo TURP for what is thought to be bladder outflow obstruction, without benefit. Women may undergo surgery for stress incontinence before the underlying neurological disorder is appreciated.

Incontinence associated with marked urgency of micturition usually occurs first, although some patients suffer predominantly from urinary stress incontinence. As the strength of detrusor contractions diminishes, the bladder fails to empty and large postmicturition residual volumes develop. Upper-tract urinary complications are rare, possibly because the residual urine remains at a low pressure.

Detrusor hyper-reflexia in MSA may result from the degeneration of areas in the midbrain and basal ganglia and the atonic bladder seen in the later stages of the disease may be due to progressive degeneration of the intermediolateral columns of the cord and the loss of cells from preganglionic neurones of the thoracolumbar and sacral spinal segment. The urethral and anal sphincters are innervated by motor neurones whose cell bodies lie in Onuf's nucleus in the ventral horn of the spinal cord at S2, S3 and S4, which also undergoes selective degeneration. Thus patients with MSA may have a weak sphincter, incomplete bladder emptying, and detrusor hyper-reflexia, i.e. several factors likely to cause incontinence.

It may be because the neural control of the bladder is affected at several different sites within the nervous system that incontinence occurs early and is so severe in patients with MSA. A retrospective study of 52 patients with MSA compared their bladder symptoms with 41 patients with idiopathic Parkinson's disease (IPD). Although urinary urgency and frequency occurred in both groups, incontinence affected 73 per cent of those with MSA but only 15 per cent of those with IPD (Chandiramani et al. 1997).

The loss of anterior horn cells in Onuf's nucleus results in EMG abnormalities of the urethral and anal sphincters. Motor units recorded from the anal and urethral sphincter are of abnormally prolonged duration and sometimes of increased amplitude, changes consistent with denervation and reinnervation. Sphincter EMG with measurement of the mean duration of 10 motor units forms the basis of a test used to detect the pathological changes characteristic, although not diagnostic, of MSA. Sphincter EMG analysis can be used to distinguish between patients with idiopathic Parkinson's disease and patients with MSA who present with atypical parkinsonism (Eardley et al. 1989; Palace et al. 1997). The test is reliable since the abnormalities that occur are so extreme, but the EMG

changes of reinnervation are not specific and results from women who have had multiple childbirth or patients who have undergone pelvic surgery must be interpreted with caution. Also, the specificity of the test for MSA amongst other neurodegenerative conditions has been questioned (Valldeoriola et al. 1995).

Treatment of urinary dysfunction in patients with MSA can be effective until the late stages of the disease—initially detrusor hyper-reflexia is the predominant abnormality and, if there is no significant residual, anticholinergic medication alone may then be helpful. Patients with MSA often develop large residual volumes in the later stages of the disease and volumes in excess of 200 ml are not unusual (Beck et al., 1994; Chandiramani et al. 1997). The algorithm shown in Fig. 30.5 should be followed if possible. Desmopressin® nasal spray administered at night is valuable in reducing nocturia and treating nocturnal enuresis. However, with progression of the disease a stage may be reached when an indwelling catheter becomes necessary.

In contrast to erectile dysfunction resulting from other neurological conditions such as multiple sclerosis, men with MSA require large doses of pharmacotherapy such as prostaglandin E if they also have hypotension. The combination of abnormal corporeal innervation and poor arterial inflow may make the erectile dysfunction of MSA relatively resistant to treatment with vasoactive substances.

Parkinson's disease

Bladder symptoms can be marked in Parkinson's disease but the nature of the bladder dysfunction is different from that which occurs in MSA. Frequency and urgency of micturition are common and although incontinence may occur, it is often less of a problem than it is in MSA (Chandiramani et al. 1997).

In animal studies the basal ganglia have been shown to exert an inhibitory effect on the bladder and loss of this central inhibition may explain the occurrence of detrusor hyper-reflexia in patients with idiopathic Parkinson's disease. Studies have been performed to examine the relationship between detrusor hyper-reflexia and the effect of anti-parkinsonian drugs in patients undergoing cystometric studies in both 'on' and 'off' states (Fitzmaurice et al. 1985). Although differences between the cystometrograms were found, the changes were unpredictable and the role of the basal ganglia in the control of micturition seems to be more complicated that simple inhibition of detrusor activity. The effect of subcutaneous apomorphine on voiding function in patients with idiopathic Parkinson's disease and urinary symptoms has been investigated. Following apomorphine injections, urinary flow rates were shown to increase and residual volumes decrease (Christmas et al. 1988). It has been proposed that there is a failure of relaxation of the urethral sphincter in patients with Parkinson's disease and, in men, apomorphine injections may be helpful in deciding whether urinary symptoms are due to prostatic enlargement or Parkinson's disease. The urethral sphincter in Parkinson's disease has been studied electromyographically and the motor units were found to be indistinguishable from those of age-matched controls (Eardley et al.1989; Valldeoriola et al. 1995). This contrasts with the highly abnormal sphincter EMG findings in the majority of patients with MSA (Palace et al. 1997).

Although there have been several reports concerning hypersexual behaviour and L-dopa therapy in patients with Parkinson's disease, there have been few studies of sexual dysfunction. In a questionnaire survey of young patients with IPD and their partners, a high level of sexual dysfunction was found, particularly in couples in which the affected partner was male. Erectile difficulties and premature ejaculation were common (Brown *et al.* 1990). A further study demonstrated a high incidence of erectile difficulties in IPD but in general the onset of erectile dysfunction follows the diagnosis of IPD and does not precede the neurological disease as in MSA (Singer *et al.* 1989; Chandiramani *et al.* 1997).

When reading the literature on urogenital symptoms in Parkinson's disease it is important to note whether or not the authors have excluded patients with MSA.

Distal autonomic neuropathy

There have been a number of reports of distal autonomic neuropathy affecting both the sympathetic and parasympathetic systems. The term pan dysautonomia has been applied to the disorder, but if only the parasympathetic system is involved is the condition is known as cholinergic dysautonomia. Painful urinary retention usually occurs in both conditions (Kirby *et al.* 1985). Other urogenital symptoms include erectile failure and, when the sympathetic nerves are involved, impairment of ejaculation.

Diabetes mellitus

Cystopathy was once considered an uncommon complication of diabetes, but the greater use of techniques for studying bladder function have shown that this is incorrect, although the condition is mostly asymptomatic and discovered incidentally. It develops gradually over several years with progressive loss of bladder sensation and impairment of bladder emptying, eventually culminating in chronic low-pressure urinary retention. Urodynamic studies demonstrate impaired detrusor contractility, reduction in the urinary flow rate, and increased postmicturition residual volume and reduction in bladder sensation. The sequence of pathophysiological events that result in diabetic neurocystopathy are uncertain, but it seems likely that there is involvement of both the vesical sensory afferent fibres, causing a reduced awareness of bladder filling, and involvement of parasympathetic efferent fibres to the detrusor, decreasing the ability of the bladder to contract. The density of acetylcholinesterasepositive-staining nerves in the bladder wall has been shown to be reduced in diabetics compared with controls (Faerman *et al.* 1973). The bladder neck, which is principally innervated by sympathetic fibres, is competent in most cases of diabetic cystopathy, suggesting that, as in the cardiovascular system, sympathetic denervation is probably a late phenomenon. Asymptomatic diabetics with cystopathy should be made aware of their disorders since having lost their normal desire to micturate, they may void infrequently. They should be advised to void at regular intervals and before going to bed at night. Symptomatic patients are best managed by clean intermittent self-catheterization.

Diabetes is one of the most common causes of erectile failure and, compared with the mostly asymptomatic condition of diabetic cystopathy, is a problem for which many diabetics seek help. Occasionally impotence may be the presenting symptom of diabetes. The incidence of erectile failure in diabetic men has been estimated at between 25 and 59 per cent (Fairburn *et al.* 1982). Affected by this problem, the diabetic usually complains of gradual progressive loss of rigidity of erection over some months until there is complete failure. This is not initially accompanied by loss of libido but decrease in sexual interest sometimes follows as a reaction to the erectile problem.

Several processes are thought to contribute to the high prevalence of erectile problems of diabetics. These include large-vessel disease, microangiography, and autonomic neuropathy, as well as psychological factors. Diabetic patients are prone to an accelerated form of atherosclerosis and the association between large-vessel disease and impotence is well recognized (Leriche's syndrome).

Although a relationship between diabetic autonomic neuropathy and impotence has long been recognized, there is still no direct means of testing the autonomic nerves that innervate the corpora. Histological study of tissue from diabetic patients has shown morphological abnormalities of the autonomic fibres of the corpus cavernosum. *In vitro* studies of the corporeal smooth muscle from impotent diabetic patients have demonstrated impaired muscle relaxation in response to autonomic nerve stimulation and also after administration of acetylcholine (Saenz de Tejada *et al.* 1989).

Electrophysiological measurement of the bulbocavernosus reflex is not contributory, but genital recordings of the sympathetic skin responses or SPACE may been absent (Fowler 1998). Diabetic patients may complain of failure of ejaculation despite normal orgasm. In these patients an autonomic neuropathy is thought to affect the sympathetic innervation of the genital tract and either ejaculation occurs in a retrograde manner or there may be failure of emission from the seminal vesicles. If retrograde ejaculation is suspected, then the urine passed after ejaculation may appear cloudy and microscopic examination may reveal spermatozoa.

Other causes of retrograde ejaculation

The sympathetic fibres that innervate the smooth muscle of the bladder neck, vas deferens, seminal vesicles, and prostate fibres arise from the anterior roots of T10–L2 and pass through the hypogastric plexus. Retrograde ejaculation occurs when there is emission of semen into the prostatic urethra and at the time of ejaculation the bladder neck fails to close so that semen is forced back into the bladder. This is a common occurrence after transurethral prostatectomy and operations on the bladder neck. Retrograde ejaculation may also result from disorders affecting the sympathetic innervation of the muscle in the region of the bladder neck. Lumbar sympathectomy and retroperitoneal lymph node dissection may cause retrograde ejaculation by interruption of the sympathetic supply to the bladder neck.

Congenital dopamine β-hydroxylase (DBH) deficiency

Congenital dopamine β-hydroxylase (DBH) deficiency (see Chapter 40) is characterized by a deficiency of noradrenaline. Men with this disorder are capable of erection but ejaculation is difficult to achieve or absent. This can be reversed by selectively replacing noradrenaline with the prodrug l-threo dihydroxyphenylserine, emphasizing the role of the α-adrenergic system in control of this function.

References

Beck, R. O., Betts, C. D., and Fowler, C. J. (1994). Genitourinary dysfunction in multiple system atrophy: clinical features and treatment in 62 cases. *J. Urol.* **151**, 1336–41.

Blaivas, J. and Chancellor, M. (1996). *Atlas of urodynamics.* Williams & Wilkins, Baltimore, USA.

Boolell, M., Gepi-Attee, S., Gingell, J. C., and Allen, M. J. (1996). Sildenafil, a novel effective oral therapy for male erectile dysfunction. *Br. J. Urol.* **78**, 257–61.

Brown, R. G., Jahanshahi, M., Quinn, N., and Marsden, C. D. (1990). Sexual function in patients with Parkinson's disease and their partners. *J. Neurol. Neurosurg. Psychiat.* **53**, 480–6.

Chandiramani, V., Palace, J., and Fowler, C. (1997). How to recognise patients with parkinsonism who should not have urological surgery. *Br. J. Urol.,* **80**, 100–4.

Christmas, T. J., Kempster, P. A., Chapple, C. R., Frankel, J. P., Lees, A. J., and Stern, G. M. (1988). Role of subcutaneous apomorphine in parkinsonian voiding dysfunction. *Lancet* **2**, 1451–3.

Dasgupta, P., Haslam, C., Goodwin, R. J., and Fowler, C. J. (1997). The Queen Square bladder stimulator; a device for emptying the neurogenic bladder. *Br. J. Urol.,* **80**, 234–7.

Delodovici, M. L. and Fowler, C. J. (1995). Clinical value of the pudendal somatosensory evoked potential. *Electroenceph. Clin. Neurophys.* **96**, 509–15.

Eardley, I., Quinn, N. P., Fowler, C. J. *et al.* (1989). The value of urethral sphincter electromyography in the differential diagnosis of parkinsonism. *Br. J. Urol.* **64**, 360–2.

Ertekin, C., Colakoglu, Z., and Altay, B. (1995). Hand and genital sympathetic skin potentials in flaccid and erectile penile states in normal potent men and patients with premature ejaculation. *J. Urol.* **153**, 76–9.

Faerman, I., Glocer, L., Celener, D. *et al.* (1973). Autonomic nervous system and diabetes, histological and histochemical study of the autonomic nerve fibres of the urinary bladder in diabetic patients. *Diabetes* **22**, 225–37.

Fairburn, C. G., Wu, F. C. W., McCulloch, D. K. *et al.* (1982). The clinical features of diabetic impotence: a preliminary study. *Br. J. Psychiat.* **140**, 447–52.

Fitzmaurice, H., Fowler, C. J., Rickards, D. *et al.* (1985). Micturition disturbance in Parkinson's Disease. *Br. J. Urol.* **57**, 652–6.

Fowler, C. J. (1998). Investigation of the neurogenic bladder. *J. Neurol. Neurosurg. Psychiat.* **60**, 6–13.

Fowler, C. J. (1993). The neurology of male sexual dysfunction and its investigation by clinical neurophysiological methods. *Br. J. Urol.* **81**, 785–95.

Fowler, C. J., Beck, R. O., Gerrard, S., Betts, C. D., and Fowler, C. G. (1994). Intravesical capsaicin for treatment of detrusor hyperreflexia. *J. Neurol. Neurosurg. Psychiat.* **57**, 169–73.

Fulgham, P. F., Cochran, J. S., and Denman, J. L. *et al.* (1998). Disappointing initial results with transurethral and prostadil for erectile dysfunction in an urology practise setting. *J. Urol.* **160**, 2041–6.

Goldstein, I., Lue, T. F., Padma-Nathan, H., Rosen, R. C., Steers, W. D., and Wicker, P. A. (1998). Oral sildenafil in the treatment of erectile dysfunction. *New Engl. J. Med.* **338**, 1397–1404.

Kirby, R. S., Fowler, C. J., Gosling, J., and Bannister, R. (1985). Bladder dysfunction in distal autonomic neuropathy of acute onset. *J. Neurol. Neurosurg. Psychiat.* **48**, 762–7.

Kirby, R. S., Carson, C. C., and Webster, G. D. (edn.) (1991). *Impotence: diagnosis and management of male erectile dysfunction.* Butterworth Heinemann, Oxford.

Mundy, A., Stephenson, T., and Wein, A. (1994). *Urodynamics: Principles, practice and applications.* Churchill-Livingstone, Edinburgh.

Palace, J., Chandiramani, V. A., and Fowler, C. J. (1997). Value of sphincter EMG in the diagnosis of Multiple System Atrophy. *Muscle Nerve* **20**, 1396–1403.

Porst, H. (1996). The rationale for prostaglandin E1 in erectile failure: a survey of worldwide experience. *J. Urol.* **155**, 802–15.

Saenz de Tejada, I., Goldstein, I., Azadzoi, K., Krane, R. J., and Cohen, R. A. (1989). Impaired neurogenic and endothelium-mediated relaxation of penile smooth muscle from diabetic men with impotence. *New Engl. J. Med.* **320**, 1025–30.

Singer, C., Weiner, W. J., Sanchez-Ramos, J. R., and Ackerman, M. (1989). Sexual dysfunction in men with Parkinson's Disease. *J. Neurol. Rehabil.* **3**, 199–204.

Stief, C. G., Djamilian, M., Anton, P., de Riese, W., Allhoff, E. P., and Jonas, U. (1991). Single potential analysis of cavernous electrical activity in impotent patients: a possible diagnostic method for autonomic cavernous dysfunction and cavernous smooth muscle degeneration. *J. Urol.* **146**, 771–6.

Valldeoriola, F., Valls-Sole, J., Tolosa, E. S., and Marti, M. J. (1995). Striated anal sphincter denervation in patients with progressive supranuclear palsy. *Movement Disorders* **10**, 550–5.

PART IV

Primary Autonomic Failure: Clinical and Pathological Studies in Pure Autonomic failure and Multiple System Atrophy

31. Clinical features and evaluation of the primary chronic autonomic failure syndromes

Roger Bannister and Christopher J. Mathias

Classification

The clinical classification of primary chronic autonomic failure adopted in this book (see Introduction Chapter) is:

1. Patients with pure autonomic failure (PAF), without associated neurological disorders, formerly known as 'idiopathic orthostatic hypotension'.

2. Patients with multiple system atrophy (MSA). MSA comprises a group of central neurological degenerations, often but not always including parkinsonism (Bannister and Oppenheimer 1972). The combination of AF and MSA was known as the Shy–Drager syndrome (Shy and Drager 1960). For brevity, in this chapter the use of the acronym MSA can be taken to mean MSA associated with autonomic failure. MSA in the form of striatonigral degeneration (SND) may occasionally occur without the symptoms of autonomic failure in life (Fearnley and Lees 1990).

3. Patients with autonomic failure (AF) associated with Parkinson's disease (PD).

Of these three primary autonomic disorders, MSA is the most common. Hughes *et al.* (1992), summarizing the results from the Parkinson's Disease Brain Bank at the Institute of Neurology, London, found that seven of the first 100 cases, supposed in life by the referring physicians to have PD, in fact had striatonigral degeneration or MSA. This is consistent with further observations (Colisimo *et al.* 1995). This means that MSA may have a prevalence rate as high as 10 per 100 000, by comparison with the prevalence rate of 100–150 per 100 000 for PD. PAF is much less common than MSA, and AF with PD rarer still.

The Consensus Panel of international experts convened by the American Autonomic Society and co-sponsored by the American Academy of Neurology (Consensus Statement 1996) defined MSA as 'a sporadic progressive adult onset disorder characterised by autonomic dysfunction, parkinsonism and ataxia in any combination' (Fig. 31.1). The features of this disorder include:

(1) parkinsonism (bradykinesia with rigidity or tremor or both), usually with poor or unsustained motor response to chronic levodopa therapy

(2) cerebellar or corticospinal signs; and

(3) orthostatic (postural) hypotension, impotence, urinary incontinence or retention, usually preceding or within 2 years after the onset of motor symptoms.

Characteristically, these features cannot be explained by medications or other disorders. Parkinsonism and cerebellar features quite commonly occur in combination. However, certain features may predominate.

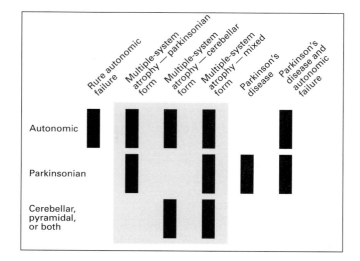

Fig. 31.1. Schematic representation of the major clinical features in the primary autonomic failure syndromes and Parkinsons disease (From Mathias (1997); adapted from Mathias and Williams (1994).)

When parkinsonian features predominate, the term striatonigral degeneration is often used (Fearnley and Lees 1990). When cerebellar features predominate, the term olivopontocerebellar atrophy or degeneration is often used. When autonomic failure predominates, the term Shy–Drager syndrome is often used. These manifestations may occur in various combinations and evolve with time.

Clinical features of primary chronic autonomic failure

The clinical features of autonomic failure can be described separately from the neurological features which are characteristic of MSA or PD.

The particular autonomic functions affected differ in degree from patient to patient but are remarkably similar in all three groups. The patients are usually middle aged or elderly. In MSA, males are affected more often than females. In men, impotence and loss of libido are commonly the first symptoms. Patients living in hot climates may complain of inability to sweat, which could lead to hyperpyrexia and collapse in the tropics but rarely causes problems in temperate countries. The most dramatic symptom, however, and the most common reason for seeking medical advice, is postural dizziness, or even fainting, on standing erect, especially in the morning or after meals or exercise.

One curious symptom of autonomic failure, which presumably reflects a phase of denervation supersensitivity, is that in some patients, over a few weeks or months, an autonomic function may appear hyperactive before failure occurs. This may, in particular, be noted in salivation or sweating and in sexual function in the male in which more frequent spontaneous erection may precede erectile failure.

Postural hypotension

The postural attacks may be 'drop' attacks resembling sudden brainstem vascular dysfunction, but more commonly there is a gradual fading of consciousness over half a minute or so while the patient is standing or walking. A neckache radiating to the occipital region of the skull and to the shoulders often precedes actual loss of consciousness. The neckache may be due to ischaemia in continuously contracting postural muscles in the neck and back in a 'coathanger' distribution (Bleasdale-Barr and Mathias 1998), but the mechanism of this common and virtually unique symptom of postural hypotension is unknown. This ache may be associated with a progressive anterior cervical flexion — anterocollis.

Occasionally, patients may complain of other symptoms suggesting muscle ischaemia. For example, some have described the classical symptoms of angina on exercise and others have described leg symptoms which have features suggestive of 'claudication' affecting the cauda equina. Perhaps surprisingly, despite a very low systolic blood pressure of under 60 mmHg during exercise at the time anginal symptoms occur, the electrocardiogram usually fails to show T-wave inversion or other signs of ischaemia, although a prolonged QT time (although without changes in QT dispersion) has been documented in primary chronic autonomic failure (Lo et al. 1996).

In the postural hypotensive attacks, usually after a visual disturbance or sensation of dizziness, the patient may then fall slowly to his knees; experience teaches him that, after lying flat, there will be recovery and loss of all symptoms, including the neckache, within a few minutes. The recovery from such transient neurological symptoms is usually complete and occlusive cerebrovascular incidents are rare, possibly because many patients, after years of postural hypotension, have not only preserved but enhanced compensatory cerebral autoregulation (Thomas and Bannister 1980). The attacks of loss of consciousness also differ from normal fainting in that the patient usually does not sweat, and there is no vagally induced bradycardia (see Chapter 44).

Symptoms are strikingly worse in the mornings, in hot weather, and also after meals and exercise, all of which cause an unfavourable redistribution of blood volume. The disease is likely to be progressive for several years before significant incapacity occurs, because autonomic compensatory mechanisms postpone overt failure. A few patients, if treated by bed rest for hypotensive symptoms, develop persistent recumbent hypertension, mainly due to loss of baroreflexes, of such severity that they may develop papilloedema with retinal haemorrhages.

Visual disturbances

Sometimes there are transient visual disturbances, scotomata, hallucinations, or tunnel vision, suggesting occipital-lobe ischaemia. The symptoms of visual disturbance may be particularly striking in some patients with autonomic failure. One observant patient was able to classify the disturbances into three kinds. First, there was a disturbance of primary colours, but particularly yellow and red, in which they became brilliant, and secondary colours, or pastel shades, appeared non-existent. Secondly, objects might appear in a photonegative form, that is dark shades being light and the light shades being dark, mostly in various shades of green. Finally, if he did not lie down promptly and had developed a severe neckache and one of the previous disturbances of vision had been present for several minutes, he would then find that his central vision was blurred. On closing his eyes he would see a very clear oval orange or yellow shape filling the whole of the central field with a dark background outside it and in the very centre what appeared to be an irregularly shaped black hole. Once this particular disturbance had occurred it might take some 30 min to subside completely.

On occasion patients describe visual disturbances accompanied by neck and even lumbar aching, brought on by physical exertion while standing, particularly after a meal. The effects of arm exercise, such as washing up after meals or using an ironing board, appear, under conditions of critically reduced systolic blood pressure, to imitate the effects of the subclavian steal syndrome. This is similar to the visual disturbances described by Ross Russell and Page (1983) in patients with critical underperfusion of the brain and retina with extensive occlusive disease of the extracranial arteries. In patients with autonomic failure, however, such symptoms are relatively benign and patients quickly learn to use them as a warning sign that they must lie down quickly to restore an adequate perfusion pressure.

Defective sweating

Defective sweating (Fig. 31.2) causes the risk of hyperpyrexia and collapse in hot climate. The testing of thermoregulatory sweating is described in Chapter 27.

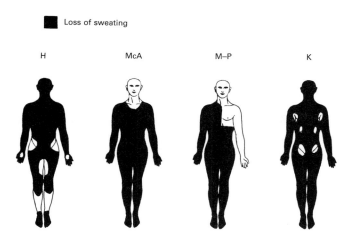

Loss of sweating

H   McA   M–P   K

Fig. 31.2. Sweating response to 1 °C rise in central body temperature in four patients with autonomic failure. From Bannister *et al.* (1967).)

Sexual function

Sexual function in the male is lost early. Failure of erection occurs first, though occasionally after an initial period with excessive erections, and later is followed by disturbance of ejaculation consistent with progressive parasympathetic and then sympathetic failure. As discussed in Chapter 30, complex techniques using pharmacological agents or electrical stimulation may enable some sexual function to be achieved for a time.

Gastro-intestinal function

As the disease advances there may be difficulties with swallowing (Mathias 1996). In combination with laryngeal paresis this may increase the risk of pulmonary infection and even sudden death. Bowel control is sometimes affected, with constipation, intermittent diarrhoea, or rectal incontinence as symptoms. A few cases of MSA with predominant bowel disturbance and cholinergic dysfunction (including salivation) have been described (Khurana *et al.* 1980; Khurana 1994). A marked disturbance of bowel function with a predominance of diarrhoea and faecal incontinence suggests the possibility of amyloid.

Clinical motor features of multiple system atrophy

Three principal forms of motor disturbance occur in MSA: (1) parkinsonian (2) cerebellar and (3) pyramidal.

Parkinsonism

The term 'striatonigral degeneration' (SND) was first used by Adams *et al.* (1964) and later by Fearnley and Lees (1990), to describe patients with a parkinsonian syndrome with special pathological distinguishing features (see Chapter 33). Often the disorder was clinically indistinguishable from PD and, with hindsight, these patients, especially if autonomic defects had been looked for and found, could probably now be classified as having MSA. In this

disease there is a predominance of rigidity without much tremor, associated with progressive loss of facial expression and limb akinesis. The limbs show rigidity on examination, without the classical 'cog wheel' or 'lead pipe' rigidity of PD. Facial expression is often less affected than in PD. The patient has difficulty in standing, walking, or turning and has difficulty in feeding himself. Salivation is reduced. As a result of akinesis, the speech becomes faint and slurred. The patient's gait becomes slow and clumsy, superficially resembling PD, with an attitude of stooping and often extreme forward cervical flexion which makes forward gaze difficult. In MSA, analysis of the dysarthia (Kluin *et al.* 1996) and of the motor disturbances, including ataxia and spasticity (Fetoni *et al.* 1997) have recently been reported.

Cerebellar

The cerebellar form of MSA associated with olivopontocerebellar atrophy (OPCA) was not included in Shy and Drager's original clinical description of only two cases. In this form there is a prominent disturbance of gait with truncal ataxia which frequently makes it impossible for the patient to stand without support. In addition, marked slurring of speech with irregularity of speed of diction has the features describe above for SND. There may also be a mild or moderate intention tremor affecting the arms and legs. This form of MSA is to be distinguished from familial OPCA in which the associated clinical features may include optic atrophy, retinitis pigmentosa, chorea, cataracts, and areflexia (Harding 1981; Gilman and Quinn 1996).

Pyramidal

In either the parkinsonian or cerebellar forms of degeneration there may be a pyramidal increase in tone, together with impaired rapid hand and foot movements and exaggerated deep-tendon jerks and bilateral extensor plantar responses. It is, of course, difficult to detect a pyramidal disturbance of tone in the presence of the extrapyramidal disturbance. Primitive reflexes such as the palmomental reflex may also be present.

Other clinical features in multiple system atrophy

Muscle wasting and neuropathy

Progressive muscle wasting not infrequently occurs (see Chapter 35) although this is not as marked as in motor neurone disease. Fasciculation occurs rarely, but on electromyographic examination there is usually some evidence of denervation with little evidence of any abnormality of peripheral nerve motor conduction. Rarely in PAF and uncommonly in MSA there is clinical and electrophysiological evidence of a mild distal sensorimotor neuropathy with the report of a mild reduction of myelinated fibre density (Cohen *et al.* 1987) and unmyelinated fibre density (Kanda *et al.* 1996).

Intellectual state

Dementia is no more common than might be expected on the basis of chance in patients of this age group, though more detailed testing of cognitive function has shown deficits in visuospatial organization and visuomotor ability, similar to those seen in PD (Testa *et al.* 1993; Pillon *et al.* 1995, Monza *et al.* 1998). It is surprising to observe preserved intellectual function in a patient who is almost totally incapacitated in terms of motor control, postural blood pressure regulation, and bladder disturbance. This is, of course, in striking contrast to the neuronal degeneration of presenile dementia (Alzheimer's disease) in which the predominant degeneration affects cortical cholinergic neurones. It is also in contrast to the intellectual impairment which is a feature of some cases of PD.

Affect

There is no evidence of a mood defect when allowance is made for the considerable disability of patients with MSA, as confirmed by detailed testing in patients with the parkinsonian forms that indicate an overall normal affective state (Pillon *et al.* 1995). This is surprising in view of the hypothesis that central catecholamine function plays a part in the preservation of normal mood and that patients with depression can be helped by augmenting central noradrenergic function.

Sensory function

In two cases out of a personal series of more than 150 patients with MSA, there was sensory loss in the legs, confirmed by loss of sural sensory action potentials in one and by post-mortem studies in the other (Bannister and Oppenheimer 1972). Nerve conduction studies in MSA confirm the presence of a mixed sensorimotor axonal neuropathy (Pramstaller *et al.* 1995).

Pupils

Abnormalities recorded in patients with MSA include Horner's syndrome, alternating anisocoria, and abnormal pupillary responses to drugs. Ponsford, Paul, and Bannister (unpublished observations) studied 16 patients with MSA and compared them with patients with PD and age-matched controls. There was alternating anisocoria in five patients. This was variable and different from the alternating resting anisocoria which was noted in a single case of acute pandysautonomia. It was concluded that in MSA the disturbance was due to a central lesion rather than to unilateral hypersensitivity to cholinergic drugs on one side and to adrenergic drugs on the contralateral side. Alternating anisocoria differs from the variable but consistently lateralized anisocoria in the patients with pandysautonomia and the pupillotonia of the Holmes–Adie syndrome which reflects the different hypersensitivity of the two pupils to circulating cholinergic drugs.

In more than half the patients with MSA or PD, with or without AF, there was an abnormal and excessive constrictor response to methacholine. The degree of constriction in the more sensitive pupils was in the same range as in the Holmes–Adie syndrome. More than half of the patients with autonomic failure, whether PAF, MSA or AF with PD, showed an abnormal sensitivity.

Ocular movements

There is frequently restriction of conjugate ocular movements in advanced MSA, but this is usually an upward rather than a downward restriction and is less severe than in progressive supranuclear palsy (PSP), in which the ocular movement disorder dominates the clinical picture. Nuchal rigidity and striatonigral features in PSP, superficially resembling MSA, may make the differential diagnosis difficult at an early stage. In due course the ocular movement disorder of PSP becomes more apparent and this, with the lack of autonomic symptoms and signs, will distinguish it from MSA.

Detailed testing of ocular movements by Dr T. J. Anderson of the National Hospital, London (personal communication) has shown that only a minority of patients with probable MSA have normal eye movements. Often the findings are similar to those of idiopathic PD, with hypometria of saccades, particularly upwards saccades. Prominent slowing of saccades is not normally seen and suggests familial OPCA or PSP. A supranuclear gaze paresis, seldom severe and usually affecting vertical more than horizontal gaze, is present in up to 20 per cent of cases. Cerebellar eye signs—particularly gaze-evoked nystagmus, saccadic dysmetria, and poor smooth pursuit and vestibulo-ocular response suppression—are often present in patients with other features of cerebellar dysfunction, but may be found in the absence of cerebellar ataxia or limb dysmetria. Down-beat nystagmus (DBN) is present in up to a third of cases of MSA. In a minority of these, the DBN is noted in the head upright (i.e. sitting) position, but in most it is only elicited on positioning the patient with the head hanging (Dix–Hallpike or Barany manoeuvre) and may be of relatively short duration.

Disturbances of breathing

Rhythm and depth control

The disturbance of breathing may occur during the day, with involuntary inspiratory gasps (Bannister *et al.* 1967) or 'cluster' breathing, apparently normal breathing interspersed with regular apnoeic periods lasting about 20 s (Lockwood 1976), which appear to have a central origin. At night the patients may develop the sleep apnoea syndrome. The sleep apnoea may be 'central' with cessation of respiratory motor activity, or 'obstructive' in which there is a disturbance of the pharyngeal and laryngeal muscles. There is, in addition, evidence of an alteration of CO_2 sensitivity MSA, probably due to the brainstem lesion. The patient of Guilleminault *et al.* (1977) with MSA also had a reduced amount of rapid eye movement (REM) sleep and had disturbed non-REM sleep. This study showed that pulmonary arterial pressure rose progressively during sleep in direct association with each apnoeic episode and related hypoxaemia and hypocapnia, but without the extreme bradycardia which occurred in the REM sleep of patients who did not have autonomic failure.

Laryngeal function

At night, stridor with consequent hypoxia may secondarily cause disturbances of brainstem function and apnoea. The laryngeal stridor is due to a bilateral defect of the laryngeal abductors (Williams *et al.* 1979; Guindi *et al.* 1980; Harcourt *et al.* 1996) with changes of denervation on laryngeal electromyography (Guindi *et al.* 1981). At post-mortem, atrophy of the posterior cricoarytenoid muscles was found, due to an unusual form of denervation (Bannister *et al.* 1981). In the only case in which the laryngeal nerve was studied at post-mortem there appeared to be a reduced number of nerve fibres, although the nucleus ambiguus, thought to be the nucleus from which neurones innervating the laryngeal abductors arise, failed to show any selective neuronal loss. Once stridor and apnoea occur, CPAP, nasal surgery, and arytenoidectomy can be considered, but usually tracheostomy cannot be long delayed. It is justified because such patients may manage well for several years before other symptoms become troublesome or incapacitating. However, sudden death during sleep remains a frequent cause of death in MSA (Munschauer *et al.* 1990).

Urinary bladder function

Bladder symptoms are a combination of urgency, frequency, and nocturia due to uninhibited detrusor activity, or incontinence due to sphincter weakness, or, later, overflow incontinence due to an atonic bladder. During attempted evacuation there may be a weak or interrupted stream or incomplete evacuation, with residual urine. At its most severe there may be a complete inability to urinate. In MSA there may be various combinations of upper and lower motor neurone lesions affecting the detrusor and internal and external sphincter muscles.

As described in Chapter 30, the degeneration of sacral autonomic neurones (Onuf's nucleus) leads to the loss of both autonomic and somatic efferents as the nucleus has a status intermediate between ordinary somatic motoneurones and autonomic neurones. The anal and urethral sphincter impairment results from the loss of both innervations. Incontinence, usually without retention, is the result. There is, in addition, detrusor instability with lack of the capacity to initiate micturition in MSA, which is probably the result of a lesion of the pontine centre for micturition. Very occasionally, reduction of the outflow resistance can be achieved surgically, although routine operations based on the common belief that the patient may have prostatism almost always make these patients worse. An appropriate operation, however, may postpone the need for the use of surgical drainage in the male. Ureteric sphincter implants are now available. In younger females with good co-ordination, intermittent self-catheterization may sometimes be an acceptable management instead of continuous drainage or the use of incontinence pads.

Biochemical investigations

The most useful investigation is the measurement of plasma noradrenaline, taken under standard resting conditions, which is in the normal range in MSA but low in PAF. In neither disorder does the level rise on tilting or standing, because of the impairment of baroreceptor pathways (see Chapter 20). The low levels also help to separate the rare syndrome of dopamine 3-hydroxylase deficiency (see Chapter 40), which may not at first appear to differ from PAF, apart from its earlier age of onset.

Other investigations

See also Chapter 20.

Computed tomography (CT) brain scanning

With the CT scan the enlargement of the cisterna ambiens associated with brainstem atrophy in MSA is visible along with atrophy of the pons and cerebral peduncles. In the cerebellar forms, atrophy of the vermis and cerebellar cortex is visible (Savoiardo *et al.* 1983; Huang and Plaitakis 1984).

Magnetic resonance imaging of the brain

The putaminal changes which are unique to multiple system atrophy can be identified by T_1 weighted magnetic resonance imaging (MRI) (Pastakia *et al.* 1987). Brown *et al.* (1987) found that MRI changes ranked with the severity of the rigidity but not the other parkinsonian features of tremor or bradykinesia. The advances in MRI have increased the precision of diagnosis of MSA. Figure 31.3 shows MRI scans of patients with MSA and PAF. Fulham *et al.* (1991) showed that the most common MRI finding in MSA, present in 82 per cent of their series, was cerebellar atrophy, which was seen in many patients whose symptoms were parkinsonian rather than cerebellar (see Fig. 31.3a. The second most common finding, present in more than half the patients in their series, was hypodensity in the posterolateral putaminal region, which matches exactly the region of cell loss found pathologically in MSA (Fig. 31.3b). Half the MSA patients have a specific further defect, anterior globose hyperintensity (Konagaya *et al.* 1994). In contrast, the MRI scans in patients with PAF were normal. An abnormal MRI scan provides a reliable method of diagnosing MSA even though the neurological signs of parkinsonism

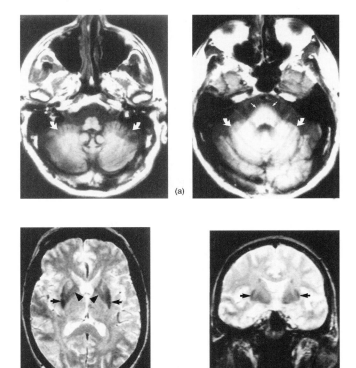

Fig. 31.3. (a) MRI axial T_1-weighted images, in two patients with MSA showing cerebellar hemispheric atrophy (curved arrows); the belly of the pons (small arrows) is flattened and atrophic. (b) Axial (on left) and coronal (on right) MRI T_2-weighted images in a patient with MSA. There is severe signal hypointensity in the posterolateral putamina (arrows) greater than in the globus pallidus (triangular arrows). (From Fulham *et al.* (1991).)

or cerebellar atrophy may be slight. Clearly, as with PD, the pathological changes in the brain in MSA may precede by some years the development of recognizable neurological clinical signs. In contrast, a normal MRI scan in a patient with severe orthostatic hypotension but without neurological symptoms strengthens the likelihood of the diagnosis of PAF. Though the MRI changes usually distinguish MSA from PD, at any rate in the late stages, MRI does not reliably distinguish between MSA and PSP (Savoiardo *et al.* 1994).

Neuroimaging studies using radioligands

The use of positron emission tomography (PET) in defining the morphological and neurochemical characteristics of the cerebral lesions in MSA and PAF are described in Chapter 32. Allied investigations include the use of single photon emission computed tomography (SPECT) (Schultz *et al.* 1994; Pirker *et al.* 1997).

Brainstem auditory evoked potentials

The usefulness of brainstem auditory evoked responses in providing an easier, non-invasive means of assessing the integrity of brainstem function in multiple sclerosis (Prasher and Gibson 1980) led us to investigate its use in patients with AF (Prasher and Bannister 1986). A group of patients with PAF and uncomplicated PD failed to show any abnormality. However, in nearly all patients with MSA there was a disruption of the brainstem responses in the pontomedullary region with delay or reduction of components of the response generated beyond this region (Fig. 31.4). The brainstem auditory evoked potentials, which are now widely available, may be helpful in distinguishing at an early stage the patients developing MSA from the patients with PAF, in whom the prognosis is so much better and the management easier. These findings have been confirmed by Vamatsu *et al.* (1987).

Cognitive events-related potentials

Cognitive event-related potentials provide a unique means of separating decision processes from motor involvement. The cerebral potentials are associated with information processing, especially the timing of sensory stimulus discrimination and categorization, together with the reaction time measures. These studies were undertaken in four patients with MSA at the National Hospital Human Movement

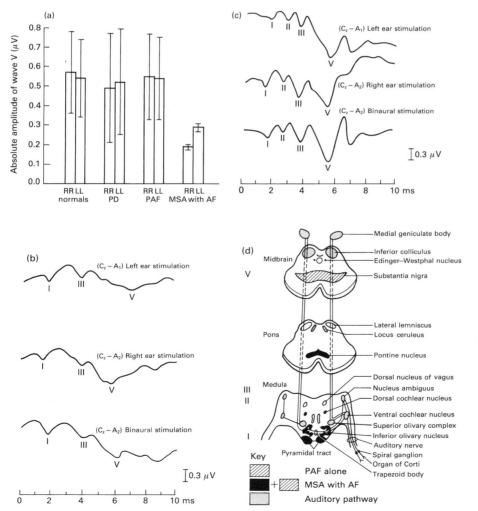

Fig. 31.4. (a) Mean and standard deviation of absolute amplitude of Wave V for the groups tested; PD, Parkinson's disease; PAF, pure autonomic failure; MSA with AF, multiple system atrophy with autonomic failure. Note the major reduction in the mean and variance of the amplitude of wave V in MSA. (b) Brainstem responses of MSA: bilateral abnormalities more severe on the left. (c) Brainstem responses of PAF: normal in amplitude and latency. (d) This diagram shows sites involved in PAF alone which clearly do not affect the brainstem auditory evoked potential. As these sites, which involve central autonomic control, are also affected in MSA it is necessary to exclude the site common to both syndrome. Therefore, by subtraction, the remaining sites in which degeneration is exclusive to the MSA component of the syndrome may be obtained. The auditory pathways are also shown with the Roman numerals indicating the generator sites of the brainstem potentials.

and Balance Unit (D. K. Prasher, personal communication). They showed normal results by comparison with patients with PD, in whom they were all delayed. These findings are of interest in view of the impression of normal intellectual function in MSA.

Distinction between MSA with striatonigral degeneration (SND) and olivopontocerebellar atrophy (OPCA)

Clearly, there are difficulties in distinguishing clinically the degree of SND and OPCA in patients with the features of both. In our experience careful attempts to elicit signs of striatonigral disease and cerebellar disease will usually give a correct diagnosis of MSA as judged by the only real criterion, the ultimate pathological verification. There may be only limited value in striving clinically to separate SND from OPCA, although we attempt to do so on the grounds of clinical signs at diagnosis. PET studies suggest that subclinical nigrostriatal involvement is present in the majority of patients with the cerebellar form of MSA (Rinne *et al.* 1995) and the ultimate pathology usually shows the changes of both MSA and OPCA (Fearnley and Lees 1990; see also Chapter 33), even though in life one form may predominate at first diagnosis and in the early stages. The association with autonomic failure, however, marks out the cerebellar form of MSA from the other progressive cerebellar syndromes, especially predominantly inherited cases, which have little relationship with SND (Gilman and Quinn 1996).

Autonomic failure and Parkinson's disease

The question of whether, and to what degree, autonomic involvement occurs in PD has been discussed for many years. The problem has been confused by the clinical description of supposed minor autonomic disturbances in PD, whose significance is difficult to assess, such as greasy skin or unequal pupils. Autonomic impairment, and in particular postural hypotension, in a patient with parkinsonism may be due to a variety of possibilities (see Table 31.1), including

Table 31.1. Possible causes of postural hypotension and autonomic dysfunction in a patient with parkinsonian features (adapted from Mathias 1996)

Multiple system atrophy

Parkinson's disease with autonomic failure

Side effects of anti-parkinsonian therapy
    including L-dopa and selegiline

Coincidental disease causing autonomic dysfunction
    such as diabetes mellitus

Concomitant administration of drugs for an allied condition
    antihypertensives (for hypertension)
    α-adrenoceptor blockers (for benign prostatic hyperplasia)

unexpected effects of drugs, as has been described recently with selegiline (Churchyard *et al.* 1997). Autonomic involvement should be defined as measurable sympathetic or parasympathetic dysfunction, assessed by physiological or biochemical means. If a battery of tests of the kind described in Chapter 20 is undertaken, a few parkinsonian patients have autonomic failure according to defined autonomic criteria. The autonomic failure syndrome associated with PD as defined by these tests is rare and very much less common than the association of autonomic failure with MSA.

Many patients with classical PD have mild postural hypotension when compared with control groups. There have been reports that resting recumbent levels of plasma noradrenaline in these patients are in a lower range than in normal controls (Turkka 1986). However, such patients do not have the abnormalities of cardiovascular reflex control which are linked with baroreceptor defects and intermediolateral column cell loss which are characteristic of autonomic failure. Gross *et al.* (1972) studied 20 patients with moderate PD, wishing to exclude abnormalities that occur with advanced parkinsonism, and compared them with controls. The only abnormality was that on head-up tilt their blood pressures were significantly lower than those of matched controls. There was, therefore, some increased impairment of cardiovascular control. This was consistent with later studies, demonstrating a small postprandial fall in supine blood pressure in PD, but without unmasking postural hypotension post-prandially (Thomaides *et al.* 1993). The conclusion drawn is that, because the cardiovascular reflexes and Valsalva tests were normal, there may be changes in the midbrain or hypothalamus associated with classical PD pathology that affect the input to the autonomic nervous system and these might well be the reason for the relatively mild abnormalities.

The clinical distinction between multiple system atrophy and Parkinson's disease

The differential diagnosis clinically between MSA and PD can sometimes be difficult. There are, however, certain clinical features that should make the clinician suspicious that the true diagnosis is MSA, and not PD. Until the diagnosis becomes unequivocal clinically, which is usually within a year or so of presentation, it may sometimes be justified to preface the diagnosis with the word 'probable'. In this group a patient with the diagnosis of probable PD may well become a patient with probable MSA. The clinical features favouring a clinical diagnosis of MSA may be listed.

1. *Marked orthostatic hypotension.* Mild orthostatic hypotension occurs in PD and this effect is exaggerated by the action of levodopa used in its treatment. The hypotension may be worse on standing or after exercise and food.

2. *Levodopa unresponsiveness.* It should, however, be remembered that about 30 per cent of patients with MSA show a significant but short-lived improvement in their akinetic-rigid symptoms on levodopa (see Chapter 37).

3. *Erectile impotence* in males, some in their forties (see Chapter 30). This symptom is unlikely to be prominent in PD, though, of course, it will be present if the autonomic failure syndrome is associated with PD.

4. *Urinary symptoms,* usually frequency, urgency, and a poor and intermittent stream (see Chapter 30). The suspicion of MSA arises when urinary symptoms occur in younger males or older males in the absence of prostatic hypertrophy or, in women, in the absence of other causes such as pelvic trauma with multiple births.

5. *Mild pyramidal or cerebellar signs* or both.

6. A parkinsonian syndrome in which *rigidity and akinesis* are more marked than tremor.

7. *Nocturnal stridor,* which may be inspiratory or expiratory and may be extraordinarily loud, sometimes likened to the braying of a donkey. The recent onset of snoring at night or sudden inspiratory gasps during the day may be a warning of more rapid progression of the disease.

It should be stressed that the diagnosis of MSA can be difficult but can only be based on clinical features and investigation. The most that can be expected is a probable diagnosis which may eventually be confirmed at post-mortem. The accuracy of diagnoses clinically at two stages, prior to death and histological confirmation, have confirmed previous impressions that MSA is underdiagnosed (Litvan *et al.* 1997).

Table 31.2. Age of onset and duration of illness in PAF and MSA patients assessed at the National Hospital for Neurology and Neurosurgery, Queen Square, London, up to 1987 (by Bannister and Mathias) and at the National Institute of Health, Bethesda (by Polinsky). Data for duration included those alive, and therefore is not an indication of survival (From Bannister *et al.* 1988)

	UK	US
PAF		
Number	24 (10 dead)	22 (2 dead)
Age (years)	58 ± 10 (38–78)	47 ± 3 (25–68)
Duration (years)	9 ± 1 (2–16)	14 ± 2 (5–31)
AF + MSA		
Number	73 (56 dead)	44 (26 dead)
Age (years)	54 ± 10 (34–74)	51 ± 1 (25–67)
Duration (years)	3 ± 2 (1–8)	8 ± 1 (2–15)

The clinical distinction between pure autonomic failure and early multiple system atrophy

There is a second area in which diagnosis can be difficult. The wrong clinical diagnosis of PAF may be made in a patient who is in fact in the earliest stage of developing MSA or, much less commonly, PD. We made this error in a 68-year-old with severe postural hypotension but no other detectable signs of a neurological disorder. We thought she had PAF. We did, however, note that her plasma noradrenaline was in the normal range which should have made us suspicious that she might be developing MSA. In fact, 2 years after postural hypotension had been diagnosed, she developed a tremor of one hand. In the course of the next 18 months she developed all the signs of an akinetic-rigid syndrome with nocturnal stridor requiring a tracheostomy; in other words she had typical MSA. After this experience we have made the plasma noradrenaline value an essential part of the investigation of all our patients.

Clinical course of primary chronic autonomic failure

The clinical progression of patients with pure autonomic failure (PAF) is relatively benign since the hypotensive symptoms can usually be controlled (see Chapter 36), so that life expectancy is only a little reduced; sphincter disturbance may be minimal. Occasionally, patients may survive from diagnosis for more than 20 years, raising the possibility that in some the lesion is nonprogressive (Table 31.2). Patients with AF and PD fare less well than patients with uncomplicated PD but, again, may survive for many years.

Patients with MSA face a distressing progression of their disability, unmitigated by any loss of insight, as their intelligence is almost always preserved. They often remain surprisingly cheerful, especially when attempts to help them with various drug regimes are pursued. The attempts are entirely justifiable since there is never any single drug regime that can be applied automatically to patients with such a variety of sites and extents of their lesions. However, within a few years, some patients with MSA can barely move, due to the extrapyramidal and pyramidal weakness, and have a sphincter disturbance that may be helped but cannot be cured. Their survival is considerably poorer than in PAF (Table 31.2). The survival curves in various series indicate a mean of 7.5 years (Testa *et al.* 1996), 8.9 (Schulz *et al.* 1994), and 9.3 (Wenning *et al.* 1994), consistent with our earlier observations. When the parkinsonian and cerebellar forms were compared, there did not appear to be a difference between the groups (Testa *et al.* 1996). Of clinical relevance is the individual survival, from 1 year to 15 years, again a wide range as we had noted previously. The preterminal development is often sleep apnoea or stridor.

Death in sleep may be due to stridor or apnoea causing hypoxia and may sometimes be a providential release. The denervation supersensitivity of α- and β-adrenoceptors of the heart may render these patients more liable to cardiac arrhythmias from which they may die, as in patients with diabetic autonomic neuropathy (Page and Watkins 1978).

Despite all the physiological, biochemical, and pharmacological investigations in patients with autonomic failure, it must be stressed that the diagnosis remains a clinical one in individual cases. The final verification of the correctness of the diagnosis lies in the post-mortem examination (see Chapter 33), but, from a practical point of view, the diagnosis in life is important because of the prognostic implications and the consideration of supportive and preventative aspects of care of the patient's acute and other disabilities. In order to help patients, their partners, relatives, and carers, support organisations have been formed, in the U.K. 'The Autonomic Disorders Association Sarah Matheson Trust', that currently focuses on MSA and the primary autonomic failure syndromes, and in the U.S.A. the Shy-Drager Association with similar interests.

Useful addresses

Autonomic Disorders Association Sarah Matheson Trust, Neurovascular Medicine Unit, Imperial College School of Medicine, St Mary's Hospital, Praed Street, London W2 1NY, UK. Tel : 0171-886-1520, Fax: 0171-886-1540.

Shy–Drager Association 1607 Silver Avenué SE, Albuquerque, NM 87106, USA. Tel : 1-800-SDS-4999.

References

Adams, R. D., van Bogaert, L., van der Eecken, H. (1964). Striato-nigral degeneration. *J. Neuropathol. Exp. Neurol.* 23, 584–608.

Bannister, R. and Oppenheimer, D. R. (1972). Degenerative diseases of the nervous system associated with autonomic failure. *Brain* 95, 457–74.

Bannister, R., Ardill, L., and Fentem, P. (1967). Defective autonomic control of blood vessels in idiopathic orthostatic hypotension. *Brain* 90, 725–46.

Bannister, R., Gibson, W., Michaels, L., and Oppenheimer, D. R. (1981). Laryngeal abductor paralysis in multiple system atrophy. *Brain* 104, 351–68.

Bannister, R., Mathias, C. J., and Polinsky, R. J. (1988). Autonomic failure : a comparison between UK and US experience. In *Autonomic failure. A textbook of disorders of the autonomic nervous system*, (2nd edn), (ed. R. Bannister and C. J. Mathias), pp. 281–8. Oxford University Press, Oxford.

Bleasdale-Barr, K. M. and Mathias, C. J. (1998). Neck and other muscle pains in autonomic failure: their association with orthostatic hypotension. *J. Roy. Sci. Med.* 91, 355–9.

Brown, R. T., Polinsky, R. J., DiChiro, G., Pastakia, B., Wener, L., and Simmons, J. T. (1987). MRI in autonomic failure. *J. Neurol. Neurosurg. Psychiat.* 50, 913–14.

Churchyard, A., Mathias, C. J., Boonkongchuen, P., and Lees, A. J. (1997). Autonomic effects of selegiline: possible cardiovascular toxicity in Parkinson's disease. *J. Neurol. Neurosurg. Psychiat.* 63, 228–34.

Cohen, J., Low, P., Fealey, R., Sheps, S., and Jiang, N.-S. (1987). Somatic and autonomic function in progressive autonomic failure and multiple system atrophy. *Ann. Neurol.* 22, 692–9.

Colosimo, C., Albanese, A., Hughes, A. J., De Bruin, V. M. S., and Lees, A. J. (1995). Some specific clinical features differentiate multiple system atrophy (striato-nigral variety) from Parkinson's disease. *Arch. Neurol.* 52, 294–8.

Consensus statement (1996). Consensus statement on the definition of orthostatic hypotension, pure autonomic failure and multiple system atrophy. *Clin. Auton. Res.* 6, 125–6.

Fearnley, J. M., Lees, A. J. (1990). Striatonigral degeneration: a clinico-pathological study. *Brain* 113, 1823–42.

Fetoni, V., Genitrini, S., Monza, D. *et al.* (1997). Variations in axial, proximal and distal motor response to L-dopa in multisystem atrophy and Parkinson's disease. *Clin. Neuropharmacol.* 20, 239–44.

Fulham, M. J., Dubinsky, R. M, Polinsky, R. J., *et al.* (1991). Computed tomography, magnetic resonance imaging and positron emission tomography with [18F] fluorodeoxyglucose in multiple system atrophy and pure autonomic failure. *Clin. Auton. Res.* 1, 27–36.

Gilman, S. and Quinn, N. P. (1996). The relationship of MSA to sporadic olivopontocerebellar atrophy and other forms of late onset cerebellar atrophy. *Neurology* 46, 1197–9.

Gross, M., Bannister, R., and Godwin-Austen, R. (1972). Orthostatic hypotension in Parkinson's disease. *Lancet* i, 174–6.

Guilleminault, C., Tilkian, A., Lehrman, K., Forno, L., and Dement, W. C. (1977). Sleep apnoea syndrome: states of sleep and autonomic dysfunction. *J. Neurol. Neurosurg. Psychiat.* 40, 718–25.

Guindi, G. M., Michaels, M., Bannister, R., and Gibson, W. (1980). Pathology of the intrinsic muscles of the larynx. *Clin. Otolaryngol.* 6, 101–9.

Guindi, G. M., Bannister, R., Gibson, W., and Payne, J. K. (1981). Laryngeal electromyography in multiple system atrophy with autonomic failure. *J. Neurol. Neurosurg. Psychiat.* 44, 49–53.

Harcourt, J., Spraggs, P., Mathias, C., and Brookes, G. (1996). Sleep-related breathing disorders in the Shy-Drager syndrome. Observations on investigation and management. *Eur. J. Neurol.* 3, 186–90.

Harding, A. E. (1981). Idiopathic late onset cerebellar ataxia. A clinical and genetic study of 36 cases. *J. Neurol. Sci.* 51, 259–71.

Huang, Y. O. and Plaitakis, A. (1984). Morphological changes of olivopontocerebellar atrophy in computed tomography and comments on its pathogenesis. *Adv. Neurol.* 41, 39–85.

Hughes, A. J., Daniel, S. E., Kilford, L., and Lees, A. J. (1992). The accuracy of clinical diagnosis of idiopathic Parkinson's disease: a clinical pathological study of 100 cases. *J. Neurol. Neurosurg. Psychiat.* 55, 181–2.

Kanda, T., Tsukagoshi, H., Oda, M., Miyamoko, K., and Tanabe, H. (1996). Changes of unmyelinated fibres in sural nerve in ALS, PD and MSA. *Acta Neuropath. Berlin* 91, 145–54.

Khurana, R. K. (1994). Cholinergic dysfunction in Shy–Drager syndrome: effect of the parasympathomimetic agent, bethanechol. *Clin. Auton. Res.* 4, 5–13.

Khurana, R. K., Nelson, E., Azzarelli, B., and Garcia, J. H. (1980). Shy–Drager syndrome: diagnosis and treatment of cholinergic dysfunction. *Neurology, Minneapolis* 30, 805–9.

Kluin, K. J., Gilman, S., Lohman, M., and Junck, L. (1996). Characteristics of dysarthria of multiple system atrophy. *Arch. Neurol.* 53, 545–8.

Konagaya, Y., Konagaya, M., and Iida, M. (1994). Clinical and magnetic resonance imaging study of extrapyramidal syndromes in multiple system atrophy. *J. Neurol. Neurosurg. Psychiat.* 57, 1528–31.

Litvan, I., Goetz, C. G., Jankovic, J. *et al.* (1997). What is the accuracy of the clinical diagnosis of multiple system atrophy? *Arch. Neurol.* 54, 937–44.

Lo, S. S., Mathias, C. J, and St. John Sutton & M. (1996). QT interval and dispersion in primary autonomic failure. *Heart* 75, (5), 498–501.

Lockwood, A. H. (1976). The Shy–Drager syndrome with abnormal respiration and antidiuretic hormone release. *Arch. Neurol., Chicago* 33, 292–5.

Mathias, C. J. (1996). Gastrointestinal dysfunction in multiple system atrophy. *Sem. Neurol.* 16, 251–8.

Mathias, C. J . (1997). Autonomic disorders and their recognition. *New Engl. J. Med.* 10, 721–4.

Mathias, C. J. (1996). Disorders affecting autonomic function in parkinsonian patients. In: *Parkinson's Disease*, (ed. L. Battistin, G. Scarlato, T. Caraceni, and S. Ruggieri.) *Advances in Neurology*, 69, pp. 383–91, Lippincott-Raven, Philadelphia.

Mathias, C. J. and Williams, A. C. (1994). The Shy Drager syndrome (and multiple system atrophy). In *Neurodegenerative diseases*, (ed. Donald B. Calne), Chapter 43, pp. 743–68. W. B. Saunders, Philadelphia.

Monza, D., Soliveri, P., Radice, D. *et al.* (1998). Cognitive dysfunction and impaired organization of complex motility in degenerative parkinsonian syndromes. *Arch. Neurol.* 55, 372–8.

Munschauer, F., Loh, L., Bannister, R., and Newsom Davis, J. (1990). Abnormal respiration and sudden death during sleep in multiple system atrophy with autonomic failure. *Neurology* 40, 677–9.

Page, M. McB. and Watkins, P. J. (1978). Cardiorespiratory arrest and diabetic autonomic neuropathy. *Lancet* i, 14–16.

Pastakia, B., Polinsky, R., DiChiro, G., Simmons, J. T., Brown, R., and Wener, L. (1987). Multiple system atrophy (Shy–Drager syndrome) MR imaging. *Radiology* 159, 499–502.

Pillon, B., Gouider-Khouja, N., Deweer, B. *et al.* (1995). Neuropsychological pattern of striatonigral degeneration: comparison with Parkinson's disease and progressive supranuclear palsy. *J. Neurol. Neurosurg. Psychiat.* 58, 174–9.

Pirker, W., Asenbaum, S., Wenger, S. *et al.* (1997). Iodine 123-Epidepride-SPECT: Studies in Parkinson's disease, multiple system atrophy and Huntington's disease. *J. Nucl. Med.*, 38, 1711–17

Pramstaller, P. P., Wenning, G. K., Smith, S. J., Beck, R.O., Quinn, N. P., and Fowler, C. J. (1995). Nerve conduction studies, skeletal muscle EMG and sphincter EMG in multiple system atrophy. *J. Neurol. Neurosurg. Psychiat.* 58, 618–21.

Prasher, D. K., Bannister, R. (1986). Brainstem auditory evoked potentials in patients with multiple system atrophy with progressive autonomic failure (Shy–Drager syndrome). *J. Neurol. Neurosurg. Psychiat.* **49**, 278–89.

Prasher, D. K. and Gibson, P. R. (1980). Brainstem auditory evoked potentials. A comparative study of monaural vs binaural stimulation in the detection of multiple sclerosis. *J. Clin. Neurophysiol.* **50**, 247–53.

Rinne, J. O., Burn, D. J., Mathias, C. J., Quinn, N. P., Marsden, D. C., and Brooks, D. J. (1995). Positron emission tomography studies on the dopaminergic system and striatal opiod binding in the olivopontocerebellar atrophy variant of multiple system atrophy. *Ann. Neurol.* **37**, 568–73.

Ross Russell, R. W. and Page, N. G. R. (1983). Critical perfusion of brain and retina. *Brain* **106**, 419–34.

Savoiardo, J. W., Bracchi, M., Passerini, A., Visciani, A., DiDonato, S., and Cocchinni, F. (1983). Computed tomography of olivopontocerebellar atrophy. *Am. J. Neuroradiol.* **4**, 509–12.

Savoiardo, M. *et al.* (1994). Magnetic resonance imaging in progressive supranuclear palsy and other parkinsonian disorders. *J. Neurol. Transm.* Suppl. **42**, 93–110.

Schulz, J. B., Klockgether, T., Petersen, D. *et al.* (1994). Multiple system atrophy: natural history, MRI morphology, and dopamine receptor imaging with [123]IBZM-SPECT. *J. Neurol. Neurosurg. Psychiat.* **57**, 1047–56.

Shy, G. M., and Drager, G. A. (1960). A neurological syndrome associated with orthostatic hypotension. *Arch. Neurol. Chicago* **3**, 511–27.

Testa, D., Fetoni, V., Soliveri, P., Musicco, M., Palazzini, E., and Girotti, F. (1993). Cognitive and motor performance in multiplesystem atrophy and Parkinson's disease compared. *Neuropsychologia* **31**, 207–10.

Testa, D., Filippini, G., Farinotti, M., Palazzini, E., and Caraceni, T. (1996). Survival in multiple system atrophy: a study of prognostic factors in 59 cases. *J. Neurol.* **243**, 401–4.

Thomaides, T., Bleasdale-Barr, K., Ray Chandhuri, K., Pavitt, D., Marsden, C.D., and Mathias, C. J. (1993). Cardiovascular and hormonal responses to liquid food challenge in idiopathic Parkinsons' disease, multiple system atrophy, and pure autonomic failure. *Neurol.* **43**, 900–4.

Thomas, D. J. and Bannister, R. (1980). Preservation of autoregulation of cerebral blood flow in autonomic failure. *J. Neurol. Sci.* **44**, 205–12.

Turkka, J. (1986). Autonomic dysfunction in Parkinson's disease. *Acta universitatis Ouluensis* **D142**, 15–66.

Vamatsu, D., Hamada, J., and Gotoh, F. (1987). Brainstem auditory evoked responses and CT findings in multiple system atrophy. *J. Neurol. Sci.* **77**, 161–71.

Wenning, G. K., Ben Shlomo, Y., Magalhaes, M., Daniel, S. E., and Quinn, N. P. (1994). Clinical features and natural history of multiple system atrophy. An analysis of 100 cases. *Brain* **117**, 835–45.

Williams, A., Hanson, D., and Calne, D. B. (1979). Vocal cord paralysis in the Shy–Drager syndrome. *J. Neurol. Neurosurg. Psychiatr.* **42**, 151–3.

32. Neuroimaging and allied studies in autonomic failure syndromes

David J. Brooks

Introduction

Neurodegenerative conditions associated with autonomic failure include Parkinson's disease (PD), multiple system atrophy (MSA), and pure autonomic failure (PAF). The pathological hallmark of PD is generally agreed to be degeneration of pigmented and other brainstem nuclei (substantia nigra compacta, locus ceruleus, dorsal nuclei of the vagus, nucleus accumbens, and nucleus basalis of Meynert) associated with neuronal Lewy inclusion bodies (Jellinger 1987). The Lewy body is an eosinophilic inclusion containing degenerating neurofilaments showing ubiquitin immunoreactivity. This loss of cells from the substantia nigra in PD results in profound dopamine depletion in the striatum, ventral projections to putamen being more affected than dorsal projections to head of caudate (Spokes *et al.* 1979; Fearnley and Lees 1991).

The pathology of MSA is associated with argyrophilic neuronal and glial inclusions and targets the nigra and striatum, brainstem and cerebellar nuclei, and intermediolateral columns of the cord (Papp and Lantos 1994). In contrast to PD, the loss of nigrostriatal dopaminergic projections is more uniform in MSA, leading to a greater involvement of caudate (Spokes *et al.* 1979; Fearnley and Lees 1990). In its early stages MSA may present as autonomic failure, an akinetic-rigid syndrome (the parkinsonian form; MSA-P) or as progressive ataxia (the cerebellar forms MSA-C). Around 50 per cent of patients with the akinetic-rigid variant show an initial respone to levodopa, making it difficult to distinguish them from PD on clinical criteria alone (Fearnley and Lees 1990). About 10 per cent of cases initially thought to have Parkinson's disease are later found to have MSA at autopsy (Colosimo *et al.* 1995).

The few PAF patients who have come to autopsy have shown either degeneration of the intermediolateral columns of the spinal cord similar to that found in MSA or Lewy bodies in the substantia nigra and sympathetic ganglia (Vanderhaegen *et al.* 1970). It can be seen, therefore, that the reported pathology of PAF has overlap features with both MSA and PD.

Clinically the syndromes of PD, MSA, and PAF also overlap. All three are associated with autonomic failure, though this is rarely a presenting feature of PD. MSA and PD result in an akinetic-rigid syndrome which is levodopa responsive in most of the former and some of the latter. A second area of clinical confusion is over whether MSA-P and MSA-C are distinct syndromes or simply comprise part of the spectrum of MSA. At post-mortem, patients clinically diagnosed as MSA-P (previously known as striatonigral degeneration) are often found to have subclinical cerebellar degeneration, while patients diagnosed as sporadic MSA-C (previously known as olivoponto-cerebellar atrophy) show subclinical striatal and nigral degeneration. Argyrophilic neuronal and glial inclusions characteristic of MSA have been reported in both the isolated akinetic rigid and cerebellar variants (Papp and Lantos 1994).

Structural imaging has not proved helpful in differentiating the different neurodegenerative disorders associated with autonomic failure. Frequently MRI is normal in PD, MSA, and PAF. Occasionally, PD patients may show increased signal from the substantia nigra on T_2-weighted MRI (Rutledge *et al.* 1987). If additional striatal or cerebellar degeneration is present, suggestive of MSA, reduced T_2-weighted lentiform nucleus signal and evidence of brainstem and cerebellar atrophy may be found (Rutledge *et al.* 1987). These differential MRI findings, however, are unreliable.

Functional imaging provides a more sensitive means of detecting and characterizing regional changes in brain metabolism and receptor binding in disorders of autonomic function. There are three main approaches to functional imaging: positron emission tomography (PET) allows quantitative examination of regional cerebral blood flow (rCBF), glucose and oxygen metabolism (rCMRGlc, rCMRO$_2$), and brain pharmacology. Single photon emission tomography (SPECT) gives semi-quantitative estimates of rCBF and receptor binding. Proton magnetic resonance spectroscopy allows *in vivo* measurements of brain metabolism and pH. The bulk of reports concerning *in vivo* brain function in autonomic disorders have, to date, concerned PET and so this chapter will concentrate on this technique, but compare SPECT and proton MRS findings where relevant.

Metabolic studies

PET measurements of regional cerebral glucose metabolism with ^{18}F-2-fluoro-2-deoxy-D-glucose ([18]FDG) primarily reflect the metabolic activity of synaptic vesicles in nerve terminals. Consequently, levels of basal ganglia glucose metabolism provide a measure of metabolic activity of interneurones and afferent projections to those nuclei, but do not reflect activity of basal ganglia efferent projections. In levodopa-responsive hemiparkinsonian patients with early disease, [18]FDG PET shows increased lentiform nucleus glucose metabolism contralateral to the affected limbs while PD patients with more long-standing bilateral disease have normal levels of striatal metabolism (Brooks 1993).

[18]FDG PET studies in patients with mixed sporadic MSA show reduced levels of striatal, cerebellar, and brainstem glucose metabolism (rCMRGlc) (Gilman *et al.* 1994). In patients with clinically probable MSA-P (levodopa-resistant parkinsonism without autonomic failure or ataxia) levels of striatal glucose metabolism have also been reported

to be reduced (De Volder *et al.* 1989; Otsuka *et al.* 1991; Eidelberg *et al.* 1993). Eidelberg *et al.* 1993 found that 8 out of their 10 levodopa non-responsive akinetic-rigid patients had reduced striatal metabolism, in contrast to 20 levodopa-responsive PD cases where metabolism was normal or raised. These workers also reported that akinetic-rigid patients with low levels of striatal glucose metabolism, irrespective of levodopa response, showed little improvement after pallidotomy (Eidelberg *et al.* 1996). In another series comprising five cases of probable MSA-P and two cases of mixed MSA, reduced levels of putamen and caudate glucose metabolism were found in all seven subjects while the two patients with ataxia showed additional reductions in cerebellar metabolism (De Volder *et al.* 1989). Otsuka *et al.* 1991 reported significantly reduced striatal glucose metabolism in eight cases of probable MSA-P, while striatal glucose metabolism was preserved in their eight PD patients. ^{18}FDG PET, therefore, provides a means of detecting the presence of striatal degeneration in MSA in around 80 per cent of cases where atypical parkinsonism is suspected.

Fulham *et al.* (1991) examined ^{18}FDG uptake in seven sporadic MSA-C patients with autonomic failure and in eight pure autonomic failure patients (clinical disease duration 5–26 years). They found significantly reduced cerebellar and frontal glucose utilization in the MSA-C patients but normal levels of rCMRGlc in PAF. These findings suggest that PET may provide a potential means of delineating whether patients presenting with isolated autonomic failure have PAF or a multisystem disturbance.

Dopaminergic dysfunction

After its intravenous administration, ^{18}F-dopa is taken up by the terminals of the nigrostriatal dopaminergic projections and converted to ^{18}F-dopamine and subsequently dopamine metabolites. The rate of striatal ^{18}F accumulation reflects both transport of ^{18}F-dopa into striatal vesicles and its subsequent decarboxylation by dopa decarboxylase. ^{11}C-nomifensine binds to dopamine reuptake sites on nigrostriatal terminals and so also provides a measure of integrity of nigrostriatal projections (Salmon *et al.* 1990).

In patients with probable MSA-P the function of both the pre- and postsynaptic dopaminergic systems is impaired. Specific putamen ^{18}F-dopa and ^{11}C-nomifensine uptake is reduced to around 50 per cent of normal levels in established MSA-P and individual levels of putamen ^{18}F-dopa uptake correlate with locomotor function (Brooks *et al.* 1990*a*,*b*; Salmon *et al.* 1990). This is also true of patients with levodopa-responsive PD, but patients with MSA show significantly greater reductions of caudate ^{18}F-dopa and ^{11}C-nomifensine uptake than PD cases (Brooks *et al.* 1990*b*; Otsuka *et al.* 1991; Fig. 32.1). These PET findings confirm that the nigra is more uniformly involved by the pathology of MSA than PD (Spokes *et al.* 1979; Fearnley and Lees 1990). Relative levels of caudate and putamen ^{18}F-dopa uptake can be used to discriminate MSA-P from PD with around 70 per cent specificity (Burn *et al.* 1994) though ^{18}FDG PET and proton MRS appear to provide greater specificity than ^{18}F-dopa PET for this purpose. At least five different subtypes of dopamine receptors have now been described but broadly they fall into D_1-type (D_1, D_5) which are adenyl cyclase dependent, and D_2-type (D_2, D_3, D_4) which are not. Postsynaptic striatal D_1 and D_2 receptors are primarily involved in modulating locomotor function. Overall, PET and SPECT findings suggest that in untreated PD, putamen D_2 binding is normal or mildly upregulated while caudate

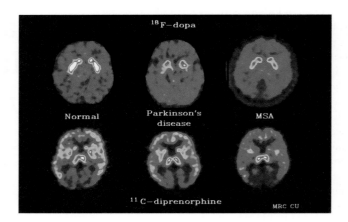

Fig. 32.1. PET images of striatal ^{18}F-dopa and ^{11}C-diprenorphine uptake in a normal subject and patients with Parkinson's disease and MSA. The PD patient shows a greater reduction in putamen than caudate ^{18}F-dopa signal and preserved ^{11}C-diprenorphine uptake. Striatal ^{18}F-dopa signal is uniformly reduced in the MSA patient, as is ^{11}C-diprenorphine uptake. (Courtesy of D. J. Burn.)

D_2 binding is normal (Playford and Brooks 1992). In chronically treated PD, putamen D_2 binding is normal while caudate binding is mildly decreased (Turjanski *et al.* 1997).

Striatal dopamine D_1 binding has been studied with ^{11}C-SCH23390 PET and D_2 binding with ^{11}C-raclopride and ^{11}C-methylspiperone PET in MSA-P (Shinotoh *et al.* 1990, 1993; Brooks *et al.* 1992). Mild, though significant, reductions in both mean putamen D_1 and D_2 binding have been reported, although a significant overlap between MSA-P, normal, and PD ranges is evident with all three tracers. Postsynaptic dopamine receptor binding, therefore, does not provide a sensitive discriminator of MSA-P from PD. In support of this viewpoint, Schwarz *et al.* (1992) found reduced striatal D_2 binding with ^{123}I-IBZM SPECT in only 8 out of their 12 parkinsonian patients with a negative apomorphine response. As a significant number of parkinsonian patients who respond poorly to levodopa retain normal levels of striatal D_2 binding, it seems likely that degeneration of downstream brainstem and pallidal rather than striatal projections is responsible for their poor response to levodopa.

Opioid dysfunction

The basal ganglia are rich in opioid peptides and their binding sites, and these are differentially affected in MSA and PD (Goto *et al.* 1990). ^{11}C-Diprenorphine is a non-specific opioid antagonist binding with equal affinity to μ, κ, and δ sites. In non-dyskinetic PD patients, caudate and putamen ^{11}C-diprenorphine uptake is preserved whereas putamen uptake is significantly reduced in patients with MSA (Burn *et al.* 1995; Fig. 32.1).

The overlap between PAF, MSA-C, and MSA-P

In order to determine the overlap between PAF and MSA, groups of these patients have been studied with PET and proton MRS. In a series of seven PAF patients, putamen ^{18}F-dopa uptake was found to be abnormal in two, suggesting that subclinical nigral dysfunction was present (Brooks *et al.* 1990*b*). One of these patients subsequently developed MSA. In a series of 10 sporadic MSA-C patients with autonomic failure, seven revealed reduced putamen ^{18}F-dopa uptake while four had reduced putamen ^{11}C-diprenorphine binding, indicative of the presence of subclinical MSA-P (Rinne *et al.* 1995). Reduced levels of striatal ^{18}F-dopa uptake (Otsuka *et al.* 1994), striatal glucose metabolism (Gilman *et al.* 1994), and lentiform *N*-acetyl aspartate (NAA) : creatine signal (Davie *et al.* 1995) have also been reported in other series of sporadic MSA-C cases. It would seem, therefore, that the majority of sporadic MSA-C cases with autonomic failure show functional imaging evidence of subclinical striatonigral dysfunction.

Conclusions

Patients with MSA show reduced striatal, cerebellar, and brainstem glucose metabolism and striatal dopamine and opioid binding. The presence of reduced striatal metabolism also distinguishes MSA-P from PD in cases where clinical doubt exists. Sporadic MSA-C patients show reduced cerebellar and brainstem glucose metabolism and the majority also have evidence of subclinical nigral and striatal dysfunction, as evidenced by reduced striatal ^{18}F-dopa and ^{11}C-diprenorphine uptake, glucose metabolism, and levels of *N*-acetyl aspartate. This suggests that isolated MSA-C and MSA-P are indeed part of an MSA spectrum, in line with recent pathological findings. The majority of PAF patients have an intact nigrostriatal dopaminergic system, arguing against this condition being a variant of PD or MSA despite some pathological overlap. PET is capable, however, of detecting subclinical nigrostriatal dysfunction in occasional PAF patients when this is present.

References

Brooks, D. J. (1993). Functional imaging in relation to parkinsonian syndromes. *J. Neurol. Sci.* 115, 1–17.

Brooks, D. J. Ibañez, V. Sawle, G. V. *et al.* (1990*a*). Differing patterns of striatal ^{18}F-dopa uptake in Parkinson's disease, multiple system atrophy and progressive supranuclear palsy. *Ann. Neurol.* 28, 547–55.

Brooks, D. J. Salmon, E. P. Mathias, C. J., *et al.* (1990*b*). The relationship between locomotor disability, autonomic dysfunction, and the integrity of the striatal dopaminergic system, in patients with multiple system atrophy, pure autonomic failure, and Parkinson's disease, studied with PET. *Brain* 113, 1539–52.

Brooks, D. J. Ibanez, V. Sawle, G. V. *et al.* (1992). Striatal D$_2$ receptor status in Parkinson's disease, striatonigral degeneration, and progressive supranuclear palsy, measured with ^{11}C-raclopride and PET. *Ann. Neurol.* 31, 184–92.

Burn, D. J., Sawle, G. V., and Brooks, D. J. (1994). The differential diagnosis of Parkinson's disease, multiple system atrophy, and Steele–Richardson–Olszewski syndrome: discriminant analysis of striatal ^{18}F-dopa PET data. *J. Neurol. Neurosurg. Psychiat.* 57, 278–84.

Burn, D. J., Rinne, J. O., Quinn, N. P., Lees, A. J., Marsden, C. D., and Brooks, D. J. (1995). Striatal opioid receptor binding in Parkinson's disease, striatonigral degeneration, and Steele–Richardson–Olszewski syndrome: An ^{11}C-diprenorphine PET study. *Brain* 118, 951–8.

Colosimo, C. Albanese, A., Hughes, A. J., de Bruin, V. M., and Lees, A. J. (1995). Some specific clinical features differentiate multiple system atrophy (striatonigral variety) from Parkinson's disease. *Arch. Neurol.* 52, 294–8.

Davie, C. A., Wenning, G. K., Barker, G. J. *et al.* (1995). Differentiation of multiple system atrophy from idiopathic Parkinson's disease using proton magnetic resonance spectroscopy. *Ann. Neurol.* 37, 204–10.

De Volder, A. G., Francard, J., Laterre, C. *et al.* (1989). Decreased glucose utilisation in the striatum and frontal lobe in probable striatonigral degeneration. *Ann. Neurol.* 26, 239–47.

Eidelberg, D., Takikawa, S., Moeller, J. R. *et al.* (1993). Striatal hypometabolism distinguishes striatonigral degeneration from Parkinson's disease. *Ann. Neurol.* 33, 518–27.

Eidelberg, D., Moeller, J. R., Ishikawa, T. *et al.* (1996). Regional metabolic correlates of surgical outcome following unilateral pallidotomy for Parkinson's disease. *Ann. Neurol.* 39, 450–9.

Fearnley, J. M. and Lees, A. J. (1990). Striatonigral degeneration: A clinicopathological study. *Brain* 113, 1823–42.

Fearnley, J. M. and Lees, A. J. (1991). Ageing and Parkinson's disease: substantia nigra regional selectivity. *Brain* 114, 2283–301.

Fulham, M. J. Dubinsky, R.M., Polinsky, R. J. *et al.* (1991). Computed tomography, magnetic resonance imaging, and positron emission tomography with [^{18}F]fluorodeoxyglucose in multiple system atrophy and pure autonomic failure. *Clin. Auton. Res.* 1, 27–36.

Gilman, S., Koeppe, R. A., Junck, L., Kluin, K. J., Lohman, M., and St Laurent, R. T. (1994). Patterns of cerebral glucose metabolism detected with positron emission tomography differ in multiple system atrophy and olivopontocerebellar atrophy. *Ann. Neurol.* 36, 166–75.

Goto, S., Hirano, A., and Matsumoto, S. (1990). Met-enkephalin immunoreactivity in the basal ganglia in Parkinson's disease and striatonigral degeneration. *Neurology* 40, 1051–6.

Jellinger, K. (1987). The pathology of parkinsonism. In *Movement disorders 2*, (ed. C. D. Marsden and S. Fahn), pp. 124–65. Butterworths, London.

Otsuka, M., Ichiya, Y., Hosokawa, S. *et al.* (1991). Striatal blood flow, glucose metabolism, and ^{18}F-dopa uptake: difference in Parkinson's disease and atypical parkinsonism. *J. Neurol. Neurosurg. Psychiat.* 54, 898–904.

Otsuka, M., Ichiya, Y., Kuwabara, Y. *et al.* (1994). Striatal ^{18}F-Dopa uptake and brain glucose metabolism by PET in patients with syndrome of progressive ataxia. *J. Neurol. Sci.* 124, 198–203.

Papp, M. I. and Lantos, P. L. (1994). The distribution of oligodendroglial inclusions in multiple system atrophy and its relevance to clinical symptomatology. *Brain* 117, 235–43.

Playford, E. D. and Brooks, D. J. (1992). *In vivo* and *in vitro* studies of the dopaminergic system in movement disorders. *Cerebrovasc. Brain Metab. Rev.* 4, 144–71.

Rinne, J. O., Burn, D. J., Mathias, C. J., Quinn, N. P., Marsden, C. D., and Brooks, D. J. (1995). PET studies on the dopaminergic system and striatal opioid binding in the olivopontocerebellar atrophy variant of multiple system atrophy. *Ann. Neurol.* 37, 568–73.

Rutledge, J. N., Hilal, S. K., Silver, A. J., Defendini, R., and Fahn, S. (1987). Study of movement disorders and brain iron by MR. *Am. J. Radiol.* 149, 365–79.

Salmon, E. P., Brooks, D. J., Leenders, K. L. *et al.* (1990). A two-compartment description and kinetic procedure for measuring regional cerebral [^{11}C]nomifensine uptake using positron emission tomography. *J. Cereb. Blood Flow Metab.* 10, 307–16.

Schwarz, J., Tatsch, K., Arnold, G. *et al.* (1992). ^{123}I-iodobenzamide-SPECT predicts dopaminergic responsiveness in patients with de-novo parkinsonism. *Neurology* 42, 556–61.

Shinotoh, H., Aotsuka, A., Yonezawa, H. *et al.* (1990). Striatal dopamine D$_2$ receptors in Parkinson's disease and striato-nigral degeneration determined by positron emission tomography. In *Basic, clinical, and therapeutic advances of Alzheimer's and Parkinson's diseases*, Vol. 2, (ed. T. Nagatsu *et al.*), pp. 107–110. Plenum Press, New York.

Shinotoh, H., Inoue, O., Hirayama, K., *et al.* (1993). Dopamine D$_1$ receptors in Parkinson's disease and striatonigral degeneration: a positron emission tomography study. *J. Neurol. Neurosurg. Psychiat.* 56, 467–72.

Spokes, E. G. S., Bannister, R., and Oppenheimer, D. R. (1979). Multiple system atrophy with autonomic failure. Clinical, histological, and neurochemical observations on four cases. *J. Neurol. Sci.* **43**, 59–62.

Turjanski, N., Lees, A. J., and Brooks, D. J. (1997). PET studies on striatal dopaminergic receptor binding in drug naive and L-dopa treated Parkinson's disease patients with and without dyskinesia. *Neurology*, **49**, 171–23.

Vanderhaegen, J. J., Perier, O., and Sternon, J. E. (1970). Pathological findings in idiopathic orthostatic hypotension: its relationship with Parkinson's disease. *Arch. Neurol.* **22**, 207–14.

33. The neuropathology and neurochemistry of multiple system atrophy

Susan E. Daniel

Introduction

Multiple system atrophy (MSA) is a primary degenerative disease of the nervous system that is histologically defined by the presence of cellular inclusions occurring predominantly in oligodendrocytes (Papp *et al.* 1989). The discovery of these inclusions has enabled a clear definition of MSA that no longer includes familial examples or cases of odd, multi-system degenerations (Graham and Oppenheimer 1969). The condition is further characterized by neurodegeneration involving widespread but apparently linked groups of neurones, in the absence of any as yet identified genetic (Plante-Bordeneuve *et al.* 1995; Cairns *et al.* 1997*a*) or environmental influence. Major sites affected include putamen, substantia nigra, basis pontis, inferior olives, cerebellar folia, spinal cord intermediolateral column, and Onuf's nucleus (Table 33.1).

MSA can be subclassified according to the predominant clinical signs of parkinsonism (the parkinsonian form (MSA-P) with striatonigral degeneration (SND)), or cerebellar involvement (the cerebellar form (MSA-C) with olivopontocerebellar atrophy (OPCA), or a combination of the two (the mixed form (MSA-M)) (Mathias 1997). Patients with parkinsonism show a preponderance of pathology in the striatonigral system, while equal involvement of the striatonigral and olivopontocerebellar systems is more unusual. Patients with predominant cerebellar signs are less common, and in these cases the principal pathology occurs in the olivopontocerebellar system with variable SND. No difference in survival rate has been found between the two groups (Ben-Shlomo *et al.* 1997). In all varieties of MSA there is usually involvement of the autonomic nervous system and the term Shy–Drager syndrome was used for patients in whom autonomic dysfunction is prominent (Shy and Drager 1960; Consensus Statement 1996; Chapter 31). Autonomic signs may be a presenting feature, alternatively there can be pathology in the autonomic nervous system in the absence of clinical symptoms (Oppenheimer 1980).

Gross neuropathology of MSA

External examination of the brain may be normal; however, when there is significant involvement of the olivopontocerebellar system the appearances are characteristic. The cerebellum is small, with the hemispheres far from covering the occipital poles. The pons is reduced in size with a wedge-shaped appearance, and there is atrophy of the middle cerebellar peduncles (Fig. 33.1). In the medulla, the protruberance of the inferior olives may be reduced.

Table 33.1. Neuronal degeneration in MSA

Site	Severity	Reference[a]
Putamen	+++	
Caudate	+	
Pallidum	+	
Thalamus	±	Martin (1975); Borit *et al.* (1975)
Subthalamic nucleus	±	Andrews *et al.* (1970)
Hypothamalus	±	Shy and Drager (1960) Nakamura *et al.* (1996)
Cerebral cortex	+	Papp and Lantos (1994) Robbins *et al.* (1992)
Substantia nigra	+++	
Edinger–Westphal nucleus	±	Shy and Drager (1960)
Pontine neurones	+++	
Locus ceruleus	+++	
Vestibular nuclear complex	+	
Cerebellar cortex	+++	
Dentate nucleus	±	Mizutani *et al.* (1988)
Dorsal vagal nucleus	++	
Inferior olives	+++	
Arcuate nuclei	±	Takei and Mirra (1973)
Optic nerve/tract	±	Buonanna *et al.* (1975)
Intermediolateral cells	+++	
Onuf's nucleus	+++	
Anterior horn cells	±	Konno *et al.* (1986)
Clarke's nucleus	±	Sung *et al.* (1979)
Pyramidal tracts	+	
Sympathetic ganglia	±	Chapter 34
Sensory ganglia	±	Bannister and Oppenheimer (1972)
Peripheral nerves	±	Bannister and Oppenheimer (1972)

±, Loss in only some cases; +, commonly affected; ++, nearly always affected; +++, always affected.

[a]Reference cited only where involvement is infrequently or recently documented.

Brain weight is usually normal for age, or only slightly reduced. The percentage weight of the detached brainstem and cerebellum to that of the whole brain is a useful indicator to the site of major pathology. In MSA with predominant SND, the proportion of brainstem and cerebellum to whole-brain weight remains normal and comprises about 10 per cent; conversely, with significant OPCA this percentage is considerably less.

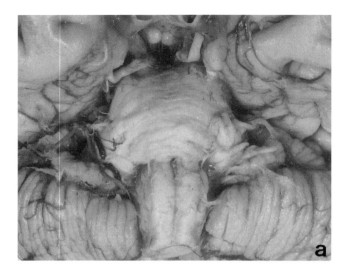

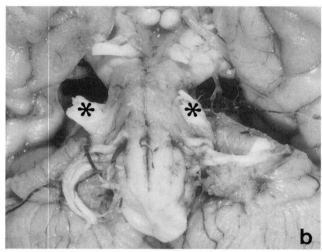

Fig. 33.1. Macroscopic appearance of the brainstem. When compared with normal (a) in MSA (b) the pons and middle cerebellar peduncles are atrophic and the trigeminal nerves (*) are prominent.

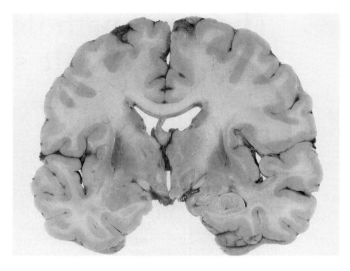

Fig. 33.2. Coronal slice of cerebrum at the level of mamillary bodies. The putamena are symmetrically shrunken. Pallida are also atrophic.

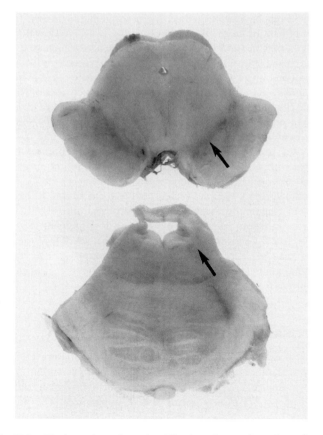

Fig. 33.3. Horizontal cut through midbrain and pons shows loss of pigment in substantia nigra and locus ceruleus (arrows).

Usually, the diagnosis of MSA is evident when the brain is cut, although the extent of the disease cannot be fully appreciated before microscopic examination. Pathology is symmetrical (Oppenheimer 1984), with only occasional cases showing asymmetry of involvement in striatum and substantia nigra. In SND the putamina are shrunken with grey–green discoloration (Fig. 33.2) and when pathology is severe there may be a cribriform appearance resembling *état lacunaire*; atrophy and discoloration of the caudate nuclei and pallida are less common. The substantiae nigrae invariably show decreased pigmentation and the loci cerulei may also appear pale (Fig. 33.3).

In OPCA the basis pontis (Fig. 33.4) and middle cerebellar peduncles are reduced, while in the cerebellum white matter appears grey and the folia atrophic. Occasionally, macroscopic abnormality is confined to the brainstem pigmented nuclei and in these instances it is impossible to make a distinction from idiopathic Parkinson's disease (PD) on naked-eye appearances alone.

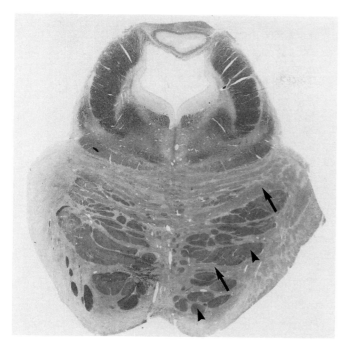

Fig. 33.4. Section of pons stained for myelin with luxol fast blue–Nissl. There is atrophy of basis pontis and pallor of transverse pontocerebellar fibres (arrows) when compared with corticospinal tracts (arrowheads).

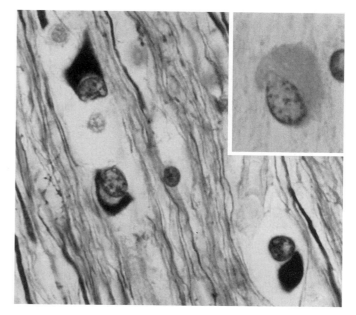

Fig. 33.5. Photomicrograph showing appearance of oligodendrocyte glial cytoplasmic inclusions with modified Bielschowsky silver impregnation and immunocytochemistry for α-tubulin (insert). Frontal cortex, ×1250.

Microscopic neuropathology in MSA

Cellular inclusions

Glial and neuronal cytoplasmic and nuclear inclusions have now been described extensively in MSA. Oligodendroglial cytoplasmic inclusions (GCIs) (Papp et al. 1989) are most ubiquitous and readily identified with silver impregnation in interfascicular, satellite, and perivascular oligodendrocytes. Additional staining with antibodies against ubiquitin, α- and β-tubulin, and tau, indicate an origin from cytoskeletal proteins (Fig. 33.5) while the recent observation of synnclein immunopositivity indicates some features in common with Lewy bodies (Wakabayashi et al. 1998). Accompanying cytoplasmic inclusions in oligodendrocytes there may also be rod-like nuclear inclusions (Papp and Lantos 1992).

Several rewarding findings have emerged from detailed study of GCIs. Their specificity for MSA when present in large numbers is undisputed and they provide a pathological hallmark for definition of the condition. Furthermore, GCIs have served as an indicator of pathology in areas previously considered unaffected. Thus, their finding in large numbers in the suprasegmental motor system and supraspinal autonomic nervous system and their targets provides the basis for system involvement and an explanation for symptomatology such as cognitive disturbance (Robbins et al. 1992) and autonomic dysfunction. Oligodendroglial cytoplasmic inclusions are also numerous in areas showing overt pathology, including putamen, caudate, globus pallidus, basis pontis, middle cerebellar peduncle, and cerebellar white matter (Papp and Lantos 1994).

Nuclear and cytoplasmic inclusions also occur in neurones and are ubiquitinated but distinguishable from those in obligodendrocytes by a lack of immunoreactivity for cytoskeletal proteins. They occur in largest numbers in the affected basis pontis where nuclear inclusions precede those of cell cytoplasm. Similar inclusions are also found in significant numbers in small putaminal neurones (Papp and Lantos 1992). In common with other neurodegenerative diseases, there are dystrophic neurites in heavily affected areas, but in MSA these processes are ubiquitinated only.

Despite the different immunohistochemical reactions of the various inclusions described, electron microscopy shows a common structure comprising 20–30 μm tubules, indicating a likely derivation from the microtubular system (Papp and Lantos 1992).

Striatonigral degeneration (SND)

This condition was first described by Adams et al. (1964). The striatonigral system is the main site of pathology but less severe degeneration can be widespread (Table 33.1) and usually includes the olivopontocerebellar system (Wenning et al. 1996). In early stages the putaminal lesion shows a distinct topographical distribution with a predilection for the caudal and dorsolateral regions (Kume et al. 1993). Glial cytoplasmic inclusions predominate while nerve cell loss and gliosis can be difficult to identify without the aid of glial fibrillary acidic protein (GFAP) immunostaining. The majority of reports indicate that the small neurones, which normally outnumber the large by about 170 to 1, are preferentially affected (Papp and Lantos 1992; Kume et al. 1993). Later on during the course of disease, the entire putamen is usually affected with the result that bundles of striatopallidal fibres are narrowed and poorly stained for myelin (Fig. 33.6). When atrophy is severe, the neuropil becomes rarefied with very few remaining nerve cells lying among hypertrophic astrocytes (Fig. 33.7). Brown pigment granules accumulate in astrocytes, macrophages, and around blood vessel walls; they have been identified as containing lipofuscin, neuromelanin, and iron.

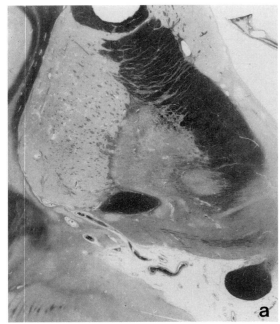

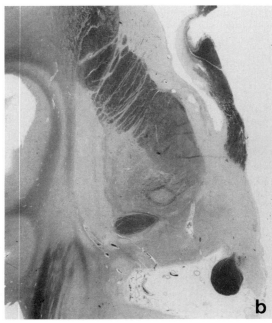

Fig. 33.6. Coronal section of striatum and globus pallidus stained for myelin. (a) Normal, with bundles of myelinated fibres identifiable in caudate and putamen; (b) in MSA myelinated bundles are unidentifiable and the pallidus is atrophic.

Borit *et al.* (1975) suggest that the neuromelanin may be derived from polymerization of dopamine in axon terminals of the nigrostriatal pathway, implying that the striatal lesion precedes nigral involvement. The amount of pigment may be quite variable but is usually greater than that associated with age and other neurodegenerative conditions, in particular PD; furthermore, in these conditions pigment occurs predominantly in a perivascular distribution.

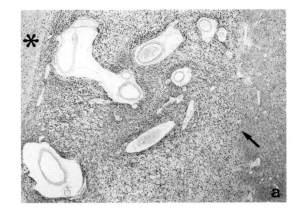

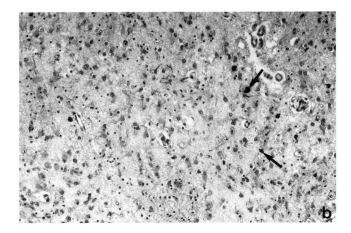

Fig. 33.7. Microscopic appearance of atrophic putamen. (a) Perivascular spaces are widened and there is gliosis extending from the lateral border with external capsule (*) medially to the globus pallidus (arrow). Immunocytochemistry for GFAP, ×17. (b) The neuropil is comprised of hypertrophic astrocytes and granules of pigment (arrows) with no nerve cells remaining in this field. Haematoxylin and eosin, ×142.

In the caudate nucleus there is nerve cell loss and gliosis but rarely to the extent of that found in putamen; the dorsomedial region is usually most noticeably affected with gliosis extending through the striatal bridges. The globus pallidus may appear uninvolved or show a reduction of myelinated fibres with gliosis and variable neuronal depletion, which is usually most severe in the ventrolateral region. The ansa lenticularis and lenticular fascicularis may appear narrowed. Pallidal atrophy is generally considered to be secondary to loss of putaminal efferents (Ito *et al.* 1996); however, in occasional cases where there is definite neuronal degeneration, this may represent a trans-synaptic effect or primary involvement.

Degeneration of pigmented nerve cells occurs in the substantia nigra zona compacta (Fig. 33.8), while non-pigmented cells of the pars reticulata are reported as normal. The caudolateral region is most severely affected with neuronal depletion, astrocytic and microglial hyperplasia, and granules of neuromelanin lying free in the neuropil and within macrophages. The appearances are usually of a more active type of degeneration when compared with that of PD; the neuropil is often vacuolated and occasionally there are microglial nodules and

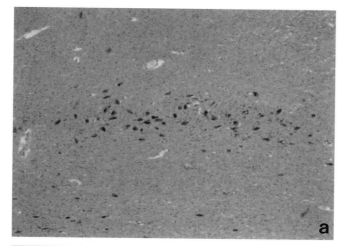

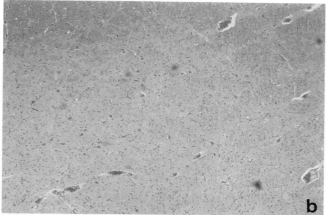

Fig. 33.8. (a) Normal population of pigmented neurones in substantia nigra which is depleted in MSA (b). Haematoxylin and eosin, ×20.

evidence of neuronophagia in addition to a diffuse increase of microglia. The topographical patterns of neurodegeneration involving the motor neostriatum, efferent pathways, and nigral neurones, reflect their anatomical relationship and suggest a common denominator or 'linked' degeneration (Kume *et al.* 1993).

Olivopontocerebellar atrophy (OPCA)

The original description of the pathology of sporadic OPCA was made by Dejerine and Thomas in 1900. The brunt of pathology is in the olivopontocerebellar system while involvement of striatum and substantia nigra is less severe. The basis pontis is atrophic, with loss of pontine neurones and transverse pontocerebellar fibres. In sections stained for myelin, the intact descending corticospinal tracts stand out against the degenerate transverse fibres and middle cerebellar peduncles (Fig. 33.4). Many authors report a disproportionate depletion of fibres from the middle cerebellar peduncles compared with the loss of pontine neurones, an observation which led to the suggestion of a 'dying-back' process (Oppenheimer 1984).

In MSA, cerebellar atrophy is often stated to be greatest in the neocerebellum whereas the palaeocerebellum is involved in primary cerebellar cortical degenerations. However, in several examples of MSA pathology is most severe in the vermis (Takei and Mirra 1973;

Wenning *et al.* 1996) or, alternatively, vermis and hemispheres may be equally affected. There is loss of Purkinje nerve cells (Fig. 33.9) and accompanying Bergmann astrocytosis resulting in isomorphic gliosis in the molecular layer. The site of degenerate Purkinje cells is marked by the presence of empty basket formations (Fig. 33.10a); and persistence of these structures provides a useful distinguishing feature from cerebellar anoxic change, where Purkinje and basket cells are both vulnerable. In the granule cell layer it is usual to find some neuronal depletion together with axon torpedoes of degenerating Purkinje cells (Fig. 33.10b). Both the folial and central hemispheric white matter is reduced in amount while that around the dentate nucleus and within the hilus is well preserved. Due to the loss of Purkinje cell axon terminals increased gliosis occurs in the dentate nucleus but there is usually no neuronal depletion at this site.

In medulla there is loss of neurones in the inferior (Fig. 33.11) and accessory olivary nuclei with increased gliosis. The olivary hilum is collapsed and there is pallor of myelin staining in olivocerebellar pathways. A lack of topographic relationship between neuronal cell loss in inferior olives and cerebellar cortex suggests that these may be primary unrelated degenerations (Wenning *et al.* 1996).

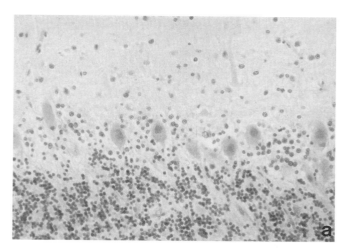

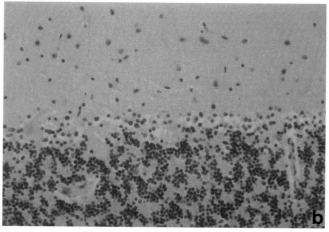

Fig. 33.9. Cerebellar cortex. In (a) there is a normal number of Purkinje cells lying between molecular layer and granule cells. In MSA (b) there is considerable Purkinje cell depletion. Haematoxylin and eosin, ×88.

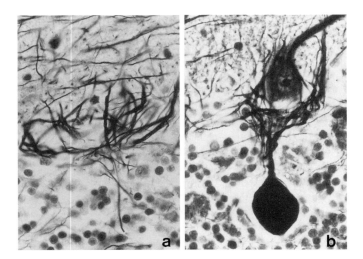

Fig. 33.10. Evidence of Purkinje cell degeneration in MSA. (a) Appearance of empty basket formations at sites where Purkinje cells are lost. (b) Axons of degenerating Purkinje cells form swellings or torpedoes in the granule cell layer. Modified Bielschowsky, ×350.

Autonomic failure

A supraspinal contribution to the autonomic failure of MSA is now well established. Cell loss is reported in dorsal motor nucleus of the vagus (e.g. Sung *et al.* 1979) and involves catecholaminergic neurons of ventrolateral medulla (Bellarroch *et al.* 1998). It has also been described for the Edinger–Westphal nucleus and posterior hypothalamus (Shy and Drager 1960) including the tuberomamillary nucleus (Nakamura *et al.* 1996). Most importantly, Papp and Lantos (1994) have shown marked involvement of brainstem pontomedullary reticular formation with GCIs, providing a supraspinal histological counterpart for impaired visceral function.

Degeneration of sympathetic preganglionic neurones in the intermediolateral column of the thoracolumbar spinal cord is considered contributory to orthostatic hypotension. Oppenheimer (1980) has stressed the importance of a quantitative assessment before excluding

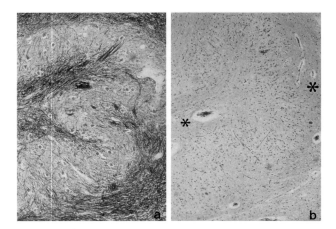

Fig. 33.11. Inferior olives in (a) normal and (b) MSA. In MSA nerve cells are depleted and there is pallor of white matter both surrounding and within the olivary hilum (*). Luxol fast blue–Nissl, ×35.

involvement of this site in MSA; most of the cells lie within the lateral horn of grey matter where they are irregularly distributed and prone to shrink according to agonal state and post-mortem fixation. Several investigators have found, using quantification, a 50 per cent depletion of intermediolateral cells in cases which were previously thought to be normal. If one considers only those reports in which formal cell counts have been made, with very few exceptions all cases of MSA with predominant pathology in either the striatonigral or olivopontocerebellar system show loss of intermediolateral cells. Oppenheimer (1980) examined 21 cases of MSA and found that lateral horn cell counts in patients with autonomic failure were on average 25 per cent of the controls, while in cases without autonomic failure there was about a 50 per cent depletion, with some overlap occurring between the two groups.

Disordered bladder, rectal, and sexual function in SND and OPCA have been associated with cell loss in parasympathetic preganglionic nuclei of the spinal cord. These neurones are localized rostrally in Onuf's nucleus between sacral segments S2 and S3 and more caudally in the inferior intermediolateral nucleus chiefly in the S3 to S4 segments (Konno *et al.* 1986). Although neurones of Onuf's nucleus resemble somatic motor neurones morphologically, the sparing of this cell column in motor neurone disease and its involvement in MSA supports the view that it is part of the parasympathetic system concerned with innervation of the anal and urethral sphincters.

In the peripheral component of the autonomic nervous system, Bannister and Oppenheimer (1972) have described atrophy of the glossopharyngeal and vagus nerves. No pathology has been reported in the visceral enteric plexuses or in the innervation of glands, blood vessels, or smooth muscles. The sympathetic and parasympathetic ganglia are discussed in Chapter 34.

Additional sites of pathology

A variety of other neuronal populations are noted to show cell depletion and gliosis with considerable differences in vulnerability from case to case. These sites are listed in Table 33.1 and only some of the reported lesions are discussed here. In addition to the recent recognition of marked involvement of motor cortex with cytoplasmic inclusions (Fig. 33.5), cell loss and astrocytosis involving deep laminae are also described (Fujita *et al.* 1993). These observations may well correlate with the sometimes detected myelin pallor of central and spinal motor pathways. Furthermore, anterior horn cells may show some depletion but not to the same extent as that occurring in motor neurone disease (Konno *et al.* 1986). Martin (1975) describes thalamic degeneration occurring in 15 of 108 cases of 'multiple system atrophy' with the centrum medianum most frequently affected; unfortunately, the cases include a wide variety of system degenerations and the number of SND and OPCA is not detailed. The vestibular nuclear complex, notably the medical component, often shows neuronal depletion; however, what influence this may have on clinical signs remains undetermined. Laryngeal stridor is a common feature of MSA and may occur as a presenting sign (Wu *et al.* 1996) or, more often, in later stages of the disease. Depletion of large myelinated nerve fibres in the recurrent laryngeal nerve which innervates intrinsic laryngeal muscles has been demonstrated in MSA patients with vocal cord palsy (Hayashi *et al.* 1997). The neuropathological background of abnormal eye movements in MSA is ill-defined, although Mizutani *et al.* (1988)

describe degeneration in the pathways concerned with the cerebellar fugal control of ocular movement.

Differential diagnosis

The levodopa response may contribute to an erroneous clinical diagnosis of Parkinson's disease. However, recent figures from the Parkinson's Disease Society Brain Research Centre indicate that MSA is now a much better-recognized clinical entity (Ansorge *et al.* 1997*a*). Patients who remain responsive to levodopa often show relative preservation of putamina and the striatal efferent woolly fibre arrangement in the globus pallidus (Ito *et al.* 1996).

From a neuropathological viewpoint, there is little cause for confusion of MSA with other neurodegenerative conditions. The GCI is the hallmark that accompanies signs of degeneration involving striatonigral and olivopontocerebellar systems. Similar inclusions have been described in several other diseases, including progressive supranuclear palsy (PSP), corticobasal degeneration (CBD) (Daniel *et al.* 1995), and familial OPCA (Berciano and Ferrer 1996); however, they are infrequent and require careful search. Furthermore, preliminary results suggest that for at least the glial inclusions of PSP and CBD there are distinct differences in tau profile when compared with those of MSA (Cairns *et al.* 1997*b*).

Rarely MSA may be combined with additional pathologies. Lewy bodies have been reported in 8–10 per cent of MSA cases and show a distribution comparable with that of PD. This frequency is similar to that of controls and suggests an incidental finding related to ageing and/or presymptomatic PD. Isolated reports of unusual clinicopathological cases occur and include overlap of MSA with progressive supranuclear palsy/corticobasal degeneration, MSA with Alzheimer's disease and PD (Ansorge *et al.* 1997*b,c*), and MSA with atypical Pick's disease (Horoupian and Dickson 1991).

The neurochemistry of MSA

Neurochemical studies have shown alterations consistent with sites of major pathology. Calcineurin, a marker for medium-sized spiny neurones, is decreased in striosomes of the putamen and in the efferent pathway of the globus pallidus and substantia nigra (Goto *et al.* 1989). Ito *et al.* (1996) also report that regardless of clinical presentation (SND, OPCA, or Shy–Drager syndrome) there is reduced immunoreactivity for additional markers of the striatal efferent system, including met-enkephalin, substance P, and calbindin. In the substantia nigra, tyrosine hydroxylase (TH) containing dopaminergic neurones are depleted. Similar neurones in the C1 and A2 regions of the medulla also show reduced TH activity, which has been associated with orthostatic hypotension (Kato *et al.* 1995).

Biochemical analyses have found only minor differences in reduced striatal and nigral dopamine content in MSA when compared with PD (Brucke *et al.* 1997). However, unlike PD, mitochondrial respiratory chain function in the substantia nigra is normal in MSA (Gu *et al.* 1997). An increase in total iron content appears to reflect sites of primary damage and occurs in both PD and MSA substantia nigra, as well as in MSA striatum (Dexter *et al.* 1991). Decreased noradrenaline levels are reported in septal nuclei, nucleus accumbens, hypothalamus, and locus ceruleus, while a consistent deficit of choline acetyltransferase is found in red nucleus, dentate, pontine, and inferior olivary nuclei, with variable involvement of the striatum and additional areas (Pokes *et al.* 1979). Cerebellar and, in particular, Purkinje cell damage, has been indicated by reduced levels of glutamate dehydrogenase (Plaitakis *et al.* 1993), amino acid binding sites (Price *et al.* 1993), and cerebrospinal fluid calbindin-D (Kiyosawa *et al.* 1993).

Pathogenesis

Despite recent advances, the pathogenesis of MSA remains speculative. The finding of widespread involvement of oligodendrocytes suggests that the interrelationship between glia and neurones is significant. Oligodendrocytes may die by apoptosis while neurons undergo a secondary non-apoptopic cell death (Probst Cousin *et al.* 1998). It is also likely that at some sites transneuronal degeneration is contributory, either when fibres afferent to neurones are lost (anterograde or transsynaptic degeneration), or when the cells that neurones project to malfunction (retrograde degeneration). In the olivopontocerebellar system, for example, degeneration of inferior olives, pontine neurones, and Purkinje cells occurs in MSA as well as in a variety of other conditions, and a linked degeneration is postulated; however, neither the site of initial pathology (axon or nerve cell) nor the direction of degeneration is known. In comparison, lesions of the striatonigral system in MSA show an anatomical correlation, but there is no convincing evidence to suggest that this is due to transneuronal degeneration; in several conditions, for example PD or postencephalitic parkinsonism, nigral degeneration occurs without significant involvement of the striatum. Concerning the autonomic nervous system, it remains uncertain whether linked degeneration occurs.

Additional mechanisms of diverse patterns of neurodegeneration include the possibility that affected nerve cell groups share physiological and/or biochemical properties that render them susceptible to an aetiological agent. From both the clinical and pathological findings, it is unlikely that the different neuronal populations are involved either simultaneously or in a regularly reproducible manner. The diversity of human genotype and phenotypic expression, combined with a range of compensatory mechanisms, confound understanding of disease patterns and their categorization.

References

Adams, R. D., van Bogaert, L., and vander Eecken, H. (1964). Striato-nigral degeneration. *J. Neuropathol. Exp. Neurol.* 23, 584–608.

Andrews, J. M., Terr, R. D., and Spataro, J. (1970). Striatonigral degeneration: clinical–pathological correlations in response to stereotaxic surgery. *Arch. Neurol. Chicago*, 23, 319–29.

Ansorge, O., Lees, A. J., and Daniel, S. E. (1997*a*). The neuropathological spectrum of clinically diagnosed idiopathic Parkinson's disease: a reappraisal. *Neuropath. Appl. Neurobiol.* 23, 181.

Ansorge, O., Lees, A. J., Brooks, D. J., and Daniel, S. E. (1997*b*). Multiple system atrophy presenting as progressive supranuclear palsy and vice-versa: two unusual cases. *Movement Disorders* 12, (Suppl. 1), 96.

Ansorge, O., Lees, A. J., and Daniel, S. E. (1997*c*). Pathological overlap of Alzheimer's disease, Parkinson's disease and multiple system atrophy. *Neuropath. Appl. Neurobiol.* 23, 179.

Bannister, R. and Oppenheimer, D. R. (1972). Degenerative diseases of the nervous system associated with autonomic failure. *Brain*, 95, 57–74.

Benarroch, E. E., Smithson, I. L. S., Low, P. A., and Parisi, J. E. (1998). Depletion of catecholaminergic neurons of the rostral ventrolateral medulla in multiple system atrophy with autonomic failure. *Ann. Neurol.* 43, 156–63.

Ben-Shlomo, Y., Wenning, G. K., Tison, F., and Quinn, N. P. (1997). Survival of patients with pathologically proven multiple system atrophy: a meta-analysis. *Neurology* **48** (2), 384–93.

Berciano, J. and Ferrer, I. (1996). Glial and neuronal cytoplasmic inclusions in familial olivopontocerebellar atrophy. *Ann. Neurol.* **40**, 819.

Borit, A., Rubinstein, L. J., and Urich, H. (1975). The striatonigral degenerations, putaminal pigments and nosology. *Brain* **98**, 101–12.

Brucke, T., Asenbaum, S., Pirker, W. *et al.* (1997) Measurement of the dopaminergic degeneration in Parkinson's disease with *123*I beta-CIT and SPECT. Correlation with clinical findings and comparison with multiple system atrophy and progressive supranuclear palsy. *J. Neural Transm. (Suppl.)* **50**, 9–24.

Buonanno, F., Nardelli, E., Ounis, L., and Rizzuto, N. (1975). Striatonigral degeneration. Report of a case with an unusually short course and multiple system degenerations. *J. Neurol. Sci.* **26**, 545–53.

Cairns, N. J., Atkinson, P. F., Kovacs, T., Lees, A. J., Daniel, S. E., and Lantos, P. L. (1997*a*). Apolipoprotein E e4 allele frequency in patients with multiple system atrophy. *Neurosci. Lett.* **221**, (2–3), 161–4.

Cairns, N. J., Mackay, D., Daniel, S. E., and Lantos, P. L. (1997*b*). Tau-pathology of oligodendroglial inclusions in multiple system atrophy, progressive supranuclear palsy and corticobasal degeneration. *Neurosci. Lett.* **230**, (1), 49–52.

Daniel, S. E., Geddes, J. F., and Revesz, T. (1995). Glial cytoplasmic inclusions are not exclusive to multiple system atrophy. *J. Neurol. Neurosurg. Psychiat.* **58**, 262.

Dejerine, J. and Thomas, A. (1900). L'atrophie olivo-ponto-cérébelleuse. *Nouvelle Iconographie Salpêtrière*, **13**, 330–70.

Dexter, D. T., Carayon, A., Javoy-Agid, F. *et al.* (1991). Alterations in the levels of iron, ferritin and other trace metals in Parkinson's disease and other neurodegenerative diseases affecting the basal ganglia. *Brain* **114**, 1953–75.

Fujita, T., Doi, M., Ogata T., Kanazawa, I., and Mizusawa, H. (1993). Cerebral cortical pathology of sporadic olivopontocerebellar atrophy. *J. Neurosci.* **116**, 41–6.

Goto, S., Hirano, A., and Rojas-Corona, R. R. (1989). Calcineurin immunoreactivity in striatonigral degeneration. *Acta Neuropath. Berlin* **78**, (1), 65–71.

Graham, J. G. and Oppenheimer, D. R. (1969). Orthostatic hypotension and nicotine sensitivity in a case of multiple system atrophy. *J. Neurol. Neurosurg. Psychiat.* **32**, 28–34.

Gu, M., Gash, M. T., Cooper, J. M. *et al.* (1997). Mitochondrial respiratory chain function in multiple system atrophy. *Movement Disorders* **12**, (2), 418–22.

Horoupian, D. S. and Dickson, D. W. (1991). Striatonigral degeneration, olivopontocerebellar cerebellar atrophy and 'atypical' Pick disease. *Acta Neuropath. Berlin* **81**, 287–95.

Hayashi, M., Isozaki, E., Oda, M., Tanabe, K., and Kimura, J. (1997). Loss of large myelinated nerve fibres of the recurrent laryngeal nerve in patients with multiple system atrophy and vocal cord palsy. *J. Neurol. Neurosurg. Psychiat.* **62**, (3), 234–8.

Ito, H., Kusaka, H., Matsumoto, S., and Imai, T. (1996). Striatal efferent involvement and its correlation to levodopa efficacy in patients with multiple system atrophy. *Neurology*, **47**, (5), 1291–9.

Kato, S., Oda, M., Hayashi, H. *et al.* (1995). Decrease of medullary catecholaminergic neurons in multiple system atrophy and Parkinson's disease and their preservation in amyotrophic lateral sclerosis. *J. Neurol. Sci.* **132**, (2), 216–21.

Kiyosawa, K., Mokono, K., Murakami, N. *et al.* (1993). Cerebrospinal fluid 28-kDa calbindin-D as a possible marker for Purkinje cell damage. *J. Neurol. Sci.* **118**, (1), 29–33.

Konno, H., Yamamoto, T., Iwasaki, Y., and Iizuka, H. (1986). Shy–Drager syndrome and amyotrophic lateral sclerosis: cytoarchitectonic and morphometric studies of sacral autonomic neurons. *J. Neurol. Sci.* **73**, 193–204.

Kume, A., Takahashi, A., and Hashizume, Y. (1993) Neuronal cell loss of the striatonigral system in multiple system atrophy. *J. Neurol. Sci.* **117**, (1–2), 33–40.

Mathias, C. J. (1997). Autonomic disorders and their recognition. *New Eng. J. Med.* **36**, 721–4.

Martin, J. J. (1975). Thalamic degenerations. In *Handbook of clinical neurology*, Vol. 21, (ed. P. J. Vinken and G. W. Bruyn), pp. 587–605. Elsevier Science, Amsterdam.

Mizutani, T., Satoh, J., and Morimatsu, Y. (1988). Neuropathological background of oculomotor disturbances in olivopontocerebellar atrophy with special reference to slow saccade. *J. Neurol. Neurosurg. Psychiat.* **7**, 53–61.

Nakamura, S., Ohnishi, K., Nishimura, M. *et al.* (1996). Large neurons in the tuberomammillary nucleus in patients with Parkinson's disease and multiple system atrophy. *Neurology* **46**, (6), 1693–6.

Oppenheimer, D. (1980). Lateral horn cells in progressive autonomic failure. *J. Neurol. Sci.* **46**, 393–404.

Oppenheimer, D. (1984). Diseases of the basal ganglia, cerebellum and motor neurons. In *Greenfield's neuropathology*, (4th edn), (ed. J. H. Adams, J. A. N. Corsellis, and L. W. Duchen), pp. 699–747. Wiley, New York.

Papp, M. I. and Lantos, P. L. (1992). Accumulation of tubular structures in oligodendroglial and neuronal cells as the basic alteration in multiple system atrophy. *J. Neurol. Sci.* **107**, 172–82.

Papp, M. I. and Lantos, P. L. (1994). The distribution of oligodendroglial inclusions in multiple system atrophy and its relevance to clinical symptomatology. *Brain* **117**, 235–43.

Papp, M. I., Kahn, J. E., and Lantos, P. L. (1989). Glial cytoplasmic inclusions in the CNS of patients with multiple system atrophy (striatonigral degeneration, olivopontocerebellar atrophy and Shy–Drager syndrome). *J. Neurol. Sci.* **94**, 79–100.

Plaitakis, A., Flessas, P., Natsiou, B. A., and Shashidharan, P. (1993). Glutamate dehydrogenase deficiency in cerebellar degenerations: clinical, biochemical and molecular genetic aspects. *Can. J. Neurol. Sci. Supplement 3*, S109–6.

Plante-Bordeneuve, V., Bandmann, O., Wenning, G., Quinn, N. P., Daniel, S. E., and Harding, A. E. (1995). CYP2D6-debrisoquine hydroxylase gene polymorphism in multiple system atrophy. *Movement Disorders* **10**, (3), 277–8.

Price, R. H., Albin, R. L., Sakurai, S. Y., Polinsky, R. J., Penney, J. B., and Young, A. B. (1993). Cerebellar excitatory and inhibitory amino acid receptors in multiple system atrophy. *Neurology*, **43**, (7), 1323–8.

Probst Cousin, S., Rickert, C. H. Schmid, K. W. and Gullotta, F. (1998). Cell death mechanisms in multiple system atrophy. *J. Neuropath. Exp. Neurol.* **57**, 814–21.

Robbins, T. W., James, M., Lange, K. W., Owen, A. M., Quinn, N.P., and Marsden, D. (1992). Cognitive performance in multiple system atrophy. *Brain*, **115**, 271–91.

Shy, G. M. and Drager, G. A. (1960). A neurological syndrome associated with orthostatic hypotension. A clinicopathological study. *Arch. Neurol. Chicago* **2**, 511–27.

Spokes, E. G. S., Bannister, R., and Oppenheimer, D. R. (1979). Mulitple system atrophy with autonomic failure—clinical, histological and neurochemical observations on four cases. *J. Neurol. Sci.* **43**, 59–82.

Sung, J. H., Mastri, A. R., and Segal, E. (1979). Pathology of Shy–Drager syndrome. *J. Neuropath. Exp. Neurol.* **38**, 353–68.

Takei, Y. and Mirra, S. (1973). Striatonigral degeneration: a form of multiple system atrophy with clinical parkinsonism. In *Progress in neuropathology*, Vol. 2, (ed. H. M. Zimmermann), pp. 217–51. Grune & Stratton, New York.

Wakabayashi, K., Hayashi, S., Kakita, A. *et al.* (1998). Accumulation of α-synuclein NACP is a cytopathological feature common to Lewy body disease and multiple system atrophy. *Acta Neuropath.* **96**, 445–52.

Wenning, G. K., Tison, F., Elliott, L., Quinn, N. P., and Daniel, S. E. (1996). Olivopontocerebellar pathology in multiple system atrophy. *Movement Disorders*, **11**, (2), 157–62.

Wu, Y. R., Chen, C. M., Ro, I., Chen, S. T., and Tang, L. M. (1996). Vocal cord paralysis as an initial sign of multiple system atrophy in the central nervous system. *J. Formosa Med. Assoc.* **95**, (10), 804–6.

34. Autonomic ganglia and preganglionic neurones in autonomic failure

Margaret R. Matthews

Introduction: classes of autonomic failure

Autonomic failure may arise as a secondary consequence of more general disorders involving the nervous system, as in multiple sclerosis, or in toxic or diabetic peripheral neuropathy, described elsewhere in this volume, or it may arise as a specific feature of certain primary degenerative disorders of the nervous system. These include importantly multiple system atrophy (MSA), pure autonomic failure (PAF), and the autonomic failure that may occur in Parkinson's disease (PD with AF). The neuropathological and neurochemical changes associated with these conditions will be considered here.

As is outlined in the introduction to this volume, the neurones and pathways of the autonomic nervous system, in each of its divisions (sympathetic, parasympathetic and enteric), comprise the following hierarchy: ganglionic neurones and their postganglionic axons innervating effectors (cardiac muscle, smooth muscle and gland cells) in the periphery; innervation of the ganglia from preganglionic neurones in the brainstem (parasympathetic) or the spinal cord (sympathetic at thoracolumbar, parasympathetic at sacral levels); and higher levels of control mediated via the cerebral cortex, the limbic system including the amygdala and septal area, the hypotalamus, and nuclei of the brainstem reticular formation. Autonomic failure may be associated with dysfunction or pathological changes at any of several levels in these pathways; thus, it may result from derangements of the postganglionic axons, as in peripheral neuropathies, or of ganglionic neurones, or of preganglionic neurones. Disorders of the central pathways involved in control of the preganglionic neurones may also lead, or contribute, to autonomic failure. More than one of these levels is often found to be involved on post-mortem examination in a particular case, even though the initial defect may have been more restricted, and the likely explanation for this is that secondary, transneuronal changes may become superimposed upon a primary lesion in this highly interdependent system. There is therefore a problem in establishing what may have been the first site or sites of the disorder.

Clinical studies come closest to revealing this, since they may be undertaken as soon as the diagnosis is suspected. Tests are available that explore differentially the integrity of postganglionic axons, the efficacy of preganglionic control, and the function of central pathways (Chapters 20 and 24). The evidence from clinical evaluation points to a primarily preganglionic and central lesion in MSA and a primarily postganglionic or ganglionic lesion in PAF. Thus, it is typical to find in patients showing orthostatic hypotension that the level of resting supine plasma noradrenaline is within normal limits in MSA but low in PAF, although in neither condition does it rise during head-up tilt; and the respective responses to injected tyramine and to the cholinomimetic edrophonium indicate integrity of peripheral noradrenergic nerve endings and of ganglionic neurones in MSA but not in PAF. In MSA, however, a selective deficit may develop in ganglionic sudomotor neurones (Kumazawa *et al.* 1989; Low and Fealey 1992). Clonidine demonstrates central involvement in MSA but not in PAF. In PD with AF, where the onset of autonomic failure tends to occur relatively late in the disease, both central and peripheral lesions may already coexist and may contribute in different ways to the autonomic failure, leading either to orthostatic hypotension via peripheral sympathetic neurocirculatory failure (Goldstein *et al.* 1997) or to urinary and gastrointestinal dysfunction, in which the respective roles of peripheral and central lesions are uncertain (Magaelhaes *et al.* 1995).

It has, in this way, become increasingly evident that there are important differences between the type of autonomic failure that occurs in MSA and that which occurs in PAF, or in PD with AF, and that these differences reflect differences in site of the primary lesion and therefore perhaps in aetiology. Neuropathological studies reinforce this distinction. None the less, the identity of the primary cause or causes of the neuronal changes underlying the autonomic failure in either group of cases, as also in Parkinson's disease, still remains elusive.

Neuropathological changes in autonomic failure

Preganglionic neurones and central pathways

Neuropathological studies in autonomic failure, notably by Oppenheimer (1980), who also reviewed earlier work, have strongly supported the possibility of a primary lesion at sympathetic preganglionic level in MSA, by showing that there is, in almost all cases of MSA with AF, considerable loss of thoracolumbar intermediolateral column (IML) neurones, amounting to 75 per cent or more of control numbers. Cases of PD with AF, however, also showed severe loss of IML neurones, and moderate loss has been found in PD without AF. Oppenheimer's work has emphasized the importance of systematic counting of neurones in samples of adequate extent, with age-matched controls for comparison. More recent series have produced similar results (see, for example, Gray *et al.* 1988; Low and Fealey 1992). It was already apparent that in the IML a loss of 50 per cent of neurones may be overlooked if no adequate counts are made, and it is now confirmed that 50 per cent or even more of IML neurones may be lost without overt AF. In PAF, however, a ganglionic lesion may coexist with a loss of up to 50 per cent of IML neurones (Low and Fealey 1992; van Ingelghem *et al.* 1994).

Counts of preganglionic parasympathetic neurones at sacral spinal levels have likewise shown severe neurone loss in MSA (Konno *et al.* 1986). Consistent neurone loss is also present in Onuf's nucleus of the sacral cord, from which the external urethral and anal sphincter muscles are innervated, in cases of MSA with sphincter disturbances (Konno *et al.* 1986); and sphincter electromyography gives clear evidence of denervation and reinnervation in such patients (Beck *et al.* 1994), so consistently that an instance of abnormal sphincter EMG in a subject with PAF raises the suspicion that this presages the future development of MSA (Bajaj *et al.* 1996). Loss of neurones has also been reported in the dorsal motor nucleus of the vagus, both in MSA (Gray *et al.* 1988) and in PD with AF (Forno 1996); and in PD this nucleus consistently shows Lewy bodies, typical of the disease, in common with other pigmented nuclei of the brainstem (Hughes *et al.* 1993; Forno 1996). Similar Lewy bodies have sometimes been seen in the IML in PD, including the sacral IML (Oyanagi *et al.* 1990). Severe depletion of catecholaminergic C1 neurones in the ventrolateral medulla and of A2 neurones in the dorsomedial medulla (region of dorsal vagal nucleus) has been observed in MSA, and some depletion, but less severe, in PD (Gai *et al.* 1993; Kato *et al.* 1995). Other parasympathetic central nuclei are less consistently examined, but in MSA there have been occasional reports of neurone loss in the Edinger–Westphal nucleus, and loss of facial and glossopharyngeal central parasympathetic neurones has also been suspected. In PD Lewy bodies have regularly been found in the Edinger–Westphal nucleus (Forno, 1996).

In the nucleus ambiguus in MSA, apart from possible loss of its periambigual parasympathetic neurones (Chapter 6) there may be loss of neurones innervating the abductors of the vocal cords, the posterior crico-arytenoid muscles, seen in terms of neurogenic atrophy of the muscles and neurone loss and gliosis in the nucleus ambiguus (Hayoshi *et al.* 1997). This is the basis of the potentially life-threatening state of laryngeal stridor. Muscles of the palatopharyngeal isthmus may be similarly affected (Lapresle and Annabi 1979). Neither the nucleus ambiguus nor Onuf's nucleus shows involvement in PD. The neurones in these groups, which share vulnerability in MSA, innervate striated muscles regulating entry to and exit from the tracts derived developmentally from the endoderm, i.e. the laryngeal and oesophageal, and anal and urethral, orifices. The relevant neurones in the nucleus ambiguus are branchiomotor neurones. It seems very possible that their common susceptibility in MSA might be founded in common factors in their development and, or, environment.

Although some of the same cell groups may show involvement in PD and in MSA, the regular occurrence of Lewy bodies in PD and their general absence in MSA assists in distinguishing the two conditions centrally. Some neurones in MSA show cytoplasmic inclusions, but these are relatively few and lack the characteristic, distinctively concentric features of Lewy bodies. A consistent positive discriminator in central nervous pathways in MSA is, however, an abundance of oligodendroglial cytoplasmic inclusions, which are argyrophilic and ubiquitinated, containing loosely arranged, granule-associated coarse filaments resembling microtubules. These are found in affected neuronal groups before the cell loss becomes severe, and also profusely in tracts of nerve fibres presynaptic to these (Papp and Lantos 1994; Chapter 33).

Ganglia and ganglionic neurones

Sympathetic ganglia have not often been examined in pathological studies of AF, and have seldom been described quantitatively. Enteric and parasympathetic ganglia have been studied in only a few instances. Here also, however, there emerges a distinction between two types of AF.

In MSA with AF (Table 32.1 of Matthews 1992*a*) it has been typical to report either no obvious abnormality in sympathetic ganglia, or some foci of gliosis and possible loss of neurones, or sometimes neuronophagia, not quantified. Spokes *et al.* (1979), in silver preparations, noted some depletion of nerve fibres, and argentophil debris. Gliosis could of itself indicate loss of nerve fibres and terminals, and not exclusively loss of neurones: gliosis may be seen in the globus pallidus in MSA in conjunction with severe loss of neurones from the putamen. Any morphological changes reported in sympathetic ganglionic neurones in MSA have tended to be non-specific, falling within the normal age-related range of appearances, and published micrographs and counts have indicated at least a moderate density, and sometimes quite a high density, of surviving neurones. Four (27 per cent) of the MSA cases reported by Gray *et al.* (1988), which had severe AF, are unusual in showing 'marked neuronal loss' in sympathetic ganglia.

In PAF, however, and in PD, it has been characteristic to find Lewy bodies (and often numerous Lewy body-like 'eosinophilic bodies' of bizarre, serpiginous form, now regarded as intraneuritic Lewy bodies) in the sympathetic ganglia, with or without obvious neuronal loss (Table 32.1 of Matthews 1992*a*), just as in the pigmented neurones of the brainstem in PD. Rajput and Rozdilsky (1976) found Lewy bodies in sympathetic ganglia in five of six PD cases, with 'axonal swellings' in the other, and reported (without formal counting) slight to severe loss and atrophy of the ganglionic neurones, roughly correlated with the degree of orthostatic hypotension, in the three cases of PD which also showed AF. The subject with severest AF and greatest loss of sympathetic neurones showed only 'minimal reduction' of neurones in the IML, whereas a subject with MSA and AF was judged to have moderate loss of IML neurones and no more than slight neurone loss in the sympathetic stellate ganglion. Recently, Goldstein *et al.* (1997) found no demonstrable cardiac uptake of ^{18}F-6-fluorodopamine on thoracic PET scan, coupled with other indices of peripheral sympathetic cardiac denervation, in two PD patients with orthostatic hypotension. Hague *et al.* (1997), in a subject with PAF of long standing, have reported the presence of Lewy bodies both in central neurones (in substantia nigra, locus ceruleus, substantia innominata) and in sympathetic ganglionic neurones, including peripheral autonomic (presumptive sympathetic) axons at distal sites: in the epicardial fat, in peri-adrenal tissue, and in the muscularis of the urinary bladder. Such findings have suggested the possibility of a primary lesion in PD, and now also in PAF, affecting in common neurones of similar or related phenotypes. The disease process is, however, not restricted to catecholaminergic, or monoaminergic, neurones, either centrally, where the cholinergic nucleus basalis is regularly involved, or peripherally. Wakabayashi *et al.* (1993), while confirming the consistency of occurrence of Lewy bodies in sympathetic ganglia in cases of PD, have reported in 12 such cases (and also in five non-parkinsonian subjects with many Lewy bodies in the central nervous system) an increased incidence of Lewy bodies in enteric neurones and in neurones of cardiac and pelvic plexuses, in comparison with an extensive control series. Takeda *et al.* (1993) found Lewy bodies, both intrasomatic and intraneuritic, in the submandibular ganglion as well as in myenteric ganglia in a case of Parkinson's disease. Thus, there may be widespread involvement of peripheral autonomic neurones, sympathetic, parasympathetic and enteric, by the pathological process which leads to the formation of Lewy bodies in PD and in diffuse Lewy body disease or the pre-parkinsonian state; and the latter may include PAF, since it is now reported that central as well as peripheral neurones may develop Lewy bodies in this condition also (Hague *et al.* 1997).

Since the autonomic ganglia appear to differ distinctively in these two forms of AF, it is clearly important to examine them carefully for any further evidence that may throw light on the pathological processes involved.

Why is it so difficult to be sure about the underlying changes? There are various reasons, some of which are common to all neuropathological studies while others are peculiar to the autonomic nervous system. First, the basic defect may be biochemical, metabolic, or regulatory, and may not express itself in gross structural terms. Secondly, the condition may be well advanced before it presents clinically. This is perhaps particularly true of the autonomic nervous system, which, unlike the somatic motor system, shows no clearly defined functional demarcation between an upper (higher centres) and a lower motor neurone (IML) lesion. In this context the fact that the earliest symptom in MSA is often sphincter disturbance from involvement of Onuf's nucleus, which innervates striated muscle, offers a valuable cue to immediate and follow-up evaluation of autonomic functions. There are both divergence and convergence of preganglionic neurones on to ganglionic neurones, and the latter may receive multiple inputs which have the characteristic that they are subthreshold, requiring coincidence of several inputs to bring the neurone to the threshold for firing. The peripheral effectors are smooth or cardiac muscle and gland cells; neuroeffector contacts are typically not close; and electrotonic coupling in the effector organ is frequent or invariable. The interstitial dropping-out of peripheral sympathetic nerve endings may be initially compensated by diffusion of transmitter, since fewer nerve endings mean less high-affinity reuptake, by increase in receptor density, and by electrotonic coupling, until the changes have become extreme. Moreover, collateral sprouting of residual preganglionic nerves in the ganglia (cf. Liestøl *et al.* 1986) and also of postganglionic nerves in the periphery is further able to compensate to a remarkable extent. A slowly progressive change may thus not become clinically evident until the underlying pathological changes are severe, as in the case of IML neurone loss in MSA with AF (Oppenheimer 1980).

By this time, secondary trophic and degenerative changes may well have occurred, involving not only neurones but also satellite or Schwann cells, supporting tissues, and vasculature. As far as the neurones are concerned, these secondary changes are likely to be transneuronal in character, but could be either anterograde or retrograde. Much knowledge has accrued latterly concerning retrograde trophic influences on neurones, and this has arisen largely from studies of autonomic and sensory ganglia, relating to nerve growth factor and, more recently, to brain-derived, ciliary, and other tissue-derived neurotrophic factors, which govern the development and maintenance of peripheral ganglion cells (Thoenen 1991). A similar control may be expected to apply in the case of the preganglionic neurones. Survival and phenotypic specification may be governed by different factors, and a neurone may be induced to change its phenotype by target-derived factor(s) after it has reached and innervated the target, as in the case of the sympathetic sudomotor neurone, which is initially adrenergic but undergoes a cholinergic transformation after it has innervated the sweat glands. Anterograde influences may also be important, as is well exemplified by the striated muscle fibre: trophic maintenance is influenced by activation, and in its absence shrinkage and a varying degree of dedifferentiation may occur. Whether in the long term denervation may lead to neuronal death is uncertain: it depends strongly on age, on the type of neurone, and the presence or absence of other inputs.

From the time of onset of autonomic failure a patient may survive for several or even many years. The availability of biopsy is strictly limited, e.g. to the peripheral autonomic terminals as seen in muscle or skin biopsies, since the removal of ganglia would be too destructive; and the possibility of early biopsy is virtually ruled out by the lateness of presentation. Post-mortem changes may preclude the finer aspects of the eventual analysis, and agonal changes, involving intense nervous discharges, may also have supervened, as the terminal event is often apparently asphyxial.

Desiderata for studying the ganglia post-mortem

These include early chilling of the body and early removal of tissues, to optimize tissue preservation; extensive sampling within the autonomic nervous system; the obtaining of adequate age-matched control material for comparison; and the use of appropriate fixation schedules: for example, buffered 4 per cent formaldehyde followed by paraffin embedding for conventional histology, including neurone counting, or by cryostat or frozen sections for enzyme histochemistry and immunohistochemistry; buffered 3 per cent glutaraldehyde followed by resin-embedding for electron microscopy and for light microscopy of 1 μm sections; or alternatively, especially where little tissue is obtainable, Bouin's fluid, or Zamboni's fixative (buffered 2 per cent formaldehyde with 15 per cent saturated picric acid), which is compatible with both immunohistochemistry and electron microscopy as well as conventional histology. In practice, for various reasons, it may only be possible to fulfil a limited number of these criteria.

Experimental observations

Matthews (1992*a*) reported a study of sympathetic ganglia from six subjects dying with MSA and AF, aged 46–77 years, two subjects dying with clinically pure AF, aged 58 and 70 years, and ganglia from 10 subjects dying of other causes, aged 16–98 years.

Light microscopy

No Lewy bodies were found in any ganglia from the control or MSA subjects. The ganglia of subjects with MSA were well populated with neurones which resembled those of control ganglia in size, general cytology, and packing density. Almost all neurones had conspicuous aggregates of lipofuscin granules. Nissl material was, however, relatively scanty. In silver-stained preparations many neurones were seen to have well-preserved dendritic arborizations (Fig. 34.1). Some

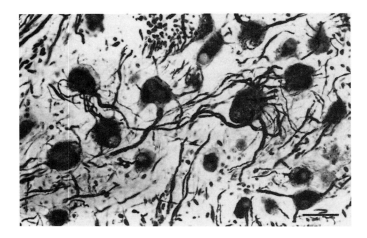

Fig. 34.1. Neurones of a thoracic sympathetic ganglion from a subject with MSA. Silver preparation (Glees and Marsland). Scale bar, 50 μm.

of these dendritic patterns were perhaps unusually complex and profuse, and some processes unusually stout, but no gross distortions were observed. Some of the smaller neurones showed no stainable arborizations; but failure to stain processes in this material cannot necessarily be taken to imply their absence.

Semi-quantitative cytological comparisons were made in 1-μm resin-embedded sections from comparable mid-ganglion levels (Fig. 34.2). In superior cervical ganglia (SCGs) of three control subjects (ages 16, 64, 98 years), the mean packing density of neurones in areas of neuropil averaged 7.1 nucleated neuronal profiles (NNP) in a standard reference area (range of means 5.6–8.3). In SCGs of three subjects with MSA (ages 59, 60, 77 years) the corresponding average was 8.9 NNP (range of means 6.8–10.4). This hardly suggests

neuronal loss, but might indicate compaction consequent on reduction of other elements such as preganglionic nerve fibres and extent of dendritic trees. Schmidt *et al.* (1993) found no decrease of neuronal packing density with age in sympathetic ganglia of control, non-diabetic subjects.

In the control ganglia, a mean of 91 per cent of NNP (range 84–95 per cent) showed distinct Nissl granules. In all three MSA subjects, fewer NNP (37, 46, and 72 per cent) showed distinct Nissl granules. Heavy clumps or masses of lipofuscin bodies were relatively few in the youngest control subject (35 per cent of NNP) but their incidence differed little between the other two (87 and 84 per cent) and the subjects with MSA (range 78–93 per cent, mean 84 per cent). The proportion of NNP showing centrally situated, rather than eccentric, nuclei was similar in the two groups (control mean l5 per cent, range 11–24 per cent; MSA mean 13 per cent, range 8–18 per cent). The mean diameters of the five to eight largest and smallest neurones were compared, for two subjects from each group, and were not found to differ markedly.

Thus, in the MSA group of subjects with AF, the principal observed difference from the controls lay in the reduced incidence of distinct Nissl granules in the neuronal cell bodies. No consistent abnormalities were noted in the vasculature or in adventitious cells in the ganglia; but in one MSA subject there was some perivenular lymphocytic infiltration, part of a generalized distribution associated with a long-standing leukaemic condition (Waldeström macroglobulinaemia).

In sympathetic ganglia from the two subjects with PAF, the packing densities of NNP in the neuropil were strikingly reduced, to means of 3.4 and 2.2 per standard reference area, and there was similar heavy depopulation of neurones, with scattered evidence of neuronophagia, in all ganglia studied. Lewy bodies were seen in both subjects, with mean incidences of 1.1 and 1.25 per NNP; these were sometimes in neuronal somata and sometimes in enlarged neuronal processes. In the surviving neurones, however, the mean incidence of visible Nissl granules was high (92 and 93 per cent of NNP), and the proportions of NNP which showed massed lipofuscin bodies (82 per cent in each case) resembled those reported above for the MSA and control subjects. In these ganglia, therefore, the salient and distinctive features were the evidence of loss of neurones and the presence of Lewy bodies. In the younger PAF subject an entire SCG was available for neurone-counting in serial paraffin sections. Corrected counts of all neuronal nuclei in every fiftieth section, of 10-μm thickness, yielded an estimate of 214 002 neurones in the entire ganglion. When compared with the mean figure of approximately 937 000 (range 760 370–1 041 652) obtained from four ganglia of young adults by Ebbesson (1963), this suggests a loss of over 75 per cent of neurones, which is much greater than might be expected to occur with age in normal subjects.

Histochemistry, immunohistochemistry, in situ hybridization

In frozen sections of a thoracic ganglion from the younger PAF subject specific acetylcholinesterase activity was demonstrable, after prolonged incubation, with a normal distribution in the few surviving neuronal cell bodies and in parts of the surrounding neuropil, but not in nerve bundles.

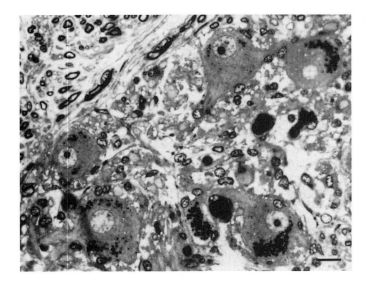

Fig. 34.2. 1-μm section of an Araldite-embedded thoracic ganglion of a subject with MSA, stained with methylene blue and Azur II. Most of the neurones have eccentric nuclei and contain arcs or masses of darkly stained lipofuscin bodies, but also contain some distinct Nissl material (intermediate grey clumps). Scale bar, 20 μm.

Immunofluorescence histochemistry by the indirect method was performed on sections from ganglia of two subjects with MSA (males aged 56 and 77 years) and one with PAF (female, aged 58 years, from whom neurone counts were made in the SCG), in comparison with ganglia from three young (ages 17–27 years) and four older male control subjects (ages 57–85 years), with the following results.

Sensory nerve collaterals

In the control subjects prevertebral ganglia (coeliac–superior mesenteric; CSMG) contained perineuronal networks of finely varicose nerve fibres immunoreactive for substance P (SP), and likewise for calcitonin-gene-related peptide (CGRP), which surrounded individual neurones or clusters of neurones. Both these peptides are found in primary sensory neurones, in many of which they coexist, and the intraganglionic networks are attributable to collateral terminal branches of sensory nerve fibres from the viscera which traverse the prevertebral ganglia *en route* to the dorsal root ganglia and spinal cord (Matthews *et al.* 1987). In thoracic and lumbar paravertebral ganglia only occasional, solitary varicose trails were seen which were immunoreactive for SP or CGRP. No obvious differences were found between the younger and older control subjects. Similar networks in a prevertebral ganglion, resembling those in the controls both in distribution and in density, and occasional solitary fibres in paravertebral ganglia, were found in one of the MSA subjects (Fig. 34.3b, c). (No prevertebral ganglion was available from the other MSA subject.) The coeliac ganglion of the subject with PAF showed localized baskets of SP- and CGRP-immunoreactive varicosities surrounding some of the residual neurones, but not those with Lewy bodies or dystrophic neurites. These findings suggest that such trophic interactions as may be required for the maintenance of these sensory collateral networks are still present and operative, not only

in older control subjects equally with younger subjects, but also in MSA, and in relation to some surviving neurones in PAF.

Neuromedin B (NMB) immunoreactivity in ganglia (Matthews 1992*b*)

In the CSMG of control subjects NMB immunoreactivity was observed in finely varicose nerve fibres and pericellular networks surrounding many groups of neurones. Paravertebral ganglia showed only very occasional NMB-immunoreactive (-IR) fibres. A similar distribution of NMB-IR fibres was found in the MSA subjects, and some remnants of NMB networks also persisted in the CSMG of the PAF subject. Additionally, ileal myenteric ganglia of three control subjects were found to contain occasional NMB-IR neurones, and networks of NMB-IR fibres were observed surrounding some of the ganglionic neurones. In contrast, only scanty NMB-IR nerve fibre networks were found in spinal-cord sections, in superficial laminae of the dorsal horn. It cannot be excluded that the intraganglionic NMB-IR nerve networks in the CSMG are collateral branches of sensory nerve fibres, but it is also possible that they may originate from neurones in the enteric nerve plexuses and that, like sensory nerve collaterals, they may persist in MSA and to some extent in PAF.

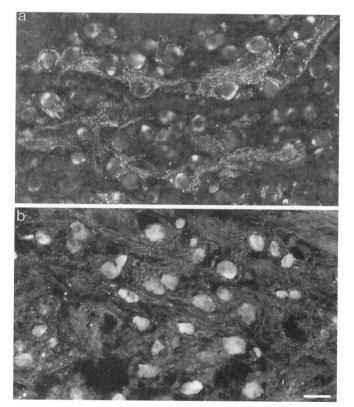

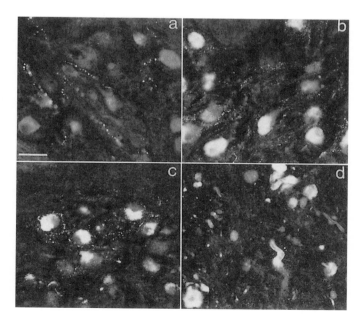

Fig. 34.3. Immunofluorescent staining for neuropeptides in the coeliac ganglion: (a) enkephalin, (b) substance P, (c) CGRP, all from a case of MSA; (d) neuropeptide Y in dystrophic neurites, from a case of pure autonomic failure. Scale bar, 50 μm. Some neurones in (b) and (c) show intensely autofluorescent lipofuscin masses.

Fig. 34.4. Immunofluorescent staining for enkephalin in thoracic paravertebral ganglia: (a) from a young control subject, (b) from a case of MSA. Very few trails of fine enkephalin-immunoreactive fibres are present in (b). Most of the solitary bright points in this field represent lipofuscin autofluorescence. Scale bar, 50 μm.

Enkephalin-immunoreactive elements

In the control prevertebral ganglia, equally in younger and older subjects, short trails and perineuronal arcs of coarse enkephalin-immunoreactive varicosities were scantily distributed from place to place. Similar enkephalin-immunoreactive nerve elements, similarly distributed, were found in the prevertebral ganglion of the MSA subject (Fig. 34.3a) and occasionally, near to some of the surviving neurones, in the PAF subject.

In the paravertebral ganglia of all the control subjects, profuse pericellular networks of finely varicose, slender, enkephalin-immunoreactive nerve fibres were seen, surrounding clusters of neurones from place to place throughout the ganglia (Fig. 34.4a). In the two MSA subjects, although the post-mortem intervals (10 h, 13 h) had been shorter than for any of the controls (21–48 h, mean 31 h), only slight and scanty enkephalin-immunoreactive networks were found in thoracic and lumbar paravertebral ganglia (Fig. 34.4b). In a thoracic ganglion of the PAF subject, no enkephalin-immunoreactive fibres or varicosities could be detected. This could have either of two causes: (1) ante-mortem loss, through degeneration, or (2) post-mortem degradation of these very fine nerve fibres, since in this case the post-mortem interval was long (84 h), although cooling had been begun early. The question must remain open.

The fine enkephalin-immunoreactive networks in the paravertebral ganglia are attributable to preganglionic nerve fibres. Clearly, these do not represent all the preganglionic nerve endings, since not all neurones are surrounded by them. In the rat, enkephalin and choline acetyltransferase, the acetylcholine-synthesizing enzyme, have been shown to coexist in some of the preganglionic sympathetic neurones (Kondo *et al.* 1985). The severe depletion of enkephalin-immunoreactive networks in paravertebral ganglia in MSA suggests, first, that the corresponding IML neurones are heavily depleted, and secondly, that this loss has not been fully compensated by whatever intraganglionic sprouting may have occurred from the nerve endings of surviving enkephalin-immunoreactive neurones. The same could well also apply to the other, non-enkephalin-immunoreactive preganglionic neurones. In the PAF subject, absence of enkephalin-immunoreactive networks could indicate retrograde transneuronal loss of the preganglionic neurones from target deprivation, consequent upon the severe neurone depopulation of the ganglion. It is appropriate to consider whether death of preganglionic neurones from target deprivation could contribute to the loss of enkephalin-immunoreactive nerve networks in the MSA subjects, since there is evidence for selective loss of sudomotor ganglionic neurones in this condition (Low and Fealey 1992). Upon this point, however, the available evidence is conflicting, one study (Schmitt *et al.* 1988) suggesting that presumptive sudomotor neurones in human paravertebral sympathetic ganglia are not innervated by enkephalin-immunoreactive nerve fibres and another (Järvi and Pelto-Huikko 1990) indicating the contrary.

Neuropeptide Y (NPY) immunoreactivity in ganglia

A proportion of sympathetic ganglionic neurones contains NPY-immunoreactive material in addition to noradrenaline. These include vasoconstrictor neurones, and neurones innervating the heart and vas deferens, *inter alia*. In the young control subjects many ganglionic neurones showed moderate immunoreactivity for NPY, and a few short varicose trails and somewhat larger foci of more intense

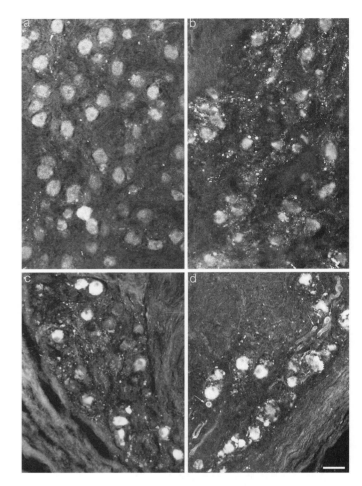

Fig. 34.5. Immunofluorescent staining for NPY in the coeliac ganglion: (a) From a young control subject, aged 17 years, (b) from a case of MSA, subject aged 77 years, (c) from an old control subject, aged 85 years. NPY immunoreactivity is visible in most of the neurones in (a) and (b), but in (c) is partly obscured by lipofuscin masses. Irregular varicose trails and larger foci of bright immunofluorescence are much more numerous in (c) than in (a) and are particularly conspicuous in (b). Section (d) is from the case of PAF illustrated also in Fig. 34.3d, and shows the prevalence of Lewy bodies and dystrophic neurites, some with strong peripheral NPY immunoreactivity (arrows), in a region unusually well populated with surviving neurones. Scale bar, 50 μm.

immunoreactivity were seen in the surrounding neuropil (Fig. 34.5a). In older subjects these additional foci of more intense immunoreactivity were more numerous and widespread, and the NPY immunoreactivity of the cell bodies also appeared more intense (Fig. 34.5c). In the ganglia of the MSA subjects this difference was at least as strongly marked, and possibly greater, placing them in sharp contrast with the ganglia of the younger subjects (Fig. 34.5b). The additional foci may represent NPY-rich short intracapsular dendrites or additional dendritic branches of the neurones, which increase with age, and might be particularly profusely developed, or strongly charged with NPY, in the MSA subjects, there perhaps reflecting low recruitment and engorgement with undischarged secretory material, and perhaps the formation of local collateral sprouts and synapses (cf. Ramsay and Matthews 1985). In the PAF subject, many of the

Lewy bodies and dystrophic neurites showed NPY immunoreactivity in their peripheral zone, marginal to the halo (Fig. 34.5d).

Tyrosine hydroxylase immunoreactivity

Tyrosine hydroxylase (TH) is a cytoplasmic enzyme of the sympathetic neurone which is of interest as being the rate-limiting enzyme in catecholamine synthesis. It is also subject to up-regulation via incoming nerve impulses. A low cytoplasmic level of immunofluorescent signal for TH, approximately 1.8 × primary-antibody blank level, was demonstrable in neurones of a ganglion from a young control subject by image densitometry of film micrographs exposed for a standard interval. Similar measurements in the corresponding ganglion of an MSA subject gave a value of approximately 1.2 × antibody blank level. These measurements were made with precautions to avoid deposits of lipofuscin in the neurones. They indicate that TH-like material and a presumptive catecholamine productive capacity may persist in sympathetic ganglionic neurones in MSA despite a severe degree of decentraliza-

tion, which harmonizes with the observation of normal supine plasma noradrenaline levels in this condition.

In situ hybridization for tyrosine hydroxylase mRNA

Cryostat sections of ganglia of the same two MSA subjects and the PAF subject and ganglia from three younger and three older male control subjects, all from the above series, were examined by *in situ* hybridization for TH mRNA (Foster *et al.* 1990). Sections from MSA subjects and both older and younger controls showed similar levels of binding of the 35S-labelled TH mRNA antisense oligonucleotide probe used (Fig. 34.6a, c; Fig. 34.7a). In contrast, sections from the PAF subject showed very low levels of probe binding over the few remaining neurones (Fig. 34.6b; Fig. 34.7b); neurones containing Lewy bodies did not differ noticeably from those without such inclusions. All the sections studied showed low levels of

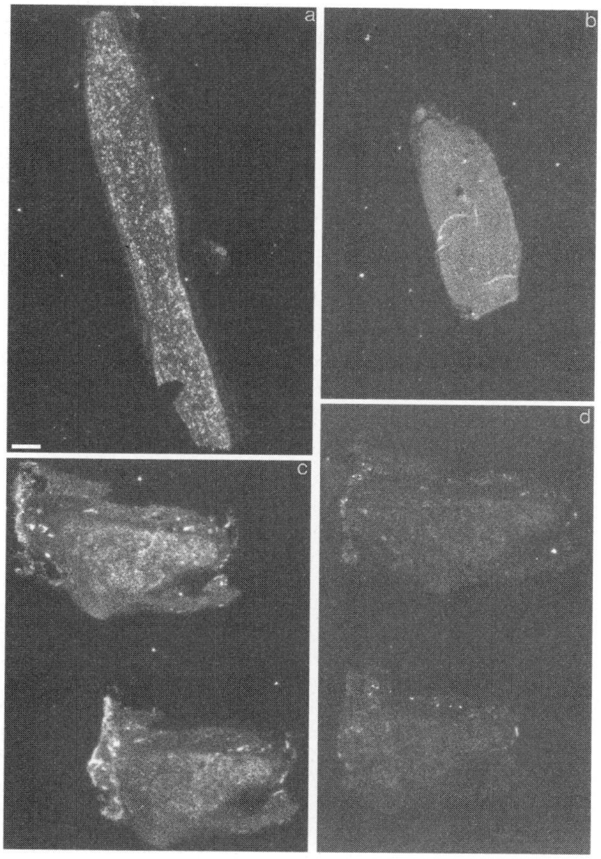

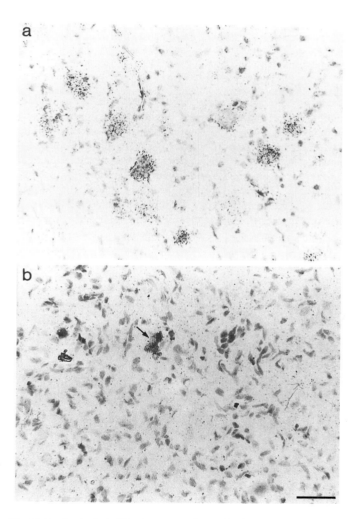

Fig. 34.6. *In situ* hybridization autoradiographs (reverse phase) from slide-mounted cryostat sections: (a) paravertebral (lumbar) ganglion from a case of MSA, (b) coeliac ganglion from a case of PAF, (c) stellate ganglion from a control subject aged 66 years, all showing extent of binding of the antisense probe for tyrosine hydroxylase mRNA; (d) coeliac ganglion of the same control subject, adjacent section to that in (c), showing low level of non-specific binding of the sense probe. Scale bar, 1 mm.

Fig. 34.7. In situ hybridization autoradiographs, lightly counterstained with toluidine blue, light micrography. Scale bar, 50 µm. (a) Lumbar ganglion of a 66-year-old control subject, showing heavy binding of antisense probe for tyrosine hydroxylase mRNA over ganglionic neurones; (b) coeliac ganglion of the PAF subject showing some binding of the same probe over a neuron containing a Lewy body (arrow) but little or no binding elsewhere; the binding in this specimen did not differ appreciably from the non-specific binding of the sense probe.

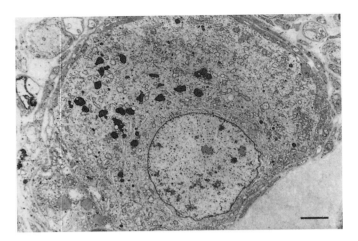

Fig. 34.8. Electron micrograph of a neurone from the SCG of a subject with MSA. The nucleus is markedly eccentric. The cytoplasm shows numerous lipofuscin bodies and little rough endoplasmic reticulum (Nissl material). At the lower right, the satellite sheath of the neurone is very thin and in places deficient (cf. Fig. 34.12). Scale bar, 5 μm.

hybridization to a TH sense probe, employed to reflect non-specific binding (Fig. 34.6d). Binding of this probe was localized almost exclusively to collections of lipofuscin in the ganglionic neurones. This study indicated that TH mRNA is detectable post-mortem in human sympathetic neurones by *in situ* hybridization. The finding that TH probe binding was similar in MSA and in control ganglia suggests that TH biosynthetic pathways may be functioning normally in the ganglionic neurones of MSA subjects, despite the deficiencies in preganglionic pathways. In the case of PAF studied, the low level of TH antisense probe binding did not differ appreciably from the level of non-specific binding indicated by the sense probe. Any conclusion that TH biosynthesis in surviving neurones was reduced in this case must, however, be tentative because of the long post-mortem delay of over 80 h, already noted.

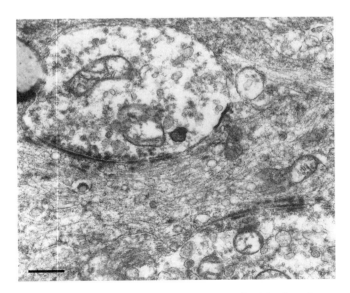

Fig. 34.9. Two synapses of cholinergic type on a dendrite from the SCG of a control subject aged 16. Scale bar, 0.5 μm.

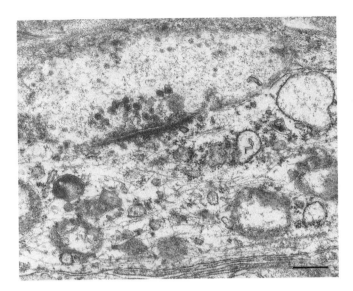

Fig. 34.10. Axodendritic synapse from the SCG of a subject with MSA. The presynaptic profile is heavily depleted of synaptic vesicles and shows evidence of numerous coated vesicles, suggesting recent extensive liberation of transmitter. Scale bar, 0.5 μm.

Electron microscopy

Not all the material was sufficiently well preserved to be informative. Questions addressed included general neuronal cytology (Fig. 34.8), the presence and type of synapses, the completeness of satellite cell cover of the neurones, and the state of the pre- and postganglionic nerve fibres.

In the youngest control subject, synapses were readily localizable with an incidence of approximately 6–10 per grid square of side 100 μm; they were of cholinergic preganglionic type (Fig. 34.9; Matthews 1983) and were mostly axodendritic. In the subjects with MSA similar synapses were present (Fig. 34.10), occurring in clusters in areas of dendritic neuropil, but were much less frequent, and tended to be greatly expanded and depleted of vesicles. This appearance was not necessarily just a post-mortem artefact, since it appeared equally in

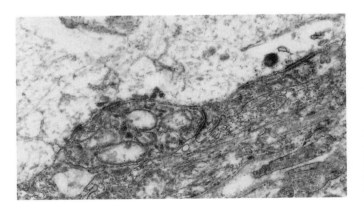

Fig. 34.11. Two synapses of possible adrenergic type from the same presynaptic profile, one axodendritic and the other probably axosomatic, from the SCG of a subject with MSA (same ganglion as Fig. 34.10). On the right the dendrite is linked with the presumptive soma by an attachment plaque. ×21 000.

ganglia fixed within 8 h and over 36 h post-mortem: it recalled the appearance of nerve endings heavily overstimulated by black widow spider venom, and could possibly have reflected intense sympathetic discharges in surviving preganglionic endings in the ante-mortem period. In addition, occasional synapses were seen containing tubular vesicles with a relatively electron-dense content (Fig. 34.11); these resemble a type of adrenergic nerve ending and could be intrinsic synapses, which can increase appreciably in incidence in denervated (and presumably in partly denervated) ganglia (Ramsay and Matthews 1985).

Neuro-neuronal attachment plaques were seen both in control and in MSA ganglia (Fig. 34.11).

Neurone–satellite relations did not seem to differ markedly between control and MSA ganglia. In both, neurones or their dendrites could show short, sometimes multiple, regions of their surfaces devoid of satellite cell cover (Fig. 34.12); these appeared to be at least as frequent in the MSA ganglia. There was possibly some tendency for the enveloping satellite cell processes to be thinner in the MSA ganglia; but further study, of material better matched as to age and preservation, would be required to clarify this question.

In one MSA subject the pre- and postganglionic nerve fibres were sufficiently well preserved for study. Among the preganglionic nerve fibres there was evidence of loss of axons, in the form of collagen-filled Schwann cell channels; myelinated fibres were few, and other Schwann–axon units contained each only one or two non-myelinated axons. The indications of fibre loss are consistent with the well-documented loss of IML neurones in MSA. Some of the non-myelinated axons were singly ensheathed and of relatively large diameter, up to 4 μm, which suggests possible demyelination, or hypertrophy without accompanying myelination. These axons were well populated with longitudinally oriented microtubules and neurofilaments, and did not appear to be pathologically swollen. Among the postganglionic fibres in the internal carotid trunk there was also some suggestion of fibre loss, in the form of collagen-filled channels in Schwann cells, and here also there was a wide range of diameters of non-myelinated axons, suggesting possible denervation atrophy of some neurones and hypertrophy of others. The number of fibres per Schwann unit was not unduly high, ranging mostly from 2 to 6; thus, there was little evidence of axon sprouting at this level.

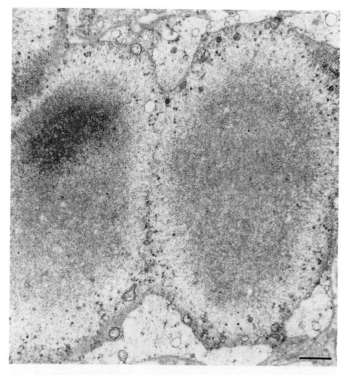

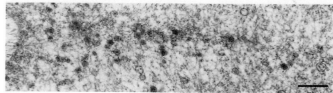

Fig. 34.13. Electron micrograph of two Lewy bodies filling adjacent parts of a neurite, possibly an axon, from the SCG of a subject with PAF. Scale bar, 2 μm. Below is shown at higher magnification part of the periphery of the Lewy bodies, where dense-cored vesicles are associated with the margins of the fibrillary masses. Scale bar, 0.5 μm.

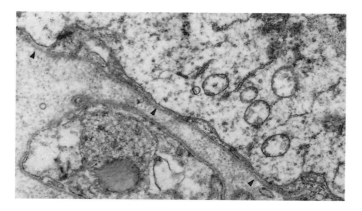

Fig. 34.12. Arrowheads indicate short deficiencies in the satellite sheath of a neurone, from the SCG of a subject with MSA. ×13 000.

In the older subject with PAF, although preservation of the interneuronal neuropil was poor, information was obtained on the nature of the Lewy bodies in these sympathetic neurones (Fig. 34.13): a mass of densely fibrillar material with an amorphous denser core was surrounded by a rim of dense-cored vesicles, which were associated with radiating marginal filaments of the mass (cf. Forno and Norville 1976). Densely packed lysosomal bodies in addition to much lipofuscin were seen in some neurones; but otherwise the surviving neurones, apart from those containing Lewy bodies, did not look grossly abnormal.

Conclusions and comment

This study in sympathetic ganglia has indicated a clear difference in ganglionic pathology, and hence presumably in underlying cause of the autonomic failure, between multiple system atrophy and pure autonomic failure.

In MSA the neurones of sympathetic ganglia are not in general severely reduced in number and do not exhibit major abnormalities, apart from a relative lack of Nissl material which might indicate a partial denervation atrophy of long standing. There is confirmatory evidence of the loss of preganglionic nerve fibres, and there is evidence suggesting that, despite any regenerative sprouting from surviving fibres, by the time autonomic failure supervenes there is a severe deficiency of preganglionic nerve endings in the ganglia. The loss of preganglionic nerve endings appears to be selective, since other demonstrable fibre systems, for example sensory collateral nerve networks, seem at least as profuse as in normal subjects. It has not so far proved feasible to determine whether they may actually be increased in MSA ganglia, by some mechanism of sprouting in response to the partial denervation. It is possible however that NPY-immunoreactivity in neurones and their processes may be increased in these ganglia, by more than the increment with age which this study has revealed in control subjects. Tyrosine hydroxylase and its mRNA may still be demonstrable in these sympathetic neurones, in MSA with AF.

In PAF, on the other hand, the packing density of ganglionic neurones may be severely reduced; and counts in one complete SCG have indicated a neuronal loss of over 75 per cent, which resembles the proportional loss of IML neurones at which AF becomes severe (Oppenheimer 1980). Some of the surviving ganglionic neurones show Lewy bodies, many display eosinophilic Lewy-like bodies in distorted, dystrophic neurites, and some show evidence of an intense lysosomal activity, but almost all of the remainder show well-defined Nissl granules and do not appear grossly abnormal for the age of the subject.

It therefore seems reasonable to assume, as a working hypothesis, that the prime determinants of these two forms of AF are, respectively, the loss of preganglionic and of ganglionic neurones. To this must be added, in MSA, the losses of branchiomotor neurones and of caudal sphincteric motoneurones (Onuf's nucleus) which underlie the development of laryngeal and sphincter problems; and in PD with AF, and possibly also in PAF (Hague et al. 1997), the as yet incompletely defined contribution of the involvement of central as well as peripheral neurones. The initial causes of these losses of neurones remain obscure, although they evidently differ: in both 'Lewy body disease' and MSA abnormal intraneuronal accumulations of material occur which are evidently derived from modified cytoskeletal elements, but these are not identical in composition. In both cases the material may be ubiquitinated, but this is a non-specific sign of non-lysosomal protein degradation. It is not clear in either case whether the same metabolic dysfunction causes the fibrillar or filamentous accumulations and also leads to neuronal death. Neurones containing Lewy bodies may still, if catecholaminergic, exhibit tyrosine hydroxylase; and their nuclei and cytoplasmic organelles usually appear intact (Forno 1996). The apparently short-lived stage of intraneuronal granulofilamentous accumulations in MSA is possibly a more direct precursor of neuronal death, since few such accumulations are seen at stages when neuronal loss has become pronounced. It remains to be confirmed by counting to what extent there may be loss of ganglionic neurones in the AF which can develop in Parkinson's disease; but it seems possible that PAF, PD, and PD with AF are different manifestations of the same disease process. The ramifications of the secondary consequences remain likewise to be unravelled. As Oppenheimer (1980) clearly showed, loss of IML

neurones in PAF, or in AF with PD, can be quite as severe as that found in MSA. This could be a retrograde neuronal death, consequent upon target deprivation and related to the profundity and duration of the latter. Indeed, the loss of IML neurones in MSA might itself be due to disruption of a retrograde trophic influence from the ganglionic neurones, which might arise, for example, from inadequate production or release of essential neurotrophic factor(s), without overt morphological changes in the ganglionic neurones. The demonstration of apparently normal prevertebral sensory collateral nerve networks in MSA suggests, however, that any deficiency of trophic substance must be highly specific for the preganglionic neurones.

The observations reported here denote some advances to date but also present challenges for verification and questions for exploration. The wider range of approaches and techniques now available offers renewed hope of progress in resolving the basic problems of causation, and hence possibly of prevention, in these devastatingly disabling conditions of autonomic failure.

Acknowledgements

This work received MRC support. Thanks are due to Mr P. J. Belk and Mr M. Masih for technical assistance and to Mr B. Archer and Mr C. Beesley for photographic work. Generous gifts of primary antibodies from A. C. Cuello (SP, Enk, TH) and J. M. Polak (CGRP, NPY, NMB) are gratefully acknowledged. The author is indebted to the late Dr D.R. Oppenheimer, Professor M. M. Esiri, Drs J. R. Ponsford, M. Rossi, N. D. Francis and F. Scaravilli for assistance in obtaining ganglia, and to the late Professor L. W. Duchen for access to paraffin-embedded material.

References

Bajaj, N. P. S., Fowler, C., and Chaudhuri, K. R. (1996). Pure autonomic failure with abnormal sphincter electromyography: a case report. Clin. auton. Res. 6, 279.

Beck, R. O., Betts, C. D., and Fowler, C. J. (1994) Genitourinary dysfunction in multiple system atrophy: clinical features and treatment in 62 cases. J. Urol. 151, 1336–41.

Ebbesson, S. O. E. (1963). A quantitative study of human superior cervical sympathetic ganglia. Anat. Rec. 146, 353–6.

Forno, L. S. (1996). Neuropathology of Parkinson's disease. J. Neuropath. Exp. Neurol. 55, 259–72.

Forno, L. S. and Norville, R. L. (1976). Ultrastructure of Lewy bodies in the stellate ganglion. Acta neuropath. Berlin 34, 183–97.

Foster, O. J. F., Matthews, M. R., Lightman, S. L., and Bannister, R. (1990) In situ hybridisation studies of sympathetic ganglia in multiple system atrophy and pure autonomic failure. J. autonom. nerv. Syst. 31, 171.

Gai, W. P., Geffen, L. B., Denoroy, L., and Blessing, W. W. (1993). Loss of C1 and C3 epinephrine-synthesizing neurons in the medulla oblongata in Parkinson's disease. Ann. Neurol. 33, 357–67.

Goldstein, D. S., Holmes, C., Cannon, R. O. III, Eisenhofer, G., and Kopin, I. J. (1997). Sympathetic cardioneuropathy in dysautonomias. New Engl. J. Med. 336, 696–702.

Gray, F., Vincent, D., and Hauw, J. J. (1988). Quantitative study of lateral horn cells in 15 cases of multiple system atrophy. Acta neuropath. Berlin 75, 513–18.

Hague, K., Lento, P., Morgello, S., Caro, S., and Kaufmann, H. (1997). The distribution of Lewy bodies in pure autonomic failure: autopsy findings and review of the literature. *Acta neuropath. Berlin* 94, 192–6.

Hayoshi M., Isozaki, E., Oda, M., Tanabe, H., and Kimura, J. (1997). Loss of large myelinated fibres of the recurrent laryngeal nerve in patients with multiple system atrophy and vocal cord palsy. *J. Neurol. Neurosurg. Psychiat.* 62, 234–48.

Hughes, A. J., Daniel, C. J., and Lees, A. J. (1993). A clinico-pathological study of 100 cases of Parkinson's disease. *Arch. Neurol.* 50, 140–8.

Järvi, R. and Pelto-Huikko, M. (1990). Localization of neuropeptide Y in human sympathetic ganglia: correlation with met-enkephalin, tyrosine hydroxylase and acetylcholinesterase. *Histochem. J.* 22, 87–94.

Kato, S., Oda, M., Hayashi, H. *et al.* (1995). Decrease of medullary catecholamine neurons in multiple system atrophy and Parkinson's disease and their preservation in amyotrophic lateral sclerosis. *J. Neurol. Sci.* 132, 216–21.

Kondo, N., Kuramoto, H., Wainer, B. H., and Yanaihara, N. (1985). Evidence for the coexistence of acetylcholine and enkephalin in the sympathetic preganglionic neurons of rats. *Brain Res.* 335, 309–14.

Konno, H., Yamamoto, T., Iwasaki, Y., and Iizuka, H. (1986). Shy–Drager syndrome and amyotrophic lateral sclerosis: cytoarchitectonic and morphometric studies of sacral autonomic neurons. *J. neurol. Sci.* 73, 193–204.

Kumazawa K., Sobue, G., Nakao, N., and Mitsuma, T. (1989). Postganglionic sudomotor function in multiple system atrophy. *Rinsho Shinkeigaku, Japan* 29, 1357–63. (English abstract).

Lapresle, J. and Annabi, A. (1979). Olivopontocerebellar atrophy with velopharyngolaryngeal paralysis: a contribution to the somatotopy of the nucleus ambiguus. *J. Neuropath. Exp. Neurol.* 38, 401–6.

Liestøl, K., Maehlen, J., and Njå, A. (1986). Selective synaptic connections: significance of recognition and competition in mature sympathetic ganglia. *Trends Neurosci.* 9, 21–4.

Low, P. A. and Fealey, R. D. (1992). Pathological studies of the sympathetic neuron. In *Autonomic failure. A textbook of disorders of the autonomic nervous system*, (ed. R. G. Bannister and C. J. Mathias), (3rd edn.) pp. 586–592. OUP, Oxford.

Magaelhaes, M., Wenning, G. K., Daniel, S. E., and Quinn, N. P. (1995). Autonomic dysfunction in pathologically confirmed multiple system atrophy and idiopathic Parkinson's disease—a retrospective comparison. *Acta neurol. scand.* 91, 98–102.

Matthews, M. R. (1983). The ultrastructure of junctions in sympathetic ganglia of mammals. In *Autonomic ganglia*, (ed. L.-G. Elfvin), pp. 27–66. John Wiley, Chichester.

Matthews, M. R. (1992a). Autonomic ganglia in multiple system atrophy and pure autonomic failure. In *Autonomic failure. A textbook of disorders of the autonomic nervous system*, (ed. R. G. Bannister and C. J. Mathias), (3rd edn.) pp. 593–621. OUP, Oxford.

Matthews, M. R. (1992b). Neuromedin B immunoreactive networks are present in human sympathetic ganglia and may persist in autonomic failure. *Clin. auton. Res.* 2, 71.

Matthews, M. R., Connaughton M., and Cuello, A. C. (1987). Ultrastructure and distribution of substance P immunoreactive sensory collaterals in the guinea pig prevertebral sympathetic ganglia. *J. comp. Neurol.* 258, 28–51.

Oppenheimer, D. R. (1980). Lateral horn cells in progressive autonomic failure. *J. neurol. Sci.* 46, 393–404.

Oyanagi, K., Wakabayashi, K., Ohama, E., Takeda, S., Horikawa, Y., Morita, T., and Ikuta, F. (1990). Lewy bodies in the lower sacral parasympathetic neurons of a patient with Parkinson's disease. *Acta neuropath. Berlin* 80, 558–9.

Papp, P. L. and Lantos, M. I. (1994). The distribution of oligodendroglial inclusions in multiple system atrophy and its relevance to clinical symptomatology. *Brain* 117, 235–43.

Rajput, A. H. and Rozdilsky, B. (1976). Dysautonomia in Parkinsonism: a clinico-pathological study. *J. Neurol. Neurosurg. Psychiat.* 39, 1092–100.

Ramsay, D. A. and Matthews, M. R. (1985). Denervation-induced formation of adrenergic synapses in the superior cervical sympathetic ganglion of the rat and the enhancement of this effect by postganglionic axotomy. *Neuroscience* 16, 997–1026.

Schmidt, R. E., Plurad, S. B., Parvin, S. A., and Roth, K. A. (1993). Effect of diabetes and aging on human sympathetic autonomic ganglia. *Am. J. Pathol.* 143, 143–53.

Schmitt, M., Kummer, W., and Heym, C. (1988). Calcitonin gene-related peptide (CGRP)-immunoreactive neurons in the human cervico-thoracic paravertebral ganglia. *J. chem. Neuroanat.* 1, 287–92.

Spokes, E. G. S., Bannister, R., and Oppenheimer, D. (1979). Multiple system atrophy with autonomic failure—clinical, histological and neurochemical observations on four cases. *J. neurol. Sci.* 43, 59–82.

Takeda, S., Yamazaki, K., Miyakawa, T., and Arai, H. (1993). Parkinson's disease with involvement of the parasympathetic ganglia. *Acta neuropath. Berlin* 86, 397–8.

Thoenen, H. (1991). The changing scene of neurotrophic factors. *Trends Neurosci.* 14, 165–70.

van Ingelghem, E., van Zandijcke, M., and Lammens, M. (1994). Pure autonomic failure: a new case with clinical, biochemical and autopsy data. *J. Neurol. Neurosurg. Psychiat.* 57, 745–7.

Wakabayashi, K., Takahashi, H., Ohama, E., Takeda, S., and Ikuta, F. (1993). Lewy bodies in the visceral autonomic nervous system in Parkinson's disease. *Adv. Neurol.* 60, 609–12.

35. Histological studies of skeletal and smooth muscle in autonomic failure

Roger Bannister, Marjorie Ellison, and John Morgan-Hughes

Introduction

Muscle wasting was reported in the original description by Shy and Drager of two cases of the syndrome which now bears their name, autonomic failure with multiple system atrophy. Since then there have been no systematic studies of muscle biopsy changes but a few isolated reports of electromyographic studies and nerve and muscle biopsies. There are several reports of electromyographic signs of degeneration in MSA (Montagna *et al.* 1983). Reports of nerve biopsies in MSA are rare but Toghi *et al.* (1982) found selective loss of small myelinated and unmyelinated fibres in three cases of MSA by comparison with control patients with olivopontocerebellar degeneration without autonomic dysfunction. Galassi *et al.* (1982) described loss of both large and small fibres in a sural-nerve biopsy in a single case of MSA. An anterior tibial muscle biopsy showed chronic neurogenic changes with large fields of atrophic fibres of the same histological type. However, loss of anterior horn cells has been reported in half the neuropathological reports of MSA (see Chapter 33). There is also evidence that, rarely, the muscle wasting in MSA may be part of a mild distal sensorimotor neuropathy (Cohen *et al.* 1987). In the hope of throwing some light on this aspect of the curiously selective degeneration of neurones in MSA, advantage was taken of a previous investigation into the catecholamine fluorescence and electron microscopy of muscle blood vessels (Bannister *et al.* 1981) to study striated muscle, taking advantage of modern histochemical techniques.

Muscle biopsy findings

The biopsies of the quadriceps femoris muscle were examined in 10 patients with MSA, using a battery of histochemical reactions. Fibre diameters were measured with a digitized pit pad on an image analyser. Three patients showed atrophy of type 2a and type 2b fibres, one patient showed selective type 2b atrophy, and in a fifth case the type 1 and type 2b fibres were atrophic (Figs 35.1 and 35.2). The variation in selective fibre-type atrophy could not be correlated with the clinical features of the patients nor with their age. The muscle biopsy appearances and fibre-diameter histograms were entirely normal in the remaining five cases, except that one case showed early grouping of the type 1 muscle fibres. Again this patient was not in any other way atypical of the entire group. The morphometric changes were not related to age, as the patients with the selective fibre-type atrophy were generally younger than those with normal fibre diameters.

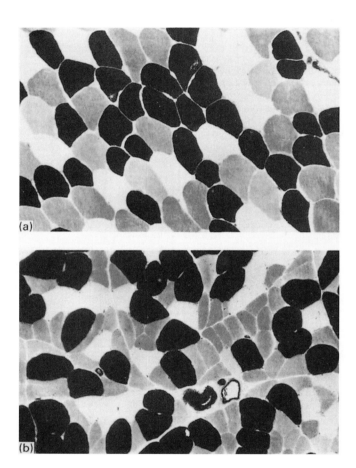

Fig. 35.1. Transverse sections of the vastus lateralis muscle from (a) a normal human control and (b) a patient with MSA, stained with the ATPase reaction at pH 4.35. The type 1 fibres are dark, the type 2a fibres are light, and the type 2b fibres are intermediate. Note the presence of type 2a and type 2b muscle-fibre atrophy in the patient.

A biopsy was taken from only one patient with PAF. The patient was a 68-year-old man who had had postural hypotension for 20 years, without other significant neurological symptoms or signs apart from impotence. His muscle biopsy was studied by the same histochemical techniques as used for the patients with MSA and there were no abnormalities.

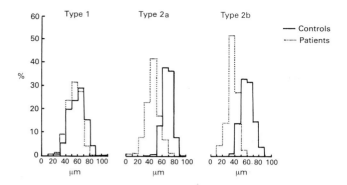

Fig. 35.2 Fibre diameter histograms from three patients with multiple system atrophy to show selective atrophy of the type 2a and type 2b fibres (interrupted line). Three age-matched controls are shown for comparison (continuous lines). Between 400 and 450 muscle fibres were measured in each case.

Discussion

The pattern of histochemical muscle fibre responses in human quadriceps is well established (Mahon *et al.* 1984; Dorriguzzi *et al.* 1986). The type of selective fibre atrophy seen in half the patients with MSA is quite abnormal. It is unlike the large-group atrophy or small-group atrophy seen in motor neurone disease, a disease with which, in some clinical respects, it might be thought to have some similarities (Dubowitz 1981; Jennekens 1982). Nor is there a suggestion of type grouping with large clusters of different fibre types adjacent to each other as occurs in regeneration as a result of sprouting. Perhaps a closer parallel is the selective fibre-type atrophy which sometimes occurs in myasthenia gravis (Aström and Adams 1981). Selective fibre atrophy itself is a rather non-specific type of change seen in a range of diverse disease pathologies from steroid or alcoholic myopathy to collagen vascular disease.

It could be argued that in MSA there is a preferential selective involvement of type 2a and 2b neurones by a process that in general seems to spare type 1 neurones and is not associated with sprouting

and reinnervation. The morphological appearances of the anterior horn cells giving rise to each type of motor unit are not known. The number of neurones which need to be affected to produce changes of this type may be small, in that up to 1000 muscle fibres in the human quadriceps may be innervated from a single neurones. In MSA the anterior horn cells have not been systematically counted in the same way as intermediolateral column cells and so mild reductions in the number of these cells may have been missed.

References

Aström, K. E. and Adams, R. D. (1981). Pathology of human skeletal muscle. In *Disorders of voluntary muscle*, (ed. J. N. Walton), pp. 151–208. Churchill Livingstone, Edinburgh.

Bannister, R., Crowe, R., Eames, R., and Burnstock, G. (1981). Adrenergic innervation in autonomic failure. *Neurology, Minneapolis* 31, 1501–6.

Cohen, J., Low, P., Fealey, R., Sheps, S., and Jiang, N-S. (1987). Somatic and autonomic function in progressive autonomic failure. *Ann. Neurol.* 22, 692–9.

Dorriguzzi, C. P., Palmucci, L., Mongini, T., Leone, M., Gagnor, E., Gagliano, A., and Schiffer, D. (1986). Quantitative analysis of quadriceps muscle biopsy. *J. Neurol. Sci.* 72, 201–9.

Dubowitz, V. (1981). Histochemistry of muscle disease. In *Disorders of voluntary muscle*, (ed. J. N. Walton), pp. 261–95. Churchill Livingstone, Edinburgh.

Galassi, G., Nemni, R., Baraldi, A., Gibertoni, M., and Columbo, A. (1982). Peripheral neuropathy in multiple system atrophy with autonomic failure. *Neurology, NY* 32, 1116–20.

Jennekens, F. G. I. (1982). Muscle histochemistry. In *Skeletal muscle pathology* (ed. F. L. Mastaglia and J. N. Walton), pp. 204–34. Churchill Livingstone, London.

Mahon, M., Toman, A., Willian, P. L. T., and Bagnall, K. M. (1984). Variability of the histochemical and morphometric data from needle biopsy specimens of human quadriceps. *J. Neurol. Sci.* 63, 85–100.

Montagna, P., Martinelli, P., Rizzuto, N., Salviati, A., Rasi, F., and Lugaresi, E. (1983). Amyotrophy in Shy–Drager syndrome. *Acta Neurol. Belg.* 83, 142–57.

Toghi, H., Tabuchi, M., Tomonaga, M., and Izumiyana, N. (1982). Selective loss of small myelinated and unmyelinated fibres in Shy–Drager syndrome. *Acta Neuropathol., Berlin* 57, 282–6.

36. Management of postural hypotension

Roger Bannister and Christopher J. Mathias

General principles

The treatment of postural (orthostatic) hypotension due to autonomic failure is fraught with difficulties, many caused by inaccurate localization of the sites of the lesions. Treatment requires targetting; as Ehrlich commented on chemotherapy, 'we must learn to aim and aim in a chemical sense'. In autonomic failure, treatment has to be directed to overcoming precisely identified defects. This chapter focuses on the management of orthostatic hypotension due to primary autonomic failure but many of the principles outlined here are applicable to postural hypotension due to other causes.

In secondary autonomic failure there may be special factors, which are covered in other chapters. Some examples of these include:

(1) insulin affecting postural hypotension in diabetes (see Chapter 39);

(2) difficulties in managing postural hypotension in tetraplegics as pressor drugs can lead to severe hypertension (see Chapter 51);

(3) the aggravating effects of hypoalbuminaemia due to protein loss in amyloidosis, making treatment with fludrocortisone very difficult; and

(4) the successful treatment of postural hypotension in dopamine β-hydroxylase deficiency, with the replacement prodrug, dihydroxyphenylserine (see Chapter 40).

Some principles of management are common to all patients.

Cerebral blood flow

It is important not to be overconcerned about a low standing blood pressure if the patient is without symptoms. Some patients can tolerate a standing systolic blood pressure as low as 70 mmHg without dizziness or syncope, probably because cerebral blood flow is maintained at an adequate level because of the capacity of the cerebral circulation for autoregulation. Several studies have attempted to clarify whether in autonomic failure there is a reduced fall of cerebral blood flow for a standard fall of mean arterial pressure. In five patients with multiple system atrophy (MSA), autoregulation was preserved down to a systolic blood pressure close to 60 mmHg which is well below the 80 mmHg at which autoregulation fails in normal subjects (Thomas and Bannister 1980). Results in a further three patients with pure autonomic failure (PAF) showed a similar trend. A shift of autoregulation to the left in autonomic failure almost certainly occurs and the reason some have failed to record it is probably that, when cerebral blood flow was measured during tilt, the

arterial pressure may have been transiently much lower than the recorded pressure. There was evidence of this in one patient with autonomic failure who developed symptoms of cerebral ischaemia when his systolic pressure fell transiently to 40 mmHg and the clearance curve changed (Fig. 36. 1), implying a transient fall in flow (Thomas and Bannister 1980). The change in autoregulation may be the result of prolonged exposure to lower than normal arterial pressure, causing some changes in the response of normally innervated vessels, or because cerebral vessels are partially or completely sympathectomized in autonomic failure. It has been suggested that the major sympathetic innervation is to the extraparenchymal vessels, the intraparenchymal vessels being under myogenic and metabolic control. If this is so, the sympathetic innervation at the lower level of autoregulation may normally reduce cerebral blood flow by constricting extraparenchymal vessels. Whatever the explanation, it is

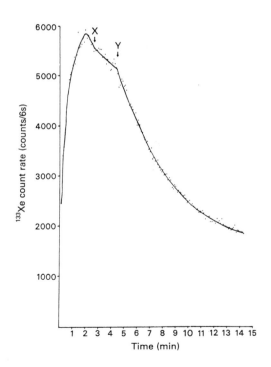

Fig. 36.1. Cerebral ^{133}Xe count rates/6 s in patient G. K. with pure autonomic failure tilted to 45°. At point X, the blood pressure fell suddenly to a systolic pressure of 40 mmHg. The rate of ^{133}Xe clearance decreased and the patient developed symptoms of cerebral ischaemia. At point Y, the tilt table was lowered, blood pressure rose, and the rate of clearance increased. (From Thomas and Bannister (1980).)

certain that patients with autonomic failure have a remarkable tolerance to low blood pressure without developing postural hypotensive symptoms.

Recumbent (supine) hypertension

A second principle that has to be considered in treatment is the tendency of patients with autonomic failure to develop recumbent hypertension owing principally to defective baroreceptor reflexes, supersensitivity, and treatment with drugs such as fludrocortisone. Clearly, this may result in a reactive increase of cerebrovascular resistance, leading to the likelihood of cerebral ischaemic symptoms when such patients stand suddenly. Some patients, if nursed lying flat, may develop severe hypertension and run the risk of developing complications such as papilloedema, other features of hypertensive retinopathy, and cerebral haemorrhage. There is concern about using antihypotensive agents in such patients. Nocturnal antihypertensive therapy has been suggested but this has potential dangers in patients who often have nocturia and thus run undue risks from hypotension if they need to arise from bed to empty their bladder at night. More information on the effects of the treatment will emerge from 24-hour blood pressure monitoring, as in the case of the peptide release inhibitor octreotide that reduces postprandial and postural hypotension but does not increase nocturnal hypertension (Alam *et al.* 1995).

Control of blood volume

A third principle is that, although loss of baroreflexes determines the immediate response of blood pressure to standing, control of blood volume is the long-term and more important adjustment to postural hypotension in autonomic failure. Blood volume is influenced by various factors, including low-pressure receptors, the kidney and various hormones such as antidiuretic hormone, atrial natriuretic peptides, and the renin–angiotensin–aldosterone system.

Limitations of treatment

All methods of treatment, directly or indirectly, aim either at reducing the vascular volume into which pooling occurs on standing, or increasing the volume of blood available for pooling. A reduction of the volume into which the blood may pool by pressor drugs has its limitations. Unless the drugs increase the responsiveness of vessels to small amounts of noradrenaline that still can be liberated, they will aggravate the tendency to recumbent hypertension. An increase in blood volume runs the risk of overloading the circulation, thus leading to cardiac failure and peripheral oedema. Many patients with autonomic failure have defects of renal preservation of sodium when recumbent and are sensitive to sodium depletion, which leads to a reduction of intravascular and extracellular fluid volume. Though we are aware that many patients continue to receive a variety of treatments in different medical centres, it is probable that any treatment with pressor drugs that temporarily enables a patient to become more mobile will improve the patient's other homeostatic responses to standing. Hence, an improvement, even if sustained, may be erroneously attributed to a particular form of treatment when it might, under controlled conditions, be possible to withdraw or replace it with a safer method.

Testing of drugs

There has been a series of reports of treatment with many different drugs, usually given empirically for a short uncontrolled trial, often in patients with an imprecise diagnosis of autonomic failure. It may reasonably be asked whether any pressor drug is effective if so many different treatments have been proposed. It is also reasonable to question whether the effect of drugs can be monitored, when the lack of baroreceptor reflexes in autonomic failure leads to marked fluctuations with changes of posture and other events, such as food ingestion, over the course of 24 h, so that adequate maintenance of blood pressure is as difficult as targetting in a video space game. In any attempt to measure the benefit of a drug in autonomic failure, the recumbent and standing blood pressure must be taken under standard conditions, preferably four times a day by trained staff. A number of factors, in addition to postural change, can influence blood pressure, including food ingestion and even moderate exercise (Alam *et al.* 1995; Mathias 1995); these need to be both considered and incorporated into the assessment protocols. There is increasing use of non-invasive, 24-hour ambulatory blood pressure and heart rate recorders, and some are reliable at low blood pressures, thus providing useful information for therapeutic studies (see Chapter 20). As blood pressure of patients with autonomic failure usually continues to fall when they stand; the duration of standing has to be recorded. Ideally, the blood pressure should be recorded 2 min after the onset of standing, because intra-arterial recordings have shown that by then any fall in pressure will be clearly apparent. Another approach is to record the duration of standing (standing time), but this may not be practical especially in those with additional neurological deficits, and other disabilities in whom there may be further reasons for difficulties in standing and mobility. Prior to drug treatment it is advisable to have an equilibrium period of a week on a standard daily sodium diet of 150 mmol with monitoring of position and physical activity during the day and consistent head-up tilt at night. The ideal would be to measure the haematocrit, plasma protein, urea, creatinine, and electrolytes every 3 days, weigh the patient on accurate scales twice daily, measure day and night fluid balance and urinary sodium and potassium excretion, and measure blood pressure at least four times a day while lying and standing before meals and exercise.

Drug combinations

Since patients with autonomic failure often have lesions at more than one site, it should always be considered whether a combination of drugs may be more effective than a single drug. For example, drugs with central, ganglionic, and postganglionic effects may have synergistic actions. At the sympathetic terminals, drugs that increase noradrenaline release may be combined with drugs that reduce re-uptake of the transmitter or increase the sensitivity of receptors. Similarly, drugs that affect intravascular and extracellular fluid volume (such as fludrocortisone and desmopressin), release of vasodilatatory hormones (such as octreotide), or other factors influencing blood pressure, may be of value in combination.

Approaches to treatment

Advice on factors that influence blood pressure

A number of factors have now been defined, which can considerably lower blood pressure and thus enhance the postural fall and therefore the symptoms accompanying postural hypotension. The pathophysiological mechanisms accounting for a number of these have been worked out, and in a number of situations avoidance measures can be instituted. Therefore, patients should be advised on these factors.

Diurnal changes in blood pressure

The supine blood pressure in patients with autonomic failure is lowest in the morning and rises gradually during the day. This has been confirmed by non-invasive measurements and also by using continuous ambulatory intra-arterial blood pressure recordings (Fig. 36.2). The circadian changes in blood pressure are the reverse of those in normal subjects, in whom the blood pressure falls during sleep and rises prior to awakening. The low level of blood pressure in the morning appears to be the result of nocturnal polyuria and natriuresis, which can result in a substantial overnight weight loss, at times over 1 kg (Mathias *et al.* 1986). The reduction in extracellular fluid volume is likely to contribute to the low blood pressure as it is improved by administration of desmopressin (see below). The low supine blood pressure aggravates the symptoms of postural hypotension in the morning, and some patients find it extremely difficult

to conduct their normal activities for a few hours after waking. Methods of preventing morning postural hypotension are described below.

Straining during micturition and defaecation

A number of patients suffer from either urinary bladder problems or from constipation. Straining might result in a Valsalva manoeuvre being performed; this can result in a substantial reduction in blood pressure without the recovery mechanisms that normally come into play. Episodes of hypotension in some situations may be particularly dangerous, for example when patients lose consciousness while propped against a lavatory wall and may not fall to the ground and thus automatically correct their low blood pressure.

Exposure to a warm environment

Patients exposed to tropical or subtropical temperatures tend to have greater symptoms for a variety of reasons. They often lack the ability to sweat, and their core temperature therefore can rise. Uncompensated vasodilatation often ensues and the blood pressure may fall. Adequate precautions therefore should be taken by patients travelling to warm countries or in tropical areas, who should be aware of the possible worsening of postural hypotension. Patients should be warned of the probability of a deterioration after a hot bath, especially if prolonged.

Effect of food and alcohol

The majority of patients with autonomic failure have substantial postprandial hypotension (see Chapter 29). This occurs soon after food ingestion and may last for up to 3 h after a standard meal. The supine blood pressure can be lowered to levels of 80/50 mmHg even in the supine position and therefore these patients often exhibit increased symptoms of postural hypotension. Carbohydrate appears to be the major component causing the hypotension, and this may be linked to the release of insulin and other gastrointestinal hormones which have vasodilatatory properties. Vasodilatation in the gut, not compensated for by defective sympathetic reflexes, is the probable cause of the reduction in pressure. Food ingestion enhances postural hypotension in PAF and MSA (Mathias *et al.* 1991). The pathophysiology and management of postprandial hypotension is described in Chapter 29. Alcohol has the potential to cause mesenteric vasodilatation and will lower blood pressure in these patients.

Effect of exercise

It is now recognized that the majority of patients with autonomic failure have exercise-induced hypotension (Smith *et al.* 1995a); the fall in blood pressure may occur even during relatively mild forms of exertion, such as walking upstairs or even while on level ground. The symptoms and circumstances vary between individual patients (see Chapter 20). Exercise-induced hypotension occurs even while supine, and can compound the hypotensive effects of postural change during and even after the cessation of exercise (Smith and Mathias 1995). The hypotension is presumably due to vasodilatation in exercising muscle that is not accompanied by adequate compensatory changes in different vascular regions as occur normally (Puvi-Rajasingham *et al.* 1997).

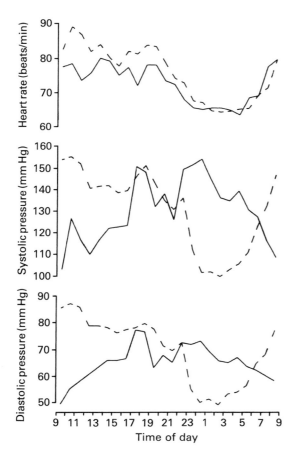

Fig. 36.2. Overall trend in heart rate and systolic and diastolic pressures of six subjects with autonomic failure (——) compared with those derived from a matched group of six subjects with normal or elevated blood pressure (– – –). Lines join pooled hourly means. (From Mann *et al.* (1983).)

Effect of drugs with vasoactive properties

Both the patient and the physician should be aware that drugs with vasoactive properties, even if only a minor action of the agent, may result in substantial vascular and blood pressure changes because of supersensitivity. The responses to pressor agents and particularly sympathomimetics, have already been described (Chapter 20). Vasopressor responses may occur to a variety of agents acting on receptors other than adrenoceptors. An example is the drug Saralasin, which has an immediate pressor response because of its initial agonist activity on angiotensin II receptors (Mathias *et al.* 1984), despite being an angiotensin II antagonist. Even drugs administered via the intraocular or intranasal route may have clinically important effects; an example is the use of β-adrenoceptor blockers for glaucoma which occasionally can cause bradycardia and lower blood pressure (Vahidassr *et al.* 1997). Drugs used for non-autonomic features also may unmask or enhance postural hypotension and an example is hypotension induced by L-dopa in certain parkinsonian patients; its hypotensive effects may at times draw attention to underlying autonomic failure and the diagnosis of MSA. Marked hypotension may also occur with drugs which have vasodilatory properties. An example is glyceryl trinitrate, which routinely is used sublingually in patients with angina pectoris; when given to patients with autonomic impairment even in the supine position, it can result in severe hypotension.

Head-up tilt at night

The first line of treatment in a patient with autonomic failure is to attempt to increase the patient's blood volume by the use of head-up tilt at night. Figure 36.3 shows the change in lying and standing blood pressure and body weight in a patient placed in the head-up position at night (Bannister *et al.* 1969). The increase of 2.6 kg in body weight points to a progressive increase in extracellular fluid volume, which was reversed on the one night when the patient slept flat. The effect of this procedure was studied further in one patient followed on a

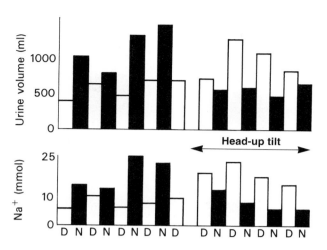

Fig. 36.4. Diurnal changes in water and sodium excretion in a patient with autonomic failure and multiple system atrophy during 5 days lying flat at night and 5 days of head-up tilt at night. D, day; N, night.

90 mmol per day sodium diet in whom water and sodium balance was monitored. As shown in Fig. 36.4, the patient was losing more sodium and water during the night than during the day for each of 5 days until head-up tilt at night was introduced, when the nocturnal loss of sodium and water was reversed over the subsequent 5 days. Head-up body tilt at night is likely to operate by reducing renal arterial pressure and promoting renin release with consequent angiotensin II formation, leading to aldosterone release, and thus increasing blood volume for patients with autonomic failure who can still release renin (Bannister *et al.* 1977). Patients with autonomic failure have complex defects of renal sodium conservation (see Chapter 18) that can result in excessive nocturnal polyuria. Some patients with PAF, with incapacitating postural hypotension until the introduction of head-up tilt, have been maintained satisfactorily for years solely by this form of treatment.

Positions and manoeuvres to raise blood pressure

A number of positions and manoeuvres have been increasingly recognized as being helpful to patients with severe orthostatic hypotension. The beat-by-beat recording of blood pressure with the Finapres and the Portapres has enabled evaluation of the magnitude of rise induced by many of these manoeuvres (Wieling *et al.* 1993). The term 'physical countermeasures' has been used, and these include crossing the legs while standing, squatting, abdominal compression, bending forward, placing one foot on a chair and stooping as if to tie shoe laces (Fig. 36.5). They appear to raise blood pressure either by raising vascular resistance or by increasing venous return. The effect of leg muscle pumping and tensing (Ten Harkel *et al.* 1994) may be of particular value in subjects with exercise-induced hypotension, who are at their worst on ceasing exercise, presumably because of lower limb pooling (see Chapter 20).

External support to prevent pooling

The application of graduated pressure to the lower half of the body and legs reduces the amount of blood pooling in the legs on standing

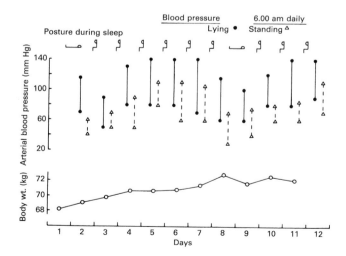

Fig. 36.3. The change in the early morning blood pressure (lying and standing) in a patient (H) with autonomic failure and MSA studied when he slept in the sitting position for 10 days with one interruption. The changes in blood volume and body weight are also shown. (From Bannister *et al.* (1969).)

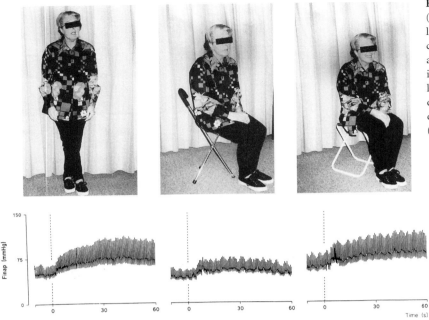

Fig. 36.5. The effect on finger arterial blood pressure (Finapres) of standing in the crossed leg position with leg muscle contraction (left), and sitting on a derby chair (middle), or fishing chair (right) in a patient with autonomic failure. Orthostatic symptoms were present initially when standing and disappeared on crossing legs and sitting on the fishing chair. Sitting on the derby chair caused the least rise in blood pressure and did not relieve completely the patient's symptoms. (From Smit *et al.* (1997).)

and so temporarily improves central blood volume and left ventricular filling. However, there must be concern that this treatment is in danger of reducing the intrinsic myogenic reaction of smooth muscle in response to stretch caused by increased intravascular pressure on standing, in addition to preventing other compensatory hormone and other responses to a low blood pressure. Thus the patient with orthostatic hypotension is more vulnerable than ever when *not* wearing the support garment. In practice, a support garment may be necessary temporarily in order to achieve mobility in a patient who has been recumbent as a result of severe postural hypotension for some time, or because of an intercurrent illness. Then, as the effect of head-up tilt and drugs such as fludrocortisone produce a benefit, a counterpressure garment may be abandoned.

Originally, antigravity suits devised for aviators were used; these were certainly effective (Fig. 36.6), but were uncomfortable. The graded counterpressure support garments of the Jobst type (Sheps 1976) are more comfortable. Elastic pressure stockings are often recommended but are often not patient-acceptable, and do not appear to provide the value they should. The use of abdominal binders may provide benefit; this may be in the form of a corset, or an inflatable abdominal band, as has been demonstrated in children (Tanaka *et al.* 1997).

Cardiac pacing

There have been reports of benefit obtained by implantation of a cardiac pacemaker and elevation of heart rate during postural change. The benefit noted by Moss *et al.* (1980) occurred in a patient who apparently had an incomplete autonomic lesion, and therefore had the potential to vasoconstrict at times. In patients with more severe lesions, in whom there are low plasma noradrenaline levels at rest and in response to tilt, there appears to be no benefit. Beneficial effects of tachypacing are unlikely in patients who have maximal arteriolar and venous dilatation, as cardiac output is dependent upon venous return which is often considerably reduced in such patients.

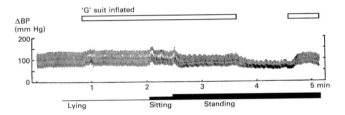

Fig. 36.6. The effect of an antigravity suit on the changes of brachial arterial blood pressure (ΔBP) which occur on sitting and standing in a patient with pure autonomic failure. (From Bannister *et al.* (1969).)

Occasionally, cardiac pacing may be needed to prevent excessive bradycardia in response to elevation of blood pressure by drugs, as described in a patient in whom atrial demand pacing was needed to protect against vagal overactivity in the presence of a severe sympathetic autonomic neuropathy (Bannister *et al.* 1986). In this patient administration of drugs to raise blood pressure resulted in severe bradycardia and consequent dysrhythmias (Fig. 36.7). Assessment was initially made with atropine, which raised the heart rate but resulted in unacceptable side-effects. Atrial pacing was performed, initially with a temporary pacemaker which was clearly beneficial, and later with permanent implantation. This enabled effective use of pressor agents without the fear of development of either cardiac arrest or a serious dysrhythmia (Fig. 36.8).

Noradrenaline infusion device

One potential future advance may be the utilization of devices which are closely linked to blood pressure control and postural change and which administer short-acting pressor agents. One such device was described by Polinsky *et al.* (1983). They used an electromechanical

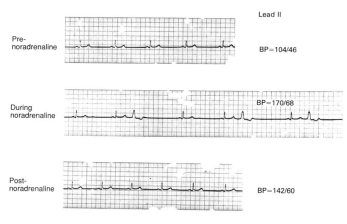

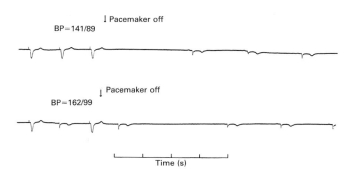

Fig. 36.7. ECG tracings before, during and after intravenous infusion of noradrenaline. Sinus bradycardia and coupled beats occur when the blood pressure (BP) is elevated to 170/68 mmHg. This is reversed when the BP returns to normal. (From Bannister *et al.* (1986).)

Fig. 36.8. EBCG tracings, initially with pacemaker off, on upper trace. There are pacemaker triggered complexes followed by a pause and then sinus bradycardia. During noradrenaline infusion (lower trace) with the BP elevated, there are alternating pacemaker-induced and intrinsic complexes. Following exclusion of the pacemaker there is a longer pause before endogenous rhythm takes over. The elevation in BP appears to enhance sinus node suppression. (From Bannister *et al.* (1986).)

device, utilizing the arterial transducer to record blood pressure from one arm while controlling the rate of an intravenous infusion of noradrenaline into the opposite arm (Fig. 36.9). There do not appear to have been further developments, although advances in drug administration, using either implantable devices or mini-infusion pumps, linked to the ability to non-invasively measure blood pressure on a beat-by-beat basis, should lead to further advances. This will be of especial benefit to severely impaired patients in whom multiple drug therapy has failed.

Drugs in postural hypotension

A variety of agents has been used to reduce postural hypotension. In Table 36.1 an attempt has been made to classify these agents on the basis of their main actions in helping postural hypotension.

Plasma volume expansion and reduction of natriuresis

Fludrocortisone

Fludrocortisone is the most commonly used drug treatment and has multiple pharmacological effects (Chobanian *et al.* 1979). In an initial dose of 0.1 mg at night, in some patients with autonomic failure, fludrocortisone approaches most closely to the ideal of a drug which increases effective vasoconstriction on standing, by augmenting the action of noradrenaline released by some remaining normal sympathetic efferent activity but without aggravating recumbent hypertension. In normal subjects, fludrocortisone also sensitizes vascular receptors to pressor amines (Schmidt *et al.* 1966). Fludrocortisone may also increase the fluid content of vessel walls, so increasing their resistance to stretching (Tobian and Redleaf 1958).

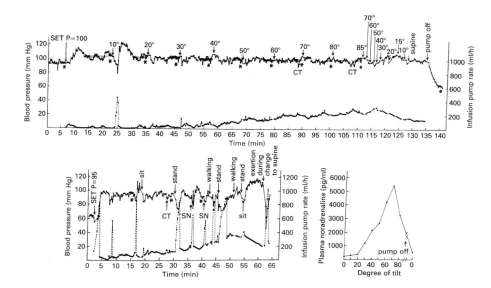

Fig. 36.9. Mean blood pressure (upper trace in each record), noradrenaline infusion rate (lower trace in each record), and plasma noradrenaline levels during clinical trial of a sympathetic neural prosthesis. The * indicates points at which blood samples were obtained. CT, clear throat; SN, sneeze. (From Polinsky *et al.* (1983).)

Table 36.1. Drugs used in the treatment of postural hypotension

Site of action	Drugs	Predominant action
Plasma volume: expansion	Fludrocortisone	Mineralocorticoid effects— increased plasma volume Sensitization of α-adrenoceptors
Kidney: reducing diuresis	Desmopression	Vasopressin$_2$-receptors on renal tubules
Vessels: vasoconstriction (adrenoceptor-mediated) Resistance vessels	Ephedrine	Indirectly acting sympathomimetic
	Midodrine*, phenylephrine, methylphenidate Tyramine Clonidine Yohimbine DL-DOPS and L-DOPS	Directly acting sympathomimetics Release of noradrenaline Postsynaptic α_2-adrenoceptor agonist Presynaptic α_2-adrenoceptor antagonist Pro-drug resulting in formation of noradrenaline
Capacitance vessels	Dihydroergotamine	Direct action on α-adrenoceptors
Vessels: vasoconstriction (non-adrenoceptor mediated)	Triglycyl-lysine-vasopressin (glypressin)	Vasopressin$_1$-receptors on blood vessels
Vessels: prevention of vasodilatation	Propranolol Indomethacin Metoclopramide	Blockade of β_2-adrenoceptors Prevents prostaglandin synthesis Blockade of dopamine receptors
Vessels: prevention of postprandial hypotension	Caffeine Octreotide	Blockade of adenosine receptors Inhibits release of vasodilator gut/pancreatic peptides
Heart: stimulation	Pindolol, xamoterol	Intrinsic sympathomimetic action
Red cell mass: increase	Erythropoietin	Stimulates red cell production

* Through its active metabolite.

In a study of MSA, 0.1 mg of fludrocortisone daily did not increase body weight but caused a shift to the left of the noradrenaline infusion sensitivity curve and a significant rise in standing blood pressure (Davies *et al.* 1979). This effect may be less apparent in patients with PAF (Chobanian *et al.* 1979). It was speculated that fludrocortisone might either increase the number of α-adreno-receptors, change their structure, or decrease the clearance rate by the uptake-2 mechanism by smooth muscle of blood vessels. There is an increase in the α-adrenoreceptors of platelets and β-adrenoreceptors of lymphocytes in autonomic failure and these changes are increased further after treatment with fludrocortisone (Bannister *et al.* 1981; Davies *et al.* 1982). In autonomic failure there also is an increase in the pressor response to angiotensin II which is not affected by fludro-cortisone, indicating a probable change in angiotensin vascular receptors as well as α-adrenoceptors (Davies *et al.* 1979).

In higher doses with careful supervision, fludrocortisone can expand the blood volume, improve cardiac output, and so reduce postural hypotension. Patients with autonomic failure have a normal or slightly low plasma volume when supine but this does not, as in normal subjects, fall on standing owing to the lack of vasoconstriction, probably because the lowered arterial pressure compensates for the raised hydrostatic pressure in the legs on standing. Patients with autonomic failure lose twice as much body weight as control subjects when on a low-sodium diet, with a corresponding increase in their postural hypotension. The resting plasma renin activity in autonomic failure is usually low, with a reduced rise on standing, though this is increased by sodium restriction or by dopamine infusion. This suggests that renin synthesis and storage are intact but release may be defective. Aldosterone secretion may be reduced in autonomic failure but it is unclear whether the defect is the result of a chronic reduction

of angiotensin stimulation of aldosterone secretion rather than an adrenal defect. The dose of fludrocortisone likely to increase the blood volume by replacing aldosterone levels without overloading the circulation requires delicate and continuous adjustment probably because of the baroreflex defect, in contrast to the situation in a patient with Addison's disease. As with other forms of treatment, each patient shows variations in response which are the result of the different types of lesion present in each patient. The combination of fludrocortisone (0.1 mg) with head-up tilt at night and a high salt diet (150–200 mmol sodium/day) is an effective means of improving postural hypotension (Ten Harkel *et al.* 1992), and symptoms are reduced with only minimal side-effects (such as ankle oedema) and without the causation of hypokalaemia.

Desmopressin

Desmopressin (DDAVP) is a vasopressin analogue which acts specifically upon the V$_2$ receptors on the renal tubules, which are responsible for the antidiuretic effects of vasopressin (antidiuretic hormone). It has virtually no activity on the V$_1$ receptor, which is responsible for the vasoconstriction induced by vasopressin. In patients with autonomic failure, nocturnal polyuria, overnight weight loss, and the subsequent reduction in extracellular fluid volume and intravascular volume, account for the low morning blood pressures and for the increased severity of symptoms from postural hypotension. Intramuscular DDAVP prevents nocturnal polyuria and reduces overnight weight loss, and raises the supine blood pressure in the morning, thus improving symptoms resulting from postural change (Mathias *et al.* 1986; Fig. 36.10). Because of the lack of direct vascular effects of DDAVP an increased tendency to supine hypertension is not present. Studies with intranasal DDAVP indicate that it is equally effective in the short term and also in the long term; doses between 5 and 40 μg given at bedtime as a single dose are of benefit both in relation to preventing nocturia (which can also be a problem especially in those with bladder involvement) and also in morning postural hypotension. An oral form of DDAVP is available and should have advantages over the intranasal form. Tablets of 200 μg have been used successfully in adolescents and adults with nocturnal enuresis (Janknegt *et al.* 1997); 400 μg tablets are also available.

However, DDAVP has the potential to cause side-effects. Some patients, and in particular those with PAF, may be exquisitely sensitive to its action and hyponatraemia can readily ensue (Mathias *et al.* 1986). In these patients, low starting doses of intranasal DDAVP should be administered under careful supervision to ensure that hyponatraemia does not occur, before stabilization. In some patients, natriuresis continues as before and occasionally is in excess and DDAVP needs to be combined with fludrocortisone and sodium supplements to ensure that the patient remains in sodium balance. We have treated patients with intranasal DDAVP for many years with regular monitoring of plasma osmolality or plasma sodium levels and with no long-term side-effects.

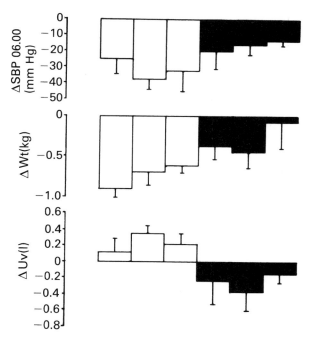

Fig. 36.10. Desmopressin (DDAVP) in the treatment of autonomic failure. From above, morning postural hypotension, difference between sitting and lying systolic pressure (ΔSBP), change in body weight overnight (ΔWt), and change in urine volume between night and day (ΔUv). The open rectangles show the changes during a 3-day control period and the closed rectangles the changes after 2 μg of intramuscular DDAVP each evening for 3 days. The mean results in five patients with autonomic failure show after DDAVP a reduction in postural hypotension and a gain in extracellular and intravascular fluid volume as measured by the reduction in nocturnal weight loss and nocturnal urinary volume.

Drugs causing vasoconstriction

Drugs acting as vasoconstrictors can be divided broadly into those working through the sympathetic nervous system and/or its receptors and those with actions on non-adrenergic receptors. Examples of the latter include vasopressin and its analogue, glycopressin, acting on V_1 receptors. The majority of these drugs act on resistance vessels and will be described below, along with dihydroergotamine, which acts predominantly on capacitance vessels.

Directly acting agents

A variety of agents have been used which act directly on α-adrenoceptors. These include agents such as phenylephrine, phenylpropanolamine, methylphenidate, and midodrine. A factor to be kept in mind is the potential of these agents to cause severe constriction in peripheral vessels. This might be a disadvantage, especially in the elderly who are more likely to have peripheral vascular abnormalities.

Of the sympathomimetic vasoconstrictor agents, midodrine has been studied extensively (Kaufmann *et al.* 1988; Jankovic *et al.* 1993; Fouad-Tarazi *et al.* 1995; Low *et al.* 1997). Midodrine is a prodrug that is metabolized to the active form, desglymidodrine, which acts on α_1-adrenoceptors to cause constriction of both arterial resistance and venous capacitance vessels. It is absorbed fairly rapidly, with peak concentrations within 20–40 min and with a short half-life, in the region of 30 min. It is administered in doses of 2.5–10 mg given three times daily. Its side-effects include goose skin (cutis anserina), tingling of the skin and pruritis, especially of the scalp; the pruritis can be severe in some patients. Impaired urine flow, hesitancy, and urinary retention may occur, especially in the male, presumably because of its adrenoceptor agonist effects on the internal sphincter. It may be of particular value in patients with severe postural hypotension and in those with peripheral lesions, as in PAF. Surprisingly, some patients on midodrine become worse, for reasons that are unclear; in these patients there may be a reduction in intra- and extravascular fluid volume, as manifested by weight loss (Kaufmann *et al.* 1988).

Indirectly acting agents

Ephedrine acts by both releasing noradrenaline and also by acting directly on adrenoceptors. This drug may have a role in patients with central lesions (such as in multiple system atrophy) and in patients with incomplete lesions, where a combination of its direct effects and the release of noradrenaline may be of benefit. As with other agents, there is the potential to cause supine hypertension. The value of the drug in patients with severe sympathetic lesions is probably minimal. The starting dose is 15 mg three times daily. With larger doses of ephedrine (in excess of 30 mg, three times daily), side-effects such as tachycardia or tremulousness may occur, in part due to central stimulation.

Drugs predominantly releasing noradrenaline

Tyramine is an agent that raises blood pressure by the release of noradrenaline from the sympathetic nerve endings. In some patients with autonomic failure there may be sufficient sparing of nerve endings for this to be achieved, and the effects of tyramine can be potentiated by the concurrent administration of a monoamine oxidase inhibitor. This applies even to the newer selective monamine oxidase inhibitors, as has been reported in a case treated with moclobemide (Karet *et al.* 1994). A number of foods, especially

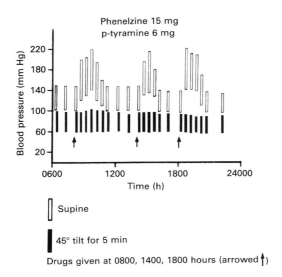

Fig. 36.11. Blood pressure and heart rate before and after treatment of a patient with pure autonomic failure with phenelzine and *p*-tyramine. (From Davies *et al.* (1978).)

certain cheeses and Bovril, contain *p*-tyramine and this may have been partially responsible for the erratic blood responses, except that these were also obtained using chemically pure *p*-tyramine when studied in combination with phenelzine (Fig. 36.11; Davies *et al.* 1978); in these studies the marked fluctuation of blood pressure that occurred along with pronounced supine hypertension made such treatment potentially hazardous. The improvement in postural hypotension caused by this combination appears to be less effective than that caused by midodrine or ephedrine, and its use largely has been abandoned.

α_2-Adrenoceptor agonists

Clonidine is an α_2-adrenoceptor agonist, which is highly lipophilic and has actions both centrally and peripherally. Its central actions, which result in withdrawal of sympathetic tone, are responsible for the fall in supine blood pressure in both normal subjects and hypertensive patients. In tetraplegics, therefore, with a decentralized sympathetic nervous system, clonidine does not lower resting blood pressure (Mathias *et al.* 1979); however, it is capable of attenuating the pressor response to urinary bladder stimulation, indicating that it may have effects either on spinal sympathetic neurones or on presynaptic α_2-adrenoceptors in the periphery (see Chapter 51). When given intravenously to tetraplegics there is an initial pressor response (Mathias and Frankel, unpublished observations) which results from its normally transient peripheral postsynaptic effects causing vasoconstriction. These are probably a combination of both postsynaptic α_1- and α_2-adrenoceptor effects. These effects are probably the basis for the observations of the benefit of clonidine in some patients with autonomic failure. Our own experience with the use of clonidine in the management of postural hypotension in autonomic failure patients has not been favourable, and it may be that the drug is only of benefit in those with complete lesions involving postganglionic fibres where there is extreme pressor sensitivity to α-adrenoceptor agents. This is consistent with the observations of Thomaides *et al.*

(1992) who studied the systemic and regional haemodynamic responses to intravenous clonidine (2 μg/kg body weight) in MSA and PAF; blood pressure fell in MSA but rose in PAF.

Presynaptic α_2-adrenoceptor antagonists

Yohimbine is an α_2-adrenoceptor antagonist which can act both centrally and peripherally. The blockade of presynaptic α_2-adrenoceptors may facilitate the release of noradrenaline at nerve terminals. The drug has been used in single doses with benefit in autonomic failure with probable partial lesions, thus resulting in accentuation of noradrenaline release (Onrot *et al.* 1987). The drug may have a role in patients with autonomic failure with central lesions, as reported in MSA (Senard *et al.* 1993*a*); it does not appear to be effective in parkinsonian patients with autonomic failure of presumed peripheral origin (Senard *et al.* 1993*b*). It has not been evaluated in the long term and it is not known whether it has advantages over ephedrine and midodrine.

Increased production of noradrenaline

The prodrug, dihydroxyphenylserine (DOPS) in the laevo form (L) or racemic mixture (DL), raises levels of plasma noradrenaline when decarboxylated, as described in the management of postural hypotension in dopamine β-hydroxylase deficiency (see Chapter 40). Since 1980, DOPS has been used, often with success, in hypotension associated with a variety of disorders (Table 36.2). It has been used in doses of 250–500 mg twice daily. The mechanisms by which DL and L-DOPS raise blood pressure in autonomic failure are unclear. This may be through the rise in plasma noradrenaline levels and thus direct stimulation of peripheral postsynaptic adrenoceptors. If so, it could be more effective in patients with PAF (who have a greater degree of pressor supersensitivity), than patients with MSA, although this has not been the observation in two separate studies (Hoeldtke *et al.* 1984; Kaufmann *et al.* 1991), albeit in a small number of patients. The administration of DOPS has been shown, using microneurographic techniques, to increase sympathetic nerve activity in a patient with MSA (Kachi *et al.* 1988) and also in normal subjects (Iwase *et al.* 1992). DOPS has the ability to enter the central nervous system, and enhancing sympathoneural activity may be a factor in raising blood pressure, especially in patients with MSA who usually have preserved postganglionic sympathetic pathways. The value of L-DOPS in the management of orthostatic hypotension in PAF and MSA is being evaluated currently in a pan-European multicentre trial.

Dopaminergic agents

A dopaminergic prodrug, ibopamine, that also has weak α- and β-adrenoceptor agonist activity, has been studied in three patients with pure autonomic failure (Rensma *et al.* 1993). Within 10–30 min after administration there was substantial improvement in orthostatic tolerance, that lasted for 20–50 min. These effects were reversed by the α-adrenoceptor blocker phentolamine, favouring a predominant effect on these receptors. The pharmacokinetic profile was highly variable, and in one patient there was severe hypertension and tachycardia. There have been no further reports on the use of this agent.

Table 36.2. Examples of disorders with orthostatic intolerance and postural hypotension in whom either DL or L-DOPS has been used

Disorder	Reference	Effect on hypotension
Familial amyloidosis	Suzuki *et al.* (1980)	+
	Suzuki *et al.* (1982)	+
	Ando *et al.* (1995)	+
	Carvalho *et al.* (1997)	+
Diabetic autonomic neuropathy	Hoeldtke *et al.* (1984)	−
Dialysis-induced hypotension	Iida *et al.* (1994)	+
Spinal lesion—T4	Muneta *et al.* (1992)	+
Children with orthostatic intolerance	Tanaka *et al.* (1996)	+
Parkinson's disease	Birkmayer *et al.* (1983)	+
Pure autonomic failure	Hoeldtke *et al.* (1984)	−
	Kaufmann *et al.* (1991)	+
Multiple system atrophy	Kachi *et al.* (1988)	+
	Kaufmann *et al.* (1991)	+
Postprandial hypotension	Freeman *et al.* (1996)	+

Also included are studies in dialysis-induced and postprandial hypotension. Studies in the latter were in patients with pure autonomic failure and multiple system atrophy.

The benefit (+) or lack of effect (−) of DOPS is indicated for each study.

Predominantly venoconstrictor agents with direct action on α-adrenoceptors

Dihydroergotamine has a long history in treatment of postural hypotension since reports by Nordenfelt and Mellander (1972). It acts as a direct α-adrenoceptor agonist, stimulating venous capacity vessels although resistance vessels may even show slight dilatation when normally innervated. It increases central blood volume by about 120 ml with only a slight rise in venous pressure. Nordenfelt and Mellander (1972) studied patients with intact sympathetic function but liable to syncope (so-called 'sympathotonic' orthostatic hypotension) and their results are not directly applicable to autonomic failure. When there is sympathetic denervation as in autonomic failure, dihydroergotamine almost certainly causes constriction of resistance vessels (Bevegard *et al.* 1974). It is highly effective after venous injection and abolishes postural hypotension almost completely for half an hour even in severe cases of autonomic failure, sometimes temporarily improving the Valsalva response, these benefits being obtained at the price of severe recumbent hypertension. The effectiveness of intravenous dihydroergotamine was confirmed by Jennings *et al.* (1979) in two patients with PAF and two with MSA. They showed reduction of the excessive fall of central blood volume on standing. An oral dose of 30 mg daily was needed in three out of four patients to improve their postural hypotension, and the addition of fludrocortisone resulted in further improvement.

The major disadvantage of dihydroergotamine is its poor bioavailability. One approach has been to combine it with oral glyceryl trinitrate, which was reported to increase its bioavailability and thus increase its efficacy. However, studies in our unit, using such a combination in our patients with autonomic failure, did not provide any evidence of beneficial effect when dihydroergotamine with placebo was compared with dihydroergotamine in combination with 0.5 mg of glyceryl trinitrate. In some patients there may even have been a fall in blood pressure, presumably because of the vasodilator effects of

glyceryl trinitrate. Increasing the daily oral dose of dihydroergotamine may be of benefit in some patients, keeping in mind the potential complication of peripheral vasoconstriction. Dihydroergotamine can also be given parenterally, either subcutaneously or intramuscularly, as in the prevention of thromboembolic complications. It has been used with benefit intramuscularly in autonomic failure resulting from alcoholism and diabetes. Other ergot derivatives have also been assessed in patients with autonomic failure; ergotamine tartrate can be given orally, and has been used in doses of 2–5 mg daily with some benefit.

Vasopressin$_1$-receptor agonists

Stimulation of V$_1$-receptors in blood vessels results in constriction. The drug triglycyl-lysine-vasopressin (glypressin), an analogue of vasopressin with predominant V$_1$ effects, results in constriction of arteries, mainly in the splanchnic and skin circulation, and may reduce postural hypotension (Rittig *et al.* 1991). Further studies using this approach are awaited.

Prevention of vasodilatation

A variety of drugs has been used on the premise that blood pressure control can be improved by preventing vasodilatatory mechanisms.

β-Adrenoceptor blockade

Propranolol was introduced in the treatment of autonomic failure on the grounds, despite the obvious α-adrenoceptor defect, that β-adrenoceptor agonist induced vasodilatation might also contribute to the orthostatic hypotension and should be reversed by the β-adrenoceptor blocking properties of propranolol. It may also act on presynaptic β-adrenoceptors and so reduce the release of noradrenaline. Chobanian *et al.* (1977) reported beneficial effects in four patients with PAF on oral propranolol in doses of 40–240 mg daily but, as they were already taking 0.3–0.5 mg fludrocortisone daily and had an excessive salt intake, no clear conclusion can be drawn. They later withdrew propranolol in one patient because it caused severe recumbent hypertension and they reported that in two patients episodes of 'syncope' still occurred in the early morning when orthostatic intolerance was most severe. In practice propranolol has not proved sufficiently encouraging for other trials to be reported.

Other forms of postural intolerance and hypotension have been treated with propranolol. Some patients do not appear to have autonomic failure, but have orthostatic tachycardia or a hyperadrenergic orthostatic response leading to postural hypotension, partially due to a decreased cardiac output. The tachycardia is probably emotionally determined and is accompanied by a mounting sense of anxiety when standing, associated with overbreathing, and then sometimes, paradoxically, increasing bouts of vagally induced bradycardia, which may eventually lead to syncope. Propranolol reduces the initial tachycardia and may benefit such patients. Some patients with autonomic failure or diabetes mellitus, and in whom there is sparing of cardiac sympathetic efferents but impaired sympathetic tone to the vascular bed, have a compensatory tachycardia and deteriorate if this compensatory mechanism is blocked by propranolol.

Prostaglandin synthetase inhibitors

Indomethacin was first proposed on the theoretical basis that some prostaglandins are potent vasodilators and their effect may be inhibited by indomethacin, which also may have several other effects that modify pressor responses. Improvement with indomethacin was reported in four patients with postural hypotension (Kochar and Itskovitz 1978). However, the diagnosis was uncertain in one of them, in that the standing blood pressure was within the normal range for her age and, in all, the diagnosis of autonomic failure and MSA was based on clinical features without the benefit of physiological tests. Oral indomethacin (50 mg three times daily) increased sensitivity to infused noradrenaline and angiotensin II in four patients with MSA but the pressor effect was only significant on recumbent blood pressure, probably because the hydrostatic stresses on standing require compensatory constriction of different blood vessels in different vascular beds (Davies et al. 1980). Inhibition of prostaglandin synthesis may be a factor because urinary prostaglandin excretion was greater than in normal subjects and was decreased by indomethacin. The lack of improvement in the standing blood pressure might also have been due to a decrease in plasma renin activity due to indomethacin. Benefit has been reported from the combined effect of fludrocortisone and flurbiprofen in PAF (Watt et al. 1981). Since both prostaglandin inhibitors and fludrocortisone have pressor effects, we have decided, in some cases failing to respond to fludrocortisone alone, to add indomethacin because both substances appear to increase smooth muscle sensitivity to noradrenaline and, in larger doses, may increase blood volume. Drugs such as indomethacin have side-effects, including gastric–duodenal ulceration.

Dopamine antagonists

Metoclopramide, a dopamine antagonist, has been used on the basis that it blocks the vasodilator effects of dopamine. In a single patient with postural hypotension after an extensive sympathectomy, Kuchel et al. (1980) reported an improvement in postural hypotension. They postulated that this was the result of the drug inhibiting the vasodilator and natriuretic effects of the excess dopamine released. In four patients with PAF, in whom plasma dopamine levels were similar to those of normal subjects, intravenous metoclopramide (10 μg) caused a small but significant fall in blood pressure. A similar dose given to patients with dopamine β-hydroxylase deficiency, in whom plasma dopamine levels were elevated, lowered blood pressure substantially (see Chapter 40). These observations do not favour a role for these drugs in the treatment of postural hypotension, except in situations where concurrent drug therapy (such as with L-dopa or apomorphine) elevates peripheral dopamine levels and stimulates vasodilatatory dopaminergic receptors. However, caution is necessary in patients with supersensitivity of central dopamine receptors who may be vulnerable to the extrapyramidal side-effects, and antagonists with mainly peripheral effects, such as domperidone, may be preferable.

Drugs preventing postprandial hypotension (see Chapter 29)

Dilatation within the splanchnic circulation following a meal is probably the cause of the marked postprandial fall in blood pressure in patients with autonomic failure. Splanchnic vasodilatation may result from the release of vasodilatatory neuropeptides. Drugs such as dihydroergotamine seem to have minimal effects in preventing postprandial hypotension. The beneficial use of other agents, particular octreotide, is discussed in Chapter 29. It should be noted that octreotide also reduces postural hypotension (Armstrong and Mathias 1991) and may provide some benefit in exercise-induced hypotension (Smith et al. 1995b).

Drugs acting on the heart

Pindolol

Pindolol has additional partial β-adrenoceptor agonist activity (so-called intrinsic sympathomimetic activity) which should cause less reduction in resting heart rate than a pure β-blocker might be expected to cause. The initial encouraging report was by Frewin et al. (1980) on two patients with diabetic autonomic neuropathy who probably had supersensitivity to noradrenaline. It was followed by Man in't Veld and Schalekamp (1981), who showed benefits in three patients with autonomic failure, two of whom had amyloidosis and one following acute autonomic neuropathy. They argued that, when receptor occupancy is low as is assumed in the postganglionic lesion of autonomic failure, there was a strong possibility that even a partial β-agonist would act as a full agonist and its agonist effect would be enhanced by denervation hypersensitivity and lack of baroreflexes. They also raised the possibility that pindolol might have an effect on β-adrenoceptors in veins and, like dihydroergotamine, might increase venous tone. They showed that the improvement in postural hypotension was due to an improvement in cardiac output but vascular resistance was unchanged. Their patients had an increase in cardiac rate. However, this enthusiasm was premature. Davies et al. (1981) reported briefly on five patients studied under standard conditions after a control period. Pindolol was given in an adequate dose, gauged by the heart rate response to intravenous isoprenaline, but did not increase blood pressure or cause symptomatic benefit at any dose level. The trend was towards a decrease in lying and standing pressure. Pindolol did not have a chronotropic action and there was instead a tendency for the pulse rate to decrease with increasing doses of pindolol. Two patients had raised jugular venous pressure after 3 days on 15 mg daily and frank cardiac failure after 45 mg daily for 3 days. Pindolol causes a rightward shift of the isoprenaline dose–response curve so that, although in theory pindolol acts more as a sympathetic agonist than a competitive antagonist, its β-blocking action was still pronounced. In our patients there was evidence of increased receptor numbers and denervation supersensitivity to noradrenaline. Therefore, the view put forward by Man in't Veld and Schalekamp (1981), that their patients responded because of the partial agonist effect of pindolol may not be the only explanation.

Prenalterol and xamoterol

Two other β-blockers with α_1-adrenoceptor partial agonist effects have been assessed in AF. Prenalterol was found to be effective (Goovaerts *et al.* 1984). Xamoterol has also been shown in a number of patients to benefit postural hypotension (Mehlsen and Trap-Jensen 1985; Mathias *et al.* 1990). However, xamoterol, like pindolol, has the potential to cause cardiac failure and has been withdrawn.

Erythropoietin

Erythropoietin is a polypeptide that is produced mainly in the kidney. It stimulates red blood cell production. The level of oxygen to the kidney is a key factor in its synthesis as stimuli such as hypoxia, blood loss, or chronic anaemia increase erythropoietin levels. The role of the sympathetic nervous system in erythropoietin synthesis is unclear; previously we had noted low haemoglobin levels, with normocytic, normochromic anaemia, mainly in pure autonomic failure patients. Further studies indicate that in autonomic failure the anaemia is not associated with an appropriate increase in erythropoietin levels, as otherwise would be expected (Biaggioni *et al.* 1994).

Erythropoietin is now produced using recombinant techniques, and it was first used in postural hypotension by Hoeldtke and Streeten (1993), in a dose of 50 units/kg body weight, three times a week for 6–8 weeks. It raised haemoglobin levels and red cell volume, but it had no effect on plasma volume in eight patients with postural hypotension, of whom four had diabetic autonomic neuropathy, three PAF, and one sympathotonic orthostatic hypotension. Following erythropoietin, there was a rise in both systolic and diastolic blood pressure with an improvement in postural hypotension and symptoms. Erythropoietin in primary chronic autonomic failure has since been used successfully by other groups (Biaggioni *et al.* 1994; and Perera *et al.* 1995). It may be of particular value in autonomic failure where anaemia may be a complication, as in diabetic autonomic neuropathy with renal failure (see Chapter 39). It is not known whether erythropoietin will be effective in reducing postural hypotension in the large number of patients with autonomic failure who are not anaemic.

Summary of management approaches

The management of postural hypotension entails consideration of a large number of factors. Some of these include the marked lability of blood pressure (at times with supine hypertension), the variability of

Table 36.3. Outline of non-pharmacological and pharmacological measures used in the management of postural hypotension due to neurogenic failure (adapted from Mathias 1995 and Mathias and Kimber 1998)

Non-pharmacological measures

To be avoided
Sudden head-up postural change (especially on waking)
Prolonged recumbency
Straining during micturition and defaecation
High environmental temperature (including hot baths)
'Severe' exertion
Large meals (especially with refined carbohydrate)
Alcohol
Drugs with vasodepressor properties

To be introduced
Head-up tilt during sleep
Small, frequent meals
High salt intake
Judicious exercise (including swimming)
Body positions and manoeuvres

To be considered
Elastic stockings
Abdominal binders

Pharmacological measures

Starter drug: fludrocortisone
Sympathomimetics: ephedrine, midodrine
Specific targeting: octreotide, desmopressin, erythropoietin

It should be emphasized that non-neurogenic factors, such as fluid loss due to vomiting or diarrhoea (see Chapter 20), may substantially worsen neurogenic postural hypotension and will need to be rectified.

symptoms despite a similar blood pressure fall, and the effects of activities in daily life that can worsen postural hypotension substantially. The patient must be made aware that the treatment, even with a combination of drugs, is unlikely to be a substitute for the rapid and complex responses of the autonomic nervous system. The physician, and in many situations the patient also, should be aware that various non-neurogenic factors that lower blood pressure (see Chapter 20) can worsen postural hypotension; an example is even modest fluid loss induced by vomiting or diarrhoea. The management, therefore, is dependent upon an integrated approach, with education of the patient of particular importance. A summary is provided in Table 36.3, outlining the non-pharmacological and pharmacological approaches that we use.

The non-pharmacological approaches are an important component of the patient's contribution to management. Awareness of the various factors that worsen hypotension are important, together with the means to avoid these. Some are readily definable, while others, such as exercise, need to be related specifically to the individual as the severity of exertion causing symptomatic hypotension will vary. The patient, often with the help of the partner or carers, will need to implement measures to reduce postural hypotension. Some, such as increasing salt intake either by the liberal addition of salt at meals or salt tablets, often may need explanation, as the risks of high salt intake have been so well publicized that a low intake is often erroneously adhered to. Exercise is needed to maintain an adequate muscle mass and improve circulatory control. The type of, and even position during, exercise will need to be modified, depending upon the degree of hypotension and associated neurological and musculoskeletal disabilities. Thus, in some patients it may need to be performed while lying flat. There may be advantages in swimming, because the subject is semi-supine with the supportive external pressure of water. An important component is the utilization of various positions and manoeuvres to raise blood pressure in different circumstances, that again need to be tailored to the patient's associated disabilities.

Drugs should be used when it is clear that non-pharmacological approaches alone are not beneficial. A valuable starter drug with minimal side-effects is low-dose fludrocortisone. This can be followed by the sympathomimetic drugs, ephedrine (especially in those with central or incomplete lesions) or midodrine (in those with peripheral lesions). If the combination of fludrocortisone and sympathomimetics does not produce the desired effects, then selective targetting is needed, depending upon the pathophysiological disturbances. Thus, octreotide may be of value in those with postprandial hypotension, desmopressin in those with nocturnal polyuria, and erythropoietin in those with associated anaemia. The drug treatment, therefore, needs to be individually tailored.

Finally, the management of postural hypotension in each patient will need to be linked to non-autonomic features and any other medical disorder, and must be relevant to their life style. Thus the treatment of parkinsonism and introduction of L-DOPA may necessitate changes in dosage or frequency of drugs to control hypotension. In the cerebellar form of MSA there may be marked truncal ataxia, and exercise and walking programmes will need to be modified; such patients may, in due course, be safer in a wheelchair to reduce the risk of falling and trauma. The laboratory evaluation of postural hypotension also needs consideration, as blood pressure measurements are made usually with passive change (such as head-up tilt) or while standing still, precisely the measures that we encourage our patients to avoid. The evaluation of standing time, advocated by some, is often irrelevant in practice, as this will be influenced by many factors that worsen postural hypotension in daily life, and also by the additional neurological disabilities, as in patients with MSA. However, measurements of blood pressure are necessary for evaluation, and have their value, although in the individual patient symptoms and the ability to function independently are the crucial factors. The increasing availability of home blood pressure monitors should, in general, be discouraged, as unfortunately there are many patients shackled to monitors that inadvisedly have been recommended; these are not even a poor second to the patient's symptoms! The key aims, therefore, in the management of postural hypotension are to ensure that the patient is appropriately mobile and functional, is on low-risk therapy that prevents falls and associated trauma, and is able to maintain a suitable quality of life.

References

Alam, M., Smith, G. D. P., Bleasdale-Barr, K., Pavitt, D. V., and Mathias, C. J. (1995). Effects of the peptide release inhibitor, Octreotide, on daytime hypotension and on nocturnal hypertension in primary autonomic failure. *J. Hypertension.* 13, 1664–9.

Ando, Y., Gotoh, T., Kawaguchi, Y., Tanaka, Y., Sakashita, N., and Ando, M. (1995). Intranasal L-threo-3,4,-dihydroxyphenylserine in treating diarrhea associated with familial amyloidotic polyneuropathy. *Pharmacotherapy* 15, 345–9.

Armstrong, E. and Mathias, C. J. (1991). The effects of the somatostatin analogue, octreotide, on postural hypotension, before and after food ingestion in primary autonomic failure. *Clin. Auton. Res.* 2, 135–40.

Bannister, R., Ardill, L., and Fentem, P. (1969). An assessment of various methods of treatment of idiopathic orthostatic hypotension. *Q. J. Med.* 38, 377–95.

Bannister, R., Sever, P., and Gross, M. (1977). Cardiovascular reflexes and biochemical responses in progressive autonomic failure. *Brain* 100, 327–44.

Bannister, R., Boylston, A. W., Davies, I. B., Mathias, C. J., Sever, P. S., and Sudera, D. (1981). Beta-receptor numbers and thermodynamics in denervation supersensitivity. *J. Physiol. London* 319, 369–77.

Bannister, R., Da Costa, D. F., Hendry, W. G., Jacobs, J., and Mathias, C. J. (1986). Atrial demand pacing to protect against vagal overactivity in sympathetic autonomic neuropathy. *Brain* 109, 345–56.

Bevegard, S., Castenfors, J., and Lindblad, L.-E. (1974). Haemodynamic effects of dihydroergotamine in patients with postural hypotension. *Acta Med. Scand.* 196, 473–7.

Biaggioni, I., Robertson, D., Krantz, D. S., Jones, M., and Hale, V. (1994). The anaemia of primary autonomic failure and its reversal with recombinant erythropoietin. *Ann. Int. Med.* 121, 181–6.

Birkmayer, W., Birkmayer, G., Lechner, H., and Riederer, P. (1983). DL-3, 4-threo-DOPS in Parkinson's disease: effects on orthostatic hypotension and dizziness. *J. Neural Transmission* 58, 305–13.

Carvalho, M. J., van den Meirackers, A. H., Boomsma, F. *et al.* (1997). Improved orthostatic tolerance in familial amyloidotic polyneuropathy with unnatural noradrenaline precursor L-threo-3,4,-dihydroxyphenylserine. *J. autonom. nerv. Syst.* 62, 63–71.

Chobanian, A. V., Volicer, L., Liang, C. S., Kershaw, G., and Tifft, C. (1977). Use of propranolol in the treatment of idiopathic orthostatic hypotension. *Trans. Ass. Am. Physcns.* 90, 324–34.

Chobanian, A. V., Volicer, L., Tifft, C., Gavras, H., Liang, C., and Faxon, D. (1979). Mineralocorticoid-induced hypotension in patients with orthostatic hypotension. *New Engl. J. Med.* 301, 68–73.

Davies, B., Bannister, R., and Sever, P. (1978). Pressor amines and monoamine oxidase inhibitors for treatment of postural hypotension in progressive autonomic failure. Limitations and hazards. *Lancet* i, 172–5.

Davies, B., Bannister, R., Sever, P., and Wilcox, C. S. (1979). The pressor actions of noradrenaline, angiotensin 11 and saralasin in chronic autonomic failure treated with fludrocortisone. *Br. J. Clin. Pharmacol.* 8, 253–60.

Davies, B., Bannister, R., Hensby, C., and Sever, P. (1980). The pressor actions of noradrenaline, angiotensin 11 in chronic autonomic failure treated with indomethacin. *Br. J. clin. Pharmacol.* 10, 223–9.

Davies, B., Bannister, R., Mathias, C. J., and Sever, P. (1981). Pindolol in postural hypotension; the case for caution. *Lancet* i, 982–3.

Davies, B., Sudera, D., SagneHa, E. *et al.* (1982). Increased numbers of alpha-receptors in sympathetic denervation supersensitivity in man. *J. Clin. Invest.* 69, 779–84.

Fouad-Tarazi, F. M., Okabe, M., and Goran, H. (1995). α-sympathomimetic treatment of autonomic insufficiency with orthostatic hypotension. *Am. J. Med.* 99, 604–10.

Freeman, R., Young, J., Landsbert, L., and Lipsitz, L. (1996). The treatment of postprandial hypotension in autonomic failure with 3,4-DL-threo-dihydroxyphenylserine. *Neurology* 47, 1414–20.

Frewin, D. B., Leonello, P. P., Pentall, R. K., Hughes, L., and Harding, P. E. (1980). Pindolol in orthostatic hypotension: possible therapy? *Med. J. Aust.* 1, 128.

Goovaerts, J., Ver faillie, C., Fagard, R., and Knochaert, D. (1984). Effect of prenalterol on orthostatic hypotension in the Shy–Drager syndrome. *BMJ.* 288, 817–18.

Hoeldtke, R. D., Cilmi, K. M., and Mattis-Graves, K. (1984). DL-Threo-3, 4-dihydroxyphenylserine does not exert a pressor effect in orthostatic hypotension. *Clin. Pharmacol. Ther.* 36, 302–6.

Hoeldtke, R. D., and Streeten, D. H. P. (1993). Treatment of orthostatic hypotension with erythropoietin. *New Engl. J. Med.* 329, 611–15.

Iida, N., Tsubakihara, Y., Shirai, D., Imada, A., and Suzuki, M. (1994). Treatment of dialysis-induced hypotension with L-threo-3,4,-dihydroxyphenylserine. *Nephrol. Dial. Transplant* 9, 1130–5.

Iwase, S., Mano, T., Kunimoto, M., and Saito, M. (1992). Effect of L-threo-3,4,-dihydroxyphenylserine on muscle sympathetic nerve activity in humans. *J. autonom. nerv. Syst.* 39, 159–67.

Janknegt, R. A., Zweers, H. M. M., Delaere, K. P.J., Kloet, A. G., Khoe, S. G. S., and Arendsen, H. J. (1997). Oral desmopressin as a new treatment modality for primary nocturnal enuresis in adolescents and adults: a double-blind, randomized, multicenter study. *J. Urol.* 157, 513–17.

Jankovic, J., Gilden, J. L. D., Heine, B. C., *et al.* (1993). Neurogenic orthostatic hypotension: a double blind, placebo controlled study with midodrine. *Am. J. Med.* 95, 38–48.

Jennings, G., Esler, M., and Holmes, R. (1979). Treatment of orthostatic hypotension with dihydroergotamine. *BMJ.* ii, 307–8.

Kachi, T., Iwase, S., Mano, T., Saito, M., Kunimoto, M., and Sobue, I. (1988). Effect of L-threo-3,4-dihydroxyphenylserine on muscle sympathetic nerve activity in Shy–Drager syndrome. *Neurology* 38, 1091–4.

Karet, F. E., Dickerson, J. E. C., Brown, J., and Brown, M. J. (1994). Bovril and moclobemide: a novel therapeutic strategy for central autonomic failure. *Lancet* 344, 1263–5.

Kaufmann, H., Brannan, T., Krakoff, L., Yahr, M. D., and Mandeli, J. (1988). Treatment of orthostatic hypotension due to autonomic failure with a peripheral α-adrenergic agonist (midodrine). *Neurology* 38, 951–6.

Kaufmann, H., Oribe, E., and Yahr, M. D. (1991). Differential effect L-threo-3,4-dihydroxyphenylserine in pure autonomic failure and multiple system atrophy with autonomic failure. *J. Neurol. Transm.* 3, 143–8.

Kochar, M. S. and Itskovitz, H. D. (1978). Treatment of idiopathic orthostatic hypotension (Shy–Drager syndrome) with indomethacin. *Lancet* i, 1011–14.

Kuchel, O., Bun, N. T., Gutkowska, J., and Genest, J. (1980). Treatment of severe orthostatic hypotension by metoclopramide. *Ann. int. Med.* 93, 841–3.

Low, P. A., Gilden, J. L., Freeman, R., Sheng, K.-N., and McElligott, M. A. (1997). Efficacy of midodrine vs placebo in neurogenic orthostatic hypotension. A randomized, double-blind multicenter study. *J. Am. Med. Ass.* 277, 1046–51.

Man in't Veld, A. J. and Schalekamp, M. A. D. H. (1981). Pindolol acts as betaadrenoceptor agonist in orthostatic hypotension: therapeutic implications. *BMJ.* 282, 929–31.

Mann, S., Altman, D. G., Raftery, E. B., and Bannister, R. (1983). Circadian variation of blood pressure in autonomic failure. *Circulation* 68, 477–83.

Mathias, C. J., Reid, J. L., Wing, L. M. H., Frankel, H. L., and Christensen, N. J. (1979). Antihypertensive effects of clonidine in tetraplegic subjects devoid of central sympathetic control. *Clin. Sci.* 57, 425–6.

Mathias, C. J., Unwin, R. J., Pike, F. A., Frankel, H. L., Sever, P. S. and Peart, W. S. (1984). The immediate pressor response to saralarin in man: evidence against sympathetic activation and for intrinsic angiotensin II-like myotropism. *Clin. Sci.* 66, 517–24.

Mathias, C. J., Fosbraey, P., de Costa, D. F., Thorley, A., and Bannister, R. (1986). Desmopressin reduces nocturnal polyuria, reverses overnight weight loss and improves morning postural hypotension in autonomic failure. *BMJ.* 293, 353–4.

Mathias, C. J., O'kuchu, M., Raimbach, S. J., Watson, L., and Bannister, R. (1990). Xamoterol reduces postural hypotension in both pure autonomic failure and multiple system atrophy. *J. Neurol.* 237, (Suppl. 1:), s24.

Mathias, C. J., Holly, E., Armstrong, E., Shareef, M., and Bannister, R. (1991). The influence of food on postural hypotension in three groups with chronic autonomic failure: clinical and therapeutic implications. *J. Neurol. Neurosurg. Psychiat.* 54, 726–30.

Mathias, C. J. and Alam, M. (1995). The influence of certain daily activities on 24 hour ambulatory blood pressure in hypotensive, normotensive and hypertensive subjects. *Clin. Auton. Res.* 5, 321.

Mathias, C. J. (1995). Orthostatic hypotension. *Prescribers J.* 35, 125–32.

Mathias, C. J. and Kimber, J. R. (1998). Treatment of postural hypotension. *J. Neurol. Neurosurg. Psychiat.* 65, 285–9.

Mehlsen, J., and Trap-Jensen, J. (1985). Use of xamoterol, a new selective betaadrenoreceptor partial agonist, in the treatment of postural hypotension. *Proceedings of the International Symposium on Cardiovascular Pharmacotherapy, Geneva,* Abstract 73.

Moss, A. J., Glaser, W., and Topol E. (1980). Atrial tachypacing in the treatment of a patient with primary orthostatic hypotension. *New Engl. J. Med.* 302, 1456–7.

Muneta, S., Iwata, T., Hiwada, K., Murakami, E., Sato, Y., and Imamura, Y. (1992). Effect of L-threo-3,4-dihydroxyphenylserine on orthostatic hypotension in a patient with spinal cord injury. *Jap. Circ. J.* 56, 243–7.

Nordenfelt, I., and Mellander, S. (1972). Central haemodynamic effects of dihydroergotamine in patients with orthostatic hypotension. *Acta Med. Scand.* 191, 115–20.

Onrot, J., Goldberg, M. R., Biaggioni, I., Wiley, R. G., Hollister, A. S., and Robertson, D. (1987). Oral yohimbine in human autonomic failure. *Neurology* 37, 215–20.

Perera, R., Isola, L., and Kaufmann, H. (1995). Effect of recombinant erythropoietin on anemia and orthostatic hypotension in primary autonomic failure. *Clin. Auton. Res.* 5, 211–14.

Polinsky, R. J., Samaras, G. M., and Kopin, I. J. (1983). Sympathetic neural prosthesis for managing orthostatic hypertension. *Lancet* i, 901–4.

Puvi-Rajasingham, S., Smith, G. D. P., Akinola, A., and Mathias, C. J. (1997). Abnormal regional blood flow responses during and after exercise in human sympathetic denervation. *J. Physiol.* 505, 481–9.

Rensma, P. L., van den Meiracker, A. H., Boomsma, F., Man in't Veld, A. J., and Schalekamp, M. A. (1993). Effects of ibopamine on postural hypotension in pure autonomic failure. *J. Cardiol. Pharmacol.* 21, 863–8.

Rittig, S., Arentsen, J., Sorensen, K., Matthiesen, T., and Dupont, E. (1991). The hemodynamic effects of triglycyl-lysine-vasopressin (glypressin) in patients with parkinsonism and orthostatic hypotension. *Movement Disorders* 6, 21–8.

Schmidt, P. G., Eckstein, J. W., and Abboud, F. M. (1966). Effect of 9-alpha-fluorohydrocortisone on forearm vascular responses to norepinephrine. *Circulation* 34, 620–6.

Senard, J. M., Rascol, O., Durrieu, G., *et al.* (1993a). Effects of yohimbine on plasma catecholamine levels in orthostatic hypotension related to Parkinson disease or multiple system atrophy. *Clin. Neuropharmacol.* 1, 70–6.

Senard, J. M., Rascol, O., Rascol, A., and Montastruc, J. L. (1993b). Lack of yohimbine effect on ambulatory blood pressure recoding: a double-blind cross-over trial in parkinsonians with orthostatic hypotension. *Fund. Clin. Pharmacol.* 7, 465–70.

Sheps, S. G. (1976). The use of an elastic garment in the treatment of idiopathic orthostatic hypotension. *Cardiology* 62, (Suppl. 1), 271–9.

Smit, A. A. J, Hardjowijono, M. A., and Wieling, W. (1997). Are portable folding chairs useful to combat orthostatic hypotension? *Ann. Neurol,* 42, 975–8.

Smith, G. D. P., and Mathias, C. J. (1995). Postural hypotension enhanced by exercise in patients with chronic autonomic failure. *Q. J. Med.* 88, 251–6.

Smith, G. D. P., Watson, L. P., Pavitt, D. V., and Mathias, C. J. (1995a). Abnormal cardiovascular and catecholamine responses to supine exercise in human subjects with sympathetic dysfunction. *J. Physiol. London,* 485, 255–65.

Smith, G. D. P., Alam, M., Watson, L. P., and Mathias, C. J. (1995b). Effects of the somatostatin analogue, octreotide, on exercise induced hypotension in human subjects with chronic sympathetic failure. *Clin. Sci.* 89, 367–73.

Suzuki, S., Higa, S., Tsuga, I., Sakoda, S., Hayashi, A., Yamamura, Y., Takaba, Y., and Nakajima, A. (1980). Effects of infused L-threo-3,4-dihydroxyphenylserine in patients with familial amyloid polyneuropathy. *Eur. J. Clin. Pharmacol.* 17, 429–35.

Suzuki, T., Higa, S., Sakoda, S., Ueji, M., Hayashi, A., Takaba, Y., and Nakajima, A. (1982). Pharmacokinetic studies of oral L-threo-3,4-dihydroxyphenylserine in normal subjects and patients with familial amyloid polyneuropathy. *Eur. J. Clin. Pharmacol.* **23**, 463–8.

Tanaka, H., Yamaguchi, H., and Mino, M. (1996). The effects of the noradrenaline precursor, L-threo–3,4,-dihydroxyphenylserine, in children with orthostatic intolerance. *Clin. Auton. Res.* **6**, 189–93.

Tanaka, H., Yamaguchi, H., and Tamaih, H. (1997). Treatment of orthostatic intolerance with inflatable abdominal band. *Lancet* **349**, 175.

Ten Harkel, A. D. J., van Lieshout, J. J., and Weiling, W. (1994). Effect of leg muscle pumping and in tensing on orthostatic arterial pressure; a study in normal subjects and in patients with autonomic failure. *Clin. Sci.* **87**, 533–58.

Ten Harkel, A. D. J., van Lieshout, J. J., and Wieling, W. (1992). Treatment of orthostatic hypotension with sleeping in the head-up tilt position and in combination with fludrocortisone. *J. Intern. Med.* **232**, 139–45.

Thomaides, T. N., Chaudhuri, K. R., Maule, S., and Mathias, C. J. (1992). Differential responses in superior mesenteric artery blood flow may explain the variant pressor responses to clonidine in two groups with sympathetic denervation. *Clin. Sci.* **83**, 59–64,

Thomas, D. J., and Bannister, R. (1980). Preservation of autoregulation of cerebral blood flow in autonomic failure. *J. neurol. Sci.* **44**, 205–12.

Tobian, L. and Redleaf, P. D. (1958). Ionic composition of the aorta in renal and adrenal hypertension. *Am. J. Physiol.* **192**, 325–30.

Vahidassr, M. D., Foy, C. J., O'Malley, T., and Passmore, A. P. (1997). Eye drops and lethargy. *J. R. Soc. Med.* **90**, 155.

Watt, S. J., Tooke, J. E., Perkins, C. M., and Lee, M. (1981). The treatment of idiopathic orthostatic hypotension: a combined fludrocortisone–flurbiprofen regime. *Q. J. Med.* **50**, 205–12.

Wieling W, van Lieshout J. J., and van Leeuwen A. M. (1993). Physical manoeuvres that reduce postural hypotension. *Clin. Ant. Res.* **3**, 57–65.

37. The treatment of the motor disorders of multiple system atrophy

A. J. Lees

Introduction

It has become clear from recent clinicopathological studies at the United Kingdom Parkinson's Disease Society Brain Research Centre at the Institute of Neurology, Queen Square, London, that multiple system atrophy (MSA) presenting as a parkinsonian syndrome is considerably underdiagnosed. Most of the patients confirmed at post-mortem as MSA have minimal or no cerebellar signs, but involutional changes of the cerebellar folia may be demonstrable on neuroimaging. Autonomic signs and symptoms, on the other hand, are more frequent and include urgency of micturition, impotence, and symptomatic orthostatic hypotension. In many cases they are indistinguishable from Parkinson's disease (PD) in life, although a more malignant clinical course, early gait disturbances with falls, early severe dysarthria, and absence of rest tremor are helpful clinical pointers. A minority have Babinski signs which, provided cervical spondylotic myelopathy has been excluded, is incompatible with a diagnosis of PD.

Of 370 brains of patients dying with a parkinsonian syndrome seen at the UK Parkinson's Disease Society Brain Research Centre up to 1992, 35 (9.5 per cent) showed the pathological changes of multiple system atrophy. Twelve of these cases had remained misdiagnosed as PD up to the time of their death and even retrospectively reviewing the case material it was impossible in 10 of these to make a diagnosis of multiple system atrophy based on the information recorded in the notes (Ben-Shlomo *et al.* 1995). Of the first 100 cases prospectively diagnosed as having PD, seven were found to have multiple system atrophy (Hughes *et al.* 1992a). In another post-mortem study of 59 cases of parkinsonian syndrome, 13 (22 per cent) had MSA, but no information is given in this paper as to how many were correctly diagnosed in life (Rajput *et al.* 1990). A few patients have also been reported to have the pathological lesions of both PD and MSA (Gibb and Lees 1989). Striatonigral degeneration (SND) therefore probably constitutes between 5 and 10 per cent of all causes of parkinsonian syndrome due to brainstem degeneration.

Treatment of the parkinsonian syndrome in MSA

Acute challenges with oral L-dopa or subcutaneous apomorphine to assess dopaminergic responsiveness

The assessment of dopaminergic responsiveness in multiple system atrophy is of some limited value in diagnosis and helpful in determining the likelihood of a worthwhile therapeutic response to long-term L-dopa therapy. After withdrawal of oral dopaminergic drugs for 12 hours a single dose of L-dopa/dopa decarboxylase inhibitor (250/25 mg) is given in the fasting state. The motor response is assessed by timed tapping and walking tests at 15 min intervals and four-point scales for tremor and dyskinesia. A modified Webster Scale is also used at baseline and peak response to assess the amplitude of motor response. The peripheral dopamine receptor antagonist drug, domperidone, is given in a dose of 30 mg three times a day for at least 24 h before the apomorphine test, which should also be given in the fasting state using serial challenges of 1.5, 3.0, 4.5, and 7.0 mg s.c. The test is continued until either an unequivocal response occurs, intolerable side-effects are experienced, or the maximum dose is reached. One of four clinically definite MSA patients responded to both apomorphine and L-dopa and subsequently to sustained L-dopa therapy. The other three patients had negative responses to acute challenges and failed to benefit from L-dopa therapy. A further eight patients with possible MSA were tested, five of whom had negative responses to the challenges and failed to respond to L-dopa therapy. One had positive responses to both apomorphine and the L-dopa test and responded well to chronic L-dopa, and a further two patients had equivocal responses to both apomorphine and L-dopa and subsequently responded to long-term L-dopa therapy (Hughes *et al.* 1990). In contrast, however, Oertel and colleagues (1989) found that none of five patients with clinically definite MSA responded positively to apomorphine. In another study evaluating the apomorphine and oral L-dopa tests in 45 previously untreated patients with PD, nine cases failed to respond either to challenge or to long-term L-dopa therapy and one of these developed pyramidal signs and autonomic nerve dysfunction in the 12 months of follow-up, suggesting a diagnosis of MSA. One of the other patients died after a rapidly progressive akinetic-rigid syndrome, a further two developed signs strongly suggestive of Steele–Richardson–Olszewski disease, while the other five patients had physical signs still consistent with PD (Hughes *et al.* 1991). Parati *et al.* (1993) gave acute L-dopa challenges to eight clinically probable MSA cases and only four had a positive response. It has been my subjective impression that patients who turn out to have MSA tend to have more adverse events when challenged with L-dopa or subcutaneous apomorphine in the early stages, and a profound drop of blood pressure with orthostatic symptoms is particularly suggestive of early MSA.

Clinical studies with L-dopa and dopaminergic agonists

The therapeutic results of L-dopa therapy in presumed cases of MSA are difficult to interpret because of the variability. Aminoff and colleagues (1973) treated five cases of MSA with autonomic failure with doses of L-dopa between 1.25 and 3.5 g/day and four of the five got worse with respect to their parkinsonian disabilities, although two had some modest increase in the level of their standing blood pressure and three in their lying blood pressure. These were all patients with MSA and marked autonomic failure. Sharpe and colleagues (1973) treated a 58-year-old man with MSA with small doses of L-dopa and a non-selective monoamine oxidase inhibitor in an attempt to produce anti-parkinsonian benefit and a controlled improvement in postural hypotension. Worthwhile benefit occurred with respect to tremor and rigidity, but only minimal improvement in bradykinesia. Goetz and colleagues (1984) reported that 16 of 19 patients with presumed MSA treated with L-dopa obtained definite improvement in rigidity and bradykinesia, and postural tremor was improved in two. The mean duration of disease in this study was long, averaging 10 years with a range of 5–20 years. Eleven of the patients presented with a parkinsonian syndrome, six with cerebellar signs and the rest with a mixed picture. Fourteen had a definite or suspected family history of a similar condition presenting with cerebellar symptoms alone, which raised the possibility that some patients may have had a familial cerebellar degeneration. Ten of the patients experienced drug-induced chorea and five had visual hallucinations. Lang and colleagues (1986) reported three patients diagnosed initially as having PD who derived sustained benefit from L-dopa preparations with the emergence of on–off oscillations. Limb ataxia and cerebellar dysarthria developed in two of the cases and a third was unable to stand or walk within 5 years of the onset of the disease. All three had marked involutional changes of the cerebellar folia on computed axial tomography (CAT) scan. In a further study of 23 cases with possible SND (Staal et al. 1990) no response to L-dopa occurred in 15, four developed on–off effects, and four acute psychotic reactions. Wenning and colleagues (1994) reported a good or excellent response to L-dopa (300–600 mg/day) in 29 of 100 patients, but only 13 per cent maintained this response. Prominent orofacial and axial dyskinesias occurred in 52 per cent of patients in this series. A prompt and marked improvement to L-dopa is therefore a relative contraindication to the diagnosis of MSA, but does not exclude the diagnosis. In contrast, a marked response to L-dopa in progressive supranuclear palsy is so unusual that one should seriously reconsider the clinical diagnosis.

Results with the new synthetic ergolenes, lisuride and pergolide, have been even more disappointing. Goetz and colleagues (1984) using doses of 10–80 mg daily of bromocriptine, reported benefit in five patients who had responded to L-dopa and one patient who had failed to respond to L-dopa. Williams and colleagues (1979) also reported temporary benefit in an occasional patient; others, however, have had more disappointing results. Gautier and Durand (1977) in a controlled trial with lisuride (mean dose 2.4 mg daily), found that only one of seven patients with MSA and autonomic failure derived improvement in parkinsonian features and another, who had been deriving considerable benefit from L-dopa before the study began, failed to respond at all to large doses of lisuride. Severe psychiatric side-effects occurred in six patients on lisuride, with nightmares, isolated visual hallucinations, and toxic confusional states (Lees and Bannister 1981). Wenning et al. (1994) reported a response to oral dopamine agonists in 4 of 46 patients. None of 30 patients receiving bromocriptine improved, but 3 of 10 who received pergolide had some benefit. Twenty-two per cent of the L-dopa responders (2 of 9)

had good or excellent response to at least one orally active dopamine agonist in addition.

Clinicopathological studies

If one reviews the therapeutic effects of L-dopa on histologically proven cases of SND, the results are generally disappointing (Tables 37.1 and 37.2). Of the 33 patients in the literature only five derived sustained improvement (Fearnley and Lees 1990; Feve et al. 1997). Another 10, however, derived definite initial benefit lasting for periods of up to several months, and one of these patients who could not tolerate L-dopa subsequently improved in a sustained fashion on high doses of bromocriptine (Van Leuwen and Perquin, 1988). Wenning and colleagues (1997) have recently reviewed 203 pathologically confirmed cases of MSA, 82 per cent of whom had parkinsonian features in life. Twenty-eight per cent of the cases had experienced a worthwhile response to L-dopa therapy, with about a quarter developing dyskinetic side-effects. Taken alone, the results reported recently by Fearnley and Lees (Table 37.2) are somewhat better, suggesting that as many as 60 per cent of patients might derive worthwhile initial benefit. Half of these patients were misdiagnosed in life as having PD and in the responders autonomic dysfunction was not severe. Hughes and colleagues (1992b) in their review of 23 pathologically confirmed cases of MSA from the UK Parkinson's Disease Society Brain Research Centre also found that around 60 per cent of cases had initial benefit to L-dopa therapy. They drew attention to presence of dystonia in facial musculature in 11 cases and the appearance of dyskinesias in the absence of any discernible therapeutic response in other patients. A further interesting observation from this study was that the proportion of patients who appeared not to have any substantial therapeutic response to L-dopa deteriorated markedly 7–10 days after L-dopa withdrawal. Ben-Shlomo et al. (1995) have recently reviewed the therapeutic response of 35 pathologically confirmed cases of multiple system atrophy with 40 per cent having an initial therapeutic response to L-dopa, but with only 7 per cent maintaining their response at the last assessment before death. Coexisting severe autonomic dysfunction greatly reduces the chances of a worthwhile therapeutic response to L-dopa in MSA, as intolerable orthostatic hypotension may occur on initial challenge with the drug.

Non-dopaminergic therapies

A severe reduction in the levels of noradrenaline in the central nervous system also occurs in both Parkinson's disease and multiple system degeneration, but so far trials with drugs known to enhance or antagonize noradrenaline seem to be without substantial effect in either disorder. Administration of threo-3,4-dihydroxyphenylserine (L-threo-DOPS), a non-physiological amino acid which can be converted by dopa decarboxylase to noradrenaline, was shown by Birkmayer more than 20 years ago to increase standing blood pressure. In the belief that some of the refractory symptoms of PD, such as freezing, poor balance, and dysarthria, might be due to noradrenaline deficiency caused by severely lowered dopamine β-hydroxylase activity, Narabayashi and colleagues (1986) have administered first DL-threo-DOPS and then more recently L-threo-DOPS to a large number of patients with parkinsonian syndromes. These authors have shown clear penetration of L-threo-DOPS into the central nervous system but it is not yet known whether the agent is able to increase the level of noradrenaline.

Table 37.1. The therapeutic effects of levodopa on histologically proven cases of striatonigral degeneration (± autonomine failure); all patients had severe rigidity and bradykinesia

Reference	Sex	Age at onset (years)	Duration of disease (years)	Clinical features						Levodopa treatment			
				Tremor	Dysarthria	Pyramidal signs	Cerebellar signs	Postural hypotension	Sphincter dysfunction	Duration at onset (years)	Max. dosage (mg/day)	Results	Adverse effects
Izumi et al. (1971)	M	51	2			+				1	6 400	No effect	None
	F	53	3							2	2 600	No effect	None
Greer et al. (1971)	F	73	4	+						3	12 000	Marked benefit for 6 months	None
Bannister and Oppenheimer (1972)	F	48	6		+	+		+		3	3 000	No effect	Severe postural hypotension
Rajput et al. (1972)	F	56			+	+			+	7	5 000	No effect	None
	F	63	7		+		+			7	5 000	No effect	Severe postural hypotension
Trotter (1973)	F	66	8	+		+				4	8 000	Modest benefit for 3 months	Orofacial dyskinesia
Sharpe et al. (1973)	F	41	6	+	+	+				5	6 000	Modest benefit for 2 months	Nausea
Takei and Mirra (1973)	F	66	2		+					1	3 000	No effect	None
Schober et al. (1975)	F	53	3	+	+	+		+	+	1	2 000* / 3 000	Modest benefit for 6 months	Rise in erect blood pressure
Michel et al. (1976)	M	61	3		+	+			+	2	3 000	No effect	None
	F	61	2		+	+			+	1	600*	No effect	None
Boudin et al. (1976)	F	59	7		+	+			+	3	3 000 / 600*	No effect	None
	F	56	4		+	+			+	2	5 000 / 800* / 4 000	Modest benefit for 6 months	Orofacial and limb dyskinesia

Table 37.1. (*continued*)

Reference	Sex	Age at onset (years)	Duration of disease (years)	Tremor	Dysarthria	Pyramidal signs	Cerebellar signs	Postural hypotension	Sphincter dysfunction	Duration at onset (years)	Max. dosage (mg/day)	Results	Adverse effects
				Clinical features						**Levodopa treatment**			
DeLean and Deck (1976)	M	54	6	+		+		+	+	4	1 000	Modest benefit for 3 months	Rise in erect blood pressure
Rajput and Rozdilsky (1976)	M	46	5	+	+	+		+	+	4	750*	No effect	Severe postural hypotension
Fève et al. (1977)	F	61	4	+							3 000	Marked benefit for 3 years	Dyskinesias
Spokes et al. (1979)	M	70	9	+	+	+	+	+				No effect	None
	M	49	9		+	+		+	+			No effect	None
	M	51	4	+	+	+		+	+			No effect	None
	F	53	5	+	+	+		+	+			No effect	None
Van Leuwen and Perquin (1989)	M	68	4					+		2	N/S	Modest benefit for 3 months; bromocriptine 45 mg: good response for 10 months	Severe postural hypotension

*In combination with a peripheral dopa decarboxylase inhibitor.

N/S = not stated.

Table 37.2. The therapeutic effects of L-dopa on histologically proven cases of striatonigral degeneration (± autonomic failure) from the UK–PDS Brain Bank (Fearnley and Lees 1990)

| | | | Clinical features | | | | | | | Levodopa treatment | | |
Sex	Age at onset (years)	Duration of disease (years)	Tremor	Dysarthria	Pyramidal signs	Cerebellar signs	Postural hypotension	Sphincter dysfunction (years)	Duration at onset (mg/day)	Max. dosage	Results	Adverse effects
F	64	3	+	+			+	+	1	800*	Modest benefit for 3 years	Increased postural hypotension
M	47	4			+	+		+	2	500*	Modest benefit for 2 years	On-off effects and dyskinesia
M	70	8		+				+	2	600*	Modest benefit for 5 years	Dyskinesias
F	67	5	+						2	400*	Modest benefit for 3 years	Dyskinesias
F	51	5					+	+	1	300*	Mild benefit for 3 months	—
F	49	10					+		2	400	Modest benefit for 6 months	Severe postural hypotension orofacial chorea
F	51	10	+	+	+		+		2	1200	Modest benefit for 5 years	Hypotension, visual hallucinations dyskinesia
F	64	8	+					+	3	300	No response	None
M	62	6		+			+	+	2	N/K	No response	None
M	68	2		+					1	300	No response	None

*In combination with a peripheral dopa decarboxylase inhibitor.

Among the patients treated were six with MSA and autonomic failure and 20 with a condition labelled as pure akinesia by Narabayashi. This latter syndrome consists of severe akinesia with hypotonia and freezing without tremor or rigidity, but with the late emergence of supranuclear ophthalmoplegia in some patients. No post-mortem data are as yet available, but it is possible that some of these cases may turn out to have multiple system atrophy or progressive supranuclear palsy. Of the six patients with MSA and autonomic failure, three showed a slight improvement, one was unchanged, one was worse, and one was impossible to rate.

In contrast, in the pure akinesia group, two showed marked improvement, three moderate improvement, eight slight improvement, four no change, one worsened, and two were impossible to rate. The authors concluded that two-thirds of the cases with pure akinesia were benefited, with dramatic improvement in freezing in two individuals, moderate in one and relatively slight in six. Modest pressor effects were also reported in those patients with low blood pressure before medication, and in one patient with syncope considerable functional improvement occurred. Striking antidepressant effects were also noted in a proportion of patients. A number of physicians in western Europe and the United States of America have also tried this drug on a small numbers of parkinsonian patients, with generally rather disappointing results, but it seems clear from Narabayashi's study (Narabayashi et al. 1986) that patient selection is of the utmost importance and that the drug probably only substantially benefits hypotonic freezing. The author (Lees and Bannister, unpublished observations) has given DL-threo-DOPS in doses of 1–1.5 g/day to four patients with multiple system atrophy, two of whom had marked problems with freezing. No clear benefit occurred in any of the four after treatment periods lasting up to 6 weeks. One patient went into acute retention of urine during drug therapy; another temporarily improved, but this was not maintained. No significant elevations of blood pressure were recorded. Despite these generally disappointing results, interest in L-threo-DOPS, continues both for the treatment of motor disorders and autonomic failure (Kaufmann et al. 1991). Trials of other drugs which influence noradrenergic systems, such as idazoxan and yohimbine, may also be of interest.

There has been a modest resurrection of interest in the use of amantadine in the treatment of MSA and PSP unresponsive to L-dopa. This drug is believed to have non-selective NMDA antagonist effects and Wenning et al. (1994) reported a good or excellent response to the drug in 4 of 26 patients who had been treated in series of 100 patients diagnosed as probable MSA. Colosimo and colleagues (1996), however, studied five cases of MSA who were L-dopa and apomorphine unresponsive, and at doses of amantadine up to 600 mg failed to demonstrate worthwhile benefit in an open-label study. Further double-blind trials of this drug are certainly warranted as it has been my anecdotal experience that occasional patients respond quite strikingly. None of the few MSA patients who have been inadvertently grafted with adrenal medullary or fetal material into the corpus striatum have benefited.

Treatment of cerebellar symptoms

Within the large group of 'idiopathic' late-onset cerebellar ataxia are patients with a sporadic olivopontocerebellar atrophy who have striking cerebellar signs as their major disability. Some of these patients—but by no means all—go on to develop autonomic failure and mild parkinsonism. Attempts to treat the cerebellar ataxia of multiple system degeneration have so far proved fruitless. Occasional successes have been reported with cholinergic drugs, amantadine, 5-hydroxytryptophan, isoniazid, baclofen, and propranolol; for the large majority of patients these drugs proved to be ineffective. One intriguing observation is the apparent temporary exacerbation of ataxia by cigarette smoking (Spillane 1955; Graham and Oppenheimer 1969; Johnsen and Miller 1986). The tobacco sensitivity takes the form of an acute increase in unsteadiness of gait and less commonly slurring of speech; extrapyramidal symptoms are not made worse and only one patient had increased orthostatic hypotension. Spillane injected nicotine tartrate intravenously in two of his patients, documenting changes identical to those occurring with smoking. The exact mechanism of this effect is unclear, but a direct effect on the central nervous system is more probable than a secondary effect due to autonomic changes. Nicotine is known to increase the release of acetylcholine in many areas of the brain and probably also releases noradrenaline, dopamine, 5-hydroxytryptophan, and other neurotransmitters. Nicotinic systems may therefore play a role in cerebellar function. Johnsen and Miller (1986) suggested that trials with the nicotinic antagonist, dihydro-β-erythroidine, might be worthwhile in cerebellar degenerations.

Concluding remarks

Patients with MSA presenting with a parkinsonian syndrome without severe autonomic dysfunction may respond beneficially to therapeutic doses of L-dopa, but the progression of the illness is still more rapid than that seen in Parkinson's disease. There is currently no treatment of cerebellar symptoms in MSA. However, much can be done to make the life of a patient with MSA more tolerable. This includes early referral to speech and swallowing therapists, to physiotherapists, and to occupational therapists to organize home visits and wheelchair assessments. Subcutaneous gastrostomy is necessary in many patients and botulinus toxin injections may help associated blepharospasm. Inspiratory stridor may require tracheotomy or cord lateralization procedures, and prismatic spectacles may help anterocollis.

References

Aminoff, M. J., Wilcox, C. S., Woakes, M. M., and Kremer, M. (1973). Levodopa therapy for parkinsonism in the Shy–Drager syndrome. J. Neurol. Neurosurg. Psychiat. 36, 350–3.

Bannister, R. and Oppenheimer, D. R. (1972). Degenerative diseases of the nervous system associated with autonomic failure. Brain 95, 457–74.

Ben-Shlomo, Y., Magalhaes, M. Daniel, S. E., and Quinn, N. P. (1995). Clinicopathological study of 35 cases of multiple system atrophy. J. Neurol. Neurosurg. Psychiat. 58, 160–6.

Boudin, G., Guillard, A., Mikol, J., and Galle, P. (1976). Dégénérescence striatonigrique—à propos de l'étude clinique, thérapeutique et anatomique de 2 cas. Rev. Neurol. Paris 132, 137–56.

Colosimo, C., Merello, M., and Pontieri, F. E. (1996). Amantadine in parkinsonian patients unresponsive to levodopa: a pilot study. J. Neurol. 423, 422–4.

DeLean, J. and Deck, J. H. (1976). Shy–Drager syndrome—neuropathological correlation and response to levodopa therapy. *Can. J. neurol. Sci.* 3, 167–77.

Fearnley, J. M. and Lees, A. J. (1990). Striatonigral degeneration—a clinicopathological study. *Brain* 113, 1823–42.

Feve, J., Mussini, J. N., Cler, J.-L., and Nombalais M.-F. (1977). Dégénérescence striatonigrique—étude clinique et anatomique d'un cas ayant réagi très favorablement à la L-dopa. *Rev. Neurol., Paris* 133, 271–8.

Gautier, J.-C., and Durand, J. P. (1977). Traitement des syndromes parkinsonien par la bromocriptine. *Nouv. Presse Med.* 6, (3), 171–4.

Gibb, W. R. G., and Lees, A. J. (1989). The significance of the Lewy body in the diagnosis of idiopathic Parkinson's disease. *Neuropath. Appl. Neurobiol.* 15, 27–44.

Goetz, C. G., Tanner, C. A., and Klawans, H. L. (1984). The pharmacology of olivo-ponton-cerebellar atrophy. *Adv. Neurol.* 41, 143–8.

Graham, J. G. and Oppenheimer, D. R. (1969). Orthostatic hypotension and nicotine sensitivity in a case of multiple system atrophy. *J. Neurol. Neurosurg. Psychiat.* 32, 28–34.

Greer, M., Collins, G. H., and Anton, A. H. (1971). Cerebral catecholamines after levodopa therapy. *Arch. Neurol.* 25, 461–7.

Hughes, A. J., Lees, A. J., and Stern, G. M. (1990). Apomorphine test to predict dopaminergic responsiveness in Parkinsonian syndrome. *Lancet* 335, 32–3.

Hughes, A. J., Lees, A. J., and Stern, G. M. (1991). Challenge tests to predict the dopaminergic response in untreated Parkinson's disease. *Neurology* 41, 723–5.

Hughes, A. J., Daniel, S. E., Kilford, L., and Lees A. J. (1992*a*). The accuracy of clinical diagnosis of idiopathic Parkinson's disease: a clinicopathological study of 100 cases. *J. Neurol. Neurosurg. Psychiat.* 55, 181–4.

Hughes, A. J., Colosimo, C., Kleedorfer, B., Daniel, S. E., and Lees, A. J. (1992*b*). The dopaminergic response in multiple system atrophy. *J. Neurol. Neurosurg. Psychiat.* 55, 1009–13.

Izumi, K., Inoue, N., Shirabe, T., Miyazaki, T., and Kuroiwa, Y. (1971). Failed levodopa therapy in striato-nigral degeneration. *Lancet* 1, 1355.

Johnsen, J. A. and Miller, V. T. (1986). Tobacco intolerance in multiple system atrophy. *Neurology* 36, 986–98.

Kaufmann, H., Oribe, E., and Yahr, M. D. (1991). Differential effect of 3-threo-3, 4, dihydroxyphenylserine in pure autonomic failure and multiple system atrophy with autonomic failure. *J. Neural. Transm.* 3 (2), 143–8.

Lang, A. E., Birmbaum, A., Blair, R. D. G., and Kierans, C. (1986). Levodopa dose-related fluctuations in presumed olivo-ponto-cerebellar atrophy. *Movement Disorders* 1, 93–102 .

Lees, A. J. and Bannister, R. (1981). The use of lisuride in the treatment of multiple system atrophy with autonomic failure (Shy–Drager syndrome). *J. Neurol. Neurosurg. Psychiat.* 44, 347–51.

Michel, D., Tommasi, M., Laurent, B., Trillet, M. and Schott, B. (1976). Dégénérescence striato-nigrique—à propos de 2 observations anatomocliniques. *Rev. Neurol., Paris* 132, 3–22.

Narabayashi, H., Kondo, T., Yokochi, F., and Nagatsu, T. (1986). Clinical effects of L-threo-3,4-dihydroxyphenylserine in Parkinsonism pure akinesia. *Adv. Neurol.* 45, 593–602.

Oertel, W., Gasser, T., Ippisch, R., Trenkwalder, C., and Poewe, W. H. (1989). Apomorphine test for dopaminergic responsiveness. *Lancet* ii, 1261–2.

Parati, E. A., Fetoni, V., Geminiani, G. C. *et al.* (1993). Response to L-dopa in multiple system atrophy. *Clin. Neuropharmacol.* 16, (2), 139–44.

Rajput, A., Kazi, K. A., and Rozdilsky, B. (1972). Striatonigral degeneration—response to levodopa therapy. *J. Neurol. Sci.* 16, 331–41.

Rajput, A. H. and Rozdilsky, B. (1976). Dysautonomia in Parkinsonism—a clinicopathological study. *J. Neurol. Neurosurg. Psychiat.* 39, 1092–100.

Rajput, A. H., Rozdilsky, B., Rajput, A., and Ang, L. (1990). Levodopa efficacy and pathological basis of Parkinson's syndrome. *Clin. Neuropharmacol.* 13, 553–8

Schober, R., Langston, J. W., and Forno, L. S. (1975). Idiopathic orthostatic hypotension. Biochemical and pathologic observations in 2 cases. *Eur. Neurol.* 13, 177–88.

Sharpe, J. A., Rewcastle, N.B., Lloyd, K. G., Hornykiewicz, O., Hill, M., and Tasker, R. (1973) Striatonigral degeneration response to levodopa therapy with pathological and neurochemical correlation. *J. Neurol. Sci.* 19, 275–86.

Spillane, J. D. (1955). The effect of nicotine on spinocerebellar ataxia. *BMJ* 2, 1341–51.

Spokes, E. G. S., Bannister, R., and Oppenheimer, D. R. (1979). Multiple system atrophy with autonomic failure. Clinical, bistological and neurochemical observations in 4 cases. *J. neurol. Sci.* 43, 59–82.

Staal, A., Van der Meerwaldt, J. D., Van dongen, K. J., Mulder, P. G. H., and Busch, H. F. M. (1990). Non-familial degenerative disease and atrophy of brain stem and cerebellum. *J. Neurol. Sci.* 95, 259–69.

Takei, Y. and Mirra, S. A. (1973). A form of multiple system atrophy with clinical Parkinsonism. In *Progress in neuropathology*, Vol. 2 (ed. H. M. Zimmerman), pp. 217–51. Grune & Stratton, New York.

Trotter, J. (1973). Striato-nigral degeneration. Alzheimer's disease and inflammatory changes. *Neurology* 23, 1211–16.

Van Leuwen, R. V. and Perquin, W. V. M. (1988). Bromocriptine therapy in striatonigral degeneration. *J. Neurol. Neurosurg. Psychiat.* 51, 592.

Wenning, G. K., Ben-Shlomo, Y., Magalhaes, M., Daniel, S. E., and Quinn, N. P. (1994). Clinical features and natural history of multiple system atrophy: an analysis of 100 cases. *Brain* 117, 835–45.

Wenning, G. K., Tison, F., Ben-Shlomo, Y., Daniel, S. E., and Quinn, N. P. (1997). Multiple system atrophy: a review of 203 pathologically proven cases. *Movement Disorders*, 12, 133–47.

Williams, A. C., Nutt, J., Lakes, C. R. *et al.* (1979). Actions of bromocriptine in the Shy–Drager and Steele–Richardson–Olszewski syndromes. In *Dopaminergic ergots and motor control*, (ed. K. Fuxe, and D. B. Calne), pp. 271–83. Pergamon Press, Oxford.

PART V
Peripheral Autonomic Neuropathies

38. Autonomic dysfunction in peripheral nerve disease

J. G. McLeod

Introduction

The autonomic nervous system is affected to some extent in many peripheral neuropathies, although the clinical manifestations may be mild (Table 38.1). When small-diameter myelinated and unmyelinated fibres in afferent and efferent nerves are pathologically involved by the disease process (e.g. diabetes, amyloid) or when segmental demyelination affects myelinated autonomic fibres in the vagus or sympathetic pathways (e.g. Guillain–Barré syndrome, diabetes) autonomic disturbances will be present. The clinical features of this autonomic dysfunction may range from the frequent mild impairment of sweating of the extremities to the more serious postural hypotension. The mechanisms and manifestations of autonomic dysfunction in peripheral nerve diseases are summarized in this chapter, and in a recent review (McDougall and McLeod 1996).

Histology of the autonomic nervous system

Sympathetic nervous system

The sympathetic chain, white rami, and splanchnic nerve in humans consist of myelinated and unmyelinated fibres. The fibre diameter distribution of myelinated fibres is similar in all three nerves. Most of the fibres are in the range 2–6 μm but there is another distinct group of larger fibres with a peak at about 12 μm; the larger myelinated fibres and some of the smaller fibres are afferent. Internodal lengths in the sympathetic chain and in the white rami are shorter in relation to fibre diameter than those in the peripheral nervous system (Fig. 38.1). Morphometric analysis of the preganglionic neurones in the human spinal cord and of the sympathetic preganglionic fibres in the ventral roots has shown that the preganglionic fibres range in diameter from 1.5 to 4.7 μm with a peak at 2.5 μm. There is progressive reduction of numbers of both cells and fibres with age.

Parasympathetic nervous system

In the human cervical vagus nerve only a small proportion (about 20 per cent) of the afferent and efferent fibres are myelinated and most of these are 3 μm or less in diameter. The carotid sinus nerve has been studied in different animal species including man and contains myelinated fibres which range in diameter from 2 to 14 μm, most of these being in the 2–5 μm diameter range; it also contains many unmyelinated fibres. Afferent fibres from the aortic arch receptors are both myelinated and unmyelinated; the myelinated fibres in the cat range from 2 to 10 μm, although most are in the 2–6 μm range.

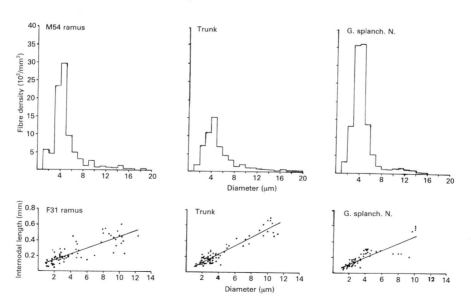

Fig. 38.1. Control subjects. (Above) diameter distribution of myelinated fibres in white ramus, sympathetic trunk, and greater splanchnic nerve. (Below) relationship between internodal length and diameter of myelinated fibres in white ramus, trunk and greater splanchnic nerve. (From McLeod (1980).)

Table 38.1. Causes of peripheral autonomic neuropathy

Acute autonomic neuropathy
  Acute idiopathic autonomic neuropathy
    Acute pandysautonomia
    Acute noradrenergic autonomic neuropathy
    Acute cholinergic neuropathy
  Acute paraneoplastic autononomic neuropathy
  Botulism
  Guillain–Barré syndrome
  Porphyria
  Drug-induced autonomic neuropathies
    Vincristine
    Cisplatin
    Taxol
    Amiodarone
    Pethexiline
  Toxic
    Heavy metals
    Organic solvents
    Hexacarbons
    Acrylamide
    Vacor
    Organophosphous canpounds

Chronic autonomic neuropathy
  Clinically important
    Diabetes
    Amyloidosis (primary amyloidosis, familial amyloid neuropathy
      type I)
    Hereditary sensory and autonomic neuropathy
      Familial dysautonomia (Riley-Day syndrome, HSAN type III)
      Swanson type (HSAN IV)
  Minor clinical importance
    Hereditary neuropathies
      Charcot–Marie–Tooth disease
      Hereditary sensory and autonomic neuropathy (HSAN type I, II)
      Fabry's disease
      Adrenomyeloneuropathy
      Navajo neuropathy
      Amyloidosis (some familial amyloid neuropathic and secondary
        amyloidosis)
    Chronic inflammatory demyelinating polyradiculoneuropathy (CIDP)
      Metabolic and nutritional disorders
      Chronic renal failure
      Chronic liver disease
      Vitamin B_{12} deficiency
      Alcoholism and nutritional disorders
    Connective tissue diseases
      Rheumatoid arthritis
      Systemic lupus erythematosus
      Mixed connective tissue disease
      Sjögren's syndrome
    Infection
      Leprosy
      HIV
      Chagas' disease
      Diphtheria
    Other systemic disorders
      Inflammatory bowel disease
      Chronic lung disease
      Multiple symmetrical lipomatosis (Madelung's)
      Amyotrophic lateral sclerosis

Manifestations of autonomic dysfunction in peripheral nerve diseases

Impaired sweating of the extremities is common and probably results from degeneration of cholinergic postganglionic sympathetic unmyelinated fibres that travel with the peripheral nerves to innervate sweat glands, or to degeneration or demyelination of preganglionic sympathetic efferent fibres. Hyperhidrosis may be seen in partial nerve injuries associated with causalgia, some toxic neuropathies, or when there is pressure on the nerve roots such as that which occurs in malignancy. When sweating is impaired in the extremities, excessive compensatory sweating may occur on trunk and face.

Orthostatic postural hypotension results from damage to the small-diameter myelinated and unmyelinated fibres in afferent and efferent nerves in the baroreflex pathways and in the splanchnic outflow. Postural hypotension is therefore most commonly seen in diseases such as diabetes and amyloidosis, in which the small fibres degenerate, and in the Guillain–Barré syndrome, in which segmental demyelination affects the myelinated autonomic fibres in the vagus and sympathetic pathways. It is more likely to occur when fibres in the splanchnic vascular bed are pathologically involved since the latter plays an important part in human blood pressure regulation. Orthostatic hypotension is uncommon in dying-back neuropathies which initially affect predominantly the large-diameter fibres of the longest nerves. Impaired heart rate control results from vagal impairment in patients with autonomic neuropathy, particularly diabetes. Bladder dysfunction, impotence, and pupillary abnormalities are other clinical manifestations of autonomic dysfunction in peripheral nerve disease.

Investigation of autonomic dysfunction in peripheral nerve diseases

The physiological and pharmacological tests of autonomic function in peripheral nerve disease are described in Chapter 20 of this volume. Biopsy techniques are not widely used in the investigation of autonomic function but have provided useful information in some conditions. In peripheral autonomic failure, such as due to diabetes, amyloidosis, chronic alcoholism, and the inflammatory neuropathies, the findings on sural nerve biopsy generally reflect the changes in the autonomic nervous system. In some cases, biopsy of the vagus or sympathetic nerves at abdominal operations has shown characteristic degenerative changes and has increased the understanding of the pathophysiology of some autonomic neuropathies. Rectal biopsy may demonstrate degenerative changes in the myenteric plexus but is rarely diagnostic. Skin biopsy may demonstrate reduction in the number of sweat glands. Muscle biopsy studied with histochemical techniques may demonstrate absence of catecholamine fluorescence in perivascular nerves in pure autonomic failure. In general, biopsy techniques have little place in the investigation of peripheral autonomic failure but in selected cases have been helpful research tools.

Acute autonomic neuropathies

Acute and subacute idiopathic autonomic neuropathy

Young and colleagues (1969) were the first to describe a definite entity of pure pandysautonomia involving both sympathetic and parasympathetic nervous systems with a subacute onset, monophasic course, and partial recovery without significant features of somatic peripheral neuropathy. There had been some earlier reports of the condition in the literature although it was not clearly defined. The disorder differs from other neurological causes of autonomic dysfunction in that normal function of the central nervous system is preserved and there are no, or only minor, features of peripheral somatic nervous system involvement. Since these first reports, a number of other patients with acute pandysautonomia have been described, as well as some cases of pure cholinergic dysautonomia. Some cases have been reported of acute dysautonomia with significant sensory disturbances; in some, but not all, of which there is electrophysiological and pathological evidence of loss of small diameter myelinated and unmyelinated fibres.

Suarez and colleagues (1994) have clarified the features of acute idiopathic autonomic neuropathy by performing clinical, neurophysiological, and follow-up studies on 27 patients at the Mayo Clinic. There is a spectrum of autonomic and somatic features, which range from pure pandysautonomia to selective noradrenergic or cholinergic failure with varying degrees of somatic nerve involvement.

Both sexes and all ages can be affected. The onset is acute or subacute and there is an antecedent viral infection in approximately one-half of the patients. Several cases have been described that follow Epstein–Barr virus (EBV) infection, in one of which EBV DNA and antibody to EBV were found in the CSF (Bennett et al. 1996). The most common presenting symptoms are orthostatic hypotension (light-headedness, dizziness, syncope), gastrointestinal (nausea, vomiting, diarrhoea, constipation, and postprandial bloating), and sudomotor (failure to sweat causing heat intolerance and flushing). Other symptoms include numbness, tingling, bladder disturbances, and impotence. Neurological examination was normal in about half the patients, the remainder having depressed reflexes and distal sensory impairment. The clinical course is monophasic and recovery is gradual and often incomplete. The CSF protein may be mildly elevated. Nerve conduction studies are normal in most cases but rarely there may be evidence of sensory neuropathy. Sural nerve biopsy in some cases has shown reduction of myelinated fibre density, predominantly of small fibres, and axonal degeneration. Autonomic function studies have demonstrated orthostatic hypotension, decreased Valsalva ratio, impaired thermoregulatory sweat tests and QSART, and normal supine noradrenaline with reduction of the expected rise on standing.

The cause of the condition remains uncertain but it is probably a form of acute idiopathic polyneuritis restricted to autonomic nerves with an immune-mediated pathogenesis similar to that of the Guillain–Barré syndrome.

The differential diagnosis includes botulism, acute autonomic neuropathy associated with Guillain–Barré syndrome, porphyria, diabetes, toxic causes, systemic lupus erythematosus, and other connective tissue diseases.

Sympathomimetic drugs and 9–α-fluorohydrocortisone have been of value in treating postural hypotension in cases of pandysautonomia. Corticosteroids are frequently used and plasmapheresis and intravenous immunoglobulin may be effective (Heafield et al. 1996; Smit et al. 1997).

Acute cholinergic neuropathy

A number of cases of pure cholinergic dysautonomia have been reported in children. Symptoms consist of blurred vision, impaired lacrimation, dry mouth, constipation, urinary retention and incontinence, and absence of sweating, but there is no postural hypotension. In the early stages of the illness, excessive salivation and sweat secretion have been reported. CSF findings are normal. Carbachol may be helpful for the management of urinary retention and impaired gastrointestinal motility.

Acute paraneoplastic autonomic neuropathy

Acute pandysautonomia may be seen as a paraneoplastic manifestation of carcinoma of the lung, lymphoma, and other malignancies. It may precede the diagnosis of the malignancy by several months. It is usually progressive, but may remit following treatment of the malignancy.

Not all paraneoplastic autonomic neuropathies are acute. Subclinical autonomic neuropathy is relatively common in lymphomas and other forms of malignancy and may also occur in paraneoplastic sensory neuropathy.

Autonomic dysfunction is present in about three-quarters of the cases of Lambert–Eaton syndrome. Autonomic symptoms indicative of cholinergic failure predominate, such as dry mouth, impaired lacrimation, sweating, impotence, constipation, and postural hypotension.

Paraneoplastic visceral neuropathy may be seen in small cell lung carcinoma and other malignancies. Symptoms of gastrointestinal pseudo-obstruction, such as progressive constipation, abdominal pain, and vomiting usually precede the diagnosis of the tumour. The pathological changes are loss of the myenteric plexus neurones, secondary axonal degeneration, and lymphocytic inflammatory cell infiltrates (Lennon et al. 1991).

Botulism

Botulism is characterized by the acute onset of ptosis, extraocular, facial and bulbar palsies, and sometimes generalized neuromuscular paralysis associated with cholinergic failure. Gastrointestinal symptoms of constipation and paralytic ileus are common and there may also be urinary retention and anhidrosis since the toxin, most commonly produced by the type B strain of Clostridium botulinum, impairs the release of acetylcholine from nerve terminals. The electrophysiological features are similar to those seen in the Lambert–Eaton syndrome. An acute cholinergic syndrome may be present without associated muscle weakness, in which circumstance the condition may be difficult to distinguish clinically from acute cholinergic neuropathy.

Acute inflammatory neuropathy (Guillain–Barré syndrome)

Disturbances of autonomic function are well recognized in the Guillain–Barré syndrome (Zochodne 1994). Tachycardia, which may remain fixed and unresponsive to postural change, has been reported

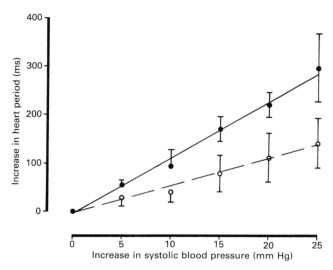

Fig. 38.2. Relationship of increase in heart period to increase in systolic blood pressure in control subjects (closed circles) and in patients with Guillain–Barré syndrome (open circles) following intravenous phenylephrine. Vertical bars represent ± 1SE. (From Tuck and McLeod (1982).)

by a number of workers. Urinary retention and incontinence, constipation, gastric paresis, paralytic ileus, and sexual dysfunction can occur in approximately 10 per cent of patients and bradycardia, asystole, and arrhythmia may also be complications. Elevated or fluctuating arterial blood pressure has been documented, as well as postural hypotension.

There are frequently abnormalities of the heart rate and of the blood pressure response to the Valsalva manoeuvre. The heart rate response to elevated arterial blood pressure induced by intravenous injection of phenylephrine may be impaired (Fig. 38.2) and the sweat test is commonly abnormal (Fig. 38.3). The abnormalities of autonomic function are variable and depend upon the site of the demyelinating lesions, which may be present in the afferent fibres in the vagus and glossopharyngeal nerves, in the arterial baroreceptors, in the efferent parasympathetic fibres in the vagus nerves, and in the sympathetic nerves that innervate the heart and control sweating and vasomotor tone. Pathological studies have demonstrated demyelinating lesions in the glossopharyngeal and vagus nerves and in the sympathetic chains and white rami. The severity of the involvement of the autonomic nervous system does not appear to be related to the degree of motor or sensory disturbance. In most patients the consequences of involvement of the autonomic nervous system are not serious, but on some occasions they can be life-threatening. Postural hypotension may lead to syncope and irreversible brain damage in a paralysed patient who is inadvertently left in a sitting position or who requires an anaesthetic; sudden death due to cardiac arrhythmias or to asystole may also occur.

Porphyria

Postural hypotension may occur in acute intermittent and variegate porphyria, although hypertension is more common and may precede the manifestation of peripheral neuropathy. Persistent tachycardia may be an early feature of an attack and may also precede the onset of

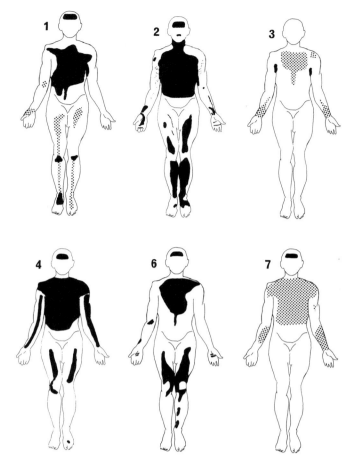

Fig. 38.3. Patterns of sweating in Guillain–Barré syndrome. Black areas indicated regions of normal sweat production; spotted areas are those in which sweating was patchy. (From Tuck and McLeod (1982).)

neuropathy. Other clinical features of autonomic neuropathy include abdominal pain, nausea and vomiting, constipation, diarrhoea, bladder distension, and disorders of sweating. Autonomic function studies have demonstrated abnormalities of sympathetic and parasympathetic function. There is pathological evidence of involvement of brainstem and spinal-cord cells and vagus and sympathetic nerves.

Drug-induced acute autonomic neuropathies

Most drugs that affect the peripheral autonomic nervous system cause an acute or subacute neuropathy but sometimes the onset may be more insidious.

Vincristine

The vinca alkaloids are cytotoxic drugs used in the treatment of lymphoma, leukaemia, and some other malignancies. Vincristine, and occasionally vinblastine, cause peripheral neuropathy, the predominant pathological change in the peripheral nerve being axonal degeneration. Postural hypotension has been reported as a neurotoxic side-effect of vincristine, and constipation, abdominal pain, paralytic ileus, urinary retention, and other bladder disturbances are well-recognized complications. Published accounts of autonomic function studies in patients with vincristine-induced autonomic neuropathy are limited but have demonstrated abnormalities of postganglionic sympathetic efferent function and abnormal Valsalva responses in patients with postural hypotension. The sympathetic nerves and ganglia were normal in two cases in whom autopsy material was examined pathologically.

Autonomic dysfunction may develop within days of commencement of vincristine therapy. The mechanism of action is not clear, although there is some evidence in humans and other animals that the primary site of damage is the unmyelinated noradrenergic fibres of the sympathetic nervous system. However, the symptoms in humans of constipation, paralytic ileus, and bladder disturbances indicate that parasympathetic fibres are also affected. Ultrastructurally, vinca alkaloids disrupt microtubules and cause an increase in the neurofilaments and the appearance of paracrystalline structures in axons. Unmyelinated fibres are more susceptible to the neurotoxin than myelinated fibres.

Cisplatin

Cisplatin is a cytotoxic agent with dose-related neurotoxic side-effects such as peripheral neuropathy, retrobulbar neuritis, and ototoxicity. An autonomic neuropathy with postural hypotension may be associated with these abnormalities (Rosenfeld and Broder 1984).

Taxol

This antineoplastic drug disrupts microtubule assembly, causing peripheral sensory neuropathy as one of its dose-limiting side-effects. It may cause an autonomic neuropathy (Jerian *et al.* 1993).

Amiodarone

Amiodarone, an antiarrhymthic agent, causes a sensorimotor neuropathy in about 10 per cent of patients. Autonomic failure with postural hypotension has been reported.

Perhexiline

Perhexiline maleate may cause a peripheral neuropathy. Some patients may also develop an autonomic neuropathy with postural hypotension and an abnormal Valsalva ratio.

Toxic causes

Heavy metals

There have been very few cases of heavy metal poisoning in which autonomic function has been adequately studied. In thallium poisoning, tachyardia and hypertension have been reported in association with peripheral neuropathy. In arsenical poisoning, excessive sweating and impairment of sweating on the extremities have been described. Subacute or chronic inorganic mercury poisoning is the cause of acrodynia, which occurs mainly in children and includes amongst its manifestations tachycardia, hypertension, and profuse sweating.

Organic solvents

Autonomic function has been shown to be disturbed in some workers who had experienced prolonged chronic occupational expo-

sure to a variety of organic solvents containing mainly aliphatic, aromatic, and other hydrocarbons, alcohols, ketones, esters, and ethers as well as to carbon disulphide and toluene. They had significant impairment of heart rate variation, respiration, and Valsalva ratio compared to controls. The most severely affected patients were those exposed to carbon disulphide. Some of the patients had clinical and electrophysiological evidence of peripheral neuropathy (Matikainen and Juntunen 1985).

Hexacarbons

Hexacarbon neuropathy may follow industrial exposure or inhalatant abuse. Inhalation of *n*-hexane and methyl-*n*-butyl-ketone may result in a rapidly progressive polyneuropathy associated with autonomic features of excessive or impaired sweating on the extremities, postural hypotension, and impotence.

Acrylamide

Acrylamide is neurotoxic in the soluble monomeric form in which it is manufactured and distributed. After transformation to a polymer it is used in industry as a flocculator for separating solids from aqueous solutions. It is also used in the preparation of grouts for the sealing of pipes and subterranean tunnels. The major toxic effect in man is a predominantly sensory polyneuropathy, often preceded by blueness and excessive sweating of the extremities due to a disturbance of sympathetic function. Other human autonomic disturbances are rarely seen, although they have been studied extensively in experimental animals.

Vacor

Vacor (*N*-3-peridylmethyl-*N*-*p*-nitraphenylurea) is a rodenticide that antagonizes nicotinamide metabolism. Accidental or deliberate ingestion results in acute hyperglycaemic ketoacidosis and an autonomic and somatic peripheral neuropathy. Autonomic manifestations include postural hypotension and gastrointestinal hypomotility.

Organophosphorus compounds

Organophosphorus esters are used as insecticides, petroleum additives and modifiers of plastic. They are acetylcholinesterase inhibitors that can cause acute cholinergic symptoms, usually within hours of exposure consisting of diarrhoea, vomiting, irritability, nervousness, fatigue, lethargy, impaired memory and other behavioural changes. There may be a delayed peripheral neuropathy most commonly seen after poisoning with tri-ortho-cresyl phosphate (TOCP) intoxication in which there is a distal axonopathy affecting both central and peripheral nervous system fibres. Epidemics of TOCP intoxication have occurred in a number of countries due to contamination of cooking oils with mineral oil containing TOCP. The peripheral neuropathy usually develops 7 to 21 days after the acute intoxication and symptoms include calf pain, paraesthesiae, weakness and muscle wasting. Pyramidal tract signs are frequently present. Autonomic dysfunction is not a significant feature of the delayed polyneuropathy.

In addition to TOCP other organophosphorus compounds known to cause distal axonopathy include leptophos, mipafox, chlorphos and trichlorfon. Some others have been shown to induce peripheral neuropathy in experimental animals (Schaumburg and Berger 1993).

Chronic autonomic neuropathies

The autonomic nervous system is affected in many peripheral neuropathies, although the clinical manifestations may be mild. Autonomic dysfunction is clinically important in the neuropathies associated with diabetes, amyloid disease, porphyria, Guillain–Barré syndrome, and some cases of hereditary sensory neuropathy, particularly the Riley–Day syndrome. In most of the other conditions it is usually of only minor clinical importance.

Clinically important chronic autonomic neuropathies

Diabetes

Autonomic neuropathies are commonly associated with diabetic peripheral neuropathy in which degenerative change can be demonstrated in the peripheral autonomic nerves. It is considered in detail in Chapter 39.

Amyloid neuropathy

The types most frequently complicated by autonomic dysfunction are primary amyloidosis and the Portuguese type of familial amyloid polyneuropathy (FAP type I). Autonomic dysfunction is much less common in FAP II (Indiana type), FAP III (Iowa type), and FAP IV (Finnish type) See Chapter 42).

Autonomic dysfunction is attributable to predominant loss of unmyelinated and small myelinated fibres in the peripheral autonomic nerves and reduction in the number of cells in the intermediolateral columns. Widespread deposition of amyloid in the autonomic nerves and ganglia has been seen frequently (Fig. 38.4).

Familial dysautonomia

Riley–Day syndrome, hereditary sensory and autonomic neuropathy (HSAN) type III), see Chapter 41.

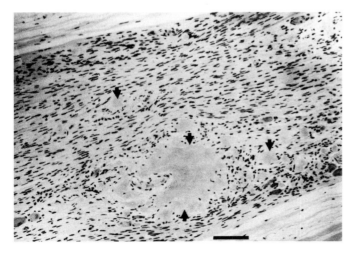

Fig. 38.4. Amyloid deposits (arrows) in thoracic sympathetic trunk of a patient with primary amyloidosis. Bar, 100 μm.

Autonomic neuropathies of minor clinical importance

Hereditary neuropathies

Charcot–Marie–Tooth disease (hereditary motor and sensory neuropathies (HMSN) types I and II)

Autonomic function has been investigated in Charcot–Marie–Tooth disease by a number of workers, with conflicting results. There is general agreement that pupillary reflexes may be abnormal and that there is impairment of sweating distally. There are only minor or no abnormalities of cardiovascular reflexes in patients with HMSN types I and II. The impairment of sweating is most probably caused by distal degeneration of postganglionic sympathetic fibres and is consistent with the hypothesis that HMSN results from neuronal atrophy, the extremities of the nerve cell being affected first and most severely.

Hereditary sensory and autonomic neuropathies, type I and II

There is impairment of sweating, but no cardiovascular autonomic dysfunctions.

Fabry's disease

Fabry's disease is an X-linked disorder with deficiency of the enzyme α-galactosidase A, causing accumulation of glycolipids, particularly ceramide trihexose. Glycolipid accumulation is found in autonomic neurones and there is loss of unmyelinated and small myelinated fibres. The principal clinical features are painful neuropathy in young boys associated with angiokeratoma of the skin. Autonomic symptoms include impaired sweating leading to complete anhidrosis, gastrointestinal dysfunction with indigestion, nausea, belching, oesophageal reflux, abdominal pain, flatus, and diarrhoea. Autonomic tests reveal pupillary abnormalities, abnormal tear and saliva production, widespread anhidrosis, reduced cutaneous flare response for scratch and intradermal histamine, and abnormal colonic motility. Cardiovascular autonomic tests are normal.

Adrenomyeloneuropathy

Postural hypotension has been reported in adrenomyeloneuropathy; this may result from adrenal insufficiency.

Navajo neuropathy

This neuropathy presents in Navajo Indians in the first 5 years of life, with corneal ulceration, infections, liver disease, and failure to thrive. Sensorimotor neuropathy is characterized by pathological changes of loss of large- and small-diameter fibres. The condition is progressive and patients become wheelchair-bound and die usually before the age of 25. Autonomic manifestations of anhidrosis and heat intolerance tend to be overshadowed by the mutilating neuropathy (Appenzeller and Oribe 1990).

Chronic inflammatory demyelinating polyradiculoneuropathy (CIDP)

In chronic inflammatory demyelinating polyradiculoneuropathy, postural hypotension and other symptoms of autonomic nervous system dysfunction are uncommon (Ingall et al. 1990). These findings are in contrast to those in acute inflammatory neuropathy, in which the more severe disturbances of autonomic function are presumed to be related to acute conduction block and possibly more extensive involvement of unmyelinated fibres in the acute stages.

Metabolic and nutritional disorders

These include diabetes (see Chapter 39), porphyria, and a number of conditions as described below.

Chronic renal failure

Impairment of autonomic function occurs in both predialysis and haemodialysis patients. There is a significant association between the degree of autonomic dysfunction and impairment of nerve conduction (Wang *et al.* 1994).

Parasympathetic cardiovascular abnormalities, such as variation in the RR interval, are more common than sympathetic abnormalities, such as postural hypotension and abnormalities of the sympathetic skin response. Impaired baroreflex function is also reported. In some patients hypotension may occur during haemodialysis. These patients have normal sympathetic efferent function but impaired baroreflex sensitivity. There may be factors other than autonomic neuropathy contributing to the severe hypotension in these patients. Renal transplantation may result in improvement of the autonomic abnormalities.

Chronic liver disease

Cardiovascular autonomic dysfunction occurs in both alcoholic and non-alcoholic chronic liver disease, the latter including chronic hepatitis and primary biliary cirrhosis. In non-alcoholic chronic liver disease parasympathetic abnormalities are more common (45 per cent of patients) than sympathetic changes (12 per cent). Patients may have abnormal autonomic function without evidence of a peripheral neuropathy. The prevalence and severity of cardiovascular autonomic dysfunction is related to the severity of hepatic damage and is independent of aetiology. The presence of autonomic neuropathy is associated with a worse long-term prognosis. The mechanism of autonomic neuropathy in chronic liver disease remains uncertain but is most likely due to damage of the peripheral autonomic nervous system resulting from nutritional and metabolic disturbances consequent upon hepatic failure, or, alternatively, due to immunoglobulin or immune complex deposition.

Vitamin B$_{12}$ deficiency

Orthostatic hypotension may rarely be the initial manifestation of pernicious anaemia. It usually responds well to replacement therapy. The pathological findings in the peripheral neuropathy of vitamin B$_{12}$ deficiency are those of axonal degeneration but this alone is unlikely to cause postural hypotension which may possibly be due to some central mechanism.

Alcoholism and nutritional disorders

Clinical manifestations of autonomic dysfunction, except for impaired sweating distally, are unusual in uncomplicated alcoholic peripheral neuropathy. Postural hypotension may occur in severely affected cases or in Wernicke's encephalopathy which is associated with central abnormalities of autonomic control. Abnormalities of cardiovascular parasympathetic tests are common but cardiovascular and sympathetic changes are much less frequent (Monforte *et al.* 1995).

Alcoholic neuropathy is a dying back neuropathy so that the distal part of the long vagal fibres of the heart are affected before the short sympathetic fibres to the splanchnic and other blood vessels. There is significant reduction in the density of myelinated fibres in the distal parts of the vagus (Fig. 38.5) and carotid sinus nerves and relative sparing of the splanchnic nerves. There is a significant relationship between the estimated total lifetime of consumption and parasympa-

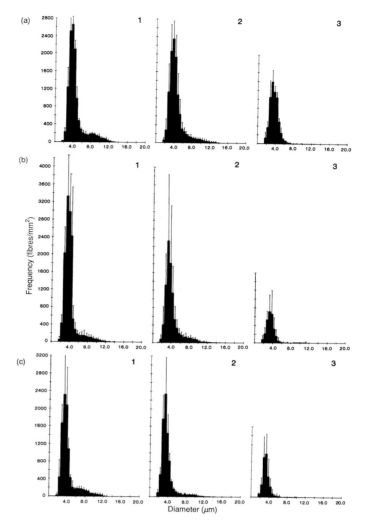

Fig. 38.5. Mean myelinated fibre density distribution of vagus nerves from: (a) controls; (b) diabetics; and (c) alcoholics at (1) midcervical; (2) lung hilum; and (3) diaphragm levels. Bars indicate one standard deviation from mean. (From Guo *et al.* (1987).)

thetic abnormalities, and there is a correlation between abnormalities of autonomic function and sensory conduction in peripheral nerves (Monforte *et al.* 1995).

Connective tissue disorders

Rheumatoid arthritis

Impairment of sweating on the extremities is relatively common in rheumatoid arthritis and is probably related in most cases to damage to postganglionic sympathetic efferent fibres in the peripheral nerves. In addition, there may be vagus nerve involvement since the heart rate response to standing, to the Valsalva manoeuvre, and to respiration may be impaired, particularly in patients with peripheral neuropathy. Rarely, autonomic neuropathy may be secondary to amyloidosis.

Systemic lupus erythematosus and mixed connective tissue diseases

Autonomic neuropathy has been reported as a complication of systemic lupus erythematosus and mixed connective tissue diseases.

Sjögren's syndrome

Autonomic neuropathy is present in patients with sensory neuropathy of Sjögren's syndrome. There is impairment of sweating due to postganglionic involvement of sympathetic fibres. Salivation is impaired and cardiac parasympathetic function is also affected (Low et al. 1988).

Infections

Leprosy

Leprosy, one of the most common causes of peripheral neuropathy, may be associated with autonomic disturbances. Loss of sweating over the skin supplied by the diseased nerves is the usual finding but, in addition, cardiac denervation, postural hypotension, decreased sweating, and impaired response to the cold pressor test, even in the absence of other features of peripheral neuropathy, have been described. Abnormalities of cardiovascular parasympathetic tests are more common and occur earlier in the illness than those of cardiovascular sympathetic tests. The severity of the autonomic dysfunction is related to the duration of the disease. Abnormalities of fingertip vasomotor reflex tests, measured with a laser Doppler flowmeter, may be an early indication of nerve damage (Beck et al. 1991).

HIV

Autonomic dysfunction is a common complication of HIV infection. The most prominent symptoms are syncope, impotence, bladder and bowel dysfunction, and anhidrosis. Abnormalities of autonomic function tests may be found in the early stage of the illness, but are more common and more severe in patients with AIDS, up to 80 per cent of this group having abnormalities (Freeman et al. 1990; Ruttimann et al. 1991).

The mechanism of autonomic dysfunction in HIV infection is uncertain. It is associated with widespread changes in the central and peripheral nervous system and the abnormalities of autonomic tests do not correlate with the presence of a peripheral somatic neuropathy. HIV-1 antigens are present in the sensory and sympathetic ganglia even when there is no peripheral evidence of peripheral nerve disease. The effects of antiretroviral therapy on HIV-associated autonomic dysfunction have not been studied systematically.

Chagas' disease

Chagas' disease is caused by infection with the protozoal parasite Trypanosoma cruzi, and is widespread in Latin America, with at least 20 million people being affected (Fernandez et al. 1992). Autonomic nervous system abnormalities, particularly those affecting the gastrointestinal tract and heart, occur in the chronic phase in the infection. There is destruction of autonomic ganglia and enteric plexus neurones throughout the digestive tract. In the heart there are pathological changes in the myocardium and conducting system as well as in autonomic ganglia and postganglionic neurones. The neuronal damage is thought to be due to a cell-mediated, delayed-type, hypersensitive immune response (Fernandez et al. 1992). Autonomic manifestations include prominent gastrointestinal motility dysfunction with dysphagia, achalasia, aperistalsis, megaoesophagus, constipation, intestinal volvulus, and megacolon. Cardiovascular autonomic changes include cardiac arrhythmias, sudden death and postural hypotension. There is ocular involvement, with parasympathetic denervation of the iris (Idiaquez 1992). Autonomic function tests show widespread abnormalities of cardiovascular reflex control.

Diphtheria

Diphtheria results in a demyelinating motor polyneuropathy in about 20 per cent of cases. The presence of parasympathetic cardiovascular reflex dysfunction may explain how tachycardia can occur in the absence of myocarditis in some cases (Solders et al. 1989). The severity of parasympathetic abnormalities may not be closely related to the severity of peripheral nerve damage. Sympathetic abnormalities have not been reported.

Other systemic disorders

Inflammatory bowel disease

Abnormalities of cardiovascular autonomic function tests have been found in a large proportion of patients with Crohn's disease and ulcerative colitis. The autonomic abnormalities do not correlate well with the severity, duration, or treatment of the bowel disease or the presence of a peripheral somatic neuropathy (Lindgren et al. 1991, 1993).

Chronic lung disease

Patients with hypoxaemic chronic obstructive pulmonary disease have some clinical abnormalities in parasympathetic cardiovascular autonomic function tests and tests of sudomotor function; sympathetic cardiovascular autonomic tests are spared (Stewart et al. 1991, 1994). It has been proposed that intraneural hypoxia may be the pathogenic mechanism for these changes.

Multiple symmetrical lipomatosis (Madelung's disease)

The characteristic feature of this condition is the formation of large symmetrical subcutaneous fat masses and the deep accumulation of adipose tissue, associated with metabolic abnormalities of adipose tissue. A peripheral sensorimotor neuropathy of variable severity is part of the condition. Autonomic symptoms include gustatory sweating, hyperhidrosis of the feet, impotence, and resting tachycardia. Abnormal cardiovascular autonomic function tests are found in most affected patients (Enzi et al. 1986).

Amyotrophic lateral sclerosis (motor neurone disease)

Symptoms of disturbed autonomic function are rare in amyotrophic lateral sclerosis but abnormal autonomic tests have been described by a number of workers in up to 40 per cent of patients (Litchy et al. 1987) and abnormal vasomotor responses causing hypertension after drug administration have been reported (Shimizu et al. 1996). The mechanism of the abnormalities of autonomic function is not clear but abnormalities in the axons to dermal vessels and sweat glands, and ultrastructural abnormalities in the sweat glands, have been reported (Provinciali et al. 1994).

Experimental autonomic neuropathy

Autonomic neuropathy has been induced in experimental animals in order to study its pathophysiology in greater detail than is possible in man. A number of different methods have been employed for inducing experimental autonomic neuropathy, including sympathectomy with 6–hydroxydopamine, nerve growth factor antiserum, and guanethidine; experimental allergic neuritis; injection of extracts of sympathetic chain; acrylamide; and diabetes.

6-hydroxydopamine sympathectomy

6-Hydroxydopamine (6-OHDA) causes selective destruction of peripheral adrenergic nerve terminals. Its effect on mesenteric vascular control was studied in cats. There was no clinical or electrophysiological evidence of peripheral neuropathy in the animals but studies of mesenteric blood flow demonstrated that neural control of the mesenteric vascular bed was abnormal. There was denervation supersensitivity to noradrenaline and phenylephrine, there was no response to intravenous tyramine, and there was a markedly impaired vasoconstrictor response to electrical stimulation of the splanchnic nerve. No morphological changes were demonstrated in the posterior tibial or splanchnic nerves. 6-OHDA therefore produces a chemical sympathectomy in animals, resulting in impaired vasomotor control, but there does not appear to be any precise counterpart in humans of the sympathetic failure seen in these animals.

Nerve growth factor antiserum

Nerve growth factor antiserum induces immunosympathectomy by causing degeneration of sympathetic ganglion cells and other postganglionic fibres. It results in impaired vasoconstriction and blood pressure control. There is no precise counterpart in humans of this experimental autonomic neuropathy.

Guanethidine-induced sympathectomy

Guanethidine causes degeneration of postganglionic sympathetic nerves. Rats treated with guanethidine have low arterial blood pressure, ptosis, loss of neurones in the cervical sympathetic ganglia, and a decreased C-fibre action potential in the cervical sympathetic trunk, while normal function is preserved in somatic and vagus nerves (Zochodne et al. 1988).

Autoimmune preganglionic sympathectomy

Injection of monoclonal antibodies to neural acetylcholinesterase in adult rats caused destruction of presynaptic fibres in sympathetic ganglia and the adrenal medulla. The animals develop ptosis, hypotension, bradycardia, and postural syncope. There is failure of ganglionic transmission when preganglionic fibres are stimulated, but there is a normal response on direct ganglionic stimulation. The preganglonic terminals are inactivated but postganglionic neurones remain intact. Parasympathetic function and motor function are normal. Morphological and histochemical studies demonstrate depleted presynaptic aceylcholinesterase and loss of presynaptic terminals with preservation of the ganglion cells. This example of preganglionic immunosympathectomy in rats may be a useful model for studying some forms of human autonomic failure (Brimijoin and Lennon 1990).

Experimental immune autonomic neuropathy

Appenzeller and colleagues (1965) sensitized rabbits with antigen extracted from human sympathetic nerves and ganglia. Although the animals were not clinically ill, they had impaired reflex vasodilatation of the ear vessels. The defect in reflex vasomotor function was attributed to involvement of efferent sympathetic cholinergic fibres. Basophils were abundant in the perivascular spaces of the ear vessels in the immunized animals but there were no abnormalities detected histologically in the sympathetic nervous system, although morphometric studies suggested regeneration of unmyelinated fibres.

Experimental allergic neuritis

Autonomic function has been studied in several animals species with experimental allergic neuritis (EAN) (Tuck et al. 1981; Morey et al. 1985). Slowed conduction and dispersion of the compound action potential were demonstrated in the splanchnic and vagus nerves of guinea pigs, and light and electron microscopy confirmed the presence of demyelination. In some animals unmyelinated fibres were also damaged. In the Lewis rat the pathological changes were mainly in the vagus nerves. Since the clinical, histopathological, and electrophysiological features of EAN and the Guillain–Barré syndrome are similar, the findings are relevant to the pathogenesis of autonomic dysfunction in the Guillain–Barré syndrome.

Acrylamide neuropathy

Acrylamide causes a distal symmetrical axonal neuropathy in man and animals. The autonomic nervous system has been studied in animals with acrylamide neuropathy in order to help understand the pathophysiology of autonomic degeneration in the common peripheral neuropathies in which axonal degeneration is the underlying pathological abnormality (e.g. alcoholic, nutritional, and toxic neuropathies). Comparison of the histological changes in the peripheral, somatic, and autonomic nerves of cats demonstrated that the longest fibres were the most profoundly damaged: the peripheral somatic nerves were more severely affected than the autonomic nerves, and the vagus nerves showed greater degrees of fibre loss than the shorter splanchnic nerves. Vasomotor control of the mesenteric vascular bed was impaired in the more severely affected animals. The findings are consistent with the clinical observations in alcoholic and other dying-back neuropathies that the earliest autonomic abnormalities are those of vagal function and that postural hypotension occurs only in the more severe peripheral neuropathies when the splanchnic nerves are likely to be involved.

Studies of baroreflexes in animals with acrylamide neuropathy have shown that aortic arch baroreceptors, innervated by the vagus nerve, are more affected than the carotid sinus baroreceptors that are innervated by the shorter carotid sinus nerves (Satchell 1990). It is likely that human blood pressure control would remain relatively normal in dying-back neuropathies until the carotid sinus and splanchnic nerves became pathologically involved.

Dogs with acrylamide neuropathy develop mega-oesophagus, which has been shown to be caused by damage to the vagally innervated oesophageal mechanoreceptors. Pulmonary stretch receptors are affected in relatively mild acrylamide neuropathy in dogs, resulting in abnormalities of respiratory reflexes. The cough reflex is also impaired. These experimental findings suggest that damage to vagal afferent fibres may contribute to respiratory complications in humans with peripheral nerve disease.

Sudomotor function has been studied in mice with acrylamide intoxication. There is a reduction in the number of pilocarpine-reactive sweat glands when high doses are administered but abnormalities of motor function are detected before those of sudomotor function, a finding consistent with damage occurring initially in large-diameter fibres (Navarro et al. 1993). Similarly, large-diameter afferent fibres from the bladder are affected before the smaller efferent fibres.

Experimental diabetic autonomic neuropathy

Autonomic neuropathy has been studied in rats with streptozotocin-induced diabetes and diabetic BB Wistar rats (Sima *et al.* 1987). The diabetic Wistar rat has clinical, pathological, and physiological evidence of sympathetic and parasympathetic dysfunction. Dystrophic axonal changes are widely distributed throughout the sympathetic nervous system, but not the parasympathetic nervous system, which is characterized by progressive axonal degeneration.

Conclusions

Disturbances of autonomic function are frequently present in patients with peripheral neuropathy, but may be mild and asymptomatic. Severe autonomic dysfunction is most likely to result from conditions such as amyloidosis and diabetes that affect the small myelinated and unmyelinated fibres in the baroreceptor afferents, the vagal innervation of the heart, and the sympathetic efferent fibres in the mesenteric vascular bed, or from the Guillain–Barré syndrome, in which there is acute segmental demyelination in the sympathetic and parasympathetic nerves, and other acute autonomic neuropathies.

References

Appenzeller, O. and Oribe, E. (1997). *The autonomic nervous system* (5th edn). Elsevier, Amsterdam.

Appenzeller, O., Arnason, B. G., and Adams, R. D. (1965). Experimental autonomic neuropathy: an immunologically induced disorder of reflex vasomotor function. *J. Neurol. Neurosurg. Psychiat.* 28, 510–15.

Beck, J. S., Abbot, P. D., Samson, P. D. *et al.* (1991). Impairment of vasomotor reflexes in the fingertips of leprosy patients. *J. Neurol. Neurosurg. Psychiat.* 54, 965–71.

Bennett, J. L., Mahalinga, M.R., Wellish, M. C., and Gilden D. H. (1996). Epstein–Barr virus-associated acute autonomic neuropathy. *Ann. Neurol.* 40, 453–5.

Brimijoin, S. and Lennon, V. A. (1990). Autoimmune preganglionic sympathectomy induced by acetylcholinesterase antibodies. *Proc. Natl Acad. Sci. USA* 87, 9630–4.

Enzi, G., Angelini, C., Negrin, P., Armani, M., Pierobon. S. and Fedele, D. (1986). Sensory, motor, and autonomic neuropathy in patients with multiple symmetric lipomatosis. *Medicine*, 64, 388–93.

Fernandez, A., Hontebeyrie, M., and Said, G. (1992). Autonomic neuropathy and immunological abnormality in Chagas' disease. *Clin. Auton. Res.* 2, 409–12.

Freeman, R., Roberts, M. S., Friedman, L. S., and Broadbridge, C. (1990). Autonomic function and human immunodeficiency virus infection. *Neurology* 40, 575–80.

Guo, Y.-P., McLeod, J. G. and Baverstock, J. (1987). Pathological changes in the vagus nerve in diabetics and chronic alcoholics. *J. Neurol. Neurosurg. Psychiat.* 50, 1449–53.

Heafield, N. T. E., Gammage, M. D., Nightingale, S., and Williams, A. C. (1996). Idiopathic dysautonomia treated with intravenous gammaglobulin. *Lancet* 347, 28–9.

Idiaquez, J. (1992). Parasympathetic denervation of the iris in Chagas' disease. *Clin. Auton. Res.* 2, 277–9.

Ingall, T. J., McLeod, J. G. and Tamura, N. (1990). Autonomic dysfunction and unmyelinated fibres in chronic demyelinating polyradiculopathy. *Muscle Nerve* 13, 70–6.

Jerian, S. M., Sarosy, G. A., Link, C. J., Fingert, H. J., Reed, E. and Kohn, E. C. (1993). Incapacitating autonomic neuropathy precipitated by taxol. *Gynaecol. Oncol.* 51, 277–80.

Lennon, V. A., Sas, D. F., Busk, M. F. *et al.* (1991). Enteric neuronal autoantibodies in pseudo-obstruction with small-cell lung carcinoma. *Gastroenterology* 100, 137–42.

Lindgren, S., Lilja, B., Rosen, I., and Sundkvist, G. (1991). Disturbed autonomic nerve function in patients with Crohn's disease. *Scand. J. Gastroenterol.* 26, 361–6.

Lindgren, S., Stewenius, J., Sjolund, K., Lilja B., and Sundkvist, G. (1993). Autonomic vagal dysfunction in patients with ulcerative colitis. *Scand. J. Gastroenterol.* 28, 638–42.

Litchy, W. J., Low, P. A., Daube, J. R., and Windebank, A. J. (1987). Autonomic abnormalities in amyotrophic lateral sclerosis. *Neurology*, 37 (Suppl. 1), 162A.

McDougall, A. J. and McLeod, J. G. (1996). Autonomic neuropathy, II: Specific peripheral neuropathies. *J. Neurol. Sci.* 138, 1–13.

McLeod, J. G. (1980). Autonomic nervous system. In *The physiology of peripheral nerve disease*, (ed. A. J. Sumner), pp. 432–83. Saunders, Philadelphia.

Matikainen, E. and Juntunen, J. (1985). Autonomic nervous system dysfunction in workers exposed to organic solvents. *J. Neurol. Neurosurg. Psychiat.* 48, 1021–4.

Montforte, R., Estruch, R., Valls-Solé, J., Nicolás, J., Villalta, J., and Urbano-Marquez, A. (1995) Autonomic and peripheral neuropathies in patients with chronic alcoholism. A dose-related effect of alcohol. *Arch. Neurol.* 52, 45–51.

Morey, M. K., Wiley, C. A., Hughes, R. A. C., and Pal, H. C. (1985). Autonomic nerves in experimental allergic neuritis in the rat. *Acta Neuropathol.* Berlin, 67, 75–80.

Navarro, X., Verdu, E., Guerrero, J., Butí, M., and Goñalons, E. (1993). Abnormalities of sympathetic sudomotor function in experimental acrylamide neuropathy. *J. Neurol. Sci.* 114, 56–61.

Provinciali, L., Cangiotti, A., Tulli, D., Carboni, V., and Cinti, S. (1994). Skin abnormalities and autonomic involvement in the early stage of amyotrophic lateral sclerosis. *J. Neurol. Sci.* 126, 54–61.

Rosenfeld, C. S. and Broder, L. E. (1984). Cisplantin-induced autonomic neuropathy. *Cancer Treat. Rep.* 68, 659–60.

Ruttimann, S., Hilti, P., Spinas, G. A., and Dubach, U. C. (1991). High frequency of human immunodeficiency-associated autonomic neuropathy and more severe involvement in advanced stages of human immunodeficiency virus disease. *Arch. Intern. Med.* 151, 2441–3.

Satchell, P. M. (1990). Baroreceptor dysfunction in acrylamide axonal neuropathy. *Brain* 113, 167–76.

Schaumburg, H. H., and Berger, A. R. (1993) Human toxic neuropathy due to industrial agents. In *Peripheral Neuropathy*. (3rd edn). (ed P. J. Dyck, P. K. Thomas, J. W. Griffin, P. A. Low, and J. F. Poduslo), pp. 1533–48. W. B. Saunders, Philadelphia.

Shimizu, T., Kato, S., Hayashi, M., Hayashi, H., and Tanabe, H. (1996). Amyotrophic lateral sclerosis with hypertensive attacks: blood pressure changes in response to drug administration. *Clin Auton. Res.* 6, 241–4.

Sima, A. A. F., Brismar, T., and Yagihashi, S. (1987). Neuropathies encountered in the spontaneously diabetic B. B. Wistar rat. In *Diabetic neuropathy*, (ed. P. J. Dyck, P. K. Thomas, A. K. Asbury, A. L. Winegrad, and D. Porte), pp. 253–9. W. B. Saunders, Philadelphia.

Smit, A. A. J., Vermenlen, M., Koelman, J. H. T. M., and Wieling, W. (1997). Unusual recovery from acute pandysautonomic neuropathy after immunoglobulin therapy. *May. Clin. Proc.* 72, 333–5.

Solders, G., Nennesmo, I., and Persson, A. (1989). Diphtheritic neuropathy. An analysis based on nerve biopsy and repeated neurophysiological and autonomic function tests. *J. Neurol. Neurosurg. Psychiat.* 2, 876–80.

Stewart, A. G., Waterhouse, J. C., and Howard, P. (1991). Cardiovascular autonomic nerve function in patients with hypoxaemic chronic obstructive pulmonary disease. *Eur. Resp. J.* 4, 1207–14.

Stewart, A. G., Marsh, F., Waterhouse, J. C., and Howard, P. (1994). Autonomic nerve dysfunction in COPD as assessed by the acetylcholine sweat-spot test. *Eur. Resp. J.* 7, 1090–5.

Suarez, G. A., Fealey, R. D. Camilleri, M., and Low, P. A. (1994). Idiopathic autonomic neuropathy: clinical neurophysiologic and follow-up studies on 27 patients. *Neurology* 44, 1675–82.

Tuck, R. R. and McLeod, J. G. (1982) Autonomic dysfunction in Guillain–Barré syndrome. *J. Neurol. Neurosurg. Psychiat.* **44**, 983–90.

Tuck, R. R., Pollard, J. D. and McLeod, J. G. (1981). Autonomic neuropathy in experimental allergic neuritis: an electrophysiological and histological study. *Brain* **104**, 187–208.

Wang, S.-J., Liao, K.-K., Liou, H.-H. *et al.* (1994). Sympathetic skin response and R-R interval variation in chronic uraemic patients. *Muscle Nerve* **17**, 411–8.

Young, R. R., Asbury, A. K., Adams, R. D. and Corbett, J. L. (1969). Pure pandysautonomia with recovery. *Trans. Am. Neurol. Ass.* **94**, 355–7.

Zochodne, D. W. (1994). Autonomic involvement in Guillain–Barré Syndrome: A review. *Muscle Nerve* **17**, 1145–55.

Zochodne, D. W., Ward, K. K. and Low, P. A. (1988). Guanethidine adrenergic neuropathy: an animal model of selective autonomic neuropathy. *Brain Res.* **461**, 10–16.

39. Diabetic autonomic failure

P. J. Watkins and M. E. Edmonds

Introduction

Diabetic neuropathy is a common condition with highly characteristic features due to the early and extensive involvement of small nerve fibres. It is the most common cause of autonomic neuropathy, causing functional defects and symptoms in a wide variety of systems. The gastrointestinal tract, the urogenital system, the heart, and blood vessels are all affected; there are abnormalities of sweating, pupillary defects, and a wide variety of metabolic disorders. Early small-fibre damage is manifested by impairment of vagally controlled heart rate variability, while diminished peripheral sympathetic tone leads to increased blood flow, which is detectable before there is clinical evidence of neuropathy. Thermal sensation (a small-fibre modality) is lost before vibration sensation (a large-fibre modality). Reduced thermal sensation is probably a very early marker of this and other neuropathies.

Causes of diabetic autonomic neuropathy

The mechanisms that underlie the development of diabetic autonomic neuropathy are still poorly understood. Studies over almost a whole decade in the Diabetes Control and Complications Trial (DCCT Research Group 1993) suggested that tight control of diabetes may slow the decline of autonomic function tests, while at a later stage of diabetes, pancreatic transplantation may halt further deterioration (Kennedy *et al.* 1990). No drug therapy convincingly alters the course of autonomic decline.

Major metabolic changes in diabetic nerves are described elsewhere in this book: their impact on neural circulation causing reduced blood flow and hypoxia could be important factors in the development of neuropathy (Stevens 1995). The idea that immunological mechanisms might underlie symptomatic autonomic neuropathy developed from our observation of an association with iritis (Guy *et al.* 1984). The presence of autoantibodies to cervical sympathetic ganglion, vagus nerve, and adrenal medulla in 20–28 per cent of patients with insulin-dependent diabetes mellitus (IDDM) lends weight to the hypothesis, and there is some association of these antibodies with autonomic neuropathy (Zanone *et al.* 1993; Ejskjaer *et al.* 1998; Watkins 1998). The presence of activated T cells has also been shown, and at autopsy, extensive cellular infiltrations (lymphocytes, macrophages, and plasma cells) in relation to autonomic tissues in ganglia and nerve bundles have been demonstrated (Watkins *et al.* 1995).

Nerve growth factor (NGF) regulates sympathetic nerve development and is required to maintain their neurotransmitter levels in animals. Antibodies to NGF can both damage autonomic nerves and cause pronounced atrophy of sympathetic ganglion cells in adult rats and mice (Ruit *et al.* 1990). The iris contains large amounts of NGF and even more when denervated. NGF (or other growth factors) accumulation might, on the one hand, provoke a cytokine-mediated inflammatory response—hence iritis—or its depletion might have major effects on neural peptides (e.g. calcitonin-gene-related peptide, vasoactive intestinal polypeptide), and nerve survival and regeneration, which are described elsewhere in this book.

Autonomic dysfunction in diabetes is common but, in sharp contrast, symptomatic autonomic neuropathy is rare. An immune attack is some cases might explain this striking difference. Abnormal cardiovascular tests are found in at least 16 per cent of a diabetic population, although others describe up to 40 per cent (Neil 1992). Higher proportions may be found if single rather than multiple tests are assessed. Sweating abnormalities have been described in as many as 84 per cent of diabetic patients, and abnormalities of pupillary function in about 14 per cent. The prevalence of symptomatic autonomic neuropathy (other than impotence) is not established, but it is uncommon. A survey by Neil *et al.* (1988) suggested that it was present in 12 per cent of IDDM patients and 0.5 per cent of patients with non-insulin-dependent diabetes mellitus (NIDDM): while we share the view that it is much more common in IDDM patients, we would estimate its prevalence to be much lower perhaps no more than 1 per cent.

Cardiac denervation

The demonstration of loss of heart rate variation during deep breathing in IDDM patients indicates the presence of vagal denervation of the heart, which becomes increasingly common with lengthening duration of diabetes. Sympathetic denervation was thought to develop after parasympathetic changes had occurred, but newer techniques suggest that sympathetic changes might occur very early in the course of diabetes. Thus, the cardiac uptake of the guanethidine analogue, meta-iodobenzyl guanidine (MIBG), assessed by single-photon emission computed tomography (SPECT), indicates early sympathetic denervation, sometimes occurring before the development of any other recognizable autonomic function tests (Schnell *et al.* 1995). Whether or not this results in impaired cardiac function is still debated, and the long-term significance of these findings needs to be determined. Total effective cardiac denervation has been described in patients with diabetic autonomic neuropathy whose heart rates are fixed and virtually unresponsive to any external agents.

Prolongation of the QT interval on the electrocardiogram is known to be a feature of diabetic autonomic neuropathy (Chambers *et al.* 1990). Development of dangerous cardiac arrhythmias, which might be expected by analogy with subjects with idiopathic prolongation of the QT intervals, has not been described in diabetes, and there is no evidence that sudden unexplained deaths in diabetic autonomic neuropathy are due to this cause.

Postural hypotension

Maintenance of blood pressure on standing depends on afferent impulses from baroreceptors (namely in the carotid sinus and aortic arch) and on efferent sympathetic impulses to the heart and blood vessels. In normal people, there is a 20 per cent fall in cardiac output on standing; about 700 ml of blood accumulates in the legs and splanchnic circulation, but compensatory mechanisms prevent a fall in blood pressure. If one or more of the pathways in this system are impaired, postural hypotension results.

Postural hypotension is an established complication of diabetic autonomic neuropathy and is chiefly due to efferent sympathetic vasomotor denervation. Recent blood-flow studies do indeed show that the reduction in foot blood flow on standing is diminished in diabetic patients with postural hypotension, although significant vasoconstriction still occurs (Flynn *et al.* 1988). Failure of cardiac acceleration and reduced cardiac output (exhibited under the stress of exercise) both contribute to the problems. Noradrenaline levels are also generally reduced in diabetics with postural hypotension, which occurs despite evidence of denervation hypersensitivity. An excess of noradrenaline is found in some patients with hypotension due to reduced intravascular volume rather than autonomic neuropathy (Cryer *et al.* 1978). Failure of renin responses on standing, though probably not responsible for acute postural hypotension, may or may not be abnormal.

Insulin is known to have cardiovascular effects (Porcellati *et al.* 1993; Bellavere *et al.* 1996; Yki-Järvinen and Utriainen 1998). It causes a reduction in plasma volume, an increase of peripheral blood flow from vasodilatation, and an increase of heart rate. In patients with autonomic neuropathy, insulin may cause or exacerbate postural hypotension to the point of fainting, whether it is given intravenously or subcutaneously, and just occasionally a blackout from hypoten-

sion may be confused with hypoglycaemia (Fig. 39.1). It has a similar effect in sympathectomized patients. These cardiovascular effects of insulin are likely to be due to the insulin itself, and not to changes in blood glucose concentration.

Failure of the splanchnic bed to vasoconstrict on standing could be a more important mechanism, as it is in primary autonomic failure, and in diabetic autonomic neuropathy, using ultrasound techniques, diminished mesenteric vasoconstriction was demonstrated (Purewal and Watkins 1995; Purewal *et al.* 1995). This was, however, no worse than in diabetics without hypotension, so that the importance of this mechanism in diabetic autonomic neuropathy remains uncertain.

Postprandial hypotension in various non-diabetic patients with autonomic neuropathy is described in Chapter 29. The raised insulin level following the meal is thought to be responsible. Observations on insulin-dependent diabetics established that while food causes a large increase in mesenteric blood flow, the latter does not coincide with an exacerbation of the hypotension (Purewal *et al.* 1995), although we have witnessed this phenomenon in one intractable case (Stevens *et al.* 1991*b*). Furthermore, in a small number of patients we have not found octreotide to be of value in the treatment of postural hypotension in diabetic autonomic neuropathy.

Patients with diabetic autonomic neuropathy, especially those with postural hypotension, lose the normal diurnal/nocturnal blood pressure variation in which night-time blood pressure is overall lower than that in the daytime. Nocturnal blood pressures in patients with diabetic autonomic neuropathy are therefore higher than in normal people. This, in turn, may be the cause of the cardiac hypertrophy known to occur in these patients, and is postulated as one possible cause of their increased mortality, though the majority also suffer nephropathy and may die from renal failure.

Postural hypotension (a fall of systolic pressure of more than 30 mmHg) occurs in diabetics with advanced neuropathy, although symptoms are infrequent and were noted in only 23 of 73 autonomic neuropathy patients described by Ewing and Clarke (1986). Disabling hypotension, when systolic pressure falls below 70 mmHg, is rare. Both hypotension and its symptoms fluctuate spontaneously to a remarkable degree, but may persist for many years without necessarily deteriorating (Sampson *et al.* 1990). The explanation for the variability is unclear, although insulin itself may be partly responsible by exacerbating the condition, and fluid retention may ameliorate it.

Treatment of postural hypotension

Few diabetics develop symptoms sufficiently severe to need treatment. When they do, it is first essential to stop any drugs that exacerbate hypotension, notably diuretics, tranquillizers and antidepressants. Simple treatments should always be tried and include raising the head of the bed and wearing full-length elastic stockings, but the benefits are slight. Anti-g suits are not helpful and are too cumbersome to be acceptable. Measures that increase plasma volume are the most effective, although oedema is a troublesome side-effect which often renders treatment unacceptable. However, a high salt intake or fludrocortisone, sometimes in high doses (up to 0.4 mg daily), can be effective. The use of an orally active adrenergic agonist, midodrine, can help; it has an exclusively peripheral pressor effect on arterial and venous capacitance vessels. Intranasal administration of an antidiuretic agent such as desmopressin (as DDAVP) can, by

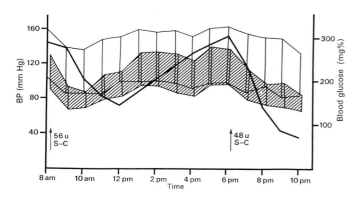

Fig. 39.1. Diurnal variation of lying and standing blood pressure in a 48-year-old man with severe autonomic neuropathy. Insulin was given subcutaneously (S-C) at times shown by the vertical arrows. The unhatched area shows supine blood pressure, the hatched area the standing blood pressure, and the continuous line the blood glucose.

reducing nocturnal diuresis, improve symptomatic postural hypotension at least in PAF, though its efficacy in diabetic autonomic neuropathy has not been demonstrated. Erythropoietin administered subcutaneously to anaemic autonomic neuropathy patients has been described (Hoeldtke and Streeton 1993) but further research of this approach needs to be undertaken.

Many other treatments have been suggested: their effectiveness is inconsistent. Some regimes are hazardous, and supine hypertension is a common sequel. These treatments include β-blockers with partial agonist activity, such as pindolol, and the use of ergotamine, caffeine, non-steroidal inflammatory drugs, clonidine, and metoclopramide (Chapter 36).

Erythropoietin depletion in autonomic neuropathy

Renal erythropoietin production is stimulated chiefly by the presence of anaemia and hypoxia. However, sympathetic innervation of the kidney appears to have a modulating influence, and experimental renal denervation leads to a reduction of stimulated erythropoiesis due to a decreased production of erythropoietin. Studies of human autonomic neuropathy with postural hypotension, including some patients with diabetes, have demonstrated erythropoietin depletion (Hoeldtke and Streeton 1993; Biaggioni et al. 1994). Our own preliminary investigations of diabetic autonomic neuropathy suggest that it may indeed, in some instances, cause both anaemia and diminished erythropoietin production in patients without renal impairment (Watkins 1998). These observations merit further research and, as reported in non-diabetic autonomic failure, administration of erythropoietin may improve symptomatic postural hypotension (Biaggioni et al. 1994).

Blood flow in the neuropathic foot

Diabetic foot problems are due to a combination of ischaemia and neuropathy, often complicated by infection. They tend to occur in insulin-dependent diabetics of moderate to long duration, and in the elderly non-insulin-dependent diabetic. In practice, there are two types of diabetic feet, the neuropathic foot and the neuroischaemic foot. In neuropathic foot, peripheral neuropathy predominates in the absence of significant large-vessel disease. In the neuroischaemic foot, there is a combination of both neuropathy and ischaemia. Although there is no significant abnormality in arterial inflow to the neuropathic foot, it may be affected by functional abnormalities of the microcirculation secondary to the neuropathy or to diabetes itself.

Circulatory changes in neuropathy

Sympathetic denervation of the peripheral arteries may occur quite early in the evolution of neuropathy and has major effects on blood flow and vascular responses, and causes structural changes in the arterial wall (Tooke 1997). Postural hypotension develops in the most advanced cases of autonomic neuropathy.

Sympathetic denervation causes loss of vasoconstrictor tone and peripheral vasodilatation, associated with opening of arteriovenous shunts. Skin blood flow increases substantially (on average, to above five times normal), and this can occur in the absence of other clinical evidence of neuropathy (Archer et al. 1984). These blood flow changes explain some of the clinical features of the neuropathic foot, notably the excessively warm skin, bounding pulses, and marked venous distension. The venous Po_2 in the feet is increased because of arteriovenous shunting. Capillary pressure is increased, and may contribute to neuropathic oedema, which can occasionally be severe and sometimes reversed by administration of ephedrine. However, nutritive capillary flow is not compromised by shunting, and has been shown directly by television microscopy to be normal or even increased (Flynn et al. 1988). Bone blood flow is also elevated in these patients, and this is thought to contribute to the osteopenia that predisposes to the development of Charcot osteo-arthropathy.

Blood-flow responses to various stimuli are also abnormal. Sympathetic stimulation (e.g. by coughing) or standing normally induce peripheral vasoconstriction. Neuropathic patients show blunting of these responses, although to a variable degree. Most strikingly, heating the skin of the neuropathic foot can induce paradoxical vasoconstriction (in contrast to the normal vasodilation), probably because neuropathy has interrupted the local axon reflex that governs this response (Fig. 39.2; Stevens et al. 1991a). Maximal vasodilation is also reduced in these patients. Although this defect is partly attributable to the effects of hyperglycaemia per se on the microvasculature, failure of nitric-oxide-dependent smooth muscle vasodilatation in neuropathy has been described (Pitei et al. 1997). Increased blood flow in the neuropathic foot may sometimes be related to the presence of pain, and a reduction in blood flow can be associated with diminution of pain in these cases (Archer et al. 1984).

Vascular sympathetic denervation can lead to degeneration of the smooth muscle of arteries, leading to medial calcification (Fig. 39.3; Mönckeberg's sclerosis) and stiffening of the arteries (Edmonds et al. 1982). This calcification may assume the histological characteristics of bone (Edmonds et al. 1995), and has a striking radiographic appearance. Vascular calcification does not usually cause major pathological effects in the feet. However, long-term progression of calcification in conjunction with atherosclerosis of the distal vessels has been associated with gangrene of the toes.

Sweating abnormalities

Defective sweating in diabetic neuropathy was described many years ago. The sweat gland is an important structure with a complex peptidergic as well as cholinergic innervation. Neuropeptide immunoreactivity, especially that of vasoactive intestinal polypeptide, is low in diabetic sudomotor nerves (Levy et al. 1989). There is a renewed interest in this field brought about by development of new techniques. Measurement of sweating in the periphery is one of the few quantitative methods for assessing cholinergic nerve function.

There are various methods for studying sweat responses. The thermoregulatory sweat test (adapted by Fealey et al. 1989) involves whole-body heating and sweating is detected by the application of alizarin red powder: this method assesses peripheral sympathetic function (pre- plus postganglionic). The quantitative sudomotor axon reflex test (QSART) stimulates sweating by iontophoresis of acetylcholine and assesses postganglionic sympathetic function by the axon reflex. Direct stimulation of sweat glands either by iontophore-

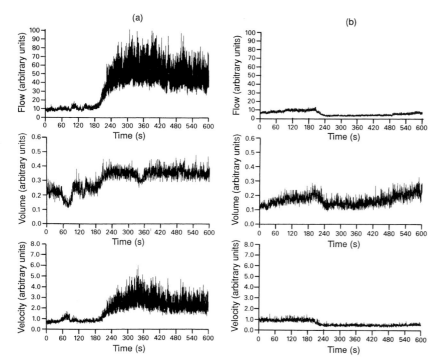

Fig. 39.2. Two typical skin blood-flow recordings of (a) a normal subject and (b) a diabetic patient with neuropathy, during local heating of the great toe. Local heating was started at 180 s after measuring basal flow for 3 min. Total skin blood flow is shown in the uppermost trace and the changes in microvascular volume and velocity are shown by the middle and lower traces, respectively.

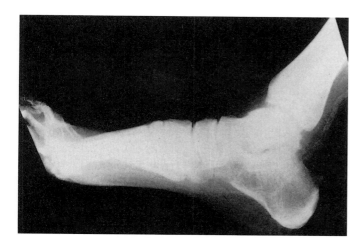

Fig. 39.3. Medial calcification in the arteries of a young, severely neuropathic, insulin-dependent diabetic.

sis of pilocarpine and counting sweat droplets on a silastic imprint or by acetylcholine injection and counting iodine starch sweat spots assesses postganglionic sweat gland denervation. Finally, the dermal sweat glands are normally activated by a sympathetic discharge and this provides the galvanic skin response. This is a biphasic charge of electrical potential that can be recorded from the skin using electrocardiogram electrodes. A recent technique can measure basal and stimulated sweating using a direct-reading computerized sudorometer, and this technique has shown that transepidermal water loss is reduced in diabetics with neuropathy and is consistent with the lack of spontaneous sympathetic activity measured by microneurography.

The most common sweating deficit is in the feet in the classical stocking distribution. There is close correlation with other autonomic defects, especially with postural hypotension, but also with cardiac vagal denervation, although the cardiovascular function tests tend to be abnormal before there is evidence of peripheral sweating loss. Abnormal responses may be found in cases of painful neuropathy, and patients with truncal mononeuropathies may have patchy sweaty defects. These tests all confirm the widespread small nerve damage that occurs in diabetic neuropathy.

Gustatory sweating is a highly characteristic symptom of diabetic autonomic neuropathy (Fig. 39.4; Watkins 1973), occurring more commonly than previously thought and seen even more frequently in those complicated by nephropathy as well (Shaw *et al.* 1996). Sweating begins soon after starting to chew tasty food, especially cheese. It starts on the forehead, and spreads to involve the face, scalp, and neck, and sometimes the shoulders and upper part of the chest, compelling patients to keep a towel at the dinner table. Distribution of the sweating is in the territory of the superior cervical ganglion. It may be of sudden onset; its cause is unknown, although aberrant nerve regeneration has been suggested. Gustatory sweating, once established, generally persists over many years, though there can be a remarkable and unexplained remission after renal transplantation (Shaw *et al.* 1996).

Gustatory sweating is occasionally sufficiently severe to need treatment: anticholinergic drugs are highly effective though side-effects may limit their use. Propantheline bromide (Pro-banthine®) can be used. It is given half an hour before meals, but may also be effective if given before single meals at social occasions. Clonidine might help. Recently, the use of glycopyrrolate cream has been described (Atkin and Brown 1996) made from glycopyrrolate powder (an antimuscarinic anticholinergic agent) as Robinul®, obtained from Wyeth UK, and made into a cream using standing cream base, Cetamacrogol A®, normally at 0.5 per cent, but 1 or 2 per cent may be more effective. The cream is applied on alternative days to the areas affected by sweating, avoiding contact with the mouth, nose and eyes. The area

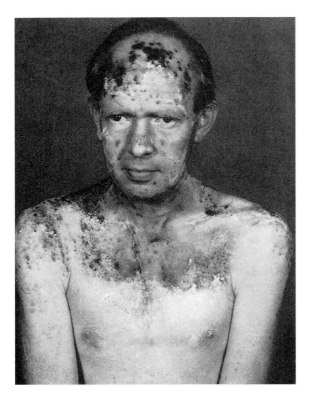

Fig. 39.4. Severe facial and shoulder sweating (gustatory sweating) seen a few minutes after eating cheese. The area of sweating is clearly delineated by the application of quinazarine powder which turns blue when moist.

should not be washed for 4 hours after the application. The only contraindication known is narrow angle glaucoma which might be exacerbated if the eye is accidently contaminated.

Diabetic diarrhoea

Diarrhoea is a very disagreeable symptom of autonomic neuropathy. Borborygmi and discomfort precede attacks of watery diarrhoea, without pain or bleeding, and usually without malabsorption. Faecal incontinence is common, especially at night, when exacerbations seem to be worse. Symptoms last from a few hours to a few days and then remit, with normal bowel action or even constipation (sometimes induced by treatment) in between attacks. Constipation is not otherwise, in our view, a particular problem experienced by neuropathic diabetics.

Intermittent attacks of diabetic diarrhoea tend to persist over many years and rarely remit completely. Very few patients suffer almost continuous diarrhoea for which no other cause is discovered, and they are very difficult to treat.

The underlying cause of diabetic diarrhoea is not established. Gut denervation probably alters gut motility (Werth *et al.* 1992) and bacterial overgrowth has been demonstrated in these cases. Yet many other mechanisms are possible and have not been well studied. Thus, gastroparesis might result in maldigestion of disaccharides and result in malabsorption of bile acids, which may in turn cause diarrhoea. Neuromuscular dysfunction might exist causing a shortened transit

time. The possibility of a secretory diarrhoea also exists, while the idea that intestinal permeability might be altered has not been studied.

Full investigation of diarrhoea in a diabetic patient is crucial in order not to overlook easily treatable causes such as coeliac disease, which may be increased in IDDM, pancreatic malabsorption, or other rarer causes. Autonomic function tests should be abnormal otherwise autonomic diarrhoea is very unlikely, and normal tests virtually exclude this as a cause. Nevertheless, the presence of abnormal autonomic function is not alone sufficient to lead to a diagnosis of diabetic diarrhoea and may thus be very deceptive. The diagnosis is most likely to be correct in long-standing IDDM patients with other autonomic symptoms, such as gustatory sweating and postural hypotension.

Tetracycline offers effective treatment in approximately half the patients, and is given in one or two doses of 250 mg at the onset of an attack, which is abruptly aborted. If this fails, a range of the antidiarrhoea remedies could be tried, notably codeine phosphate, lomotil, or loperamide (Imodium®). The use of clonidine has also been described. The use of somatostatin has been suggested and although we have not so far had any success with this approach, it merits further investigation.

Gastroparesis

Gastric emptying can be normal, accelerated, or retarded in patients with diabetes (Horowitz *et al.* 1996; Kong *et al.* 1996). Gastric stasis is a feature of autonomic neuropathy which sometimes, though rather surprisingly, not always, causes vomiting. Symptomatic gastroparesis is a rare diabetic complication. The vomiting may be due to vagal denervation of the stomach: several post-mortem studies have demonstrated loss of myelinated fibres in the vagus nerve and recently, loss of unmyelinated fibres has been shown in a vagus nerve removed at laparotomy from a patient with intractable vomiting from gastroparesis. However, there is also evidence of smooth muscle degeneration, characterized by subtotal smooth muscle cell atrophy in the muscularis propria associated with transformed smooth muscle cells undergoing a form of necrobiosis, appearing as highly distinctive, homogeneous, round eosinophilic bodies. Since vagal degeneration does not normally cause gut smooth muscle degeneration, these changes might represent an independent gastromyopathic process as the cause of gastroparesis (Watkins 1998).

The diagnosis is difficult to establish, and three approaches are needed: first, other obstructive causes should be excluded by endoscopic and barium studies; secondly, the presence of gastric stasis must be established, with videography to detect decreased or absent peristalsis; and thirdly, the presence of abnormal autonomic function should be demonstrated. Most patients with this complication also suffer other symptoms of autonomic neuropathy.

Gastric stasis must be confirmed by radioisotopic studies, using anterior and posterior cameras to exclude artefacts from stomach movements during the test. Liquids, solids, and indigestible solids are emptied by the stomach at different rates, and by different mechanisms. Radioisotope studies in diabetics with autonomic neuropathy have variously shown normal solid emptying, impairment of the usual differentiation between solid and liquid emptying, abnormal solid but normal liquid emptying, and abnormal solid and liquid emptying. Abnormal liquid emptying probably represents advanced disease. Dual phase studies should therefore be performed using two isotopes, ^{111}In-DTPA (diethylenetriaminepentaacetic acid) for liquid and ^{99}Tc-sulphur colloid for solid emptying times.

Dopamine antagonists (metoclopramide and domperidone) enhance gastric tone and emptying. They may accelerate gastric emptying in diabetic autonomic neuropathy with some effect. The motility stimulant cisapride can also be tried. These drugs form the mainstay of treatment during vomiting bouts. The use of erythromycin has been described recently (Janssens et al. 1990): this binds to motilin receptors and acts as a motilin agonist. Intravenous erythromycin causes a substantial acceleration of gastric emptying (Janssens et al. 1990); oral administration is less effective in alleviating symptoms and still needs more investigation. It should be given in a dose of 50 mg four times daily since higher doses may cause down-regulation of the receptors. Erythromycin and cisapride must not be used together because of the risk of serious cardiac arrythmias.

The very rare cases of intractable vomiting from gastroparesis may require more invasive treatments. The introduction of percutaneous endoscopic jejunostomy or gastrostomy can benefit patients in the short term: this may alleviate the problem until a natural remission of the vomiting occurs even after protracted periods of time. Sometimes a more definitive procedure is required and a two-thirds gastrectomy with a Roux-en-Y loop anastomosed 60 mm from the gastric stump, as developed by Professor E. R. Howard at King's College Hospital, has proved to be successful in carefully selected cases. However, the long-term outlook for most of these patients, who generally suffer multiple diabetic complications, is poor.

Oesophagus

Abnormal oesophageal motility has been described in diabetic autonomic neuropathy. No symptoms have been attributed to this functional abnormality.

Gallbladder

Enlargement of the gallbladder, probably due to poor contraction, may be a feature of diabetes related to autonomic neuropathy. Studies by ultrasonography have not confirmed the enlargement of the gallbladder, but do suggest impaired muscular contraction. There are no known clinical effects from this. However, administration of erythromycin does enhance gallbladder emptying.

Neurogenic bladder

Autonomic neuropathy affecting the sacral nerves causes bladder dysfunction (see Chapter 30). Bladder function tests are commonly abnormal in neuropathic diabetics but symptoms from neurogenic bladder in diabetes are relatively rare, usually occurring in diabetics who already have advanced complications. Most men with neurogenic bladder are also impotent.

Impairment of bladder function is chiefly the result of neurogenic detrusor muscle abnormality, while pudendal innervation of perineal and periurethral striated muscle is usually unaffected in diabetic neuropathy. Afferent damage results in impaired sensation of bladder filling, and leads to detrusor areflexia: thus, the bladder pressure during cystometrography fails to increase as the bladder is filled. In advanced cases, bladder emptying is reduced because of impaired detrusor activity and possibly failure of the internal sphincter to open adequately. Measurements of urine flow show that the peak flow rate is reduced and that duration of flow is increased.

There are no symptoms in the early stages, but later patients experience hesitancy during micturition, develop the need to strain, a feeble stream, and a tendency to dribble. Micturition is sometimes in short, interrupted spurts which result from straining. Patients may be aware of lengthening intervals between micturition, and also experience a sensation of inadequate bladder emptying. Gradually, residual urine volume increases and, in severe cases, gross bladder retention occurs with abdominal swelling and sometimes overflow incontinence as well. Bladder capacity may exceed 1 litre.

Diagnosis of neurogenic bladder is usually possible, especially in those patients with clinical evidence of severe neuropathy. It is, however, important to exclude bladder neck obstruction and, especially, prostatic obstruction in men. Ultrasound examination before and after emptying should be performed, and cystoscopy is usually needed: rarely, diabetic neurogenic bladder causes hydroureter and hydronephrosis. Occasionally, more sophisticated bladder function tests are needed. These include cystograms, cystometrography, and urine flow rate measurements (see Chapter 30).

The principles of treatment are to compensate for deficient bladder sensation and thus prevent the development of a high residual urine volume. For those diabetics who have few symptoms of cystopathy, education is important and may suffice. In particular, the patients should be told to void every 3 hours during the daytime. Manual suprapubic pressure can increase the efficiency of bladder emptying. With more severe symptoms, more active measures are needed. Prazosin, an α_1-adrenoreceptor blocker may help by reducing urethral resistance. Self-catheterization three times daily is now the recommended treatment for patients with chronic retention. Recurrent urinary tract infections are often troublesome in these patients, and protracted courses of antibiotics, changing monthly, may be needed to prevent this problem.

Impotence

Autonomic neuropathy is still considered to be the main aetiological factor in diabetic impotence (Chapter 30). It is due to erectile failure resulting from damage to both parasympathetic and sympathetic innervation of the corpora cavernosa. VIP-ergic nerves are also important in the vasodilatation of erection and the concentration of VIP is low in the penile corpora in diabetics with autonomic neuropathy. Failure to achieve erection may also be the result of a concomitant sensory deficit in the dorsal nerve of the penis. The onset of neuropathic impotence is usually gradual, progressing slowly over months, but complete erectile failure is usually present within 2 years of the onset of symptoms. This history contrasts with psychogenic impotence which begins suddenly and in which nocturnal erections are present.

Impotence may also be due to vascular occlusion of the branches of the internal pudendal artery. Furthermore, in rare cases, erectile failure may be caused by the Leriche syndrome.

The diagnosis of neuropathic impotence in diabetes is difficult. The use of an intracavernosal injection of prostaglandin E₁ (Caverject®, alprostadil) is to some extent useful in distinguishing neurogenic from vasculogenic impotence—it causes an erection in the former and fails to do so in the latter. This is helpful both in terms of diagnosis and giving guidance in the choice of treatment. For centres with particular interest, other techniques are available. Thus, it is possible to record nocturnal penile tumescence and rigidity during sleep: the absence of tumescence and rigidity over three successive nights is a strong indication of an organic cause of impotence. Vasculogenic impotence can be confirmed by a measurement of penile blood pressure and by comparing it with a brachial systolic pressure, thereby achieving a penile–brachial index. When the ratio of penile to brachial pressure is 0.75 or less, a diagnosis of penile vascular disease can be considered. Autonomic function tests give some guidance as to the presence of autonomic neuropathy, but they do not establish conclusively in an individual whether it is the cause of the impotence. A neuropathic cause can be more exactly defined by electrophysiological testing of reflex sexual pathways. Conduction velocity is reduced in the dorsal nerve of the penis in diabetic impotent patients, and the latency of the bulbocavernosus reflex is prolonged.

The rational treatment of diabetic impotence depends on a careful history, in particular, to evaluate any psychological component. If this factor is present, then the patient and his partner may be helped by appropriate discussion and advice. For the younger patients, rigid penile implants are often successful, especially since ejaculation is often retained. Inflatable prostheses can also be inserted, but are more prone to failure. The intracavernous injection of the vasodilator prostaglandin E₁ causes an erection in patients not suffering from severe vascular disease, and offers a treatment which some men find satisfactory: potential problems exist from infection and penile fibrosis and this treatment should not be provided under expert supervision. The use of a vacuum pump applied to a condom is less invasive, and is a technique which some patients find satisfactory, especially if they are properly instructed. In vasculogenic impotence, arterial disease is often distal and arterial reconstruction is only likely to be useful in those patients with major arterial occlusions.

New treatments using intraurethral prostaglandins, or oral treatment with Sildenafil®, a selective inhibitor of type 5 cyclic GMP-specific phosphodiesterase, are now available.

Respiratory responses and arrests

Sudden respiratory arrests have been well described in diabetes with autonomic neuropathy. In most of these episodes, there was some interference with respiration either by anaesthesia, drugs, or bronchopneumonia. These episodes are transient, and while temporary ventilation may be needed, recovery to normal health is expected. We have known one patient who had three witnessed transient respiratory arrests. Anaesthetists need to be forewarned of this possibility when symptomatic autonomic neuropathy patients require even minor surgery.

These observations have led to further investigation of the respiratory system of diabetics with autonomic neuropathy: (1) the control of ventilation in response to hypoxia and hypercapnia; (2) the pattern of respiration during sleep; and (3) the bronchial reactivity to chemical and physical agents.

The integrity of the ventilatory responses in autonomic neuropathy has been studied by measuring responses to hypoxia and hypercapnia in diabetics with and without neuropathy. The results of these investigations are conflicting. Normal increased ventilatory responses to transient hypoxia during exercise and to progressive hypoxia have been reported, implying that peripheral chemoreceptors and their afferent nerves are intact in diabetic autonomic neuropathy. However, other studies have found a defective response to hypoxia in autonomic neuropathy. The results regarding responses to hypercapnia have also been conflicting; both normal ventilatory and reduced responses have been detected (Ewing and Clarke 1986). Thus, the true importance of abnormal ventilatory responses as a cause of respiratory arrest has yet to be established.

Sleep apnoea has been reported in IDDM subjects, occasionally in association with autonomic neuropathy (Rees et al. 1981). Heart-rate responses to apnoeic episodes may also be abnormal. Uncertainty still exists, however, and in the study of Catterall et al. (1984) there was no evidence of increased sleep apnoea in diabetics with autonomic neuropathy.

The third area of study has assessed the integrity of respiratory reflexes which affect bronchomotor tone. Airways tone is mainly under vagal control and is reduced in diabetics with autonomic neuropathy, with diminished bronchodilatation in response to anticholinergic agents. Diabetics with autonomic neuropathy also show decreased bronchoconstriction during inhalation of cold air and, even more strikingly, a diminished or even absent cough reflex in response to an inhaled irritant such as citric acid (Fig. 39.5). These deficits are due to neuropathic denervation and not to any intrinsic abnormality in bronchial smooth muscle, which responds normally to direct stimulation by inhaled histamine. Whether the absence of these stimulated reflexes has any clinical implications is unknown.

The perception of respiratory sensations in diabetics has also been measured in patients breathing through a tube manifold apparatus with resistance to air flow that was randomly varied. Diminished per-

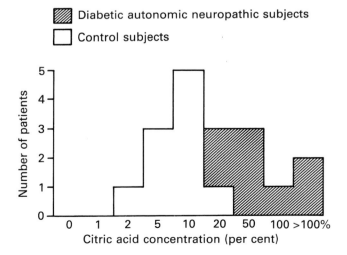

Fig. 39.5. Cough responses to inhaled citric acid in normal subjects and diabetics with severe autonomic neuropathy. The response may be impaired or even absent in autonomic neuropathy.

ception of respiratory resistance loads occurred in diabetics with neuropathy and this may render the patient prone to subclinical episodes of respiratory illness (O'Donnell *et al.* 1988).

Respiratory arrests in diabetics with autonomic neuropathy continue to be reported. Whether or not they are responsible for the sudden unexplained deaths reported in diabetic autonomic neuropathy patients (see below) is unclear, but we suspect, from clinical observation, that they might be.

Hypoglycaemia

Hypoglycaemia is a powerful stimulus of autonomic function, causing sweating, tremor, tachycardia, and an increase of pulse pressure with a notable rise of systolic blood pressure. There are also major circulatory and endocrine changes in response to hypoglycaemia.

Glucagon, adrenaline, noradrenaline, pancreatic polypeptide (PPP), somatostatin, ACTH, growth hormone, and corticosteroids all increase in response to hypoglycaemia (Hilsted 1993). The presence of autonomic neuropathy prevents the stimulated increase of PPP, and possible of somatostatin, while responses of the remaining hormones are unaffected beyond the diminished responses which occur anyway in long-term IDDM regardless of the presence of neuropathy, notably for glucagon (and adrenaline). Noradrenaline release is, of course, reduced in patients with autonomic neuropathy, but responses to hypoglycaemia are unaffected. Glucose recovery following hypoglycaemia may be impaired in IDDM, especially following repeated episodes, but this deficit is not related to the presence of autonomic neuropathy.

Loss of warning of hypoglycaemia has often, in the past, been attributed to autonomic neuropathy, but it is now established that the phenomenon occurs chiefly in those subjected to repeated hypoglycaemia, and can be reversed (Cranston *et al.* 1994). Thus, studies from Edinburgh in IDDM patients of more than 15 years' duration with and without lost warning of hypoglycaemia showed equal proportions of autonomic damage in the two groups; and furthermore, they demonstrated that patients with established autonomic neuropathy had similar autonomic and neuroglycopenic symptoms to those without autonomic neuropathy (Hepburn *et al.* 1990; Frier 1993). The DCCT study (1993) also showed a lack of relationship between loss of warning in those with tight control and the presence of autonomic neuropathy. The concept, however, that diminished autonomic symptomatic and counter-regulatory changes may occur as a result of reduced central nervous system responses to hypoglycaemia has gained substantial support but these changes are independent of the presence or absence of autonomic neuropathy itself.

The use of β-blocking drugs can, however, cause abrupt loss of warning of hypoglycaemia in delayed metabolic recovery. This occurs infrequently (perhaps in as few as 1 in 50 patients in β-blockers) yet when it occurs, it is dramatic and potentially dangerous, and patients should always by warned of this hazard.

Prognosis

Autonomic function declines with age, but in diabetes it deteriorates, on average, faster than in normal subjects. Thus, heart rate variation, which normally decreases at approximately 1 beat/min/3 years

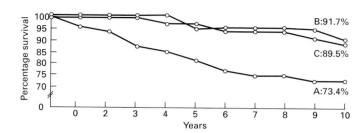

Fig. 39.6. Calculated 10-year survival (per cent) in groups A (symptomatic autonomic neuropathy; *n* = 49), B (abnormal heart rate variation; *n* = 24), and C (asymptomatic normal heart rate variation; *n* = 38). (From Sampson *et al.* (1990).)

declines about three times faster in the diabetic patients, although there is substantial variation (Sampson *et al.* 1990). Most patients who develop abnormal autonomic function do not become symptomatic. Mortality of asymptomatic patients with autonomic dysfunction may be increased (O'Brien *et al.* 1991) but the prognosis is generally good, and 90 per cent of our patients (all under 50 years old at the beginning of the study) were alive 10 years later (Fig. 39.6). In contrast, the outcome for those with symptomatic autonomic neuropathy is not as good, although even in this group, 73 per cent were still alive after a decade. Ewing and Clarke (1986) described a poorer prognosis, although patient selection was different, the patients were older and some had renal damage. Those with postural hypotension appear to have the highest mortality, perhaps because of the premature development of left ventricular hypertrophy. Most deaths in these patients are from renal failure or myocardial infarction. There are a few sudden unexplained deaths amongst autonomic neuropathy patients, which we believe are more likely to be from respiratory than cardiac arrest or arrhythmia.

Established symptoms of autonomic neuropathy including diarrhoea, vomiting from gastroparesis, and postural hypotension run a very protracted through intermittent course and rarely become disabling, even over the 10–15 years during which we have reviewed these patients. Postural hypotension fluctuates substantially with corresponding variation in the intensity of symptoms. Gustatory sweating also tends to persist without remission, though many patients describe disappearance of this symptom after renal transplantation. The general absence of progression to debilitating disease remains unexplained and contrasts with devastating and indeed fatal progression in some of the primary autonomic failure syndromes. The late Professor John Malins made many of these observations years ago when he wrote that, 'The prognosis for autonomic manifestations is poor although the disability is often surprisingly slight' (Malins 1968).

References

Archer, A. G., Roberts, V. C., and Watkins, P. J. (1984). Blood flow patterns in painful diabetic neuropathy. *Diabetologia*, **27**, 563–7.

Atkin, S. L. and Brown, P. M. (1996). Treatment of diabetic gustatory sweating with topical glycopyrrolate cream. *Diabet. Med.* **13**, 493–4.

Bellavere, F., Cacciatori, V., Moghetti, P. *et al.* (1996). Acute effect of insulin on autonomic regulation of the cardiovascular system: a study by heart rate spectral analysis. *Diabet. Med.* **13**, 709–14.

Biaggioni, I. *et al.* (1994). The anaemia of primary autonomic failure and its reversal with recombinant erythropoietin. *Ann. Int. Med.* **121**, 181–6.

Catterall, J. R. *et al.* (1984). Breathing, sleep and diabetic autonomic neuropathy. *Diabetes*, **33**, 1025–7.

Chambers, J. B. *et al.* (1990). QT prolongations in diabetic autonomic neuropathy. *Diabet. Med.* **7**, 105–10.

Cranston, I. *et al.* (1994). Restoration of hypoglycaemia unawareness in patients with long-duration insulin-dependent diabetes. *Lancet* **344**, 283–7.

Cryer, P. E. *et al.* (1978). Plasma catecholamines in diabetes: the syndromes of hypoadrenergic and hyperadrenergic postural hypotension. *Am. J. Med.* **64**, 407–16.

DCCT (Diabetes Control and Complications Trial) Research Group (1993) The effect of intensive treatment of diabetes on the development and progressive of long-term complications in insulin dependent diabetes mellitus. *New Eng. J. Med.* **329**, 977–86.

Edmonds, M. E. *et al.* (1982). Medial arterial calcification and diabetic neuropathy. *BMJ* **284**, 928–30.

Edmonds, M. E. *et al.* (1995). Diabetic tibial arteries show increased calcification associated with increased gene expression of matrix Gla protein. *Diabet. Med.* **12**, 515–16.

Ejskjaer, N., Zanone, M. M., and Peakman, M. (1998). Autoimmunity in diabetic autonomic neuropathy: does the immune system get on your nerves? *Diab. Med.* **15**, 723–9.

Ewing, D. J. and Clarke, B. F. (1986). Autonomic neuropathy: its diagnosis and prognosis. In *Clinics in endocrinology and metabolism*, (ed. P. J. Watkins), pp. 855–88. Saunders, London.

Fealey, R. D., Low, P. A., and Thomas, J. E. (1989). Thermoregulatory sweating abnormalities in diabetes mellitus. *Mayo Clin. Proc.* **64**, 617–28.

Flynn, M. E. *et al.* (1988). Direct measurement of capillary blood flow in the diabetic neuropathic foot. *Diabetologia* **31**, 652–6.

Frier, B. M. (1993). Hypoglycaemia unawareness. In *Hypoglycaemia and diabetes*, (ed. B. Frier and M. Fisher), pp. 291–3. Edward Arnold, London.

Guy, R. J. C. *et al.* (1984). Diabetic autonomic neuropathy and iritis: and association suggesting an immunological cause. *BMJ* **189**, 343–5.

Hepburn, D. A. *et al.* (1990). Unawareness of hypoglycaemia in insulin treated diabetic patients: prevalence and relationship to autonomic neuropathy. *Diabet. Med.* **7**, 711–17.

Hilsted, J. (1993). Classical autonomic neuropathy and denervation. In *Hypoglycaemia and diabetes*, (ed. B. Frier and M. Fisher), pp. 268–74. Edward Arnold, London.

Hoeldtke, R. D., and Streeton, D. H. (1993). Treatment of orthostatic hypotension with erythropoietin. *New Engl. J. Med.* **329**, 611–15.

Horowitz, M. *et al.* (1996). Gastric emptying in diabetes: an overview. *Diabet. Med.* **13**, S16–S22.

Janssens, J. *et al.* (1990). Improvement of gastric emptying in diabetic gastroparesis by erythromycin: preliminary studies. *New Engl. J. Med.* **322**, 1028–30.

Kennedy, W. R. *et al.* (1990). The effects of pancreas transplantation on diabetic neuropathy. *New Engl. J. Med.* **322**, 1031–7.

Kong, M. F. *et al.* (1996). Gastric emptying in diabetes. *Diabet. Med.* **13**, 112–19.

Levy, D. M. *et al.* (1989). Depletion of cutaneous nerves and neuropeptides in diabetes mellitus: an immunocytochemical study. *Diabetologia*, **32**, 427–33.

Malins, J. M. (1968). *Clinical diabetes mellitus*. Eyre & Spottiswoode, London.

Neil, H. A. W. (1992). The epidemiology of diabetic autonomic neuropathy. In *Autonomic failure*, (ed. R. Bannister and C. J. Mathias), pp. 682–97. Oxford Medical Publications, Oxford.

Neil, H. A. W. *et al.* (1988). Diabetic autonomic neuropathy: the prevalence of impaired heart rate variability in a geographically defined population. *Diabet. Med.* **6**, 20–4.

O'Brien, I. A. D. *et al.* (1991). The influence of autonomic neuropathy on mortality in insulin dependent diabetes. *Q. J. Med.* **290**, 495–502.

O'Donnell, C. R. *et al.* (1988). Diminished perception of inspiratory resistive loads in insulin dependent diabetics. *New Engl. J. Med.* **319**, 1369–73.

Pitei, D. L. *et al.* (1997). NO-dependent smooth muscle vasodilatation is reduced in NIDDM patients with peripheral sensory neuropathy. *Diabet. Med.* **14**, 284–90.

Porcellati F. *et al.* (1993) Mechanisms of arterial hypotension after therapeutic doses of subcutameous insulin in diabetic autonomic neuropathy. *Diabetes* **42**, 1055–64.

Purewal, T. S., and Watkins, P. J. (1995). Postural hypotension in diabetic autonomic neuropathy: a review. *Diabet. Med.* **12**, 192–200.

Purewal, T. S. *et al.* (1995). The splanchnic circulation and postural hypotension in diabetic autonomic neuropathy. *Diabet. Med.* **12**, 513–22.

Rees, P. J. *et al.* (1981). Sleep apnoea in diabetic patients with autonomic neuropathy. *J. R. Soc. Med.* **74**, 192–5.

Ruit, K. G. (1990). Nerve growth factor regulates sympathetic ganglion cell morphology and survival in the adult mouse. *J. Neurosci.* **10**, 2412–19.

Sampson, M. J. *et al.* (1990). Progression of diabetic autonomic neuropathy over a decade in insulin dependent diabetics. *Q. J. Med.* **75**, 635–46.

Schnell, O. *et al.* (1995). Scintigraphic evidence for cardiac sympathetic dysinnervation in long-term IDDM patients with and without ECG-based autonomic neuropathy. *Diabetologia*, **38**, 1345–52.

Shaw, J. E. *et al.* (1996). Gustatory sweating in diabetes mellitus. *Diabet. Med.* **13**, 1022–37.

Stevens, M. J. *et al.* (1991*a*). Influence of neuropathy on the microvascular response to local heating in the human diabetic foot. *Clin. Sci.* **80**, 249–56.

Stevens, M. J. *et al.* (1991*b*). Difficulties in the management of postural hypotension: complications in diabetic autonomic neuropathy. *Diabet. Med.* **8**, 870–4.

Stevens, M. J. (1995). Nitric oxide as a potential bridge between metabolic and vascular hypotheses of diabetic neuropathy. *Diab. Med.* **12**, 292–5.

Tooke, J. E. (1997). The microcirculation in diabetes mellitus. In *International Textbook of Diabetes.* (ed. K. G. M. M. Alberti, P. Zimmet, R. A. Defronzo, pp. 1339–48. John Wiley and Sons.

Watkins, P. J. (1973). Facial sweating after food: a new sign of diabetic autonomic neuropathy. *BMJ* **1**, 583–7.

Watkins, P. J. *et al* (1995). Severe sensory-autonomic neuropathy and endocrinopathy in insulin-dependent diabetes. *Q. J. Med.* **88**, 795–804.

Watkins, P. J. (1998). The enigma of autonamic failure in diabetes. *J. Roy. Coll. Physns.* **32**, 360–5.

Werth, B. *et al.* (1992). Non-invasive assessment of gastrointestinal motility disorders in diabetic patients with and without cardiovascular signs of autonomic neuropathy. *Gut* **33**, 1199–203.

Yki-Järvinen, H., and Utriainen, T. (1998). Insulin-induced vasodilatation: physiology or pharmacology? *Diabetologia* **41**, 369–79.

Zanone, M. M. *et al* (1993). Autoantibodies to nervous tissue structures are associated with autonomic neuropathy in type 1 (insulin-dependent) diabetes mellitus. *Diabetologia* **36**, 564–9.

40. Dopamine β-hydroxylase deficiency— with a note on other genetically determined causes of autonomic failure

Christopher J. Mathias and Roger Bannister

Introduction

Dopamine β-hydroxylase (DBH) is the enzyme that converts dopamine into noradrenaline (Fig. 40.1). It is present within vesicles in sympathetic nerve endings and within the adrenal medulla and is released stoichiometrically with noradrenaline during sympathetic stimulation. It can be measured readily in plasma, and studies in both animals and man indicate that the major contribution to circulating levels is from sympathetic nerve endings. It was once thought that it might serve as a better indicator of sympathetic nervous activity than noradrenaline. However, further studies, have indicated that there are marked differences within normal subjects and that plasma levels are largely genetically predetermined. Its half-life is probably in the region of about 30 min and is considerably longer than that of noradrenaline. This can be a disadvantage with short-lived sympathetic stimuli. Furthermore, it has a much larger molecular weight (290 kDa as compared to 169 Da for noradrenaline) and it reaches the circulation predominantly by lymphatic channels rather than through diffusion. Studies from a variety of sources indicate that in humans it is not as sensitive an indicator of short- or long-term changes in sympathetic activity as is noradrenaline (Mathias *et al.* 1976; Weinshilboum 1979).

Interest in DBH in autonomic disorders was stimulated by the lower plasma levels observed in familial dysautonomia (Weinshilboum and Axelrod 1971) and later in familial amyloid polyneuropathy (Suzuki *et al.* 1980). In the latter group, further evidence of a functional DBH deficit was provided by successful treatment of hypotension with the agent DL-dihydroxyphenylserine (DOPS), which bypassed the deficient enzymatic component (Fig. 40.2). There was a resurgence of interest in the late 1980s with the description of two patients with a congenital deficiency of DBH resulting in severe postural hypotension due to sympathetic adrenergic failure (Robertson *et al.* 1986; Man in't Veld *et al.* 1987*a*). Since then five further cases have been described, two of whom are siblings (Table 40.1).

The clinical features, autonomic deficits, and results of routine and specialized investigations, together with the management of DBH deficiency are described. There will also be a short discussion on differences from other genetically determined causes of autonomic failure and postural hypotension.

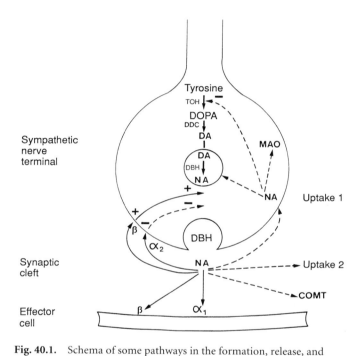

Fig. 40.1. Schema of some pathways in the formation, release, and metabolism of noradrenaline from sympathetic nerve terminals. Tyrosine is converted into dihydroxyphenylalanine (DOPA) by tyrosine hydroxylase (TOH). DOPA is converted into dopamine (DA) by dopa-decarboxylase (DDC). In the vesicles, DA is converted into noradrenaline (NA) by dopamine β-hydroxylase (DBH). Nerve impulses release both DBH and NA into the synaptic cleft by exocytosis. NA acts predominantly on α_1-adrenoceptors but has actions on β-adrenoceptors on the effector cell of target organs. It also has presynaptic adrenoceptor effects. Those acting on α_2-adrenoceptors inhibit NA release while those acting on β-adrenoceptors stimulate NA release. NA may be taken up by a neuronal (uptake 1) process into the cytosol, where it may inhibit further formation of DOPA through the rate-limiting enzyme TOH. NA may be taken into vesicles or metabolized by monoamine oxidase (MAO) in the mitochondria. NA may be taken up by a higher-capacity but lower-affinity extraneuronal process (uptake 2) into peripheral tissues such as vascular and cardiac muscle, and certain glands. NA is also metabolized by catechol-*o*-methyl transferase (COMT). NA measured in plasma is thus the overspill which is not affected by these numerous processes. (From Mathias (1996).)

Table 40.1. Details of seven patients with DBH deficiency

	USA		The Netherlands		UK		Australia
	Patient 1	Patient 2	Patient 3	Patient 4	Patient 5[a]	Patient 6[a]	Patient 7
Reference	Robertson et al. (1986)	Biaggioni et al. (1990)	Man in 't Veld et al. (1987a)	Man in 't Veld et al. (1988)	Mathias et al. (1990)	Mathias et al. (1990)	Thompson et al. (1995)
Sex	F	M	F	F	M	F	F
Origin	Scotch–Irish	Dutch, Scotch–Irish, Cherokee	Dutch[b]	Dutch[b]	English	English	Australian
Consanguinity	—	—	None		None	None	None
Siblings	1 brother	—	1 brother, 1 sister	—	1 sister	1 brother	1 brother
Family affected	No	No	No	—	Yes (sister)	Yes (brother)	No[c]
Age when postural hypotension recognized (years)	25	33	21	20	29	21	14

[a]Patients 5 and 6 are siblings.　　　　— No details provided.
[b]Presumed, as no details provided.
[c]See text.

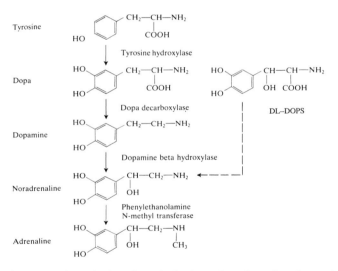

Fig. 40.2. Biosynthetic pathway in the formation of noradrenaline and adrenaline. The structure of DL-DOPS is indicated on the right. It is converted directly to noradrenaline by dopa decarboxylase, thus bypassing dopamine β-hydroxylase.

Clinical features

Presentation

Of the seven patients, five are female (Table 40.1). Except for the most recent (at 14), they were diagnosed after the age of 20, although their history was suggestive of autonomic failure from birth or early childhood. In patients 2 and 3 there were other complicating features (hypoglycaemia and probably incorrectly diagnosed epilepsy). In all, the reason for investigation and subsequent diagnosis was directly related to symptoms and signs of postural hypotension. This was recognized only in their teens or later.

Family history

In none of the cases was there a history of a similar problem in previous generations. Patient 7 had a maternal grandfather who died at an early age (less than 30 years) of a blood pressure problem, but details were not available. There was no evidence of consanguinity. The patients were of white Caucasian stock; of Scottish, Irish, Dutch, and northern English descent, except for patient 2 who also had Cherokee Indian lineage. There was a history of miscarriages in some of their parents. The brother and sister in the UK (patients 5 and 6) were the only siblings in the family. Evaluation of the parents of patients 5 and 6 confirmed normal autonomic function and catecholamine levels.

In a mouse model where gene targeting resulted in absence of dopamine β-hydroxylase, the majority of homozygous embryos died *in utero* (Thomas *et al.* 1995). Death of the embryos was due to cardiovascular failure. Treatment with dihydroxyphenylserine (DOPS) prevented foetal loss; this was reversed by the addition of a dopa decarboxylase inhibitor, carbidopa. It was thought that the survival of the embryos was dependant upon catecholamine transfer across the placenta, as all the embryos of homozygous mothers died *in utero*. The high foetal loss in these studies may explain the rarity of human dopamine β-hydroxylase deficiency.

Pre-adult manifestations

All, except for patient 5, were unwell from early childhood. Patient 7 was 4 weeks premature. There was a strong association between their symptoms, syncope, and exercise, which was avoided especially in patients 3 and 6. In patient 7, dizziness was more frequent and severe in a warm environment. As a child, patient 6 had difficulty in walking, which her mother attributed to her not trying. Epilepsy was considered in patients 2 and 3 who were unsuccessfully tried on anti-epileptic medication. At birth, patient 3 had episodes of hypoglycaemia and hypothermia. Physical growth in all appeared to be normal, and sexual maturation was not delayed. Symptoms, however, became more apparent in their teens; in patient 5, however, this only emerged at 13 years. The mother of patient 7 was mainly concerned that she did not have the energy of a normal teenager. Whether the clinical manifestations in their teens were associated with greater activity, worsening of their condition, or sharpening of their ability to associate symptoms with specific events is not clear.

Clinical manifestations at diagnosis

Autonomic function

Symptoms pointed to postural hypotension, with blurring of vision, dizziness, and at times syncope (Table 40.2). This was often worse in the morning, during exercise, and during hot weather. Postural symptoms were not worse after food ingestion except in patient 2. Patient 5 occasionally had aching in the back of the neck and shoulders after meals. In patient 6, food often reduced postural symptoms but there was no evidence of hypoglycaemia. In patients 5 and 6, precordial pain occasionally occurred during exertion, and was repro-

duced during exercise testing with electrocardiography (ECG), but without concomitant evidence of ischaemia on the ECG. They both also had weakness and paraesthesiae in the legs during exertion, suggestive of ischaemia to the spinal cord. On formal testing immediately post-exercise, no objective evidence of a neurological or vascular deficit in the periphery was obtained.

Patients 1–4 and 7 had bilateral partial ptosis, presumably related to the lack of sympathetic tone to Muller's muscle in the upper lid. Patient 1 had nasal stuffiness probably due to vasodilatation secondary to lack of sympathetic vasoconstriction, as seen in acute tetraplegia (Guttmann's sign) and after α-adrenoceptor blockers such as phenoxybenzamine. It is recorded that patients 2, 5, and 6 were aware of their ability to sweat. There were no abnormalities in relation to lacrimation or salivation. There was normal gut and large bowel function, except for intermittent diarrhoea in patients 1 and 2. Urinary bladder function was normal in all. Patient 6 had nocturia. In patient 5, erection was preserved but ejaculation took a prolonged time to achieve, or was absent. Patient 2 was originally described as impotent (Biaggioni and Robertson 1987) but was later reported to

Table 40.2. Clinical symptoms and signs in seven patients[a] with DBH deficiency

Symptoms and signs	USA		The Netherlands		UK		Australia
	Patient 1	Patient 2	Patient 3	Patient 4	Patient 5	Patient 6	Patient 7
Autonomic							
Postural symptoms	+	+	+	+	+	+	+
Postural hypotension	+	+	+	+	+	+	+
Postural rise in heart rate	+	+	+	+	+	+	+
Sweating	+	+	+	+	+	+	+
Bowels	ID	ID	N	N	N	N	N
Urinary bladder	N	N	N	N	N	N	N
Sexual							
Maturation (or menarche)	N	N	N	N	N	N	N
Erection		Impaired			N		
Ejaculation		Retro-grade			Delayed or absent		
Partial ptosis	+	+	+	+	−	−	+
Neurological	N	Reduced deep tendon reflexes	Hypotonia, facial weakness, sluggish deep tendon reflexes		N	N	
Higher function	N	N	N	N	N	N	N
Miscellaneous		Hyper extensible joints	Brachydactyly, high palate				

N, normal; +, symptom or sign present; −, symptom or sign absent; ID, intermittent diarrhoea.

[a]Patient details in Table 40.1.

have difficulty in maintaining an erection and to have retrograde ejaculation (Biaggioni *et al.* 1990).

Neurological and mental function

There were no major neurological abnormalities. Mild ptosis was present in patients 1–4 and 7. Patient 2 had reduced deep tendon reflexes. Muscle hypotonia, weakness of the facial musculature, and sluggish deep tendon reflexes were reported in patients 3 and 4. No neurological deficits were recorded in patients 5 and 6. There was no evidence of impairment of mental function and detailed psychometric examinations in patients 5 and 6 were normal.

Miscellaneous

Patients 2 and 6 had renal impairment with an elevated creatinine level (220 and 150 mmol/l, respectively). In patient 6 this was due to an episode of glomerulonephritis which had been treated successfully with steroids when she was 21, but which left her with an elevated but stable creatinine level; she had remained mildly anaemic (Hb 10 g/dl). Patients 3 and 4 had brachydactyly and a high palate. Patient 2 had atrial fibrillation and patient 3 had negative or flat T waves in the precordial leads of the ECG.

Autonomic investigations

Physiological

Cardiovascular

The investigations indicated sympathetic adrenergic failure (Table 40.3). All had severe postural hypotension, with an abnormal Valsalva manoeuvre, but with an adequate rise in heart rate when the blood pressure fell, showing preserved baroreceptor afferent and vagal efferent pathways. In patients 1, 5, and 6 there was a small rise in blood pressure and heart rate during some of the pressor tests; patient 7 was reported as having a suppressed blood pressure rise during the cold pressor test. The responses, in the absence of noradrenaline, suggested the presence of alternative although less effective mechanisms which raise blood pressure. These include vagal withdrawal, which can raise heart rate and cardiac output, and pressor effects exerted through dopamine, neuropeptides (such as neuropeptide Y), or purines (such as adenosine triphosphate) released from otherwise intact sympathetic nerve terminals. Heart-rate responses to deep breathing and hyperventilation were present, indicating functional cardiac vagus nerves.

Table 40.3. Summary of physiological autonomic investigations in seven patients[a] with DBH deficiency

Physiological investigations	USA		The Netherlands		UK		Australia
	Patient 1	Patient 2	Patient 3	Patient 4	Patient 5	Patient 6	Patient 7
Sympathetic adrenergic							
Head-up postural change-BP	↓	↓	↓	↓	↓	↓	↓
Valsalva manoeuvre							
-BP	A	A	A	A	A	A	A
-Phase IV-HR	A	A	A	A	A	A	A
Pressor tests	A	A	A	A	A	A	A
Sympathetic cholinergic							
Sweating	N	N	N	N	P	P	N
Parasympathetic							
Sinus arrhythmia	+	+	+	+	+	+	+
Hyperventilation-HR	↑	↑	↑	↑	↑	↑	
Head-up postural change-HR	↑	↑	↑	↑	↑	↑	↑
Valsalva manoeuvre Phase II-HR	↑	↑	↑	↑	↑	↑	↑
Schirmer's test					N	N	
Miscellaneous							
Food on BP					↔	↔	
Exercise on BP					↔	↔	
Nocturnal polyuria					+	+	
Nocturnal natriuresis					+	+	

BP, blood pressure; HR, heart rate; A, abnormal; N, normal; P, preserved but patchy; ↓, fall; ↑, rise; ↔, no change; +, symptom present; no symbol, not described.

[a]Patient details in Table 40.1.

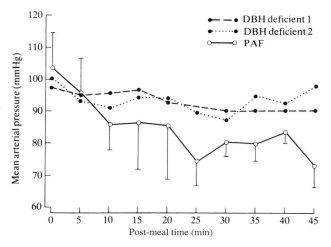

Fig. 40.3. Blood pressure before and after ingestion of a balanced liquid meal with measurements in the supine position, in five patients with pure autonomic failure (PAF) and in patients 5 and 6 with dopamine beta hydroxylase (DBH) deficiency.(1 and 2, respectively, in figure). (From Mathias *et al.* (1990).)

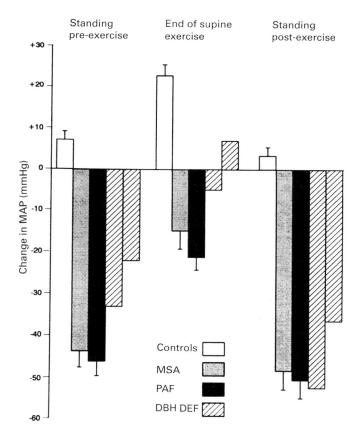

Fig. 40.4. Change in mean arterial blood pressure (MAP) at the end of 9 mins of supine exercise on a bicycle, and on standing before and after exercise in normal subjects (controls), and patients with multiple system atrophy (MSA), pure autonomic failure (PAF), and patients 5 and 6 (DBH DEF). Exercise raises supine blood pressure in normal subjects and lowers blood pressure in MSA and PAF, but with little change in patients 5 and 6. After exercise, however, blood pressure on standing falls further in both patients. (From Smith and Mathias (1995).

The responses to food ingestion were tested in patients 5 and 6. In neither was there a fall in supine blood pressure nor an accentuation of postural hypotension after food (Mathias *et al.* 1990); this differs from observations in patients with primary chronic autonomic failure due to pure autonomic failure and multiple system atrophy (Fig. 40.3). Possible mechanisms for this difference indicate their ability to influence cardiac output and to release vasoactive neurotransmitters other than noradrenaline (see Chapter 29). Neither patient 5 nor 6 had a fall in supine blood pressure with bicycle exercise, and this differed again from the patients with PAF and MSA; their blood pressure did not go up with exercise as occurs normally, consistent with their inability to increase circulating noradrenaline and adrenaline levels (Smith *et al.* 1995) (Fig. 40.4). However, when patients 5 and 6 stood up after exercise there was a marked fall in blood pressure that was considerably greater than pre-exercise (Smith and Mathias 1995). It is likely that the absence of exercise-induced hypotension while supine was due to similar mechanisms that prevented the fall in blood pressure during food ingestion in these patients. The enhanced postural hypotension after exercise presumably reflects the limitations of these secondary mechanisms, and indicates the importance of neurally mediated vasoconstriction as exerted through noradrenaline.

Spectral analysis of heart rate variability was performed in patient 7 (Fig. 40.5). At rest the high-frequency, respiratory-related variability (0.2–0.3 Hz) linked to parasympathetic activity was preserved, while the low-frequency heart rate variability (0.1 Hz) that reflects sympathetic activation was not present; with head-up tilt there was a marked reduction in high-frequency heart rate variability, suggesting vagal withdrawal.

Sweating

Sweating was preserved in all patients. The thermoregulatory sweating response was tested in patients 3–6 and was present, although in patients 5 and 6 this was patchy when compared with normals. Patient 3 sweated profusely when hypoglycaemia was induced by insulin.

Lacrimation and salivation

There were no symptoms to suggest xerostomia. Schirmer's test was normal in patients 5 and 6.

Nocturnal polyuria and natriuresis

This was recorded in patients 5 and 6. Both had nocturnal polyuria and excreted large amounts of sodium (Fig. 40.6). In patient 3, sodium output was reported as high but details were not provided.

Electrophysiological studies

Sympathetic microneurography was performed in patients 2 (Rea *et al.* 1990) and 7. This demonstrated a rise in muscle sympathetic nerve activity with pressor stimuli (despite no change in blood pressure) and a fall in nerve discharge with phenylephrine, both consistent with functional preservation of sympathetic nerve activity (Fig. 40.7a,b and Fig. 40.5).

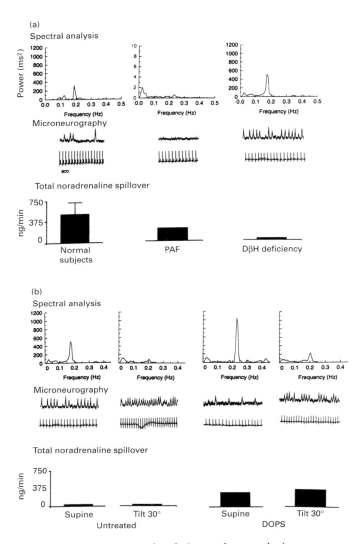

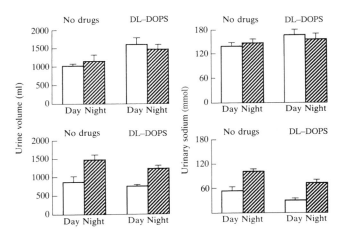

Fig. 40.6. Day (open histograms) and night (hatched histograms) urine volumes (left panels) and urinary sodium excretion (right panels) in patient 5 (upper panels) and patient 6 (lower panels) with DBH deficiency, before and after drug therapy with DL-DOPS. (From Mathias et al. (1990).)

Fig. 40.5. Heart-rate spectral analysis, muscle sympathetic nerve activity (microneurography), and total noradrenaline spillover in normal subjects, pure autonomic failure patients (PAF), and patient 7 with dopamine β-hydroxylase deficiency. (From Thompson et al. (1995).) In (a), at rest, only high-frequency respiratory-related variability (0.2–0.3 Hz; representing parasympathetic activity) was present without the low-frequency heart-rate variability (0.01 Hz; that reflects sympathetic activity); muscle sympathetic nerve activity was greater than in normals while noradrenaline spillover was extremely low. In (b), data in patient 7 alone is provided, while supine and during head-up tilt to 30° while untreated and after L-DOPS. With L-DOPS there was an increase in the high-frequency peak, but the low-frequency variability remained undetectable; muscle sympathetic nerve activity fell to within the normal range. There was an increase in noradrenaline spillover while supine but a lower than expected rise with head-up tilt

Fig. 40.7. Heart rate (HR), blood pressure (BP), and muscle sympathetic nerve activity (MSNA) recorded from the peroneal nerve in a patient with DBH deficiency (patient 2): (a) before and during isometric exercise (static handgrip); and (b) during injection of phenylephrine. Isometric exercise increases MSNA and phenylephrine decreases MSNA indicating that baroreflex pathways are intact. (From Rea et al. (1990).)

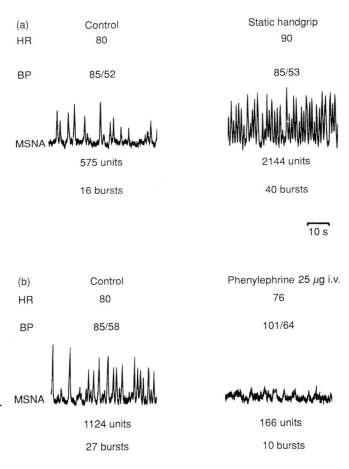

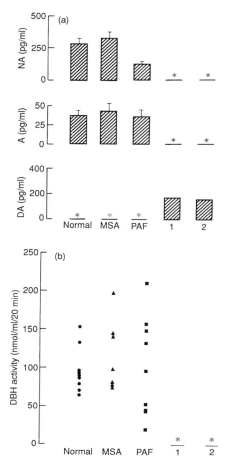

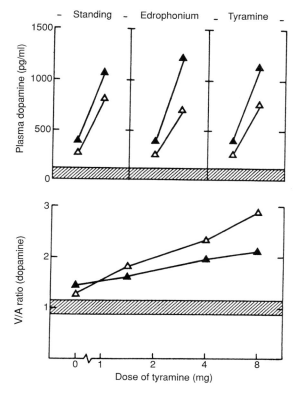

Fig. 40.9. Effect of standing, edrophonium and tyramine or plasma dopamine and the venous/arterial (V/A) ratio for dopamine in two patients (3 and 4) with congenital DBH deficiency. (Filled triangles, patient 3; open triangles, patient 4; hatched area, 95 per cent confidence intervals in normals). (From Man in't Veld *et al.* (1988).)

Fig. 40.8. (a) Mean levels (± SEM) of plasma noradrenaline (NA), adrenaline (A), and dopamine (DA) in 10 normal subjects, 12 patients with multiple system atrophy (MSA), and 8 patients with pure autonomic failure (PAF). Individual values on the first occasion in patients 5 and 6 (1 and 2, respectively, in figure) with DBH deficiency are indicated. The asterisk indicates undetectable levels, which were below 5 pg/ml for NA and A and 20 pg/ml for DA. (b) Scattergram showing DBH activity in 10 normal subjects, 7 MSA, and 9 PAF patients. In patients 5 and 6 (1 and 2, respectively, in figure) activity was undetectable. (From Mathias *et al.* (1990).)

Biochemical investigations

Plasma catecholamines

The key findings were the virtual absence of circulating levels of noradrenaline and adrenaline, with abnormally elevated levels of dopamine (Fig. 40.8a). Patient 1 was reported to have detectable plasma adrenaline levels but this was later retracted (Biaggioni *et al.* 1990) on the basis that the levels observed were probably due to cross-reactivity with high levels of dopamine. The evidence of an inability to convert dopamine to noradrenaline suggested a lack of DBH activity which was confirmed (Fig. 40.8b). In patients 2–4 the precursor substance to dopamine, dihydroxyphenylalanine, was also elevated in plasma. The high levels of dopamine suggested lack of inhibition of tyrosine hydroxylase, the rate-limiting enzyme, which is normally inhibited by intraneuronal noradrenaline. Despite these

high basal levels, definite elevations in plasma dopamine levels were associated with physiological and pharmacological stimulation (Fig. 40.9). Neither intravenous tyramine (patients 1–4), nor insulin-induced hypoglycaemia (patients 3 and 4) caused an elevation in noradrenaline or adrenaline levels (respectively), as they normally do.

Cerebrospinal fluid catecholamines

In patients 2 and 3, noradrenaline and adrenaline were not detectable in cerebrospinal fluid, while dopamine and its metabolites were elevated (Fig. 40.10). These observations are consistent with undetectable dopamine β-hydroxylase immunoreactivity in cerebrospinal fluid in such patients (O'Connor *et al.* 1994).

Urinary catecholamine measurements

The urinary metabolites of dopamine (homovanillic acid and 3–methoxy-tyramine) were normal or elevated while those of noradrenaline (normetanephrine) and adrenaline (metanephrine) were either extremely low or undetectable (Fig. 40.11). This was consistent with the observations in plasma.

Noradrenaline and adrenaline kinetics

In patient 7, total body noradrenaline and adrenaline spillover to plasma was measured using radiotracer methods (Thompson *et al.* 1995; Fig. 40.5). At rest, total body noradrenaline spillover was very

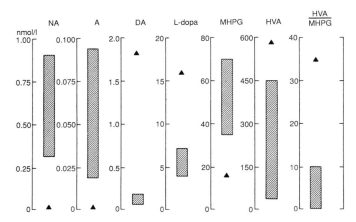

Fig. 40.10. Plasma catecholamine concentrations, 3-methoxy-4-hydroxyphenyl ethylene glycol (MHPG) and homovanillic acid (HVA) in cerebrospinal fluid (CSF) of patient 3 with DBH deficiency. NA, noradrenaline; A, adrenaline, DA, dopamine, L-dopa = L-dihydroxyphenylalanine. (From Man in't Veld *et al.* (1987*a*).)

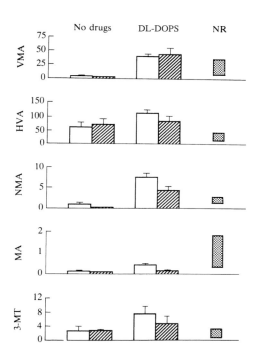

Fig. 40.11. Twenty-four hour urinary secretion of catecholamine metabolites in patient 5 (open histograms) and patient 6 (filled histograms) with DBH deficiency, before and after treatment with DL-DOPS. Bars indicate ± SEM and relate to collections over 3 consecutive days. VMA, vanillylmandelic acid; HVA, homovanillic acid; 3-MT, 3-methoxy-tyramine; MA, metadrenaline; NMA, normetadrenaline. Normal range (NR) indicated by stippled histogram on right. HVA and 3-MT are metabolites of dopamine. (From Mathias *et al.* (1990).)

low (38 ng/min) compared with normals (519 ± 43 ng/min) and patients with pure autonomic failure (251 ± 22 ng/min). Adrenaline secretion was almost undetectable. During head-up tilt in patient 7, total body noradrenaline spillover fell to 27 ng/min, with a minimal

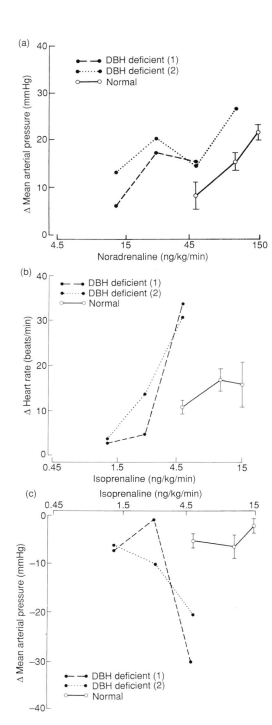

Fig. 40.12. (a) Change in mean blood pressure in normal subjects and in patients 5 and 6 (1 and 2, respectively, in figure) with DBH deficiency after incremental intravenous infusion of noradrenaline. In patient 5 the pulse rate fell to 40 beats/min after the third dose infusion and no further doses were administered. (b) and (c) Rise in heart rate (b) and fall in mean blood pressure (c) in normal subjects and in patients 5 and 6 (1 and 2, respectively, in figure) after incremental intravenous infusion of isoprenaline. (From Mathias *et al.* (1990).)

fall in adrenaline clearance (from 1.9 ng/min to 1.7 ng/min). This contrasts with normal subjects during head-up tilt, when noradrenaline spillover increases (to 677 ± 8 ng/min).

Tissue studies

Electron microscopy was performed on axillary and gluteal skin in patients 5 and 6 and did not show any structural abnormalities of sympathetic nerve terminals. In these patients, immunohistochemical staining indicated the presence of tyrosine hydroxylase but not DBH. In patient 3, immunohistochemistry of skin biopsy material was negative for DBH and noradrenaline and positive for dopamine, but no details of methodology were provided. Immunofluorescence to vasoactive intestinal polypeptide, neuropeptide Y, substance P, and calcitonin-gene-related peptide was present in patients 5 and 6, similar to that in normal subjects.

Pharmacological

A series of investigations further emphasized the enzymatic deficiency and the associated autonomic abnormalities (Table 40.4). There was pressor supersensitivity to both noradrenaline and to clonidine, emphasizing α-adrenoceptor up-regulation (Figs 40.12a, 40.13). There was a depressor response to isoprenaline with an exaggerated heart rate response, probably due to a combination of α-adrenoceptor supersensitivity and also vagal withdrawal in response to the fall in blood pressure (Fig. 40.12b,c). Tyramine did not raise levels of plasma noradrenaline in patients 1–4 (Fig. 40.14); edrophonium administration in patients 3 and 4 had no effect, but raised levels of plasma dopamine. The functional role of high circulating levels of dopamine varied; in patients 1 and 2 there was no response to oral metoclopramide, in patients 3 and 4 intravenous metoclopramide raised blood pressure, while an identical dose in patients 5 and 6 lowered blood pressure (Fig. 40.15). The reasons for these differences are not known.

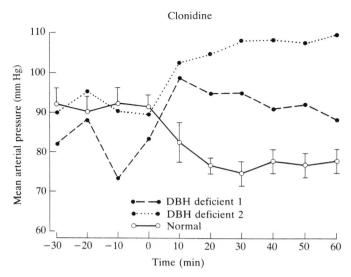

Fig. 40.13.   Blood pressure changes following intravenous clonidine given at time 0 (2 μg/kg infused over 10 min) in six normal subjects and in patients 5 and 6 (1 and 2, respectively, in figure) with DBH deficiency. In the normal subjects there is a substantial and significant fall in blood pressure after clonidine. (From Mathias *et al.* (1990).)

Other familial and hereditary autonomic disorders

The presence of the disorder at birth and the recognition of siblings with DBH deficiency places this condition among other familial and hereditary autonomic disorders, some of which are described briefly below. In the majority of these disorders there are associated neurological deficits which immediately separate them from congenital

Table 40.4.   Summary of pharmacological investigations in seven patients[a] with DBH deficiency. Responses relate to blood pressure unless otherwise stated.

Pharmacological investigations	USA Patient 1	Patient 2	The Netherlands Patient 3	Patient 4	UK Patient 5	Patient 6	Australia Patient 7
Noradrenaline	↑++	↑++	↑++	↑++	↑++	↑++	
Isoprenaline (BP)	↓++	↓++	↓++	↓++	↓++	↓++	
HR response	↑++	↑++	↑++	↑++	↑++	↑++	
Tyramine	↔[b]	↔[b]	↔[b]	↔[b]			
Clonidine	↑++	↑++	↑++	↑++	↑++	↑++	
Edrophonium			↔[b]	↔[b]			
Atropine (HR)	N	N	N	N	N	N	N
Metoclopramide	↔	↔	↑	↑	↓	↓	
DL-DOPS	↑	↑	↑		↑	↑	
L-DOPS					↑	↑	↑
L-DOPS + carbidopa					↔	↔	

BP, blood pressure; HR, heart rate; N, normal; ↑, rise; ↓, fall; ↔, no response; ++, excessive response; no symbol, not described.
[a]Patient details in Table 40.1.
[b]Includes plasma noradrenaline response.

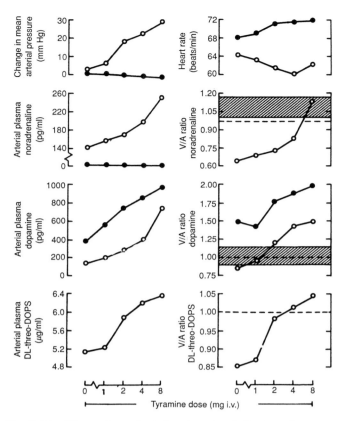

Fig. 40.14. Effects of tyramine before (●—●) and after (○—○) treatment with DOPS in patient 3. V/A venous/arterial. Hatched areas indicate 95 per cent confidence interval of V/A ratios for noradrenaline and dopamine in 30 untreated patients with borderline hypertension under basal conditions. Prior to treatment with DL-DOPS, tyramine has no effects on blood pressure and plasma noradrenaline levels. This is changed after treatment with DOPS. (From Man in't Veld *et al.* (1987*b*).)

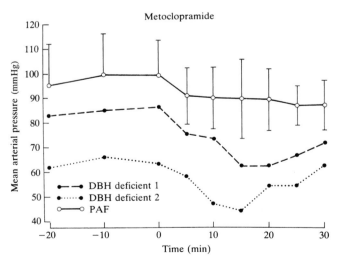

Fig. 40.15. Blood pressure changes before and after the dopamine antagonist metoclopramide (10 mg given as 2.5 mg i.v. every 2.5 minutes from time 0) in four patients with pure autonomic failure (PAF) and patients 5 and 6 (1 and 2 in figure, respectively) with DBH deficiency. (From Mathias *et al.* (1990).)

DBH deficiency. In two of the disorders (familial hyperbradykinism and adrenoleukodystrophy) there are no autonomic deficits, but there are overlapping features, such as postural hypotension.

Riley–Day syndrome (familial dysautonomia)

This is an autosomal recessive disorder with autonomic abnormalities present from birth and is described in Chapter 41.

Familial 'Shy–Drager' like-syndrome

There have been two reports of a familial syndrome with postural hypotension, sphincter involvement, and multiple neurological deficits. The age of onset, however, was the late thirties or early forties in the first family (Lewis 1964) and even later in the second (Ilson *et al.* 1982). Details of the autonomic disorder in these patients are limited.

Familial amyloidosis (familial amyloid polyneuropathy)

This is characterized by abnormal deposition of fibrillar amyloid protein predominantly into peripheral and autonomic nerves, and is described in Chapter 42.

Other hereditary peripheral neuropathies

These are described in Chapter 38, and include porphyria (the acute intermittent, variegate, and coproporphyria forms), where the inheritance is autosomal dominant. Widespread autonomic involvement may occur, including tachycardia and hypertension, that is thought to be related to baroreceptor denervation, in addition to other factors. There are a number of hereditary sensory and autonomic neuropathies (Thomas 1992) where the key feature is the sensory neuropathy. The autonomic abnormalities often include those affecting the urinary bladder and sweat glands.

Fabry–Anderson disease

This is an X-linked glycolipid lysosomal storage disease (Iannaccone and Rosenberg 1996). It results from mutation of the α-galactosidase genes situated on the X chromosome and there are a number of variants. The enzymatic deficiency results in accumulation of its main natural substrate, ceramide trihexoside, being deposited in connective tissues. Globoside, a tetrahexoside which is its major precursor, is also found in red blood cells, blood vessels, and the kidney. A characteristic of the disease is skin deposits resulting in angiokeratoma, hence the alternative name angiokeratoma corporis diffusum. In addition, the peripheral and autonomic nervous systems, the kidney, the gastrointestinal tract, and the blood vessels themselves are affected. Vascular dilatation and constriction may be impaired directly or through autonomic involvement. In a detailed study of 10 males (Cable *et al.* 1982), lacrimal and salivary secretion and abnormal pupillary responses to pilocarpine were found in half the cases. The responses to postural change and the plasma noradrenaline levels were normal in all. Impaired sweating was found in all 10 cases. Detailed studies in a single case suggest that both skin sympathetic nerve activity and sweat gland dysfunction may contribute to anhidrosis (Yamamoto *et al.* 1996).

Allgrove's syndrome

In this paediatric disorder there is alachrima, achalasia, and adreno-cortical insufficiency due to insensitivity to corticotrophin (Allgrove et al. 1978), of unknown aetiology. An autosomal recessive disorder is likely. An autonomic neuropathy may be present, as described in four children tested between 6 and 8 years of age (Gazarian et al. 1995) and two Hispanic adolescents (Chu et al. 1996); orthostatic hypotension with decreased heart rate variability and impaired responses to deep breathing, was reported. The features appear to result from progressive degeneration of cholinergic neurones, although the observations on orthostatic hypotension, if not due to cortisol deficiency, suggest additional involvement.

Mitochondrial encephalomyopathy

These are disorders in which there are structural or biochemical defects in mitochondria, thus impairing oxidative phosphorylation, and affecting a number of systems (Iannoccone and Rosenberg 1996). Abnormalities vary in different subgroups. In Leigh syndrome, vomiting and gastrointestinal abnormalities occur, as in patients with myoneural gastrointestinal encephalopathy. In Kearns–Sayre syndrome there is cardiac involvement. In mitochondrial encephalomyopathy with lactic acidosis and stroke-like episodes (MELAS) both gastrointestinal and cardiac involvement occur. Whether the abnormalities result from involvement of the autonomic nervous system is unclear. In a recent report of three children with a mitochondrial encephalomyopathy, there was gastrointestinal dysmotility, cardiac arrhythmias, decreased lachrymation, supersensitivity to methacholine, altered sweating, postural hypotension and apnoea; some of these features were attributed to autonomic dysfunction (Zelnik et al. 1996). The clinical course in these patients was variable, and differed from that of other groups with mitochondrial encephalomyopathy.

Tyrosine hydroxylase, DBH, and sensory neuropeptide deficiency

A patient with sympathetic adrenergic failure, who had preserved sweating and parasympathetic function, and thus with findings similar to those in DBH deficiency, has been described (Anand et al. 1991). In addition, she had undetectable plasma dopamine levels, with immunohistochemical evidence of absent neuronal tyrosine hydroxylase, DBH and the sensory neuropeptides, substance P and calcitonin-gene-related peptide. Dopa decarboxylase activity was present and she could convert oral L-dopa into dopamine and L-DOPS to noradrenaline. There was an impaired histamine response on skin testing. Nerve growth factor (NGF) levels in skin were subnormal. The combined autonomic and sensory neuropeptide deficit appeared related to a reduction in NGF. Thus, there were marked differences from isolated DBH deficiency.

In experimental studies using gene targetting, inactivation of tyrosine hydroxylase, when performed in mid-gestation in utero, results in death of 90 per cent of mutant embryos, probably as a result of cardiovascular failure; this can be prevented by the administration of L-dopa (dihydroxyphenylalanine), indicating the importance of catecholamines for mouse foetal development and postnatal survival (Zhou et al. 1995). This may be of relevance to this particular patient and raises the possibility that the pathological process accounting for her syndrome (that included tyrosine hydroxylase deficiency) was likely to have occurred either in the later stages of pregnancy or postpartum.

Aromatic L-amino acid decarboxylase deficiency (AADC)

Three children (including monozygotic twins) with AADC deficiency have been described (Hyland et al. 1992). The twins (1 year old) had reduced plasma dopamine, noradrenaline, and adrenaline levels, along with absent DBH in plasma. Whole-blood serotonin levels were low. Cerebrospinal fluid levels of dopamine and serotonin metabolites were reduced. AADC was not present in liver tissue and was reduced in plasma. The previous sibling had died soon after birth and limited information suggested a similar disorder. The autonomic abnormalities included temperature and blood pressure instability, excessive sweating, miosis, and ptosis. Heart-rate variation was preserved. The neurological features (oculogyric crises and abnormal movements) were consistent with a cerebral deficiency of dopamine and responded to dopamine agonists (bromocriptine) and monoamine oxidase inhibitors. The parents appeared normal, except for plasma AADC levels that were less than 20 per cent of controls. They were first cousins. The inheritance of the disorder appears to be autosomal recessive.

Fatal familial insomnia

This is an autosomal dominant condition characterized by selective degeneration of the anterior and dorsomedial thalamic nuclei. It is an inherited prion disease. It presents in the third or fourth decade with progressive insomnia, ataxia, dysarthria and myoclonus, along with hypertension, tachycardia, and sweating. The autonomic investigations suggest preserved parasympathetic, but higher background and stimulated sympathetic activity (Cortelli et al. 1991). Recent positron emission tomography scanning studies confirm hypometabolism of the thalamus and cingulate cortex although there is variable involvement of other brain regions (Cortelli et al. 1997).

Menkes' kinky hair disease (trichopoliodystrophy)

This is a focal degenerative disorder of grey matter in which there is a maldistribution of body copper with low serum copper and caeruloplasmin levels (Menkes 1995). It is transmitted as a sex-linked disorder. Variants have been described (Proud et al. 1996). There is reduced activity of DBH, which is dependent on copper as a cofactor. This results in impaired conversion of dopamine to noradrenaline. Menkes disease presents in infancy with vomiting, hypothermia, and neurological abnormalities such as hypotonia and poor head control. An important pointer to the diagnosis is the appearance of the hair, which is colourless and friable. Most infants have delayed growth and development and the mean age at death is 19 months, although survival to the age of 13 years has been recorded. Early copper replacement may be beneficial (Kaler et al. 1996).

Familial hyperbradykininism

These patients have symptoms suggestive of postural hypotension (Streeten et al. 1972). During head-up postural change the systolic (but not necessarily the diastolic) blood pressure usually fails and there is a marked rise in heart rate. Associated signs include cutaneous dilatation in the face and the lower limbs, the latter may turn purple. There are no neurological deficits. The findings have been attributed to excessive bradykinin levels. The postural hypotension, therefore, is not due to autonomic failure. These patients appear to benefit from propranolol, fludrocortisone, and the serotonin antagonist, cyproheptadine.

Adrenoleucodystrophy

This is an X-linked disorder that is related to the deposition of long-chain fatty acids (such as hexocosanoate C26 : 0) in cerebral white matter and in the adrenal cortex. This is thought to be due to an enzymatic defect in degradation of long-chain fatty acids (Iannaccone and Rosenberg 1996). There are three forms which result in adrenocortical failure (Addison's disease) and therefore may cause a low supine blood pressure and also postural hypotension; thus the latter is not the result of autonomic failure. In the childhood form, with presentation between the ages of 4 and 8 years, there may be deafness, dementia, cortical blindness, and tetraparesis. In the adult form, the presentation is usually between 20 and 30 years, with a longer life expectancy. In this form spastic paraparesis and polyneuropathy are common. A mixed form has been described. The symptomatic heterozygote form, which may occur in females, does not appear to involve the adrenal cortex.

Like hyperbradykininism, there is no evidence of autonomic failure accounting for the postural hypotension. In adrenoleucodystrophy deficiency of cortisol and aldosterone is responsible for the hypotension.

Management of DBH deficiency

The main problem in these patients is postural hypotension which in general responds unsatisfactorily to conventional approaches and drugs (see Chapter 36). In patients 1–4, details of the drug combinations used were not provided. Patient 5 improved on fludrocortisone alone but did not benefit from desmopressin at night despite having nocturnal polyuria; patient 6 needed a combination of fludrocortisone, dihydroergotamine, and desmopressin at night, which helped partially.

Metyrosine is a drug that inhibits the rate-limiting enzyme tyrosine hydroxylase and is used in patients with malignant phaeochromocytoma to prevent the formation of noradrenaline. In patient 1 it was used successfully to raise supine blood pressure and improve postural hypotension. This was thought to be due to reducing the formation of dopamine (Biaggioni et al. 1987). However, in this same patient the dopamine antagonist, metoclopramide, had no effect on blood pressure. The reasons for this difference are not clear.

The drug that has been particularly beneficial in all seven patients is dihydroxyphenylserine (DOPS). It is similar in structure to noradrenaline (Fig. 40.2), except that it has a carboxyl group as in Dopa. Therefore it is acted upon by dopa-decarboxylase, which is present both intraneurally and in a number of extraneuronal tissues, including the kidney and liver, and is converted directly into noradrenaline, thus bypassing the DBH enzymatic step. The drug crosses the blood–brain barrier, as has been demonstrated in animal studies (Kato et al. 1987). Its effects on reducing postural hypotension were described initially by Suzuki et al. (1980) in patients with familial amyloidosis (see also Chapter 36). It is available either as the racemic

mixture (DL-DOPS) or in the laevo form (L-DOPS). The L form is thought to be the active form, based on both animal studies and on observations in patients with familial amyloidosis, where it was effective in half the dosage of the DL form (Suzuki et al. 1982).

In each of the patients, DL-DOPS had remarkable effects. There were definite improvements, with an elevation of supine blood pressure and, more importantly, a reduction in postural hypotension (Fig. 40.16). There were no mood changes in patients 1 and 2. In patients 3, 5, 6, and 7 the description indicated that use of the drug effectively changed their lives. Patient 3 could cycle, climb stairs, and sit in the sun without feeling faint; she could not do this previously. Patients 5 and 6 were less tired and fatigued, especially in the morning. In patient 5, the symptoms of postural hypotension were virtually eliminated, and in patient 6 they were considerably improved. They both became far more active physically and noted perspiration to a greater extent on exertion, especially around the axillae and groins. Both noted cutis anserina (goose pimples) over the forearms and thighs, that they had not seen previously. In patient 7, symptoms of orthostatic intolerance disappeared.

The change in patient 6 improved a strained marital relationship. She was at times slightly more aggressive than previously and even challenged her mother-in-law for the first time, having previously wished to do so but having been too timid. Neither patient 5 nor 6 had difficulty in sleeping, which is consistent with observations in patients 3 and 4 (Tulen et al. 1990). After DOPS, patient 5 may have had an increase in the number of nightmares, which she had suffered from for many years. There was little doubt, however, that initially on DL-DOPS and later with L-DOPS, patients 5 and 6 were symptomatically far better than when their blood pressure was raised to an equivalent degree on the conventional therapy described above (i.e. fludrocortisone in patient 5 and fludrocortisone, dihydroergotamine, and desmopressin in patient 6). The treatment with DL-DOPS had no effect on nocturia in patient 6, and in both patients the nocturnal diuresis and natriuresis continued (Fig. 40.6). Whether the overall improvement was related to the effects of the drug (including central effects), or non-specifically to the rise in blood pressure and reduction in postural hypotension, was not entirely clear.

An additional advantage of DL- and L-DOPS in patient 5 was the improvement in sexual function, as he was able to achieve ejaculation, which had been difficult or impossible previously. The effect of DOPS on sexual function in the other male (patient 2) was not described.

Levels of plasma noradrenaline rose in each of the patients to whom DL-DOPS was administered; there was also a rise in patients 5, 6, and 7 who were also given L-DOPS. In patients 1–3 there was a further increase in plasma noradrenaline levels with postural challenge (Fig. 40.17), as occurred in patient 7. This was not consistently observed in patients 5 and 6 (Fig. 40.16a,b) when given either DL-DOPS or L-DOPS. In patients 5 and 6 this may imply inadequate intraneuronal replacement. In patient 3 the ability of tyramine to release noradrenaline after DL-DOPS was provided as evidence of intraneuronal replacement. However, noradrenaline formed extraneuronally (dopa decarboxylase is extensively distributed, especially in liver and kidneys) would have been incorporated by uptake mechanisms into the cytosol and this could have been released by tyramine, not necessarily indicating intraneuronal conversion of DL-DOPS to noradrenaline and release of noradrenaline by neuronal impulses. The data for patients 5 and 6 suggest that in these patients

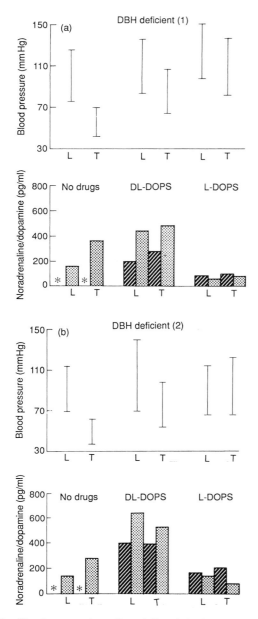

Fig. 40.16. Blood pressure (systolic and diastolic) while lying (L) and during head-up tilt (T) in (a) patient 5 and (b) patient 6 (b) with DBH deficiency (1 and 2, respectively, in figures), before and during treatment with DL-DOPS and L-DOPS. Plasma noradrenaline (hatched histogram) and dopamine (stippled histogram) levels are indicated before and during tilt. Plasma noradrenaline was undetectable (* = <5pg/ml) in both while off drugs. (From Mathias *et al.* (1990).)

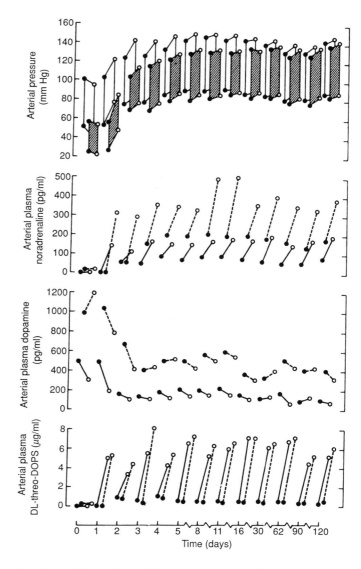

Fig. 40.17. Effects of DL-DOPS in patient 3 with DBH deficiency. Open columns and solid lines indicate values with the patient supine, hatched columns and broken lines with the patient standing. (Filled circle) 12 h after dosing: (open circle) 2 h after dosing. (From Man in't Veld *et al.* (1987*b*).)

extraneuronal formation of noradrenaline may have played a more important role. In patient 7, the noradrenaline spillover at rest was extremely low and rose to within the normal range during treatment with L-DOPS. During head-up tilt, however, the noradrenaline spillover, although initially increased by L-DOPS, remained below the normal range. Another explanation provided was that the replacement dose, although clinically satisfactory, may have not provided adequate biochemical replacement of noradrenaline. In patient 7 there was a marked increase in plasma concentration of dihydrox-

yphenyl glycol (DHPG), the intraneuronal metabolite of noradrenaline, providing evidence of noradrenaline synthesis within sympathetic nerves.

In patients 5 and 6, adrenaline remained undetectable in plasma and the metabolites of adrenaline in urine (metadrenaline) minimally changed (Fig. 40.11) after 3 months of therapy. This raised the question of abnormalities in the conversion of noradrenaline to adrenaline, either because of an atrophic adrenal medulla or because of the absence of the enzyme phenylethanolamine-*N*-methyl transferase (PNMT). A similar conclusion, based on barely detectable changes in adrenaline secretion after L-DOPS, was reported in patient 7. Further evidence of the inability to form adrenaline was obtained in patients 5 and 6 in whom insulin hypoglycaemia was induced while they were on treatment with L-DOPS. During hypoglycaemia, there was no rise in plasma adrenaline levels, and a small rise in plasma noradrenaline levels. The absence of a rise of metadrenaline excretion in urine was also noticed in patients with familial amyloidosis who were given L-DOPS (Suzuki *et al.* 1982).

In patients 5 and 6, the question of whether DOPS had direct pressor effects was tested by pre-treating them with the dopa decarboxylase inhibitor carbidopa, in a dose sufficient to prevent peripheral decarboxylation. L-DOPS was then administered and, unlike in previous studies, it had no beneficial effect either on blood pressure or on the patients' ability to stand. This was consistent with a lack of its conversion to noradrenaline, which could not be detected in plasma. Thus L-DOPS alone, even in patients with known adrenoceptor supersensitivity, has no direct pressor effects.

Another point of interest is the question of the central effects of DOPS. This has been partially discussed in relation to behavioural and mood changes and may also be relevant to the blood pressure responses. Animal studies indicate that DL- and L-DOPS enter the brain (Kato *et al.* 1987). In patients 5 and 6, L-DOPS in the same dose as DL-DOPS was equally effective; theoretically it should have been doubly effective. One possibility is greater formation of noradrenaline within the central nervous system, as has been demonstrated in animal studies, which reduces centrally induced sympathetic discharge and would thus have negated the peripheral effects of the drug (Araki *et al.* 1981). This would be consistent with the lower levels of plasma dopamine observed after L-DOPS, as compared with levels after DL-DOPS (Fig. 40.16a,b). There may also have been other effects, including a central reduction of dopamine levels. Both patients 5 and 6 felt that DL-DOPS was 'better' than L-DOPS, though this has not been quantified. In repeat studies after 10 years of treatment with L-DOPS in patients 5 and 6, there was no evidence of any neurological or behavioural impairment and they continue to benefit from the drug.

References

Allgrove, J., Clayden, G. S., and Grant, D. B. (1978). Familial glucocortoid deficiency with achalasia of the cardia and deficient tear production. *Lancet* 1, 1284–6.

Anand, P., Rudge, P., Mathias, C. J., *et al.* (1991). New autonomic and sensory neuropathy with loss of adrenergic sympathetic functions and sensory neuropeptides. *Lancet* 337, 1253–4.

Araki, H., Tanaka, C., Fujiwara, H., Nakamura, M., and Ohmura, I. (1981). Pressor effect of L-threo-3, 4–dihydroxyphenylserine in rats. *J. Pharm. Pharmacol.* 33, 772–7.

Biaggioni, I. and Robertson, D. (1987). Endogenous restoration of noradrenaline by precursor therapy in dopamine beta-hydroxylase deficiency. *Lancet* ii, 1170–2.

Biaggioni, I., Goldstein, D. S., Atkinson, T., and Robertson, D. (1990). Dopamine beta-hydroxylase deficiency in humans. *Neurology* 40, 370–3.

Cable, W. J. L., Kolodny, E. H., and Adams, R. D. (1982). Fabry disease: impaired autonomic function. *Neurology* 32, 498–502.

Chu, M. L., Berlin, D., and Axelrod, F. B. (1996). Allgrove syndrome: documenting cholinergic dysfunction by autonomic tests. *J. Pediatr.* 129, 156–9.

Cortelli, P., Parchi, P., Contin, M. *et al.* (1991). Cardiovascular dysautonomia in fatal familial insomnia. *Clin. Aut on. Res.* 1, 15–22.

Cortelli, P., Perani, D., Parchi, P. *et al.* (1997). Cerebral metabolism in fatal familial insomnia: Relation to duration, neuropathology, and distribution of protease-resistant prion protein. *Neurology* 49, 126–33.

Gazarian, M., Cowell, C. T., Bonney, M., and Grigo, W. G. (1995). The '4A' syndrome: adrenocorticol insufficiency associated with achalasia, alacrima, autonomic and other neurological abnormalities. *Eur. J. Pediatr.* 154, 18–23.

Hyland, K., Surtees, R. A., Rodeck, A. H., and Clayton, T. (1992). Autonomic effects of aromatic L-amino acid decarboxylase deficiency: Clinical features, diagnosis and treatment of a new inborn error of neurotransmitter amine synthesis. *Neurology* 42, 1980–8.

Iannaccone, S. T. and Rosenberg, R. N. (1996). Principles of molecular genetics and neurologic diseases. In *Principles of child neurology.* (ed. B. Berg), pp. 461–606. McGraw-Hill, New York.

Ilson, J., Parrish, M., Fahn, S., and Cote, L. J. (1982). Familial Shy–Drager syndrome: clinical, biochemical and pathological findings. *Neurology* 32, A160.

Kaler, S. G., Das, S., Levinson, B. *et al.* (1996). Successful early copper therapy in Menkes disease associated with a mutant transcript containing a small in-frame deletion. *Biochem. Mol. Med.* 57, 37–46.

Kato, T., Karai, N., Katsuyama, M., Nakamura, M., and Katsube, J. (1987). Studies on the activity of L-threo-3, 4–dihydroxyphenylserine (L-DOPS) as a catecholamine precursor in the brain: Comparison with that of L-DOPA. *Biochem. Pharmacol.* 36, 3051–7.

Lewis. P. (1964). Familial orthostatic hypotension. *Brain* 87, 719–28.

Man in't Veld, A. J., Boomsma, F., Moleman, P., and Schalekamp, M. A. D. H. (1987*a*). Congenital dopamine beta-hydroxylase deficiency. A novel orthostatic syndrome. *Lancet* i, 183–7.

Man in't Veld, A. J., Van den Meiracker, A. H., Boomsma, F., and Schalekamp M. A. D. H. (1987*b*). Effect of unnatural noradrenaline precursor on sympathetic control and orthostatic hypotension in dopamine beta-hydroxylase deficiency. *Lancet* ii, 1172–5.

Man in't Veld, A. J., Boomsma, F., Lenders, J. *et al.* (1988). Patients with congenital dopamine beta-hydroxylase deficiency. A lesson in catecholamine physiology. *Am. J. Hypertens.* 1, 231–8.

Mathias, C. J. (1996). Disorders of the autonomic nervous system. In *Neurology in clinical practice,* (2nd edn), (eds. W. G. Bradley, R. B. Daroff, G. M. Fenichel, and C. D. Marsden), vol. 82, pp. 1953–81. Butterworth-Heinemann, Boston.

Mathias, C. J, Smith, A. D., Frankel, H. L., and Spalding, J. K. M. (1976). Dopamine beta-hydroxylase release during hypertension from sympathetic nervous overactivity in main. *Cardiovasc. Res.* 10, 176–81.

Mathias, C. J., Bannister, R., Cortelli, P. *et al.* (1990). Clinical autonomic and therapeutic observations in two siblings with postural hypotension and sympathetic failure due to an inability to synthesize noradrenaline from dopamine because of a deficiency of dopamine beta-hydroxylase. *Q. J. Med.* 75, 617–33.

Menkes, J. H. (1995). Metabolic diseases of the nervous system. In *Textbook of child neurology,* (ed. J. H. Menkes), pp. 29–151. Williams & Wilkins, Baltimore, Maryland.

O'Connor, D. T., Cervenka, J. H., Stone, R. A., *et al.* (1994). Dopamine beta-hydroxylase immunoreactivity in human cerebrospinal fluid: properties, relationship to central noradrenergic neuronal activity and variation in Parkinson's disease and dopamine beta-hydroxylase deficiency. *Clin. Sci.* 86, 149–58.

Proud, V. K., Mussell, H. G., Kaler, S. G., Young, D. W., and Percy, A. K. (1996). Distinctive Menkes disease variant with occipital horns: delineation of natural history and clinical phenotype. *Am. J. Med. Genet.* 65, 44–51.

Rea, R., Biaggioni, I., Robertson, R. M., Haile, V., and Robertson, D. (1990). Reflex control of sympathetic nerve activity in dopamine-beta-hydroxylase deficiency. *Hypertension* 1, 107–12.

Robertson, D., Goldberg, M. R., Onrot, J. *et al.* (1986). Isolated failure of autonomic noradrenergic neurotransmission. Evidence for impaired beta-hydroxylation of dopamine. *New Engl. J. Med.* 314, 1494–7.

Smith, G. D. P. and Mathias, C. J. (1995). Postural hypotension enhanced by exercise in patients with chronic autonomic failure. *Q. J. Med.* 88, 251–6.

Smith, G. D. P, Watson, L. P., Pavitt, D. V., and Mathias, C. J. (1995). Abnormal cardiovascular and catecholamine responses to supine exercise in human subjects with sympathetic dysfunction. *J. Physiol.*, London, **485**, 255–65.

Streeten, D. H. P., Kerr, L. P., Kerr, C. B., Prior, J. C., and Dalakos, T. G. (1972). Hyperbradykininism: a new orthostatic syndrome. *Lancet*, **2**, 1048–53.

Suzuki, S., Higa, S., Tsuga, I. *et al.* (1980). Effects of infused L-threo-3, 4–dihydroxyphenylserine in patients with familial amyloid polyneuropathy. *Eur. J. Clin. Pharmacol.* **17**, 429–35.

Suzuki, S., Higa, S., Sakoda, S. *et al.* (1982). Pharmacokinetic studies of oral L-threo-3, 4–dihydroxyphenylserine in normal subjects and patients with familial amyloid polyneuropathy. *Eur. J. Clin. Pharmacol.* **23**, 463–8.

Thomas, P. K. (1992). Autonomic involvement in inherited neuropathies. *Clin. Auton. Res.* **2**, 51–6.

Thomas, S. A., Matsumoto, A. M., and Palmiter, R.D. (1995). Noradrenaline is essential for mouse fetal development. *Nature* **374**, 643–6.

Thompson, J. M., O'Callaghan, C. J., Kingwell, B. A., Lambert, G. W., Jennings, G. L., and Esler, M. D. (1995). Total norepinephrine spillover, muscle sympathetic nerve activity and heart rate spectral analysis in a patient with dopamine β-hydroxylase deficiency. *J. Autonom. Nerv. Syst.* **55**, 198–206.

Tulen, J. H. M., Mann in't Veld, A. J., Mechelse, K., and Boomsma, F. (1990). Sleep patterns in congenital dopamine beta-hydroxylase deficiency. *J. Neurol.* **237**, 98–102.

Weinshilboum, R. M. (1979). Serum dopamine beta-hydroxylase. *Pharmacol. Rev.* **30**, 133–66.

Weinshilboum, R. M. and Axelrod, J. (1971). Reduced plasma dopamine beta-hydroxylase in familial dysantonomia. *New Engl. J. Med* **285**, 938.

Yamamoto, K., Sobue, G., Iwase, S., Kumazawa, K., Mitsuma, T., and Mano, T. (1996). Possible mechanism of anhidrosis in a symptomatic female carrier of Fabry's disease: an assessment by skin sympathetic nerve activity and sympathetic skin response. *Clin. Auton. Res.* **6**, 107–10.

Zelnik, N., Axelrod, F. B., Leshinsky, E., Griebel, M. L., and Kolodny, E. H. (1996). Mitochondrial encephalomyopathies presenting with features of autonomic and visceral dysfunction. *Pediat. Neurol.* **14**, 251–4.

Zhou, Q.-Z., Quaife, C. J., and Palmiter, R. D. (1995). Targeted disruption of the tyrosine hydroxylase gene reveals that catecholamines are required for mouse fetal development. *Nature* **374**, 640–3.

41. Familial dysautonomia

Felicia B. Axelrod

Introduction

Familial dysautonomia (FD), originally termed the Riley–Day syndrome, is an autosomal recessive disorder with extensive central and peripheral autonomic perturbations. It is now appreciated that FD is one example of a group of rare disorders termed hereditary sensory and autonomic neuropathies (HSAN); (Axelrod 1996*a*). Within this classification FD is termed HSAN type III. The HSANs can be thought of broadly as entities in which normal migration and maturation of neural-crest-derived cells has been impeded, especially those destined to evolve into the sensory and autonomic populations. The genetic defect affects prenatal neuronal development so that symptoms are present from birth, although individual expression varies widely. Because the entire autonomic nervous system is affected, there is a pervasive effect on the functioning of other systems. However, with supportive treatments of the various manifestations, the prognosis for affected individuals has improved and a growing number of individuals affected with FD are surviving into adulthood.

Because the FD population is presumed to be genetically homogeneous, it serves as an excellent model with which to understand autonomic dysfunction caused by depleted unmyelinated neurones. It is anticipated that the gene for FD will be discovered shortly which will enlighten us further regarding the interrelationship of neuropathological lesions and the biochemical and physiological factors controlling the autonomic nervous system.

Genetics

FD is due to a recessive genetic defect with a remarkably high carrier frequency in individuals of Ashkenazi Jewish extraction. In this population, the carrier rate has been estimated to be 1 in 30, with a disease frequency of 1 in 3600 live births (Maayan *et al.* 1987*a*). Using genetic linkage, the defective gene was mapped to the distal long arm of chromosome 9 (q31) with sufficient DNA markers to permit prenatal diagnosis and carrier identification for families in which there has been an affected individual (Blumenfeld *et al.* 1993; Fig. 41.1) By analysing haplotypes of a large cohort of homozygous affected individuals, it was appreciated that a common ancestral mutation could be found in a closely linked marker in most of the FD chromosomes. At D9S1677, 95 per cent of FD chromosomes carried a '12' allele in contrast to only 2.7 per cent of control chromosomes. (Gusella *et al.* 1997). This finding supports the hypothesis that the ethnic bias in this disorder is due to a founder effect.

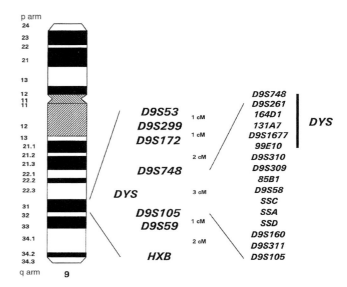

Fig. 41.1. Genetic map of the DYS region. An ideogram of human chromosome 9 is shown with the genetic map of the DYS region in 9q31. The 3 cM interval between D9S748 and D9S105 is expanded to the right to show all polymorphic markers and the location of the minimal FD candidate region.

The other HSANs do not have the same ethnic bias as FD and are presumed to have unique genotypes accounting for their subtle phenotypic differences. Because all of the HSANs affect neuronal development, possible candidates are genes that encode neurotrophins, their receptors, or any proteins that might participate in a neurotrophin-related signal transduction pathway. HSAN type IV recently has been shown to result from mutations in the gene that encodes a neurotrophin receptor, NTRK1, which is located on chromosome 1 (Indo *et al.* 1996).

Neuropathology

Although clinical manifestations suggest both central and peripheral nervous system involvement, consistent neuropathological lesions have only been described for the peripheral nervous system. Pathological findings indicate that within the peripheral sensory and autonomic systems individuals affected with FD suffer from incomplete neuronal development as well as progressive neuronal degeneration. Investigations are yet to be performed to see whether similar lesions are present in the central autonomic tracts.

Sensory nervous system

Intrauterine development and postnatal maintenance of dorsal root ganglion neurones are abnormal. The dorsal root ganglia are grossly reduced in size due to decreased neuronal population. Within the spinal cord, lateral root entry zones and Lissauer's tracts are severely depleted of axons (Pearson and Pytel 1978a). With increasing age, the numbers of neurones in dorsal root ganglia decrease more than one would expect as part of normal ageing and there is an abnormal increase in the number of residual nodules of Nageotte. In addition, loss of dorsal column myelinated axons becomes evident in older patients. Neuronal depletion in dorsal root ganglia and spinal cord is consistent with reports of decreased size of the sural nerve in FD patients. The sural nerve is reduced in area and contains markedly diminished numbers of non-myelinated axons, as well as diminished numbers of small-diameter myelinated axons. Even in the youngest subject, extensive pathology has been evident, as might be expected from the fact that this is a developmental disorder. The sural nerve findings are sufficiently characteristic for familial dysautonomia to differentiate it from other sensory neuropathies (Axelrod 1996a).

Autonomic nervous system

Consistent with an actual decrease in neuronal numbers, the mean volume of superior cervical sympathetic ganglia is reduced to 34 per cent of the normal size (Pearson and Pytel 1978a; Fig. 41.2), yet staining for tyrosine hydroxylase is enhanced in the neurones that are present in the sympathetic ganglia (Pearson et al. 1979b). Decreased

numbers of neurones in the intermediolateral grey columns. of the spinal cord suggests involvement of preganglionic neurones (Pearson and Pytel 1978a). Furthermore, autonomic nerve terminals cannot be demonstrated on peripheral blood vessels (Grover-Johnson and Pearson 1976). Lack of innervation is consistent with postural hypotension, as well as exaggerated responses to sympathomimetic and parasympathomimetic agents (Smith et al. 1965).

Other than the sphenopalatine ganglia, which are consistently reduced in size with low total neuronal counts, other parasympathetic ganglia, such as the ciliary ganglia, do not seem to be affected (Pearson and Pytel 1978b). The paucity of neurones in the sphenopalatine ganglion would explain the supersensitivity of the lacrimal gland to infused methacholine (Smith et al. 1965).

Neurophysiology

Chemoreceptor and baroreceptor dysfunction

Denervation extending to chemoreceptors and baroreceptors has never been demonstrated pathologically but is strongly suggested by physiological studies. During hypoxia (12 per cent O_2), patients with FD initially increase ventilation but with continued hypoxia, ventilation decreases (Edelman et al. 1970). These observations suggest that patients with FD have normal peripheral chemoreceptors but an inordinate central depression of ventilation by hypoxia. Furthermore,

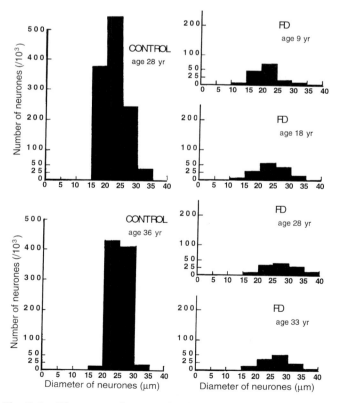

Fig. 41.2. Histograms of neurone distribution in sympathetic ganglia in patients with familial dysautonomia and controls. (From Pearson and Pytel (1978a).)

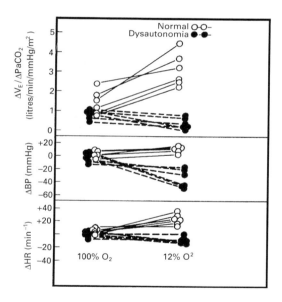

Fig. 41.3. Ventilatory and cardiovascular responses to the rebreathing of 100 per cent and 12 per cent oxygen by six dysautonomic and six normal subjects. Left-hand points: 100 per cent O_2; right-hand points: 12 per cent O_2. Upper panel: ventilatory response to CO_2 expressed as increase in ventilation per mmHg increase in $PaCO_2$ normalized for body surface area. Middle panel: each point represents the change in mean systemic blood pressure from the beginning to the end of a rebreathing period. Lower panel: each point represents the change in heart rate from the beginning to the end of a rebreathing period. In contrast to control subjects, rebreathing 12 per cent O_2 by dysautonomia subjects resulted in a lower ventilatory response to CO_2 than during 100 per cent rebreathing, bradycardia, and a substantial fall in systemic blood pressure. (From Edelman et al. (1970).)

hypoxia induces profound circulatory responses consistent with sympathetic denervation (Edelman *et al.* 1970). In contrast to controls, when FD subjects are exposed to hypoxia during rebreathing, there is a marked decrease in heart rate and systemic blood pressure (Fig. 41.3)

Studies of forearm blood flow have described inappropriate arteriolar and venous tone responses to both upright positioning and cold stimuli (Mason *et al.* 1966). In individuals with FD, vascular resistance did not increase with either stimulus. It is now well recognized that indiviuals with FD consistently manifest orthostatic hypotension without compensatory tachycardia.

Catecholamine metabolism

On measurement of urinary catecholamine metabolites, FD patients were found to have elevated levels of homovanillic acid (HVA) and

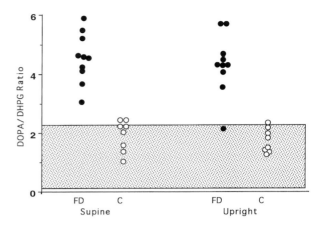

Fig. 41.5. DOPA : DHPG ratios for 10 FD and 8 control subjects. FD values (●) are averages from two to three testing sessions. Control values (o) are absolute values. The grey area indicates the normal range of this ratio in plasma (0.13–2.28). (From Axelrod *et al.* (1996).)

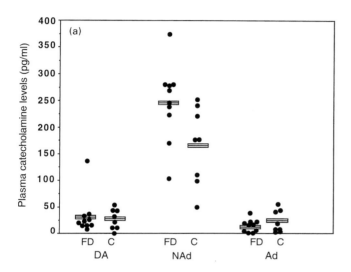

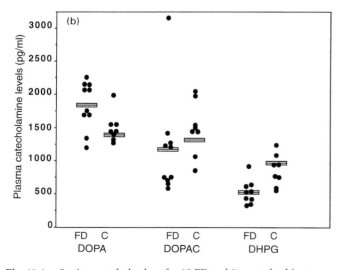

Fig. 41.4. Supine catechol values for 10 FD and 8 control subjects. FD values are averages from two to three testing sessions. Control values are absolute values. Horizontal bars are means. (a) Catecholamine: DA, dopamine; NAd, noradrenaline; Ad, adrenaline; (b) catechol metabolites: DOPA, dihydroxyphenylalanine; DOPAC, dihydroxyphenylacetic acid; DHPG, dihydroxyphenylglycol. (From Axelrod *et al.* (1996).)

normal to low levels of vanillylmandelic acid (VMA), resulting in elevated HVA : VMA ratios (Smith *et al.* 1963). These findings are consistent with the later neuropathological descriptions of a decreased sympathetic neuronal population. Although supine plasma levels of noradrenaline (NAd) are normal or elevated, FD patients, like most other patients with neurogenic orthostatic hypotension, do not have an appropriate increase in plasma levels of NAd and dopamine β-hydroxylase (DBH) with standing (Ziegler *et al.* 1976; Axelrod *et al.* 1996) In addition, FD patients appear to have a distinctive pattern of plasma levels of catechols (Fig. 41.4). Regardless of posture, plasma levels of dopa are disproportionately high and plasma levels of DHPG are low resulting in elevated plasma dopa : DHPG ratios (Fig. 41.5) which are not seen in other disorders associated with neurogenic orthostatic hypotension. The low levels of DHPG could be a consequence of either decreased availability of axoplasmic NAd or decreased sequential activity of monoamine oxidase (MAO) and aldehydic reductase on NAd. The high plasma dopa levels are consistent with FD subjects having an increased proportion of tyrosine hydroxylase in superior cervical ganglia (Pearson *et al.* 1979*b*).

When FD subjects are supine, there is a strong correlation between mean blood pressure and plasma levels of NAd, but when they are upright, the correlation is seen only with plasma dopamine levels (Fig. 41.6) suggesting that in FD patients dopamine may serve to maintain upright blood pressure. During emotional crises, plasma NAd and dopamine levels are markedly elevated and vomiting usually coincides with the high dopamine levels. The elevation of plasma NAd is attributed to peripheral conversion of dopamine by DBH. Diazepam sedates patients in crises and relieves vomiting, possibly by enhancing GABA and damping the release of dopamine.

Other vascular modulators

Supine early morning plasma renin activity is elevated in FD subjects and the release of renin and aldosterone is not co-ordinated (Rabinowitz *et al.* 1974). In FD individuals with supine hypertension, an increase in plasma atrial natriuretic peptide (ANP) has also been

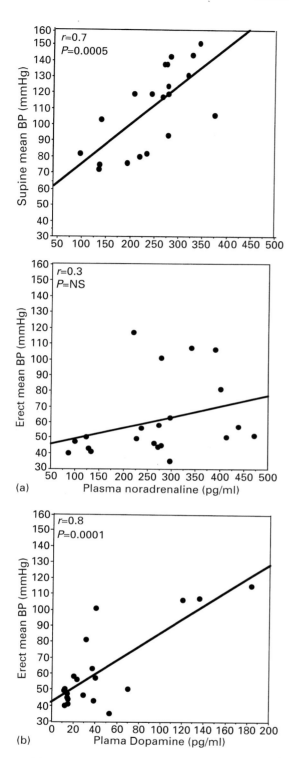

Fig. 41.6. (a) Correlation of mean blood pressure and plasma level of noradrenaline in FD subjects when supine and erect. (b) Correlation of mean blood pressure and plasma level of dopamine in FD subjects when erect.

demonstrated (Axelrod *et al.* 1994). The combination of these factors may serve to explain the exaggerated nocturnal urine volume and increased excretion of salt in some FD individuals, especially during stress and hypertension.

Clinical features and management

Diagnostic criteria

As a the specific genetic error has not yet been described for FD, diagnosis relies on clinical criteria that are based upon the ethnic bias for this disorder as well as a constellation of signs attributed to sensory and autonomic dysfunctions. Although this is a neurological disorder, the clinical features are pervasive and involve many other systems (Table 41.1). The diagnosis should be suspected by history and physical examination, which can provide much of the essential information. Confirmation is then obtained by ascertaining the presence of five 'cardinal' criteria, i.e. absence of overflow emotional tears, absent lingual fungiform papillae (Fig. 41.7), depressed patellar reflexes, lack of an axon flare following intradermal histamine (Fig. 41.8) , and documentation of Ashkenazi Jewish extraction. Further supportive evidence is provided by findings of decreased response to pain and temperature, orthostatic hypotension, periodical erythematous blotching of the skin, and increased sweating. In addition, cine-oesophagrams may reveal delay in cricopharyngeal closure, tertiary contractions of the oesophagus, gastro-oesophageal reflux, and delayed gastric emptying.

Because individuals affected with the other HSANs will also fail to produce an axon flare after intradermal histamine, careful assessment of the other clinical signs and symptoms is necessary in order to distinguish between these disorders. Because there can be extreme variability in expression, clinical criteria are not always sufficient and sural nerve biopsy may be suggested.

Table 41.1. Clinical features of familial dysautonomia

System	Common symptoms	Frequency (%)
Ocular		
	Decreased tears	>60
	Corneal analgesia	>60
Gastrointestinal dysfunction		
	Dysphagia	>60
	Oesophageal and gastric dysmotility	>60
	Gastroesophageal reflux	67
	Vomiting crises	40
Pulmonary		
	Aspirations	NA
	Insensitivity to hypoxia and hypercarbia	NA
	Restrictive lung disease	NA
Orthopaedic		
	Spinal curvature	90
	Asceptic necrosis	15
Vasomotor		
	Postural hypotension	100
	Blotching	99
	Excessive sweating	99
	Hypertensive crises	>60
Neurological		
	Decreased deep tendon reflexes	95
	Dysarthria	NA
	Decreased pain and temperature sensation	NA
	Decreased vibration (after 13 years)	NA
	Progressive ataxia (in adult years)	NA
	Less than average IQ	38

NA, Percentages not available.

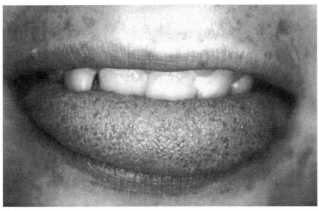

(a)

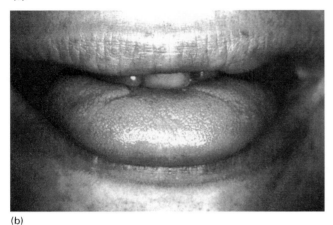

(b)

Fig. 41.7. (a) Normal tongue with fungiform papillae present on the tip; (b) dysautonomic tongue.

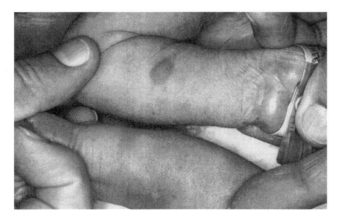

Fig. 41.8. Histamine test. Dysautonomic reaction (forearm on top) demonstrates a narrow areola surrounding the wheal. Normal reaction (lower forearm) displays diffuse axon flare around a central wheal.

Sensory system

In the younger patient, sensory abnormalities appear to be limited to the unmyelinated neuronal population, but in the older patient there is progressive involvement of myelinated neurones of the dorsal column tracts. Although pain sensation is decreased, it is not completely absent and there is usually sparing of palms, soles of feet, neck, and genital areas, with these areas often being exquisitely sensitive. Temperature appreciation, as documented by sympathetic skin responses and Thermotest readings to both hot and cold stimuli, is also affected (Hilz *et al.* 1994). With both pain and temperature perceptions, the trunk and lower extremities are more affected and older individuals have greater losses than younger (Axelrod *et al.* 1981). In the older individual, vibration sense, and occasionally joint position, become abnormal and Rombergism may be noted. Visceral sensation is intact so patients are able to perceive discomfort with pleuritic or peritoneal irritation.

Peripheral sensory deprivation makes the FD patient prone to self-injury. In addition to inadvertent trauma to joints and long bones, causing Charcot joints, aseptic necrosis, and unrecognized fractures, some patients will self-mutilate by picking at their fingers to the point of bleeding. Spinal curvature, which can be early and pernicious in its course, requires extreme care in fitting of braces to avoid development of pressure decubiti on insensitive skin.

Central sensory deficits include decreased pain perception along the branches of the trigeminal nerve, diminished corneal reflexes, and decreased taste perception, especially in recognition of sweet, flavours which corresponds to the absence of fungiform papillae on the tip of the tongue.

Although the motor system is spared, the young child with FD is frequently hypotonic, which may be due to a combination of central deficits and decreased tone of stretch receptors. Older patients are not weak but develop a broad-based and mildly ataxic gait, with special difficulties in performing rapid movements or turning. Gait abnormalities can be severe enough to require the use of walkers or wheelchairs.

Autonomic dysfunction

Pervasive autonomic dysfunction results in protean functional abnormalities affecting other systems and yielding a myriad of clinical manifestations. As the disorder has variable expression, there are individual variations. Some of these manifestations are apparent at birth and others become more prominent and problematic as a function of age.

Gastrointestinal system

Oropharyngeal incoordination is one of the earliest signs of FD. Poor sucking or discoordinated swallowing is observed in 60 per cent of infants in the neonatal period. Oral incoordination can persist in the older patient and be manifested as a tendency to drool. Cine-radiographic swallowing studies, using various food consistencies, are used to assess function and provide guidelines for therapy. Liquids are more apt to be aspirated. If dysphagia impedes maintenance of nutrition, or if respiratory problems persist, then gastrostomy is recommended.

The most prominent manifestation of abnormal gastrointestinal dysmotility in FD individuals is the propensity to vomit. Vomiting can occur intermittently as part of a systemic reaction to physical or emotional stress or it can occur daily in response to the stress of arousal. Because vomiting is often associated with hypertension, tachycardia, diffuse sweating, and even personality change, this constellation of signs has been termed the dysautonomic crisis. Diazepam is considered to be the most effective anti-emetic for the dysautonomic crisis and can be administered orally, intravenously, or rectally at 0.1–0.2 mg/kg/dose. Subsequent doses of diazepam are repeated at 3–hour intervals until the crisis resolves. If diastolic hypertension persists (>90 mm Hg) after giving diazepam, then either chloral hydrate or clonidine (0.004 mg/kg/dose) is suggested. Clonidine can be repeated at 8–hour intervals. The crisis usually resolves abruptly and is marked by return of personality to normal and return of appetite.

Gastro-oesophageal reflux (GER) is another common problem and should be considered in FD individuals with frequent vomiting. If GER is identified, medical management, including prokinetic agents and H_2 antagonists, should be tried. However, if pneumonia, heaematemesis, or apnoea occur, then surgical intervention (fundoplication) is recommended. After surgery, dysautonomic crises may continue but retching will be substituted for vomiting.

Respiratory system

Aspiration is the major cause of lung infections. Most of the lung damage occurs during infancy and early childhood when oral incoordination is extremely poor and the diet contains mostly liquids. If gastro-oesophageal reflux is present, the risk for aspiration increases.

The ventilatory response to lung infection is often altered due to insensitivity to hypoxia and hypercapnia (Edelman *et al.* 1970). Low oxygen saturations do not cause tachypnoea and can cause syncope as hypoxia induces both hypotension and bradycardia. Dysautonomic patients must be cautious in settings where the partial pressure of oxygen is decreased, such as at high altitudes or during aeroplane travel. When the aeroplane's altitude exceeds 39 000 feet (≏ 12 000 m), the cabin pressure will be equivalent to more than 6000 feet (≏ 2000 m), and supplemental oxygen probably will be necessary. Diving and underwater swimming can be potential hazards.

Cardiovascular irregularities

Consistent with sympathetic dysfunction, patients exhibit rapid and severe orthostatic decreases in blood pressure, without appropriate compensatory increases in heart rate. Clinical manifestations of postural hypotension include episodes of lightheadedness or dizzy spells. Some patients complain of 'weak legs'. On occasion, there may be syncope. Symptoms tend to be worse in the morning, in hot or humid weather, when the bladder is full, before a large bowel movement, after a long car ride, coming out of a movie theatre, or with fatigue. Symptoms referable to hypotension become more prominent in the adult years and can limit function and mobility. Postural hypotension is treated by maintaining adequate hydration, as monitored by blood urea nitrogen levels. Lower-extremity exercises are encouraged to increase muscle tone and promote venous return. Elastic stockings and fludrocortisone, a mineralocorticoid, have been of some benefit. Recently midodrine, an α-adrenergic agonist, has been tried. At an average dose of 0.25 mg/kg/day, all patients exhibited clinical improvement (Axelrod *et al.* 1995).

General anaesthesia has the potential for inducing severe hypotension. With greater attention to stabilization of the vascular bed by hydrating the patient before surgery and titrating the anaesthetic to continuously monitored arterial blood pressure, anaesthetic risk has been greatly reduced.

In the older patients, supine hypertension can become prominent despite the retention of severe responses to orthostatic challenge.

Hypertension can also occur intermittently in response to emotional stress or visceral pain, or as part of the crisis constellation. The hypertension will respond to the same medications recommended for crisis management. Hypertension can also exist without any other symptoms. Because blood pressure is so labile in individuals with FD, asymptomatic hypertension is not usually treated as the hypertension is usually transitory and appears to be better tolerated than hypotension.

Although FD subjects consistently exhibit orthostatic instability, they have variable electrocardiographic findings. As part of the progressive nature of FD, there is worsening of sympathetic dysfunction and development of parasympathetic dysfunction. Heart-rate variability studies, using power spectral analysis, indicate, that with exertion, there is inappropriate persistence of parasympathetic activity and failure to enhance sympathetic activity (Maayan *et al.* 1987*b*). Prolongation of the QTc occurs in some patients and may be an ominous sign.

Renal problems

Azotaemia is frequently prerenal in origin. Although clinical signs of dehydration may not be present, blood urea nitrogen values often can be reduced by simple hydration. Renal function appears to deteriorate with advancing age, so that about 20 per cent of adult patients

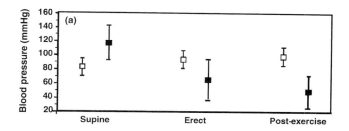

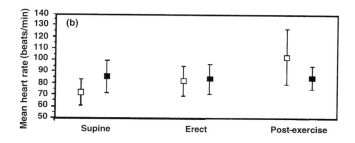

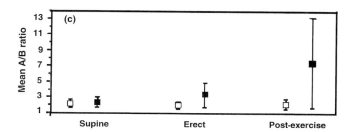

Fig. 41.9. Haemodynamic response to change in position and exercise in controls (□) and FD subjects (■). (a) Mean blood pressures with 1 SD bars, $P = 0.0001$; (b) mean heart rates with 1 SD bars, $P = 0.0002$; (c) mean A/B ratios with 1 SD bars, $P = 0.005$. (From Axelrod *et al.* (1993).)

have reduced renal function. Renal biopsies performed on individuals with uncorrectable azotaemia revealed significant ischeaemic-type glomerulosclerosis and deficient vascular innervation. Renal hypoperfusion secondary to cardiovascular instability has been suggested as the cause of the progressive renal disease. This hypothesis was supported by studies utilizing the technique of renal artery Doppler blood velocity waveform analysis (Axelrod *et al.* 1993). In contrast to controls, when FD patients assumed the erect position and exercised, renal systolic velocity decreased as reflected in an increased A/B ratio, the ratio of the peak systolic velocity (point A) to the end diastolic velocity (point B). An increase in A/B ratio can be interpreted as consistent with a decrease in the end diastolic flow (Fig. 41.9). Thus, aggressive treatment of postural hypotension appears to be justified.

Ophthalmological manifestations

Individuals with FD do not cry with overflow tears. Corneal hypaesthesia compounds the ocular status, as it results in decreased blink frequency and indifference to corneal trauma. Epithelial erosions of the exposed cornea and conjunctiva are the hallmarks of dry-eye states. These lesions may become confluent, leading to patchy areas of de-epithelialization. Early treatment of corneal epithelial erosions includes increased frequency of tear substitutes, attention to the general state of hydration, and the search for precipitating systemic factors that might have disturbed the patient's fragile catecholamine homeostasis. Persistent erosions or ulcerations may require a therapeutic soft contact lens, occlusion of the lacrimal puncta or small lateral tarsorrhaphies that limit the area exposed to surface evaporation. Corneal grafts generally have not been successful as the dry anaesthetic cornea is an unfavourable environment for a corneal graft. The importance of restoring the patient's homeostasis when treating ocular complications in familial dysautonomia cannot be overemphasized. Failure to correct dehydration or even a low-grade systemic infection can thwart the most heroic efforts at ocular therapy.

Other ophthalmological features include hyperreactivity to sympathetic and parasympathetic agents as well as tendency to myopia, optic pallor, and strabismus.

Central nervous system features (intelligence/emotion /seizures)

Emotional lability has been considered one of the prominent features of FD and was stressed in its original description (Riley *et al.* 1949). It is now appreciated that the behavioural abnormalities tend to be part of the crisis constellation and may be secondary to periodic catecholamine imbalance. The prompt normalization of personality in response to benzodiazepines supports this hypothesis (Axelrod 1996*b*).

Most affected individuals are of normal intelligence. In one study, 38 per cent of FD patients had less than average intelligence (Welton *et al.* 1979) but correlation with other systemic problems was not available. Individuals with FD usually perform well on the Similarities subtest of the WISC (Wechsler Intelligence Scale for Children), which suggests that verbal intellect is relatively spared.

About 25 per cent of FD patients have abnormal EEGs but less than 10 per cent actually have a true seizure disorder. In the population of FD patients who have had a seizure, the incidence of an abnormal EEG rises to 65 per cent. Anticonvulsant therapy should be used in these cases.

Prolonged breath-holding with crying can be severe enough to result in cyanosis, syncope, and decerebrate posturing and has been thought to represent a type of seizure activity. Breath-holding is frequent in the early years, occurring at least one time in 63 per cent of patients. This phenomenon probably is a manifestation of insensitivity to hypoxia and hypercapnia. It can become a manipulative manoeuvre with some children. In our experience, the episodes are self-limited, cease by 6 years of age, and have never been fatal.

Metabolic seizures, induced by hyponatraemia, have been observed during extremely hot weather when fluid and salt intake have failed to compensate for the excessive sweating manifested by these patients. Hyponatraemic seizures have also occurred with severe infections.

Progressive features (peripheral and central problems)

As survival has improved for the FD population (Axelrod and Abularrage 1982), an adult FD population has evolved which has confirmed the progressive nature of the disorder. Slow progressive peripheral degeneration is appreciated clinically, as the older patients exhibit further worsening of sensory loss (Axelrod *et al.* 1981), and neuropathologically, as the number of neurones in dorsal root ganglia diminish and residual nodules of Nageotte increase abnormally with age. Adult FD patients do not appear to appreciate the decline in their sensory abilities but they frequently complain of poor balance, unsteady gait, and difficulty concentrating. They are prone to depression, anxieties, and even phobias. With increasing age, sympathovagal balance becomes more precarious with worsening of orthostatic hypotension, development of supine hypertension, and even occasional bradyarrhythmias (Axelrod *et al.* 1995).

Prognosis

With greater understanding of the disorder and development of treatment programmes, survival statistics have markedly improved so that increasing numbers of patients are reaching adulthood. Survival statistics prior to 1960 reveal that 50 per cent of patients died before 5 years of age. Current survival statistics indicate that a newborn with FD has a 50 per cent probability of reaching 30 years of age (Axelrod and Abularrage 1982) Many FD adults have been able to achieve independent function. Both men and women with FD have married and reproduced. All offspring have been phenotypically normal despite their obligatory heterozygote state. Although pregnancies were tolerated well, at time of delivery blood pressures were labile.

Causes of death are less often related to pulmonary complications, indicating that aggressive treatment of aspirations has been beneficial. Of recent concern have been the patients who have succumbed to unexplained deaths which may have been the result of unopposed vagal stimulation or a sleep abnormality. A few adult patients have died of renal failure.

Future goals

Discovery of the genetic defect in FD will permit resolution of this disorder's relationship to the other HSANs, may well provide direct clues to the genetic causes of these similar disorders, and will almost certainly yield valuable insight into the processes involved in normal development and maintenance of the sensory and autonomic nervous systems. This information may serve to aid us in providing more definitive treatments to individuals affected with FD, as well as fostering innovative treatment approaches for other adult-onset or acquired autonomic disorders.

References

Axelrod, F. B. (1996a). Autonomic and sensory disorders. In *Principles and practice of medical genetics,* (3rd edn), (ed. A. E. H. Emory and D. L. Rimoin), pp. 397–411. Churchill Livingstone, Edinburgh.

Axelrod, F. B. (1996b). Familial dysautonomia. In *Current pediatric therapy* (15th edn), (ed. F. D. Burg, J. R. Ingelfinger, E. R. Wald, and R. A. Polin). pp. 91–4. W.B. Saunders, Philadelphia.

Axelrod, F. B. and Abularrage, J. J. (1982). Familial dysautonomia. A prospective study of survival. *J. Pediatr.* 101, 234–6.

Axelrod, F. B., Iyer, K., Fish, I., Pearson, J., Sein, M. E., and Spielholz, N. (1981) Progressive sensory loss in familial dysautonomia. *Pediatrics* 65, 517–22.

Axelrod, F. B., Glickstein, J. S., Weider, J., Gluck, M. C., and Friedman, D. (1993). The effects of postural change and exercise on renal haemodynamics in familial dysautonomia. *Clin. Auton. Res.* 3, 195–200 .

Axelrod, F. B., Krey, L., Glickstein, J. S. et al. (1994). Atrial natriuretic peptide and catecholamine response to orthostatic hypotension and treatments in familial dysautonomia. *Clin. Auton. Res.* 4, 311–18.

Axelrod, F. B., Krey, L., Glickstein, J. S., Weider-Allison, J, and Friedman, D. (1995). Preliminary observations on the use of midodrine in treating orthostatic hypotension in familial dysautonomia. *J. auton. nerv. Syst.* 55, 29–35

Axelrod, F. B., Goldstein, D. S., Holmes, C., Berlin, D., and Kopin, I. (1996). Pattern of plasma catechols in familial dysautonomia. *Clin. Auton. Res.* 6, 205–9.

Blumenfeld, A., Slaugenhaupt, S. A., Axelrod, F. B. et al. (1993). Localization of the gene for familial dysautonomia on Chromosome 9 and definition of DNA markers for genetic diagnosis. *Nature Genet.* 4, 160–4 .

Edelman, N. H., Cherniack, N.S., Lahiri, S., Richards, E., and Fishman, A. P. (1970). The effects of abnormal sympathetic nervous function upon the ventilatory response to hypoxia. *J. Clin. Invest.* 41, 1153–65.

Grover-Johnson, N. and Pearson, J. (1976). Deficient vascular innervation in familial dysautonomia, an explanation for vasomotor instability. *Neuropath. Appl. Neurobiol.* 2, 217–24.

Gusella, J. F., Slaugenhaupt, S. S., Blumenfeld, A., Breakefield, X. O., Maayan, Ch., and Axelrod, F. B. (1999). Familial dysautonomia. In *Advances in Jewish genetic diseases,* (ed. R. Desnick). Oxford University Press, New York in press.

Hilz, M. J., Axelrod, F. B., Schweibold, G., Neuner, I., Glorius, S., and Kolodny, E. H. (1994). Sympathetic skin response (SSR) to thermal stimulation in familial dysautonomia—an objective indicator of sensory small-fibre neuropathy. *Am. Auton. Soc. Proc.,* October 21–23, Rochester, M. N.

Indo, Y., Tsuruta, M., Hayashida, Y. et al. (1996). Mutations in the NTRKA/NGF receptor gene in patients with congenital insensitivity to pain with anhidrosis. *Nature Genet.* 13, 485–8.

Maayan, Ch., Kaplan, E., Shachar, Sh., Peleg, O., and Godfrey, S. (1987a). Incidence of familial dysautonomia in Israel 1977–1981. *Clin. Genet.* 32, 106–8.

Maayan, Ch., Axelrod, F. B., Akselrod, S., Carley, D. W., and Shannon, C. D. (1987b). Evaluation of autonomic dysfunction in familial dysautonomia by power spectral analysis. *J. Autonom. nerv. Syst.* 21, 51–8.

Mason, D. T., Kopin, I. J., and Braunwald, E. (1966). Abnormalities in reflex control of the circulation in familial dysautonomia. *Am. J. Med.* 41, 898–909.

Pearson , J. and Pytel, B. (1978a). Quantitative studies of sympathetic ganglia and spinal cord intermedio-lateral gray columns in familial dysautonomia. *J. Neurol. Sci.* 39, 47–59.

Pearson, J. and Pytel, B. (1978b). Quantitative studies of ciliary and sphenopalatine ganglia in familial dysautonomia. *J. Neurol. Sci.* 39, 123–30.

Pearson, J., Brandeis, L., and Goldstein, M. (1979b). Tyrosine hydroxylase immunohistoreactivity in familial dysautonomia. *Science* 206, 71–2.

Rabinowitz, D., Landau, H., Rosler, A., Moses, S. W., Rotem, Y., and Freier, S. (1974). Plasma renin activity and aldosterone in familial dysautonomia. *Metabolism* 23, 1–5.

Riley, C. M., Day, R. L., McL. Greeley, D., and Langford, W. S. (1949). Central autonomic dysfunction with defective lacrimation. Report of 5 cases. *Pediatrics* 3, 468–77.

Smith, A. A., Taylor, T., and Wortis, S. B. (1963). Abnormal catecholamine metabolism in familial dysautonomia. *New Engl. J. Med.* 268, 705–7.

Smith, A. A., Hirsch, J. I., and Dancis, J. (1965). Responses to infused methacholine in familial dysautonomia. *Pediatrics* 36, 225–30.

Welton, W., Clayson, D., Axelrod, F. B., and Levine, D. B. (1979). Intellectual development and familial dysautonomia. *Pediatrics* 63, 708–12.

Ziegler, M. G., Lake, R. C., and Kopin, I. J. (1976). Deficient sympathetic nervous system response in familial dysautonomia, *New. Engl. J. Med.* 294, 630–3.

42. Amyloid neuropathy

Mary M. Reilly and P. K. Thomas

Introduction

Amyloid deposition can be focal or generalized and may be derived from a variety of different molecules. Only those forms of amyloidosis that lead to neuropathy with autonomic involvement will be considered in this chapter. These are light-chain (AL) amyloidosis and familial amyloidoses related to mutations in the genes for transthyretin (TTR), apolipoprotein A-1 (Apo A-1), and gelsolin. Reactive systemic (AA) amyloidosis occurs in chronic inflammatory

(a)

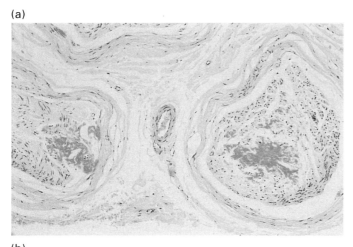

(b)

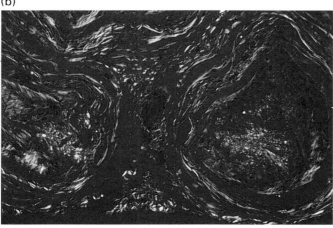

Fig. 42.1. Endoneurial amyloid deposits visualized by Congo red staining (a) and, again after Congo red staining but viewed by polarization optics (b), showing the green birefringence displayed by the deposit.

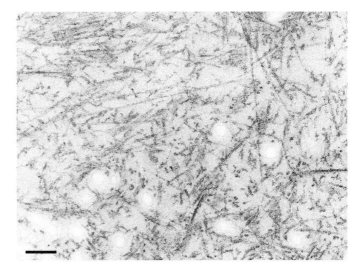

Fig. 42.2. Electron micrograph of amyloid fibrils showing the straight, unbranched, 'rigid' appearance. Bar = 0.1 μm.

disorders such as rheumatoid arthritis and in chronic infections, including syphilis, leprosy, tuberculosis, and osteomyelitis. The amyloid in this form is mainly composed of a protein, AA, which is derived by proteolysis from a serum protein SAA. Peripheral nerve involvement is exceedingly rare. In dialysis-associated amyloidosis, encountered in patients on long-term haemodialysis, the amyloid is derived from retained β_2-microglobulin. Deposits occur primarily in periarticular connective tissues and frequently lead to the carpal tunnel syndrome.

Nature of amyloid

When observed by light microscopy, amyloid consists of amorphous deposits that stain metachromatically with methyl or crystal violet. When stained with Congo red and viewed under polarization optics they exhibit apple-green birefringence (Fig. 42.1a,b). On electron microscopy, amyloid is seen to be composed of aggregates of straight unbranched, 'rigid' fibrils with a diameter of 10–15 nm (Fig. 42.2). The characteristic staining and optical properties of amyloid are related to the configuration of the major protein from which it is derived, which is in the form of a β-pleated sheet. The deposits are also regularly associated with a glycoprotein termed serum amyloid P (SAP) whatever the nature of the main component. Variable quantities of other substances, including glycosaminoglycans, are also present. Amyloid infiltrates and replaces tissue in which it is deposited and causes tissue destruction by mechanisms that are, so far, imperfectly understood.

Immunoglobulin light chain (AL) amyloidosis

In this form there is tissue deposition of amyloid derived from monoclonal immunoglobulin light chains secondary to multiple myeloma, malignant lymphoma or Waldenström macroglobulinaemia, or to a non-malignant immunocyte dyscrasia. Cases of 'primary amyloidosis' without an underlying inflammatory disorder or family history are most likely to have AL amyloidosis, although the family history may be negative in hereditary cases for a variety of reasons (see later). Amyloid develops in approximately 15 per cent of patients with myeloma and less frequently in other malignant B cell disorders. It probably occurs in about 5–10 per cent of patients with benign monoclonal gammopathy.

The amyloid is more commonly derived from λ than κ light chains and either just from the variable portion or from the complete light chain. Buxbaum and Hauser (1986), from studies on human bone marrow cells in tissue culture, produced evidence that aberrant immunoglobulin synthesis leads to the production of amyloid. The λ_{VI} subgroup comprises more than 50 per cent of those cases with light-chain amyloidosis and virtually all recognized examples of λ_{VI} light chains have been associated with amyloidosis. Apart from excessive or aberrant production of light chains, AL deposition may involve its defective degradation and removal. The way in which the amyloidosis arises is still not established but macrophages may be implicated. There is evidence of processing of light chains to produce amyloid by macrophages in cultures of myeloma-derived plasma cells (Durie *et al.* 1982).

Clinical features

Light-chain amyloidosis is more common in males and occurs predominantly in later life. In the series of cases reported by Kyle and Greipp (1983), almost two-thirds were male and 97 per cent of the patients were aged 40 years or older. The mean age at diagnosis was 65 years. It may present with non-specific symptoms such as malaise, fatigue, and weight loss or with symptoms related to renal, cardiovascular, or peripheral nerve involvement. Associated features include purpura, peripheral oedema, hepatosplenomegaly, and macroglossia. Such features can suggest the diagnosis in cases of undiagnosed neuropathy. In the experience of Kyle and Dyck (1993), approximately one-sixth of patents show evidence of peripheral nerve involvement at the time of diagnosis and the presentation can be generalized, although Kyle and Dyck found that no less than a quarter initially presented with the carpal tunnel syndrome. Focal cranial nerve involvement may also be seen.

In patients with a generalized polyneuropathy, the initial symptoms are usually sensory and begin distally in the lower limbs, later spreading to the hands. The patient experiences numbness and tingling paraesthesiae but may first notice difficulty in distinguishing hot and cold temperature. Spontaneous pain can occur, felt as burning pain, especially nocturnally, or as lancinating stabs. Autonomic involvement tends to be an early manifestation.

Symptoms include distal anhidrosis in the limbs, orthostatic hypotension, difficulty in voiding urine, and, in the male, erectile and ejaculatory impotence. Diarrhoea is often a prominent feature whether this is related to involvement of the enteric nervous system or to infiltration of the gut wall with amyloid is uncertain. Gastroparesis, giving rise to nausea and vomiting, also occurs. With advance of the neuropathy, the sensory loss extends proximally up the limbs and then becomes evident over the anterior abdominal wall, spreading laterally around the trunk. Motor involvement appears later with progressive distal wasting and weakness, beginning in the lower limbs. The symptoms therefore evolve in the manner of a distal length-related neuropathy.

Examination in the earlier stages may show selective pain and temperature sensory loss with relative preservation of large fibre sensory modalities, motor function, and the tendon reflexes. These latter features later become added. Orthostatic hypotension may be evident, as may abnormal pupillary responses. The peripheral nerves may be enlarged.

Diagnosis and investigation

Following clinical suspicion of AL amyloidosis, the diagnosis is established histologically (Fig. 42.3) by the demonstration of green birefringence after Congo red staining when viewed under polarized light (Fig. 42.1b). Confirmation that it is AL amyloid is obtained by immunohistochemical staining for λ or κ light chains. Suction biopsy of abdominal fat or a rectal biopsy can be undertaken, but in a patient who presents with neuropathy, proceeding straight to a nerve

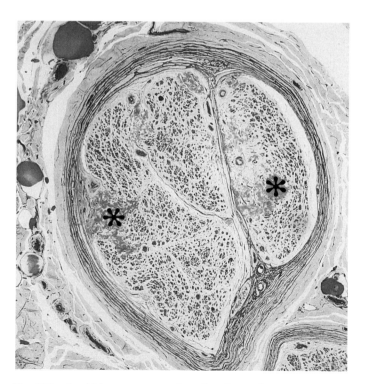

Fig. 42.3. Semithin transverse section of sural nerve biopsy specimen, showing severe loss of myelinated nerve fibres and the presence of endoneurial amyloid deposits (asterisks). Thionin and acridine orange stain; ×100.

biopsy may be preferable. The use of radiolabelled SAP, demonstrated scintigraphically, is a specific marker for amyloid, although it does not indicate its nature. This procedure may be helpful for monitoring treatment to assess the body load of amyloid.

Most cases of AL amylodosis will show Bence Jones protein in the urine and a monoclonal paraprotein band or free light chains in the serum or urine. Investigations should be undertaken for underlying myeloma or malignant lymphoma. If not detectable initially in cases of 'primary amyloidosis', support for the diagnosis may be obtained by finding a general reduction in serum immunoglobulin concentrations and increased plasma cell proportions in the bone marrow.

The presence of amyloid P component (AP) in amyloid deposits of whatever type, including those in the hereditary amyloid neuropathies, led to the introduction of radiolabelled serum amyloid component P (SAP) to reveal the presence of amyloid deposits (Hawkins *et al.* 1990; Hawkins and Pepys 1995). These are regularly demonstrated. No tissue localization or retention of the labelled SAP occurs in healthy individuals or in other diseases. The SAP is obtained by purification from donor serum and labelled with ^{123}I. The amyloid deposits are visualized by scintigraphic imaging (Fig. 42.4). The uptake of the tracer into affected organs can be quantitated and the technique can therefore be used for serial monitoring to assess responses to treatment, although scintigraphy is poor for evaluating cardiac deposits.

^{123}I has a short half-life and the injected radiolabelled SAP is rapidly catabolized and excreted in the urine. The dose of radioactivity falls well within accepted safety limits. As the technique involves the administration of a serum component, the donor individuals must be carefully screened to avoid inadvertent viral transmission. Experience to date has shown that this ^{123}I scintigraphy constitutes a valuable and safe technique but its use so far is restricted to specialized centres. Labelling of SAP with technetium (^{99}Tc^{m}) is being explored (Pepys 1996). This is an inexpensive and widely available gamma-emitting isotope.

Prognosis

Kyle and Greipp (1983) found a median survival of 12 months from the time of diagnosis in AL amyloidosis. More recently a figure of 2 years was obtained (Kyle and Dyck 1993), probably because of improved supportive measures. The prognosis differs depending on the type of presentation. Duston *et al.* (1989) found a median survival time of 35 months for patients with peripheral neuropaghy compared with 16 months for those without neuropathy. Kyle and Dyck (1993) recorded a median survival time for those with only peripheral neuropathy of more than 5 years. Death was usually because of involvement of other systems.

Hereditary amyloid neuropathies

Amyloid neuropathy derived from mutated proteins is called familial amyloid polyneuropathy (FAP). The familial amyloid polyneuropathies are a heterogeneous group of autosomal dominant disorders first described by Andrade in Portuguese patients in 1952 (Andrade 1952). FAP used to be classified into four types, based on clinical presentation: lower limb onset (FAP I) originally recognized in Portuguese (Andrade, 1952), Japanese, and Swedish families; upper-limb onset (FAP II) originally described in the Indiana/Swiss and in the German/Maryland kindreds; lower-limb neuropathy, nephropathy, and gastric ulcers (FAP III) originally described in an Iowa kinship; and the Finnish type of cranial neuropathy with corneal lattice dystrophy (FAP IV). This classification has now been replaced by a classification based on the chemical and molecular nature of the constituent proteins. The commonest fibril protein deposited as amyloid in FAP is a variant form of transthyretin (TTR) but, as already stated, FAP can also occur secondary to apolipoprotein A-1 (Apo A-1) deposition and to gelsolin deposition.

Transthyretin (TTR)-derived FAP

Costa and colleagues first showed that the fibril protein in the Portuguese type of FAP was immunologically related to TTR (Costa *et al.* 1978). The first point mutation in the TTR gene associated with FAP, methionine 30 (Met 30), was identified in 1983 (Dwulet and Benson 1983) and is still the most commonly described TTR point mutation. TTR is a tetramer (55 kDa) composed of four identical monomer units. Each monomer shows an extensive β-pleated structure with eight β-pleated sheets arranged in two parallel plates. Two monomers combine to form a dimer and the two dimers bond noncovalently to give the tetramer. Over 90 per cent of TTR is produced in the liver, the remainder being synthesized in the choroid plexus and the retina. The mature protein has two known functions. It is responsible for about 20 per cent of plasma thyroxine binding and it binds with retinol binding protein.

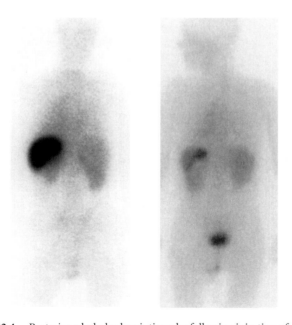

Fig. 42.4.   Posterior whole-body scintigraphy following injection of ^{123}I-labelled serum amyloid P component in a patient with TTR Met 30 associated FAP before (left) and 2 years after liver transplantation (right). The amyloid deposits in the spleen, kidneys, and adrenal glands have regressed between the two studies. (Figure kindly supplied by Dr P. N. Hawkins.)

Genetics of TTR-derived FAP

TTR is a product of a gene mapping to chromosome 18q11.2–q12.1, which contains four exons coding for a 127–amino-acid mature protein and an 18–residue signal peptide. The first exon codes for the signal peptide and the first three amino acids of the protein. No mutations have been described in this exon. Numerous point mutations have been described in the other three exons. Most of these are associated with FAP but some just cause a cardiomyopathy and others are non-pathogenic polymorphisms. The first case of FAP due to a TTR variant caused by an in-frame deletion in exon 4 of the TTR gene has been described recently (Uemichi *et al.* 1996).

Large family studies in FAP indicate that TTR-related FAP was an autosomal dominant condition with reduced penetrance, suggesting that the underlying mutations are expressed in the heterozygous state. This is true of Met 30, the first TTR point mutation associated with FAP to be described, which does exist in the heterozygous state (Dwulet and Benson 1983). This mutation was found to be associated with all the original cases of FAP described in Portugal, Sweden, and Japan, and since then has been described in association with FAP in many other countries, including Cyprus, Greece, Italy, Majorca, France, England, Germany, Turkey, Brazil, and the United States. It had been postulated that all patients with FAP TTR Met 30 were Portuguese in origin and had a common founder, because Met 30–related FAP was first described in Portuguese patients and is present in over 500 Portuguese kindreds; in addition, there are historical or trading links between Portugal and the countries where other large clusters of patients with this mutation are seen, particularly Sweden and Japan. However, haplotype studies in Portugal, Sweden, Japan, United States, France, and England using TTR intron polymorphisms have shown at least five different disease-associated haplotypes, suggesting multiple founders for this mutation. The occurrence of this mutation so commonly in FAP may be explained partly by the fact that the first nucleotide on the antisense strand of the normal Val 30 codon is a C and is the first nucleotide of a CpG dinucleotide sequence, and therefore may be more liable to mutations.

Most of the TTR point mutations were originally detected by direct sequencing and this method remains the main method used to detect new mutations. Known mutations such as TTR Met 30 are most commonly screened for using the polymerase chain reaction (PCR) and subsequent digestion by the appropriate restriction enzyme if the mutation creates or abolishes a restriction site for a known restriction enzyme (Reilly and Staunton 1996). Certain mutations do not create or eliminate a restriction site and either allele-specific PCR, where a primer is constructed so that it only causes amplification of the mutated allele, or mismatched primer PCR (MMP-PCR), where a primer is constructed with a mismatch of one or more bases so that after PCR amplification a gain or loss of a restriction site only occurs in the presence of the mutation, can be used to detect mutations. With the exception of TTR Met 30, most other TTR mutations described have only been seen in one or two families. TTR Tyr 77 has been described in a number of families but is still relatively rare. Haplotype data suggest multiple founders for this mutation also. TTR Ala 60 is the second most common TTR mutation described in different areas but haplotype data suggest a common founder for this mutation in north-western Ireland (Reilly *et al.* 1995). Nearly all mutations are inherited but penetrance is probably incomplete, explaining the occurrence of most apparently sporadic cases. There was probable evidence for a fresh mutation in a patient with the Arg 47 mutation, as neither parent carried the mutant allele.

Homozygosity has been reported for the Met 30 mutation but is neither associated with early onset disease nor more aggressive disease. Compound heterozygosity has been described for Met 30 (Met 30 and Met 119; Met 30 and Asn 90) in which it exists with other apparently non-pathogenic TTR mutations. The combination of Met 30 and Met 119 was related to a benign clinical course in some Portuguese families (Coelho 1996). Further evidence for this comes from an *in vivo* study in mice which proposed that the coexistence of these variants could exert a stabilizing influence on TTR Met 30. Compound heterozygosity has also been described for Ile 33 and Ser 6, Gly 42 and Asn 90 and Gly 54 and Ser 6, where Ser 6 and Asn 90, are thought to be non-pathogenic mutations. It is not yet known whether they can affect the phenotype in the presence of another mutation as in the case of Met 119 above.

Pathogenesis of TTR-derived FAP

The amyloidogenic potential of TTR is presumed to be partly due to its extensive β-pleated structure. Further proof of this is seen in systemic senile amyloidosis, a condition that affects approximately 25 per cent of people over the age of 80 years, in which normal transthyretin is deposited in the heart as amyloid. Presumably conformational changes in circulating TTR caused by various amino acid substitutions resulting from point mutations increase the amyloidogenic potential of TTR. There has been evidence for conformational changes shown by X-ray crystallography. The X-ray structure of TTR Met 30, when compared to normal TTR, shows minor, but significant changes (Benson *et al.* 1996). Another study comparing the X-ray crystal structures of normal, Met 30, and Thr 109 (non-pathogenic) TTR molecules showed conformational changes present in the Met 30 TTR molecule that were not found in the Thr 109 or normal TTR molecules. The Met 30 variant caused overcrowding, whereas the Thr 109 variant was easily accommodated by empty space at the centre of the TTR molecule. Another interesting observation showed that TTR Pro 55 is significantly less stable than wild-type TTR and causes a more aggressive disease. Further studies are needed to understand the effect of mutation-induced conformational changes on amyloidogenesis.

Alteration of the function of TTR has been described for some variants but has not helped our understanding of TTR amyloidogenesis significantly. Some TTR mutations, for example Met 30, cause decreased affinity for thyroxine, and others, for example Thr 109 cause increased affinity (Benson *et al.* 1996). It has been shown that the ability of TTR to form amyloid is not related to its affinity for thyroxine by studying the relative affinity of 10 different naturally occurring TTR variants.

Transgenic mice are another useful tool for studying disease pathogenesis. Transgenic mice expressing the human TTR Met 30 mutation have shown amyloid deposition starting at 6 months in the gastrointestinal tract, cardiovascular system, and the kidneys. By 24 months, the pattern of amyloid deposition was the same as that seen in autopsy cases of human FAP, except for its absence in the peripheral and autonomic nervous systems and the choroid plexus (Yi *et al.* 1991). Transgenic mice carrying the autologous TTR regulatory sequences have amyloid deposits in the choroid plexus and the meninges but not in the peripheral nerves. Further transgenic mice studies are in hand to try to understand the mechanism of TTR amyloidogenesis in peripheral nerves.

The evidence for reduced penetrance in TTR-related FAP, together with the late onset of these disorders, suggests that there are other factors involved in amyloid formation besides the amyloidogenic potential of TTR itself, although these factors have yet to be identified. The role of amyloid P component (AP) has been investigated as all types of amyloid contain AP. Transgenic mice with the human mutant TTR gene and the human SAP gene had the same clinical course and pattern of tissue amyloid deposition as the mouse with only the mutant TTR gene (Tashiro *et al.* 1992). This provides some evidence that SAP is not important for the initiation or progression of amyloid deposition.

Apolipoprotein A-1-derived FAP

One type of FAP, seen in an Iowa kindred, known as FAP type III in the old classification, was described by Van Allen in 1969 (Van Allen *et al.* 1969). The phenotype is similar to that of FAP TTR Met 30. This type of FAP has been shown to be associated with a variant of apolipoprotein A-1 in which an arginine for glycine substitution occurs at position 26 (Nichols *et al.* 1990). The gene for apolipoprotein A-1 is on chromosome 11. The amyloid fibrils are composed of an 83–residue amino terminal fragment of apolipoprotein A-1, which is part of the high-density lipoprotein complex. It is of interest to note that, although apolipoprotein A-1 itself is not likely to have an extensive β-pleated structure, the first 55 residues of the 83 amino terminal fragment referred to above are predicted to have a mostly β-pleated structure. It has been postulated that the Arg 26 point mutation may make the protein more susceptible to proteolytic cleavage, with subsequent deposition of the 83 amino acid fragment as amyloid fibrils (Nichols *et al.* 1990).

Gelsolin-derived FAP

Gelsolin-derived FAP (FAP type IV in the old classification) was first described in a Finnish kindred in 1969. Clinically it usually presents in the fourth decade of life with a corneal lattice dystrophy followed later by a progressive cranial neuropathy and a mild sensory and autonomic neuropathy. The fibril protein in this disease is an abnormal fragment of gelsolin, which begins at position 173 of plasma gelsolin. Gelsolin is a cytoskeletal and plasma protein with actin-modulating properties. The gene for gelsolin is located on chromosome 9. It codes for two separate proteins, one intracellular and one extracellular with an additional 25 amino acid residues. The amyloid fibrils in Finnish FAP are composed of a 9 kDa molecular weight fragment. There have been two point mutations in the gelsolin gene associated with this type of FAP: a substitution of asparagine for aspartic acid at residue 187 (position 15 of the amyloid protein) (Levy *et al.* 1990) and a substitution of tyrosine for aspartic acid at the same position, that is residue 187 (de le Chapelle et al. 1992). The first mutation, that is Asn 187, has now been described in over 200 Finnish kindreds but has also been reported in patients of Dutch, Japanese, and Irish–American origins. A recent haplotype study has suggested an independent genetic origin for this mutation in Japan and Finland. Two homozygotes for this mutation have been described and both were more severely affected than heterozygotes. The second gelsolin mutation, Tyr 187, has been reported in a Danish and a Czech family (de le Chapelle *et al.* 1992). The occurrence of two mutations at the same site suggests that this site represents a mutation hot spot and it is of interest that the site includes a CpG dinucleotide, which is known to be a mutational hot spot.

An aberrant 68 kDa gelsolin fragment has been demonstrated in this type of FAP and has been shown to carry the amyloid sequence on its amino terminus. It therefore probably represents a precursor for both the C-terminal 60 kDa gelsolin fragment of patients' serum and for the amyloid-forming polypeptide. Another study refined the amyloidogenic region of gelsolin to a nine-residue sequence in the highly conserved B motif and has also demonstrated that residue 187 is a critical site where a substitution of an amino acid with an uncharged (asparagine) or hydrophobic side chain (tyrosine or valine) creates a conformation that is highly amyloidogenic.

Clinical features of FAP syndromes

TTR FAP

It has become clear with the ever increasing number of pathogenic mutations in TTR that the clinical syndromes overlap and a specific clinical syndrome does not predict a particular mutation. While keeping this in mind, there are certain features more commonly associated with particular mutations and even with particular ethnic groups with the same mutation. The more commonly seen TTR clinical syndromes are described here (Met 30, Ala 60, Tyr 77, etc) together with a brief description on diagnosis of TTR-derived FAP.

FAP Met 30 (Portuguese)

The clinical features of FAP TTR Met 30 were first described by Andrade in 1952 and are similar to those of neuropathy associated with light-chain amyloidosis. Andrade gave a detailed description of 74 patients with FAP, and subsequent descriptions of the clinical features of FAP Met 30 in Portuguese patients fit well with the original observations. As stated above, TTR Met 30 is most most commonly observed in Portuguese patients but is also the common type of FAP worldwide. In Portugal, this type of FAP usually presents in the lower limbs with painful dysaesthesia and then progresses to a severe mixed but predominantly sensory polyneuropathy. There is greater small-fibre susceptibility giving rise to early lack of pain and temperature sensation, but eventually all sensory modalities are involved. Painless injury to the feet can result in ulcers, cellulitis, osteomyelitis, and Charcot joints. As the disease progresses, motor involvement is universal, characterized by wasting and weakness with progressive loss of reflexes. Upper-limb involvement occurs months to years after lower-limb manifestations. Carpal tunnel syndrome can occur in TTR Met 30 but is rarely the presenting feature. Autonomic involvement occurs frequently, can be severe and can occur early in the course of the disease. This manifests with orthostatic hypotension, alternating constipation and diarrhoea, gastric retention and distension, sexual impotence, urinary hesitancy, and dry skin. Examination may show scalloped pupils due to ciliary body denervation, postural hypotension, an abnormal Valsalva response, and a fixed pulse rate.

Neurophysiological studies confirm an axonal neuropathy. Sensory nerve action potentials may be of normal amplitude early in the course of the disease, reflecting the mainly small-fibre involvement but eventually are small or absent, initially in the lower limbs but later also in the upper limbs. Motor conduction velocities are normal or slightly reduced and electromyography shows the signs of chronic partial denervation in established cases. Sympathetic and parasympathetic autonomic nervous system dysfunction is confirmed by autonomic testing.

Cardiac involvement in Met 30 is common, presenting as an arrhythmia, heart block, or heart failure. Electrocardiographic abnormalities include widespread Q-wave and T-wave repolarization changes and various conduction disturbances. Echocardiography shows either a restrictive or a hypertrophic cardiomyopathy.

Vitreous involvement is seen in TTR Met 30 but is more commonly seen in Swedish than Portuguese patients and may be the presenting feature in the former patients.

Involvement of other systems in TTR Met 30 includes the kidneys and more rarely pulmonary or bone involvement.

FAP TTR Met 30 is characterized by marked variation, with some consistency in each major cluster of the disease, in relation both to age of onset (ranging from 17 to 78 years) and the nature of the initial presentation. Portuguese patients tend to present early with lower-limb involvement whereas Swedish patients tend to present in their late fifties and often with vitreous opacities. Variable penetrance is well documented in TTR Met 30, although a recent epidemiological study from Portugal showed a large number of families in that country approaching a full penetrance in adult life. Both Swedish and Portuguese families show more affected men than women, with women having a slightly later age of onset (35.6 years) than men (31.9 years). The same study showed that the disease has an earlier age of onset when inheritance was from an affected mother and that correlation of age at onset among sibs in higher than that between affected parents and their offspring.

Sporadic cases of Met 30 have been described. These may be due to variable penetrance or new mutations. No data on the frequency of new mutations are available but they are probably rare.

Other TTR variants with a similar phenotype (including Tyr 77)

After TTR Met 30 and Ala 60, Tyr 77 is the next most frequently described mutation in the TTR gene. This mutation was originally described in a German kindred from Illinois but since then has been reported in many countries, including France, England, America, and Spain. Haplotype data suggest multiple founders for this mutation. The clinical features of this mutation are similar to those for Met 30 and the age at presentation is most commonly in the fifties. Patients with more rarely described TTR mutations can also present with a similar clinical picture to that described in FAP TTR Met 30. These include isoleucine 33, leucine 33, asparagine 35, glycine 42, arginine 47, alanine 49, glutamine 54, lysine 61, alanine 71, glycine 97, and cysteine 114.

FAP Ala 60 (Irish/Appalachian)

This type of FAP is clinically similar to Met 30 with some differences. It was originally described in a family in the Appalachian region of the USA and subsequently in other American families but it is now apparent that the mutation originated in north-western Ireland. A cluster of families from Donegal, north-western Ireland have the same mutation and recent evidence has shown that the American families either originated from Ireland in the early nineteenth century or have a common haplotype with the Donegal families (Reilly *et al.* 1995). Families, of Irish origin, have also been described in England and Australia. The Ala 60 families therefore represent the second

largest group of families with a common mutation from different areas to be traced to a common founder, the largest being those of known Portuguese origin with FAP TTR Met 30.

The onset of disease is late, usually in the sixth or seventh decade, and both motor involvement and large-fibre sensory involvement are more prominent than in FAP Met 30. Cardiomyopathy may be the presenting feature and is often severe.

FAP Ser 84 and His 58 and others with a similar phenotype

This type of FAP usually presents in the upper limbs (FAP type II, old classification) and was originally described in two kindreds; a large family in Indiana of Swiss origin and a pedigree comprising 11 families in Maryland of German origin. Onset is most commonly in the early forties with carpal tunnel syndrome. A generalized neuropathy, mainly sensory at first, subsequently develops, initially in the upper limbs but eventually becoming generalized. Autonomic failure is common and both a cardiomyopathy and vitreous involvement are recognized.

Patients with other, more rarely described, TTR mutations have been reported as presenting either with carpal tunnel syndrome or a more generalized neuropathy starting in the upper limbs. These include serine 24, arginine 50, arginine 58, leucine 64, asparagine 70, glutamine 89, valine 107 and histidine 114.

Diagnosis of TTR-derived FAP

The diagnosis of FAP requires the diagnosis of amyloidosis in the first place, with subsequent characterization of the nature of the amyloid fibril protein. This can be done by direct examination of biopsy material from rectum, nerve, heart, or other tissues. The most widely used technique for diagnosis is a combination of alkaline Congo red and polarizing filters to demonstrate the characteristic apple-green birefringence, as described above. The nature of the amyloid fibrils is identified by immunohistochemistry (Fig. 42.5). This technique is not completely reliable because sometimes the amount of amyloid present in the biopsy is insufficient to characterize the nature of the constituent amyloid fibril protein.

As nearly all patients with TTR-derived FAP are heterozygotes, both normal and variant TTR circulate in the blood. Variant TTR can be detected in blood using radioimmunoassay (RIA) and enzyme-linked immunosorbent assay (ELISA).

TTR point mutations can be detected by the methods described above. In patients with a family history of FAP and a documented mutation or patients from an ethnic group where a particular mutation, is common (Portuguese Met 30/Irish Ala 60), diagnostic analysis is relatively straightforward. If there are no such clues, it is sensible to screen for the most common mutations first, Met 30, Ala 60, and Tyr 77. If these are not present and the patient has either immunohistochemically proven TTR amyloid or a suggestive clinical picture (a predominantly small-fibre neuropathy with autonomic dysfunction) and a positive family history, it is appropriate to sequence the TTR gene directly. Alternatively, it is possible to screen exons for mutations before sequencing by several techniques, including single-strand conformation polymorphism, but as this is not known to be 100 per cent sensitive and as it is a relatively small gene it is often easier to sequence the gene directly.

The above methods of mutation detection are suitable for diagnosis, presymptomatic and prenatal testing in the appropriate circumstances.

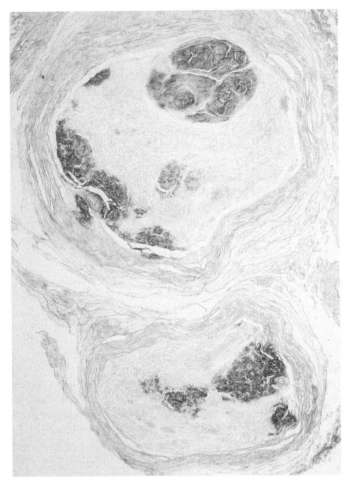

Fig. 42.5. Same patient as in Fig. 42.3, showing positive immunostaining of the endoneurial amyloid deposits for TTR. ×100.

Apolipoprotein A-1-derived FAP

One type of FAP (type III, old classification), described in an Iowa kindred, has been shown to be associated with deposition of a variant apolipoprotein A-1 in which an arginine for glycine substitution occurs at position 26 (Nichols *et al.* 1990). The phenotype is similar to that of FAP TTR Met 30 except for a higher incidence of renal amyloidosis and severe gastric ulcer disease.

Gelsolin-derived FAP

Gelsolin-derived FAP (type IV, old classification) was first described in a Finnish kindred but since then has been identified in other countries (see above). It is associated with an abnormal fragment of the plasma protein, gelsolin, in which either an asparagine or tyrosine for aspartic acid substitution occurs at residue 187. Clinically, it usually presents in the third or fourth decade with corneal lattice dystrophy, although this is often asymptomatic. This is followed by the insidious development of a progressive cranial neuropathy in the fifth or sixth decades. The most common nerve involved is the facial, which usually starts with involvement of the upper fibres, as manifested by forehead muscle weakness. Other cranial nerves that may be affected are the trigeminal, hypoglossal, and vestibulocochlear nerves. The facial skin is at first thickened but with time becomes lax. A mild sensory neuropathy may develop later in the limbs. Autonomic involvement, if present, is mild.

Neurophysiological studies confirm an axonal neuropathy. Sensory potentials show severely reduced amplitude but sensory and motor conduction velocities are normal or near normal. Carpal tunnel syndrome has been shown to be a characteristic feature electrophysiologically in Finnish patients. Gelsolin amyloid deposits in cardiac tissue have been described, although signs of cardiac involvement are rare clinically.

Electrodiagnostic features of amyloid neuropathy

Abnormalities of nerve conduction in all types of amyloid neuropathy are consistent with an axonopathy, sensory nerve action potentials being of reduced amplitude or absent and motor conduction velocities being mildly or moderately reduced. Distal motor latencies, except for the median nerve in patients with the carpal tunnel syndrome, tend to be normal or only slightly increased. Needle electromyography shows evidence of denervation in affected muscles.

Pathology and pathogenesis

The pathological changes in the peripheral nervous system are similar in AL amyloidosis and in the hereditary amyloid neuropathies. Amyloid deposits are found both diffusely in the endoneurium and epineurium and surrounding endoneurial and epineurial blood vessels. They are also present in sensory and autonomic ganglia. In milder cases there is predominant loss of small myelinated and unmyelinated axons (Dyck and Lambert 1969; Thomas and King 1974); at later stages larger myelinated fibres are also lost. The pathology is predominantly one of axonal degeneration with some regenerative activity.

The mechanism of the nerve fibre loss and the explanation for the preferential damage to small axons in the initial stages is uncertain. Amyloid deposits tend to accumulate preferentially around the satellite cells of small dorsal root ganglion cells, raising the possibility that destruction of the cell bodies contributes to the neuropathy. Dyck and Lambert (1969) observed globular endoneurial deposits of amyloid displacing axons, but a direct mechanical effect is unlikely to be an important mechanism for axonal loss. Despite the presence of amyloid around endoneurial and epineurial microvessels, neural ischaemia is also an unlikely mechanism in view of the pattern of nerve fibre damage. In general, ischaemia results in predominant damage to large myelinated fibres with relative preservation of small myelinated fibres and, in particular, of unmyelinated axons. Thomas and King (1974) observed infiltration of the basal laminae of Remak fibres by amyloid fibrils, with concomitant Schwann cell damage and axonal loss (Fig. 42.6). This raises the possibility of a direct 'toxic' action of the amyloid fibrils on Schwann cell and axonal integrity (Sommer and Schröder 1989). The distal length-related evolution of the neuropathy (Said *et al.* 1984) is presumably related to the summation of the effects of multiple amyloid deposits throughout the peripheral nervous system.

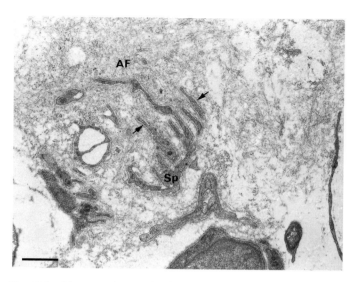

Fig. 42.6. Electron micrograph of endoneurial amyloid deposit associated with a disrupted Remak fibre. The amyloid fibrils (AF) are enmeshed in the basal laminae (arrows) of the Schwann cell processes (Sp). Bar = 1 μM.

Management

Treatment of AL amyloidosis

As the amyloid arises from immunoglobulin light chains, measures to suppress B-cell function with alkylating agents should be adopted, depending upon the clinical state and the aggressivity of the disease. Occasional patients are observed to enter clinical remission, and regression of amyloid deposits has been documented by SAP scintigraphy. Extensive cardiac or renal involvement may merit organ transplantation with significant prolongation of survival, particularly in younger individuals with selective cardiac or renal involvement. Currently, treatment by stem cell bone marrow transplantation is being explorer. As already stated, in patients who present with neuropathy, prognosis for survival is usually determined by amyloidosis affecting other organs.

Symptomatic treatment for manifestations of neuropathy

The symptoms of autonomic dysfunction that develop in AL amyloidosis and in TTR and Apo A-1 FAP, such as postural hypotension, can be treated by pharmacological and other measures. Details will be found in the relevant chapters of this book.

Spontaneous pain, related to small-fibre damage, can be a troublesome feature. As with neuropathic pain in other conditions, opiates are usually ineffective. Treatment is difficult but some benefit can be obtained from carbamazepine, tricyclic antidepressant drugs (e.g. amitriptyline, clomipramine), or mexiletine.

In patients with FAP, the early onset of pain and temperature sensory loss with initial preservation of motor function can lead to a mutilating acropathy, so much so that TTR FAP is known in Portugal as *mal dos pèsinhos* ('foot disease'). It is therefore important to instruct patients with pain and temperature sensory loss to avoid inadvertent injury to the feet and hands, for example by carefully checking footwear for protruding nails, the presence of stones, etc, and taking care to avoid burns to the hands when cooking.

Liver transplantation for TTR amyloidosis

Liver transplantation was first suggested as a potential treatment for TTR-derived FAP because over 90 per cent of TTR is produced in the liver. The first liver transplant for TTR derived FAP was performed in Sweden in 1990 and the number of treated patients has increased rapidly since then; data from 146 patients from a world registry of patients based in Sweden were presented at the Second Workshop on Liver Transplantation in FAP in 1995 (Ericzon 1996). Liver transplants in TTR-derived FAP from living-related donors have been described from Japan.

The biochemical effect of transplantation is good, as demonstrated by a dramatic reduction in variant TTR in plasma (Holmgren *et al.* 1991) and scintigraphic evidence of reduced amyloid deposits postoperatively.

There is now a large consensus that liver transplantation halts the progression of FAP. General well-being, gastrointestinal symptoms, and autonomic function are the most frequent indices reported to improve (Coelho 1996). The neuropathy has appeared to stop progressing in most reports; some studies have suggested improvement (Bergethon 1996) but others showed that the neuropathy remained stable or worsened despite evidence of a reduction in the rate of axon loss after liver transplantation (Adams *et al.* 1996). Most studies have suggested a better outcome if the transplant is carried out early in the course of the disease.

Global mortality from liver transplantation for TTR-derived FAP is 21 per cent (Ericzon 1996). Technically, surgery is not usually a problem but circulatory problems secondary to autonomic dysfunction can occur perioperatively. The need for pacemaker insertion should be assessed preoperatively as arrthymias can develop perioperatively. Death tends to occur in the first 6 months after surgery, with infections and cardiocirculatory problems being the main culprits. An advanced stage of disease has been related to mortality (Suhr *et al.* 1995). Renal dysfunction has emerged as a major problem for transplant patients. Detailed preoperative renal function assessment and careful perioperative and postoperative renal monitoring are recommended.

The optimum time for transplantation has yet to be determined, but the present studies suggest that liver transplantation should be considered when symptoms from the disease start to interfere with a normal active life, despite adequate supportive treatment (Coelho 1996). This particularly pertains to younger patients. In older patients, the duration and severity of the disease, general health of the patients, and the mortality of the procedure have all to be considered carefully before treatment is recommended.

Although many questions about liver transplantation have still to be answered, it is the first effective treatment for FAP patients and undoubtedly should be considered in affected patients.

References

Adams, D., Samuel, D., Goulon-Goeau, C. *et al.* (1996). Evaluation of liver transplantation in familial amyloid polyneuropathy. *Neuromusc. Disord.* **6**, (Suppl. 1), S76.

Andrade, C. (1952). A peculiar form of peripheral neuropathy. *Brain* 75, 408–27.

Benson, M. D., Murrel, J. R., Schormann, N., Liepnieks, J. J., and Uemichi, T. (1996). Structure, function and metabolism of transthyretin [abstract]. *Neuromusc. Disord.* 6, (Suppl. 1), S7.

Bergethon, P. R., Sabin, T. D., Lewis, D., Simms, R. W., Cohen, A. S., and Skinner, M. (1996). Improvement in the polyneuropathy associated with familial amyloid polyneuropathy after liver transplantation. *Neurology* 47, 944–51.

Buxbaum, J. and Hauser, D. (1986). Aberrant immunoglobulin synthesis in light chain amyloidosis: free light chain and light chain fragment production by human bone marrow cells in short-term tissue culture. *J. Clin. Invest.* 78, 789–96.

Coelho, T. (1996). Familial amyloid polyneuropathy: new developments in genetics and treatment. *Curr. Opin. Neurol.* 9, 355–9.

Costa, P., Figueira, A. S., and Bravo, R. R. (1978). Amyloid fibril protein related to pre-albumin in familial amyloidotic polyneuropathy. *Proc. Natl Acad. Sci. USA.* 75, 4499–503.

De le Chapelle, A., Tolvanan, R., Boysen, G. *et al.* (1992). Gelsolin derived familial amyloidosis caused by asparagine or tyrosine substitution for aspartic acid at residue 187. *Nature Genet.* 2, 157–60.

Durie, B. G. M., Persky, B. and Soehnlen, P. J. (1982). Amyloid production in human myeloma stem-cell culture, with morphological evidence of amyloid secretion by associated macrophages. *New Engl. J. Med.,* 307, 1689–92.

Duston, M. A., Skinner, M., Anderson, J., and Cohen, A. S. (1989). Peripheral neuropathy as an early marker of AL amyloidosis. *Arch. Int. Med.* 149, 358–60.

Dwulet, F. E. and Benson, M. D. (1983). Polymorphism of human plasma thyroxine binding prealbumin. *Biochem. Biophys. Res. Comm.* 114, 657–62.

Dyck, P. J. and Lambert, E. H. (1969). Dissociated sensation in amyloidosis. *Arch. Neurol.* 20, 490–507.

Ericzon, B.-G. (1996). Liver transplantation for familial amyloid polyneuropathy – report from the world register [abstract]. *Neuromusc. Disord.* 6, (Suppl. 1), 65.

Hawkins, P. N. and Pepys, M. B. (1995). Imaging amyloidosis with radiolabelled SAP. *Eur. J. Nucl. Med.* 22, 595–9.

Hawkins, P. N. Lavender, J. P., and Pepys, M. B. (1990). Evaluation of systemic amyloidosis by scintigraphy with ^{123}I-labeled serum amyloid P component. *New Engl. J. Med.* 323, 508–13.

Holmgren, G., Steen, L., Ekstedt, J. *et al.* (1991). Biochemical effect of liver transplantation in two Swedish patients with familial amyloidotic neuropathy (FAP-met30). *Clin. Genet.* 40, 242–6.

Kyle, R.A. and Dyck, P.J. (1993). Amyloidosis and neuropathy. In *Peripheral neuropathy*, (3rd edn), (ed. P. J. Dyck, P. K. Thomas, J. W.

Griffin, P. A. Low, and J. F. Poduslo), pp. 1294–307. W. B. Saunders, Philadelphia.

Kyle, R. A. and Greipp, P. R. (1983). Amyloidosis (AL): clinical and laboratory features in 229 cases. *Mayo Clin. Proc.* 58, 665–72.

Levy, E., Haltia, M., Fernandez-Madrid, I. *et al.* (1990). Mutation in gelsolin gene in Finnish hereditary amyloidosis. *J. Exp. Med.* 172, 1865–7.

Nichols, W. C., Gregg, R. E., Bryan Brewer, H., and Benson, M. D. (1990). A mutation in apolipoprotein A-1 in the Iowa type of familial amyloidotic polyneuropathy. *Genomics* 8, 318–23.

Pepys, M. B. (1996). Amyloidosis. In *Oxford textbook of medicine*, (ed. D. J. Weatherall, J. G. G. Ledingham, and D. A. Warrell) Oxford Medical Publications, Oxford.

Reilly, M. M. and Staunton, H. (1996). Peripheral nerve amyloidosis. *Brain. Pathol.* 6, 163–77.

Reilly, M., Staunton, H., and Harding, A. E. (1995). Familial amyloid polyneuropathy (TTR Ala 60) in north west Ireland: a clinical, genetic, and epidemiological study. *J. Neurol. Neurosurg. Psychiat.* 59, 45–9.

Said, G., Ropert, A., and Faux N. (1984). Length-dependent degeneration of fibers in Portuguese amyloid polyneuropathy. *Neurology* 34, 1025–32.

Sommer, C. and Schröder J. M. (1989). Amyloid neuropathy: immunocytochemical localization of intra- and extracellular immunoglobulin light chains. *Acta Neuropath.* 79, 190–9.

Suhr, O. B., Holmgren, G., Steen, L. *et al.* (1995). Liver transplantation in familial amyloidotic polyneuropathy. Follow up of first 20 Swedish patients. *Transplantation* 60, 933–8.

Tashiro, F., Yi, S., Wakasugi, S., Maeda, S., Shimida, K., and Yamamura, K. (1992). Role of serum amyloid P component for systemic amyloidosis in transgenic mice carrying human mutant transthyretin gene. *Gerontology* 37, 56–62.

Thomas, P. K. and King, R. H. M. (1974). Peripheral nerve changes in amyloid neuropathy. *Brain* 97, 395–406.

Uemichi, T., Liepnieks, J. J., Waits, R. P., and Benson, M. D. (1996). In frame deletion in the transthyretin gene (D V122) associated with amyloidotic polyneuropathy [abstract]. *Neuromusc. Disord.* 6, (Suppl. 1), 21.

Van Allen, M. W., Frohlich, J. A., and Davis, J. R. (1969). Inherited predisposition to generalised amyloidosis. Clinical and pathological study of a family with neuropathy, nephropathy and peptic ulcer. *Neurology* 19, 10–25.

Yi, S., Takahashi, K., Naito, M. *et al.* (1991). Systemic amyloidosis in mice carrying the human mutant transthyretin (MET 30) gene. Pathologic similarity to human familial amyloidotic polyneuropathy, type 1. *Am. J. Pathol.* 138, 403–12.

PART VI

Other Disorders associated with Autonomic Dysfunction

43. Introduction to neurocardiology

Martin A. Samuels

In 1942, Walter Bradford Cannon published a remarkable paper entitled '"Voodoo" death' (Cannon 1942), in which he recounted anecdotal experiences, largely from the anthropology literature, of death from fright. These often remote events, drawn from widely disparate parts of the world, had several features in common. They were all induced by an absolute belief that an external force, such as a wizard or medicine man, could, at will, cause demise and that the victim himself had no power to alter this course. This perceived lack of control over a powerful external force is the *sine qua non* for all the cases recounted by Cannon, who postulated that death was caused 'by a lasting and intense action of the sympathico-adrenal system'. Cannon believed that this phenomenon was limited to societies in which the people were 'so superstitious, so ignorant, that they feel themselves bewildered strangers in a hostile world. Instead of knowledge, they have fertile and unrestricted imaginations which fill their environment with all manner of evil spirits capable of affecting their lives disastrously'. Over the years since Cannon's observations, evidence has accumulated to support his concept that 'voodoo' death is, in fact, a real phenomenon, but far from being limited to ancient peoples, may be a basic biological principle which provides an important clue to understanding the phenomenon of sudden death in modern society as well as providing a window into the world of neurovisceral disease. George Engel collected 160 accounts from the lay press of sudden death which were attributed to disruptive life events (Engel 1971). He found that such events could be divided into eight categories: (1) the impact of the collapse or death of a close person; (2) during acute grief; (3) on threat of loss of a close person; (4) during mourning or on an anniversary; (5) on loss of status or self-esteem; (6) personal danger or threat of injury; (7) after danger is over; (8) reunion, triumph, or happy ending. Common to all is that they involve events impossible for the victim to ignore and to which the response is overwhelming excitation, giving up, or both.

In 1957, Carl Richter reported on a series of experiments aimed at elucidating the mechanism of Cannon's 'voodoo' death (Richter 1957). He studied the length of time domesticated rats could swim at various water temperatures and found that at a water temperature of 93°C these rats could swim for 60–80 min. However, if the animal's whiskers were trimmed, it would invariably drown within a few minutes. When carrying out similar experiments with fierce, wild rats, he noted that a number of factors contributed to the tendency for sudden death, the most important of which was restraint, involving holding the animals and confinement in the glass swimming jar with no chance of escape. Trimming the rats' whiskers, which destroys possibly their most important proprioceptive mechanism, contributed to the tendency for early demise. In the case of the calm, domesticated animals in which restraint and confinement were apparently not significant stressors, shaving the whiskers rendered these animals as fearful as wild rats with a corresponding tendency for sudden death. Electrocardiograms taken during the process showed a bradycardia developing prior to death, and adrenalectomy did not protect the animals. Furthermore, atropine protected some of the animals and cholinergic drugs led to an even more rapid demise. All this was taken as evidence that overactivity of the sympathetic nervous system was not the cause of the death but rather it was caused by increased vagal tone.

We now know that the apparently opposite conclusions of Cannon and Richter are not mutually exclusive, but rather that a generalized autonomic storm, occurring as a result of a life-threatening stressor, will have both sympathetic and parasympathetic effects. The apparent predominance of one over the other depends on the parameter measured (e.g. heart rate, blood pressure) and the timing of the observations in relation to the stressor (e.g. early events tend to be dominated by sympathetic effects whereas late events tend to be dominated by parasympathetic effects).

In human beings, one of the easily accessible windows into autonomic activity is the electrocardiogram. Edwin Byer and colleagues reported six patients whose ECGs showed large upright T waves and long QT intervals (Byer *et al.* 1947). Two of these patients had hypertensive encephalopathy, one had a brainstem stroke with neurogenic pulmonary oedema, one had an intracerebral haemorrhage, one had a postpartum ischaemic stroke possibly related to toxaemia, and one had no history except a blood pressure of 210/110. Based on experimental results of cooling or warming the endocardial surface of the dog's left ventricle, Byer *et al.* concluded that these ECG changes were due to subendocardial ischaemia. Levine reported on several disorders, other than ischaemic heart disease, which could produce ECG changes reminiscent of coronary disease (Levine 1953). Among these was a 69-year-old woman who was admitted and remained in coma. Her admission ECG showed deeply inverted T waves in the anterior and lateral precordial leads. Two days later, it showed ST segment elevation with less deeply inverted T waves, a pattern suggestive of myocardial infarction. However, at autopsy a ruptured berry aneurysm was found and no evidence of myocardial infarction or pericarditis was noted. Levine did not propose a specific mechanism but referred to experimental work on the production of cardiac arrhythmias by basal ganglia stimulation and ST and T-wave changes induced by injecting caffeine into the cerebral ventricle.

Burch *et al.* (1954) reported on 17 patients who were said to have 'cerebrovascular accidents' (i.e. strokes). In 14 of the 17, haemorrhage was demonstrated by lumbar puncture. It is not possible to determine which of these patients had haemorrhagic infarction, intracerebral haemorrhage and subarachnoid haemorrhage and no data about the territory of the strokes are available. The essential features of the ECG abnormalities were:

(1) long QT intervals in all patients;

(2) large, usually, inverted T waves, in all patients; and

(3) U waves in 11 of the 17 patients (Burch *et al.* 1954).

Cropp and Manning (1960) reported on the details of the ECG abnormalities in 29 patients with subarachnoid haemorrhage. Twenty-two of these patients survived. Two of those who died had no post-mortem examination, leaving five in whom autopsies confirmed the presence of a ruptured cerebral aneurysm. In three of these five, the heart and coronary arteries were said to be normal, but the details of the pathological examination are not revealed. The point is made that ECG changes seen in the context of neurological disease do not represent ischaemic heart disease but are merely a manifestation of autonomic dysregulation, possibly emanating from a lesion affecting the cortical representation of the autonomic nervous system. The authors argued that Brodmann area 13 on the orbital surface of the frontal lobe and area 24 on the anterior cingulate gyrus were the cortical centres for cardiovascular control.

In contrast to this rather inconclusive clinical data, there is clear evidence that cardiac lesions can be produced as the result of nervous system disease. The concept of visceral organ dysfunction occurring as a result of neurological stimuli can be traced to Pavlov, who may have introduced the concept of a neurogenic dystrophy. Selye, a student of Pavlov, described ESCN (electrolyte–steroid–cardiopathy with necroses) (Selye 1958). His view was that this cardiac lesion was common and often described using different names in the literature. He argued that this lesion was distinct from the coagulation necrosis which occurred as a result of ischaemic disease, but could exist in the same heart. Selye felt that certain steroids and other hormones created a predisposition for the development of ESCN, but that other factors were required for ESCN to developed. The most effective conditioning steroid was 2-α-methyl-9-α-chlorocortisol. Among the factors that led to ESCN in steroid-sensitized animals were certain electrolytes (e.g. NaH_2PO_4), various hormones (e.g. vasopressin, adrenaline, insulin, thyroxine), certain vitamins (e.g. dihydrotachysterol), cardiac glycosides, surgical interventions (e.g. cardiac reperfusion after ischaemia), and psychic or nervous stimuli (e.g. restraint, fright). The cardiac lesions could not be prevented by adrenalectomy, suggesting that the process, if related to autonomic hyperactivity, must exert its influence by direct neural connection to the heart rather than by a blood-borne route.

Cardiac lesions may be produced in rats by pre-treating with either 2-α-methyl-9-α-flourohydrocortisone (flourocortisol), dihydrotachysterol (calciferol) or thyroxine (Synthroid) and then restraining the animals on a board for 15 hours or by using cold stress (Raab *et al.* 1961). Agents that act by inhibition of the catecholamine-mobilizing reflex arc at the hypothalamic level (e.g. chlorpromazine) or by blockade of only the circulating, but not the neurogenic, intramyocardial catecholamines (e.g. dibenamine) were the least effective in protecting cardiac muscle, whereas those drugs that act by ganglionic blockade (e.g. mecamylamine) or by direct intramyocardial catecholamine-depletion (e.g. reserpine) were the most effective. Furthermore, it is clear that blood catecholamine levels are often normal but that identical ECG findings are seen with high systemic catecholamines. These clinical and pharmacological data support the concept that the cardiac necrosis is due to cate-

cholamine toxicity and that catecholamines released directly into the heart via neural connections are much more toxic than those reaching the heart via the bloodstream, though clearly the two routes could be additive in the intact, non-adrenalectomized animal. Intracoronary infusions of adrenaline reproduce the characteristic ECG pattern of neurocardiac disease which is reminiscent of subendocardial ischaemia, though no ischaemic lesion can be found in the hearts of dogs sacrificed after several months of infusions (Barger *et al.* 1961). In the years that followed, numerous reports emanated from around the world documenting the production of cardiac repolarization abnormalities in the context of various neurological catastrophes and proposing that this was due to an autonomic storm. It seemed likely that the connection between neuropsychiatric illness and the visceral organs would be provided by the autonomic nervous system.

Melville *et al.* (1963) produced ECG changes and myocardial necrosis by stimulating the hypothalamus of cats. With anterior hypothalamic stimulation, parasympathetic responses occurred, with bradycardia predominating. Lateral hypothalamic stimulation produced tachycardia and ST segment depressions. With intense bilateral and repeated lateral stimulation, persistent, irreversible ECG changes occurred and post-modern examination revealed a stereotyped cardiac lesion characterized by intense cytoplasmic eosinophilia with loss of cross-striations and some haemorrhage. The coronary arteries were normal without occlusion. Although Melville referred to this lesion as 'infarction', it is probably best to reserve that term for coagulative necrosis caused by ischaemia. This lesion is probably identical to Selye's ESCN and would now be called coagulative myocytolysis, myofibrillar degeneration or contraction band necrosis. More recently, Oppenheimer has mapped the chronotropic organizational structure in the rat insular cortex, demonstrating that sympathetic innervation arises from a more rostral part of the posterior insula then does parasympathetic innervation (Oppenheimer and Cechetto 1990).

Despite the fact that myocardial damage could definitely be produced in animals, until the mid-1960s there was little recognition that this actually occurred in human beings with acute neurological or psychiatric illness, until Koskelo *et al.* (1964) reported on three patients with ECG changes due to subarachnoid haemorrhage who were noted on post-mortem examination to have several small subendocardial petechial haemorrhages. Connor (1969) reported focal myocytolysis in 8 per cent of 231 autopsies, with the highest incidence seen in patients dying of intracranial haemorrhages. The lesion reported by Connor conforms to the descriptions of Selye's ESCN or what might now be called myofibrillar degeneration, coagulative myocytolysis or contraction band necrosis. Connor pointed out that previous pathological reports probably overlooked the lesion because of the fact that it was multifocal, with each individual focus being quite small, requiring extensive tissue sampling. It is clear now that even Connor underestimated the prevalence of the lesion and that serial sections are required to rigorously exclude its presence.

Greenshoot and Reichenbach (1969) reported on three new patients with subarachnoid haemorrhage and a review of six prior patients from the same medical centre. All nine of these patients had cardiac lesions of varying degrees of severity, ranging from eosinophilia with preservation of cross-striations to transformation of the myocardial cell cytoplasm into dense eosinophilic transverse bands with intervening granularity, sometimes with endocardial haemorrhages. Both the ECG abnormalities and the cardiac pathology could be reproduced in cats given mesencephalic reticular formation stimulation. Adrenalectomy did not protect the hearts, supporting the contention that the ECG changes and cardiac lesions are due to direct intracardiac release of catecholamines.

Hawkins and Clower (1971) injected blood intracranially into mice, thereby producing the characteristic myocardial lesions. The number of lesions could be reduced but not obliterated by pretreatment with adrenalectomy and the use of either atropine or reserpine, which suggested that the cause of the lesions was in part due to sympathetic overactivity (humorally reaching the myocardium from the adrenal and by direct release into the muscle by intracardiac nerves) and in part due to parasympathetic overactivity. This supports the concept that the cause is an autonomic storm with both divisions contributing to the pathogenesis.

Jacob *et al.* (1972) produced subarachnoid haemorrhage experimentally in dogs and carefully studied the sequential haemodynamic and ultrastructural changes that occurred. The haemodynamic changes occurred in four stages and directly paralleled the effects seen with intravenous noradrenaline injections. These stages were:

(1) dramatic rise in systemic blood pressure;

(2) extreme sinus tachycardia with various arrhythmias (e.g. nodal or ventricular tachycardia, bradycardia, atrioventricular block, ventricular premature beats, ventricular tachycardia, ventricular fibrillation with sudden death), all of which could be suppressed by bilateral vagotomy or orbital frontal resection;

(3) rise in left ventricular pressure parallel to rise in systemic pressure; and

(4) up to twofold increase in coronary blood flow.

Ultrastructurally, a series of three stereotyped events occurred which could be imitated exactly with noradrenaline injections. These were:

(1) migration of intramitochondrial granules containing Ca^{2+} to the periphery of the mitochondria;

(2) disappearance of these granules; and

(3) myofilament disintegration at the I bands while the density of the I band was increased in the intact sarcomeres (Jacob *et al.* 1972).

Partially successful efforts to modify the developments of neurocardiac lesions were made by using reserpine pre-treatment in mice subjected to simulated intracranial haemorrhage (McNair *et al.* 1970) and by Hunt and Gore (1982) who pre-treated a group of rats with propranolol and then attempted to produce cardiac lesions with intracranial blood injections. No lesions were found in the control animals, in 21 of the 46 untreated rats and in only 4 of the 22 treated rats. This suggested that neurological influences via catecholamines may be partly responsible for cardiac cell death due to ischaemic causes.

The phenomenology of the various types of myocardial cell death was finally clarified by Baroldi (1975), who pointed out that there were three main patterns of myocardial necrosis:

(1) coagulation necrosis, the fundamental lesion of infarction, in which the cell loses its capacity to contract and dies in the atonic state with no myofibrillar damage;

(2) colliquative myocytolysis, in which oedematous vacuolization with dissolution of myofibrils without hypercontraction occurs in the low-output syndromes; and

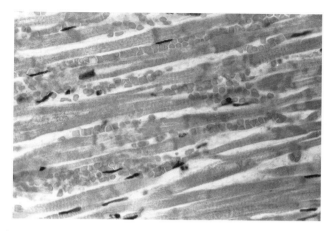

Fig. 43.1. The neurocardiac lesion: contraction band necrosis, also known as myofibrillar degeneration or coagulative myocytolysis.

(3) coagulative myocytolysis, in which the cell dies in a hypercontracted state, with early myofibrillar damage, and anomolous irregular cross-band formations.

Coagulative myocytolysis is seen in reperfused areas around regions of coagulation necrosis in transplanted hearts, in 'stone hearts', in sudden unexpected and accidental death, and in hearts exposed to toxic levels of catecholamines, such as in patients with phaeochromocytoma. This is probably the major lesion described by Selye as ESCN and is clearly the lesions seen in animals and people suffering acute neurological or psychiatric catastrophes. Although coagulative myocytolysis is probably the preferred term, the terms myofibrillar degeneration and contraction band necrosis are commonly used in the literature. This lesion tends to calcify early and to have a multifocal subendocardial predisposition (Fig. 43.1).

It is likely that the subcellular mechanisms underlying the development of coagulative myocytolysis involve calcium entry. Zimmerman and Hulsmann (1966) reported that the perfusion of rat hearts with calcium-free media for short periods of time creates a situation such that upon readmission of calcium, there is a massive contracture followed by necrosis and enzyme release. This phenomenon, known as the calcium paradox, can be imitated almost exactly with reoxygenation followed by hypoxaemia and reperfusion following ischaemia. The latter, called the oxygen paradox, has been linked to the calcium paradox by pathological calcium entry (Hearse *et al.* 1978). This major ionic shift is probably the cause of the dramatic ECG changes seen in the context of neurological catastrophe, a fact that could explain the phenomenon of sudden unexpected death (SUD) in many contexts.

Although SUD is now recognized as a medical problem of major epidemiological importance, it has generally been assumed that neurological disease rarely results in SUD. In fact, it has been taught traditionally that neurological illnesses almost never cause sudden demise, with the only exceptions being the occasional patient who dies during an epileptic convulsion or rapidly in the context of a subarachnoid haemorrhage. Further, it has been assumed that the various SUD syndromes (e.g. sudden death in middle-aged men; sudden infant death syndrome (SIDS); sudden unexpected nocturnal death syndrome (SUNDS); frightened to death ('voodoo' death); sudden death during a seizure; sudden death during natural catastrophe; sudden death associated with drug abuse; sudden death in wild and domestic animals; sudden death during asthma attacks; sudden death during the alcohol withdrawal syndrome; sudden death during grief after a major loss; sudden death during panic attacks; sudden death from mental stress; and sudden death during war are entirely separate and have no unifying mechanism. For example, it is generally accepted that sudden death in middle-aged men is usually caused by a cardiac arrhythmia (i.e. ventricular fibrillation) which results in functional cardiac arrest, while most work on SIDS focuses on respiratory failure.

However, the connection between the nervous system and the cardiopulmonary system provides the unifying link that allows a coherent explanation for most, if not all, of the forms of SUD. Powerful evidence from multiple disparate disciplines allows for a neurological explanation for SUD (Samuels 1993).

Neurogenic heart disease

Definition of neurogenic electrocardiographic changes

A wide variety of changes in the electrocardiogram (ECG) is seen in the context of neurological disease. Two major categories of change are regularly noted: (1) arrhythmias and (2) repolarization changes. It is likely that the increased tendency for life-threatening arrhythmias found in patients with acute neurological disease is due to the repolarization change, which increases the vulnerable period during which an extrasystole would be likely to result in ventricular tachycardia and/or ventricular fibrillation. Thus, the essential and potentially most lethal features of the ECG which are known to change in the context of neurological disease are the ST segment and T wave, reflecting abnormalities in repolarization. Most often, the changes are seen best in the anterolateral or inferolateral leads. If the ECG is read by pattern recognition by someone who is not aware of the clinical history, it will often be said to present subendocardial infarction or anterolateral ischaemia. The electrocardiographic abnormalities usually improve, often dramatically, with death by brain criteria.

The phenomenon is not rare. In a series of 100 consecutive stroke patients, 90 per cent showed abnormalities on the ECG, compared with 50 per cent of a control population of 100 patients admitted for carcinoma of the colon (Dimant and Grob 1977). This, of course, does not mean that 90 per cent of stroke patients have neurogenic electrocardiographic changes. Obviously, stroke and coronary artery disease have common risk factors, so that many electrocardiographic abnormalities in stroke patients represent concomitant atherosclerotic coronary disease. None the less, a significant number of stroke patients have authentic neurogenic electrocardiographic changes.

The mechanism of the production of neurogenic heart disease

Catecholamine infusion

Josue (1907) first sowed that adrenaline infusions could cause cardiac hypertrophy. This observation has been reproduced on many occasions, documenting the fact that systemically administered catecholamines are not only associated with electrocardiographic changes reminiscent of widespread ischaemia but with a characteristic pathological picture in the cardiac muscle that is dis-

tinct from myocardial infarction. An identical picture may be found in human beings with chronically elevated catecholamines, as is seen with phaeochromocytoma. Patients with stroke often have elevated systemic catecholamine levels, a fact which may, in part, account for the high incidence of cardiac arrhythmias and ECG changes seen in these patients. On light microscopy, these changes range from increased eosinophilic staining with preservation of cross-striations to total transformation of the myocardial cell cytoplasm into dense eosinophilic transverse bands with intervening granularity. In severely injured areas, infiltration of the necrotic debris by mononuclear cells is often noted, sometimes with haemorrhage.

Ultrastructurally, the changes in cardiac muscle are even more widespread than they appear to be in light microscopy. Nearly every muscle cell shows some pathological alteration, ranging from a granular appearance of the myofibrils to profound disruption of the cell architecture with relative preservation of ribosomes and mitochondria. Intracardiac nerves can be seen, identified by their external lamina, microtubules, neurofibrils, and the presence of intracytoplasmic vesicles. These nerves can sometimes be seen immediately adjacent to an area of myocardial cell damage. The pathological changes in the cardiac muscle are usually less at a distance from the nerve, often returning completely to normal by a distance of 2–4 μm away from the nerve ending (Jacob *et al.* 1972).

Myofibrillar degeneration (also known as coagulative myocytolysis and contraction band necrosis) is an easily recognizable form of cardiac injury, distinct in several major respects from coagulation necrosis, the major lesion of myocardial infarction (Baroldi 1975; Karch and Billingham 1986). In coagulation necrosis, the cells die in a relaxed state without prominent contraction bands. This is not visible by any method for many hours or even days. Calcification occurs only late and the lesion elicits a polymorphonuclear cell response. In stark contrast, in myofibrillary degeneration the cell die in a hypercontracted state with prominent contraction band (Fig. 43.1). The lesion is visible early, perhaps within minutes of its onset. It elicits a mononuclear cell response and may calcify almost immediately (Rona 1985; Karch and Billingham 1986).

Stress plus or minus steroids

A similar, if not identical, cardiac lesion can be produced using various models of 'stress'. This concept was applied to the heart when Selye published his monograph *The Chemical Prevention of Cardiac Necrosis* in 1958. He found that cardiac lesions probably identical to those described above could be produced regularly in animals that were pretreated with certain steroids, particularly 2-α-methyl-9-α-fluorohydrocortisone (fluorocortisol), and then subjected to various types of stress. Other hormones, such as dihydrotachysterol (calciferol) and thyroxine, could also sensitize animals for stress-induced mycardial lesions, but less potently than fluorocortisol. This so-called stress could be of multiple types, including restraint, surgery, bacteraemia, vagotomy, toxins, and others. He believed that the 'first mediator' in translating these widely disparate stimuli into a stereotyped cardiac lesion was the hypothalamus and that it, by its control over the autonomic nervous system, caused the release of certain agents that were toxic to the myocardial cell. Since Selye's original work, similar experiments have been repeated in many different types of laboratory animals, with comparable results. Although the administration of exogenous steroids facilitates the production of cardiac lesions, it is clear that stress alone can result in the production of morphologically identical lesions.

Whether a similar pathophysiology could ever be operable in human beings is, of course, of great interest. Many investigators have speculated on the role of 'stress' in the pathogenesis of human cardiovascular disease and, in particular, on its relationship to the phenomenon of sudden unexpected death. A few autopsies on patients who experienced sudden death have shown myofibrillar degeneration. Cebelin and Hirsch (1980) reported on a careful retrospective analysis of the hearts of 15 victims of physical assault who died as a direct result of the assault, but without sustaining internal injuries. Eleven of the 15 individuals showed myofibrillar degeneration. Age- and cardiac disease-matched controls showed little or no evidence of this change. This appears to represent a human stress cardiomyopathy. Whether or not such assaults can be considered murder has become an interesting legal correlate of the problem.

Since the myofibrillar degeneration is predominantly subendocardial, it may involve the cardiac conducting system, thus predisposing to cardiac arrhythmias. This lesion, combined with the propensity of catecholamines to produce arrhythmias even in a normal heart may well raise the risk of a serious arrhythmia. This may be the major immediate mechanism of sudden death in many neurological circumstances, such as subarachnoid haemorrhage, stroke, epilepsy, head trauma, psychological stress, and increased intracranial pressure. Even the arrhythmogenic nature of digitalis may be largely mediated by the central nervous system. Further evidence for this is the antiarrhythmic effect of sympathetic denervation of the heart for cardiac arrhythmias of many types.

Furthermore, it is known that the stress-induced myocardial lesions can be prevented by sympathetic blockade using many different classes of antiadrenergic agents, most notably, ganglionic blockers such as mecamylamine and catecholamine-depleting agents such as reserpine (Raab et al 1961). This suggests that catecholamines, either released directly into the heart by sympathetic nerve terminals or reaching the heart through the bloodstream after release from the adrenal medulla, may be excitotoxic to myocardial cells.

Nervous system stimulation

Nervous system stimulation produces cardiac lesions histologically indistinguishable from those just described for stress and catecholamine-induced cardiac damage. It has been known for a long while that stimulation of the hypothalamus can lead to autonomic cardiovascular disturbances, and many years ago, lesions in the heart and gastrointestinal tract has been produced using hypothalamic stimulation. It has been demonstrated clearly that stimulation of the lateral hypothalamus produces hypertension or electrocardiographic changes reminiscent of those seen in patients with central nervous system damage of various types. Furthermore, this effect on the blood pressure and ECG can be completely prevented by C2 spinal section and stellate ganglionectomy, but not by vagotomy, suggesting that the mechanism of the electrocardiographic changes is sympathetic rather than parasympathetic or humoral. Stimulation of the anterior hypothalamus produces bradycardia, an effect that can be blocked by vagotomy. Unilateral hypothalamic stimulation does not result in histological evidence of myocardial damage by light microscopy, but bilateral prolonged stimulation regularly produces myofibrillar degeneration indistinguishable from that produced by catecholamine injections and stress, as previously described (Melville et al. 1963).

Other methods of producing cardiac lesions of this type include stimulation of the limbic cortex, the mesencephalic reticular formation, the stellate ganglion, and region known to elicit cardiac reflexes such as the aortic arch. Experimental intracerebral and subarachnoid haemorrhages can also result in cardiac contraction band lesions. These neurogenic cardiac lesions will occur even in an adrenalectomized animal, although they will be somewhat less pronounced (Hawkins and Clower 1971). This evidence argues strongly against an exclusively humoral mechanism in the intact organism. High levels of circulating catecholamines exaggerate the electrocardiographic findings and myocardial lesions, but high circulating catecholamine levels are not required for the production of pathological changes. These electrocardiographic abnormalities and cardiac lesions are stereotyped and identical to those found in the stress and catecholamine models already outlined. They are not affected by vagotomy and are blocked by manoeuvres that interfere with the action of the sympathetic limb of the autonomic nervous system, such as C2 spinal section, stellate ganglion blockage, and administration of antiadrenergic drugs such as propranolol.

The histological changes in the myocardium range from normal muscle on light microscopy to severely necrotic (but not ischaemic) lesions with secondary mononuclear cell infiltration. The findings on ultrastructural examination are invariably more widespread, often involving nearly every muscle cell, even when the light microscopic appearance is unimpressive. The electrocardiographic findings undoubtedly reflect the total amount of muscle membrane affected by the pathophysiological process. Thus, the ECG may be normal when the lesion is early and demonstrable only by electron microscopy. Conversely, the ECG may be grossly abnormal when only minimal findings are present by light microscopy, since the cardiac membrane abnormality responsible for the electrocardiographic changes may be reversible. Cardiac arrhythmias of many types may also be elicited by nervous system stimulation along the outflow of the sympathetic nervous system.

Reperfusion

The fourth, and last, model for the production of myofibrillar degeneration is reperfusion, as is commonly seen in patients dying after a period of time on a left ventricular assist pump for cardiac surgery. Similar lesions are seen in hearts which were reperfused using angioplasty or fibrinolytic therapy. The mechanism by which reperfusion of ischaemic cardiac muscle produces myofibrillar degeneration involves entry of calcium after a period of relative deprivation (Braunwald and Kloner 1985).

Sudden calcium influx by one of several possible mechanisms (e.g. a period of calcium deficiency with loss of intracellular calcium, a period of anoxia followed by reoxygenation of the electron transport system, a period of ischaemia followed by reperfusion, or opening of the receptor-operated calcium channels by excessive amounts of locally released noradrenaline) may be the final common pathway by which the irreversible contractures occur, leading to myofibrillar degeneration. Thus reperfusion-induced myocardial cell death may be a form of apoptosis (programmed cell death) analogous to that seen in the central nervous system wherein excitotoxicity with glutamate results in a similar, if not identical, series of events (Gottlieb et al. 1994).

The precise cellular mechanism for the electrocardiographic change and the histological lesion may well reflect the effects of large volumes of noradrenaline released into the myocardium from sympathetic nerve terminals (Eliot *et al.* 1979). The fact that the cardiac necrosis is greatest near the nerve terminals in the endocardium and is progressively less severe as one samples muscle approaching the epicardium provides further evidence that catecholamine toxicity produces the lesion (Greenshoot and Reichenbach 1969). This locally released noradrenaline is known to stimulate synthesis of adenosine 3′, 5′-cyclic phosphate, which in turn results in the opening of the calcium channel with influx of calcium and efflux of potassium. This efflux of potassium could explain the peaked T waves (a hyperkalaemic pattern) often seen early in the evolution of neurogenic electrocardiographic changes (Jacob *et al.* 1972). The actin and myosin filaments interact under the influence of calcium but do not relax unless the calcium channel closes. Continuously high levels of noradrenaline in the region may result in failure of the calcium channel to close, leading to cell death, and finally to leakage of enzymes out of the myocardial cell. Free radicals released as a result of reperfusion after ischaemia or by the metabolism of catecholamines to the known toxic metabolite adrenochrome may contribute to cell membrane destruction, leading to leakage of cardiac enzymes into the blood (Singal *et al.* 1982; Meerson 1983). Thus, the cardiac toxicity of locally released noradrenaline would represent a continuum ranging from a brief reversible burst of electrocardiographic abnormalities to a pattern resembling hyperkalaemia and then, finally, to an irreversible failure of the muscle cell with permanent repolarization abnormalities, or even the occurrence of transmural cardiac necrosis with Q waves seen on the ECG.

Histological changes would also represent a continuum ranging from complete reversibility in a normal heart through mild changes seen best with electron microscopy to severe myocardial cell necrosis with mononuclear cell infiltration and even haemorrhages. The level of cardiac enzymes released and the electrocardiographic changes would roughly correlate with the severity and extent of the pathological process. This explanation, summarized in Fig. 43.2 would tie together all the observations in the catecholamine infusion, stress plus or minus steroid, nervous system stimulation, and reperfusion models.

Concluding remarks

In conclusion, there is powerful evidence suggesting that overactivity of the sympathetic limb of the autonomic nervous system is the common phenomenon that links the major cardiac and pulmonary pathologies seen in neurological catastrophes. These profound effects on the heart and lungs may contribute in a major way to the mortality rates of many primarily neurological conditions such as subarachnoid haemorrhage, status epilepticus, and head trauma. These phenomena may also be important in the pathogenesis of sudden unexpected death in adults, sudden infant death, sudden death during asthma attacks, cocaine- and amphetamine-related deaths, and sudden death during the alcohol withdrawal syndrome, all of which may be linked by stress and catecholamine toxicity.

Investigations aimed at altering the natural history of these events using catecholamine receptor blockade, calcium-channel blockers, free-radical scavengers, and antioxidants are continuing in many centres around the world and are summarized in Fig. 43.3.

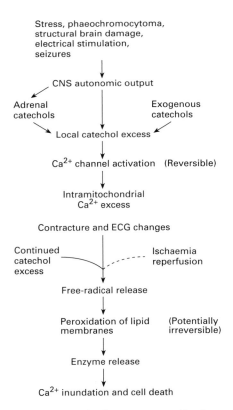

Fig. 43.2. Cascade of events leading to neurocardiac damage.

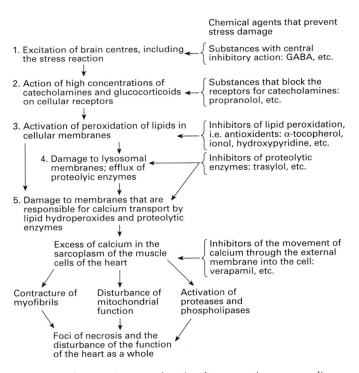

Fig. 43.3. Therapeutic approaches aimed at preventing neurocardiac damage.

References

Barger, A. C., Herd, J. A., and Liebowitz, M. R. (1961). Chronic catherization of coronary artery induction of ECG pattern of myocardial ischaemia by intracoronary epinephrine. *Proc. Soc. Exp. Biol. Med.* 107, 474–7.

Baroldi, F. (1975). Different morphological types of myocardial cell death in man. In Fleckstein A., Rona G., eds. *Recent advances in studies in cardiac structure and metabolism. Pathophysiology and morphology of myocardial cell alteration*, (ed. A. Fieckstein and G. Rona), Vol. 6, pp. 385–97. University Park Press, Baltimore.

Braunwald, E. and Kloner, R. A. (1985). Myocardial reperfusion: a double-edged sword? *J. Clin Invest.* 76, 1713–19.

Burch, G. E., Myers, R., and Adildskov, J. A. (1954). A new electrocardiographic pattern observed in cerebrovascular accidents. *Circulation* 9, 719–26.

Byer, E., Ashman, R., and Toth, L. A. (1947). Electrocardiogram with large upright T wave and long Q-T intervals. *Am. Heart J.* 33, 796–801.

Cannon, W. B. (1942). 'Voodoo' death. *American Anthropologist*.

Cebelin, M. and Hirsch, C. S. (1980). Human stress cardiomyopathy. *Hum. Pathol.* 11, 123–32.

Connor, R. C. R. (1969). Myocardial damage secondary to brain lesions. *Am. Heart J.* 78, 145–8.

Cropp, C. F. and Manning, G. W. (1960). Electrocardiographic change simulating myocardial ischaemia and infarction associated with spontaneous intracarnial haemorrhage.

Dimant, J. and Grob, D. (1977). Electrocardiographic changes and myocardial damage in patients with acute cerebrovascular accidents. *Stroke* 8, 448–55.

Eliot, R. S., Todd, G. L., Pieper, G. M., and Clayton, F. C. (1979). Pathophysiology of catecholamine-mediated myocardial damage. *J. S. Carolina Med. Assoc.* 75, 513–18.

Engel, G. (1971). Sudden and rapid death during psychological stress. *Ann. Int. Med.* 74, 771–82.

Gottlieb, R., Burleson, K. O., Kloner, R. A. *et al.* (1994). Reperfusion injury induces apoptosis in rabbit cardiomyocytes. *J. Clin. Invest.* 94, 1621–8.

Greenshoot, J. H. and Reichenbach, D. D. (1969). Cardiac injury and subarachnoid haemorrhage. *J. Neurosurg.* 30, 521–31.

Hawkins, W. E. and Clower, B. R. (1971). Myocardial damage after head trauma and simulated intracranial haemorrhage in mice: the role of the autonomic nervous system. *Cardiovasc. Res.* 5, 524–9.

Hearse, D. J., Humphrey, S. M., and Bullock, G. R. (1978). The oxygen paradox and the calcium paradox: two facets of the same problem? *J. Mol. Cell. Cardiol.* 10, 641–68.

Jacob, W. A., Van Bogaert, A., and DeGroot-Lasseel, M. H. A. (1972). Myocardial ultrastructural and haemodynamic reactions during experimental subarachnoid haemorrhage. *J. Mol. Cell. Cardiol.* 4, 287–98.

Josue, O. (1907). Hypertrophie cardiaque causee par l'adrenaline et la toxine typhique. *C. R. Soc. Biol. (Paris)* 63, 285–7.

Karch, S. B. and Billingham, M. E. (1986). Myocardial contraction bands revisited. *Hum. Pathol.* 17, 9–13.

Koskelo, P., Punsar, S. O., and Sipila, W. (1964). Subendocardial haemorrhage and ECG changes in intracranial bleeding. *BMJ* 1, 1479–83.

Levine, H. D. (1953). Non-specificity of the electrocardiogram associated with coronary heart disease. *Am. J. Med.* 15, 344–50.

McNair, J. L., Clower, B. R., and Sanford, R. A. (1970). The effect of reserpine pretreatment on myocardial damage associated with stimulated intracranial haemorrhage in mice. *Eur. J. Pharmacol.* 9, 1–6.

Meerson, F. Z. (1983). Pathogenesis and prophylaxis of cardiac lesions in stress. *Adv. Myocardiol.* 4, 3–21.

Melville, K. I., Blum, B., Shister, H. E. *et al.* (1963). Cardiac ischemic changes and arrhythmias induced by hypothalamic stimulation. *Am. J. Cardiol.* 12, 781–91.

Oppenheimer, S. M. and Cechetto, D. F. (1990). Cardiac chronotropic organization of the rat insular cortex. *Brain Res.* 533, 66–72.

Raab, W., Stark, E., MacMillan, W. H. *et al.* (1961). Sympathogenic oriin and anti-adrenergic prevention of stress-induced myocardial lesions. *Am. J. Cardiol.* 8, 203–11.

Richter, C. P. (1957). On the phenomenon of sudden death in animals and man. *Psychosom. Med.* 19, 191–8.

Rona, G. (1985). Catecholamine cardiotoxicity. *J. Mol. Cell. Cardiol.* 17, 291–306.

Samuels, M. A. (1993). Neurally induced cardiac damage. *Neurol. Clin.* 11, 273–92.

Selye, H. (1958). *The chemical prevention of cardiac necrosis.* Ronald Press, New York.

Singal, P. K., Kapur, N., Dhillon, K. S., Beamish, R. E., and Dhalla, N. A. (1982). Role of free radicals in catecholamine-induced cardiomyocaphy. *Can. J. Physiol. Pharmacol.* 60, 1390–7.

Zimmerman, A. N. A. and Hulsmann, W. C. (1966). Paradoxical influence of calcium ions on the permeability of the cell membranes of the isolated rat heart. *Nature* 211, 616–47.

44. Syncope and fainting: classification and pathophysiological basis

Roger Hainsworth

Introduction

Syncope or fainting refers to a transient loss of consciousness usually resulting from a temporarily inadequate cerebral blood flow. A syncopal attack is frequently preceded by sweating, pallor, blurring of vision, dizziness, and nausea. It is uncommon in supine subjects and usually when subjects become supine as the result of syncope they rapidly recover consciousness. There is a wide variation in the susceptibility of individuals to syncope. The fainting of pregnant women or soldiers standing motionless on hot parade grounds is well known. On the other hand, patients in heart failure rarely, if ever, faint. Syncope does not necessarily point to organic disease, although it is clearly important to exclude diseases such as epilepsy, autonomic neuropathies, cerebrovascular disease, and cardiac and endocrine disorders. Most healthy individuals can precipitate at least presyncopal symptoms if, particularly in a warm environment (causing skin vasodilatation), they hyperventilate (to constrict cerebral blood vessels), and after having been in a crouching position suddenly stand (to allow abdominal blood vessels to fill with blood and to increase the height to which blood must be pumped to the brain).

The onset of syncope can be gradual with ample warning signs, or it may be quite abrupt. Usually preceding the faint there is increased activity of the sympathetic nervous system, leading to a maintained or sometimes increased blood pressure accompanied by increases in heart rate and vascular resistance. Then there is a profound fall in arterial blood pressure, inadequate cerebral perfusion, and loss of consciousness. Often the syncopal attack is accompanied by vasodilatation and bradycardia. This is the vasovagal attack, a term introduced in 1932 by Sir Thomas Lewis.

In this chapter, the main causes of syncope are first categorized. The control of cerebral blood flow and its inadequacy in causing loss of consciousness is then discussed, followed by discussion of the factors leading to vasodilatation and to bradycardia and the consequences of these responses for the maintenance of blood pressure. Cardiac and neurological causes of syncope are described in Chapter 46. This Chapter concentrates on fainting due to unexplained hypotension and, in particular, on vasovagal syncope.

Causes of syncope

Syncope is a transient loss of consciousness resulting from cerebral dysfunction due usually to cerebral hypoperfusion, although sometimes from metabolic disorders. Cerebral hypoperfusion may result from an abnormally high cerebral vascular resistance or from an inadequate cerebral perfusion pressure. In some cases the cause of syncope may be identified as being secondary to some recognizable clinical condition, such as cardiac arrhythmias or autonomic failure. However, in many cases the cause is not immediately apparent but it

Table 44.1. Causes of syncope

Low arterial blood pressure

Low cardiac output
    Inadequate venous return—due either to excessive venous pooling or to low blood volume
    Cardiac causes—tachyarrhythmias, bradyarrhythmias, valvular disease, bradycardia
Low total peripheral vascular resistance
    Vasovagal attacks
    Widespread cutaneous vasodilatation in thermal stress
    Reflex causes—vasovagal attacks, 'carotid sinus syndrome', visceral pain reflexes (may cause vasodilatation or vasoconstriction), decreased stimulation of visceral stretch receptors (e.g. voiding distended bladder)
    Vasodilator drugs
    Autonomic neuropathies

Increased resistance to cerebral blood flow

Cerebral vasoconstriction
    Low Pa_{CO_2}, due to hyperventilation
    Cerebral vasospasm (?)
Vascular disease—either extracranial of intracranial arteries.

Other causes of cerebral dysfunction

Epilepsy—may confuse with simple faints
Metabolic and endocrine disorders—hypoglycaemia, Addison's disease, hypopituitarism
Electrolyte disorders—may be associated with hypovolaemia or pre dispose to cardiac arrhythmias

---

occurs when in the upright position, often accompanied by vasodilatation and sometimes bradycardia. These faints are often referred to as vasovagal attacks or neurocardiogenic syncope.

The causes of syncope have been listed in Table 44.1 and have been classified on a pathophysiological basis. Cerebral hypoperfusion may result from systemic hypotension. Since blood pressure is dependent on cardiac output and total peripheral vascular resistance, any factor that decreases either variable must decrease blood pressure.

The most important physiological factor determining cardiac output is venous filling, since the heart can never pump more out than flows in. Therefore, excessive pooling of blood in dependent veins or a small blood volume predisposes to syncope. Occasionally cardiac output may be impaired due to bradyarrhythmias, tachyarrhythmias, or valvular disease. These disorders are discussed in detail in Chapter 46. Rarely, cardiac output may be reduced due to vagally induced bradycardia in vasovagal syncope or 'carotid sinus syncope'. These are discussed later in this chapter.

Widespread and excessive vasodilatation causes blood pressure to fall. This is the main reason for the sudden fall in blood pressure in the vasovagal attack. Vasodilatation also occurs during thermal stress and in response to some reflex stimuli, as well as when vasoactive drugs are given. Normal vasoconstrictor responses are impaired in autonomic neuropathies.

Cerebral blood flow may be reduced as the result of cerebral vasoconstriction due to low blood levels of carbon dioxide. There is some recent evidence suggesting that there may be cerebral vasoconstriction preceding the onset of syncope (see Chapter 45.). Vascular disease involving extracranial and/or intracranial arteries may also predispose to syncope.

Syncope may result from cerebral dysfunction due to causes other than hypoperfusion. An obvious cause to consider is epilepsy, which may be misdiagnosed in cases of vasovagal attacks because of the tonic clonic movements that are sometimes seen. Metabolic disorders, notably hypoglycaemia, can also lead to loss of conciousness. Syncope may also occur in various other endocrine disorders, particularly Addison's disease and hypopituitarism, probably mainly due to low blood volume. Severe electrolyte disturbances may cause impaired consciousness or predispose to syncope from low blood volume or cardiac dysrhythmias.

Cerebral blood flow

The blood flow to the human brain normally remains relatively constant. Unlike tissues such as muscle or glands, in which changes in metabolic activity result in large changes in blood flow, changes in cerebral activity result in changes in flow that are usually too localized and, overall, too small to be apparent in estimates of total flow. Typical values of cerebral blood flow are 50–60 ml/min 100 g brain tissue or, about 15 per cent of the resting cardiac output.

The brain cannot withstand more than a few seconds of total interruption of flow without loss of consciousness; interruption for longer periods results in irreversible damage.

Regulation of cerebral blood flow

Cerebral blood flow shows marked autoregulation. That means that cerebral blood flow remains almost constant over a wide range of perfusion pressures. Two mechanisms are postulated for causing relaxation of arteriolar smooth muscle to maintain a constant flow to a region when perfusion pressure decreases: response to decreased stretch (the myogenic theory), and relaxation in response to an increase in local concentrations of vasodilator metabolites following a transient decrease in flow (the metabolic theory). In the brain it seems likely that metabolic factors predominate, although there may also be a myogenic component.

Changes in the level of carbon dioxide in the arterial blood are particularly effective in causing changes in cerebral blood flow. At normal levels of arterial pressure, an increase in P_{CO_2} from 5.3 to 7 kPa approximately doubles cerebral flow, whereas a decrease to 4 kPa halves it. The level of CO_2 in the perfusing blood also influences the autoregulation of cerebral blood flow. Autoregulation is abolished during hypercapnia; during hypocapnia cerebral blood flow is low at all perfusion pressures (Fig. 44.1).

Cerebral blood vessels are innervated to some extent by sympathetic vasoconstrictor nerves. These are thought to be relatively unimportant in most circumstances. However, recent work, using transcranial Doppler estimates of middle cerebral arterial flow, has

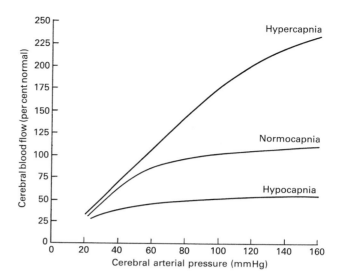

Fig. 44.1. Schematic diagram showing autoregulation of cerebral blood flow. The flow at normal cerebral perfusion pressure and normal arterial P_{CO_2} is taken at 100 per cent. Cerebral perfusion pressure (cerebral arterial pressure minus intracranial pressure) is 5–10 mmHg less than cerebral arterial pressure. Above a pressure of about 60 mmHg the flow is largely independent of pressure. During hypercapnia the autoregulation is largely lost. During hypocapnia blood flow is only about 50 per cent of the normal value, at all levels of CO_2.

shown that there may be quite marked cerebral vasoconstriction just before the onset of syncope (see Chapter 45).

Cerebral blood flow during hypotension

It must first be appreciated that in the upright position cerebral arterial pressure is 15–30 mm Hg lower than that in the aortic arch and the difference is even greater compared with that in a dependent arm (Fig. 44.2). Consciousness starts to be lost when cerebral blood flow falls below about 25 ml/min/100 g, half the normal flow. This level can be reached by severe hypocapnia (P_{CO_2} less than 4 kPa) achieved by hyperventilation, or by cerebral arterial pressure falling below about 40 mmHg (Fig. 44.1). Note that in the upright position the critical level of cerebral arterial pressure would correspond to a mean brachial arterial pressure of about 70 mmHg; for example 90/60 mmHg (mean pressure is approximately diastolic plus 1/3 pulse pressure). Syncope is much less likely to occur when subjects are supine, partly because cerebral arterial pressure is then the same as aortic pressure and partly because there is less pooling of blood in dependent veins.

Vasodilatation

Poiseuille's equation states that flow through a tube is proportional to pressure and the fourth power of the radius. By rearranging Poiseuille's equation, arterial pressure, P, can be seen to be dependent on cardiac output, and a term r, relating to the radius of resistance vessels:

$$P \alpha \dot{Q}/r^4.$$

Thus, the effect of vasodilatation on blood pressure depends on whether the change in r^4 is greater than the change in $\dot{Q}$.

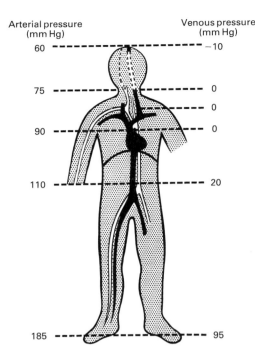

Arterial pressure
(mm Hg)

Venous pressure
(mm Hg)

Fig. 44.2. Effects of gravity on arterial and venous blood pressures in an erect, motionless man. Arterial and venous pressures in the lower part of the body are increased and in the upper part of the body decreased. Note that cerebral arterial pressure is about 15 mmHg lower than aortic root pressure. Because the brain is enclosed by rigid skull, the venous pressures may be below atmospheric. This results in a relatively constant arterial-venous pressure difference in different parts of the brain. (From Hainsworth (1985).)

Vasodilatation can be particularly pronounced in skeletal muscle during exercise. At rest in a comfortable environment, the cardiac output (typically about 5.5 litres/min) is distributed so that less than 20 per cent of it perfuses skeletal muscle, even though muscle comprises nearly half the tissue mass. During severe exercise total muscle blood flow may increase from 1 to 20 litres/min and it then forms the major part of the cardiac output. This intense vasodilatation, however, is usually associated with an increase rather than a fall in blood pressure. The main reason for this is that the contracting muscles and increased respiratory activity return blood rapidly back to the heart, and this, together with an increased activity in cardiac sympathetic nerves, increases cardiac output. The same effect does not occur when there is vasodilatation in the absence of increased muscular activity. Thus administration of vasodilator drugs, such as sodium nitroprusside, or pharmacologically blocking sympathetic vasoconstrictor activity, results in vasodilatation with relatively little accompanying increase in cardiac output, so that the change in r^4 is greater than the change in $\dot{Q}$ and this results in a decrease in blood pressure.

Blood flow in the skin has been estimated to lie between as little as 20 ml/min for the entire skin during cooling of both skin and body core, to as much as 3 litres/min during severe heat load. Thermally induced vasodilatation results in a decrease in total vascular resistance and an increased volume of blood in cutaneous veins, and this may decrease blood pressure and predispose to fainting.

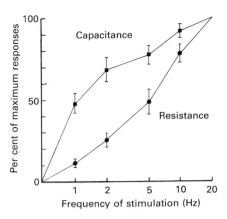

Fig. 44.3. Capacitance and resistance responses in abdominal circulation of anaesthetized dogs to stimulation of splanchnic nerves at various frequencies. Responses expressed as percentages of the changes at 20 Hz. Values are means ± SE from 14 dogs. Note that at 1 Hz the capacitance response was nearly 50 per cent of maximal whereas the resistance response was only about 10 per cent maximal. Above 2 Hz there was little further response of capacitance but larger responses of resistance. (Modified from Karim and Hainsworth (1976).)

Mechanisms of vasodilatation

The diameter of blood vessels can change in response to neural, chemical and mechanical influences.

Sympathetic vasoconstrictor (noradrenergic) nerves increase the contraction of smooth muscle in both arterioles and veins. Resting discharge rate is quite low (<1 Hz) but this may increase up to about 10 Hz during severe stresses or baroreceptor unloading. Capacitance vessels have been shown to be more sensitive to low levels of sympathetic activity (Hainsworth 1986) (Fig. 44.3) and moderate levels of hypotension result in baroreceptor-mediated responses which maintain blood pressure more by capacitance vessel constriction than by increases in vascular resistance.

Blood flow to most regions of the body is regulated so that it is appropriate for the level of metabolic activity. This is achieved through the formation of metabolic products which dilate resistance vessels. Flow is thus a balance between neurally mediated vasoconstriction and metabolically mediated vasodilatation. In circumstances, such as orthostatic stress, in which the degree of sympathetic activity is high, flow is reduced and metabolic products consequently accumulate. Abrupt removal of the normal vasoconstrictor activity would therefore result in a transient reactive hyperaemia and a fall in blood pressure. This is illustrated in Fig. 44.4 in which it can be seen that during constant pressure perfusion of a dog's hind-limb, stimulation of the efferent sympathetic nerves decreased the blood flow. Immediately after switching off the stimulator, blood flow increased transiently to well above the steady-state value seen before stimulation.

Is flow also controlled by vasodilator nerves?

The importance of sympathetic adrenergic nerves in the control of blood pressure is undisputed. However, it has also been proposed that blood flow, particularly to skeletal muscle, is also under the influence of sympathetic cholinergic vasodilator nerves.

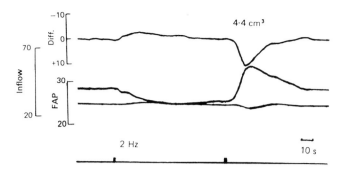

Fig. 44.4. Reactive hyperaemia in response to cessation of sympathetic efferent activity. A dog's hind-limb was perfused at constant pressure and efferent sympathetic nerves to the limb were stimulated at 2 Hz for 90 s. Traces from above down are of the electronically subtracted difference between outflow of blood from the limb and inflow in ml/min (an upward deflection indicates that outflow exceeds inflow and so the volume decreases), inflow in ml/min, and femoral arterial perfusion pressure in kPa (1 kPa = 7.5 mmHg). Stimulation of sympathetic nerves caused a decrease in flow to the limb and a decrease in the volume of blood in the limb. After cessation of the stimulus the flow increased and was initially much greater than the steady-state value in absence of stimulation. The increase in flow also resulted in the retention of blood within the limb. (From Hainsworth *et al.* (1983).)

The importance of these nerves was thought to lie not only with their supposed ability to increase flow at the onset of exercise, but also that they might mediate the vasodilatation that precedes syncope.

The evidence in support of cholinergic vasodilator responses in humans comes from experiments of fainting in which there was seen to be an increase in limb blood flow just before the onset of syncope and this was prevented by sympathetic block (Barcroft and Edholm 1945) and reduced by intra-arterial atropine (Blair *et al.* 1959). There is, however, considerable evidence against the existence of a cholinergic vasodilator supply to muscle in man. First, Uvnas (1966) looked for these nerves in many animals and found them only in some sub-primate species and not in any of several primates studied; their existence in humans therefore seems unlikely. Secondly, the observation that flow in an innervated limb increases transiently to become greater than that in a sympathectomized limb is not evidence for active vasodilatation because it is likely that there would have been reactive hyperaemia following abrupt withdrawal of sympathetic tone (e.g. Fig. 44.4). The evidence in support of cholinergic vasodilatation provided by the administration of atropine is also not conclusive because, although atropine blocks the bradycardia occurring during a vasovagal attack, the fall in blood pressure is not prevented (Lewis 1932). Any small effect of atropine in human limbs may be an effect on the cutaneous circulation since thermally induced vasodilatation may be a cholinergic response associated with sweating. Further evidence against active muscle vasodilatation was provided by Wallin and Sundlof (1982) who recorded activity in efferent sympathetic nerves in two humans during vasovagal fainting. They observed an abrupt cessation of nervous activity with the onset of the hypotension, but there was no suggestion of any increase in other nervous activity which might have been expected if vasodilator nerves had become active.

Bradycardia

Heart rate is controlled mainly by the activity in the vagus and sympathetic nerves, although it is also influenced by body temperature and the concentrations of various hormones, particularly catecholamines. At rest there is tonic vagal activity. Intense vagal activity causes profound bradycardia and can even result in asystole although vagal 'escape' usually prevents a potentially dangerous prolonged arrest.

Effect of heart rate on cardiac output

Cardiac output is equal to the product of heart rate and stroke volume. Although this equation is mathematically unarguable, it can be misleading because stroke volume is not independent of heart rate. Figure 44.5 illustrates the effect of changes in heart rate when venous

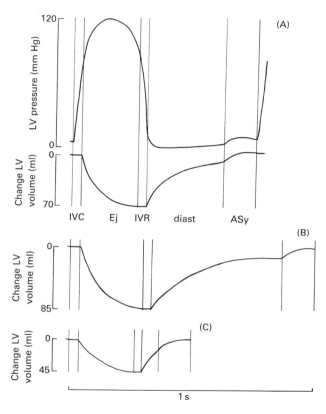

Fig. 44.5. Diagrammatic representation of left ventricular (LV) pressures and volumes during the cardiac cycle and the influence of heart rate. IVC, isovolumic contraction phase; Ej, ejection phase; IVR, isovolumic relaxation phase; diast, ventricular and atrial diastole; ASy, atrial systole. (A) Pressure and volume changes at heart rate of 80 beats/min (cycle length 0.75 s). Note the rapid ventricular filling during early diastole and the small contribution of atrial systole. Stroke volume is 70 ml and cardiac output is 5.6 l/min. (B) Volume changes at a heart rate of 60 beats/min (cycle length 1.0 s). Diastole is prolonged and there is a period of diastasis during which ventricular filling virtually ceases. Stroke volume increases to 85 ml and cardiac output is only slightly reduced at 5.1 l/min. (C) Volume changes at a heart rate of 120 beats/min (cycle length 0.5 s). The shortening is mainly at the expense of diastole which is greatly reduced. Atrial systole now makes a major contribution to ventricular filling. Stroke volume decreases to 45 ml and cardiac output again remains almost unchanged at 5.4 l/min.

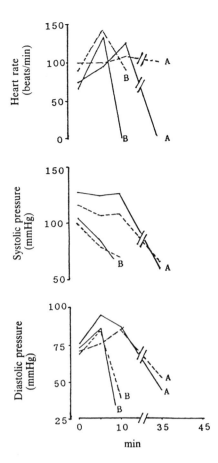

Fig. 44.6. Responses in two patients (A and B) to head-up tilting before (continuous lines) and after (interrupted lines) implantation of atrioventricular pacemakers. The pacemakers successfully prevented the asystole, but had no effect on the blood pressure change or on the time to onset of syncope. (From El-Bedawi *et al.* 1994.)

filling of the heart is not enhanced. A moderate decrease in heart rate, say to 60 beats/min, results in longer time for cardiac filling so that the effect of the bradycardia is offset by an increase in stroke volume.

The effect of a change in heart rate on cardiac output depends on the rate of venous filling and also on whether it is accompanied by a change in the inotropic state. During exercise, an increase in heart rate is accompanied by a positive inotropic change which reduces the duration of systole and so preserves diastolic filling time. Venous filling pressure is high and this results in a large increase in output. On the other hand, during orthostatic stress venous filling pressure would be low and changes in heart rate would then have little effect on cardiac output.

The unimportance of bradycardia in contributing to syncope caused by orthostatic stress has been demonstrated in studies of the effects of cardiac pacemakers. Figure 44.6 shows the effects of head-up tilting in two patients before and after implanting atrioventricular pacemakers. The pacemakers successfully prevented bradycardia but had no effect on the hypotension or on the time at which it occurred.

Vasovagal syncope

Lewis (1932) described fainting attacks as being vasovagal because they were accompanied by hypotension and bradycardia. He consid-

ered that bradycardia usually was not the main cause of the faint since heart rate rarely fell to very low levels (less than 40 beats/min) and the hypotension was little affected by the administration of atropine which prevented the bradycardia.

Barcroft *et al.* (1944) performed an illuminating study in which they induced fainting in healthy subjects by bleeding and application of tourniquets to the legs. They observed that, before the onset of the faint, heart rate increased and there was also an increase in vascular resistance shown by blood pressure being relatively little changed despite a decrease in cardiac output. During the faint, blood pressure decreased abruptly, accompanied by decreases in heart rate and vascular resistance, but no further fall and perhaps even a small increase in cardiac output. Subsequent investigators have also made similar observations, of a fall in vascular resistance but no further fall in cardiac output during fainting.

Barcroft and Edholm (1945) reported an increase in forearm blood flow during fainting (Fig. 44.7) and suggested that the hypotension was due mainly to dilatation of vessels in skeletal muscle. More recent work, however, has suggested that vasodilatation in hypotensive haemorrhage may be more widespread (Morita and Vatner 1985).

Emotional stress leads to increases in heart rate and blood pressure with little change in total vascular resistance. However, if a vasovagal faint occurs, blood pressure, heart rate and forearm vascular resistance decrease abruptly.

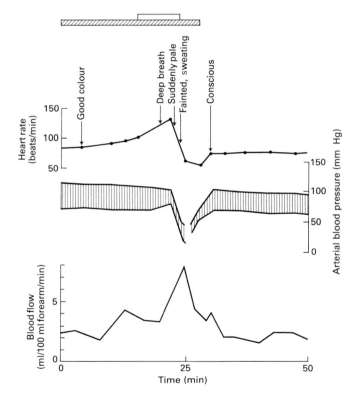

Fig. 44.7. Heart rate, arterial blood pressure, and forearm blood flow in a human subject during a haemorrhagic faint. Shaded bar: venous return impeded by application of tourniquets to both thighs; open bar: venesection. Note that initially blood pressure was relatively well maintained but that heart rate was increased. Then heart rate slowed and blood pressure fell. This was accompanied by an increase in forearm blood flow. (From Barcroft and Edholm 1945.)

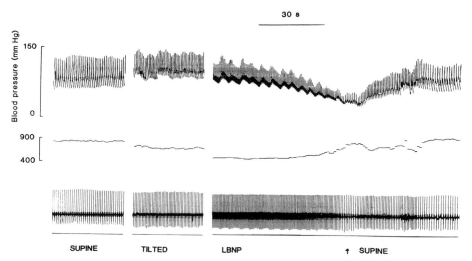

Fig. 44.8. Vasovagal syncope in a healthy subject. Traces are of arterial blood pressure (Finapres—finger at heart level), pulse interval, and ECG. Head-up tilting alone for 20 min caused an increase in diastolic pressure and a decrease in pulse interval. Addition of lower-body negative pressure (LBNP) while still tilted caused a further decrease in pulse interval accompanied by a decrease in blood pressure, particularly systolic. Subsequently, blood pressure fell, with a small pulse pressure and an increase in pulse interval. The subject experienced symptoms of pre-syncope. (From El-Bedawi and Hainsworth 1994).)

Thus a vasovagal attack is usually preceded by evidence of increased sympathetic and decreased vagal activity. During this stage blood pressure is maintained or, particularly in emotional faints, increased. The vasovagal attack is characterized by sudden onset of hypotension and bradycardia. The main cause of the hypotension is vasodilatation due to inhibition of sympathetic vasoconstrictor activity. The bradycardia is usually relatively unimportant because heart rate is seldom greatly slowed and cardiac output does not usually decrease with the onset of the faint. Furthermore, prevention of bradycardia by pacing the heart does not necessarily prevent or even delay syncope (Fig. 44.6).

Patients with histories suggestive of fainting attacks are frequently investigated by determining the effects of head-up tilting, either alone or accompanied by administration of a vasodilator drug such as isoprenaline. We use a stress that combines head-up tilting with application of progressive lower-body suction (El-Bedawi and Hainsworth 1994) and have been able to induce syncope in all volunteer subjects tested if the stress is great enough. Figure 44.8 shows responses obtained in a volunteer subject during the combined test. Head-up tilt alone did not induce hypotension but during the combined stress there were decreases in blood pressure and heart rate with symptoms of presyncope. It is important to note that vasovagal syncope is not necessarily an abnormal response. It is just that some people are more susceptible than others. The stages of the stress which are required to induce presyncope in volunteer subjects and in patients with suspected orthostatic intolerance are compared in Fig. 44.9. It can be noted that tilting with lower-body suction at −40 mmHg induces syncope in most subjects but that at −20 mmHg syncope is much more likely in the patients than in volunteers.

Many factors may be involved in the initiation of syncope and these are listed earlier in this chapter. The cardiac and neurological disorders leading to syncope are dealt with elsewhere. Most other fainting attacks seem to be associated with a reduction in the return of blood to the heart. Thus, when patients faint they are almost invariably standing or sitting up, when dependent veins become distended with blood. The effects of posture are enhanced by performing the Valsalva manoeuvre. In this, intrathoracic and intra-abdominal pressures are increased by expiring against a resistance or a closed glottis. Initially, the Valsalva results in an increase in arterial blood pressure as the thoracic and abdominal arteries are compressed. After a few seconds, owing to a decreased venous return

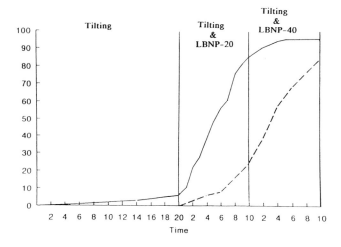

Fig. 44.9. Cumulative incidence of presyncope in volunteers (interrupted line) and patients with attacks of unexplained syncope (continuous line) to an orthostatic stress test of 20 min of 60° head-up tilt, followed while still tilted by lower body suction at −20 and −40 mmHg for 10 min at each. Note that tilting alone did not induce syncope in many subjects of either group and that before the end of the test most subjects had developed syncope. The best discrimination between the groups was at the end of the first level of suction, when 85% of patients but only 20% of volunteers had developed symptoms. (From Hainsworth and El-Bedawi (1994).)

into the abdomen and thorax due to the high pressures, cardiac output and blood pressure fall, possibly resulting in syncope. Two clinical manifestations of this are cough syncope and micturition syncope.

Paroxysms of coughing are effectively a Valsalva manoeuvre, but in addition, there may be reflex vasodilatation from stimulation of lung receptors (Daly *et al.* 1967). If sufficiently intense or prolonged, syncope may result.

Micturition syncope is particularly interesting as many diverse mechanisms seem to operate. Usually the problem occurs when a man stands to micturate after leaving a warm bed. His cutaneous circulation is dilated and therefore peripheral vascular resistance is low.

He stands motionless so the muscle pump mechanism does not operate and the dependent capacitance vessels distend leading to a decrease in venous return. He may have an enlarged prostate and have to perform a Valsalva type of strain. Relief of bladder distension may also result in reflex vasodilatation as the result of a reduced stimulus to bladder stretch receptors (Mary 1989).

Physiological mechanisms and factors predisposing to vasovagal syncope

Although there have been several analyses of the haemodynamic changes that occur before and during the faint, the mechanism responsible for suddenly switching the apparently appropriate responses of vasoconstriction and tachycardia to the inappropriate ones of vasodilatation and bradycardia remains a matter for speculation. A number of possibilities have been suggested.

An abnormal baroreceptor reflex

It has been suggested that vasovagal syncope might be triggered by stimulation of baroreceptors. In emotional syncope the faint is usually preceded by an increase in blood pressure. This, however, does not usually happen in orthostatic syncope. Furthermore, baroreceptors normally function as a stabilizing negative feedback system and would not be expected to induce sufficient vasodilatation to lower blood pressure abnormally.

In the so-called carotid sinus syndrome, syncope is thought to be caused by an exaggerated baroreceptor reflex. The original classical case was attributed to pressure on the sinus by a stiff winged collar, although the stimulus in present cases is uncertain. The condition is usually diagnosed by excessive bradycardia or even asystole in response to carotid sinus massage. However, when we have studied such patients using a neck chamber to apply a controlled carotid baroreceptor stimulation we have never seen syncope or asystole. Part of the explanation for this apparent anomaly may be that some patients who are susceptible to orthostatically induced syncope have brisk baroreceptor responses (Wahbha et al. 1989; El-Sayed and Hainsworth 1995). Thus, many of the patients diagnosed as having carotid sinus syndrome may actually have poor orthostatic tolerance associated with brisk baroreceptor responses. It is interesting to note that patients who were treated successfully so that orthostatic tolerance improved also consistently showed decreases in baroreceptor sensitivity (El-Sayed and Hainsworth 1996).

Stimulation of cardiac receptors

Another theory, which has been popular for several years, is that the vasodilatation and bradycardia are a type of Bezold–Jarisch reflex resulting from stimulation of cardiac ventricular receptors (for references, see Hainsworth 1991). The postulated mechanism was that, following haemorrhage or orthostasis, the ventricle would be contracting powerfully at a small volume and this would strongly stimulate ventricular mechanoreceptors. The basis for this was the observation by Oberg and Thoren (1972) that some ventricular non-myelinated afferents in the cat became excited under these conditions. The possible cardiac origin of syncope forms the rationale for infusing isoprenaline to subjects during othostatic tests and for the use of β-blocking drugs in treatment. However, it is very unlikely that stimulation of ventricu-

lar afferents has any significant part to play. First, in the original report of discharge in ventricular afferent nerves, only a few of them were actually excited under these conditions; in most the activity decreased. Secondly, other animal studies, in which the sympathetic nerves were stimulated and the heart bypassed, failed to show either vasodilatation or bradycardia (Al-Timman and Hainsworth, 1992). Thirdly, recent studies have been carried out on humans with transplanted, and therefore denervated, ventricles and these showed that orthostatic stress could also cause vasodilatation, hypotension, and syncope (Fitzpatrick et al. 1993). The effect of isoprenaline infusion is probably related to some other property of the drug, possibly its action as a β_2 vasodilator. Furthermore, it is almost as effective in inducing syncope in normal subjects as in patients susceptible to fainting attacks (Kapoor and Brant 1992).

Emotional stress

Many people faint at the sight of blood or the feel or sight of an intravenous needle. Also, and of particular relevance to orthostatic stress testing, people faint much earlier during head-up tilt if any intravascular instrumentation is employed (Stevens 1966). The mechanism for inducing vasodilatation and bradycardia during emotional stress is unknown.

Central mechanisms

Animal studies have defined a region in the hypothalamus which, when activated either by electrical stimulation or exposure of the animal to prey or predator, initiates a response called the 'defence reaction'. This response may include vasodilatation, particularly in muscle, and bradycardia. It may also be related to the 'playing dead' response seen in some animals. It is has also been suggested that emotionally induced fainting in humans may be comparable to activation of the hypothalamic defence area in animals. However, the mechanisms inducing vasodilatation seem to be different and there is no evidence for defence area involvement in human syncope.

Although the precipitating factors are not known, there is evidence that some central nervous mechanisms are involved. Opioids, probably of the delta subtype, may be implicated in the initiation of vasodilatation. Administration of naloxone has been shown to prevent the vasodilatation in rabbits, dogs, and rats (Morita and Vatner 1985) but has not yet been shown to have the same effect in people. This may be because far greater doses were given to the animals. It has also recently been suggested that serotonergic mechanisms may also be involved (see Chapter 45).

Relation to plasma volume

Orthostatic stress results in a decrease in return of blood to the heart and a consequent decrease in cardiac output. This effect is enhanced by the loss of fluid from the plasma to the tissues in dependent regions. When cardiac output falls to below about half the supine value, syncope becomes very likely (El-Bedawi and Hainsworth 1994). It is conceivable therefore, that a person's susceptibility to syncope might be related to his plasma or blood volume, and this indeed was shown to be the case (El-Sayed and Hainsworth 1995). The role of plasma volume has been further examined in patients by interventions designed to increase plasma volume. Several of these may be effective, including salt loading (El-Sayed and Hainsworth 1996), exercise training (Mtinangi et al. 1997) and sleeping head-up at 10°. Results have shown that *changes* in plasma volume were correlated with changes in orthostatic tolerance (Fig. 44.10).

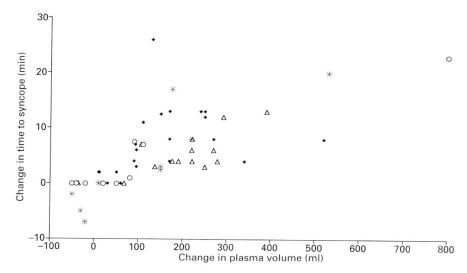

Fig. 44.10. Relationship between changes in orthostatic tolerance and changes in plasma volume. Orthostatic tolerance is assessed in terms of the time for which the progressive test of head-up tilt and lower-body suction (see Fig. 44.8) is endured. Interventions employed are administration of placebo tablets (○), salt loading (◆), sleeping with bed head raised 10° (✳) , exercise training (△). Note that changes in plasma volume, however induced, are accompanied by directionally similar changes in orthostatic tolerance.

Summary

Vasovagal syncope is a transient loss of consciousness, due to temporarily inadequate cerebral blood flow, followed by a full recovery. Syncope usually occurs when the subject is upright and blood 'pools' in dependent vessels and gravity causes cerebral perfusion pressure to be lower than elsewhere. Most of the time, orthostatic stress does not result in hypotension because of the effects of reflexes, particularly baroreceptors. However, if the stress becomes too great, and this may occur earlier in particularly susceptible individuals, the normal sympathetic activity ceases and blood pressure falls. The hypotension is usually associated with a slowing of the heart rate, although this is rarely sufficient to make an important contribution to the syncope.

Several factors may predispose to syncope. Straining manoeuvres which impede venous return may initiate an attack and this, together with standing still with a warm dilated cutaneous circulation, may explain micturition syncope. Hypovolaemia also seems to be an important factor and procedures which increase blood volume are of benefit in increasing orthostatic tolerance and preventing fainting.

The actual trigger mechanism which turns off sympathetic activity remains unknown. There have been suggestions that it is caused by inappropriate stimulation of baroreceptors or ventricular receptors. However, this is very unlikely and the responsible mechanism remains one of the continuing mysteries in cardiovascular physiology.

References

Al-Timman, J. K. A. and Hainsworth, R. (1992). Reflex vascular responses to changes in left ventricular pressures, heart rate and inotropic state in dogs. *Exp. Physiol.* 77, 455–69.

Barcroft, H. and Edholm, O.G. (1945). On the vasodilatation in human skeletal muscle during post-haemorrhagic fainting. *J.Physiol.* 104, 161–75.

Barcroft, H., McMichael, J. and Sharpey-Schafer, E.P. (1944). Post haemorrhagic fainting. Study by cardiac output and forearm flow. *Lancet* i, 289–91.

Blair, D. A., Glover, W. E., Greenfield, A. D. M., and Roddie, I. S. (1959). Excitation of cholinergic vasodilator nerves to human skeletal muscles during emotional stress *J. Physiol.* 148, 633–47.

Daly, M.de.B., Hazzledine, J. L., and Ungar, A. (1967). The reflex effects of alterations in lung volume on systemic vascular resistance in the dog. *J. Physiol.* 188, 331–51.

El-Bedawi, K. M. and Hainsworth, R. (1994) Combined head-up tilt and lower body suction: a test of orthostatic tolerance. *Clin. Auton. Res.* 4, 41–7.

El-Bedawi, K. M. Wahbha, M. M. A. E., and Hainsworth, R. (1994). Cardiac pacing does not improve orthostatic tolerance in patients with vasovagal syncope. *Clin. Auton. Res.* 4, 233–7.

El-Sayed, H. and Hainsworth, R. (1995) Relationship between plasma volume, carotid baroreceptor sensitivity and orthostatic tolerance. *Clin. Sci.* 88, 463–70.

El-Sayed, H. and Hainsworth, R. (1996). Salt supplement increases plasma volume and orthostatic tolerance in patients with unexplained syncope. *Heart* 75, 134–40.

Fitzpatrick, A. P., Banner, N., Cheng, A., Yacoub, M., and Sutton, R. (1993). Vasovagal reactions may occur after orthotopic heart transplantation. *J. Am. Coll. Cardiol.* 21, 1132–7.

Hainsworth, R. (1985). Arterial blood pressure. In *Hypotensive anaesthesia*, (ed. G. E. H. Enderby), pp. 3–29. Churchill Livingstone, Edinburgh.

Hainsworth, R. (1986). Vascular capacitance: its control and importance. *Rev. Physiol. Biochem. Pharmacol.* 105, 101–73.

Hainsworth, R. (1991). Reflexes from the heart. *Physiol. Rev.* 71, 617–58.

Hainsworth, R. and El-Bedawi, K. M. (1994). Orthostatic tolerance in patients with unexplained syncope. *Clin. Auton. Res.* 4, 239–44.

Kapoor, W. N. and Brant, N. (1992). Evaluation of syncope by upright tilt testing with isoproterenol, a nonspecific test. *Ann. Int. Med.* 116, 358–63.

Hainsworth, R., Karim, F., McGregor, K. H., and Wood, L. M. (1983). Hind-limb vascular-capacitance responses in anaesthetized dogs. *J. Physiol.* 337, 417–28.

Karim, F. and Hainsworth, R. (1976). Responses of abdominal vascular capacitance to stimulation of splanchnic nerves. *Am. J. Physiol.* 231, 434–40.

Lewis, T. (1932). Vasovagal syncope and the carotid sinus mechanism. *BMJ* 1, 873–6.

Mary, D. A. S. G. (1989). The urinary bladder and cardiovascular reflexes. *Int. J. Cardiol.* 23, 11–17.

Morita, H. and Vatner, S. F. (1985). Effects of haemorrhage on renal nerve activity in conscious dog. *Circ. Res.* 57, 788–93.

Mtinangi, B. L. and Hainsworth, R. (1998). Increased orthostatic tolerance following moderate exercise training in patients with unexplained syncope. *Heart* 80, in press.

Oberg, B. and Thoren, P. (1972). Increased activity in left ventricular receptors during haemorrhage or occlusion of the caval veins in the cat. A possible cause of vasovagal reaction. *Acta Physiol. Scand.* **85**, 164–73.

Stevens, P. M. (1966). Cardiovascular dynamics during orthostasis and influence of intravascular instrumentation. *Am. J. Cardiol.* **17**, 211–18.

Uvnas, B. (1966). Cholinergic vasodilator nerves. *Fed. Proc.* **25**, 1618–22.

Wahbha, M. M. A. E., Morley, C. A., Al-Shamma, Y. M. H., and Hainsworth, R. (1989). Cardiovascular reflex responses in patients with unexplained syncope. *Clin. Sci.* **77**, 547–5 3.

Wallin, B. G and Sundlof, G. (1982). Sympathetic outflow to muscle during vasovagal syncope. *J. autonom. nerv. System.* **6**, 287–91.

45. Neurally mediated syncope

Blair P. Grubb and Barry Karas

Introduction

Syncope, the transient loss of consciousness and postural tone with spontaneous recovery, is one of the most challenging and at the same time frustrating medical problems encountered in clinical practice. Derived from the Greek work '*synkoptein*' (to cut short) the vast number of possible aetiologies and the difficulties inherent in determining an exact cause renders the evaluation of the patient with recurrent syncope a particularly daunting enterprise. Over the past decade there has been a tremendous increase in our knowledge of one cause of recurrent fainting, the condition known as neurocardiogenic (also called vasovagal or neurally mediated) syncope. This chapter will attempt to provide some basic background material on syncope, that is relevant to the following discussion on current understanding of the pathophysiology of neurocardiogenic syncope, and addresses the most recent concepts in both diagnosis and management of this and related disorders.

The problem of syncope

Syncope is a quite common occurrence. Each year in the United States alone syncope accounts for 3 per cent of all emergency room visits and up to 6 per cent of all hospital admissions. Recurrent episodes of unpredictable syncope frequently provoke a profound sense of anxiety in both patient and physician. This sense of foreboding is further enhanced by the knowledge that recurrent syncope may be the only symptom that precedes an episode of sudden death. However, even when the underlying cause of the syncope is in itself benign, the consequences of suddenly falling due to loss of consciousness may not be. As the American humorist Will Rogers once observed, 'it's not the fall that hurts, it's that sudden stop at the end'. The falls that occur from syncope may result in subdural haematomas and lead to fractures of the face, skull and extremities. Syncope while driving can endanger not only the life of the patient, but the lives of others as well. Linzer and colleagues have found that these sudden unpredictable syncopal spells place a tremendous psychological burden on both patients and their families, causing a degree of functional impairment not dissimilar to that seen with chronic debilitating diseases such as rheumatoid arthritis (Linzer *et al.* 1991). Patients with recurrent syncope often find that their social, education and employment opportunities are severely limited.

Until relatively recently the patient with recurrent syncope was frequently subjected to a long, tedious, expensive and often unrewarding routine series of tests and examinations aimed at disclosing a possible cause. This series would usually include a 24-hour ambula-tory electrocardiogram (Holter monitor), computed axial tomographic and/or magnetic resonance scans of the brain, in addition to electroencephalography. In some centres coronary angiography and cardiac electrophysiological testing were not infrequently employed. Yet, despite this battery of examinations (which could cost up to US$16 000 per patient) an identifiable cause of syncope was disclosed in only 40 per cent of patients (Calkins *et al.* 1993). This would place the cost of syncope evaluation in the United States alone at more than US$800 million annually.

Over the years several investigators had felt that a number of these episodes occurred due to the sudden transient periods of autonomically mediated hypotension and bradycardia. However, until relatively recently these speculations could not be confirmed as there existed no effective modality for reproducing a syncopal episode which could thereby confirm the diagnosis.

To be able to determine a particular individual's predisposition towards episodes of neurocardiogenic (or neurally mediated) hypotension and bradycardia, investigators postulated that a strong orthostatic stimulus (such as prolonged upright posture) be utilized. Following the initial paper describing its use as a method of provoking syncope (Kenny *et al.* 1989), head-upright tilt-table testing has been widely reported by a number of centres as a safe and effective modality for uncovering an individual's predisposition toward these neurocardiogenic events. In addition, the advent of head-upright tilt-table testing has been permitted the ability to provoke these episodes in a controlled environment, and allowed a unique opportunity to observe directly the sequence of events that occurs during syncope, thereby greatly enhancing our understanding of these disorders.

Pathophysiological aspects

The manner in which the human body responds to various changes in position has been the subject to scientific inquiry since the 1940s. During this period tilt table testing was first utilized as a controlled method with which the body's response to incremental changes in position could be carefully measured (Allen *et al.* 1995). These observations established the fact that in normal subjects about one-quarter of the circulating blood volume is contained in the thorax. The assumption of upright posture leads to a gravity-mediated displacement of approximately 300–800 ml of blood (or roughly 6–8 ml/kg) to the abdominal area and the lower extremities. This therefore results in a 25 per cent drop in volume, with about half of this fall occurring within seconds of standing. This peripheral pooling leads to a fall in venous return to the heart. Since the heart cannot pump what it does not receive, there is a corresponding fall in cardiac stroke volume by as much as 40 per cent. This process causes the cardiac mechanoreceptors (or C fibres), located in the basilar portions of the right and left ventricles, to decrease their frequency of afferent impulse formation due to less stretch on the receptors themselves. These C fibres communicate centrally to the dorsal vagal nucleus of the medulla, and as their afferent output decreases a reflex increase in sympathetic output occurs (Smith *et al.* 1991). This results in an increase in heart rate, inotropy and peripheral vascular resistance. Thus the normal response of an individual upon assumption of upright posture is an increased heart rate, an increased diastolic pressure, and an unchanged or slightly decreased systolic pressure.

Sir Thomas Lewis is usually credited with originating the term 'vasovagal syncope' (Lewis 1932). Although the exact pathophysiology is still being elaborated, a basic understanding of the process has gradually evolved (Kosinski *et al.* 1995). It is believed that in some predisposed individuals there is an excessive degree of peripheral venous pooling that produces a sudden drop in central venous return. This abrupt fall in ventricular filling allows for exceptionally vigorous ventricular contractions, which are sufficiently forceful so as to cause the activation of a large number of mechanoreceptors that would normally respond only to mechanical stretch. The resultant surge in afferent neural traffic to the brainstem appears to somehow mimic the conditions seen with hypertension, and thus there is elicited an apparently 'paradoxical' reflex bradycardia along with a further reduction in peripheral vascular resistance. Echocardiographic recordings performed at the time of upright tilt-induced neurocardiogenic syncope have tended to demonstrate an increase in ventricular fractional shortening, a decrease in end-systolic area, and an increase in intracavitary pressure as compared to normal nonsyncopal subjects during upright tilt.

This theory has been questioned by Fitzpatrick *et al.* (1992) who demonstrated that head-up tilt was able to provoke neurocardiogenic hypotensive episodes in 7 of 10 patients who had previously undergone cardiac transplantation (whose heart had technically been denervated). However, C fibres similar to the ventricle mechanoreceptors have also been identified in the atria and pulmonary arteries. Thus, the aforementioned observations do not entirely exclude a cardiac contribution to the process causing neurocardiogenic hypotension and bradycardia.

Although the initial term employed to describe this sequence of events was 'vasovagal' syncope, more recent evidence has demonstrated that although parasympathetically mediated hypotension and bradycardia may occur, the principal contributing process is that of vasodilatation with resultant hypotension. Early on investigators realized that administration of atropine or rate support with cardiac pacing are often ineffective in preventing syncope. Several studies have advanced the concept that alterations in sympathetic tone were of primary importance. This was initially proposed by Chosy and Graham, who, by means of a microneurographic technique, offered evidence that sympathetic withdrawal from skeletal muscle occurs during neurocardiogenic syncope. Details of this process are covered in other chapters.

Perhaps one of the more intriguing, (and at the same time perplexing) aspects of neurocardiogenic syncope is the nature of the events that occur in the central nervous system at the time of an episode (Rea and Thames 1993). Most of the research has required an animal model of syncope, with most investigators employing an induced form of haemorrhagic shock. This is based on the observa-

tion that even a relatively small, but rapid, loss of blood volume during haemorrhage can result in a sudden, paradoxic sympathoinhibition with resultant profound hypotension and bradycardia. As has been observed in neurocardiogenic syncope, serum adrenaline levels will increase as noradrenaline levels fall in the setting of haemorrhagic shock. At the time of the paradoxic bradycardia associated with hypotension, animal studies have found that there is an increase in adrenal nerve activity as well as a decline in renal sympathetic nerve activity.

A series of insightful studies using the model have shown that abrupt alterations in the central nervous system levels of serotonin (5-hydroxytryptamine) appears to be the signal that initiates sympathetic withdrawal (Grubb and Kosinski 1996). It has also been shown that this sequence of events may be blocked by the central serotonin receptor blocker, methylsergide (Elam *et al.* 1985). Further studies reported by Abboud have shown that the intracerebroventricular administration of serotonin results in hypotension, excitation of adrenal sympathetic nerve activity, and inhibition of renal sympathetic nerve activity (Abboud 1993). Taken together, these observations would seem to suggest that a precipitous surge in central serotonin levels plays an important role in the process of sympathetic withdrawal seen in neurocardiogenic syncope. This idea has been given some support by observations made following the use of serotonin reuptake inhibitors in patients with refractory neurocardiogenic syncope (Grubb *et al.* 1994). The agents known as serotin reuptake inhibitors function by inhibiting the presynaptic reuptake in serotonin, thereby causing a progressive increase in intrasynaptic serotonin levels. This progressive increase in intrasynaptic serotonin levels has been shown to result in a postsynaptic reduction (downregulation) in serotonin receptor density. It is postulated that the process of postsynaptic down-regulation may have a similar effect to drugs that directly block receptor sites (i.e. methylsergide). Thus, the response elicited by a sudden surge in serotonin would be blunted. As will be mentioned later, clinical trials with various serotonin reuptake inhibitors (fluoxetine hydrochloride, sertraline and nefazodone) in patients with otherwise refractory neurocardiogenic syncope have shown a consistent response rate of greater than 50 per cent.

More recent investigations have demonstrated that there are at least seven major families of serotonin receptors, for each of which there are subreceptors (Grubb and Kosinski 1996). These various receptors and receptor subtypes not only control different responses in different parts of the central nervous system, but some receptor subtypes appear directly to antagonize the effects of others (a system that appears to be similar to that of the prostaglandins) (Matzen *et al.* 1993). At the present time research is continuing in an attempt to determine the specific receptor subtypes at work in the development of neurocardiogenic syncope and to ascertain the effects of pharmacological agents directed at these receptor subtypes.

Another set of substances that has received attention as potential mediators in neurocardiogenic syncope are the endogenous opiates (Hasser *et al.* 1989). Using the haemorrhagic shock model referred to previously, it has been shown that inhibition of renal sympathetic nerve activity follows opiate receptor antagonist administration. Additional research using a rabbit model has shown that the intracisternal administration of naloxone (a drug that is an antagonist of opiate receptor sites) can block the vasodilatory component of acute haemorrhagic shock. Further observations in human subjects have found that the administration of naloxone augments the cardiopulmonary baroreflex excitation of sympathetic activity. Others have found that plasma β-endorphin levels increase in patients during tilt-induced syncope. Yet, despite the aforementioned observations, administration of the opioid antagonists has not proven effective in preventing the onset of neurocardiogenic syncope provoked during lower-body negative pressure. Recently some investigators have suggested that nitric oxide may also play a role.

The possible contributing role of the cerebral vasculature to the development of neurocardiogenic syncope has been a recent focus of investigation. Based on work done a number of years ago, it had been felt that autoregulation of cerebral blood flow took place solely at the focal cerebral arteriolar level in response to changes in systemic pressure. Arteriolar vasodilation would take place after decreases in systemic blood pressure, while vasoconstriction would occur if the systemic pressure rose, a process that would maintain cerebral blood flow at a constant level. However, using transcranial Doppler ultrasonography several different sets of investigators have found that cerebral vasoconstriction (as opposed to the expected vasodilation) would occur during tilt-induced syncope in the face of increasing hypotension (Grubb et al. 1991a). These findings have been confirmed by several investigators, who have also found that the response is not noted in normal subjects. Interestingly, a similar degree of paradoxical vasoconstriction in the setting of sudden hypotension induced by trimethopan has been seen, while at the same time others found a corresponding amount of cerebral vasoconstriction during normotensive hypovolaemia induced by lower-body negative pressure. Others have described abnormal cerebral haemodynamics in children during head-upright tilt-induced neurocardiogenic syncope. These apparently 'paradoxic' changes would seen to suggest that sudden alterations in cerebrovascular resistance (i.e. arteriolar vasoconstriction) may have a role in producing loss of consciousness during neurocardiogenic syncope. Indeed, recent reports have found that on some occasions syncope may occur on the basis of cerebral vascular changes alone in the absence of systemic hypotension. Further studies will be necessary to better understand the role of the cerebrovasculature in these disorders.

Clinical aspects

As was alluded to previously, neurocardiogenic syncope can have a wide range of presentations. Actually, there seem to be a number of potential triggers that may each ultimately result in an episode of neurocardiogenic hypotension and bradycardia. Not only upright posture, but also the postprandial state, sodium restriction on diuretic use, vigorous exercise in warm environments, as well as emotional stress are but a few of the possible triggers to consider. Alcohol consumption is well known to increase an individual's predisposition to these events.

The most evident aspect of these autonomically mediated periods of orthostatic intolerance is syncope, the transient loss of consciousness usually associated with hypotension and bradycardia. On occasion the bradycardia aspects may be quite pronounced and may result in long periods of asystole (referred to by some investigators as the 'malignant' form of neurocardiogenic syncope; Sutton 1992). In either case the hypotension or bradycardia results in diffuse cerebral ischaemia which may culminate in loss of consciousness.

One of the most frequently overlooked, yet at the same time most important, aspects of the syncope evaluation is taking a complete history. When did these events first begin? What were the circumstances surrounding the episodes? How often do they occur? Was there a clear prodrome or a postictal-like state? Were there any witnesses to an episode, and if so how do they describe them? What did the patient look like (i.e. pale, sweaty) and was there convulsive activity? Was there full of loss of consciousness, and if so, for how long? In addition to obtaining a complete past medical history (especially of cardiac problems) it is important to enquire if there is any history of sudden death among other members of the family. A careful history and physical examination will often provide much more useful information than the mindless ordering of multiple laboratory tests.

The patient will usually, although not always, report that syncopal events have occurred while standing (and on occasion while sitting). By the time a patient seeks medical attention they will often have experienced several syncopal episodes. An episode can be divided into three distinct phases, consisting of: (1) prodrome or aura; (2) loss of consciousness; and (3) a postsyncopal period. A number of patients will relate that there are quite specific events or conditions which predispose to syncope. These include extreme emotional stress, heat, acute physical pain (or in some instances even the anticipation of pain or discomfort such as the sight of a needle or of blood). During the prodromal period patients often report experiencing a sense of weakness (44 per cent), headache and visual disturbances (33 per cent), diaphoresis (33 per cent), nausea and abdominal discomfort (29 per cent), and vomiting (Wayne 1961). The duration of the aura may be anywhere from seconds to minutes, and if properly identified by the patient may allow sufficient time to abort an event by assuming a recumbent position. While recumbent, the absence of the gravitational stress added by standing or sitting will often prevent cerebral perfusion from falling to a point where cerebral hypoxia can occur.

The actual loss of consciousness itself is commonly associated with amnesia. Bystanders will often describe the patient as being quite pale and ashen in complexion, with profuse diaphoresis and dilated pupils. There may on occasion be urinary (and rarely faecal) incontinence. Often the most disturbing and anxiety-provoking sign during an event will be tonic-clonic convulsive muscular motions. The convulsive activity that may accompany neurocardiogenic syncope occurs because the anoxic threshold of the brain has been exceeded, and this produces a form of acute 'decortication', resulting in cortical disinhibition with excessive tonic brainstem motor activity. This process is not unique to neurocardiogenic syncope, rather it may be seen in any hypotensive event. Detailed observation of tilt-induced convulsive syncope have allowed for a specific sequence of movements to be described. With the onset of profound hypotension the patient will display a startled appearance as well as cessation of any other action in progress (such as speech). This is followed by a sudden loss of postural tone after which is noted extension and tonic contraction of the legs. There is usually a simultaneous extension of the arms in adduction. The head elevates and is thrown backwards (opisthotonos) after which are small short, jerking movement of the arms. This form of muscle activity usually (but not always) will not follow the classic sequence of increasing and decreasing amplitude that is a distinguishing feature of the tonic-clonic grand mal seizure activity seen in epilepsy. In the majority of patients with convulsive syncope the ictal phase itself is usually quite brief, followed by a rapid recovery. Long postictal periods are not common (but may occur). The postsyncope period is usually characterized by extreme fatigue (that may persist for up to a day) as well as headache, dizziness, nausea, and a sense of nervousness.

It should be kept in mind that while the aforementioned descriptions are true for the majority of patients, there are those in whom atypical presentations may occur. Grubb *et al.* (1991*b*) have observed that during tilt-induced neurocardiogenic syncope (performed with concomitant electroencephalographic monitoring) occasional patients may display convulsive activity that appears remarkably similar to that seen during grand mal seizures. At the same time it was noted that some patients could display significant postictal phenomena.

It was realized early on that the development of some method for reproducing these events in a controlled laboratory setting was of paramount importance, not only for confirmation of one's clinical suspicions as to the nature of the syncope, but also in order to better understand the pathophysiology of these disorders. This led investigators to explore a number of different vagal manoeuvres as methods of triggering episodes in susceptible individuals, which included Valsalva's manoeuvre, Weber's manoeuvre, carotid sinus stimulation, hyperventilation, and ocular compression. However, each of these tests fell into disuse over time due to poor sensitivity and reproducibility, as well as safety concerns and a low correlation with clinical events.

Head-upright, tilt-table testing

As was noted earlier in the discussion, tilt-table testing was first employed by physiologists who saw it as a way of providing a controlled gravitational stimulus whereby the body's adaptation to positional change could be observed carefully. Later, similar techniques were used to investigate responses to the stresses of aerospace travel. While pursuing these studies, Stevens and co-workers observed that occasional test subjects would suddenly develop hypotension, bradycardia and loss of consciousness. However, it was not until the mid 1980s that Kenny *et al.* (1989) thought to employ head-upright tilt as a method to provoke syncope in predisposed individuals by providing a continuous passive orthostatic stress, resulting in decreased venous return and increased catecholamine levels (Abi Samra *et al.* 1987). Since these initial reports, head-upright tilt-table testing has gone on to become a widely employed modality to assess a person's susceptibility to neurocardiogenically mediated hypotension and bradycardia.

Prior to proceeding it would seem helpful to consider some points concerning the nature of this sort of provocative testing. Many of the tests employed in medicine could be described as 'descriptive' in nature. This form of examination evaluates a relatively fixed (often anatomical) substrate that changes only slowly over time. A radiograph of a leg or angiography of the coronary arteries are both types of examinations which describe a specific area or condition. By contrast, provocative testing attempts to evaluate dynamic (often physiological) systems, which by their very nature may be highly variable over much briefer periods of time. Therefore, it would seem that provocative testing would tend to show a higher degree of variability than would descriptive testing. Cardiac electrophysiological studies using programmed electrical stimulation represent a form of provocative testing.

Several observations have given credence to the assertion that a positive head-upright tilt-table test corresponds reasonably closely to those events that are known to occur during spontaneous neurocardiogenic syncope. First among these is that both spontaneous and tilt-induced syncope are associated with similar prodromal signs and symptoms, among which are lightheadedness, nausea, diaphoresis, pallor, and loss of postural tone. Secondly is that the sequence of heart rate and blood pressure changes seen are identical to those seen during spontaneous syncopal events. Finally, the changes seen in serum catecholamines and other hormones are essentially the same during spontaneous and head-upright tilt-induced episodes. Indeed, with regard to the last observation that serum catecholamine levels increase markedly prior to the onset of syncope, a number of investigators have proposed that a concomitant isoproterenol infusion be used in conjunction with head-up tilt as a means of increasing the sensitivity of the test. Yet at the same time others have expressed concerns that the injudicious use of isoproterenol may achieve higher levels of sensitivity at the expense of specificity. Recently a number of other provocative agents have been used during head-upright tile-table testing, including edrophonium, nitroglycerin and adenosine triphosphate.

Two principal methods of performing tilt-table testing have evolved. The first uses head-upright tile alone to produce gravity-mediated dependent venous pooling and thereby provoke the aforementioned reflexes in susceptible individuals. The second method employs head-up tilt in combination with some type of provocative agent, most commonly intravenous isoproterenol.

When head-upright tilt-table testing is employed alone (in the absence of provocative stimuli other than gravity) it appears to be able to distinguish between symptomatic patients and asymptomatic controls with a level of accuracy that is comparable to other clinically useful testing procedures. To review all the available data supporting this claim is somewhat beyond the scope of this chapter, and the interested reader is directed toward several more extensive reviews on the subject. Some representative examples, however, will be reviewed. Concerning the issue of specificity, it has been found that during a 60° tilt for 45 minutes only 7 per cent of control subjects experienced syncope, while others reported that no syncope was provoked among a group of 35 controls after 60° tilt for a duration of 45 minutes. Grubb and co-workers have reported an equally low false positive rate among both paediatric and geriatric patients (Grubb *et al.* 1992*b*). With respect to the use of isoproterenol in conjunction with tilt-table testing, Natale *et al.* (1995) have made extensive investigations into the influence of various tilt angles as well as isoproterenol doses in a group of 150 control subjects who had no history of syncope. They found that tilt-table testing at either 60°, 70°, or 80° provided specificities of 92, 92, and 80 per cent when used with a concomitant low-dose isoproterenol infusion.

A similar study by Morillo *et al.* (1995) compared these groups of patients: 120 consecutive patients with recurrent unexplained syncope, 30 healthy patients in a control group, and 30 patients with documented syncope not due to a neurocardiogenic cause. Each group underwent head-up tilt at 60° for 15 minutes, followed by a low-dose isoproterenol infusion of no syncope was initially induced. Acute reproducibility was also assessed. They found that the overall sensitivity of the tilt-table test using this protocol was 61 per cent with a specificity of 93 per cent and a reproducibility of 86 per cent.

When taken together, the literature would suggest that when upright tilt-table testing is used without pharmacological provocation at angles between 60° and 80°, it has a specificity of approximately 90 per cent. If the test is employed with a concomitant low-dose isoproterenol infusion, the majority of studies indicated a specificity of between 80 and 90 per cent. It should be kept in mind, however, that the exact sensitivity is difficult to determine accurately as there is no actual 'gold standard' against which it can be compared. During any discussion on the sensitivity of tilt-table testing it should be remembered that the test is dependent on the physiological mechanisms that culminate in neurocardiogenic syncope. These physiological changes, that were elaborated earlier, could theoretically occur in virtually any individual if a sufficiently strong stimulus were delivered for a long-enough period. Thus, tilt-table testing does not identify a fixed pathological substrate (i.e. descriptive testing), instead it uncovers an exaggerated susceptibility to what is an otherwise normal reflex (i.e. provocative testing). The real sensitivity of tilt-table testing may actually be underestimated, as the otherwise healthy control subjects who demonstrate a 'false-positive' response during tilt-table testing may in fact be more susceptible to clinical syncopal episodes than other people. This idea has been supported by the observation that normal control subjects with tilt-induced syncope (false positives) have later gone on to experience spontaneous clinical episodes of neurocardiogenic syncope.

Although quite a bit of variation continues to exist, some standardization in the methodology of tilt-table testing seems to be coming about slowly. At our institution head-upright tilt-table testing is performed during the morning hours after an overnight fast. An intravenous line is established and the patient allowed to rest for 15–20 minutes. The patient is then placed on a mechanized tilt table with a footboard made for weight bearing, and connected to a standard electrocardiographic monitor for continuous evaluation of heart rate and rhythm. Blood pressures are recorded either by a plethysmographic finger recording device or by a standard sphygmomanometer. Transcranial Doppler recordings are also performed continuously. The patient is then slowly inclined to an angle of 70°, and maintained there for a period of 30 minutes. If syncope occurs, the patient is lowered to the supine position and test concluded. If no syncope occurs, the patient is lowered to the supine position and an infusion of intravenous isoproterenol is started, usually at 1 μg/min. The dosage is then titrated so that a heart rate 20 per cent above the baseline supine rate is achieved. The patient is again slowly inclined to an angle of 70° and maintained there for 15–20 minutes.

Uses of, and responses to, upright tilt-table testing

The American College of Cardiology has issued an expert consensus statement on the use of head-upright tilt-table testing for assessing syncope (Benditt et al. 1996). A table of these indications is provided (Table 45.1).

In the course of evaluations of subjects with recurrent syncope it became evident that a variety of response patterns could identified. At the same time it was realized that there were several uses for tilt-table testing in addition to recurrent unexplained syncope.

With respect to the different response patterns observed during upright tilt-table testing we have found it useful to define five sub-groups (Sutton and Peterson 1995) (Fig. 45.1). It must be realized,

Table 45.1. Indications for tilt-table testing (modified from Benditt et al. 1996)

General agreement
  A. Recurrent syncope or single syncope episode in a high-risk patient, whether or not the history indicates a neurocardiogenic cause, and
    (i) no evidence of structural heart disease, or
    (ii) structural heart disease is present, but other causes of syncope have been excluded by appropriate testing
  B. In-department evaluation of patients in whom an apparent cause of syncope is identified (i.e. AV block, asystole) but in whom demonstration of a neurocardiogenic component would affect therapy
  C. As a part of the evaluation of exercise-induced or associated syncope

Reasonable differences of opinion exist
  A. Differentiating convulsive syncope from epileptic seizures
  B. Recurrent unexplained falls (especially in the elderly)
  C. Evaluation of recurrent dizziness or presyncope
  D. Evaluation of unexplained syncope in peripheral neuropathy and dysautonomia
  E. The follow-up assessment of therapy

Emerging indications
  A. Recurrent idiopathic vertigo
  B. Recurrent transient ischaemia attacks
  C. Chronic fatigue syndrome
  D. Sudden infant death syndrome (SIDS)

Tilt-table testing not warranted
  A. Single syncopal episode, without injury and not in a high-risk setting with evident neurocardiogenic features
  B. Syncope where a specific cause has already been established and where demonstrating a neurocardiogenic component would not alter treatment plans

however, that any attempt to classify natural phenomena is, by its very nature, somewhat arbitrary and open to subsequent modification. We construct memory in the present, and by constructing memory we create our current concept of reality.

The first pattern described is the classic neurocardiogenic (or vasovagal) response that was referred to earlier in this chapter. These patients tend to demonstrate a relatively abrupt onset of hypotension that may occur with (or sometimes without) concomitant bradycardia. Between episodes of syncope these patients are, for the most part, normal and offer no complaints. They tend to be younger, in fact many are adolescents (although we have encountered elderly patients who display this pattern as well). We have postulated that these individuals have a 'hypersensitive' autonomic nervous system, in whom syncope can be provoked by a variety of vagal stimuli. These include carotid sinus stimulation, mechanical stimulation of the rectum and oesophagus, cough, and micturition. At times these patients will display prolonged periods of asystole during clinical syncopal episodes and those induced during head-up tilt. In North America these patients are referred to as having a 'malignant' form of neurocardiogenic syncope which may, on occasion, either mimic or lead to sudden death. Upright tilt-table testing in this group may indeed provoke prolonged periods of asystole and hypotension (that do not end with resumption of the recumbent position) which can require prolonged resuscitative

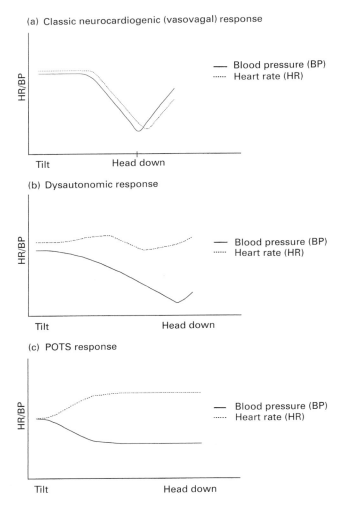

(a) Classic neurocardiogenic (vasovagal) response

Blood pressure (BP)
Heart rate (HR)

(b) Dysautonomic response

Blood pressure (BP)
Heart rate (HR)

(c) POTS response

Blood pressure (BP)
Heart rate (HR)

Fig. 45.1. Response patterns during upright tilt-table testing.

efforts to end. The author has personally had to perform cardiopulmonary resuscitation on patients in the tilt lab, and has reviewed litigation against several physicians stemming from deaths that have occurred during tilt-table testing. Tilt testing has provoked polymorphic ventricular tachycardia requiring defibrillation (Engle 1978).

The second response pattern is classed as 'dysautonomic'. Here the patient displays a gradual parallel fall in both systolic and diastolic blood pressure which ultimately end in loss of consciousness. The heart rate may increase slightly but usually remains unchanged. More often these patients are older adults; however, we have also noted this pattern in young people and occasionally in children. In distinction from the neurocardiogenic group, fainting is only one of a multitude of complaints, with the patient often describing a state of generalized malaise. They, not uncommonly, will manifest other signs of autonomic dysfunction, such as abnormal sweating and thermoregulatory instability and heat intolerance. Some older patients with dysautonomic patterns may display a combination of supine hypertension and upright hypotension.

Several groups have described a third response pattern which has come to be known as the postural orthostatic tachycardia syndrome (or POTS). During tilt these patients demonstrate an increase at least 30 beats/minute (or a maximum heart rate of >120 beats/minute)

within the first 10 minutes of upright tilt, and is usually not associated with profound hypotension (Grubb *et al.* 1997). It is felt that these patients suffer from a milder form of autonomic dysfunction wherein there is an inability to properly regulate peripheral vascular resistance, which in turn is compensated for by an apparently excessive increase in heart rate. These individuals may, on occasion, be misdiagnosed as having an 'inappropriate' sinus tachycardia. Our centre has been referred several of these patients, who had undergone radiofrequency modification of the sinoatrial node and, while having a resolution of their tachycardia, were left with profound orthostatic hypotension. Other than palpitations, POTS patients most commonly complain of extreme fatigue and exertional intolerance. It is becoming increasingly evident that there may be a large amount of overlap between POTS and the chronic fatigue syndrome (Bou-Holaigh *et al.* 1995).

The fourth pattern seen during tilt table testing was noted during use of transcranial Doppler ultrasonography (TCD) to investigate cerebral blood flow patterns during syncope. As was alluded to before, during tilt-induced neurocardiogenic syncope there is evidence for cerebral arteriolar vasoconstriction that occurs concomitant with (or on occasion precedes) the development of hypotension and syncope. Several sets of investigators have independently found occasional patients in whom tilt-induced loss of consciousness can occur associated with cerebral vasoconstriction alone (as observed by TCD) in the absence of systemic hypotension. This pattern has come to be known as 'cerebral syncope'.

The fifth response pattern has been labelled as the psychogenic or psychosomatic response pattern (Grubb *et al.* 1992a). These patients experience syncope during head-upright tilt-table testing that is not associated with any significant change in blood pressure, heart rate, transcranial blood flow pattern, or encephalographic tracing. These patients will often be found to be suffering from severe underlying psychiatric disturbances that run the gamut from anxiety disorders to conversion reactions and major depression. It is imperative to remember that patients who suffer from conversion reactions are not consciously aware of their actions at these moments. Many of the young people (especially young women) will upon psychiatric evaluation be found to have been the victims of past physical and/or sexual abuse. This form of syncope in the abused child or adolescent may represent the only way they can 'cry for help'. Their cries for help should not land upon deaf ears.

An alternative system for the classification of tilt-induced syncopal responses based upon haemodynamic and heart rate behaviour has been developed by a European Working Group (Sutton *et al.* 1992).

Reproducibility of tilt-table testing

Information concerning the reproducibility of tilt-table testing is necessary in investigating the pathophysiology of these disorders, the investigation of their natural histories, and also for the evaluation of potential prophylactic therapeutic agents. With respect to prolonged passive head-upright tilt-table testing, the reproducibility of a positive response has been reported to range from 62–80 per cent when performed over a time period of 3–7 days. When head-up tilt is used in conjunction with a low-dose isoproterenol infusion (as assessed by different investigators using various protocols), the reproducibility of a positive response has ranged between 67 and 88 per cent when performed at times varying from 30 minutes to 2 weeks from the original test (Grubb *et al.* 1992*b*). The reproducibility of an initial negative test ranges from 85 to 100 per cent. In aggregate these data would suggest that the overall reproducibility of an initial test is approximately 80 per cent. The same data would also support the idea that an initially negative study has a low probability of becoming positive on repeat testing. It is important to remember that there is some degree of day-to-day variability in test results (as would be anticipated with any form of provocative testing); this is roughly consistent with the amount of variability seen with cardiac electrophysiological testing.

Some variables seem to have differing degrees of reproducibility. In isoproterenol tilt-table testing the time until presyncope and the lowest blood pressure within groups show good reproducibility. However, on a patient-by-patient basis it is the time to lowest heart rate and blood pressure that demonstrate the most consistent reproducibility. Prolonged asystole, certainly the most dramatic response seen during tilt-table testing, appears to have a reproducibility of approximately 80 per cent.

Therapeutic approaches

The therapeutic approach to any patient with recurrent neurocardiogenic syncope must be individualized to the needs of that person. The severity of the condition varies greatly, as does its frequency. In many, syncope will occur only occasionally, and even then under exceptional circumstances. Therefore the first step in therapy is to educate the patient and family as to the nature of the condition and to caution the patient to avoid known predisposing factors such as extreme heat, dehydration, and drugs known to exacerbate syncope (Table 45.2). Often younger patients experience a definitive prodrome and can be advised to lie down when they feel that an episode is imminent. In occasional young patients, merely augmenting their fluid and salt intake may be adequate to prevent further episodes.

None the less there are, not infrequently, patients in whom syncope is recurrent, sudden, unpredictable, and occurs with little or no warning. In these individuals, in particular those who have sustained severe bodily injury or had episodes while driving, some form of prophylactic pharmacotherapy is often required.

A variety of different therapeutic agents has been employed to prevent recurrent neurocardiogenic syncope (Table 45.3). Among the

Table 45.2. Presyncopal agents—drugs that may produce or exacerbate syncope

Alcohol
β Blockers
Hydralazine
Prazosin
Tricyclic antidepressants
L-Dopa
Calcium-channel blockers
Angiotensin-converting enzyme inhibitors

first agents used to treat these disorders were the β_1-adrenergic blockers. Initially it was presumed that these agents exerted their effects because of their negative inotropic activities, which prevent the previously described increase in inotropy that leads to mechanoreceptor activation. While there are numerous reports that these agents can be effective in preventing syncope, there are also reports that in some patients they may actually exacerbate syncope (Cox *et al.* 1995; Davgovlan *et al.* 1992). At least one group has found that β-blockade is most effective in those patients who require provocation with isoproterenol during tilt-table testing, as opposed to those who faint during upright tilt alone.

Transdermal scopolamine was reported by some to be effective, however it is no longer available in North America.

Disopyramide has been found by some to be an effective therapy, felt to work because of its combination of negative inotropic anticholinergic and direct peripheral vasoconstrictive effects. However, one study has questioned the utility of this agent.

A compound that we frequently use in the therapy of these patients is hydrofludrocortisone. A mineral corticoid substance, it promotes sodium retention and volume expansion. In addition, it also seems to cause a peripheral vasoconstrictive effect by sensitizing α-receptors. The drug seems to be most effective in younger patients and in patients with a dysautonomic response on tilt-table testing.

Due to the fact that the major problem in these disorders seems to be a failure of peripheral vascular resistance to increase properly, it would seem logical to employ peripheral vasoconstricting substances

Table 45.3. Potential treatment options for recurrent neurocardiogenic syncope

Modality	Dosage or use	Limitations
Elastic support hose	Should provide at least 30 mmHg ankle counterpressure and be waist high	Expensive, hot, difficult to put on
Metoprolol	50–100 mg orally, twice a day	Prosyncope, bradycardia, impotence, fatigue
Hydrofludrocortisone	0.1 mg orally, twice a day	Hypokalaemia, hypomagnesaemia, oedema
Disopyramide	150–200 mg SR form, twice a day	Dry mouth, urinary retention, blurred vision
Theophylline	200 mg SR form, twice a day	Nausea, tremor, CNS stimulation
Methylphenidate	5–15 mg orally, three times a day. Give last dose before 6 p.m.	Insomnia, headache, nausea, dependence
Midodrine	2.5–10.0 mg orally, three times a day	Scalp itching, nausea, supine hypotension
Sertraline hydrochloride	50–100 mg orally, every day	Nausea, insomnia
Nefazodone hydrochloride	100–150 mg orally, twice a day	Nausea, dry mouth, somnolence
Pseudoephedrine	60 mg orally, four times a day	CNS stimulation, tolerance

in therapy. A number of different agents have been employed. The methylated xanthine substances, theophylline in particular, cause peripheral adenosine receptor blockade with an increase in peripheral vascular tone. However, the dosages of these agents required to be effective are seldom well tolerated.

Pseudoephedrine has been reported to be effective, particularly in children. However, we frequently find that there is a rapid tachyphylaxis to its effects. The use of dextroamphetamine in the treatment of refractory patients was first reported in 1993, but safety concerns prevented it from becoming employed widely. Later, our investigations found that oral methylphenidate was a safe and effective agent in the treatment of otherwise refractory cases, yet similar concerns about dependency and abuse have limited its use.

The new α-stimulating agent, midodrine, offers many of the advantages of the amphetamines without many of the drawbacks. Because it does not cross the blood–brain barrier, it does not possess central nervous system stimulant effects. Its relatively short half-life makes its onset of action rapid and requires it be given three to four times a day. It seems to be particularly effective if used in combination with hydrofludrocortisone.

After initial anecdotal observations, Grubb and colleagues began to explore the potential use of the serotonin reuptake inhibitors in the treatment of patients with severe recurrent syncope who were intolerant of, or unresponsive to, other forms of therapy. In separate studies using the agents fluoxetine hydrochloride and sertraline hydrochloride in patients with otherwise refractory neurocardiogenic syncope, a beneficial effect was noted in 50 per cent (Grubb et al. 1994, 1996). Thereafter the more selective serotonin altering agent nefazodone hydrochloride was found to have a 60 per cent response rate. As was mentioned previously, it is presently thought that the serotonin reuptake inhibitors exhibit these effects due to their ability to prevent rapid shifts in central serotonin levels, which thereby blunt the cerebral triggers that result in sympathetic withdrawal. Interestingly, recent findings have suggested that the β-adrenergic blockers may also display significant effects on central serotonin activity, an activity that may possibly contribute to their therapeutic effects (Hjorth 1992).

In patients with dysautonomic response patterns on upright tilt, elastic support hose may be useful. However, to be effective they should generate at least 30 mmHg ankle counter pressure and preferably be waist (or at least thigh) level. Recent reports have suggested that biofeedback can serve as a very useful adjuvant to pharmacotherapy. It appears to be most helpful in those individuals who suffer from 'situational syncope' where definite psychological triggers to episodes can be identified.

One of the more controversial therapies that have arisen for the treatment of recurrent syncope has been permanent cardiac pacing. It tends to be effective only in those patients in whom syncope is associated with significant bradycardia or asystole. Of patients with a neurocardiogenic response pattern during tilt-table testing, about 25 per cent will have only modest amounts of bradycardia and thus would not be good candidates for permanent cardiac pacing.

In the very first paper on tilt-table testing, Kenny et al. (1989) also first reported on the use of dual-chamber cardiac pacing for the prevention of neurocardiogenic syncope. A short time thereafter Fitzpatrick and Sutton observed that dual-chamber cardiac pacing could prevent symptoms in 10 of 20 patients they evaluated. Fitzpatrick later found that the use of temporary dual-chamber cardiac pacing during head-upright tilt-induced syncope (using a DVI pacemaker with surge hysteresis) could abort almost 85 per cent of tilt-induced episodes (Fitzpatrick et al. 1992). These findings were confirmed by others.

The concept of pacing was later challenged by Sra and colleagues, in a study where 22 patients with tilt-induced syncope (20 were in normal sinus rhythm and two in atrial fibrillation) were evaluated (Sra et al. 1993). Repeat tilt-table testing was performed with temporary pacing at a rate that exceeded the resting heart rate by 20 per cent. The authors reported that cardiac pacing did not prevent the onset of syncope any better than pharmacotherapy, yet at the same time they observed a statistically significant reduction in the rate of fall in arterial pressure during pacing as compared with the findings during baseline tilt. Petersen et al. (1995) have been the only ones to report on the long-term effects of permanent cardiac pacing in patients with recurrent neurocardiogenic syncope. Their study followed 37 patients who underwent dual-chamber permanent pacemaker insertion and found that over a 50 eg. 24-month period, 89 per cent had reported a significant reduction in their symptoms while 27 per cent had a complete resolution of symptoms. The overall frequency of syncopal events was reported to have fallen from 136 to 11 episodes per year.

It should be kept in mind that in the majority of patients with neurocardiogenic syncope the fall in blood pressure precedes the fall in heart rate. Therefore, pacing algorithms based upon rate criteria alone may end up being 'too little too late'. Cardiac pacemakers that come equipped with sensors that could provide either direct or indirect measurement of blood pressure could provide a more effective therapy. Grubb et al. have found that a pacemaker equipped with a sensor capable of sensing right ventricular pre-ejection interval was able to sense and pace adequately in response to positional changes in a patient with severe refractory orthostatic hypotension. Similar cardiac sensors may prove quite useful in patients with severe neurocardiogenic syncope.

At our institution we do not consider permanent pacing as first-line therapy, as the majority of patients will respond to medical therapy. None the less, in patients with a significant bradycardic component who have failed drug therapy, permanent pacing can often significantly prolong the time from the onset of symptoms to syncope and in some patients prevent syncope altogether (Benditt et al. 1995). This can be especially useful in those patients who seem to experience little or no warning prior to loss of consciousness, who report their episodes as 'drop attacks'. Here cardiac pacing may produce a more gradual decline in blood pressure than previously, which is then perceived as a 'prodrome' and permits patients to take evasive actions, such as assuming a recumbent position, at its onset. It should be noted that we perform tilt-table testing with a temporary dual-chamber pacemaker in place in any patient being considered for permanent cardiac pacing. In the majority of patients, pacing alone will not be completely effective and will need to be combined with some form of pharmacotherapy.

The determination of the effectiveness of any form of therapy can be performed by noting a decrease or elimination of the patient's clinical episodes, or alternatively by observing the response during repeat tilt-table testing. Several studies have suggested that the failure to provoke syncope during repeat tilt-table testing is a reasonable predictor of long-term clinical responses (Gamachie et al. 1991). However, some have questioned the overall utility of follow-up studies.

The wide range of therapeutic options available and the diverse nature of the disorder may leave many practitioners confused over how to initiate a rational treatment programme for patients suffering from one of the recurrent neurocardiogenic syncope syndromes. Perhaps the best way to begin is by realizing that at the present time treatment is somewhat more of an art than a science. This having been said, we will offer some suggestions on therapy based on our experiences with these patients. First, the physician must take into consideration any associated disorders or conditions that the patient might have, so as to assure the compatibility of any planned therapy. Next, we review the patient's response pattern exhibited during head-upright tilt-table testing. In the young patient who exhibits either a classic neurocardiogenic or dysautonomic response pattern, we often start treatment with hydrofludrocortisone and continue it for 2–3 weeks. If there is no response or a partial effect, we will add a second agent, a serotonin reuptake inhibitor. We have found that low-dose combination therapy is often more effective and better tolerated than high-dose monotherapy. While β-blockers may be useful in patients with a classic neurocardiogenic or POTS response, they tend to be much less effective (or may even worsen symptoms) in patients with a dysautonomic pattern. In occasional patients with severe symptoms, a third agent may be required. Most often we will employ a vasoconstrictor, such as methylphenidate or midodrine (both of which are very effective in the POTS variant of these disorders).

In the course of pursuing long-term management of these patients, the physician should be mindful of the fact that the human body constitutes a dynamic substrate that alters over time. Thus, any therapy may also have to be altered over time to keep abreast of these changes. It should also be remembered that the majority of adolescent patients will 'grow out of' the condition after a few years. In this group the major thrust should be to get them safely through their symptomatic period and then to wean them off therapy. Due to the fact that most young people grow out of the problem, we are reluctant to resort to permanent pacing in this group, and do so only if we feel that patient's life is in jeopardy. Treatment can be safely stopped in about 80 per cent of adolescents after around 2 years. This is not the case in most older patients where therapy may have to be continued indefinitely.

Reflex syncope

Hypotension and bradycardia due to sudden autonomically mediated withdrawal may be triggered by stimuli other than orthostatic stress. The previously described series of events that take place during classic neurocardiogenic syncope can be provoked by mechanoreceptor stimulation in a number of different organ systems (and may also arise from the brain itself). While the exact structure of the afferent limb varies for each of these reflex syncopes syndromes, the type of input into the cardiovascular control centres of the brainstem appears to be similar, eliciting similar responses that are mediated through similar efferent pathways, with the end product being sympathetic inhibition and parasympathetic predominance. Several illustrative examples will be discussed.

Carotid sinus syncope

The carotid sinus is an area of dilatation in the internal carotid artery at the level of the carotid bifurcation. A number of both myelinated and non-myelinated sensory fibres arise from this area (the carotid sinus nerve of Herring). While some will interconnect with the hypoglossal, vagus, and cervical sympathetic nerves, the majority will unite with the glossopharyngeal nerve. This afferent limb of the carotid sinus leads to the tractus solitarius area of the medulla. The efferent aspect involves the sympathetic system innervating the heart and vasculature as well as the cardiac vagus nerve. The carotid sinus serves as a sort of high-pressure baroreceptor, as the sensory nerve endings located in its walls are activated by stretch resulting from changes in arterial blood pressure.

Carotid sinus hypersensitivity represents an exaggerated response to stimulation of the carotid sinus area. It is determined by measuring the responses of heart rate and blood pressure to carotid sinus massage. At best the technique has a number of drawbacks, is hard to quantify and is prone to a wide degree of both intra- and interobserver variability. The test should be approached with great caution or avoided in patients with known cerebrovascular disease or carotid bruits so as to avoid neurological complications (and resultant lawsuits). Carotid sinus hypersensitivity syndrome is diagnosed when carotid sinus hypersensitivity is demonstrated in a patient suffering from otherwise unexplained syncope. Three principal response patterns have been identified. First is the cardioinhibitory form, characterized by a period of ventricular asystole of at least 3 seconds in duration. The second is the vasodepressor form, where there is a fall of at least 30 mmHg in systolic blood pressure associated with symptoms (or more than 50 mmHg fall in the absence of symptoms). A third, or mixed, form is described when both responses are present. Some investigators have described a fourth response in which facial pallor and symptoms of cerebral hypoperfusion occur in the absence of any haemodynamic change. This so-called 'cerebral subtype' of carotid sinus syndrome has been attributed to cerebral vasoconstriction, and sounds remarkably similar to the 'cerebral syncope' described earlier.

Carotid sinus syndrome is principally a disease of the elderly, rarely if ever occurring before the age of 50. Men tend to have the disorder more frequently than women. As might be expected, there seems to be a strong association between carotid sinus syndrome and other hypotensive disorders such as neurocardiogenic and dysautonomic syncope, reinforcing the notion that there is a common underlying pathophysiology to these disorders.

Symptoms are classically associated with actions that result in mechanical stimulation of the carotid sinus, such as rapid head turning especially with a tight collar. However, in a significant number of patients no specific precipitating event can be identified.

Therapy for highly symptomatic patients was, at one point in time, centred around denervation of the carotid sinus by means of either surgery or radiation. However, both techniques have been largely abandoned due to unacceptable complication rates. Cardiac pacing has enjoyed wide use in patients with any sort of cardioinhibitory component. However, while preventing bradycardia, it does little for the vasodilation-related hypotension. Investigations at our centre have found that the serotonin reuptake inhibitors can prevent symptoms in patients with carotid sinus hypersensitivity, and that these agents could also be effective as first-line agents (Grubb and Kosinski 1996). Both these observations suggest that neurocardiogenic syncope and carotid sinus hypersensitivity share a common central mechanism.

Gastrointestinal stimulation

Syncope may sometimes occur in an otherwise healthy person after swallowing a bolus of food. This can, on occasion, be the presenting sign of an oesophageal structure, malignancy or diverticulum. Thus, anyone complaining of 'swallow syncope' needs to be evaluated for these possibilities. One especially potent 'vagal' stimulus producing syncope appears to be the consumption of a very cold drink when the individual is overheated. This has been reported to cause not only oesophageal spasm, atrial fibrillation, bradycardia, atroventricular block, asystole and on occasion, death. Indeed, popular wisdom cautions against the sudden consumption of cold fluid as potentially dangerous:

> Fully many a man, both young and old
> has gone to his sarcophagus
> through pouring water, ice cold, down
> his too hot oesophagus.

Sudden hypotension resulting in syncope may also be observed after lower bowel stimulation. Rectal examinations have provoked such reactions, while the more intense stimulation seen during procedures such as colonoscopy can produce hypotension and bradycardia so profound that cardiac arrest may ensue. Syncope may occur either during or immediately after defaecation.

In each of the aforementioned circumstances, syncope is felt to occur due to sudden and intense activation of mechanoreceptors located in the gut that communicate with the tractus solitarius of the medulla.

Syncope related to increased intrathoracic pressure

A sudden increase in intrathoracic pressure diminishes venous return to the heart. As the pressure within the thorax increases, the autonomic nervous system compensates for the decreased venous return through the mechanisms alluded to earlier in this chapter. However, if these changes are insufficient to maintain cerebral perfusion, syncope can result. Examples of activities that can provoke syncope via this mechanism include cough syncope, trumpet playing, weight lifting, or intentional Valsalva manoeuvre. Sneezing has also been reported to cause syncope. In young children, breath holding may produce hypotension and bradycardia so intense that both syncope and convulsive activity may occur.

Treatment of the reflex syncopes

The treatment of the reflex syncopes is aimed principally at removing the inciting cause (such as an oesophageal malignancy). However, this may not always be feasible. Recurrent syncope during micturition or defaecation may not only result in serious injury but may also lead to social embarrassment and/or emotional stress. However, unlike neurocardiogenic syncope and its variants, our experience in treating these disorders is more limited. None the less, our anecdotal observations have suggested that the serotonin reuptake inhibitors may be useful in patients with these disorders. We postulate that, as in neurocardiogenic syncope, these drugs prevent the sudden fluctuation in central serotonin levels that appear to be the signal for sympathetic withdrawal. However, further studies will

be necessary to determine the optimal therapeutic approaches in these disorders.

Summary

The group of disorders once known as 'vasovagal' syncope actually represent a heterogeneous group of conditions which share a common underlying pathology, namely a failure of the autonomic nervous system to maintain adequate sysemic blood pressure and cerebral perfusion. Once shrouded in mystery, head-upright tilt-table testing has greatly expanded our understanding of these disorders, while at the same time providing a mechanism for their diagnosis and classification. Further studies are continuing which will further advance our understanding of these forms of autonomic disturbance, while at the same time elucidating better therapeutic options.

References

Abboud, E. M. (1993). Neurocardiogenic syncope. *New Engl. J. Med.* **328**, 1117–19.

Abi-Samra, F. Maloney, J., Fouad, F. M. and Castbe, L. (1987). Usefulness of head up tilt table testing and hemodynamic investigations in the workup of syncope of unknown origin. *PACE* **10**, 406–10.

Allen, S. C., Taylor, C. L., Hall, V. E. (1945). A study of orthostatic insufficiency by the tilt board method. *Am. J. Physiol.* **143**, 11–20.

Benditt, D., Petersen, M. E., Lurie, K. *et al.* (1995). Cardiac pacing for prevention of recurrent vasovagal syncope. *Ann. Int. Med.* **122**, 204–9.

Benditt, D., Ferguson, D., Grubb, B. P. *et al.* (1996). Tilt table testing for assessing syncope and its treatment: An American College of Cardiology Consensus document. *J. Am. Coll. Cardiol.* **28**, 263–75.

Bou-Holaigh, I., Rowe, P., Kan, J. and Calkins, H. (1995). The relationship between neurally-mediated hypotension and the chronic fatigue syndrome. *J. Am. Med. Ass.* **274**, 961–7.

Calkins, H., Byrne, M., El-Atassi, R., Kalbfleish, S., Langley, J. J., and Morady, F. (1993). The economic burden of unrecognized vasodepressor syncope. *Am. J. Med.* **95**, 473–9.

Cox, M. M., Perlman, B., Mayor, M. R. *et al.* (1995). Acute and long term Beta adrenergic blockade for patients with neurocardiogenic syncope. *J. Am. Coll. Cardiol.* **26**, 1293–8.

Davgovian, M., Jarardilla, R., and Frumin, H. (1992). Prolonged aystole during head upright tilt table testing after B blockage. *PACE* **15**, 14–16.

Elam, R. F., Bergman, F., and Feverstein, G. (1985). The use of antiserotonergic agents for the treatment of acute hemorrhagic shock in cats. *Eur. J. Pharmacol.* **107**, 275–8.

Engle, G. L. (1978). Psychologic stress, vasodepressor (vasovagal) syncope and sudden death. *Ann. Int. Med.* **89**, 403–12.

Fitzpatrick, A., Theodorakis, G., Travill, C., and Sutton, R. (1992). Incidence of the malignant vasovagal syndrome in patients with recurrent syncope. *Eur. Heart J.* **12**, 389–94.

Gamachie, C., Janosik, D., Redd, R. *et al.* (1991). Long-term outcome of head up tilt guided therapy in patients with neurally-mediated syncope. (Abstract). *PACE* **14**, 4663.

Grubb, B. P., Gerard, G., Roush, K. *et al.* (1991*a*). Cerebral vasoconstriction during head upright tilt-induced vasovagal syncope. A paradoxic and unexpected response. *Circulation* **84**, 1157–64.

Grubb, B. P., Gerard, G., Roush, K. *et al.* (1991*b*). Differentiation of convulsive syncope and epilepsy with head up tilt table testing. *Ann. Int. Med.* **115**, 871–6.

Grubb, B. P., Wolfe, D., Gerard, G. *et al.* (1992*a*). Syncope and seizures of psychogenic origin: Identification with upright tilt table testing. *Clin. Cardiol.* **15** 839–42.

Grubb, B. P., Wolfe, D., Temesy-Armos, P., *et al.* (1992*b*). Reproducibility of head upright tilt table test results in patients with syncope. *PACE* 15, 1477–81.

Grubb, B. P., Samoil, D., Kosinski, D., *et al.* (1994). The use of sertraline hydrochloride in the treatment of refractory neurocardiogenic syncope in children and adolescents. *J. Am. Coll. Cardiol.* 24, 490–4.

Grubb, B. P. and Kosinski, D. (1996). Serotonin and syncope: An emerging connection? *Eur. J. Cardiac Pacing Electrophysiol.* 5, 306–14.

Grubb, B. P., Kosinski, D., Boehm, K., and Kip, K. (1997). The postural orthostatic tachycardia syndrome: A neurocardiogenic variant identified during head up tilt table testing. *PACE*, 20, 2205–13.

Hasser, E., Schadt, J., and Grove, K. (1989). Serotonergic and opioid interactions during acute hemorrhagic hypotension in the conscious rabbit (Abstract). *FASEB J.* 3, A1014.

Hjorth, S. (1992). Penbutolol as a blocker of central 5HT1A receptor-mediated responses. *Eur. J. Pharmacol* 222, 121–7.

Kenny, R. A., Ingram, A., Bayless, J., and Sutton, R. (1989). Head up tilt: A useful test for investigating unexplained syncope. *Lancet* 1, 1352–5.

Kosinski, D., Grubb, B. P., and Temesy-Armos, P. (1995). Pathophysiological aspects of neurocardiogenic syncope. *PACE* 18, 716–21.

Lewis, T. (1932). A lecture on vasovagal syncope and the carotid sinus mechanism: with comments on Gower's and Nothnagel's syndrome. *BMJ* 1, 873–6.

Linzer, M., Pontinen, M. and Gold, G. T. (1991). Impairment of physical and psychosocial function in recurrent syncope. *J. Clin. Epidemiol.* 44, 1037–43.

Matzen, S., Secher, N. H., Knigge, U. *et al.* (1993). Effect of serotonin receptor blockade on endocrine and cardiovascular responses to upright tilt in humans. *Acta Physiol. Scand.* 149, 163–76.

Morillo, C. A., Klein, G., Zandri, S., and Yee, R. (1995). Diagnostic accuracy of a low dose isoproterenol head up tilt protocol. *Am. Heart J.* 129, 901–6.

Natale, A., Akhtar, M., Jazayeri, M. *et al.* (1995). Provocation of hypotension during head up tilt testing in subjects with no history of syncope or presyncope. *Circulation* 92, 54–8.

Petersen, M. E., Chamberlain-Webben, R., Fitzpatrick, A. P. *et al.* (1994). Permanent pacing for cardioinhibitory malignant vasovagal syndrome. *Br. Heart J.* 71, 274–81.

Rea, R. and Thames, M. (1993). Neural control mechanisms and vasovagal syncope. *J. Cardiovasc. Electrophysiol.* 4, 587–95.

Smith, M. L., Carlson, M. D. and Thames, M. D. (1991). Reflex control of the heart and circulation: Implications for cardiovascular aelectrophysiology. *J. Cardiovasc. Electrophysiol.* 2, 441–9.

Sra, J., Jazayeri, M., Avitall, B. *et al.* (1993). Comparison of cardiac pacing with drug therapy in the treatment of neurocardiogenic syncope with bradycardia or asystole. *New Engl. J. Med.* 328, 1085–90.

Sutton, R. (1992). Vasovagal syndrome: Could it be malignant? *Eur. J. Cardiac Pacing Electrophysiol.* 2, 89.

Sutton, R. and Peterson, M. (1995). The clinical spectrum of neurocardiogenic syncope. *J. Cardiovasc. Electrophysiol.* 6, 569–76.

Sutton, R., Peterson, M., Brignole, M. *et al.* (1992). Proposed classification for tilt-induced vasovagal syncope. *Eur. J. Cardiac Pacing Electrophysiol.* 2, 180–3.

Wayne, H. H. (1961). Syncope: Physiologic considerations and an analysis of the clinical characteristics in 510 patients. *Am. J. Med.* 30, 418–38.

46. Cardiac causes of syncope

Juha E. K. Hartikainen and A. John Camm

Introduction

Syncope is defined as sudden and transient loss of consciousness, usually accompanied by inability to maintain postural tone. A milder disorder without loss of consciousness is termed presyncope. It is characterized by transient weakness, lightheadedness, faintness, fading awareness of surroundings, and inability to interact.

Syncope is common disorder—in the Framingham Study, 3 per cent of men and 3.5 per cent of women had experienced at least one episode of syncope (Savage *et al.* 1985). Milder symptoms, presyncopal episodes and dizziness, have been reported in as high a proportion as 48 per cent of young individuals. It has been estimated that complaints of syncope account for about 1 per cent of all hospital admissions and about 3 per cent of admissions to acute or emergency departments (Day *et al.* 1982).

The prevalence of syncope increases markedly with ageing; in patients over 75 years of age the annual incidence of syncope can be 6–7 per cent (Lipsitz *et al.* 1986). In addition, the cause of syncope depends on the age of the patients. In young patients, syncope is often of non-cardiac origin, whereas with ageing the proportion with a cardiac cause increases.

The disorders responsible for a syncopal episode are divergent, ranging from benign fainting, resulting from emotional stress, uncomfortable environment, or pain, to the other extreme—life-threatening arrhythmias potentially leading to sudden cardiac death.

Syncope can be classified into three categories based on the cause of syncope; cardiac, non-cardiac, and undetermined types. Cardiac syncope accounts for approximately 20 per cent of patients admitted to hospital with syncope (Levis et al. 1994). In almost 50 per cent of cases the reason for syncope turns out to be non-cardiac and in 30 per cent the reason for syncope remains undetermined.

After a single syncopal episode the prognosis of an individual depends on the underlying cause. A cardiac aetiology for syncope is associated with a worse prognosis; one-year mortality is 19–30 per cent (Kapoor *et al.* 1983). This is significantly higher that the mortality related to non-cardiac causes (0–12 per cent) and mortality associated with syncope of undetermined origin (6 per cent). Thus, to assess the prognosis of a patient with a history of syncope, the cause of syncope should be identified. This Chapter will concentrate on cardiac causes of syncope.

Pathophysiology of syncope

The brain constitutes 3 per cent of total body weight. However, it receives about 15 per cent of cardiac output and its oxygen consumption represents approximately 20 per cent of whole-body oxygen consumption. To maintain sufficient oxygen supply and perfusion, cerebral blood flow is under very effective control. One of the most important regulatory mechanisms of cerebral blood flow is autoregulation.

Autoregulation adjusts cerebral blood flow according to the metabolic needs of the brain. If blood pressure falls, cerebral arteries dilate so that sufficient blood flow can be maintained. Proper autoregulatory function requires that cerebral perfusion pressure remains within the autoregulatory range, approximately 60–150 mmHg. However, autoregulation may fail if perfusion pressure falls below 60 mmHg. In this case cerebral blood flow becomes linearly related to perfusion pressure.

Syncope results from transient reduction in cerebral blood flow, which compromises the ability of brain areas subserving consciousness to extract sufficient oxygen. Studies on humans have shown that acute cerebral anoxia results in syncope after 5–15 seconds. A more prolonged cerebral ischaemia (>15 seconds) is associated with tonic spasms and incontinence.

Syncope of cardiac origin

In patients with syncope of cardiac origin, syncope usually results from sudden reduction in cardiac output. This can be accounted for by two major mechanisms; obstruction of cardiac output due to factors restricting the emptying or filling of the ventricles (obstructive syncope) or disturbances in cardiac rhythm (arrhythmic syncope). More rarely, cardiogenic syncope may occur if an embolus originating from the heart reaches the brain, obstructing cerebral blood flow (cardiogenic embolism). All these can be influenced by additional factors, such as myocardial ischaemia, status of peripheral vasodilative state, the extent of hypoxia and hypercapnia, drugs, etc. Occasionally, obstructive disorder, arrhythmias, or cardiogenic embolism coexist or one disorder may accentuate another.

Obstructive syncope

Obstructive syncope—also called mechanical syncope—refers to diseases that restrict the emptying or filling of either left or right ventricle. Because of obstruction, cardiac output is more or less fixed and does not rise normally or even decreases during exercise. In addition, arterial vasodilation and decrease in peripheral vascular resistance occur during exercise. The decrease in vascular resistance is normally compensated for by increased cardiac output maintaining arterial pressure and sufficient cerebral blood flow. However, because of

Table 46.1. Cardiac disorders associated with obstructive syncope.

Aortic stenosis

Hypertrophic cardiomyopathy

Mitral stenosis

Myxoma

Pulmonary hypertension

Pulmonary stenosis
   Isolated
   Related to tetralogy of Fallot

Right-to-left shunts
   Ventricular septal defect
   Tetralogy of Fallot

Pulmonary embolism

Cardiac tamponade

Prosthetic valve malfunction

obstruction, cardiac output may not increase adequately and a fall in cerebral perfusion pressure and blood flow ensue. Indeed, exertional syncope is a clinical finding that should lead to suspicion of obstructive syncope or cardiac arrhythmia.

The heart is an organ with two hydraulic pumps that function in series. Thus, sudden decrease in cardiac output can result from pump failure of either the left or right side of the heart. Cardiac disorders resulting in obstructive syncope are listed in Table 46.1.

Aortic stenosis

The most common reason for obstructive syncope is aortic stenosis (Fig. 46.1). Up to 42 per cent of patients with severe aortic stenosis present with a history of syncope (Grech and Ramsdale 1991). Not infrequently, syncope is the first clinical manifestation of aortic stenosis. Typically, syncope occurs with physical effort. An additional possible mechanism is arrhythmia—ventricular tachycardia, paroxysmal atrioventricular block and atrial fibrillation—which are frequently seen in patients with aortic stenosis. Myocardial ischaemia and increase in sympathetic tone during exercise are other features likely to induce arrhythmias in these patients.

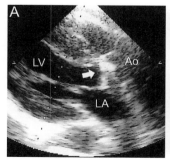
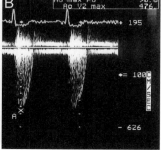

Fig. 46.1. Aortic stenosis. (a) A thickened, calcified aortic valve (arrow). LV = left ventricle, LA = left atrium, AO = aorta; (b) continuous-wave Doppler recording of the ascending aorta. The peak velocity (476 cm/s) corresponds to a pressure gradient of 90.6 mmHg across the aortic valve.

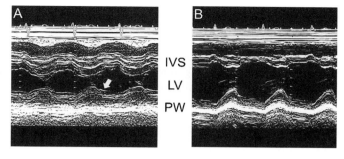

Fig. 46.2. M-mode echocardiographic scan of left ventricle (LV) from: (A) a patient with hypertrophic cardiomyopathy (HCM) and (B) a healty subject. HCM patient shows marked hypertrophy of the interventricular septum (IVS) and posterior wall (PW), diminished diameter of left ventricular (LV) lumen (volume) and reduced rate of diastolic relaxation and filling (arrow).

The use of vasodilator drugs in patients with aortic stenosis can result in a drop in peripheral vascular resistance and worsen the tendency of syncope. Patients with severe aortic stenosis often have left ventricular hypertrophy. A hypertrophied left ventricle is stiff and diastolic filling of the ventricle is critical for proper systolic function. A decrease in preload caused by vasodilator drugs may result in inadequate diastolic filling and also renders these patients vulnerable to syncope.

Syncope has prognostic significance in patients with aortic stenosis. Without valve replacement, the average survival is 3–4 years after the first episode (Ross and Braunwald 1968).

Hypertrophic cardiomyopathy

Hypertrophic cardiomyopathy (Fig. 46.2) is also associated with exertional syncope, particularly if obstruction of left ventricular outflow is present (hypertrophic obstructive cardiomyopathy). Syncope has been reported in up to 30 per cent of these patients (Fananapazir *et al.* 1989). Patients with hypertrophic obstructive cardiomyopathy are prone to experience syncope during exercise or when vasodilator drugs are administered to reduce afterload (vasodilation). This is due to inability of cardiac output to increase adequately to compensate for the decrease in peripheral resistance (Frenneaux *et al.* 1990). In addition, due to abnormal ventricular relaxation and diastolic filling, a decrease in pulmonary venous pressure caused by vasodilator drugs (decrease in preload) may severely impair diastolic filling of the left ventricle and result in fall in cardiac output.

Left ventricular obstruction associated with hypertrophic obstructive cardiomyopathy is not structural but dynamic (caused by systolic anterior movement of the mitral valve and contact with the hypertrophied ventricular septum). Thus, factors that increase myocardial contractility (e.g. exercise, inotropic drugs, etc.) increase the degree of obstruction and therefore should be avoided.

Because of abnormalities in left ventricular relaxation and diastolic filling, a loss of atrioventricular synchrony—as in the case of atrial fibrillation—can result in sudden decrease of cardiac output and syncope. Hypertrophic cardiomyopathy is also associated with sinus node disease, abnormalities in atrioventricular conduction and propensity to ventricular tachyarrhythmias, which must be born in mind as one possible mechanism of syncope in these patients (Fananapazir *et al.* 1989).

Sudden cardiac death is the most common form of death in patients with hypertrophic cardiomyopathy. Particularly, this is true for children and young adults. Indeed, hypertrophic cardiomyopathy has been identified as the most common structural heart disease among young athletes suffering from sudden cardiac death (Maron *et al.* 1996). Whether cardiomyopathy in these patients is genetically transmitted or represents undesirable consequences of 'athletes heart' is not known. Many of the patients are asymptomatic prior to sudden death. History of syncope or cardiac arrest have been found to be one of the best predictors of risk of sudden death in patients with hypertrophic cardiomyopathy (Fananapazir *et al.* 1992).

Mitral stenosis

Mitral stenosis does not obstruct left ventricular systolic pumping, but influences left ventricular filling during diastole. Impaired ventricular filling, in turn, results in decreased cardiac output. In the case of tachycardia, the duration of diastole shortens. As a result of combination of short diastole and mitral stenosis left ventricular diastolic filling may be severely impaired. Thus, mitral stenosis can result in an abrupt fall in left ventricular filling during paroxysmal tachyarrhythmias.

Left ventricular filling in the setting of mitral stenosis is also largely dependent on pressure of pulmonary veins and left atrium. A decrease in pulmonary venous pressure caused by vasodilator drugs may result in abrupt reduction of diastolic flow through the stenosed mitral valve and lead to impaired diastolic filling of the left ventricle.

Myxoma

Myxoma is a benign tumour of the heart (Fig. 46.3). Most (75 per cent) are located to the left atrium but they can also be found in the right atrium (18 per cent) or rarely in the ventricles. Myxoma may prolapse through the mitral (tricuspid) valve, obstruct mitral (tricuspid) flow and impair left (right) ventricular diastolic filling. Most often this leads to symptoms of cardiac failure, but also syncope. Myxoma may prolapse through the atrioventricular valve during standing and return into the atrium when the patient assumes the recumbent position. Thus, in addition to neurogenic postural

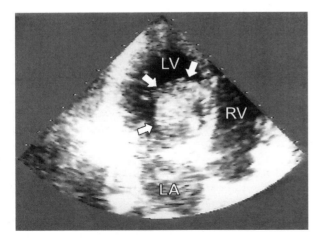

Fig. 46.3. Left atrial myxoma (arrows). The tumour mass has prolapsed into the left ventricle (LV) through the mitral valve during atrial contraction. RV, right ventricle; LA, left atrium.

hypotension, syncope related to change in body position is suggestive of myxoma (Raynen 1995).

Myxoma embolization occurs in 40–50 per cent of patients. Syncope is a rare manifestation of myxoma embolization of the central nervous system.

Pulmonary hypertension

Pulmonary hypertension can be primary or secondary. Most cases of pulmonary hypertension are secondary to cardiac or pulmonary diseases or disorders leading to alveolar hypoventilation. Pulmonary hypertension is complicated by syncope in up to 30 per cent of patients (Fuster *et al.* 1984). Usually syncope related to pulmonary hypertension is effort related. The mechanism of syncope is limitation of right ventricular outflow.

Pulmonary stenosis

Pulmonary stenosis—isolated or related to tetralogy of Fallot—is one of the most common congenital heart diseases. It accounts for about 20 per cent of congenital heart defects (Mitcell *et al.* 1971). Syncope associated with pulmonary stenosis is typically exertional. The mechanism is an obstruction to right ventricular outflow and inability to increase cardiac output during exercise. With severe obstruction, right ventricular damage can ensue over the years, rendering patients vulnerable to heart failure and arrhythmias, which may cause syncope and sudden death in adults with pulmonary stenosis (Mody 1975).

Right-to-left shunts

In patients with large communications between the left and right sides of the heart (ventricular septal defect, tetralogy of Fallot, etc.), right ventricular pressure tends to increase and can equal or exceed the pressure in the left ventricle and aorta. This reverses the left-to-right shunt to right-to-left shunt. A decrease in systemic vascular resistance, e.g. exercise induced, increases shunting from right-to-left. As a result, systemic oxygen saturation falls worsening systemic hypoxia associated with these diseases, and may precipitate a syncopal episode (Guntheroth *et al.* 1965).

Pulmonary embolism

Acute pulmonary embolism results in syncope in 10–15 per cent of patients (Thames *et al.* 1969). The mechanism of syncope is reduction of cardiac output due to development of acute right ventricular failure. Pulmonary embolism is also associated with arterial hypoxia and secondary hypocapnia, which both are prone to worsen the tendency of syncope. In addition, chronic or recurrent pulmonary embolism can result in secondary pulmonary hypertension (cor pulmonale).

Cardiac tamponade

Acute cardiac tamponade decreases cardiac output by restricting the dilation of cardiac chambers during diastole, i.e. it impairs cardiac diastolic filling. The most common cause for acute tamponade leading to syncope is acute aortic dissection. Syncope is reported in 5 per cent of these patients (Desanctis *et al.* 1987). If tamponade develops slowly, a decrease in cardiac output produces shortness of breath, rather than syncope. However, if a patient with latent tamponade develops tachyarrhythmia, diastolic filling of the heart is further impaired and syncope may ensue.

Prosthetic valve malfunction

Most often a prosthetic valve is implanted into aortic or mitral position. Even when functioning normally, prosthetic valves may have relatively high gradients. This is particularly true for small aortic prostheses. In addition, the size of gradient increases with the rate of blood flow. Thus, the gradient increases during exercise. In the case of rapid tachyarrhythmias, patients with prosthetic valves may experience syncope. In addition, malfunction of a prosthetic valve, e.g. thrombotic obstruction, can result in sudden impairment to cardiac output and syncope. Finally, a thrombotic embolization to the central nervous system can result in syncope.

Arrhythmic syncope

In patients of all age groups with unexplained syncope, arrhythmias are the most frequent identifiable cause (Rahimtoola *et al.* 1987). The most common single arrhythmia responsible for syncope is ventricular tachycardia, but supraventricular tachyarrhythmias and bradyarrhythmias are also frequently uncovered (Table 46.2).

Usually cardiac arrhythmia *per se* is not associated with sufficient haemodynamic deterioration to cause syncope, but this is rather due to either very slow or very high heart rate. In patients with severely impaired diastolic filling, loss of atrial contraction and atrioventricular synchrony as a result of, for example, atrial fibrillation can lead to haemodynamic collapse even if heart rate would otherwise be tolerable. Although cardiac arrhythmias are associated with syncope as a direct cause, they can also be a part of complicated reflex response as in the case of neurocardiogenic syncope (bradyarrhythmias). The latter is discussed separately (Chapter 45).

Bradyarrhythmias

As heart rate slows, the number of ventricular contractions per unit time decreases and the cardiac output tends to fall. At the same time, however, the duration of diastole lengthens and stroke volume increases, which compensate for the reduction of cardiac output resulting from a low heart rate. In a normal individual heart rates above 35–40 beats/min should not reduce cerebral flow significantly or result in syncope.

Bradyarrhythmias result from sinus node or atrioventricular node dysfunction. They have been estimated to account only for less than 5 per cent of syncopal episodes. However, identification of bradyarrhythmia is important, because syncope can be prevented by appropriate pacemaker therapy.

Sinus node dysfunction

Sinus node dysfunction is a relatively common finding in all age groups, but the prevalence of this disorder increases with advancing age. Sinus node dysfunction is usually structural—due to replacement of sinoatrial cells by fibrous tissue—caused by ischaemic heart disease, cardiomyopathy, trauma secondary to cardiac surgery or inflammation (Shaw *et al.* 1987). However, it may also be associated with extracardiac factors which are possibly curable, such as electrolyte abnormalities, hypothyroidism, hypothermia, drugs (e.g. β-

Table 46.2. Cardiac disorders associated with arrhythmic syncope

Bradyarrhythmia
  Sinus node dysfunction
    Sinus bradycardia
    Sinus arrest
    Brady-tachy syndrome
  Atrioventricular conduction defect
    First-degree AV block (associated with markedly prolonged PR interval or bifascicular block)
    Type I second-degree AV block (Wenckebach type)
    Type II second-degree AV block (Mobitz type)
    Third-degree AV block

Tachyarrhythmia
  Supraventricular tachyarrhythmia
    Atrioventricular nodal re-entrant tachycardia
    Atrioventricular tachycardia associated with WPW syndrome
    Atrial tachycardia
    Atrial flutter
    Atrial fibrillation
  Ventricular tachyarrhythmia
    Monomorphic ventricular tachycardia
    Polymorphic ventricular tachycardia
    Ventricular fibrillation

Pacemaker malfunction
  Bradycardia due to
    End of battery life
    Generator failure
    Electrode dysfunction
    Interference
      myopotential interference
      electromagnetic interference
    Inappropriate programming
  Tachycardia due to
    Pacemaker-mediated tachycardia
    Other arrhythmias
  Pacemaker syndrome

WPW, Wolff–Parkinson–White

blockers, calcium antagonists, digitalis), and high vagal tone. Sinus node dysfunction can be divided into three subgroups: sinus bradycardia, sinus arrest, and brady-tachy syndrome.

Sinus bradycardia is common in healthy subjects, especially during the night in young individuals with high vagal tone. In most cases sinus bradycardia does not produce any symptoms. If symptoms occur, they are most often fatigue, lethargy, and signs of heart failure rather than syncope. Thus, sinus bradycardia should not be considered as a cause of syncope unless demonstrated during a syncopal attack.

Sinus arrest (Fig. 46.4a) results either from impaired automaticity of the sinus node or impaired conduction from the sinus node to the right atrium. These two cannot be distinguished from each other based on surface ECG recording. Also sinus arrest is a common finding in ambulatory ECG recordings. Sinus pauses with duration of 2 seconds or more have been reported in 6 per cent of healthy subjects undergoing an ambulatory ECG recording and even more commonly—up to 37 per cent—in trained athletes (Viitasalo *et al.* 1982; Mazuz and Friedman 1983). In the latter group, this is related to high

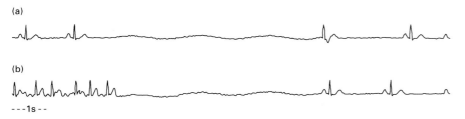

(a)

(b)

- - - 1s - -

Fig. 46.4. Sinus node dysfunction: (a) sinus arrest; (b) brady-tachy syndrome.

vagal tone. In one study, 22 patients out of 6470 (0.3 per cent) had sinus pauses of 3 seconds or more during ambulatory ECG recording, but only 10 per cent of the patients were symptomatic during the pause (Hilgard *et al.* 1985). On the other hand, in another study 85 per cent of patients with pauses of longer than 3 seconds, had symptoms (Ector *et al.* 1983). The duration of a pause has not been found to predict the occurrence of death (Mazuz and Friedman 1983; Hilgard *et al.* 1985). Sinus arrest without symptoms need not be treated and one has to be cautious when interpreting it as a cause of syncope without demonstrating sinus arrest concomitantly with syncope.

Brady-tachy syndrome is one form of sinus node dysfunction with the highest incidence of syncope (Short 1954). In brady-tachy syndrome a prolonged sinus arrest follows immediately upon the termination of an atrial tachyarrhythmia—atrial flutter, atrial fibrillation or atrial tachycardia (Fig. 46.4b). In addition to sinus node dysfunction, a prolonged arrest implies impaired function of lower pacemakers that should assume cardiac pacemaker function in the case of sinus bradycardia or sinus arrest. Concomitant impairment of sinus node function and atrial tachyarrhythmias may imply that sinus node dysfunction is produced by the same pathological process, e.g. idiopathic fibrosis, that causes atrial tachycardias. In these patients tachyarrhythmia often follows an episode of sinus bradycardia. Thus, implantation of a pacemaker not only prevents syncope, but may also reduce the incidence of tachyarrhythmic episodes.

Atrioventricular conduction defect

An intermittent high-degree atrioventricular (AV) block is a common cause of dizziness and syncope. However, because AV block can be transient and infrequent, it is sometimes difficult to demonstrate despite repeated ambulatory ECG recordings. Indeed, in one study of patients with unexplained syncope, only 3 per cent had high-degree AV block that was considered the cause of the syncope (Kapoor *et al.* 1987).

The clinical significance of an AV conduction defect depends on the site and the degree of the block. The site of conduction defect can be located within the AV node, the bundle of His or the infra-His structures. The degree of AV block is divided into first-degree, second-degree, and third-degree AV blocks.

In first-degree AV block, impulse transmission from atria to ventricles is 1 : 1 although conduction is prolonged, i.e. all P waves are conducted, but PR interval is prolonged. The normal PR interval is defined as a range of 120–200 ms. The delay in the AV conduction is most commonly in the AV node, although it can be located also to the atrium, to the bundle of His and to infra-His structures. Normally, first-degree AV block does not produce bradycardia or syncope and does not require therapy. However, if PR interval is markedly prolonged (300–500 ms), atrial contraction may occur immediately after the preceding ventricular systole, against closed AV valves. This functional AV dissociation can manifest with hypotension, dizziness, and even syncope. In these cases, restoration of AV synchrony by permanent dual-chamber pacemaker should be considered. In addition, a prolonged PR interval associated with bifascicular block (left bundle branch block or right bundle branch block + left anterior or posterior hemiblock) indicates greater involvement of the conduction system and can predict progression to higher-grade AV block (Kaul *et al.* 1988).

In second-degree block AV impulse transmission is intermittent. It is further divided into Types I and II. Type I (Wenckebach type) is characterized by progressive prolongation in AV conduction time followed by a blocked P wave (Fig. 46.5a). It can be precipitated in almost all individuals by rapid atrial pacing. It also prevents development of too rapid ventricular rate during atrial tachyarrhythmias, such as atrial tachycardia, atrial flutter, and atrial fibrillation. It can be produced by drugs, e.g. digitalis, β-blockers, and calcium-channel blockers. Wenckebach type AV block located into the AV node is typical for trained young adults in the presence of high vagal tone, particularly during rest and sleep. It is unlikely to produce syncope and it does not merit pacemaker therapy. However, if Wenckebach type AV block occurs in situations not associated with a high level of vagal tone, and particularly if it occurs in the presence of sympathetic activation (during activity), it is suggestive of location of the block to the bundle of His or infra-His structures. In these cases Type I second-degree block may precede development of higher-grade AV block and therefore permanent pacemaker therapy is recommended.

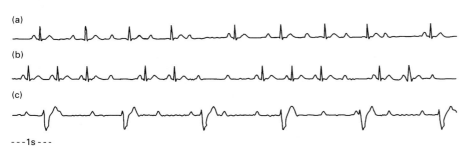

(a)

(b)

(c)

- - - 1s - - -

Fig. 46.5. Atrioventricular conduction defect: (a) Type I (Wenckebach) second-degree AV block; (b) Type II (Mobitz) second-degree AV block; (c) third-degree AV block.

In Type II (Mobitz type) second-degree AV block, a sudden failure in impulse transmission from atria to ventricles occurs without alteration in conduction time before the block (Fig. 46.5b). Type II block indicates a conduction defect in the His bundle or infra-His conduction system. It does not respond to changes in autonomic tone or drugs. The clinical implication of Type II block differs also from Type I block. Often, patients with Type II second-degree AV block are symptomatic with recurrent syncope. This is usually due to paroxysmal progression to complete AV block (see below). Thus, permanent pacemaker implantation is recommended in Mobitz-type AV blocks.

Third-degree block (complete heart block, Fig. 46.5c) implies that there is no impulse transmission from the atria to the ventricles. It can occur in the AV node, in the bundle of His or in the infra-His conduction system. Congenital heart block is a typical example of third-degree block located to the AV node. The subsidiary pacemaker is in the His bundle, the escape rhythm has narrow QRS complexes, a rate of 40–60/min, and it is usually responsive to alterations in autonomic tone and drugs influencing AV node function. Thus, syncope is rarely a presenting symptom in these patients. An acquired complete heart block is most often due to coronary artery disease, degenerative processes, or drug toxicity. In an acquired complete heart block the block is usually located to the bundle of His or infra-His conduction system, resulting in an escape rhythm with wide QRS complexes. Because the escape rhythm is slow and often unreliable, syncope is a common symptom in this setting. The block is usually unresponsive to autonomic tone and drugs (atropine, isoprenaline). Permanent pacemaker therapy is mandatory in these patients. Between syncope episodes AV conduction can be completely normal. Thus, it may not be possible to demonstrate complete heart block despite repeated ambulatory ECG recordings.

Tachyarrhythmias

Whether tachycardia is associated with hypotension and syncope depends on the rate of tachycardia, the underlying cardiac disease, posture, and the responsiveness of compensatory mechanisms (autonomic reflexes). An increase in heart rate tends to increase cardiac output. However, at the same time the duration of diastolic filling shortens (Fig. 46.6). Thus, stroke volume decreases with increasing heart rate. In healthy individuals, a heart rate not exceeding 180 beats/minute should not result in syncope. However, in patients with diastolic dysfunction (e.g. left ventricular hypertrophy) cardiac filling can be very vulnerable to shortening of diastole. As a result, stroke volume and cardiac output start to decrease even at relatively low heart rates. Correspondingly, acute myocardial ischaemia can damage myocardial function and induce arrhythmias, which together may result in syncope.

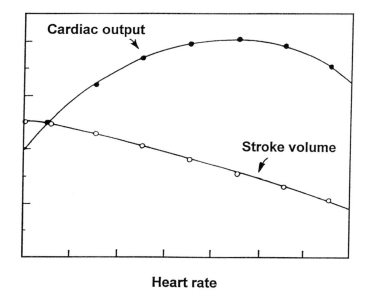

Fig. 46.6. Effect of heart rate on stroke volume and cardiac output.

Supraventricular tachyarrhythmias

Supraventricular tachycardias are common arrhythmias. In young patients these are usually caused by congenital structures creating re-entrant circuits between the atria and the ventricles. The most common form is AV nodal re-entrant tachycardia, in which the re-entrant circuit is caused by splitting of the connection between right atrium and AV node into two pathways. Wolff–Parkinson–White (WPW) syndrome is the second most common form of supraventricular arrhythmia in young patients. The re-entrant circuit is due to one or multiple accessory pathways between the atria and the ventricles. If the conduction from the atria to the ventricles conducts through the accessory pathway, the QRS complex becomes pre-excitated, i.e. a delta wave is seen at the beginning of QRS complex (Fig. 46.7). However, if the conduction takes place through the AV node, the QRS complex is narrow. During the typical form of supraventricular tachycardia associated with WPW syndrome the impulse conducts from atrium to ventricle over the normal AV node/His bundle and returns from the ventricle to atrium over the accessory pathway, producing a narrow QRS complex.

In patients at an older age, atrial flutter, atrial tachycardia, and, particularly, atrial fibrillation are typical supraventricular tachyarrhythmias. These can be caused by single or multiple ectopic atrial foci or by re-entrant circuits secondary to fibrous tissue caused by mitral valve disease, congenital heart disease, cardiomyopathy, and scars resulting form earlier cardiac surgery.

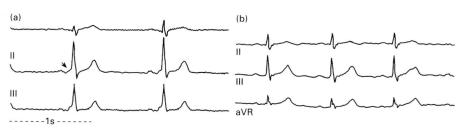

Fig. 46.7. (a) A patient with WPW syndrome caused by an accessory pathway between left atrium and left ventricle. Due to inhomogeneous ventricular depolarization, the QRS complexes are pre-excitated and have a delta wave (arrow). (b) Same patient after radiofrequency ablation of the accessory pathway. The delta wave has disappeared and the QRS complex is narrow.

(a)

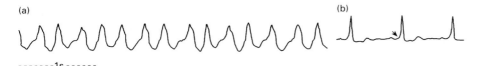

(b)

- - - - - - 1s - - - - - -

Fig. 46.8.   (a) Rapid atrial fibrillation (220 beats/min) in a patient with WPW syndrome; (b) ECG of the same patient during sinus rhythm reveals delta waves (arrow).

Most commonly supraventricular arrhythmias are accompanied by mild symptoms such as palpitations and dizziness, only rarely with syncope. If syncope develops, there is often concomitant sinus node dysfunction and syncope is due to sinus arrest at the moment when tachycardia terminates, or there is some other precipitating heart disease that renders the patients vulnerable to even less rapid heart rates. If atrial flutter or fibrillation develop in a patient with WPW syndrome and an antegradely conducting accessory pathway (pre-excitation) there is a risk of a very rapid ventricular rate (Fig. 46.8) leading to syncope or sudden death. This must be considered if a patient with syncope presents with pre-excitation during sinus rhythm.

Supraventricular tachycardias are often transient and infrequent. Thus, they may be difficult to demonstrate despite repeated ambulatory ECG recordings. However, syncope related to supraventricular tachycardia is almost invariable preceded by a sensation of rapid heart rate and palpitations, which should lead to suspicion of arrhythmic syncope mechanism. Pre-excitation during sinus rhythm is suggestive of rapidly conducting accessory pathways as discussed above. If an arrhythmic mechanism is likely, electrophysiological study can usually help to determine the type of arrhythmia. In addition, during the same procedure, radiofrequency ablation often can be performed to provide a curative therapy.

Ventricular tachyarrhythmias

Ventricular tachyarrhythmias are the most common arrhythmias responsible for syncope. These include sustained or non-sustained ventricular tachycardias and ventricular fibrillation.

According to the QRS morphology, a ventricular tachyarrhythmia is classified as monomorphic ventricular tachycardia, polymorphic ventricular tachycardia, or ventricular fibrillation. Monomorphic tachycardia is characterized by uniform and stable QRS morphology (Fig. 46.9a), whereas polymorphic tachycardia is characterized by a changing morphology, often with no isoelectric baseline (Fig. 46.10b).

Ventricular tachyarrhythmia is considered sustained if it lasts 30 seconds or more, or requires emergency intervention, and nonsustained if it consists of three or more consecutive ventricular beats at a rate of 100/minute or more with duration of less than 30 seconds.

Ventricular tachyarrhythmias occur most often in patients with some organic cardiac disease. The most common disorder is coronary artery disease, especially a postinfarction patient with a ventricular aneurysm. In this setting tachycardia is usually due to the development of fibrosis separating areas of viable myocardium,

which causes slow impulse conduction, and creates a substrate for re-entry. The typical clinical manifestation is monomorphic ventricular tachycardia (Fig. 46.9a). About 70–80 per cent of patients with monomorphic ventricular tachycardia have coronary artery disease. The tachycardia associated with coronary artery disease can also have (but less often) polymorphic morphology. Reduced left ventricular systolic function, spontaneous non-sustained ventricular arrhythmias, late potentials on signal-averaged ECG, and reduced heart rate variability predict ventricular tachyarrhythmias in postinfarction patients (Hartikainen *et al.* 1996).

Ventricular arrhythmias—most often monomorphic but also polymorphic—are found in patients with cardiomyopathies, arrhythmogenic right ventricular dysplasia, congenital heart disease (especially after repair of tetralogy of Fallot), valvular heart disease, and digoxin toxicity, but they can occur also in patients without any apparent structural abnormality of the heart. In the latter case, however, the symptom is typically palpitation rather than syncope.

A particular type of polymorphic ventricular tachycardia characterized by beat-to-beat variability of amplitude and polarity of the QRS complexes is termed torsade de pointes (Fig. 46.10b). It is often self-terminating but occasionally degenerates into ventricular fibrillation. Torsade de pointes is usually associated with long QT syndrome (LQTS) (Fig. 46.10a). LQTS can be either congenital or acquired. The congenital LQTS is caused by mutations in genes encoding cardiac ion channels resulting in delayed depolarization and a prolonged QT interval (Keating et al. 1991; Jiang et al. 1994; Schott *et al.* 1995). The onset of torsade de pointes can follow two patterns. In the bradycardia-dependent type, slowing of heart rate results in marked QT prolongation, rendering the patients susceptible to tachycardia. In the second type of LQTS, QT prolongation is associated with sympathetic activation. In these patients tachycardia is typically initiated during emotional or physical stress. The mortality of untreated patients with syncope associated with congenital LQTS exceeds 20 per cent in the year following the first syncopal episode (Schwartz 1985). β-Blockers have been reported to prevent new syncopal episodes in 75 per cent of patients. Left cardiac sympathectomy is recommended for patients with recurrence of syncope despite -blocker therapy. In patients with bradycardia- or pause-dependent torsade de pointes, a permanent pacemaker is indicated. If these therapies fail, a cardioverter-defibrillator should be considered. In the acquired type of LQTS, QT prolongation is caused by drugs (Table 46.3), bradycardia (complete heart block, sick sinus syndrome), hypothermia, metabolic disorders (hypokalaemia, hypomagnesaemia, and hypocalcaemia), myocardial

(a)

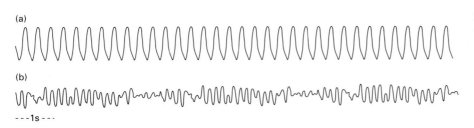

(b)

- - - 1s - - -

Fig. 46.9.   (a) Monomorphic ventricular tachycardia; (b) ventricular fibrillation.

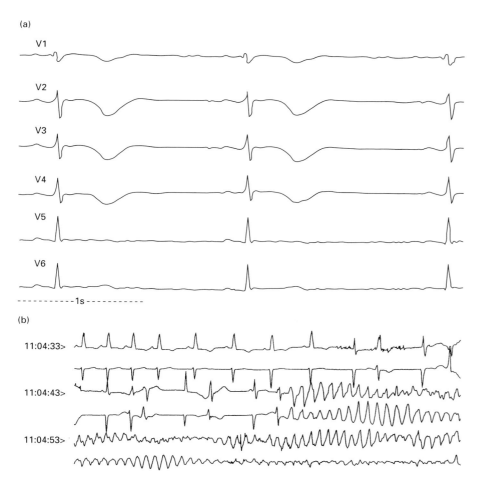

(a)

V1

V2

V3

V4

V5

V6

- - - - - - - - - - 1s - - - - - - - - - -

(b)

11:04:33>

11:04:43>

11:04:53>

Fig. 46.10. A patient with acquired long QT syndrome caused by thioridazine overdosing. (a) The ECG shows markedly prolonged QT interval, QT 0.70 s. (b) Same patient during ECG monitoring. QT interval is 0.62 s. Ventricular premature beats followed by a pause are seen, and finally torsade de pointes ventricular tachycardia develops.

ischaemia, myocarditis, or abnormal nutritional status (e.g. anorexia nervosa or intense weight reduction that involves the use of liquid protein diet). The tachycardia is usually initiated by a premature ventricular beat following a pause. In the acquired forms of LQTS, the underlying cause should be eliminated. In the acute phase, electrical defibrillation is used for termination of the tachycardia. Recurrences can often be eliminated by acceleration of the heart rate by temporary pacing of isoprenaline infusion.

Ventricular fibrillation (Fig. 46.9b) is often triggered by myocardial ischaemia. It can also result from ventricular premature beat, abrupt change in autonomic tone, or degeneration of rapid monomorphic or polymorphic ventricular tachycardia or atrial fibrillation into ventricular fibrillation. Usually, once ventricular fibrillation develops it results in sudden death. Thus, although ventricular fibrillation provokes syncope, most patients die before seeking medical advise.

In conclusion, patients experiencing a syncope caused by ventricular tachyarrhythmia have an unfavourable clinical outcome. If untreated, the recurrence of ventricular tachycardia is 30–60 per cent per year (Shenasa *et al.* 1993). In addition, without the exception of β-blocker therapy in LQTS patients, there is no evidence that the prognosis can be improved sufficiently by antiarrhythmic therapy. The best therapy is if the trigger (e.g. ischaemia, electrolyte abnormality) or the substrate (e.g. infarct scar) can be identified and eliminated. If this is not possible, the patient should be treated with an implantable cardioverter-defibrillator (ICD), which has been shown

to reduce the incidence of arrhythmic death to less than 1 per cent per year (Schlepper et al. 1995). Recently, the AVID (Antiarrhythmics vs. implantable defibrillators) Trial—the first prospective randomized study comparing survival rates between ICD and antiarrhythmic drugs for patients with life-threatening arrhythmias—was stopped because the ICD group experienced a significant reduction in mortality compared to the antiarrhythmic drug group (National Institute of Health 1997). Another recently published study showed that in patients with prior myocardial infarction and high risk for ventricular tachycardia, prophylactic therapy with ICD leads to improved survival compared to conventional drug therapy (Moss *et al.* 1996).

Syncope related to pacemaker malfunction

Permanent pacing should prevent syncope related to bradyarrhythmias. Thus, syncope occurring in a patient with a pacemaker indicates that syncope was not associated with bradycardia at all or alternatively that syncope is due to malfunction of the pacemaker system.

In general, pacemaker generators are reliable and problems occur only rarely. If the generator battery runs to its end of life and the patient is dependent on the pacemaker, rhythm syncope can ensue. However, this should not happen if the patients attend for appropriate follow-up, because the end of life of the battery can be detected early enough to schedule generator change in good time. In addition, in most cases the pacemaker does not stop abruptly at the time of end of life, but it

Table 46.3. Drugs associated with prolongation of QT interval and/or torsade de pointes ventricular tachycardia

Antiarrhythmic drugs
  Quinidine
  Disopyramide
  Procainamide
  Flecainide
  Mexiletine
  Lidocaine
  Amiodarone
  Sotalol
  Ajmaline

Psychoactive agents
  Phenothiazines
  Tricyclic antidepressants
  Other antidepressants
  Lithium

Antimicrobial agents
  Macrolide antibiotics
  Chloroquine
  Pentamidine
  Amantadine

Other agents
  Organophosphates
  Cocaine
  Antihistamines

switches into a simple backup function mode, which may influence the quality of life of the patient but should not result in syncope.

Electrode dysfunction is the most common problem with permanent pacemaker therapy. During the first months after implantation this is due to electrode dislocation or poor electronic contact between the electrode and myocardial tissue. In the longer run, the problem tends to be a failure of the electrode, caused by mechanical fracture or insulation break. In a recent study, based on the Danish pacemaker register, 25 per cent of bipolar ventricular electrodes did not function properly after 8 years and needed replacement (Moller and Arnsbo 1996). Electrode malfunction can result in loss of pacing (exit block, Fig. 46.11a) or inappropriate sensing of spontaneous cardiac activity.

A pacemaker electrode—particularly, a unipolar atrial electrode—may sense non-cardiac myopotentials which are erroneously interpreted by the pacemaker as spontaneous cardiac activity (myopotential interference), resulting in temporary pacemaker inhibition (Fig. 46.11b). In addition, environmental noise (e.g. digital mobile telephones) can cause electromagnetic interference with pacemakers and inhibit pacemaker function, trigger rapid paced rhythms or asynchronous pacing (Naegeli et al. 1996). Although the dysfunction is only transient, temporary pacemaker inhibition in pacemaker-dependent patients can be long enough to provoke syncope.

Even if the generator and the electrode are functioning properly, a successful pacemaker therapy requires that the pacemaker is programmed correctly. Inappropriate programming of the pacing and sensing functions can result in bradycardia due to loss of capture (exit block) or oversensing of non-cardiac myopotentials.

About 15 per cent of patients with complete heart block have retrograde conduction from ventricles to atria. A combination of dual-chamber pacemaker and retrograde conduction can result in pacemaker-mediated tachycardia (PMT). PMT is usually started by a retrogradely conducted ventricular premature beat which is sensed by the atrial electrode and erroneously interpreted as a normal P wave. If the pacemaker is programmed to pace the ventricles after a P wave is recognized (DDD or VDD modes), the retrogradely con-

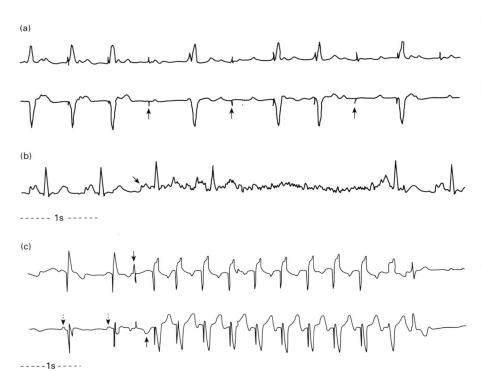

(a)

(b)

------ 1s ------

(c)

-----1s-----

Fig. 46.11. Pacemaker malfunction. (a) Exit block in a patient with a ventricular pacemaker (VVI). Some pacing spikes (arrows) are not followed by ventricular capture. (b) Myopotential interference in a patient with an atrial pacemaker. The pacemaker interprets noise caused by muscular activity as spontaneous cardiac activity, resulting in pacemaker inhibition. An atrial pacing spike is denoted with an arrow. (c) Pacemaker-mediated tachycardia. Two first P waves are sensed correctly and they trigger ventricular pacing. A ventricular ectopic beat (arrow down) is conducted retrogradely (arrow up). This is sensed by the atrial electrode and interpreted as a normal P wave. Thus, ventricular pacing is triggered which is further conducted retrogradely and pacemaker-mediated tachycardia develops.

ducted activation triggers a ventricular response and starts PMT (Fig. 46.11c). Heart rate during PMT usually corresponds to the maximum programmed rate of the pacemaker. Most often PMT results in palpitations, but syncope may also ensue. In addition, in a patient with a dual-chamber pacemaker, atrial tachyarrhythmias (atrial fibrillation, flutter, or atrial tachycardia) can be sensed by the pacemaker and activate ventricles at the maximum programmed rate, producing PMT. Usually PMTs can be prevented by appropriate programming of the pacemaker.

In a patient with complete heart block and normal sinus rhythm, use of ventricular pacing results in loss of AV synchrony and may also result in conduction of ventricular activation to the atria. As a consequence, the atria may contract against closed AV valves, which stimulates atrial and pulmonary venous stretch receptors. This may induce reflex peripheral vasodilation and hypotension, causing dizziness, presyncope, or even syncope, a clinical status referred to as pacemaker syndrome. Pacemaker syndrome can be prevented/treated by assuming AV synchrony with dual-chamber pacemaker.

If syncope occurs in a patient with a permanent pacemaker, the status of the pacemaker generator, electrode(s), and programming must be checked. In addition, the appropriate pacing mode should be verified.

Cardiogenic brain embolism

Cerebral complications may occur when abnormal material is pumped from the heart into circulation reaching the brain. Abnormal material can be a thrombus, bacterial vegetation, myxomatous tissue, or a calcified plaque. Typically, the symptoms develop suddenly and are maximal at onset. The symptoms usually indicate a deficit of function in a certain region of the brain thus arising suspicion of cerebrovascular ischaemic attack. However, sometimes embolization occurring in the vertebrobasilar area may be very transient, and presyncope—rarely also syncope—may be the only clinical manifestation of the attack.

A cardiac embolus can be related to cardiac wall abnormalities, valvular disorders or arrhythmias (Table 46.4).

Table 46.4. Cardiac disorders associated with brain embolism.

Cardiac wall abnormalities
    Akinesia/dyskinesia of left ventricle
    Left ventricular aneurysm
    Atrial septal aneurysm
    Atrial septal defect
    Myxoma

Valvular disorders
    Calcified aortic or mitral valve
    Endocarditis
    Thrombosis of a prosthetic valve

Arrhythmias
    Atrial fibrillation
    Sick sinus syndrome

Cardiac wall abnormalities

Cardiac wall abnormalities precipitate thrombus formation. This is typical for areas of regional akinesis or dyskinesis resulting from acute myocardial infarction. The incidence of stroke complicating acute myocardial infarction is c. 1 per cent (Behar et al. 1991). In addition, postinfarction ventricular aneurysm, dilated cardiomyopathy, and atrial septal aneurysm are associated with increased risk of thrombus formation and systemic embolization. Systemic myxoma embolization may also occur (see above). Venous thrombi may result in systemic embolization in the presence of defects between right and left sides of the heart (paradoxical embolization). In a patient with diagnosed thrombus or high risk of thrombus formation, anticoagulant therapy is recommended.

Valvular disorders

Calcification of mitral or aortic annulus is an important cause of systemic embolism (Benjamin et al. 1992). This may be due to ulceration and extrusion of calcium or thrombus formation. Valvular disorders increase the risk of infective endocarditis, which is associated with a 30 per cent incidence of central nervous complications (Francioli 1991). Thrombi and endocarditis may also complicate prosthetic valves (see above). There is also evidence that mitral valve prolapse is associated with a risk of cardiogenic brain embolism, although the risk seems to be extremely low (Hanson et al. 1980).

Arrhythmias

Atrial fibrillation and sick sinus syndrome are associated with increased risk of embolization of cardiac origin. The SPAF study identified three risk factors for thromboembolism: recent congestive heart failure, history of hypertension, and previous thromboembolism (SPAF 1991). Anticoagulation therapy is indicated if any of the above risk factors are present in a patient with atrial fibrillation.

Cardiac embolism as the cause of brain embolism is underdiagnosed. This is due to lack of exact criteria for the diagnosis of cardiac embolism. In addition, diagnostic investigations have their limitations. Echocardiography—transthoracic and transoesophageal—has been found to be very useful in the detection of cardiac causes of systemic embolism. However, small particles capable of blocking major brain arteries can be beyond the resolution of echocardiography technology. In addition, after thromboembolization any residual thrombus may not be present until a new clot reforms. Finally, because most of the patients with ischaemic attacks are elderly, almost half of patients with potential cardiac embolism had moderate or severe stenoses proximal to brain infarct areas (Bogousslawsky et al. 1991).

The risk of an individual with a risk factor may be difficult to address, because it depends often on multiple factors, such as age and concomitant cardiac diseases. However, even in the absence of detection of a thrombus, anticoagulation should be considered in a patient with suspected cardiac embolism and the presence of strong predictors of stroke (see above). In addition, in the presence of a valvular disorder or a prosthetic valve, prophylaxis of infective endocarditis is recommended.

Evaluation of a patient with a suspicion of syncope of cardiac origin

The goal of the diagnostic evaluation is to identify the probable cause for the syncope in order to assess the risk for future events and death as well as determine further management of the patient. The following principles should be borne in mind when a patient with a history of syncope is evaluated.

The prognosis of a patient depends on the underlying cause of the syncope. The subgroup with highest risk for recurrence of syncope and mortality are patients with syncope of cardiac origin, particularly those with ventricular tachyarrhythmias and complete heart block. Cardiac origin of syncope occurs almost invariably in patients with some underlying heart disease. Most of these are acquired, but some are congenital. Thus, the clinical evaluation of the patient—obtaining of history, physical examination, and non-invasive and invasive investigations—is focused on identification of the possible cardiac disorder.

History

Historical information includes previous cardiac diagnoses and symptoms; a family history of arrhythmias, pacemaker therapy, syncope and sudden death; use of medications; symptoms preceding and following the syncope, such as palpitations, chest pain, and drowsiness; the relationship of syncope to exertion, micturition, and changes in the body position.

Physical examination

Physical examination is focused to detect cardiac abnormalities associated with obstructive syncope. This includes palpation of the chest, cardiac auscultation, and examination of arterial pulse (carotid pulse).

Laboratory examinations

A 12–lead ECG may define the cause of syncope if the arrhythmia responsible for the syncope is present at the time of ECG recording. This is the case only rarely. However, certain findings may raise the suspicion of a specific diagnosis. Q waves are indicative of prior myocardial infarction or the ECG recording may reveal left ventricular hypertrophy, both suggestive of ventricular tachyarrhythmia as the mechanism of syncope. Sinus bradycardia, AV conduction defects, or bifascicular block raise the possibility of bradycardia-mediated syncope. Pre-excitation of QRS complexes and prolonged QT interval lead to the suspicion of tachycardia as the origin of syncope.

Serum sodium, potassium, calcium, and magnesium screening is essential. In addition, haemoglobin and blood glucose readings, and when appropriate serum drug concentrations, are to be screened.

Non-invasive testing

Echocardiogram investigation is useful for the evaluation of ventricular function, estimation of pulmonary artery pressure, the status of cardiac valves, and prosthetic valves and for the detection of

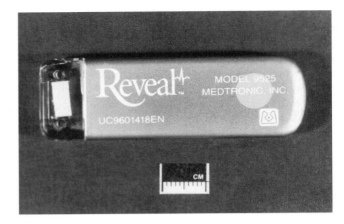

Fig. 46.12. An implantable loop recorder (ILR), positioned under the skin, can be kept implanted for several months, even years prior to battery exhaustion. The device analyses cardiac rhythms continuously and saves analysed data. The patients can also activate the device to store some raw electrocardiograms for subsequent retrieval. Initial experience in the evaluation of syncope are very encouraging.

aneurysms, congenital defects, aortic dissection, and risk factors of cardiac embolization.

Ambulatory 24–hour ECG recording may reveal bradyarrhythmias and tachyarrhythmias. Because causality of an arrhythmia and syncope is not always clear, and because syncope attacks are usually infrequent and unpredictable, it may be difficult to confirm the relationship between suspected arrhythmia and syncope despite repeated ambulatory ECG recordings. In one study, findings considered to be diagnostic were found only in 39 per cent of ambulatory ECG recordings performed for evaluation of syncope (Gibson and Heitzman 1984). In these cases an event recorder may be useful. It can be installed for several days or weeks and once the syncopal episode occurs, the recording is activated by the patient or by the arrhythmia. Recently, implantable loop recorders (ILR) have become available. They are small devices implanted subcutaneously for several months or even years (Fig. 46.12). They analyse cardiac rhythm continuously in their loop memory and when activated by the patient they can store raw ECG recordings for subsequent review.

The signal-averaged electrocardiogram is a computer-processed surface ECG to detect low-amplitude potentials at the end of the QRS complex. The presence of late potentials is suggestive of slow conduction in the ventricular myocardium and thus, a substrate for re-entrant arrhythmias. Absence of late potentials, on the other hand, predicts non-inducibility of monomorphic ventricular tachycardia in invasive electrophysiological study with an accuracy of 89–98 per cent (Winters *et al.* 1987), but is of no use in assessing the risk of arrhythmias of non-reentrant mechanisms.

Electrophysiological studies

Electrophysiological testing is the procedure of choice in patients with a high probability of an arrhythmic cause of syncope that remains undiagnosed with non-invasive evaluation. A comprehensive electrophysiological test consists of assessment of sinus node function, atrioventricular conduction, and inducibility of supraventricular and ventricular arrhythmias.

In the evaluation of syncope, a positive electrophysiological study has been found in 12–70 per cent of patients with a history of unexplained syncope. This wide range indicates that the value of electrophysiological testing in the setting of syncope depends on the criteria used to select patients for the investigation. In general, electrophysiological testing is highly recommended for all patients with a history of syncope and organic heart disease if the non-invasive tests remain negative.

References

Behar, S., Tanne, D., Abinader, E. *et al.* The SPRINT study group (1991). Cerebrovascular accident complicating acute myocardial infarction: Incidence, clinical significnce and short- and long-term mortality rates. *Am. J. Med.* **91**, 45–50.

Benjamin, E. J., Plehn, J. F., D'Agostino, R. B. *et al.* (1992). Mitral annular calcification and the risk of stroke in and elderly cohort. *New Engl. J. Med.* **327**, 374–9.

Bogousslawsky, J., Cachin, C., Regli, F., Despland, P. A., Van Melle, G., and Kappenberger, L. (1991). Cardiac sources of embolism and cerebral infarction – clinical consequences and vascular concomitants: The Lausanne Stroke Registry. *Neurology* **41**, 855–9.

Day, S. C., Cook, E. F., Funkenstein, H. and Goldman, L. (1982). Evaluation and outcome of emergency room patients with transient loss of consciousness. *Am. J. Med.* **73**, 15–23.

DeSanctis, R. W., Doroghazi, R. M., Austen, W. G. and Buckley, M. J. (1987). Aortic dissection. *New Engl. J. Med.* **317**, 1060–7.

Ector, H., Rolies, L., and De Geest, H. (1983). Dynamic electrocardiography and ventricular pauses of 3 seconds and more: etiology and therapeutic implications. *PACE* **6**, 548–51.

Fananapazir, L., Chang, A. C., Epstein, S. E., and McArevey, D. (1992). Prognostic determinants in hypertrophic cardiomyopathy. Prospective evaluation of a therapeutic strategy based on clinical, Holter, hemodynamic, and electrophysiological findings. *Circulation* **86**, 730–40.

Fananapazir, L., Tracy, C. M., Leon, M. B. *et al.* (1989). Electrophysiologic abnormalities in patients with hypertrophic cardiomyopathy. A consecutive analysis in 155 patients. *Circulation* 1259–68.

Francioli, P. (1991) Central nervous system complications of infective endocarditis. In *Infections of the central nervous system*, (ed. W. M. Scheld, R. J., Whitley, and D. T. Durack) p. 515. Raven Press, New York.

Frenneaux, M. P., Counihan, P. J., Caforio, A. L. P, Chikamori, T. and McKenna, W. J. (1990). Abnormal blood pressure response during exercise in hypertrophic cardiomyopathy. *Circulation* **82**, 1995–2002.

Fuster, V., Steele, P. M., Edwards, W. D., Gersh B. J., McGoon, M. D., and Frye, R. L. (1984). Primary pulmonary hypertension: Natural history and the importance of thrombosis. *Circulation* **70**, 580–7.

Gibson, J. C. and Heitzman, M. R. (1984). Diagnostic efficacy of 24–hour electrocardiographic monitoring for syncope. *Am. J. Cardiol.* **53**, 1013–17.

Grech E. D. and Ramsdale, D. R. (1991). Exertional syncope in aortic stenosis. *Am Heart J.* **121**, 603–6.

Guntheroth, W. G., Morgan, B. C., and Mullins, G. L. (1965). Physiologic studies of paroxysmal hyperpnea in cyanotic congenital heart disease. *Circulation* **31**, 70–6.

Hanson, M. R., Conomy, J. P., and Hodgman, J.R. (1980). Brain events associated with mitral valve prolapse. *Stroke* **11**, 499–506.

Hartikainen, J. E., Malik, M., Staunton, A., Poloniecki, J., Camm, A. J. (1996). Distinction between arrhythmic and nonarrhythmic death after acute myocardial infarction based on heart rate variability, signal-averaged electrocardiogram, ventricular arrhythmias and left ventricular ejection fraction. *J. Am. Coll. Cardiol.* **28**, 296–304.

Hilgard, J., Ezri, M. D., and Denes, P. (1985). Significance of ventricular pauses of three seconds or more detected on twenty-four hour Holter recordings. *Am. J. Cardiol.* **55**, 1005–8.

Jiang, C., Atkinson, D., Towbin, J. A. *et al.* (1994). Two long QT syndrome loci map to chromosomes 3 and 7 with the evidence for further heterogeneity. *Nature Genet.* **8**, 141–7.

Kapoor, W. N, Cha, R., Peterson, J. R., Wieand, H. S., and Karpf, M. (1987). Prolonged electrocardiographic monitoring in patients with syncope. *Am. J. Med.* **82**, 20–8.

Kapoor, W., Karpf, M., Wilband, H. S., Peterson, J., and Levey, G. (1983). A prospective evaluation and follow-up of patients with syncope. *New Engl. J. Med.* **309**, 197–204.

Kaul, U., Dev, V., Narula, J., Malhotra, A. K., Talwar, K. K., and Bahatia, M. L. (1988). Evaluation of patients with bundle branch block and 'unexplained' syncope: A study based on comprehensive electrophysiologic testing and ajmaline stress. *PACE* **11**, 289–97.

Keating, M. T., Atkinson, D., Dunn, C., Timothy, K., Vincent, G. M., and Leppert, M. (1991). Linkage of a cardiac arrhythmia, the long QT syndrome, and the Harvey ras-1 gene. *Science* **252**, 704–6.

Levis, R. P., Budoulas, H., Schaal, S. F., and Weissler, A. M. (1994). Diagnosis and management of syncope. In *Hurst's The Heart: arteries and veins*. (8th edn), (ed. R. C. Schlant and R. W Alexander), p. 928. McGraw-Hill, New York.

Lipsitz, L. A., Pluchino, F. C., Wei, J. Y. and Rowe, J. W. (1986). Syncope in institutionalized elderly: The impact of multiple pathological conditions and situational stress. *J. Chron. Dis.* **39**, 619–30.

Maron, B. J., Shirani, J., Poliac, L. C., Mathenge, R., Roberts, W. C., and Mueller, F. O. (1996). Sudden death in young competitive athletes. Clinical, demographic, and pathological profiles. *J. Am. Med. Ass.* **276**, 199–204.

Mazuz, M. and Friedman, H. S. (1983) Significance of prolonged electrocardiographic pauses in sinoatrial disease: Sick sinus syndrome. *Am. J. Cardiol.* **52**, 485–9.

Mitcell, S. C., Korones, S. B., and Berebdes, H. W. (1971). Congenital heart disease in 56,109 births. Incidence and natural history. *Circulation* **43**, 323–32.

Mody M. R. (1975). The natural history of uncomplicated valvular pulmonic stenosis. *Am. Heart J.* **90**, 317–21.

Moller, M. and Arnsbo, P. for the Danish Pacemaker Register (1996). Appraisal of pacing lead performance from the Danish Pacemaker Register. *PACE* **19**, 1327–36.

Moss, A. J., Hall, J. H., Cannom, D. S. *et al.* for the Multicenter Automatic Debibrillator Implantation Trial Investigators. (1996). *New Engl. J. Med.* **335**, 1933–40.

Naegeli, B., Osward, S., Deola, M., and Burkart, F. (1996). Intermittent pacemaker dysfunction caused by digital mobile telephones. *J. Am. Coll. Cardiol.* **27**, 1471–7.

National Institute of Health (1997) News Release, 14 April.

Rahimtoola, S. H., Zipes, D. P., Akhtar, M. *et al.* (1987). Consensus statement of the conference on the state of the art of electrophysiologic testing in the diagnosis and treatment of patients with cardiac arrhythmias. *Circulation* **75**, 1113–11.

Raynen K. (1995). Cardiac myxomas. *New Engl. J. Med.* **333**, 1610–17.

Ross J. Jr and Braunwald, E. and (1968). Aortic stenosis. *Circulation* **38**, (Suppl. 5), 61–7.

Savage, D. D., Corwin, L., McGee, D. L., Kannell, W. B., and Wolfe, P. A. (1985). Epidemiologic features of isolated syncope: the Framingman study. *Stroke* **16**, 626–9.

Schlepper, M., Nauzner, J., and Pitschner, H. (1995). Implantable cardioverter defibrillator: effect on survival. *PACE* **18**, 569–78.

Schott, J. J., Charpentier, F., Peltier, S. *et al.* (1995). Mapping of a gene for long QT syndrome to chromosome 4q25–27. *Am. J. Hum. Genet.* **57**, 1114–22.

Schwartz, P. J. (1985). Idiopathic long QT syndrome: progress and questions. *Am. Heart J.* **109**, 399–411.

Shaw, D. B., Linker, N. J., Heaver, P. A., and Evans, R. (1987). Chronic sinoatrial disorder (sick sinus syndrome): a possible result of cardiac ischemia. *Br. Heart J.* **58**, 598–607.

Shenasa, M., Borgreffe, M., Haverkamp, W., Hindricks, G., and Breithard, G. (1993). Ventricular tachycardia. *Lancet* **34**, 1512–19.

Short, D. S. (1954). The syndrome of alternating bradycardia and
    tachycardia. *Br. Heart J.* **16**, 208–15.

SPAF (Stroke Prevention in Atrial Fibrillation) Investigators (1991). The
    stroke prevention in atrial fibrillation trial: Final results. *Circulation* **84**,
    527–39.

Thames, M. D., Alpert, J. S., and DaLen, J. E. (1969). Syncope in patients
    with pulmonary embolism. *J. Am. Med. Ass.* **238**, 2509–11.

Viitasalo, M. T., Kala, R., and Eisalo, A. (1982). Ambulatory
    electrocardiographic recording in endurance athletes. *Br. Heart J.* **47**,
    213–20.

Winters, S. L., Steward, D., and Gones, J. A. (1987). Signal averaging of the
    surface QRS complex predicts inducibility of ventricular tachycardia in
    patients with syncope of unknown origin: a prospective study. *J. Am. Coll.
    Cardiol* **10**, 775–81.

47. Shock and its management

John Ludbrook

Introduction

One of the more difficult tasks in writing on the subject of shock is to define that word. What do the many clinical conditions that will be discussed, and which are summarized in Table 47.1, have in common? From the haemodynamic point of view, many are associated with an abnormally low cardiac output and all with a low arterial pressure. All are life-threatening, some immediately, others only in the longer term. However, it is the origins of the low blood pressure state of shock that are important, not the low blood pressure itself. Unless these are identified in individual patients, therapy is likely to be misdirected or even dangerous.

A classification of shock states

A conventional, very broad, and not necessarily all-inclusive, classification is given in Table 47.1. Its strength is that it focuses on causation. Its weaknesses are that in clinical practice the cause of shock in an individual patient may not be immediately obvious, and the division into mutually exclusive categories is somewhat artificial. More often than not, the origins of an individual patient's state of shock are multifactorial. For example, sepsis and hypovolaemia often coexist, so-called cardiogenic shock is as likely to originate from nocuous reflexes as from failure of the cardiac pump, and anaphylactic shock and envenomation are often indistinguishable.

The involvement of the autonomic nervous system in the shock states listed in Table 47.1 is variable. It is very direct in the cases of hypovolaemic and some causes of cardiogenic shock. But even in shock states in which hypotension is a terminal feature, hypotension always indicates a failure of the autonomic reflex control mechanisms to maintain blood pressure.

Table 47.1. A classification of shock states according to origins

- Hypovolaemic
- Septic
- Cardiogenic
- Neurogenic
- Heat stroke
- Anaphylactic
- Venoms
- Poisons

Shock states: causes and management

Acute hypovolaemia

The three most common causes of acute reduction in blood volume are acute blood loss, acute plasma loss, and depletion of extracellular fluid volume. There are also circumstances in which central blood volume is reduced rather than blood volume as a whole, as in prolonged standing or foot-down tilting, crucifixion, exposure to increased gravity, and application of negative pressure to the lower body.

Acute blood loss

There may be external haemorrhage, due to accidental or deliberate wounding with a sharp instrument or firearm. Or the haemorrhage may be internal and concealed, as with spontaneous rupture of an arterial aneurysm or damage to a major artery from a fractured bone.

When humans are bled under controlled conditions in the laboratory, or when an acute reduction of central blood volume is produced by foot-down tilting or the application of lower-body negative pressure (LBNP), there is a clear-cut biphasic haemodynamic response. This was first reported by Barcroft and his colleagues during the Second World War when they subjected human volunteers to venesection of a litre or more of blood (Barcroft *et al.* 1944) (Fig. 47.1), and has been repeatedly confirmed in human volunteers by venesection, foot-down tilting and LBNP (Ludbrook 1993). A similar biphasic response has been described in all laboratory mammals that have been studied unanaesthetized (dogs, sheep, swine, rabbits, rats) (Schadt and Lumbrook 1991). In Phase I, *pari passu* with a progressive fall in central blood volume and cardiac output there is progressive systemic vasoconstriction so that arterial blood pressure is well maintained. Animal experiments have demonstrated that the systemic vasoconstriction is accounted for almost exclusively by an increase in sympathetic vasoconstrictor drive as a reflex effect of unloading the arterial baroreceptors (Schadt and Ludbrook 1991). In humans, it has been suggested that the reflex effects of unloading cardiac or cardiopulmonary receptors may also make a contribution, though the evidence is indirect and inconclusive (Ludbrook 1993). The unloading of arterial baroreceptors also causes a progressive rise in heart rate, though this appears to contribute little to the maintenance of cardiac output or blood pressure because pharmacological blockade of cardiac nerves has little effect on these variables. When blood volume has fallen by 20–35 per cent, or cardiac output by 40–50 per cent, a second phase abruptly supervenes. At the onset of this Phase II, sympathetic vasoconstrictor drive vanishes

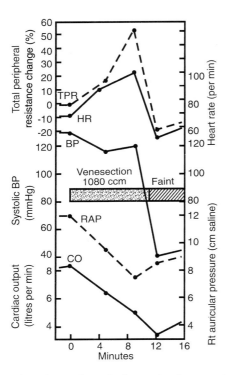

Fig. 47.1. Biphasic haemodynamic changes in a human volunteer during a venesection of 1080 ml. RAP, right atrial pressure; CO, cardiac output; BP, systolic blood pressure; TPR, calculated total peripheral resistance; HR, heart rate. (Redrawn from Barcroft *et al.* (1944).)

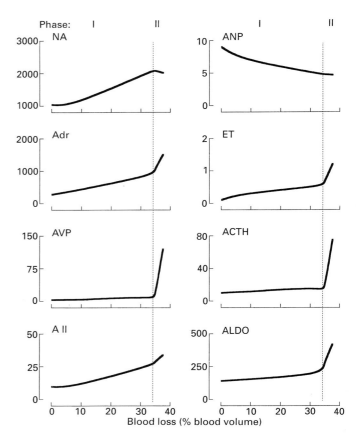

Fig. 47.2. Biphasic changes of plasma concentrations of hormones during progressive central hypovolaemia in humans. NA, noradrenaline; Adr, adrenaline; AVP, arginine vasopressin; AII, angiotensin II; ANP, atrial natriuretic peptide; ET, endothelin; ACTH, adrenocorticotrophic hormone; ALDO, aldosterone. All units in pg/l. (From Ludbrook (1993).)

abruptly and arterial blood pressure falls to very low levels (Fig. 47.1). In humans, there is also a marked vagal bradycardia, though this is not so prominent in laboratory animals. The origin of the dramatic changes of Phase II is still not clear. Barcroft and his colleagues (1944) suggested they might be due to a reflex emanating from the empty heart. From animal experiments, there has been a good deal of support for the notion that Phase II is precipitated by a sudden afferent input from cardiac vagal C-fibre afferents although animal experiments also suggest that inputs from other afferents may contribute.

There are also characteristic humoral responses to acute central hypovolaemia (Fig. 47.2). During Phase I, there is a steady increase in plasma noradrenaline concentration, as would be expected from the great increase in sympathetic drive, and there are slow and parallel increases in plasma renin activity and angiotensin II (AII) concentration. From the onset of Phase II, there is a steep rise in the plasma concentrations of arginine vasopressin (AVP), adrenocorticotrophic hormone (ACTH), aldosterone, and adrenaline. However, the plasma concentration of noradrenaline takes a downturn as sympathetic vasoconstrictor drive is cut off.

In summary, the short-term, biphasic, haemodynamic and humoral changes that occur with acute reduction in central blood volume are neural in origin. The initial, baroreflex-mediated, compensatory, systemic vasoconstriction maintains blood pressure during Phase I. But if central hypovolaemia progresses, there is obliteration of the arterial baroreflex because of a vasodepressor afferent input, perhaps from the heart. The central integration of these neural mechanisms takes place chiefly in the brainstem, although there is evidence

of contributions from higher centres such as the periaqueductal grey matter, the hypothalamus, and even the cerebral cortex. This last may tie in with the close resemblance between the events of acute hypovolaemia and those of emotional syncope (see Chapter 44).

The neural pathways and neurotransmitters in the brainstem and spinal cord concerned with the arterial baroreflex, and therefore Phase I of acute hypovolaemia, have been the subject of intense investigation, and are now beginning to be worked out (Dampney 1994). A good deal of work has also been done on the central nervous mechanisms of Phase II. Early on, an opioid-receptor mechanism was postulated (Schadt and Ludbrook 1991). This postulate has been confirmed and extended, so that it now seems that Phase II is dependent on a brainstem opioid receptor mechanism, probably a δ-receptor, and possibly of the δ_1-subtype (Ludbrook and Ventura 1994). There is thus the prospect that a specific δ_1-receptor antagonist could be used prophylactically or therapeutically to prevent or reverse Phase II without blunting the pain-relieving effects of morphine, provided the δ_1-antagonist could cross the blood–brain barrier (and this has not yet been demonstrated). However, the story has become progressively more complicated. For instance, there is evidence that μ-agonists such as morphine can prevent the occurrence of Phase II. There is also evidence that intravenous ACTH can act within the

Table 47.2. Blood volume expanders for the emergency treatment of acute hypovolaemia; 1898–1997

Era	Blood volume expander
Spanish-American War (1898)	Subcutaneous or rectal saline
Pre-First World War	Intravenous physiological saline, direct blood transfusion
First World War (1914–18)	Fresh citrated blood, gum acacia solution
Spanish Civil War (1936–39)	Citrated bank blood
Second World War (1939–45)	Large-pool citrated plasma, concentrated albumin
Korean War (1950–53)	Unmatched O-negative blood, citrated small-pool plamsa
1950–55	Polyvinyl pyrrolidone (PVP)
1950 to present	Modified gelatin solutions Hydroxyethyl starch solutions Dextran solutions (varying molecular weights)
1970 to present	Liquid or lyophilized 5% human albumin (pasteurized) Plasma protein solution (PPS) (pasteurized)
1970 to 1990	'Balanced' electrolyte solutions (e.g. lactated Ringer's)
1980 to present	Hypertonic NaCl solution (7.5%) Hypertonic NaCl plus dextran solution (HSD)

brainstem to prevent Phase II (Ludbrook and Ventura 1995). ACTH also acts as a direct peripheral vasodilator, so the idea that large doses of ACTH (1–24) could be used as a first-aid measure in hypo-volaemic shock is an attractive one (Bertolini 1995), though no prospective clinical trial has yet been conducted.

The obvious therapy for acute blood loss is to arrest the bleeding and restore blood volume by transfusion. During this century, the popularity of various blood volume expanders has waxed and waned, the process having been dictated more often by military requirements and commercial pressures than by science (Table 47.2). In particular, there has been a search for optimal artificial solutions, colloid or crystal-loid, as substitutes for blood or blood products. This search was origi-nally prompted by the economics of supply and demand for blood and its products, but has intensified as the hazards of transmitting hepatitis and HIV infection have been recognized. The popular, semi-synthetic, colloid solutions are modified gelatin, hydroxyethyl starch and dextrans of various molecular weights. Currently, there is a great enthusiasm for administering small volumes of hypertonic saline, either on its own or in combination with dextran, as a first-aid measure. One strong impetus for this is the goal of developing a universal and standard resus-citatory protocol for military and civilian injuries, and there are obvious logistic advantages of such a regimen (small volumes, long shelf-life, low risk, low cost). The logic that underlies this approach is in part that hypertonic solutions can drag fluid into the bloodstream from both extravascular and intracellular compartments, and in part that associ-ated brain injury is likely to benefit from intravascular hypertonicity. Prospective clinical trials have been supportive of these strategies (Younes *et al.* 1992; Vassar *et al.* 1993). On the scientific front, it is worth noting that hypertonic solutions have the capacity to stimulate pul-monary C-fibre afferents and engage vasodepressor reflexes (Pisarri *et al.* 1991), and that hypertonic saline has actions within the CNS via the circumventricular organs which may in part account for its beneficial effects (Hjelmqvist *et al.* 1992).

The above discussion refers principally to the first-aid treatment of victims of mechanical trauma involving blood loss, in a civilian or

military setting. In the case of burns, the rate at which hypovolaemia and hypotension occur is slower, and the loss is not of whole blood but of plasma. The case for using albumin-containing solutions, at least in the medium term, is therefore much stronger. In cases of shock due to profound salt and water depletion, the obvious therapy is salt and water replacement.

It is clear that prevention or rapid reversal of the hypotensive Phase II of acute central hypovolaemia is potentially important. But what if the degree of central hypovolaemia responsible for Phase II should persist? Provided blood loss is arrested, movement of fluid from the extravascular to the vascular compartment can partially restore central blood volume. But if central blood volume is not restored, does the sympathoinhibition of Phase II persist? For obvious reasons there is not much evidence on this point from human studies, though it is worth noting that death from crucifixion was too pro-longed to be accounted for by persistent sympathoinhibition. In our laboratory, we have shown that in conscious rabbits in which Phase II has occurred, even if cardiac output and central blood volume are held low there is recovery of systemic vascular resistance within a few minutes. But we do not yet know whether this is due to recovery of sympathetic vasoconstrictor drive, perhaps from a central action of the massive output of AII and ACTH, or to the direct vasoconstrictor actions of vasoactive hormones such as AVP or AII (Fig. 47.2).

In the 1950s, the term 'irreversible shock' was coined. This referred to rather crude experiments in laboratory animals (usually dogs) which showed that if blood volume was held at a low level for some hours, then retransfusion did not prevent death. At autopsy, there was evidence of disseminated intravascular coagulation (DIC) and damage to many organs. Fine (1965) proposed that these changes were due to absorption of bacterial endotoxins, though many of his contempor-aries criticized his evidence. Nowadays, death from 'pure' hypo-volaemia (other than by instant exsanguination) almost never occurs. But one wonders whether Fine was right, after all, and that late death from an episode of prolonged hypovolaemia may be contributed to by Gram-negative endotoxaemia and its consequences (see below).

Septic shock

The convention of categorizing septic shock according to whether the micro-organism responsible is Gram-negative or Gram-positive will be followed, although the pathophysiological basis of the two forms is similar.

Gram-negative bacteraemia or septicaemia

Bacteraemia, without an overt preceding infection, can occur after endoscopy of the urinary or biliary tracts; from a chronically placed intravascular catheter, especially in patients whose immune defences are compromised because of immunosuppressive therapy for organ transplantation or chemotherapy for cancer; and, rarely, from infusion of infected blood. If there is preceding infection, it is usually in the form of peritonitis or intraperitoneal abscesses resulting from spontaneous or traumatic perforation of a hollow viscus, especially the large intestine; infection of the biliary tree, especially with consequent intraperitoneal or intrahepatic abscesses; and pyonephrosis, especially in association with urinary calculous disease. The micro-organisms responsible are commonly a mixture of members of the *Escherichia*, *Aerobacter*, *Klebsiella*, *Proteus*, or *Pseudomonas* groups, though sometimes there is a primary infection with, for instance, the resurgent *Neisseria meningitidis*. The toxic agent is the endotoxin released by Gram-negative organisms, especially its lipopolysaccharide A moiety. The mortality rate in cases of Gram-negative septic shock is about 50 per cent, and hospital deaths from this condition are steadily increasing, partly because of the efficiency of intensive care units in keeping seriously ill patients alive, and partly because of the increasing use of immunosuppressive agents and anticancer chemotherapy (Parrillo 1993). To make matters more complicated, the effects of the endotoxaemia are often confounded by the hypovolaemia, fluid and electrolyte disturbances, and respiratory abnormalities that are so often found in this class of patient. The 'pure' effects of endotoxin have been studied, in small doses in human volunteers and in lethal or sublethal doses in subhuman primates (Ludbrook 1993). The initial responses include fever, high cardiac output, widespread systemic vasodilatation, and hypotension. The fever is attributable to the release of endogenous pyrogens. The hyperdynamic cardiovascular responses can be explained by the induction of nitric oxide synthase (NOS) and the effects of NO on vascular smooth muscle, so that blood flow and conductance are increased in almost every vascular bed (Meyer *et al.* 1994). With high dose or continuing infusion of endotoxin, more sinister changes occur. These include lactacidaemia, disseminated intravascular coagulation (DIC), multiple organ failure (especially hepatic and renal failure), adult respiratory distress syndrome (ARDS), and mental confusion.

The mainstays of therapy have been antibiotics, restoration of blood volume, and surgical drainage of abscesses with alimentary tract diversion if indicated. Until recently, the administration of massive doses of corticosteroids was popular. This empirical treatment has finally been abandoned because no benefit was demonstrated in three large, prospective, clinical trials (Ludbrook 1992; Parrillo 1993). It is still currently popular to administer positive inotropic agents such as dopamine, in the belief that there is toxic damage to the myocardium. However, though there is experimental and clinical evidence that endotoxaemia can cause myocardial dysfunction, it seems unlikely to be an important cause of death. For instance, in patients with septic shock in whom cardiac filling pressure is maintained at normal or supranormal levels, cardiac output remains normal or high until death (Ludbrook 1992).

It is now clear that one of the principal targets of the Gram-negative endotoxin is the macrophage, and that most of the features of Gram-negative septic shock can be accounted for by the release of a cascade of cytokines from macrophages, other cells of the immune system, and vascular endothelial cells (Fig. 47.3). Cytokines thought to be important in septic shock are tumour necrosis factor (TNF-α), interleukin-1 (IL-1), γ-interferon (γ-IFN), interleukin 6 (IL-6), and platelet aggregating factor (PAF). Identification of these factors has led to a surge of scientific and commercial enthusiasm for developing anti cytokine agents for prophylaxis against, or treatment for, septic shock. These include monoclonal antibodies directed against lipoprotein A or cytokines, specific cytokine receptor antagonists, and the administration of soluble, cloned receptors in an attempt to mop up

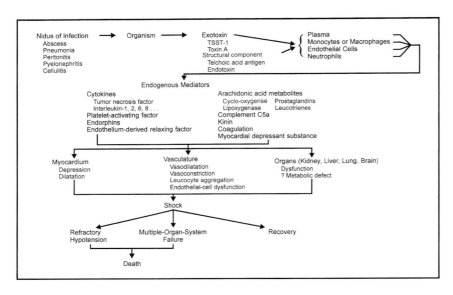

Fig. 47.3. Postulated sequence of events in septic shock. TSST-1, toxic shock toxin 1; Toxin A, Pseudomonas aeruginosa toxin A. (Redrawn from Parrillo (1993).)

the nocuous receptor ligands. Another strategy has been to enhance the resistance to infection of immunosuppressed patients by administering colony stimulating factors (CSF). But though the results of animal experiments with these new agents have sometimes been promising, those of prospective clinical trials have been either negative or equivocal (Ludbrook 1992; Parrillo 1993). Even in laboratory animals, those agents that have conferred benefit have done so only if administered before septic shock has occurred. There is some scientific and commercial optimism (though whether it will turn out to be true or false is problematic), that combinations of anti cytokines agents may be effective.

Attention has already been drawn to the role of NO in the hyperdynamic changes of endotoxaemia or severe sepsis. In conscious sheep infused with endotoxin (Meyer *et al.* 1994), and in patients with severe sepsis (Petros *et al.* 1994), administration of a NOS inhibitor brings down the high cardiac output, reduces the high regional and systemic vascular conductances, and restores arterial pressure. However, it is yet to be demonstrated that NOS inhibition will increase patient survival.

Another mediator that may contribute to the inflammatory response in severe infection is bradykinin. However, a prospective, double-blind, multicentre clinical trial of a competitive antagonist of the B$_2$ subclass of bradykinin receptors showed no overall beneficial effects on survival except in one subgroup of patients at the highest dose (Fein *et al.* 1997).

Gram-positive toxaemia

In the late 1970s a new clinical condition was recognized commonly known as the toxic shock syndrome (TSS). This chiefly affected healthy young women, and was ultimately traced to the use of vaginal tampons that had been forgotten and which had, *propter hoc* or *post hoc*, been infected by *Staphylococcus aureus* so that a toxic shock syndrome toxin 1 (TSST-1) entered the bloodstream. The haemodynamic and pathological effects of TSST-1 are very similar to those of Gram-negative endotoxin, especially in triggering the cytokine cascade and in inducing NO synthase (Zembowicz and Vane 1992), though with the additional clinical features of skin reddening and desquamation. The management of this condition is similar in principle to that of Gram-negative toxic shock: a search for and removal of the source of infection, appropriate antibiotics, and maintenance of blood volume.

Cardiogenic shock

This topic is given little space because it has already been covered in Chapter 46. The origins of cardiogenic shock can be divided into primary failure of the cardiac pump, secondary failure of the pump, and nocuous reflexes originating from cardiac receptors. There is also a condition of pseudocardiogenic shock.

Primary failure of the cardiac pump

The common sources of this are gross myocardial damage. This usually takes the form of massive myocardial infarction resulting from acute coronary artery occlusion on an atherosclerotic basis or, rarely, on aortic dissection in association with Marfan's syndrome. Occasionally, life-threatening myocardial damage can occur from envenomation, toxic drugs, or myocarditis.

Secondary failure of the cardiac pump

There are several other reasons why the heart may be unable to maintain a level of output which is compatible with life. These include cardiac tamponade (especially from haemorrhage into the pericardial sac), and sudden cardiac arrhythmias (especially ventricular tachycardia or fibrillation).

Cardiogenic reflexes

These have been discussed in detail by Hainsworth (1991). In brief, infarction of the left ventricle or obstruction to aortic outflow can excite vagal cardiac C-fibre afferents and result in reflex vasodepression and bradycardia with profound hypotension.

Pseudocardiogenic shock

One cannot resist the temptation to mention this unmentionable topic. Inexperienced surgeons have often been misled by the statement of a cardiologist that the cause of postoperative shock in a given patient is myocardial infarction. More often than not, the electrocardiographic changes which have led a cardiologist to make this diagnosis result from hypotension due to hypovolaemia—in other words, surgically correctable, concealed, postoperative bleeding.

Neurogenic shock

This topic is discussed in Chapters 44 and 45. In terms of physiology, it is a relatively clear-cut syndrome. Any physical lesion that divides or damages the central nervous system at or below the pontomedullary junction inevitably results in hypotension. This is because the final common pathway for sympathetic vasoconstrictor drive commences in the rostral ventrolateral medulla, specifically in the sub-retrofacial nucleus (Dampney 1994). The lower the lesion, the less the hypotension. Yet complete abolition of sympathetic vasoconstrictor drive, though inevitably resulting in postural hypotension, is not of itself lethal. For instance, massive doses of ganglion-blocking drugs have been administered to supine human volunteers with no untoward results, and the problem of postural hypotension is a relatively insignificant one in acute tetraplegia. The management of neurogenic shock requires little more than maintenance of the horizontal posture in the short term, and the control of postural hypotension in the longer term has been described in Chapter 36.

Heat stroke

The consequences of exposure to an excessively hot, and often humid, environment, especially during severe physical exercise, can result in death (Ludbrook 1993). Classical examples are marathons run by relatively untrained and inexperienced but enthusiastic subjects, and pilgrimages to Mecca undertaken by devout but unfit and unacclimatized subjects. The precipitating factor is hyperthermia. The lethal factor is unknown. Prodromal features are mental confusion and hyperthermia. The ante- and post-mortem syndromes include the above, plus lactacidaemia, evidence of disseminated intravascular coagulation (DIC), and more or less terminal hypotension. There is little doubt that the competition for a cardiac output which is approaching its maximum, which arises from the demands for increased skin blood flow required for thermoregulation and the demands for increased muscle blood flow required by exercising muscles, results in a diversion of blood flow away from non-exercising vascular beds. In particular, there is a marked reduction in blood flow to the gastrointestinal tract, so that the defences against entry of bacterial endotoxins into the bloodstream may be impaired.

This last prediction now seems to have been confirmed. In human subjects suffering from heat stroke, there is endotoxaemia and very high plasma concentrations of TNF-α and IL-1α, convincing evidence that Gram-negative endotoxin has entered the systemic circulation and has stimulated the cytokines cascade (Bouchama et al. 1991). This suggests that the hyperthermia may be contributed to by endogenous pyrogens as well as by heat-exposure, and that the life-threatening elements of heat stroke may result from endotoxaemia.

The mainstays of managing heat stroke are body cooling and replacement of salt and water loss. In view of the evidence of endotoxaemia, it might be prudent to administer an antibiotic effective against Gram-negative-organisms.

Anaphylactic shock

This scarcely falls within the ambit of this chapter, because although hypotension can be a feature of anaphylactic shock, the most immediate threat to life is usually respiratory obstruction. Anaphylaxis is an acute and dramatic phenomenon associated with re-exposure to a variety of allergens, ranging from penicillin to bee venom.

The reagins responsible for anaphylactic shock, members of the immunoglobulin E family, cause massive mast cell degranulation with release of potent agents such as histamine (and, in rodents, serotinin). In a classical case, there is rapidly developing oedema of the lips, tongue and other elements of the upper respiratory tract, and bronchoconstriction. Treatment consists of injecting a β-adrenoceptor agonist (classically, adrenaline), antihistamine drugs (H$_1$-antagonists), and perhaps oral corticosteroids.

Envenomation

Mammals, marsupials, snails, snakes, scorpions, spiders, ticks, ants, marine organisms, and even plants can muster an enormous range of potentially lethal venoms containing pharmacologically potent but often not clearly identified toxins. However, there are few, if any, that produce acute shock states in the sense of causing life-threatening hypotension as a primary rather than terminal, event. For the most part, the active ingredients of the venoms are neurotoxins that can produce respiratory paralysis, or substances that cause local skin necrosis (Hodgson 1997). However, a number of venoms are reported to cause prolonged hypotension. Among those of which the author is aware are the venoms of the Australian funnel-web spider (Atrax robustus), the blue-ringed octopus (Hapalochaena maculosa), the stonefish (genus Synanceja), the Japanese puffer fish (genus Sphaeroides), and poisonous marine snails (genus Conus). In each of these, the most prominent feature of massive envenomation is respiratory paralysis, due to blockade of sodium ion channels by tetrodotoxin, or of calcium channels by ω-conotoxin. However,

autonomic paralysis and hypotension seem to be late and relatively unimportant phenomena. Massive envenomation from the nematocysts of the multiple tentacles of the box jellyfish (sea wasp) (Chironex fleckeri) and related jellyfish of the cnidarian family can cause shock from massive skin oedema, respiratory obstruction, and, possibly, cardiotoxicity. These features are shared by anaphylactic shock.

Poisons and other toxins

There is an enormous variety of poisonous substances which, if ingested, injected, or inhaled, accidentally or deliberately, can cause rapid death. Several of these can affect the autonomic nervous system, notably anticholinesterases and sodium- or calcium-channel blockers. But there are few, if any, in which the cause of death is autonomic failure.

References

Barcroft, H., Edholm, O. G., McMichael, J., and Sharpey-Schafer, E. P. (1994). Lancet i, 489–91.

Bertolini, A. (1995). The opioid/anti-opioid balance in shock: a new target for therapy in resuscitation. Resuscitation 30, 29–42.

Bouchama, A., Parhar, R. S., El-Yazigi, A., Sheth, K., and Al-Sediary, S. (1991). Endotoxemia and release of tumor necrosis factor and interleukin 1α in acute heatstroke. J. Appl. Physiol. 70, 2640–4.

Dampney, R. A. L. (1994). Functional organization of central pathways regulating the cardiovascular system. Physiol. Rev. 74, 323–64.

Fein, A. M., Bernard, G. R., Criner, G. J. et al., for the CP-0127 SIRS and Sepsis Study Group (1997). Treatment of severe systemic inflammatory response syndrome and sepsis with a novel bradykinin antagonist Deltibant (CP-0127). J. Am. Med. Ass. 277, 482–7.

Fine, J. (1965). Shock and peripheral circulatory insufficiency. In Handbook of Physiology, Section 2, Vol. 3, (ed. W. F. Hamilton), pp. 2037–69. American Physiological Society, Bethesda.

Hainsworth, R. (1991). Reflexes from the heart. Physiol. Rev. 71, 617–58.

Hjelmqvist, H., Ullman, J., Gunnarson, U., Hamberger, R., and Rundgren, M. (1992). Increased resistance to haemorrhage induced by intracerebroventricular infusion of hypertonic NaCl in conscious sheep. Acta Physiol. Scand. 145, 177–86.

Hodgson, W. C. (1997). Pharmacological action of Australian animal venoms. Clin. Exp. Pharmacol. Physiol. 24, 10–17.

Ludbrook, J. (1992). New therapies for shock associated with gram-negative sepsis? Aust. N.Z. J. Surg. 62, 913–15.

Ludbrook, J. (1993). Haemorrhage and shock. In Cardiovascular reflex control in health and disease (ed. R. Hainsworth and A. L. Mark), pp. 463–490. W. B. Saunders, London.

Ludbrook, J. and Ventura, S. (1994). The decompensatory phase of acute hypovolaemia in rabbits involves a central δ_1-opioid receptor. Eur. J. Pharmacol. 252, 113–16.

Ludbrook, J. and Ventura, S. (1995). ACTH-(1-24) blocks the decompensatory phase of the haemodynamic response to acute hypovolaemia. Eur. J. Pharmacol. 275, 267–75.

Meyer, J., Hinder, F., Stothert, J. et al. (1994). Increased organ blood flow in chronic endotoxemia is reversed by nitric oxide synthase inhibition. J. Appl. Physiol. 76, 2785–93.

Parrillo, J. E. (1993). Pathogenetic mechanisms of septic shock. New Engl. J. Med. 328, 1471–7.

Petros, A., Lamb, G., Leone, A., Moncada, S., Bennett, D., and Vallance, P. (1994). Effects of a nitric oxide synthase inhibitor in humans with septic shock. Cardiovasc. Res. 28, 34–9.

Pisarri, T. E., Jonzon, A., Coleridge, H. M., and Coleridge, J. C. G. (1991). Intravenous injection of hypertonic NaCl solution stimulates pulmonary C-fibers in dogs. *Am. J. Physiol.* **260**, H1522–H1530.

Schadt, J. C. and Ludbrook, J. (1991) Hemodynamic and neurohumoral responses to acute hypovolaemia in conscious mammals. *Am. J. Physiol.* **260**, H305–H318.

Vassar, M. J., Fischer, R. P., O'Brien, P. E. *et al.* and the Multicenter Group for the Study of Hypertonic Saline in Trauma Patients (1993) *Arch. Surg.* **128**, 1003–13.

Younes R. N., Aun, f., Accioly, C. Q., Casale, L. P. L., Szajnbok, I., and Birolini, D. (1992). Hypertonic solutions in the treatment of hypovolaemic shock: a prospective, randomized study in patients admitted to the emergency room. *Surgery* **111**, 380–5.

Zembowicz, A. and Vane, J. R. (1992). Induction of nitric oxide synthase activity by toxic shock syndrome toxin 1 in a macrophage–monocyte cell line. *Proc. Nat. Acad. Sci. USA* **89**, 2051–5.

48. Sympathetic neural mechanisms in hypertension

Virend K. Somers and Krzysztof Narkiewicz

The sympathetic nervous system is an integral mechanism in the overall regulation of blood pressure. While sympathetic contributions to acute blood pressure increases are well established, the role of sympathetic activation in chronic hypertension is less clear-cut. This is due to several factors, including the heterogeneity of characteristics of essential hypertension, the evolution of the haemodynamics of hypertension from the 'early' to the 'established' phase, and the multiple other aetiological mechanisms that have been implicated in the genesis of hypertension. This chapter examines, firstly, the potential importance of the sympathetic nervous system in hypertension; secondly, the evidence that hypertension is accompanied by sympathetic activation; and thirdly, the mechanisms by which sympathetic activity may be increased in hypertension. The review focuses primarily on human hypertension. Emphasis is placed on more recent findings, particularly those involving microneurography, noradrenaline 'spillover', and studies examining central neural mechanisms in hypertension.

Potential importance of the sympathetic nervous system

That sympathetic activation, by way of tachycardia and vasoconstriction, should increase blood pressure, is self-evident. The sympathetic nervous system may also contribute to blood pressure levels in the long term by other mechanisms, by its effects on the kidney, on blood vessel growth and permeability, and via resetting of the arterial baroreflex.

First, increased renal efferent sympathetic traffic promotes sodium retention and renin release, in the absence of any effects on renal blood flow or glomerular filtration (DiBona 1992). Furthermore, while increases in arterial pressure promote natriuresis, even low levels of renal sympathetic activity attenuate the natriuretic response to an increase in arterial or renal perfusion pressure. This sympathetic-mediated shift in the pressure–natriuresis curve could favour the maintenance of hypertension by interfering with the ability of renal homeostatic mechanisms to compensate for an increase in blood pressure through pressure natriuresis.

Secondly, the sympathetic nervous system, like the renin–angiotensin system, promotes growth of vascular muscle. The effects of sympathetic activity on vascular growth are independent of haemodynamic effects. These trophic effects on blood vessels appear to be greatest during growth and development. This may be important because sympathetic overactivity appears to occur particularly during the early stages of hypertension, when it is most likely to influence the

structure of vessels and, thus, the long-term regulation of arterial pressure. Structural changes in blood vessels increase vascular resistance and the response to vasoconstrictor stimuli so that the effects of the sympathetic nervous system on vasomotor tone and vascular structures interact to increase vascular resistance and arterial pressure.

Thirdly, studies in spontaneously hypertensive rats suggest a role for the sympathetic nervous system in promoting abnormalities in vascular membrane permeability (Abel and Hermsmeyer 1981). The spontaneously hypertensive rat has an increase in passive permeability of vascular muscle to sodium, which results in augmented vasoconstrictor responsiveness to noradrenaline. This abnormality in membrane permeability appears to be related to a genetically determined trophic influence of the sympathetic nervous system. Thus, genetically determined sympathetic influences acting during development may cause long-term alterations in membrane properties that could contribute to hypertension.

Fourthly, sustained sympathetic-induced increases in blood pressure may contribute to baroreflex resetting. Increases in arterial pressure activate baroreceptors located in the carotid sinuses and aortic arch, triggering reflex inhibition of sympathetic activity, causing vasodilation and bradycardia which oppose the rise in pressure. An important mechanism that allows sympathetic and arterial pressure to increase is baroreflex resetting (Chapleau and Abboud 1993). Baroreflex resetting refers to a shift in the relationship between blood pressure changes and the efferent autonomic response (e.g. sympathetic nerve activity or heart rate). Sustained increases in pressure cause a resetting of the operating point of the reflex to a higher level of pressure, i.e. the baroreflex loses much of its ability to buffer the rise in pressure and actually functions to maintain pressure at the higher level. Hypertension-induced resetting of the baroreflex may be caused by both 'baroreceptor resetting' (shift in pressure–afferent baroreflex activity relationship) and by 'central resetting' (shift in afferent baroreflex–efferent autonomic relationship) (Chapleau and Abboud 1993). Thus sympathetic-mediated pressor responses, for example in situations of environmental stress, may, by resetting of the arterial baroreflexes, allow the development of higher long-term blood pressure levels.

Evidence for sympathetic hyperactivity in hypertension
Essential hypertension

Many studies have evaluated sympathetic activity in human hypertension using measurements of plasma catecholamine levels and responses to adrenergic antagonists. Goldstein (1983) reviewed studies of plasma catecholamine levels in patients with essential hypertension and in normotensive controls, and concluded that most studies demonstrated elevated plasma noradrenaline levels in young hypertensive patients.

Using adrenergic blocking agents to probe the role of the sympathetic nervous system, Julius and Esler (1975) found that the elevated heart rates and stroke volumes of young, mildly hypertensive patients returned to normal after autonomic blockade. Egan et al. (1987) subsequently combined measurements of plasma catecholamines and responses to adrenergic antagonists and agonists in mildly hypertensive humans. These investigators found that mildly hypertensive individuals had elevated plasma noradrenaline levels, augmented decreases in vascular resistance in response to α-adrenergic blockade, and no increase in α-receptor sensitivity as assessed by responses to noradrenaline. Their study demonstrated that young, mildly hypertensive humans have augmented sympathetic vasoconstrictor activity and strongly suggested that this increase in sympathetic vasoconstriction results from increased sympathetic neural release of noradrenaline and not from augmented α-adrenergic response to the neurotransmitter.

There is increasing evidence that hypertension, in particular 'early' hypertension, may be characterized by increased sympathetic traffic not only to the heart and blood vessels, but also to the kidneys. The sympathetic nervous system has the capacity for selective increases in efferent discharge to different subdivisions. Wallin et al. (1996) have recently demonstrated, however, that in healthy human subjects, resting sympathetic nerve traffic is similar, or proportional, in sympathetic nerves to both muscle blood vessels and the kidney.

There is evidence of uniformity of sympathetic activation to the heart and kidney in early hypertension. Using measurements of noradrenaline spillover, Esler et al. (1989) found that noradrenaline was elevated in hypertensive patients, particularly in young hypertensives, and that the increased spillover emanated mainly from the heart and kidneys. These observations may help explain the haemodynamic profile of the 'hyperdynamic circulation' of early human hypertension, which is characterized by increased heart rate, cardiac output, and renal vasoconstriction.

There is also functional evidence for heightened sympathetic neural influences on the kidney in essential hypertension (Oparil 1986). Renal vascular resistance is increased in essential hypertension. This renal vasoconstriction appears to be mediated, at least in part, by the sympathetic nervous system. α-Adrenergic blockade with phentolamine increases renal blood flow and reverses renal angiographic abnormalities in patients with essential hypertension but has no effect on renal blood flow in sodium-replete, normal individuals. Splanchnic neural blockade increases renal blood flow in patients with essential hypertension but not in normotensive controls. Since renal vascular responses to intravenous noradrenaline are normal in patients with essential hypertension, these findings suggest that increased renal vascular resistance in essential hypertension is mediated, in part, by increased activity of the renal sympathetic nerves.

Microneurographic recordings of resting sympathetic nerve activity to muscle blood vessels in humans have provided conflicting evidence for increased sympathetic neural activity in human essential hypertension. In early studies, Wallin and Sundlof (1979) reported no increase in muscle sympathetic nerve activity in hypertensive versus normotensive individuals after accounting for age (sympa-

thetic nerve activity increases with age). Several other authors (Somers et al. 1988, Rea and Hamdan 1990) also did not detect elevated resting muscle sympathetic nerve activity in hypertensive humans. In contrast, other studies have found an increased level of resting muscle sympathetic nerve activity in humans with essential hypertension (Anderson et al. 1989; Miyajima et al. 1991). For example, Anderson et al. (1989) found an increased level of muscle sympathetic nerve activity in young, mildly hypertensive men. A high-salt diet reduced muscle sympathetic nerve activity in both groups, but on both low-salt and high-salt diets, sympathetic nerve activity was higher in the mildly hypertensive group than in the normotensive group.

In a study of patients with accelerated hypertension, Matsukawa et al. (1993) have shown an increase in muscle sympathetic nerve activity, compared to patients with benign hypertension. This increase appeared to be closely related to activation of the renin–angiotensin system. In these patients, who had diastolic blood pressures of greater than 130 mmHg, accompanied by retinal changes, treatment with angiotensin-converting enzyme inhibitors lowered blood pressure and decreased muscle sympathetic activity. Thus, interactions between the renin–angiotensin system and the sympathetic nervous system may be implicated in the rapid progression of hypertension severity.

The explanation for the finding of high levels of resting muscle sympathetic nerve activity in hypertensives in some, but not all, studies is not clear, but several factors may be pertinent. The first is sodium intake, which has a profound influence on sympathetic nerve activity. Grassi and colleagues (1997) suggested that sodium restriction not only increases resting sympathetic activity, but may also impair baroreflex sensitivity in hypertension. Secondly, obesity may contribute to increased sympathetic neural activity by promoting insulin resistance and hyperinsulinaemia. The third factor is a buffering influence of cardiopulmonary baroreceptors. Rea and Hamdan (1990) suggested that elevated levels of sympathetic neural drive in human mild hypertensives may be partially masked in the supine position because of a heightened sympathetic-inhibitory influence originating in cardiopulmonary baroreceptors.

In summary, neurochemical, neurophysiological, and haemodynamic studies indicate heightened sympathetic neural activity in human essential hypertension. This is particularly notable in young, mildly hypertensive humans and may contribute to the haemodynamic profile of early human hypertension and, perhaps, to the development of structural vascular changes. The heightened sympathetic drive also appears to involve the kidney and could thereby contribute to long-term elevation of arterial pressure and to accelerated hypertension.

Secondary hypertension

The most obvious sympathetic-mediated form of secondary hypertension is that due to phaeochromocytoma, where the hypertension is principally due to intermittent release of catecholamines. Sympathetic neural mechanisms may, however, also contribute to chronic mild elevations of blood pressure in patients with phaeochromocytoma due to sustained adrenaline-mediated facilitation of noradrenaline release from peripheral adrenergic nerve terminals.

Heightened sympathetic activation is also a factor in renovascular hypertension. The evidence is described by Oparil (1986) and

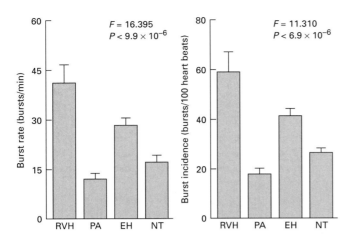

Fig. 48.1. Muscle sympathetic nerve activity in normotensive subjects (NT) and in patients with renovascular hypertension (RVH), primary aldosteronism (PA), and essential hypertension (EH). Sympathetic burst frequency was higher in both renovascular hypertension and essential hypertension than in normal individuals. Sympathetic activity was, however, decreased in patients with primary aldosteronism. (From Miyajima *et al.* (1991), with permission.)

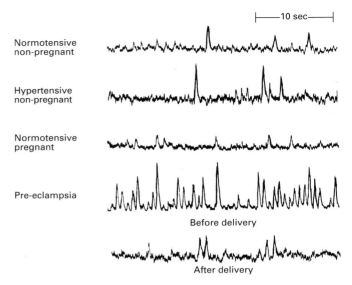

Fig. 48.2. Recordings of sympathetic nerve activity in a normotensive non-pregnant woman, a hypertensive non-pregnant woman, a normotensive pregnant woman, and a woman with pre-eclampsia (before and after delivery). Sympathetic nerve activity was similar in the two non-pregnant women and the normotensive pregnant woman, but was much higher in the patient with pre-eclampsia. After delivery blood pressure and sympathetic activity returned towards baseline in this patient. (From Schobel *et al.* (1996), with permission.)

includes increased levels of plasma and urine noradrenaline and its metabolites in patients with renovascular hypertension. Miyajima *et al.* (1991) demonstrated that in patients with renal vascular hypertension, the increases in plasma renin activity and angiotensin II are accompanied by a striking increase in muscle sympathetic nerve activity (Fig. 48.1). Furthermore, muscle sympathetic nerve activity, plasma renin activity, and angiotensin II concentration decreased several days after successful percutaneous renal angioplasty. These neurophysiological observations support previous reports that renovascular hypertension is accompanied by increased plasma levels of noradrenaline. These observations, as well as those by Matsukawa *et al.* (1993) in accelerated hypertension, suggest the concept that activation of the renin–angiotensin system increases arterial pressure, in part, by increasing sympathetic neural activity. Angiotensin II may increase post–ganglionic sympathetic neural activity by acting on the central nervous system or sympathetic ganglia or by inhibiting arterial baroreflex modulation of sympathetic nerve activity (Matsukawa *et al.* 1988).

The interplay between the kidney and the sympathetic nervous system may also be implicated in hypertension associated with renal failure. In patients receiving haemodialysis, in whom the native kidneys were still present, sympathetic nerve traffic was more than twofold the levels recorded in haemodialysis patients who had undergone bilateral nephrectomy (Converse *et al.* 1992). These findings suggest the presence of an afferent signal from the native kidneys that acts centrally to increase sympathetic outflow.

An iatrogenic form of secondary hypertension associated with cyclosporin therapy may also involve increased levels of sympathetic nerve activity (SNA). Patients receiving cyclosporin as immunosuppressive therapy have a high incidence of hypertension. Scherrer *et al.* (1990) have shown an impressive association between direct measurements of sympathetic nerve traffic and hypertension in these patients. The hypertensive effects of increased SNA would be potentiated by cyclosporin-mediated augmentation of noradrenaline-

induced vasoconstriction. Kaye and colleagues (1993), however, in studies utilizing combined measurements of renal blood flow, renal and whole-body noradrenaline spillover, and microneurography, have reported that while cyclosporin therapy in humans causes acute renal vasoconstriction, these effects were not due to increased sympathetic activation. In their subjects, cyclosporin A did not cause an increase in either muscle sympathetic activity or in total body or renal noradrenaline spillover rates. Reasons for the inconsistency regarding cyclosporin effects on sympathetic activity are not clear.

Schobel *et al.* (1996) have recently provided important new information regarding the role of the sympathetic nervous system in pre-eclampsia. Patients with pre-eclampsia had higher blood pressures and vascular resistance than normal pregnant women and had sympathetic nerve traffic three times greater than that seen in control subjects (Fig. 48.2). Sympathetic activity was also twice that seen in non-pregnant women with hypertension. After delivery, both blood pressure and sympathetic activity decreased towards normal levels in the patients with pre-eclampsia.

Mechanisms of increased sympathetic activity: implications for hypertension

Arterial baroreflex

Probably the most extensively studied of the possible aetiologies of sympathetic overactivity in hypertension are depressor and pressor autonomic reflexes. The traditional concepts hold, first, that arterial baroreflexes are abnormal in hypertension, with a higher threshold for activation and a reduction in sensitivity, and, secondly, that these alterations result from chronic increases in arterial pressure. In recent years, two new concepts have emerged regarding alterations in arterial baroreflexes in hypertension. First, it has been found that Dahl salt-sensitive rats fed a rigorously low salt diet have abnormalities in baroreceptor afferent mechanisms that occur in the absence of an increase in arterial pressure (Mark 1991). This suggests that some alterations in arterial baroreflexes in hypertension could be related to genetic abnormalities that precede and are independent of the increase in arterial pressure. This genetic influence on baroreflex sensitivity is supported by work in humans by Parmer and colleagues (1992), discussed later. Secondly, it is now known that abnormalities in baroreflex control of parasympathetic activity (heart rate) do not necessarily predict alterations in baroreflex control of sympathetic nerve activity and vascular resistance (Rea and Hamdan 1990). Indeed, there is evidence from both experimental animals and humans that baroreflex control of sympathetic activity, vascular resistance, and arterial pressure may be preserved in early or mild hypertension despite impairment of baroreflex control of heart rate. This dissociation appears to result from a greater central nervous system 'reserve' for maintaining baroreflex control of sympathetic versus parasympathetic activity. In so far as hypertension is concerned, the baroreflex-mediated sympathetic and vascular resistance responses to blood pressure changes are obviously of greater haemodynamic significance than the heart rate responses.

Cardiopulmonary baroreflex

Borderline hypertensive patients with a family history of hypertension show an augmented increase in sympathetic activity and vascular resistance in response to lower-body negative pressure (simulating orthostatic stress; Rea and Hamdan 1990; Fig. 48.3). These findings may help to explain the exaggerated diastolic blood pressure increase with upright tilt in borderline hypertension. Importantly, this sympathetic hyper-reactivity to non-hypotensive lower-body negative pressure occurred despite no detectable abnormality in arterial baroreflex regulation of sympathetic nerve responses to raising and lowering blood pressure. In addition, the augmented sympathetic nerve response to orthostatic stress occurred in the absence of an increased baseline sympathetic activity in the borderline hypertensives in the supine position. Two conclusions emerge from these studies. First, the exaggerated sympathetic response to simulated orthostatic stress suggests that mild hypertensives have a potentiated sympathetic neural drive, but in the supine position this elevated drive is masked by an augmented sympathoinhibitory effect of the cardiopulmonary baroreflex (Fig. 48.4). Secondly, the heightened sympathetic neural drive in mild hypertensives can occur in the absence of impairment of arterial baroreflex modulation of sympathetic activity. This strengthens the view that central neural mechanisms may be responsible for enhanced sympathetic nerve activity in early or mild hypertension.

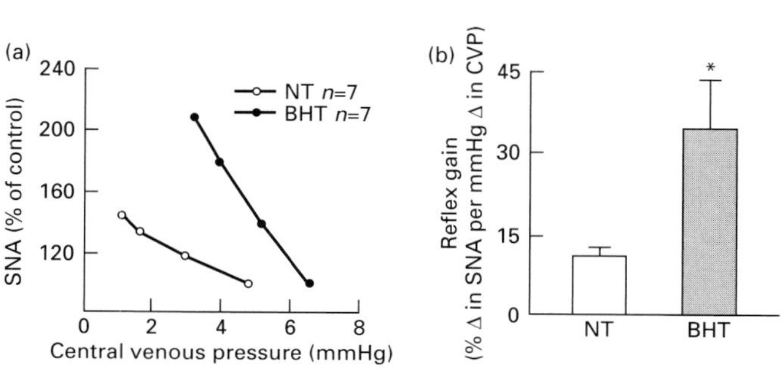

Fig. 48.3. (a) Plot of mean values of central venous pressure (CVP) versus sympathetic nerve activity (SNA) at rest and during three levels of lower-body negative pressure in normotensive (NT) and borderline hypertensive (BHT) subjects. Baseline CVP was higher in BHT, but reductions in CVP produced by lower-body negative pressure were similar in both groups. Levels of SNA were greater at each level of CVP in BHT subjects, resulting in a steeper CVP–SNA slope. These findings indicate, first, heightened sympathetic neural drive and, second, an exaggerated cardiopulmonary baroreflex sensitivity in borderline hypertensive subjects. (b) Bar graph showing mean gain of cardiopulmonary baroreflexes in NT and BHT subjects, indicating a significantly greater reflex gain in the borderline hypertensives (*, $p < 0.05$). (From Rea and Hamdan (1990), with permission.)

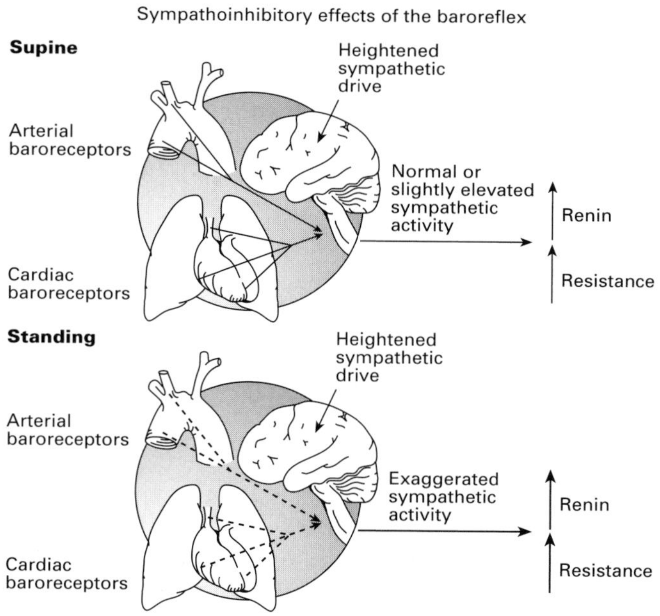

Fig. 48.4. Increased cardiopulmonary baroreflex control of sympathetic activity and its interaction with heightened central sympathetic drive may explain the reflex adjustment to changes in posture in mild hypertensive individuals. The heightened central neural sympathetic drive is attenuated by cardiopulmonary baroreflex activation when subjects are in the supine position, so that sympathetic activity, plasma renin levels, and vascular resistance may be normal or only slightly increased. When subjects are standing, however, decreased cardiac filling pressure eliminates that cardiopulmonary baroreflex buffering, allowing the heightened central sympathetic drive to manifest itself as exaggerated reflex increases in sympathetic nerve activity, plasma renin levels, and vascular resistance. (From Mark (1990), with permission.)

Chemoreflex

The role of the chemoreceptors in determining sympathetic nerve discharge as well as ventilation has recently received considerable attention. Hypoxic stimulation of the peripheral chemoreceptors triggers sympathetic excitation. This chemoreceptor reflex may be exaggerated in spontaneously hypertensive rats and hypertensive

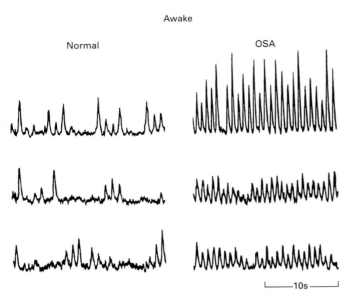

Fig. 48.5. Recordings of sympathetic nerve activity in age- and gender-matched normal subjects compared to patients with obstructive sleep apnoea. Sympathetic nerve recordings were obtained when subjects were awake, in the absence of any breathing abnormalities or oxygen desaturation. Sympathetic activity even during wakefulness was much greater in patients with obstructive sleep apnoea. (From Somers *et al.* (1995), with permission.)

humans. Young human hypertensives have an increased inspiratory drive when exposed to hypoxic conditions (Trzebski *et al.* 1982). Sympathetic nerve discharge during hypoxia is also potentiated in borderline hypertensive men (about twice the response seen in age- and weight-matched normotensives; Somers *et al.* 1988). This potentiation is especially marked during voluntary apnoea (about tenfold the response in normotensives), when the sympathetic-inhibitory influence of breathing and thoracic afferent activity is eliminated. These findings have two important implications. First, heightened resting sympathetic discharge in early hypertension may be explained by an augmented tonic chemoreflex-mediated sympathetic excitation even during normoxia. Secondly, the strong association between hypertension and sleep apnoea may be explained by chronic sympathetic excitation and consequent blood pressure elevation during sleep, triggered by episodes of hypoxia, hypercapnia, and apnoea. These frequent elevations in sympathetic nerve activity and blood pressure during episodes of sleep apnoea may have functional and structural consequences and may contribute to daytime sympathetic excitation and blood pressure elevation.

Although patients with sleep apnoea have high sympathetic activity when awake (Fig. 48.5), sympathetic activity increases even further during sleep (Fig. 48.6) (Somers *et al.* 1995). In contrast to sleep in normal subjects, blood pressure does not fall during sleep in patients with obstructive sleep apnoea. Treatment with continuous positive airway pressure prevents apnoea, and reduces sympathetic activity and blood pressure during sleep (Fig. 48.6).

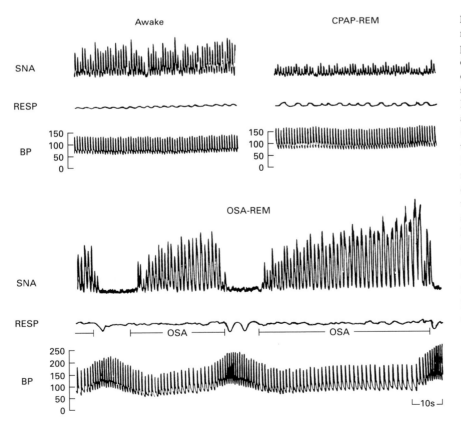

Fig. 48.6. Recordings of sympathetic activity, respiration, and intra-arterial blood pressure in a patient with sleep apnoea on no medications and free of other diseases. Measurements were obtained during wakefulness (top left), during obstructive sleep apnoea in REM sleep (bottom), and during REM sleep after treatment of obstructive sleep apnoea with continuous positive airway pressure (CPAP). During wakefulness sympathetic activity was high and blood pressure was approximately 130/60 mmHg. During REM sleep, repetitive apnoeas resulted in hypoxia and chemoreflex stimulation with consequent sympathetic activation. The vasoconstriction resulting from sympathetic activation causes marked surges in blood pressure, to levels as high as 250/110 mmHg at the end of apnoea, mmHg because of increases in cardiac output at termination of apnoea. Treatment of sleep apnoea and elimination of apnoeic episodes by CPAP resulted in stabilization and lower levels of both blood pressure and sympathetic activity during REM sleep. (From Somers *et al.* (1995), with permission.)

Environmental stress

Environmental or behavioural factors may be involved in the initiation and maintenance of sympathetic overactivity in hypertension. Mental stress tasks in the laboratory trigger transient elevations in sympathetic activity and blood pressure. Chronic stress may be related to the onset of hypertension in animals. Haemodynamic and catecholamine responses to acute mental stress are more marked in children with a family history of hypertension. During mental challenge, the increase in noradrenaline spillover into arterial blood is increased in patients with essential hypertension, as compared to normotensive control subjects.

Environmental stress increases renal sympathetic nerve activity in SHR and DOCA salt hypertensive, but not WKY rats (DiBona 1992). High salt diet augments the influence of behavioural stress on renal sympathetic nerve activity in SHR, suggesting an interaction between environmental, genetic, and dietary factors in the regulation of sympathetic responses. The sympathetic and haemodynamic response to mental stress is able to override the sympathetic-inhibitory effect of simultaneous baroreceptor stimulation. Chronic or repetitive stressful stimuli may conceivably result in sustained sympathetic activation and hypertension in susceptible persons. This response may be augmented by baroreflex resetting and by the sustained sympathetic neural effects of adrenaline uptake by nerve terminals during stressful stimuli, as discussed later.

Exercise

There has been considerable interest in the influence of physical conditioning on blood pressure and sympathetic mechanisms. We have previously demonstrated that unilateral forearm physical conditioning attenuates the increases in sympathetic nerve activity during isometric exercise of the conditioned arm. Jennings et al. (1986), using neurochemical indices of sympathetic activity, reported that a supervised daily exercise programme decreased resting sympathetic activity, but this decrease was not observed in individuals exercising only 3 days/week. Thus, physical conditioning attenuates the sympathetic nerve responses during exercise, and intensive chronic endurance exercise training lowers resting sympathetic activity in humans.

In contrast, there is increasing evidence that a single bout of endurance exercise, particularly in hypertensive subjects, is associated with a post-exercise decrease in sympathetic activity and blood pressure. Floras and Senn (1991) found that the decrease in blood pressure that occurs after a single bout of endurance exercise in borderline hypertensives is accompanied by a post-exercise decrease in muscle sympathetic nerve activity. These post-exercise decreases in muscle sympathetic nerve activity and blood pressure were not observed in normotensive individuals. These observations suggest that the decrease in blood pressure that occurs for several hours after a single bout of exercise in hypertensive subjects may be due, in part, to a transient suppression of central sympathetic neural outflow.

The mechanisms of the post-exercise and training-induced decreases in sympathetic nerve activity in hypertensive humans are not known. Somers et al. (1991) have shown that baroreflex sensitivity is increased and baroreflex set point and blood pressure are lower in hypertensive humans, both after acute exercise and after an endurance training programme. Thus, it may be that increases in baroreflex gain may mediate, in part, the lower blood pressure and

sympathetic activity associated with the post-exercise period and with endurance training.

Adrenaline

In linking the sympathetic system and hypertension, neural actions of adrenaline have been proposed. Circulating adrenaline is taken up by adrenergic nerve terminals, with subsequent sustained neural release as a co-transmitter with noradrenaline. Neurally released adrenaline stimulates prejunctional β-receptors on adrenergic nerve terminals, thereby facilitating further release of neural noradrenaline. Several studies have reported increased levels of plasma adrenaline in hypertensive patients. Infusion of adrenaline for 6 hours can result in a sustained elevation of ambulatory blood pressure for up to 18 hours after the infusion (Blankestijn et al. 1988). Floras et al. (1990) have demonstrated that intra-arterial infusion of adrenaline facilitates neurogenic vasoconstriction in borderline hypertensive humans. Tachycardia after adrenaline infusion persists even when plasma adrenaline levels return to normal. Pre-treatment with desipramine, which inhibits neuronal uptake of adrenaline, prevents the tachycardia. Thus, uptake and subsequent release of adrenaline, with facilitation of noradrenaline release at the level of the adrenergic nerve terminals may contribute to increases in sympathetic activity and reflex responsiveness in hypertensive patients, and to a 'hyperkinetic' circulatory state. It may be that repetitive adrenomedullary stimulation and adrenaline release during stress in subjects prone to developing hypertension could promote a sustained facilitation in neurally released noradrenaline which, over many years, could contribute to sustained hypertension.

Insulin

The importance of insulin in sympathetic activation and hypertension has aroused great interest. Obesity, particularly upper-body obesity, is associated with insulin resistance and hyperinsulinaemia. Hypertension is also associated with a state of insulin resistance and hyperinsulinaemia, independent of obesity or diabetes mellitus. Interestingly, the insulin resistance which occurs in obesity and hypertension affects actions of insulin on glucose uptake in skeletal muscle, but actions of insulin on the sympathetic nervous system and the kidney are preserved (Mark 1990). Thus, it has been postulated that the hyperinsulinaemia that occurs in insulin resistance causes renal sodium retention, heightened sympathetic activity, and increased vascular resistance and arterial pressure. Euglycaemic hyperinsulinaemia (insulin <400 μU/ml) results in increases in plasma noradrenaline and modest increases in blood pressure in normotensive humans. Lower levels of insulin (approximately 75–150 μU/ml), within the physiological postprandial range, result in increases in muscle sympathetic nerve activity, but produce vasodilation (not the expected sympathetic vasoconstriction), and do not increase blood pressure in normal humans (Anderson et al. 1991). Thus, it appears that insulin elicits both pressor (sympathetic-excitatory) and depressor (vasodilator) actions. At high levels of plasma insulin, exceeding the physiological range, the pressor effect is predominant. However, with physiological levels in normal humans the sympathetic-excitatory and vasodilator actions are balanced and blood pressure does not increase. It is possible that the presence of other factors, such as structural vascular changes, insulin resistance, or genetic predisposition to hypertension, could augment the sym-

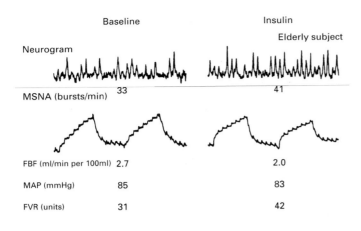

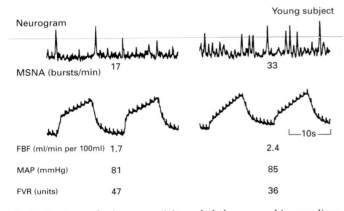

Fig. 48.7. Sympathetic nerve activity and plethysmographic recordings during baseline and after 90 minutes of insulin-infusion in an elderly subject (top) and in a young subject (bottom). Baseline sympathetic activity (MSNA) was higher in the elderly subject but the insulin induced increase was smaller than in the young subject. Forearm flow (FBF) decreased in the elderly subject, whereas it increased in the young subject, with insulin. Since mean arterial pressure (MAP) did not change significantly in either subject, forearm vascular resistance (FVR) increased with insulin in the elderly and decreased in the young subject. (From Hausberg *et al.* (1997), with permission.)

pathetic (pressor) action of insulin or attenuate the vasodilator (depressor) action, thereby permitting insulin to produce a sympathetically mediated increase in arterial pressure.

Hausberg *et al.* (1997) provide precedent for this concept of differential responses in their recent study of the effects of insulin in young versus elderly healthy subjects. While insulin caused the expected vasodilation in young subjects, elderly subjects responded to insulin by vasoconstriction (Fig. 48.7). This vasoconstriction was not explained by greater sympathetic activation, since the increase in sympathetic activity in the elderly subjects was less than that seen in the young subjects.

Renin-angiotensin system

The interactions between the renin–angiotensin system and the sympathetic nervous system are considerable, and may be especially important in renal and renovascular hypertension as discussed

earlier. Angiotensin II acts on the sympathetic nervous system at the central, ganglionic, and nerve terminal levels, as well as at the adrenal medulla to increase sympathetic nerve activity. Angiotensin II also facilitates release of noradrenaline, reduces its reuptake, and sensitizes blood vessels to the effects of noradrenaline. Infusion of exogenous angiotensin II in humans augments sympathetic mediated vasoconstriction. The reductions in sympathetic nerve traffic and heart rate observed when blood pressure is increased by infusions of angiotensin II are significantly less than those seen with equivalent blood pressure elevations using phenylephrine (Matsukawa *et al.* 1988), suggesting that angiotensin II inhibits baroreflex control of both sympathetic activity as well as heart rate in humans. Conversely, angiotensin-converting enzyme inhibition in animals blunts the vascular responses to exogenous noradrenaline as well as to electrical stimulation of the sympathetic nerves. Acute angiotensin-converting enzyme inhibition in hypertensive humans is associated with arterial baroreceptor resetting and facilitation of parasympathetic reflex responsiveness. These angiotensin–autonomic–baroreflex interactions may explain the ability of angiotensin-converting enzyme inhibitors to reduce both vascular resistance and blood pressure without any reflex increase in heart rate.

In studies in patients with heart failure, Dibner-Dunlap *et al.* (1996) report that angiotensin-converting enzyme inhibition reduced blood pressure, central venous pressure and muscle sympathetic nerve activity, and enhanced the sensitivity of arterial and cardiopulmonary baroreflexes. Thus, the renin–angiotensin system may influence sympathetic activity by actions at a central and ganglionic level, by increasing noradrenaline release, by potentiating the vasoconstrictor effects of noradrenaline, and by modulating important reflex mechanisms; angiotensin may also influence the relative balance between vagal and sympathetic drives.

Central mechanisms

Oparil *et al.* (1995) and Esler and colleagues (1995) have reviewed recently the evidence for central causes of excessive sympathetic discharge in hypertension. There may be a subgroup of hypertensive patients in whom the posterior inferior cerebellar artery and/or the vertebral artery causes compression of cardiovascular regulatory centres in the region of the ventrolateral medulla. Microvascular decompression of this region has been reported to decrease blood pressure significantly.

Using jugular vein noradrenaline spillover measurements, Ferrier *et al.* (1992) have reported that higher sympathetic activity in hypertension may be explained by increased cerebral noradrenaline release. These investigators subsequently reported that subcortical noradrenaline release was linked with both total body noradrenaline spillover as well as renal noradrenaline spillover.

Genetic factors

While the genetic contribution to essential hypertension is widely recognized, there is surprisingly little information on the heritability of sympathetic neural outflow and the factors that regulate sympathetic drive.

For example, alterations in arterial baroreflexes in hypertension could be related to genetic abnormalities that precede, and are independent of, the increase in arterial pressure. Parmer *et al.* (1992) measured baroreflex control of heart rate in patients with essential hypertension

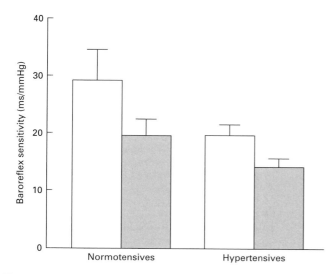

Fig. 48.8. Baroreflex sensitivity measured using phenylephrine bolus injections in normotensive and hypertensive subjects stratified by the presence (shaded bars) or absence (open bars) of a family history of hypertension. Both hypertension and a family history of hypertension was associated with significant reductions in baroreflex sensitivity. (From Parmer *et al.* (1992), with permission.)

and in normotensive humans, grouped by the presence or absence of family history of hypertension (Fig. 48.8). Baroreflex sensitivity assessed by injection of phenylephrine was 29 ± 6 ms/mmHg in normotensives without a family history of hypertension, 19 ± 3 ms/mmHg in normotensives with a family history, 19 ± 2 ms/mmHg in hypertensives with no family history, and 14 ± 1 ms/mmHg in hypertensives with a family history of hypertension. Analysis of variance showed significant effects on baroreflex sensitivity of blood pressure status and of family history of hypertension. After controlling for effects of age, mean arterial pressure, and body weight, the effect of family history of hypertension and baroreflex sensitivity was still highly significant, suggesting that impairment in baroreflex sensitivity in humans is, in part, genetically determined and may represent a hereditary component in the pathogenesis of essential hypertension.

With respect to sympathetic activity itself, Williams *et al.* (1993) in a study of over 100 twin pairs, concluded that genetic influences contributed to more than half the variability in noradrenaline levels. In a study using microneurography, Wallin *et al.* (1993) found that levels of sympathetic traffic were very similar in monozygotic twins, as compared to unrelated controls subjects. Thus, the heritability of blood pressure may be explained, in part, by the heritability of levels of sympathetic nerve traffic and/or the factors that govern it.

Summary and conclusions

There is clearly a genetic predisposition to essential hypertension, probably polygenic in origin. It is, therefore, unlikely that a single physiological abnormality can explain all cases of hypertension. Many factors, including environmental stressors and diet, may be involved, as exemplified by the so-called 'salt-sensitive subset' of essential hypertension. Further complicating the scenario is that hypertension is itself a dynamic entity, progressing from one haemodynamic and structure/function profile to another, making it difficult to establish whether any isolated finding is a cause or consequence of raised arterial pressure levels. With this magnitude of disease heterogeneity it is not surprising, therefore, that there is some lack of consensus in the literature with regard to the various reflex, cellular, and other abnormalities that have been described. It is likely that the genesis and maintenance of hypertension is multifactorial, with different abnormalities exerting different degrees of influence in various subsets of essential hypertension.

The weight of evidence, though not unequivocal, strongly suggests that sympathetic overactivity is important in the aetiology and maintenance of hypertension. This appears to be especially true for the early stages of hypertension. In the later stages of hypertension, the sympathetic nervous system may continue to be important in augmenting the vascular and myocardial dysfunction and structural damage that ensue from chronic elevations in arterial pressure.

Acknowledgements

Virend Somers is supported by an American Heart Grant-in-Aid, NIH HL14388, and an NIH Sleep Academic Award. Krzysztof Narkiewicz, a visiting research scientist from the Department of Hypertension and Diabetology, Medical University of Gdansk, Poland, is supported by an NIH Fogarty Fellowship (NIH 3F05 TW05200). The authors thank Linda Bang for superb secretarial assistance. The authors also acknowledge their colleagues at the University of Iowa who have made substantial contributions to the work described in this review.

References

Abel, P. W. and Hermsmeyer, K. (1981). Sympathetic cross-innervation of SHR and genetic controls suggests a trophic influence on vascular muscle membranes. *Cir. Res.* **49**, 1311–18.

Anderson, E. A., Sinkey, C. A., Lawton, W. J., and Mark A. L. (1989). Elevated sympathetic nerve activity in borderline hypertensive humans: evidence from direct intraneural recordings. *Hypertension* **14**, 177–83.

Anderson, E. A., Hoffman, R. P., Balon, T. W., Sinkey, C. A., and Mark, A. L. (1991). Hyperinsulinemia produces both sympathetic neural activation and vasodilation in normal humans. *J. Clin. Invest.* **87**, 2246–52.

Blankestijn, P. J., Man in't Veld, A. J., Tulen, J. *et al.* (1988). Support for adrenaline-hypertension hypothesis: 18 hour pressor effect after 6 hours adrenaline infusion. *Lancet.* **2**, 1386–9.

Chapleau, M. W. and Abboud, F. M. (1993) Mechanism of adaptation and resetting of the baroreceptor reflex. In *Cardiovascular reflex control in health and disease*, (ed. R.Hainsworth and A. L. Mark), pp. 165–93. W. B. Saunders, London.

Converse, R. L., Jacobsen, T. N., Toto, R. D. *et al.* (1992). Sympathetic overactivity in patients with chronic renal faiulre. *New Engl. J. Med.*, **327**, 1912–18.

Dibner-Dunlap, M. E., Smith, M. L., Kinugawa, T., and Thames, M. D. (1996). Enalaprilat augments arterial and cardiopulmonary control of sympathetic nerve activity in patients with heart failure. *J. Am. Coll. Cardiol.* **27**, 358–64.

DiBona, G. F. (1992). Sympathetic neural control of the kidney in hypertension. *Hypertension* **19**, 128–35.

Egan, B., Panis, R., Hinderliter, A., Schork, N., and Julius, S. (1987). Mechanism of increased alpha adrenergic vasoconstriction in human essential hypertension. *J. Clin. Invest.* **80**, 812–17.

Esler, M., Jennings, G., and Lambert, G. (1989). Noradrenaline release and the pathophysiology of primary human hypertension. *Am. J. Hypertens.* **2**, S140–6.

Esler, M. D., Lambert, G. W., Ferrier, C. *et al.* (1995). Central nervous system noradrenergic control of sympathetic outflow in normotensive and hypertensive humans. *Clin. Exp. Hypertens.* 17, 409–23.

Ferrier, C., Essler M. D., Eisenhofer, G. *et al.* (1992). Increased norepinephrine spillover into the jugular veins in essential hypertension. *Hypertension* 19, 62–9.

Floras, J. S. and Senn, B. L. (1991). Absence of post exercise hypotension and sympathoinhibition in normal subjects: additional evidence for increased sympathetic outflow in borderline hypertension. *Can. J. Cardiol.* 7, 253–8.

Floras, J. S., Aylward P. E., Mark, A. L., and Abboud, F. M. (1990). Adrenaline facilitates neurogenic vasocontriction in borderline hypertensives. *J. Hypertension* 8, 443–8.

Goldstein, D. S. (1983). Plasma catecholamine and essential hypertension: an analytical review. *Hypertension*, 5, 86–99.

Grassi, G., Cattaneo, B. M., Seravalle, G., Lanfranchi, A., Bolla, G., and Mancia, G. (1997). Baroreflex impairment by low sodium diet in mild or moderate essential hypertension. *Hypertension* 29, 802–7.

Hausberg, M., Hoffman, R. P., Somers, V. K., Sinkey C. A., Mark, A. L., and Anderson, E. A. (1997). Contrasting autonomic and hemodyanmic effects of insulin in healthy elderly versus young subjects. *Hypertension* 29, 700–5.

Jennings, G., Nelson L., Nestel, P., Esler, M., Korner, P., Burton, D., and Bazelmans, J. (1986). The effects of changes in physical activity on major cardiovascular risk factors, hemodynamics, sympathetic function and glucose utilization in man: a controlled study of four levels of activity. *Circulation* 73, 30–40.

Julius, S. and Esler, M. (1975) Autonomic nervous cardiovascular regulation in borderline hypertension. *Am. J. Cardiol.* 36, 685–96.

Kaye, D., Thompson, J., Jennings, G., and Esler, M. (1993). Cyclosporine therapy after cardiac transplantation and renal vasoconstriction without sympathetic activation. *Circulation* 88, 1101–9.

Mark, A. L. (1990). Regulation of sympathetic nerve activity in mild human hypertension. *J. Hypertension* 8, S67–75.

Mark, A. L. (1991). Sympathetic neural contribution to salt induced hypertension in Dahl rats. *Hypertension* 17, 186–90.

Matsukawa, T., Gotoh, E., Miyajima, E. *et al.* (1988). Angiotensin II inhibits baroreflex control of muscle sympathetic nerve activity and the heart rate in patients with essential hypertension. *J. Hypertension* 6, S501–4.

Matsukawa, T., Mano, T, Gotoh, E., and Ishii, M. (1993). Elevated sympathetic nerve activity in patients with accelerated essential hypertension. *J. Clin. Invest.* 92, 25–8.

Miyajima, E., Yamada, Y., Yoshida, Y. *et al.* (1991). Muscle sympathetic nerve activity in renovascular hypertension and primary aldosteronism. *Hypertension* 17, 1057–62.

Oparil, S. (1986). The sympathetic nervous system in clinical and experimental hypertension. *Kidney Int.* 30, 4437–52.

Oparil, S., Chen, Y., Berecek, K. H., Calhoun, D. A., and Wyss, J. M. (1995). The role of the central nervous system in hypertension. In *Hypertension: pathophysiology, diagnosis, and management*, (ed. J. H. Laragh and B. M. Brenner), pp. 713–40. Raven Press, New York.

Parmer R. J., Cervenka, J. H. and Stone, R. A. (1992). Baroreflex sensitivity and heredity in essential hypertension. *Circulation* 85, 497–503.

Rea, R. F. and Hamdan, M. (1990). Baroreflex control of muscle sympathetic nerve activity in borderline hypertension. *Circulation* 82, 856–62.

Scherrer, U., Vissing, S. F., Morgan, B. J. *et al* (1990). Cyclosporine-induced sympathetic activation and hypertension after heart transplantation. *New Engl. J. Med.* 323, 693–9.

Schobel, H. P., Fischer, T., Heuszer, K., Geiger, H., and Schmieder, R. E. (1996). Preeclampsia–a state of sympathetic overactivity. *New Engl. J. Med.* 335, 1480–5.

Somers, V. K., Mark, A. L., and Abboud, F. M. (1988). Potentiation of sympathetic nerve responses to hypoxia in borderline hypertensive subjects. *Hypertension* 11, 608–12.

Somers, V. K., Conway, J., Johnston, J., and Sleight, P. (1991). Effects of endurance training on baroreflex sensitivity and blood pressure in borderline hypertension. *Lancet* 337, 1363–8.

Somers, V. K., Dyken, M. E., Clary, M. P., and Abboud, F. M. (1995) Sympathetic neural mechanisms in obstructive sleep apnea. *J. Clin. Invest.* 96, 1897–904.

Trzebski, A., Tafil, M., Zoltowski, M., and Przybylski, J. (1982). Increased sensitivity of the arterial chemoreceptor drive in young men with mild hypertension. *Cardiovasc. Res.* 16, 163–72.

Wallin, B. G. and Sundlof, G. (1979). A quantitative study of muscle nerve sympathetic activity in resting normotensive and hypertensive subjects. *Hypertension* 1, 67–77.

Wallin, B. G., Kunimoto, M. M., and Sellgren, J. (1993). Possible gentic influence on the strength of human muscle nerve sympathetic activity at rest. *Hypertension* 22, 282–4.

Wallin, B. G., Thompson, J. M., Jennings, G. L., and Esler M. D. (1996). Renal noradrenaline spillover correlates with muscle sympathetic activity in humans. *J. Physiol.* 491, 881–7.

Williams, P. D., Puddey, I. B., Beilin, L. J., and Vandongen, R. (1993). Genetic influences on plasma catecholamines in human twins. *J. Clin. Endocrinol. Metab.* 77, 794–9.

49. Cardiac failure and the autonomic nervous system

Gary S. Francis and Jay N. Cohn

Introduction

Heart failure has now emerged as an important public health problem within the Western world. It is estimated that as many as 10 per cent of the population beyond age 65 will develop heart failure, a complex clinical syndrome characterized by circulatory congestion and reduced flow to vital organs in the advanced stages. Although numerous clinical trials have led to advances in the management of patients with heart failure, the mortality remains high and the morbidity is substantial.

A new model of how we conceptualize heart failure has emerged throughout the past 20 years. Originally envisioned as a simple problem of pump dysfunction, it now has become clear that the neuroendocrine responses to left ventricular dysfunction occur early in the syndrome (Francis et al. 1990), are responsible for many of the findings observed at the bedside, and are responsible for much of the pathophysiological derangement. In support of this contention, therapy designed to block excessive neuroendocrine responses, such as angiotensin-converting enzyme (ACE) inhibitors and β-adrenergic blockers, have proven to be much more effective than drugs designed to chronically stimulate the inotropic state of the heart. Although the precise mechanisms whereby altered neuroendocrine adaptation occurs is still not clear, it is believed by many investigators that abnormal baro- and cardiac reflex abnormalities make some contribution toward this end.

In the 1950s Brigden and Sharpey-Schaeffer reported that there were abnormal postural changes in peripheral blood flow observed in patients with heart failure (Brigden and Sharpey-Schafer 1950). Patients with heart failure demonstrated a limited activation of the sympathetic nervous system in response to the upright posture. Since then numerous studies have demonstrated that both patients and animals with experimental chronic heart failure have abnormal reflex control of the cardiovascular system (Covell et al. 1966; Eckberg et al. 1971; Higgins et al. 1972; Vatner et al. 1974; White 1981; Levine et al. 1983; Ferguson et al. 1984). These abnormalities of reflex control involve both arterial baroreflexes and cardiac reflexes. It is now believed that reflex control disturbances can have profound effects on patients with reduced cardiac output. New techniques for assessing reflex control mechanisms have aided investigators, although the precise mechanisms whereby these abnormalities occur remains uncertain. The use of power spectral analysis of heart rate (Saul et al. 1988) and microneurographic measurements of sympathetic traffic to skeletal muscles (Leimbach et al. 1986), as well as the study of chronically instrumented animals with various models of heart failure (Coleman et al. 1971; Higgins et al. 1973; Zucker et al. 1995), have provided enlightenment regarding reflex control abnormalities

in heart failure. Early studies by Eckberg et al. in 1971 documented a reduced bradycardic response to heightened pressor activity of intravenous injections of phenylephrine in patients with heart disease, while Vatner et al. in 1974, using a model of low output failure in dogs, demonstrated an abnormal response to hypotension as well. These studies indicated that both sympathetic and parasympathetic components of the autonomic nervous system were responsible for the modest tachycardia sometimes observed in the untreated syndrome of heart failure.

Treatment with ACE inhibitors partially reverses abnormal reflex control mechanisms in heart failure (Cody et al. 1982). Likewise, cardiac transplantation tends to reverse reflex control abnormalities found in heart failure to some extent (Levine et al. 1986; Ellenbogen et al. 1989), although patients with heart transplantation continue to demonstrate some disturbances in autonomic function (Banner et al. 1990). The purpose of this chapter is to review abnormalities of the sympathetic and parasympathetic nervous system as they relate to both clinical and experimental heart failure. Emphasis will be placed on the relevance of these abnormalities to the clinical pathophysiology of the syndrome.

Normal physiological conditions

The moment-to-moment control of blood pressure, heart rate, and regional blood flow is partially under control of various baroreceptor and cardiopulmonary reflexes. These systems provide negative feedback control, so that haemodynamics remain relatively constant despite short-term pertubations. The ultimate physiological goal is always one of circulatory homeostasis (Abboud et al. 1976).

The arterial baroreflexes include an afferent limb, a central neural component, and autonomic neuroeffector components. Sensory information from the arterial baroreceptors originates from mechanosensitive cells in the carotid sinus and the aortic arch. Activation of these sensors allows information to travel to the central nervous system, usually via the glossopharyngeal and vagus nerve. The afferent neurones synapse in the nucleus tractus solitarius, from which there are numerous projections to areas in the brainstem, particularly the medulla.

Increases in arterial pressure activate primary afferent neurones, resulting in increased vagal efferent outflow to the heart. This leads to reduced sympathetic outflow to the heart and the peripheral circulation. The vagal efferent outflow originates from neurones in the nucleus ambiguous, whereas the sympathetic neural influences are controlled from the rostral and caudal ventral lateral medulla. When arterial blood pressure is normal, the prevailing level of arterial baroreceptor discharge is such that vagal efferent activity is tonically excited and sympathetic activity is tonically inhibited. This affords a 'breaking' mechanism on the heart and the circulation.

Other important sensory fibres originate from receptors in the cardiopulmonary region. These fibres travel over the vagal nerves to the nucleus tractus solitarius and exert influence on both vagal and sympathetic outflow to the heart and circulation. This presumably occurs in a manner similar to that of the arterial baroreceptors. The cardiopulmonary sensory receptors are located throughout the heart and lungs, although they are believed to occur particularly in the left ventricle. When active, these cardiopulmonary sensory nerve endings are tonically active and exert a restraining influence on the heart and circulation.

The objective of the reflex control mechanisms is immediate production of circulatory homeostasis. For example, during exercise there may be sensory receptors in the skeletal muscles that are activated leading to reflex sympathoexcitation and vagal withdrawal. This lead to an appropriate increase in blood pressure, heart rate, and peripheral vasoconstriction to redirect blood flow to appropriate vascular beds. The arterial baroreceptors reflexes moderate this response.

Heart failure

Conditions such as heart failure, which are accompanied by abnormalities in reflex control mechanisms, may compromise the patient's ability to adjust to physiological stresses. Moreover, abnormalities in reflex control mechanisms in heart failure can lead to a reduction in tonic restraining influences on the sympathetic nervous system. The restraining influence over the heart and the circulation is thus removed, which tends to favour the development of a neurohumoral excitatory state with an increase in heart rate and sympathetically mediated vasoconstriction.

Heart failure is a syndrome characterized by a reduction in pump function with an ultimate diminishment in cardiac output. The actual cause of the failure is somewhat irrelevant to the discussion of peripheral adjustments. The adjustments take place in order to maintain pressure and blood flow. A number of compensatory mechanisms are responsible for supporting the circulation in the face of a fall in cardiac output. These include augmentation of the sympathetic nervous system with an increase in heart rate and peripheral vascular resistance, as well as neuroendocrine activation and release of atrial natriuretic peptide, arginine vasopressin, renin, endothelin and many other neurohormones and cytokines. Sympathetic tone is usually increased, whereas skeletal muscle blood flow and exercise tolerance are diminished. Activation of the renin-angiotensin-aldosterone system leads to salt and water reabsorption and an enhancement of plasma volume, adding further complexity to reflex control adjustment. This expansion of central blood volume might normally be expected to inhibit sympathetic stimulation by activation of inhibiting afferent receptors, but this inhibitory reflex appears to be suppressed in the presence of heart failure.

Although many of these compensatory mechanisms allow for adaptation toward short-term circulatory homeostasis, eventually their persistent activation leads to further deterioration of myocardial function. For example, excessive sympathoexcitation is directly toxic to the myocardium (Rona 1985; Jiang and Downing 1990;

Mann *et al.* 1992), as is a very high and persistent level of angiotensin II stimulation (Tan *et al.* 1991). Ultimately, systemic vascular resistance rises and myocardial performance diminishes, leading to exacerbation of heart failure.

Increased sympathetic outflow has been documented both by direct measurements of sympathetic nerve activity in humans, as well as through measurement of plasma levels of noradrenaline. There is a widely held notion that the sustained increase in neurohumoral drive in heart failure is mediated by the blunted arterial baroreflex and cardiopulmonary reflexes (Hirsch *et al.* 1987).

Studies from both humans and animals with various types of heart failure have provided direct evidence for impaired baroreflex control of both heart rate and sympathetic nerve activity. Eckberg and colleagues demonstrated that the heart rate response to a bolus injection of phenylephrine was depressed in patients with underlying heart disease. That is, the cardiac vagus failed to slow the heart rate in response to an increase in blood pressure. More recently, Ferguson and colleagues (1984) have demonstrated that skeletal muscle nerve activity is augmented in patients with heart failure and that baroreflex sensitivity is depressed. Animal studies by Zucker and colleagues (1995) using a canine model of heart failure that entails chronic cardiac pacing demonstrated that peak discharge from baroreceptors is significantly depressed in the dogs with heart failure. The depressed baroreceptor sensitivity is not due to a reduction in carotid sinus compliance or structural changes in carotid sinus nerve fibres (Wang *et al.* 1996), but might be due to augmented Na+K+-ATPase activity. The relationship between carotid sinus nerve stimulation and mean arterial pressure is blunted in heart failure. However, there does not appear to be a central abnormality of baroreflex control of sympathetic outflow.

Baroreflex-mediated regional circulatory redistribution in heart failure

Activation of vasoconstrictive mechanisms may provide an important contribution to the redistribution of the total cardiac output in patients with heart failure. It is well known that the fractional distribution of blood flow to the limbs, kidneys, and splanchnic beds decreases in heart failure, whereas blood flow to the heart and brain is preserved (Zelis *et al.* 1975). Although this alteration tends to maintain acute circulatory homeostasis, ultimately it may be responsible for the deleterious cardiac and peripheral end-organ responses (Goldsmith *et al.* 1983*b*). Diminished exercise capacity could be a result of chronically reduced flow to skeletal muscles. Renal hypoperfusion and altered intrarenal haemodynamics may contribute to the retention of sodium and water, a common feature of heart failure. Although limb flow may be normal at rest in patients with heart failure, it is also found to be moderately reduced in many patients. The relationship of limb blood flow to baroreceptor dysfunction is evidenced by the attenuation or absence of forearm vasoconstriction in response to orthostasis or lower-body negative pressure in patients with heart failure (Ferguson *et al.* 1984). It is very likely that altered baroreceptor sensitivity in systemic, humoral, and local metabolic factors contribute to the reduced dilator response of peripheral vessels found in patients with heart failure. Patients with heart failure have an attenuated sympathetic response to upright tilt (Levine *et al.* 1983) and have a significantly smaller increase in cardiac sympathetic activity in response to a pharmacologically induced vasodilated state (Newton and Parker 1996*b*). There is now very clear evidence for reduced baroreflex control of sympathetic activity in patients with heart failure.

Although renal blood flow normally remains relatively constant over a wide range of perfusion pressures from 60 to 180 mmHg, this control mechanism is due to a highly complex autoregulatory feature that remains intact even in the face of denervation. In patients with heart failure, this autoregulatory mechanism is insufficient to maintain normal renal arterial blood flow and intrarenal haemodynamics (Ichikawa *et al.* 1987, 1990). Patients with heart failure often have a decline by half in renal blood flow. That is, renal vasoconstriction occurs out of proportion to the vasoconstriction found in other circulations. The glomerular filtration fraction is initially preserved because of an enhancement in postglomerular arteriolar tone (Ichikawa *et al.* 1984; Packer *et al.* 1986). Glomerular filtration is generally maintained until the end stages of heart failure. This ratio of enhanced glomerular filtration despite reduced renal blood flow favours increased peritubular oncotic pressure, thereby promoting proximal tubular sodium reabsorption. Patients with heart failure also demonstrate a blunted renal vasoconstrictor response to orthostasis. Excessive levels of arginine vasopressin may decrease free water clearance, thus contributing to some extent to hyponatraemia (Goldsmith *et al.* 1983*a*). Vasopressin is not suppressed by hyponatraemia in these patients and may contribute to a hypo-osmolar state (Pruszczynski *et al.* 1984).

In conclusion, patients with heart failure demonstrate excessive vasoconstriction and sodium retention which is fundamental to the pathophysiology of heart failure. Evidence now exists that implicates abnormal cardiopulmonary and arterial baroreceptor function as one of several possible mechanisms of activation of the sympathetic nervous system, the renin-angiotensin system, and the secretion of excess vasopressin in heart failure.

Myocardial β-adrenoceptors

The membrane-bound β-adrenoceptor–G–protein–adenylate cyclase complex is a powerful regulator of cardiac contractility in both the non-failing and failing heart (Fig. 49.1). The β_1- and β_2-adrenergic cell surface membrane receptors, parts of which protrude into the extracellular space, interact with a number of messengers, including the neurotransmitter noradrenaline (NAd). By coupling to stimulatory guanine-nucleotide-binding proteins (G$_s$-proteins), the membrane β-adrenoceptors mediate stimulation of adenylate cyclase. Cyclic adenosine monophosphate (cAMP) is generated from adenosine triphosphate (ATP) via adenylate cyclase, and cAMP in turn catalyses a number of phosphorylation reactions mediated by protein kinase A. These reactions include phosphorylation of calcium channels, leading to a greater increase in calcium influx, and phosphorylation of phospholamban, leading to enhanced calcium uptake in the sarcoplasmic reticulum and subsequent augmented release of calcium to the myofilaments. The net result is an increase in myocardial contractility.

The non-failing human heart primarily relies on β_1-adrenoceptors. Approximately 80 per cent of the total pool of β-receptors are of the β_1 variety. β_2-adrenoceptors generate relatively little cAMP.

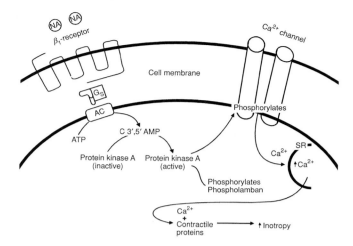

Fig. 49.1. The membrane-bound β-adrenergic receptor-G-protein-adenylate cyclase complex. The signal (i.e. noradrenaline) engages the membrane-bound β_1-receptor, which is coupled to a guanine nucleotide regulatory protein (G$_s$-protein). The G$_s$-protein dissociates from the receptor and activates the enzyme adenylate cyclase (AC). Adenosine triphosphate (ATP) is converted to cyclic 3', 5' AMP, which in turn catalyses inactive protein kinase A to active protein kinase A (PKA). PKA then phosphorylates a number of highly specialized proteins, including membrane-bound calcium channels to allow the influx of Ca^{2+} into the cell. Ca^{2+} is transported into the intracellular Ca^{2+} storage depots called sarcoplasmic reticulae (SR). The SR then provides Ca^{2+} for interaction with contractile proteins. Contraction of the myofilaments is dependent on phosphorylation by PKA of phospholamban, a specialized protein.

The cDNA for the human β_1-receptor has been cloned, and its primary amino acid structure has been elucidated. In 1982 Bristow and colleagues reported that myocardial β-adrenoceptors measured in failing human ventricles were markedly subsensitive to stimulation by the non-selective agonist isoproterenol. The alteration of the inotropic response appeared to be explicable by a decrease in the total pool of membrane-bound β-adrenoceptors as assessed by maximal ^{3}H-dihydroalprenolol binding. These authors demonstrated a highly significant reduction in isoproterenol-stimulated adenylate cyclase activity in the left ventricles of hearts removed from patients about to undergo heart transplantation (Fig. 49.2). Later studies from this same group demonstrated that 'down-regulation' of the total β-receptor population appears to begin early in mild heart failure, with some hearts showing a 60–70 percent reduction in β_1-receptor density when heart failure was more advanced. Of interest, papillary muscles from these failing hearts still responded normally with a positive inotropic response to calcium, thus implying that the primary lesion is reduced β-adrenoceptor density and/or receptor uncoupling rather than contractile protein deficiency. Since β_2-receptor density remains unchanged in the failing heart, the selective loss of β_1 receptors leads to a change in β_1/β_2 subtype ratio from approximately 80 : 20 to 60 : 40 in failing hearts. However, despite increased membrane density, the β_2-receptor is 'uncoupled' to some extent in the failing heart. The β_2-uncoupling may be related to increased G$_i$-protein activity, which inhibits the stimulation of cAMP.

It is likely that more than one mechanism is responsible for the down-regulation of β_1-adrenoceptors that occurs in heart failure.

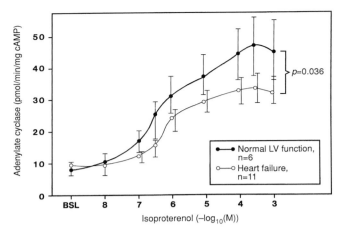

Fig. 49.2. The influence of L-isoproterenol on myocardial tissue isolated from the left ventricles (LV) of patients with severe congestive heart failure who later received a heart transplant (open circles) and from normal hearts of potential heart donors (closed circles). The failing myocardial tissue is unable to generate a normal amount of adenylate cyclase in response to L-isoproterenol. BSL, baseline. (Taken with permission from Bristow *et al.* (1982).)

Although the failing myocardium is depleted of NAd, cardiac-derived NAd (as measured from the coronary sinus) is increased in heart failure. There may also be a decrease in NAd uptake by cardiac sympathetic nerves. Increased local concentration of NAd may thereby reduce the density of membrane-bound β_1-receptors, reducing the sensitivity of the myocardium to NAd. However, it is difficult to reconcile increased local concentration of NAd when the myocardium is known to be depleted of NAd. The precise mechanism of β_1-receptor density 'down-regulation' remains unclear, but it appears to be a reversible phenomenon, as treatment with the semi-selective β-blocking agent, metoprolol, can restore both the β_1-receptor density and the responsiveness to the β_1-agonist dobutamine. The reduction in myocardial membrane-bound β_1-receptors is a marker of the adrenergic compensatory process, but it also could play a direct role in the pathophysiology of heart failure by interfering with the myocardial response to increased workloads.

There is heterogeneity in the β_2-adrenoceptor throughout the human population. At least six different phenotypes have been recognized due to genetic polymorphisms within the coding block of the receptor gene. Site-directed mutagenesis and recombinant expression have shown that some of these variances have distinct pharmacological and biochemical phenotypes. The concept of desensitization of β-adrenoceptors is probably defined as a dampening of the response despite continuing presence of the stimulus. This phenomenon is a recurrent theme in many signal transduction systems and probably represents an adaptation to intense stimuli. In that sense, it may be an adaptive phenomenon that is useful in protecting the effector organ. The desensitization that occurs after brief or minimal exposure to agonists is characterized by an uncoupling of the receptor from the G_s-protein without any change in the localization of the receptor. This rapid form of uncoupling is likely due to modification of the receptor biphosphorylation. Exposure to agonist for several minutes leads to internalization of the receptor below the cell membrane, from which it is no longer available for agonist binding. This process is usually maximal after 30 minutes of agonist exposure and is

independent of G_s coupling or the production of second messenger such as cAMP. Finally, prolonged exposure to agonists over several hours leads to reduced expression of the β-receptor, and this is termed 'down-regulation'. Receptor degradation also plays a part in down-regulation of the receptor. It is likely that sequesterization is the first step of the down-regulation process.

Plasma noradrenaline levels measured at rest

The radioenzymatic technique of measuring plasma NAd levels was an important step in bringing to the bedside a rapid and precise method of detecting heightened 'sympathetic activity' in patients with heart failure. It now seems clear that the sympathetic nervous system is activated progressively as the signs and symptoms increase over time. Patients with left ventricular dysfunction (ejection fraction ≤35 per cent) without overt signs and symptoms of heart failure have increased levels of plasma NAd as well as increased levels of atrial natriuretic peptide arginine vasopressin (Francis *et al.* 1990). In general, those patients with more advanced heart failure have the greatest increment in plasma NAd. The normal resting value of NAd is age-dependent and is generally in the range of 150–300 pg/ml. Patients with congestive heart failure have values of plasma NAd in the range of 300–3000 pg/ml, but typically average about 500–660 pg/ml.

The cause of the increase in plasma NAd in patients with congestive heart failure is poorly understood. The sympathetic nervous system and renin-angiotensin system are likely activated in a presumed attempt to maintain circulatory homeostasis in the face of a falling cardiac output (Francis *et al.* 1984), but the actual signal and how it is processed have remained elusive. Directly measured sympathetic nerve 'traffic' using a microneurographic technique has been found to be increased in the peroneal nerve of patients with heart failure (Leimbach *et al.* 1986). The correlation between directly measured nerve traffic and plasma NAd is quite good, suggesting that plasma NAd is a reasonable index of generalized sympathetic activity in the context of heart failure. Using tritiated NAd, Hasking and colleagues (1986) have demonstrated that both 'spillover' from sympathetic neurones and delayed clearance from the circulation are important contributors to increased levels of NAd in patients with heart failure (Fig. 49.3). The correlation between resting level of NAd and haemodynamic measurements such as cardiac output, systemic vascular resistance, and blood pressure are rather modest. Moreover, plasma NAd correlates only poorly with plasma renin activity and arginine vasopressin, thus suggesting that these neurohormones are under separate control mechanisms.

The parasympathetic nervous system is also abnormal in patients with heart disease (Eckberg *et al.* 1971). For any given increase in blood pressure, there is less than the usual degree of heart rate slowing. Moreover, patients with heart failure demonstrate less respiratory variation in heart rate than healthy control subjects. The cause of this relative withdrawal of vagal tone is unclear, but the reduced variation in heart rate may have prognostic significance. Of interest, the variation in RR interval is improved, but not normalized, following orthotopic heart transplantation (Sands *et al.* 1989).

Direct recordings of efferent sympathetic nerve activity from peripheral nerves in intact human subjects have been made possible by the technique of microneurography, originally developed by Valbo

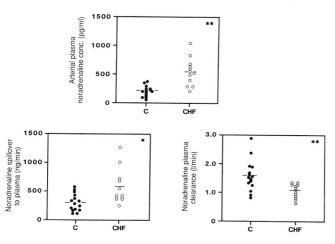

Fig. 49.3. Plasma noradrenaline concentration and its determinants in subjects with and without congestive heart failure (CHF). *, $P < 0.02$; **, $P < 0.002$. Using radioactive tracer techniques, patients with CHF demonstrate enhanced 'spillover' of NAd from synaptic clefts into plasma and reduced clearance of NAd from the circulation. Both mechanisms could contribute to increased plasma concentrations of NAd in patients with CHF. C, controls. (Taken with permission from Hasking *et al.* (1986).)

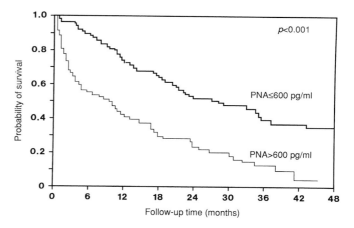

Fig. 49.4. The relationship between probability of survival and plasma noradrenaline (PNA) in 217 patients with congestive heart failure. A cut-off value of 600 pg/ml provides the most prognostic information as determined by multivariate regression analysis of survival times. (Taken with permission from Rector *et al.* (1987).)

and colleagues (1979). Studies by Ferguson *et al.* (1990) noted that the marked increase in microneurographically measured sympathetic nerve activity in patients with heart failure was significantly and inversely correlated with left ventricular stroke work index ($r = -0.86$) and positively correlated with left-sided cardiac filling pressure ($r = -0.82$). There was no correlation between sympathetic activity and left ventricular ejection fraction or mean arterial pressure. Similarly to the observations of Levine and associates (1982) using plasma NAd, Ferguson *et al.* (1990) demonstrated a correlation between cardiac performance and microneurographic efferent sympathetic nerve activity in patients with moderate-to-severe heart failure. The correlation between resting efferent nerve activity and resting levels of plasma NAd was 0.72 in the Ferguson study. Plasma NAd or directly measured nerve activity can separate mildly ill patients from those with severe disease, but these measurements do not clearly discriminate between patients with intermediate forms of heart failure, i.e. between New York Heart Association functional classes II and III.

In 1984 Cohn *et al.* reported that plasma NAd levels provide a better guide to prognosis in patients with heart failure than other commonly measured indices of cardiac performance. In this study plasma NAd was the best independent prognostic variable among several haemodynamic and biochemical measurments as determined by multivariate regression analyses of survival times. Although an update of this analysis (Rector *et al.* 1987) indicated that a cut-off value of 600 pg/ml provided the most prognostic information (Fig. 49.4), a much larger database from V-HeFT confirmed that prognosis was related to three tertiles of plasma NAd: less than 600 pg/ml, 600–900 pg/ml, and greater than 900 pg/ml. The idea of using plasma NAd to determine prognosis has been very valuable when evaluating patients for heart transplantation, where conventional haemodynamic measurements, such as ejection fraction, cardiac output, and left ventricular filling pressure, are uniformly abnormal and therefore

not discriminatory. A markedly increased plasma NAd level (i.e. greater than 900 pg/ml) is rather consistently associated with a poor prognosis.

It is believed that β-adrenoceptor blockers reduce cardiac sympathetic activity in heart failure by antagonizing β-adrenoreceptors that normally facilitate sympathetic outflow to the heart. Newton and Parker (1996a) have recently demonstrated in patients with heart failure that the administration of a β_1-selective antagonist is associated with increased cardiac adrenaline spillover. In contrast, the administration of a non-selective β-adreno blocker at similar haemodynamics results in a reduction in adrenaline spillover. These observations would suggest that there may be some advantage to non-selective β-adrenoceptor blockade in terms of inhibition of cardiac sympathetic activity. Such observations are consistent with recent findings that relatively non-selective β-blockers such as carvedilol may have some efficacy in inhibiting the progression of heart failure (Packer *et al.* 1996; Australia/New Zealand Heart Failure Research Collaborative Group 1997).

Plasma noradrenaline levels measured during exercise

Early studies using a fluorometric technique to measure plasma NAd in patients with heart failure demonstrated a greater than normal augmentation during exercise. However, careful analysis of these data indicates that patients simply stopped exercising sooner and achieved a peak total body oxygen consumption at an earlier point in time. Francis and colleagues (1982), using the more sensitive radioenzymatic technique to measure plasma NAd, confirmed the finding of early augmentation of sympathetic nervous system activity during exercise in patients with heart failure (Fig. 49.5). It is apparent from both of these studies that patients with heart failure and normal control subjects were not exercising in the same physiological framework. At relatively mild workloads patients with heart failure might have already become exhausted and achieved these peak oxygen

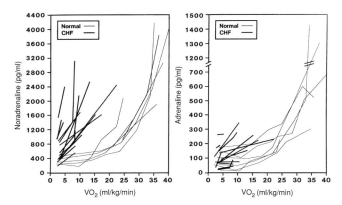

Fig. 49.5. Plasma noradrenaline response to exercise during graded bicycle ergometry is shown in thin lines for normal subjects and in thick lines for patients with congestive heart failure (CHF). VO_2, total body oxygen consumption. (Taken with permission from Francis *et al.* (1982).)

consumption, whereas control subjects were still exercising well below their anaerobic threshold.

To normalize the data so that both patients and control subjects could be compared in the same physiological framework, Francis *et al.* (1985) performed progressive bicycle ergometry and sequential plasma NAd measurements at each stage of exercise. For identical levels of exercise (defined as the percentage of peak VO_2), patients with heart failure demonstrated an attenuation of the NAd response as measured by a significantly flatter plasma NAd upward curve during exercise (Fig. 49.6). However, a subsequent study by Hasking

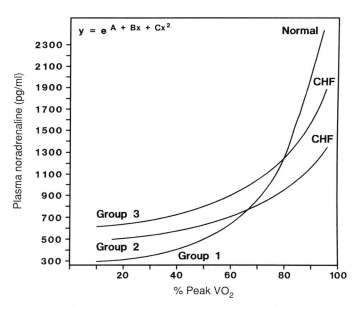

Fig. 49.6. The plasma noradrenaline response to dynamic upright exercise is plotted as a function of relative work intensity, expressed by per cent peak oxygen uptake (% peak VO_2). There is no difference in slope between group 2 (mild heart failure) and group 3 (severe heart failure). Group 1 (normal) has a steeper slope than that in groups 2 and 3 ($P = 0.002$), indicating that, at relative work intensities, normal subjects have augmented sympathetic drive. (Taken with permission from Francis *et al.* (1985).)

and colleagues (1988) using titriated NAd kinetics demonstrated increased 'spillover' of NAd during exercise in patients with heart failure compared with control subjects. In recent studies Rundqvist *et al.* (1997*a*) have demonstrated attenuated cardiac sympathetic responsiveness to exercise. The variance of these studies may have to do with differences in patient populations, techniques, etc. What remains clear is that patients with heart failure demonstrate an abnormality of the sympathetic nervous system during exercise. Such patients show an early abrupt rise in plasma NAd accompanied by an inability to mount a normal heart rate response and a failure to reduce peripheral vascular resistance to the same extent as normals. It is possible that these abnormalities contribute to their inability to perform a high level of physical activity. It is likely that some of the peripheral vascular abnormalities represent structural remodelling of the vasculature, but even these structural changes may represent a response to abnormal neurohormonal activity.

Disturbed baroreceptor function

Cardiopulmonary receptors located in the heart and lungs and baroreceptors in the great vessels normally respond to changes in pressure and volume by altering the activity of the sympathetic and parasympathetic nervous systems. In humans, heart failure is associated with abnormal autonomic responses, but the precise mechanisms underlying these abnormalities have not been completely defined. Many clinical studies have demonstrated that patients with heart failure have altered peripheral vascular and neuroendocrine responses to postural changes and orthostatic stress. Such patients demonstrate a failure to increase plasma NAd (and peripheral vascular constriction) in response to a decrease in cardiac filling pressure (so-called 'unloading' of cardiopulmonary baroreceptors) (Fig. 49.7).

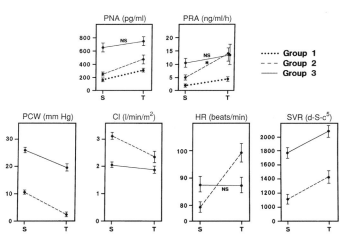

Fig. 49.7. Measurements of plasma noradrenaline (PNA) and plasma renin activity (PRA) during supine rest (S) and 60° orthostatic tilt (T) in normal subjects (group 1), patients with symptoms of heart failure but normal resting haemodynamics (group 2), and patients with heart failure and abnormal resting haemodynamics (group 3). The haemodynamic responses to tilt for groups 2 and 3 are shown in the lower panel. Pulmonary capillary wedge pressure (PCW), cardiac index (CI), and systemic vascular resistance (SVR) all changed significantly. Heart rate (HR) increased significantly in group 2, but did not change in group 3. (Taken with permission from Levine *et al.* (1983).)

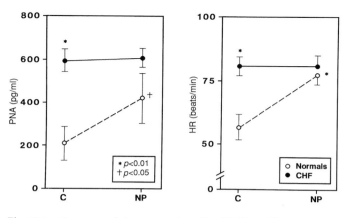

Fig. 49.8. Response of plasma noradrenaline (PNA) and heart rate (HR) to nitroprusside infusion (NP) in five normal subjects (open circles) and 46 patients with congestive heart failure (CHF) (closed circles). Symbols above the control columns (C) indicate significant difference between normal subjects and patients with congestive heart failure; symbols in NP columns indicate significant changes from control during nitroprusside infusion. *, *P* (probability) < 0.01; †, *P* < 0.05. Mean values ± standard error of the mean are shown. (Taken with permission from Olivari *et al.* (1983).)

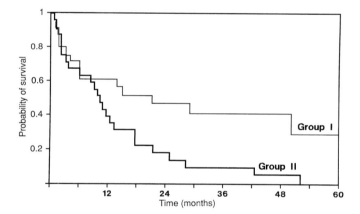

Fig. 49.9. Wilcoxon life table analysis of 21 patients in group I and 25 in group II. Group I and group II denote patients with and without a rise in plasma noradrenaline, respectively, during nitroprusside infusion. (Taken with permission from Olivari *et al.* (1983).)

Occasionally, there is even a paradoxical vasodilatory response to such orthostatic stress. While normal subject develop marked increases in sympathetic neural activity during modest nitroprusside-induced decreases in arterial and cardiac filling pressures, this response is significantly blunted in patients with heart failure (Fig. 49.8). The prognosis of patients with heart failure is poorer when they fail to activate the sympathetic nervous system during nitroprusside-induced vasodilatation (Fig. 49.9).

Patients with heart failure also have a reduced tachycardia response to blood loss. Lowering of blood pressure by the technique of lower-body negative pressure to 'unload' low-pressure cardiopulmonary baroreceptors fails to cause the expected increase in peripheral vasoconstriction (Fig. 49.10; Ferguson *et al.* 1984). These observations support the hypothesis that an impairment of car-

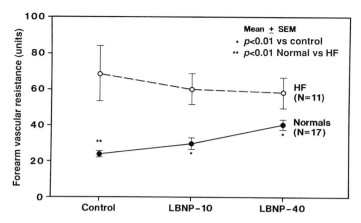

Fig. 49.10. Responses of normal subjects and patients with heart failure (HF) to unloading (deactivation) of baroreceptors with orthostatic stress produced by lower-body negative pressure (LBNP) at −10 mmHg (LBNP, −10) and at −40 mmHg (LBNP, −40). Control forearm vascular resistance (venous occlusion plethysmography) was significantly higher in the heart failure patients than in the normal subjects. Normal subjects developed significant forearm vasoconstriction during LBNP (manifested by an increase in forearm vascular resistance). In contrast, patients with heart failure failed to vasoconstrict and tended to experience paradoxical vasodilation during LBNP. (Taken with permission from Ferguson *et al.* (1984).)

diopulmonary baroreflex mechanism is at least one of the primary abnormalities responsible for the abnormal orthostatic responses observed in patients with heart failure. The abnormal response to upright tilt can be improved with therapy (angiotensin-converting enzyme inhibitors) (Cody *et al.* 1982) and the blunted heart rate lowering response to pressor activity is rapidly normalized following cardiac transplantation (Ellenbogen *et al.* 1989), suggesting that these are 'functional' disturbances rather than due to structural abnormalities. Ferguson and colleagues (1989) have reported that acute digitalization can reduced microneurographically measured efferent sympathetic nerve activity in patients with heart failure and tends to normalize that response to lower-body negative pressure. Evidence that the sympatho-inhibitory effect of digitalis is not solely related to reflex sympathetic withdrawal secondary to improved cardiac output was provided by a lack of directly measured sympathoinhibition with dobutamine, a powerful positive inotropic agent (Ferguson *et al.* 1989). It is possible that digitalis acutely sensitizes tonically active cardiac and atrial baroreceptors, thereby improving their response to changes in pressure and volume.

One of the hallmarks of congestive heart failure is chronically elevated sympathetic nervous system activity. It is possible that abnormalities of baroreflex control contribute to the heightened sympathetic drive (Fig. 49.11; Hirsch *et al.* 1987). Baroreceptors are sensory endings that normally respond to change in mechanical deformation. Using the canine pacing model of low cardiac output heart failure, Dibner-Dunlap and Thames (1989) have recorded from baroreceptor fibres and found the sensitivity of these receptors to be diminished. Dogs with chronic heart failure induced by an aortocaval fistula also demonstrate a reduced neural discharge rate from left atrial receptors during volume expansion. There appears to be a defect in transduction of the pressure stimulus, such that there is

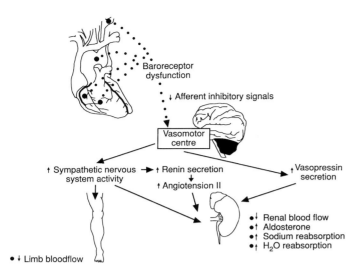

Fig. 49.11. Relationship of abnormal baroreceptor function in neurohormonal activation and regional blood flow in congestive heart failure. Increases in artrial and ventricular filling pressures and increased mean arterial or pulse pressure normally stimulate cardiopulmonary and arterial baroreceptors. Baroreceptor activation sends inhibitory signals to the medullary vasomotor centre, with suppression of sympathetic efferent activity and increased vagal efferent activity (not shown). Baroreflex inhibition is blunted in heart failure, with consequent increased activation of sympathetic and renin-angiotensin systems, and with increased neurohypophyseal release of vasopressin. Limb and renal vasoconstriction ensue, as well as renal retention of sodium and water. (Taken with permission from Hirsch *et al.* (1987).)

reduced baroreceptor input for any given arterial pressure. Preliminary studies suggest that this defect may be caused by cellular alterations in Na^+, K^+ Pump activity, since this attenuation in sensitivity is partially reversed by ouabain, a digitalis-like drug that blocks Na^+, K^+ATPase action.

Impaired baroreflex abnormalities may contribute to the pathophysiology of heart failure by increasing sympathetic nervous system activity (in itself a likely detrimental finding), by causing a suboptimal heart rate response to changes in blood pressure, and by causing an inappropriate response to orthostatic stress. Attenuation of cardiopulmonary and arterial baroreceptor function may also contribute to renal vasoconstriction, and thereby enhance sodium and water retention. Baroreceptor dysfunction may also promote activation of the renin-angiotensin system and the release of arginine vasopressin, and can be associated with dilutional hyponatraemia. It may not be coincidental that two of the principal markers for an unfavourable prognosis in patients with heart failure—increased plasma NAd concentration and hyponatraemia—share baroreceptor dysfunction as a common theme.

Autonomic dysfunction following cardiac transplantation

Following heart transplantation there is usually normalization of resting plasma NAd levels (Olivari *et al.* 1987), normalization of regional sympathetic hyperactivity (Rundqvist *et al.* 1997*b*), reduc-

tion of muscle sympathetic nerve traffic (Rundqvist *et al.* 1997*c*), and reversal of some but not all baroreceptor reflex abnormalities. However, disturbances in sensitivity to catecholamines persist and cardiopulmonary baroreflex control of forearm vascular resistance remains impaired. Experimental chronic denervation in dogs results in 'up-regulation' of β-adrenoceptor and 'down-regulation' of muscarinic receptors. A 'supersensitivity' to catecholamines develops. The major mechanism of denervation supersensitivity to NAd appears to involve lack of neuronal NAd re-uptake. Despite animal data to the contrary, recent data from human orthotopic cardiac allografts indicate that myocardial β-adrenergic receptors are not increased. Moreover, there is no direct evidence of β-receptor-mediated supersensitivity of postsynaptic origin in patients. The β-adrenergic supersensitivity is likely to be presynaptic in origin.

Patients with heart transplants generally exhibit a relative resting tachycardia (90–110 beats/minute) and demonstrate little or no increase in heart rate within 30 seconds of standing up. There is also a characteristic delayed rate of acceleration during dynamic and isometric exercise, and also a delayed deceleration at the end of exercise. Carotid sinus massage and the Valsalva manoeuvre do not affect the heart rate in the donor heart. Of interest, heart-transplant patients do demonstrate a marked tachycardia (130–140 beats/minute) in response to fever (Francis and Cohn, personal observations).

There has been a general consensus that the human donor heart is not reinnervated. Histochemical studies have failed to demonstrate reinnervation beyond the suture line following transplantation. In contrast with humans, the transplanted hearts of experimental animals have been shown to exhibit functional extrinsic reinnervation. The distinction between reinnervation in humans and animals may represent either a species difference or variations between allografts and autografts, since many of the animal experiments involved autotransplantation. Following human heart transplantation, myocardial catecholamines are undetectable in tissue biopsies for up to 5 years, indicating that, at least soon after transplantation, the adrenergic responses of these hearts probably depend mainly on variations in plasma catecholamines or presynaptic supersensitivity.

Recent evidence now suggests that some patients have functional reinnervation developing 2 or more years following heart transplantation. Wilson and colleagues (1991) have demonstrated clear increases in NAd flowing from the coronary sinus of orthotopically transplanted human hearts when tyramine is given systematically or directly into the coronary arteries. Tyramine is known to displace NAd from sympathetic neurones, and should increase NAd efflux only if there is functional reinnervation. Moreover, evidence is now accumulating that functional reinnervation may occur in a minority of heterotopic allografts. A recent study identified one case out of nine in which electrocardiographic and indirect clinical evidence of functional reinnervation was obtained 33 months after orthotopic cardiac transplantation. We have seen occasional patients with orthoptic cardiac transplantation who have developed severe coronary artery disease and classic angina pectoris, although, typically, coronary disease remains clinically silent in the transplant population.

In summary, heart transplant and heart–lung transplant will reverse some of the autonomic deficiencies observed in preceding severe heart failure, but patients may continue to demonstrate some autonomic abnormalities, including presynaptic supersensitivity to catecholamines, a blunted response to upright posture and exercise, and reduced heart rate variation. These persistent abnormalities do not keep them from leading a nearly normal life style. Although mainly dependent soon after transplantation on circulating catecholamines, new data are emerging suggesting that reinnervation occurs in some cases.

Role of the autonomic nervous system in the clinical syndrome

Still unresolved is whether the protean abnormalities in afferent and efferent sympathetic nervous system function in heart failure are fundamental to the clinical manifestations of the syndrome or are merely epiphenomena indicative of the severity of the physiological derangement. It is clear that at least some of the clinical signs—tachycardia, cool extremities, diaphoresis—are at least in part due to sympathetic activation. Other manifestations—renal sodium conservation, ventricular arrhythmia—are probably aggravated by the sympathetic nervous system. Other important complications of the disease—exercise intolerance, sudden death, ventricular hypertrophy and remodelling, atrial fibrillation, renin stimulation, etc.—could be in part related to autonomic dysfunction but the evidence for this relationship is not yet persuasive.

It is now clear that there is a fundamental abnormality in reflex control mechanisms in the syndrome of heart failure. It is generally acknowledged that these disturbances contribute, at least in part, to excessive sympathetic activity that has repeatedly characterized the syndrome. There is growing evidence that disturbances of sympathetic nervous system activity occur early, when there is left ventricular dysfunction, but no overt heart failure, and therefore may be implicated in the pathogenesis of the syndrome. Furthermore, the relationship between plasma NAd and mortality and the evidence that plasma NAd increases progressively in patients with heart failure regardless of therapy raises the possibility that inhibition of that presumed progressive sympathetic activation might favourably affect the course of the syndrome.

A number of pharmacological approaches have been entertained to induce chronic inhibition of sympathetic nervous system activity. In V-HeFT II the ACE inhibitor, enalapril, exerted shortterm (one-year) suppression of plasma noradrenaline compared to treatment with hydralazine and isosorbide dinitrate. β-Blockers have been studied in several trials, with additional multicentre studies already under way. Centrally acting sympathetic inhibitors such as clonidine and moxonidine are undergoing clinical studies. Furthermore, plasma NAd is being utilized in these and other trials as a surrogate marker for inhibiting the progression of heart failure.

References

Abboud, F. M., Heistad, D. D., Mark, A. L., and Schmid, P. G. (1976). Reflex control of the peripheral circulation. *Prog. Cardiovasc. Dis.* XVII, 371–403.

Australia/New Zealand Heart Failure Research Collaborative Group (1997). Randomised, placebo-controlled trial of carvedilol in patients with congestive heart failure due to ischaemic heart disease. *Lancet* 349, 375–80.

Banner, N. R., Williams, T. D. M., Patel, N., Chalmers, J., Lightman, S. L., and Yacoub, M. H. (1990). Altered cardiovascular and neurohumoral responses to head-up tilt after heart–lung transplantation. *Circulation* 82, 863–71.

Brigden, W. and Sharpey-Schafer, E. P. (1950). Postural changes in peripheral blood flow in cases with left heart failure. *Clin. Sci.* 9, 93–100.

Bristow, M. R., Ginsburg, R., Minobe, W. *et al.* (1982). Decreased catecholamine sensitivity and β-adrenergic-receptor density in failing human hearts. *New Engl. J. Med.* 307, 205–11.

Cody, R. J., Franklin, K. W., Kluger, J., and Laragh, J. H. (1982). Mechanisms governing the postural response and baroreceptor abnormalities in chronic congestive heart failure: Effects of acute and long-term converting-enzyme inhibition. *Circulation* 66, 135–42.

Cohn, J. N., Levine, T. B., Olivari, M. T. *et al.* (1984). Plasma norepinephrine as a guide to prognosis in patients with chronic congestive heart failure. *New Engl. J. Med.* 311, 819–23.

Coleman, H. N., Taylor, R. R., Pool, P. E., Whipple, G. H., Covell, J. W., Ross, J. R. Jr, and Braunwald, E. (1971). Congestive heart failure following chronic tachycardia. *Am. Heart J.* 81, 790–8.

Covell, J. W., Chidsey, C. A., and Braunwald, E. (1966). Reduction of the cardiac response to postganglionic sympathetic nerve stimulation in experimental cardiac failure. *Circ. Res.* 19, 51–6.

Dibner-Dunlap, M. E. and Thames, M. D. (1989). Reflex control of renal sympathetic nerve activity is preserved in heart failure despite reduced arterial baroreceptor sensitivity. *Circulation Res.* 65, 1526–35.

Eckberg, D. L., Drabinsky, M., and Braunwald, E. F. (1971). Defective cardiac parasympathetic control in patients with heart disease. *New Engl. J. Med.* 265, 877–83.

Ellenbogen, K. A., Mohanty, P. K., Szentpetery, S., and Thames, M. D. (1989). Arterial baroreflex abnormalities in heart failure. *Circulation* 79, 51–8.

Ferguson, D. W., Berg, W. J., Sanders, J. S., Roach, P. J., Kempf, J. S., and Kienzle, M. G. (1989). Sympathoinhibitory responses to digitalis glycosides in heart failure patients. *Circulation* 80, 65–77.

Ferguson, D. W., Abboud, F. M., and Mark, A. L. (1984). Selective impairment of baroreflex-mediated vasoconstrictor responses in patients with ventricular dysfunction. *Circulation* 69, 451.

Francis, G. S., Goldsmith, S. R., Ziesche, S. M., and Cohn, J. N. (1982). Response of plasma norepinephrine and epinephrine to dynamic exercise in patients with congestive heart failure. *Am. J. Cardiol.* 49, 1152–6.

Francis, G. S., Goldsmith, S. R., Levine, T. B., Olivari, M. T., and Cohn, J. N. (1984). The neurohumoral axis in congestive heart failure. *Ann. Int. Med.* 101, 370–7.

Francis, G. S., Goldsmith, S. R., Ziesche, S., Nakajima, H., and Cohn, J. N. (1985). Relative attenuation of sympathetic drive during exercise in patients with congestive heart failure. *J. Am. Coll. Cardiol.* 5, 832–9.

Francis, G. S., Benedict, C., Johnstone, D. E. *et al.* (1990). Comparison of neuroendocrine activation in patients with left ventricular dysfunction with and without congestive heart failure: A substudy of studies of left ventricular dysfunction (SOLVD). *Circulation* 82, 1724–9.

Goldsmith, S. R., Francis, G. S., Cowley, A. W., Levine, T. B., and Cohn, J. N. (1983*a*). Increased plasma arginine vasopressin levels in patients with congestive heart failure. *J. Am. Coll. Cardiol.* 1(6), 1385–90.

Goldsmith, S. R., Francis, G. S., Levine, T. B., and Cohn, J. N. (1983*b*). Regional blood flow response to orthostasis in patients with congestive heart failure. *J. Am. Coll. Cardiol.* 1(6), 1391–5.

Hasking, G. J., Ester, M. D., Jennings, G. L., Burton, D. and Korner, P. I. (1986). Norepinephrine spillover to plasma in patients with congestive heart failure: evidence of increased overall and cardiorenal sympathetic nervous activity. *Circulation* 73(4), 615–21.

Hasking, G. J., Esler, M. D., Jennings, G. L., Dewar, E., and Lambert, G. (1988). Norepinephrine spillover to plasma during steady-state supine bicycle exercise. *Circulation* 78(3), 1–7.

Higgins, C. B., Vatner, S. F., Franklin, D., and Braunwald, E. (1972). Effects of experimentally produced heart failure on the peripheral vascular response to severe exercise in conscious dogs. *Circulation* 31, 186–94.

Higgins, C. B., Pavelec, R., and Vatner, S. F. (1973). Modified technique for production of experimental right-sided heart failure. *Cardiovasc. Res.* 7, 870–7.

Hirsch, A. T., Dzau, V. J., and Creager, M. A. (1987). Baroreceptor function in congestive heart failure: effect on neurohumoral activation and regional vascular resistance. *Circulation* **75**, (Suppl. IV), IV-36–IV-48.

Ichikawa, I., Pfeffer, J. M., Pfeffer, M. A., Hostetter, T. H., and Brenner, B. M. (1984). Role of angiotensin II in the altered renal function of congestive heart failure. *Circ. Res.* **55**, 669–75.

Ichikawa, I., Kon, V., Pfeffer, M. A., Pfeffer, J. M. and Brenner, B. M. (1987). Role of angiotensin II in the altered renal function of heart failure. *Kidney Int.* **31**, S-213–15.

Ichikawa, I., Yoshioka, T., Fogo, A., and Kon, V. (1990). Role of angiotensin II in altered glomerular hemodynamics in congestive heart failure. *Kidney Int.* **38**, S-123–6.

Jiang, J. P. and Downing, S. E. (1990). Catecholamine cardiomyopathy: review and analysis of pathogenetic mechanisms. *Yale J. Biol. Med.* **63**, 581–91.

Leimbach, W. N., Wallin, B. G., Victor, R. G., Aylward, P. E., Sundlof, G., and Mark, A. L. (1986). Direct evidence from intraneural recordings for increased central sympathetic outflow in patients with heart failure. *Circulation* **73**, 913–19.

Levine, T. B., Francis, G. S., Goldsmith, S. R., Simon, A. B., and Cohn, J. N. (1982). Activity of the sympathetic nervous system and renin–angiotensin system assessed by plasma hormone levels and their relation to hemodynamic abnormalities in congestive heart failure. *Am. J. Cardiol.* **49**, 1659–66.

Levine, T. B., Francis, G. S., Goldsmith, S. R., and Cohn, J. N. (1983). The neurohumoral and hemodynamic response to orthostatic tilt in patients with congestive heart failure. *Circulation* **67**, 1070–5.

Levine, T. B., Olivari, M. T., and Cohn, J. N. (1986). Effects of orthotopic heart transplantation on sympathetic control mechanisms in congestive heart failure. *Am. J. Cardiol.* **58**, 1035–40.

Mann, D. L., Kent, R. L., Parsons, B., and Cooper, G. (1992). Adrenergic effects on the biology of the adult mammalian cardiocyte. *Circulation* **85**, 790–804.

Newton, G. E. and Parker, J. D. (1996a). Acute effects of β_1-selective and nonselective β-adrenergic receptor blockade on cardiac sympathetic activity in congestive heart failure. *Circulation* **94**, 353–8.

Newton, G. E. and Parker, J. D. (1996b). Cardiac sympathetic responses to acute vasodilation. *Circulation* **94**, 3161–7.

Olivari, M. T., Levine, B., and Cohn, J. N. (1983). Abnormal neurohumoral response to introprusside infusion in congestive heart failure. *J. Am. Coll. Cardiol.* **2**(3), 411–17.

Olivari, M. T., Levine, T. B., Ring, W. S., Simon, A., and Cohn, J. N. (1987). Normalization of sympathetic nervous system function after orthotopic cardiac transplant in man. *Circulation* **75**, V62–V64.

Packer, M., Lee, W.-H., and Kessler, P. D. (1986). Preservation of glomerular filtration rate in human heart failure by activation of the renin–angiotensin system. *Circulation* **74**, 766–74.

Packer, M., Bristow, M. R., Cohn, J. N. *et al.* for the U.S. Carvedilol Heart Failure Study Group (1996). The effect of carvedilol on morbidity and mortality in patients with chronic heart failure. *New Engl. J. Med.* **334**, 1349–55.

Pruszczynski, W., Vahanian, A., Ardaillou, R., and Acar, J. (1984). Role of antidiuretic hormone in impaired water excretion of patients with congestive heart failure. *J. Clin. Endocrinol. Metab.* **58**, 599–605.

Rector, T. S., Olivari, M. T., Levine, T. B., Francis, G. S., and Cohn, J. N. (1987). Predicting survival for an individual with congestive heart failure using the plasma norepinephrine concentration. *Am. Heart J.* **114**, 148–52.

Rona, G. (1985). Catecholamine cardiotoxicity. *J. Mol. Cell. Cardiol.* **17**, 291–306.

Rundqvist, B., Eisenhofer, G., Elam, M., and Friberg, P. (1997a). Attenuated cardiac sympathetic responsiveness during dynamic exercise in patients with heart failure. *Circulation* **95**, 940–5.

Rundqvist, B., Elam, M., Eisenhofer, G., and Friberg, P. (1997b). Normalization of total body and regional sympathetic hyperactivity in heart failure after heart transplantation. *Circulation* **15**, 516–26.

Rundqvist, B., Casale, R., Bergmann-Sverrisdottir, Y., Friberg, P., Mortara, A., and Elam, M. (1997c). Rapid fall in sympathetic nerve hyperactivity in patients with heart failure after cardiac transplantation. *J. Cardiac Fail.* **3**, 21–6.

Sands, K. E. F., Appel, M. L., Lilly, L. S., Schoen, F. J., Mudge, G. H. Jr and Cohen, R. J. (1989). Power spectrum, analysis of heart rate variability in human cardiac transplant recipients. *Circulation* **79**, 76–82.

Saul, J. P., Arai, Y., Berger, R. D., Lilly, W. S., Colucci, W. S., and Cohen, R. J. (1988). Assessment of autonomic regulation in chronic congestive heart failure by heart rate spectral analysis. *Am. J. Cardiol.* **61**, 1292–9.

Tan, L.-B., Jalil, J. E., Pick, R., Janicki, J. S., and Weber, K. T. (1991). Cardiac myocyte necrosis induced by angiotensin II. *Circ. Res.* **69**, 1185–95.

Valbo, A. B., Hagbarth, K. E., Torebjork, H. E., and Wallin, B. G. (1979). Somatosensory, proprioceptive and sympathetic activity in human peripheral nerves. *Physiol. Rev.* **59**, 919–57.

Vatner, S. J., Higgens, C. B., and Braunwald, E. (1974). Sympathetic and parasympathetic components of reflex tachycardia induced by hypotension in conscious dogs with and without heart failure. *Cardiovas. Res.* **8**, 153–61.

Wang, W., Han, H.-Y., and Zucker, I. H. (1996). Depressed baroreflex in heart failure is not due to structural change in carotid sinus nerve fibers. *J. Autonom. Nerv. Syst.* **57**, 101–8.

White, C. W. (1981). Abnormalities in baroreflex control of heart rate in canine failure. *Am. J. Physiol.* **241**, H778–82.

Wilson, R. F., Christensen, B. V., Simon, A., Olivari, M. T., White, C. W., and Laxsan, D. D. (1991). Evidence for structural sympathetic reinnervation after orthotopic cardiac transplantation in humans. *Circulation* **83**, 1210–20.

Zelis, R., Nellis, S. H., Longhurst, J., Lee, G., and Mason, D. T. (1975). Abnormalities in the regional circulations accompanying congestive heart failure. *Prog. Cardiovasc. Dis.* **XVIII**, 181–99.

Zucker, I. H., Wang, W., Brandle, M., Schultz, H. D., and Patel, K. P. (1995). Neural regulation of sympathetic nerve activity in heart failure. *Prog. Cardiovasc. Dis.* **37**, 397–414.

50. Autonomic disorders affecting cutaneous blood flow

Peter D. Drummond

Introduction

The thermoregulatory and protective functions of skin require a finely tuned cutaneous blood supply. At the local level this is achieved by autoregulatory mechanisms, driven to a large extent by interaction between chemicals in the bloodstream and the vascular endothelium, and by neurogenic inflammatory responses. Responses requiring wider co-ordination, such as thermoregulatory adjustments and exercise, are regulated by sympathetic vasodilator and constrictor nerves. In specialized parts of the body surface such as the mouth, nose, eyes, and sexual organs, a parasympathetic vasodilator supply adds another level of control over the cutaneous circulation. When this complex regulatory system breaks down, the body attempts to restore function by repairing or replacing faulty nerves or by increasing vascular sensitivity; unfortunately, however, these attempts often fail to restore normal function. In this chapter, the normal control of skin blood flow is outlined briefly, followed by examples of what can happen after normal control fails.

Normal control of skin blood flow

Cutaneous vasomotor reflexes help to regulate body temperature during the extremes of heat and cold, contribute to the maintenance of blood pressure during changes of posture and blood volume, participate in fight–flight responses, and help to dissipate body heat produced by exercise. These reflex drives are regulated by sympathetic adrenergic nerves which apply a tonic vasoconstrictor influence on arterioles and veins in cool surroundings, and by a mechanism that actively dilates cutaneous blood vessels when body temperature rises (Rowell 1977). Fluctuations in sex hormones during menopause apparently lower the threshold for active sympathetic vasodilatation (Lomax and Schönbaum 1993), leading to flushing reactions at comparatively low body temperatures. Superimposed on these tonic influences are transient sympathetic vasoconstrictor and dilator responses to painful and stressful stimuli (Krogstad *et al.* 1995). Curiously, the dilator response predominates when the skin is cool, but vasodilatation competes with vasoconstriction when the skin is warm. The mechanism of the dilator response is uncertain, but could involve an active mechanism or segmental release of sympathetic vasoconstrictor tone in precapillary resistance vessels (Blumberg and Wallin 1987). Vasoconstrictor traffic closely regulates blood flow through high-capacity arteriovenous shunts in the glabrous skin of the hands, feet, and face, and decreases blood flow through these shunts in response to pain, stress, and cold. In cool surroundings, vasoconstrictor activity regulates blood flow through the resistance vessels of hairy skin; however, vasoconstrictor responses to pain and stress are weak or absent in hairy skin regardless of ambient temperature, presumably because there are few arteriovenous shunts (Krogstad *et al.* 1995).

Before and during the early stages of exercise, an increase in vasoconstrictor tone moves blood away from the skin to exercising muscles (Kenney and Johnson 1992). The increase in body temperature during prolonged exercise provokes competition between cutaneous vasoconstriction and active sympathetic dilatation to accomodate the need for heat loss. The mechanism of active sympathetic vasodilatation is uncertain, but might involve a substance released from sweat glands or nitric oxide released from peripheral nerve endings or the vascular endothelium (Taylor and Bishop 1993).

Injury or painful stimulation of the skin initiates local neurogenic inflammation. An axon reflex mechanism discharges neuropeptides such as substance P and calcitonin-gene-related peptide from the cutaneous terminals of unmyelinated and thinly myelinated nociceptive fibres; in addition, vasoactive inflammatory mediators are released from mast cells and injured tissue (Holzer 1992). Among other functions, neuropeptides increase the calibre and permeability of blood vessels, thereby releasing plasma proteins and white blood cells into the extracellular fluid to combat infection and to begin repair. Non-painful heat stimulation evokes axon reflexes in nociceptive afferents (Magerl and Treede 1996), raising the possibility that axon reflexes also have a protective function by dispersing heat or by diluting potentially harmful substances. Local cold stimulation appears to release noradrenaline directly from sympathetic vasoconstrictor terminals, but simultaneously evokes axon reflexes in nociceptive afferents; thus, the drive to prevent heat loss from the cooled site competes with the drive to prevent tissue injury (Pergola *et al.* 1993).

The vascular endothelium produces vasodilating and vasoconstricting substances in response to local physiological factors (e.g. changes in blood flow and oxygenation) and in response to vasoactive substances manufactured by the endothelium itself or released from perivascular nerves (Burnstock and Ralevic 1994). For example, neuropeptides such as substance P induce vascular endothelial cells to synthesize a vasodilating substance (thought to be nitric oxide). Substance P released from perivascular nerves is normally partitioned from the vascular endothelium by the vessel wall; however, endothelial cells themselves produce substance P (Burnstock and Ralevic 1994). During injury and inflammation, neuropeptides and neurotransmitters gain access to the vascular endothelium, and provoke the release of endothelium-dependent relaxing or constricting factors.

Table 50.1. Some causes of facial flushing

Stimulus	Postulated mechanism
Emotion	Active sympathetic vasodilatation and activation of vascular adrenoceptors by circulating catecholamines
Heat	Active sympathetic vasodilatation and release of sympathetic vasoconstriction. Fluctuations in sex hormones during menopause apparently lower the hypothalamic set-point for thermoregulatory flushing
Endogenous vasodilators	These include vasoactive substances (e.g. serotonin, bradykinin, prostaglandins, histamine) synthesized during inflammation or by carcinoid tumours, neuropeptides (e.g. substance P, calcitonin-gene-related peptide, vasoactive intestinal polypeptide) secreted during neurogenic inflammation, and nitric oxide released from the vascular endothelium
Facial pain	Local neuropeptide release from peripheral nociceptor terminals supplements parasympathetic vasodilatation in response to ocular, nasal, or oral pain (e.g. dental pain). Sympathetic denervation supersensitivity may augment facial flushing during attacks of cluster headache
Drugs	Direct vasodilatation (e.g. calcium channel antagonists), or indirect vasodilatation (e.g. to metabolites of alcohol)
Taste, ocular pain	Postganglionic parasympathetic secretory fibres cross-innervate denervated sympathetic pathways after local injury to sympathetic nerves (e.g. in the auriculotemporal and submental syndromes), or preganglionic sympathetic secretory fibres cross-innervate denervated sympathetic neurones in the superior cervical ganglion (e.g. in preganglionic Horner's syndrome, harlequin syndrome, and Ross's syndrome)

The facial circulation

The facial circulation participates in the preliminary stages of injestion and digestion of food, helps to protect the membranes of the eyes, nose, and mouth against injury and infection and, by adding colour to emotional reactions, and can shape social behaviour. Not surprisingly, the neural control of facial blood flow is more complex than mechanisms of control in most other cutaneous regions. Some of the possible causes of normal and pathological facial flushing are summarized in Table 50.1.

Sympathetic control of the facial circulation

As in other parts of the body, thermoregulatory responses in the face are mediated by changes in sympathetic vasoconstrictor tone and by active sympathetic vasodilatation. Vasoconstrictor innervation is greatest in the most exposed parts of the face, such as the ears, nose, lips, and eyes (Fig. 50.1). Blood vessels in other parts of the face constrict weakly if at all during body cooling; however, blocking the sympathetic supply to the face immediately increases blood flow and skin temperature in blocked areas, indicating release of tonic vasoconstrictor activity. The facial circulation participates in general vasoconstrictor responses, but constriction is often overshadowed by simultaneous local vasodilatation. For example, vasoconstriction competes with active sympathetic vasodilatation in facial vessels during moderate exercise (Drummond 1997); the vasoconstrictor influence can be blocked by pretreatment with the α-adrenergic antagonist phentolamine (Fig. 50.2).

In most parts of the face, blood vessels dilate actively during body heating and emotions such as embarrassment (Fig. 50.1). This response involves more than the passive release of sympathetic vasoconstrictor tone, because increases in facial blood flow during body heating far outweigh the modest increases resulting from vasoconstrictor blockade (Drummond and Finch 1989). Nordin (1990) reported that bursts of sympathetic activity in the supraorbital nerve preceded vasodilator and galvanic skin responses in the forehead during body heating, mental stress, and arousal stimuli (electric shocks over the median nerve at the wrist). He concluded that discharge of sudomotor or vasomotor fibres provokes active sympathetic vasodilatation in the forehead circulation during thermal stress

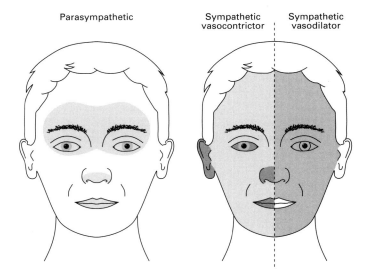

Fig. 50.1. Distribution of sympathetic vasoconstrictor innervation and sympathetic and parasympathetic vasodilator innervation in the face. Vasoconstrictor innervation is greatest in the lips, ears, eyes, and nose, whereas active sympathetic vasodilatation occurs in other parts of the face. Parasympathetic vasodilator fibres supply the respiratory and gastrointestinal tracts and large cranial blood vessels; the parasympathetic supply spills over to the facial circulation in the lips, nostrils, and forehead.

and psychological stimuli. This dilator response may be more apparent in the face than elsewhere because vasoconstrictor tone is weak.

Interrupting the sympathetic pathway to the face reduces emotional blushing (Yilmaz et al. 1996), as does the β-adrenergic antagonist propranolol (Drummond 1997). Propranolol probably blocks the vasodilator action of circulating adrenaline in facial vessels (Drummond 1996), because β-adrenoceptors are more responsive to adrenaline than to noradrenaline. Bilateral cervicothoracic sympathectomy may prevent active sympathetic vasodilatation when blushing, but this approach is limited by the prospect of postoperative complications such as pathological gustatory sweating and flushing (see below).

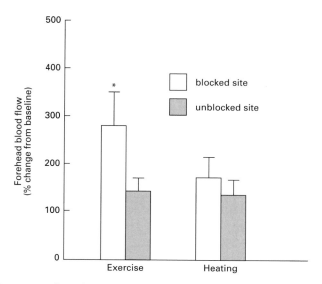

Fig. 50.2. Effect of α-adrenergic blockade with phentolamine on forehead blood flow during exercise and body heating. Phentolamine was administered by iontophoresis to a small area of the forehead before exercise. Skin blood flow was monitored at this site and at a similar site on the other side of the forehead with a laser Doppler flowmeter. Subjects pedalled as fast as they could for 1 minute on an exercise bicycle, then pedalled at 50 per cent of this rate for the next 10 minutes. Subjects were then wrapped in blankets and heated with hot air for the next 5 minutes. Blood flow measured during the last 2 minutes of exercise and the last 3 minutes of heating was expressed as the percentage change from baseline flow. During exercise, increases in flow were greater at the blocked site than at the unblocked site ($*p < 0.05$), indicating that an increase in vasoconstrictor tone during exercise normally opposes facial flushing. Bars represent the standard error of responses. (From Drummond (1997).)

Parasympathetic vasodilator reflexes and neurogenic vasodilatation in the face

Parasympathetic vasodilator fibres innervate blood vessels that supply the lacrimal and salivary glands and the secretory glands of the nose. Activation of these fibres increases the local supply of blood to enable the rapid production of secretory products. Parasympathetic vasodilator innervation extends beyond the secretory glands to surrounding tissue in the nose, eyes and mouth, and to the lips and forehead (Fig. 50.1). The primary stimulus for parasympathetic vasodilation in nonglandular parts of the face seems to be irritation of the mucosal lining of the eyes, nose, or mouth. However, other intense and possibly harmful stimuli which make the eyes water, such as bright light, might also induce cutaneous parasympathetic vasodilatation.

The glandular secretions help to dilute and wash away potentially harmful substances from the sensitive lining of the eyes, nose, and mouth. Injury elsewhere in the face initiates neurogenic vasodilatation, mediated by release of vasoactive peptides from peripheral terminals of the trigeminal nerve. The trigeminal nerve innervates large extracranial and intracranial blood vessels, and probably initiates neurogenic inflammation and parasympathetic vasodilatation in these vessels and in the facial microcirculation during migraine and cluster headache (Drummond 1994). The therapeutic effect of vasoconstrictive drugs such as ergotamine and sumatriptan depends, at

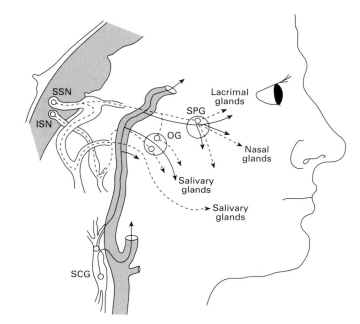

Fig. 50.3. Parasympathetic pathways to the lacrimal and salivary glands. Lacrimal and vasodilator centres near the superior salivatory nucleus (SSN) distribute fibres through the facial nerve to supply the sphenopalatine ganglion (SPG). Postganglionic fibres project from the SPG to innervate the lacrimal glands, nasal mucosa, and palatine glands. In addition, the SPG distributes parasympathetic vasodilator fibres to large cranial vessels and to the cutaneous vascular supply of the forehead. Salivatory neurones from the SSN proceed with the facial nerve and chorda tympani to supply the submandibular and sublingual ganglia. Salivatory neurones originating in the ISN leave the medulla with the glossopharyngeal nerve and follow a tortuous route to arrive at the otic ganglion (OG). Postganglionic salivatory fibres from the OG supply the parotid gland via the auriculotemporal nerve. In addition, parasympathetic vasodilator fibres from the OG innervate oral tissues and large cranial arteries. Postganglionic sympathetic fibres project from the superior cervical ganglion (SCG) to follow the internal and external carotid arteries. Sympathetic fibres branch from the internal carotid plexus to join parasympathetic nerves, but pass through the SPG and OG without synapsing.

least to some extent, on counteracting vasodilatation in large cranial vessels during headache. Vasodilator drugs, metabolic by-products of alcohol, and endogenous vasodilators that find their way into the systemic circulation may all induce facial flushing (Ray and Williams 1993).

Parasympathetic vasodilator fibres are distributed to target organs and the facial skin via two major pathways which originate in the superior and inferior salivatory nuclei; they supply the sphenopalatine, otic, and submandibular ganglia via the the facial and glossopharyngeal nerves (Fig. 50.3). Noxious stimulation of the mouth can induce lacrimation and parasympathetic vasodilatation in the forehead (mediated by the facial nerve) as well as salivation and vasodilatation in oral tissue (mediated by the glossopharyngeal nerve) (Drummond 1995a), indicating that the two vasodilator pathways can act in concert. The trigeminal nerve supplies the afferent limb for both of these parasympathetic reflexes.

Effects of nerve injury

After peripheral nerve injury, many neurones with injured or transected fibres die; cell death may progress trans-synaptically in the spinal cord. The injured fibres of surviving neurones attempt to grow back to their original destination but are sometimes unable to do so if their perineurial sheath has been damaged or destroyed. In these circumstances, collateral twigs sprout from nearby fibres in response to the high concentration of nerve growth factor produced by the injured and denervated tissue. These collateral sprouts occupy the empty perineurial sheath (Diamond *et al.* 1992) and can eventually make functional but sometimes quite inappropriate connections with the denervated tissue. Sympathetic, parasympathetic, and sensory fibres compete for nerve growth factor, so that injury to one category of fibre causes sprouting from other fibres in the vicinity (Kessler 1985). To make matters worse, supersensitivity often develops in denervated tissue (Koltzenburg *et al.* 1995), either through the removal of prejunctional constraints (e.g. presynaptic autoreceptors or neurotransmitter enzymes) or through the development of postjunctional supersensitivity (e.g. by increasing receptor density or receptor-neurotransmitter affinity, or by upregulating postreceptor activity). As described below, these responses to injury sometimes produce quite bizarre autonomic disturbances.

Pathological gustatory sweating and flushing

Painful gustatory stimulation normally induces parasympathetic vasodilatation in the forehead which is opposed by sympathetic vaso-constrictor activity, and may also induce sympathetic sudomotor activity (Fig. 50.4). After injury to pre- or postganglionic sympathetic fibres, stimuli that induce salivation sometimes provoke facial sweating and flushing in the distribution of sympathetic denervation. In the *preganglionic syndrome*, aberrant connections apparently develop between salivatory fibres and denervated vasomotor and sudomotor neurones in the superior cervical ganglion (Fig. 50.4); cross-innervation lower down in the stellate ganglion can also produce autonomic disturbances in the sympathetically denervated arm (e.g. piloerection while eating). In the *postganglionic syndrome*, collateral sprouts from parasympathetic salivatory fibres apparently make functional connections with sympathetically denervated sweat glands and blood vessels (Fig. 50.4). Because postganglionic sympathetic and parasympathetic fibres are distributed to the salivary glands and skin with sensory nerves, the postganglionic syndrome is often limited to the terminal distribution of an injured sensory nerve (e.g. in the auriculotemporal syndrome and the submental syndrome). Surgical section of the tympanic branch of the glossopharyngeal nerve in the middle ear interrupts pathological gustatory sweating in the auriculotemporal syndrome (Walsh and Hoyt 1969), implying that salivatory fibres originating in the inferior salivatory nucleus are responsible for autonomic disturbances in this syndrome (Fig. 50.3).

Pathological lacrimal sweating and flushing

Noxious stimulation of the eyes, nose, and mouth can induce sweating and flushing in sympathetically denervated parts of the face. The mechanism of this response is probably similar to that proposed above for gustatory sweating and flushing. In the postganglionic syn-

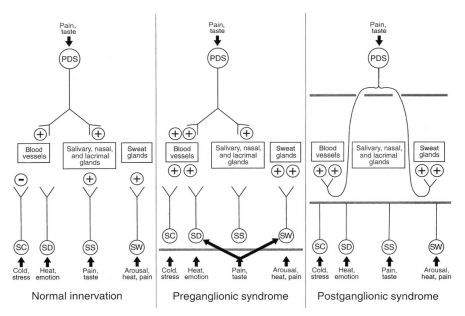

Fig. 50.4. Mechanisms of normal and pathological gustatory flushing. SC, sympathetic postganglionic vasoconstrictor neurone; SD, sympathetic postganglionic vasodilator neurone; SS, sympathetic postganglionic secretory neurone; SW, sympathetic postganglionic sudomotor neurone; PDS, parasympathetic postganglionic vasodilator and secretory neurones. In *normally innervated skin*, gustatory flushing to painful stimulation of the mouth is mediated by parasympathetic vasodilator neurones and inhibited by sympathetic vasoconstrictor discharge. Sweating during painful gustatory stimulation is mediated by sympathetic sudomotor fibres. In the *preganglionic syndrome*, connections develop between preganglionic secretory fibres and postganglionic sympathetic vasodilator and sudomotor neurones in the superior cervical ganglion. Denervation supersensitivity may also develop to neurotransmitters released from postganglionic sympathetic vasodilator and sudomotor fibres (shown as ++). In the *postganglionic syndrome* (e.g. the auriculotemporal and submental syndromes), collateral sprouts from parasympathetic fibres occupy vacant sympathetic pathways to supersensitive sweat glands and blood vessels. Nerve injury is shown as a solid line that cuts across the normal pathway of the nerve.

drome, collateral fibres sprouting from parasympathetic vasodilator and secretory fibres supplying the lacrimal glands apparently occupy sympathetically denervated pathways to the forehead, so that stimuli that normally make the eyes water provoke sweating and flushing in sympathetically denervated parts of the forehead (Drummond and Lance 1992). Lacrimal sweating and flushing were detected in one patient with a *preganglionic* sympathectomy, suggesting that aberrant connections can develop between preganglionic lacrimal fibres and denervated sudomotor and vasomotor neurones in the superior cervical ganglion (Drummond and Lance 1992). Denervation supersensitivity may contribute to pathological lacrimal flushing, because abnormal flushing was detected in patients with a central sympathetic lesion as well as those with a more peripheral site of lesion. Intense discharge of the trigeminal nerve during attacks of cluster headache probably provokes pathological lacrimal sweating and flushing in sympathetically denervated parts of the face (Drummond and Lance 1992).

The mirror-image of pathological lacrimal sweating and flushing was recently described in patients with a preganglionic lesion of parasympathetic fibres supplying the lacrimal gland. The dry eye of these patients was found to water during body heating, presumably because of cross-innervation of denervated parasympathetic neurones in the sphenopalatine ganglion by sympathetic sudomotor and vasomotor fibres which pass through the ganglion on their way to the forehead (Drummond 1995*b*). A gusto-lacrimal reflex ('crocodile tears') can also develop after injury to the facial nerve, probably because of cross-innervation of denervated lacrimal neurones in the sphenopalatine ganglion by preganglionic salivatory fibres sprouting from the tympanic branch of the glossopharyngeal nerve (Walsh and Hoyt 1969).

Horner's syndrome and harlequin syndrome

The ocular, sudomotor, and vasomotor deficit that results from injury to the sympathetic innervation of the face is known as Horner's syndrome. The distribution of sweating and flushing deficit depends upon the site of injury. A lesion of pre- or postganglionic fibres proximal to the bifurcation of the common carotid artery causes hemifacial loss of sweating and flushing. Postganglionic fibres to the forehead, the eye and to a lesser extent the cheek follow the internal carotid artery, whereas fibres to other parts of the face follow the external carotid artery (Fig. 50.5); thus, injury to fibres that follow the internal carotid artery (e.g. by an aneurysm of this vessel) disrupts sweating and flushing in the forehead to a greater extent than in other parts of the face. Using this rule of thumb, loss of thermoregulatory sweating and flushing limited to the forehead and sometimes the cheek in cluster headache patients points to an injury to fibres following the internal carotid artery, a conclusion convergent with simultaneous postganglionic pupillary deficit (Drummond and Lance 1992).

Most sympathetic oculomotor fibres leave the spinal cord before vasomotor and sudomotor fibres; thus, hemifacial loss of sweating and flushing without ocular signs of sympathetic deficit would indicate an injury of preganglionic sympathetic fibres below the first thoracic root (Fig. 50.5). This pattern of sympathetic deficit is produced by preganglionic sympathectomy below the first thoracic segment and is mimicked by patients with harlequin syndrome (loss of sweating and flushing on one side of the face without the ocular signs of Horner's syndrome). Despite the grossly normal appearance of the

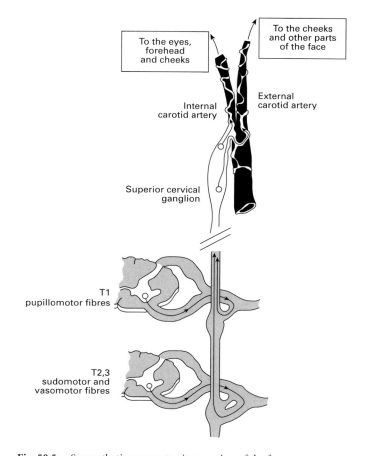

Fig. 50.5. Sympathetic vasomotor innervation of the face. Vasoconstrictor, vasodilator, and sudomotor fibres probably all follow much the same course to the face because injury affects all functions simultaneously. The development of excessive sweating on the paralysed side of the body after a stroke indicates the presence of a central inhibitory contralateral influence on sweating; however, a similar inhibitory influence on vasomotor reactions has not been described. Sympathetic vasomotor neurones projecting from the hypothalamus and higher centres synapse ipsilaterally with preganglionic neurones in the thoracic region of the spinal cord. Most preganglionic sudomotor and vasomotor fibres leave the cord in the second, third, and fourth thoracic roots, and then synapse with postganglionic neurones in the superior cervical ganglion. Fibres from the rostral part of the ganglion follow the internal carotid artery and cranial nerves to be distributed to the forehead and sometimes the cheek. Fibres from the caudal part of the ganglion follow the external carotid artery before projecting to the cheeks and other parts of the face. (Reprinted with permission from Drummond (1994).)

pupils in harlequin syndrome, most patients show pupillary signs of denervation supersensitivity to sympathetic and parasympathetic agonists (Drummond and Lance 1993). Occasionally, the tonic pupil of Holmes–Adie syndrome is associated with sympathetic deficit in the face and elsewhere (termed Ross's syndrome, Wolfe *et al.* 1995). Thus, the pathological process that attacks parasympathetic ciliary ganglia and dorsal root ganglia in Holmes–Adie syndrome might also attack sympathetic ganglia in Ross's syndrome and in the harlequin syndrome. The nature of the pathogen is uncertain, but might be a slow virus or an autoimmune reaction.

Patients sometimes seek treatment for asymmetrical sweating and flushing, for cosmetic reasons. Unfortunately, restoration of normal flushing to sympathetically denervated parts of the face is not possible; at the risk of side-effects such as postoperative gustatory sweating and flushing, cervical sympathectomy on the normally flushing side restores symmetry (Lance *et al.* 1988).

Erythromelalgia and Raynaud's disease

Erythromelalgia refers to painful, swollen, hot red hands or feet. Ochoa (1993) whimsically described erythromelalgia as the 'angry, backfiring C-nociceptor' (ABC) syndrome, because antidromic release of neuropeptides from sensitized nociceptors probably causes the swelling and hot skin. Erythromelalgia is sometimes associated with high red blood cell and platelet counts, or with diabetic autonomic neuropathy or other diseases, but most often develops by itself for unknown reasons. The burning pain of erythromelalgia appears to result from cutaneous ischaemia, despite increased flow through arteriovenous shunts rendered immobile by loss of sympathetic vasoconstrictor innervation (Rauck *et al.* 1996); it is relieved by cooling the symptomatic part, consistent with sensitization of cutaneous nociceptors. Endothelial damage, vascular swelling, and sympathetic denervation supersensitivity in superficial resistance vessels may cause chronic neurogenic inflammation, sensitization of nociceptors, and nutritional insufficiency in erythromelalgia (Cline *et al.* 1989; Rauck *et al.* 1996). A similar mechanism might account for the red ear syndrome, a painful condition which is often brought on by exercise, exposure to heat, touch, chewing, or neck movement (Lance 1996).

Parallels between the symptoms of erythromelalgia and those of complex regional pain syndrome (CRPS; causalgia and reflex sympathetic dystrophy) make one wonder whether similar mechanisms might underlie vascular disturbances and pain in these conditions. Like erythromelalgia, the increase in blood flow through the affected extremity in the warm stage of CRPS is associated with signs of sympathetic denervation (Kurvers *et al.*, 1994); in addition, blood vessels in the affected limb are supersensitive to noradrenaline (Arnold *et al.*, 1993). Perhaps an adrenoceptor disturbance that increases the excitability of cutaneous nociceptors (Drummond *et al.*, 1996) causes burning pain in both conditions.

In certain respects, Raynaud's disease is the antithesis of erythromelalgia. Raynaud's phenomenon is characterized by episodic vasospasm in the fingers or toes in response to cold, vibration or emotion; occasionally it is associated with occlusive arterial disease or connective tissue diseases such as scleroderma which narrow the lumen of digital arteries and decrease capillary blood flow. During attacks, the affected digits turn white then cyanotic, and feel numb; later on, during the stage of reactive hyperaemia, throbbing pain may develop as sensation returns (Coffman 1993). An increased sensitivity of α-adrenoceptors in digital arteries might increase susceptibility to these attacks (Freedman *et al.*, 1989).

Painful sensitivity to cold can also develop after peripheral nerve injury. Ochoa and Yarnitsky (1994) identified the coexistence of impaired cold perception with pain to more intense cold in patients with peripheral nerve disease from various causes; in addition, the symptomatic skin was abnormally cold in most patients. They suggested that partial loss of cold-specific afferent fibres releases inhibition of nociceptor input centrally, so that cold induces burning pain. Ochoa and Yarnitsky postulated that sympathetic denervation resulting from the peripheral neuropathy provokes denervation supersensitivity and vasospasm to circulating catecholamines. The cold skin might then activate nociceptors and cause pain.

Conclusions

Much still needs to be learnt about the normal control of the cutaneous circulation, and about the pathophysiology of disorders that involve disturbances in skin blood flow. The sympathetic nervous system seems to contribute to vascular disturbances and pain in poorly understood pain syndromes such as reflex sympathetic dystrophy, which often start after minor peripheral nerve injury; the relevance of aberrant cross-innervation and denervation supersensitivity for these syndromes needs to be investigated. During vascular headache, the sensory supply of cranial vessels probably initiates neurogenic inflammation which then recruits parasympathetic vasodilator reflexes, in a vicious circle. Recent advances in treatment help to prevent the escalation of this cycle, but do not stop the cycle from repeating itself during the next attack. Finally, little is known about the pathophysiology of age-related changes that cause gradual loss of normal cutaneous vasoregulation. Insights into this process might help to combat cutaneous infections and promote wound healing in elderly people.

References

Arnold, J. M. O., Teasell, R. W., MacLeod, A. P., Brown, J. E., and Carruthers, S. G. (1993). Increased venous alpha-adrenoceptor responsiveness in patients with reflex sympathetic dystrophy. *Ann. Int. Med.* **118**, 619–21.

Blumberg, H. and Wallin, B. G. (1987). Direct evidence of neurally mediated vasodilatation in hairy skin of the human foot. *J. Physiol.* **382**, 105–21.

Burnstock, G. and Ralevic, V. (1994). New insights into the local regulation of blood flow by perivascular nerves and endothelium. *Br. J. Plast. Surg.* **47**, 527–43.

Cline, M. A., Ochoa, J. L., and Torebjork, H. E. (1989). Chronic hyperalgesia and skin warming caused by sensitized C nociceptors. *Brain* **112**, 621–47.

Coffman, J. D. (1993). Raynaud's phenomenon. *Curr. Opin. Cardiol.* **8**, 821–8.

Diamond, J., Holmes, M. and Coughlin, M., (1992). Endogenous NGF and nerve impulses regulate the collateral sprouting of sensory axons in the skin of the adult rat. *J. Neurosci.* **12**, 1454–66.

Drummond, P. D. (1994). Sweating and vascular responses in the face: normal regulation and dysfunction in migraine, cluster headache and harlequin syndrome. *Clin. Auton. Res.* **4**, 273–85.

Drummond, P. D. (1995*a*). Mechanisms of physiological gustatory sweating and flushing in the face. *J. autonom. nerv. Syst.* **52**, 117–24.

Drummond, P. D. (1995*b*). Lacrimation induced by thermal stress in patients with a facial nerve lesion. *Neurology* **45**, 1112–14.

Drummond, P. D. (1996). Adrenergic receptors in the forehead microcirculation. *Clin. Auton. Res.* **6**, 23–7.

Drummond, P. D. (1997). The effect of adrenergic blockade on blushing and facial flushing. *Psychophysol* **34**, 163–8.

Drummond, P. D. and Finch, P.M. (1989). Reflex control of facial flushing during body heating in man. *Brain.* **112**, 1351–8.

Drummond, P. D. and Lance, J.W. (1992). Pathological sweating and flushing accompanying the trigeminal–lacrimal reflex in patients with cluster headache and in patients with a confirmed site of cervical sympathetic deficit: evidence for parasympathetic cross-innervation. *Brain* **115**, 1429–45.

Drummond, P. D. and Lance, J.W. (1993). Site of autonomic deficit in harlequin syndrome. *Ann. Neurol.* **34**, 814–19.

Drummond, P. D., Skipworth, S., and Finch, P.M. (1996). α_1-Adrenoceptors in normal and hyperalgesic skin. *Clin. Sci.* **91**, 73–7.

Freedman, R. R., Sabharwal, S.C., Desai, N., Wenig, P., and Mayes, M. (1989). Increased α-adrenergic responsiveness in idiopathic Raynaud's disease. *Arthritis Rheumatism* **32**, 61–5.

Holzer, P. (1992). Peptidergic sensory neurons in the control of vascular functions: mechanisms and significance in the cutaneous and splanchnic and vascular beds. *Rev. Physiol. Biochem. Pharmacol.* **121**, 49–146.

Kenney, W. L. and Johnson, J. M. (1992). Control of skin blood flow during exercise. *Med. Sci. Sports Exerc.* **24**, 303–12.

Kessler, J. A. (1985). Parasympathetic, sympathetic, and sensory interactions in the iris: nerve growth factor regulates cholinergic ciliary ganglion innervation *in vivo*. *J. Neurosci.* **5**, 2719–25.

Koltzenburg, M., Habler, H. J., and Janig, W. (1995). Functional reinnervation of the vasculature of the adult cat paw pad by axons - originally innervating vessels in hairy skin. *Neurosci.* **67**, 245–52.

Krogstad, A. L., Elam, M., Karlsson, T., and Wallin, B. G. (1995). Arteriovenous anastomoses and the thermoregulatory shift between cutaneous vasoconstrictor and vasodilator reflexes. *J. autonom. nerv. Syst.* **53**, 215–22.

Kurvers, H. A. J. M., Jacobs, M. J. H. M., Beuk, R. J. *et al.* (1994). Reflex sympathetic dystrophy: result of autonomic denervation? *Clin. Sci.* **87**, 663–9.

Lance, J. W. (1996). The red ear syndrome. *Neurology* **47**, 617–20.

Lance, J. W., Drummond, P.D., Gandevia, S. C., and Morris, J. G. L. (1988). Harlequin syndrome: the sudden onset of unilateral flushing and sweating. *J. Neurol. Neurosurg. Psychiat.* **51**, 635–42.

Lomax, P. and Schönbaum, E. (1993). Postmenopausal hot flushes and their management. *Pharmacol. Ther.* **57**, 347–58.

Magerl, W. and Treede, R. D. (1996). Heat-evoked vasodilatation in human hairy skin: axon reflexes due to low-level activity of nociceptive afferents. *J. Physiol.* **497**, 837–48.

Nordin, M. (1990). Sympathetic discharges in the human supraorbital nerve and their relation to sudo- and vasomotor responses. *J. Physiol.* **423**, 241–55.

Ochoa, J. L. (1993). The human sensory unit and pain: new concepts, syndromes, and tests. *Muscle and Nerve* **16**, 1009–16.

Ochoa, J. L. and Yarnitsky, D. (1994). The triple cold syndrome: cold hyperalgesia, cold hypoaesthesia and cold skin in peripheral nerve disease. *Brain* **117**, 185–97.

Pergola, P. E., Kellogg, D. L., Johnson, J. M., Kosiba, W. A., and Solomon, D. E. (1993). Role of sympathetic nerves in the vascular effects of local temperature in human forearm skin. *Am. J. Physiol.* **265**, H785–H792.

Rauck, R. L., Naveira, F., Speight, K. L., and Smith, B. P. (1996). Refractory idiopathic erythromelalgia. *Anaesth Analg.* **82**, 1097–101.

Ray, D. and Williams, G. (1993). Pathological causes and clinical significance of flushing. *Br. J. Hosp. Med.* **50**, 594–8.

Rowell, L. B. (1977). Reflex control of the cutaneous vasculature. *J. Invest. Dermatol.* **69**, 154–66.

Taylor, W. F. and Bishop, V. S. (1993). A role for nitric oxide in active thermoregulatory vasodilation. *Am. J. Physiol.* **264**, H1355–H1359.

Walsh, F. B. and Hoyt, W. F. (1969). *Clinical neuro-ophthalmology*, Vol. 1. (3rd edn). Williams and Wilkins, Baltimore, MD.

Wolfe, G. I., Galetta, S. L., Teener, J. W., Katz, J. S., and Bird, S. J. (1995). Site of autonomic dysfunction in a patient with Ross' syndrome and postganglionic Horner's syndrome. *Neurology* **45**, 2094–96.

Yilmaz, E. N., Dur, A. H. M., Cuesta, M. A., and Rauwerda, J. A. (1996). Endoscopic versus transaxillary thoracic sympathectomy for primary axillary and palmar hyperhidrosis and/or facial blushing: 5–year-experience. *Eur. J. Cardio-thoracic Surg.* **10**, 168–72.

51. Autonomic disturbances in spinal cord lesions

Christopher J. Mathias and Hans L. Frankel

Introduction

The integrity of the spinal cord is of particular importance to the normal functioning of the autonomic nervous system, as the entire sympathetic outflow (from Tl to L2/3) and a proportion of the parasympathetic outflow (the sacral parasympathetic) traverse and synapse in the spinal-cord before they supply their target organs. In patients with spinal cord injuries therefore, there are varying degrees of autonomic involvement, depending upon the site and extent of the lesion. In patients with cervical cord transection, if complete, the entire sympathetic and sacral parasympathetic outflow is separated from cerebral control. This results in a variety of abnormalities affecting the cardiovascular, thermoregulatory, gastrointestinal, urinary, and reproductive systems. In patients with transection, which is common after traumatic injuries to the spinal cord, despite destruction of one or more segments, the distal portion of the spinal cord often retains function, although independently of the brain. This results, in certain situations, in additional autonomic abnormalities. In incomplete lesions the functional deficits will vary. This chapter will concentrate on patients with cervical and high spinal cord injuries, as these patients often have major clinical problems resulting from autonomic dysfunction. The principles apply to other diseases affecting the spinal cord, such as due to syringomyelia or transverse myelitis, with the autonomic impairment depending on the site and extent of the lesion.

Recently injured versus chronically injured

There are differences between the autonomic problems affecting recently and chronically injured patients following a spinal lesion. Soon after transection there is initially a transient state of hypoexcitability of the isolated cord, described as 'spinal shock'. This is partially analogous to cerebral shock, as observed in the early stages after a hemisphere lesion. In spinal shock there is flaccid paralysis of the muscles, with lack of tendon reflexes. Spinal autonomic function is also impaired; the urinary bladder and large bowel are usually atonic, there is dilatation of blood vessels particularly in the skin, and spinal autonomic reflexes cannot be elicited. This stage of spinal cord depression may last from a few days to a few weeks, after which isolated activity of the spinal cord usually returns. This heralds the onset of a different range of autonomic abnormalities, which are often the result of autonomic reflex activity at a spinal level, without the normal control from higher centres in the brain.

The biochemical and molecular basis of spinal shock is not known. A range of possibilities has been proposed over the years, ranging from alterations in monoamine and neuropeptide transmitters, to abnormalities involving free oxygen radicals, lipid peroxidation, and calcium ions. Previously promising work in animals using the opiate antagonist, naloxone, and the endogenous antagonist, thyrotrophin-releasing hormone, have not been fulfilled in man. Some benefit has been shown with methylprednisolone, raising a number of possibilities which include the deleterious effects of lipid peroxidation and hydrolysis, and breakdown of cell membranes. This, however, is more likely to be related to neuronal damage and its prevention, rather than to the understanding of the mechanisms of spinal shock. The reversal of the processes causing spinal shock is of clinical importance, as a reduction in skeletal muscle flaccidity and neural activation of the vasculature is probably beneficial in preventing deep venous thrombosis; furthermore, postural hypotension which occurs in the early stages is less likely to be a problem and the return of activity to the urinary bladder and bowel should help speed up the overall rehabilitation process.

The descriptions below largely relate to the chronic stage of spinal-cord injuries, unless specifically stated. They will apply to both tetraplegies and high thoracic spinal cord lesions, unless otherwise indicated.

The cardiovascular system

Basal blood pressure and heart rate

The recently injured

The basal supine blood pressure in recently injured tetraplegics in spinal shock is usually lower than normal, and this applies particularly to the diastolic blood pressure (57 mm Hg in tetraplegics and 82 mmHg in normal subjects; Mathias *et al.* 1979*a*). The extent and the duration of the hypotension varies, as it is dependent upon a number of factors including complicating trauma and drug therapy. A subnormal basal blood pressure and low levels of both plasma noradrenaline and adrenaline (Fig. 51.1) may occur from the second day after injury. It is likely that the level of blood pressure is secondary to the marked diminution in sympathetic nervous activity, that normally accounts for about 20 per cent of vascular tone. It is unlikely that skeletal muscle paralysis alone contributes, as patients with tetraplegia due to poliomyelitis often have normal or even higher levels of blood pressure.

In tetraplegics in spinal shock the basal heart rate is usually below 100 beats/min, unlike in patients with low spinal-cord injuries in whom the heart rate is often higher. This is probably due to a reduction in neural and hormonal sympathetic-mediated chronotropic

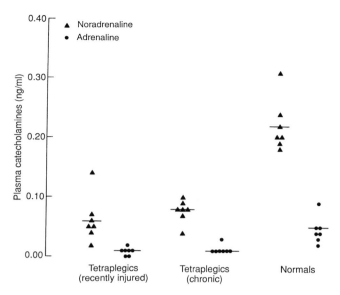

Fig. 51.1. Resting levels of plasma noradrenaline and adrenaline in recently injured tetraplegics in spinal shock, in chronic tetraplegics, and in normal age-matched subjects. The horizontal bar indicates the mean value. Basal catecholamines in both recently injured and chronic tetraplegics are a third or less than normal levels. (From Mathias *et al.* (1979*a*).)

influences in the tetraplegics. The efferent cardiac parasympathetic pathways, however, are intact and the absence of sympathetic activation may predispose susceptible patients to vagal overactivity. This may result in bradycardia and cardiac arrest, as has been noted during tracheal stimulation.

The chronically injured

In the chronic stage, the basal level of both systolic and diastolic blood pressure in high lesions is lower than in normal subjects (Fig. 51.2; Frankel *et al.* 1972; Mathias *et al.* 1976*a*). Non-invasive ambulatory 24-hour recordings indicate loss of the nocturnal circadian fall in blood pressure, as occurs normally (Nitsche *et al.* 1996; (Fig. 51.3). Basal levels of plasma noradrenaline and adrenaline in tetraplegics, in the absence of stimulation from below the lesion, remain low as in the stage of spinal shock, reflecting absent tonic supraspinal sympathetic impulses and diminished peripheral sympathetic activity. This has been confirmed in tetraplegics using microneurography to detect skin and muscle sympathetic nerve activity (Stjernberg *et al.* 1986). Patients with spinal-cord injury,

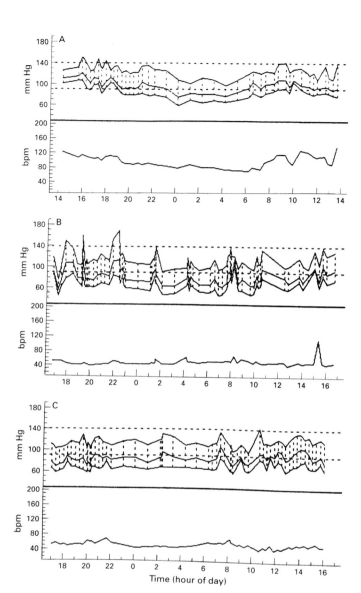

Fig. 51.3. Ambulatory blood pressure measurements demonstrating (a), a normal profile with a preserved physiological fall in blood pressure at night between midnight and 04.00 hours, (b) multiple episodes of autonomic dysreflexia in a complete tetraplegic; and (c) the same patient as in (b) after effective treatment of autonomic dysreflexia with the antihypertensive drug nifedipine. Despite improvement in (c), the loss of the circadian regulation of blood pressure persists. (From Curt *et al.* (1997).)

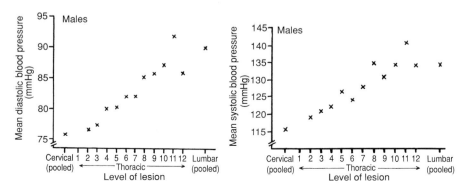

Fig. 51.2. Relationship between systolic and diastolic blood pressure in male patients with spinal-cord lesions at differing levels. Tetraplegics have the lowest resting blood pressure. (From Frankel *et al.* (1972).)

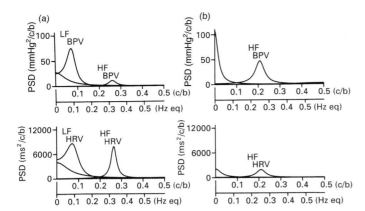

Fig. 51.4. Individual autoregressive power spectral density (PSD) components showing systolic blood pressure variabilities (BPV) (upper panel) and heart-rate period as RR interval variabilities (HRV) (lower panel) in a healthy subject (a) and a complete tetraplegic (b) at rest while supine. In the healthy male (a) there were two major spectral components; the low-frequency (LF; LF_{BPV} or LF_{HRV}) component and the high-frequency (HF; HF_{BPV} or HF_{HRV}) component. In the tetraplegic (b), the HF (HF_{BPV} and HF_{HRV}) component was present, but there was no LF (LF_{BPV} or LF_{HRV}) component. (From Inoue *et al.* (1991).)

however, are prone to renal damage and renal failure which may account for sustained hypertension in some.

In the absence of adequate resting sympathetic tone, a number of secondary mechanisms, particularly hormonal, attempt to compensate for and help maintain blood pressure. An important component is the renin–angiotensin–aldosterone system which, through the direct pressor effects of angiotensin II and the salt-retaining effects of aldosterone, helps raise blood pressure. This is particularly evident when drugs that interfere with the system are used; the angiotensin-converting enzyme inhibitor, captopril, substantially lowers supine blood pressure in tetraplegics. Even small doses of diuretics, which cause salt loss and lower intravascular fluid volume, may cause a catastrophic fall in supine blood pressure. A low salt diet lowers blood pressure, despite the ability of tetraplegics to reduce salt excretion as do normal subjects (Sutters *et al.* 1992). In tetraplegics recumbency itself may induce a diuresis but not a natriuresis; this differs from patients with primary autonomic failure, who also have nocturnal polyuria (Chapter 20), and in whom recumbency causes both diuresis and natriuresis (Kooner *et al.* 1987). The difference may relate to

the ability of the tetraplegics to mount an adequate hormonal response to oppose natriuresis, unlike the autonomic failure patients in whom these responses are often muted (Chapter 18). These observations have practical importance, as a period of recumbency in high spinal lesions will often result in accentuation of postural hypotension. This may be reduced or prevented by head-up tilt.

In chronic high lesions, the basal heart rate may be marginally lower than, or no different from, that of normal subjects. Twenty-four-hour ambulatory recordings of heart rate indicate preservation of the circadian fall at night (Nitsche *et al.* 1996). Power spectral analytical techniques in tetraplegics indicate a diminished low-frequency (presumed sympathetic) component with preservation of the high frequency (presumed parasympathetic) component (Inoue *et al.* 1991) (Fig. 51.4). There are changes in heart rate and RR intervals (heart periods) which occur when baroreceptor afferents are influenced either by a rise or a fall in blood pressure (such as by phenylephrine or nitroprusside respectively; Fig. 51.5), that results in reciprocal changes in vagal efferent activity (Koh *et al.* 1994). Various observations, therefore, suggest preservation of cardiac vagal function.

Cardiovascular responses to physiological stimuli

In tetraplegics with physiologically complete transection the brain is functionally separated from the peripheral sympathetic nervous system. This may cause a number of abnormalities, when cardiovascular responses are the result of cerebral initiation or modulation. Depending on the level and extent of the lesion, there are varying disturbances.

Postural change

Patients with high spinal-cord lesions are prone to hypotension, which commonly occurs during postural change from the horizontal to the upright position. This occurs in both recently injured patients in spinal shock and in chronically injured patients, especially in the early stages during rehabilitation. Their mobility, even in a wheelchair, can be considerably impeded. The fall in blood pressure is accompanied by symptoms mainly related to diminished cerebral perfusion (Table 51.1). The symptoms can vary in nature and intensity and are not necessarily related to the degree of hypotension.

During head-up postural change, as on a tilt table, there is usually an immediate fall in both systolic and diastolic blood pressure. The pressure may fall to extremely low levels, but usually there is no loss of consciousness except in recently injured tetraplegics or in chronic

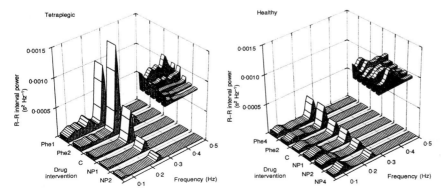

Fig. 51.5. Heart period (RR interval) power spectrum in a tetraplegic patient (left) and healthy subject (right) in the control (C) phase and during drug intervention with increasing doses of phenylephrine (Phe 1 and Phe 2) to raise blood pressure, and sodium nitroprusside (NP1, NP2 and NP4) to lower blood pressure. There is a rise in the high-frequency spectrum after phenylephrine and an increase in blood pressure in both subjects; the rise is greater in the tetraplegic. With a fall in blood pressure after nitroprusside, the low-frequency (presumed sympathetic) spectrum is elevated in the normal subject but not in the tetraplegic patient. The insets represent low-frequency (0.05–0.15 Hz) RR interval spectral power displayed at identical high gains. (From Koh *et al.* (1994).)

Table 51.1.   Clinical manifestations of postural hypotension*

Giddiness, buzzing, and ringing in ears

Blurring, greying out, and loss of vision

Facial pallor

Syncope

Hypotension and elevation in heart rate

Venous pooling and cyanotic discoloration of lower limbs

Reduced urine secretion

*Other symptoms as described in autonomic failure (Mathias (1995)) may also occur. (See Chapter 20)

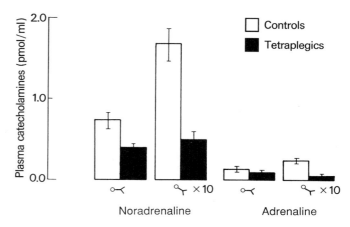

Fig. 51.7.   Plasma noradrenaline and adrenaline levels in controls (normal subjects) and chronic tetraplegic patients at rest and during head-up tilt to 45° to 10 min. There is a rise in plasma noradrenaline in the control subjects but little change in the tetraplegics. The bars indicate ± SEM.

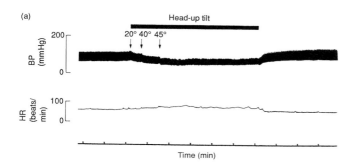

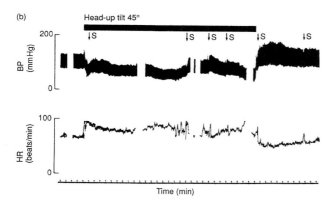

Fig. 51.6.   (a) Blood pressure (BP) and heart rate (HR) in a tetraplegic patient before and after head-up tilt, in the early stages of rehabilitation, when there were few muscle spasms and minimal autonomic dysreflexia. (From Mathias and Frankel (1992).) (b) Blood pressure (BP) and heart rate (HR) in a tetraplegic patient before, during and after head-up tilt to 45°. Blood pressure promptly falls but with partial recovery, which in this case is linked to skeletal muscle spasms (S) inducing spinal sympathetic activity. Some of the later oscillations may be due to the rise in plasma renin, which was measured where there are interruptions in the intra-arterial record. In the later phases of tilt, skeletal muscle spasms occur more frequently, and further elevate the blood pressure. On return to the horizontal, blood pressure rises rapidly above the previous level, and then slowly returns to the horizontal. Heart rate usually moves in the opposite direction, except during muscle spasms, where there is an increase. (From Mathias and Frankel (1988).)

tetraplegics following a period of recumbency. This tolerance to a low cerebral perfusion pressure is similar to that of patients with chronic autonomic failure, who are also able to autoregulate their cerebral circulation despite an extremely low perfusion blood pressure (Chapter 11). The precise mechanisms responsible for this are unclear.

Following the initial fall in blood pressure, the subsequent responses vary. In some patients, especially in the early stages, blood pressure continues to fall (Fig. 51.6a). There is no rise in levels of plasma noradrenaline in the early phases following head-up postural change (Fig. 51.7), consistent with their inability to reflexly increase sympathetic nervous activity in response to postural change, as occurs normally. In many chronically injured patients, however, if tilt is prolonged, the blood pressure tends to partly recover, often with oscillations (Fig. 51.6b). This recovery may be related to activation of the renin–angiotensin–aldosterone system. The release of renin appears to be independent of sympathetic stimulation and may be secondary to renal baroreceptor stimulation from the fall in renal perfusion pressure (Fig. 51.8a). Renin results in the formation of the peptide angiotensin II, which has powerful direct vasoconstrictor effects, may facilitate peripheral noradrenaline release and activity, and also stimulates the release of aldosterone from the adrenal cortex (Fig. 51.8b). The salt- and water-retaining effects of aldosterone have slower but important effects in increasing intravascular volume. These various actions of the renin–angiotensin–aldosterone system help to raise blood pressure. A further mechanism contributing to blood pressure recovery during tilt is the activation of spinal reflexes either from stimulation of the skin, the skeletal muscles, or the viscera. This is more likely to account for the reduction in peripheral blood flow and rise in occluded venous pressure observed during head-up tilt in tetraplegics than the spinal postural reflexes that were previously proposed. Local sympathetic reflexes (veno-arteriolar reflexes) may operate in high lesions during postural change.

During head-up postural change the fall in blood pressure is accompanied by a reduction in central venous pressure, stroke volume, and cardiac output, which is probably the result of venous pooling, diminished venous return, and the inability to increase sympathetic cardiac inotropic activity. Venous pooling often causes cyanotic discoloration of the legs and may account for ankle oedema, as

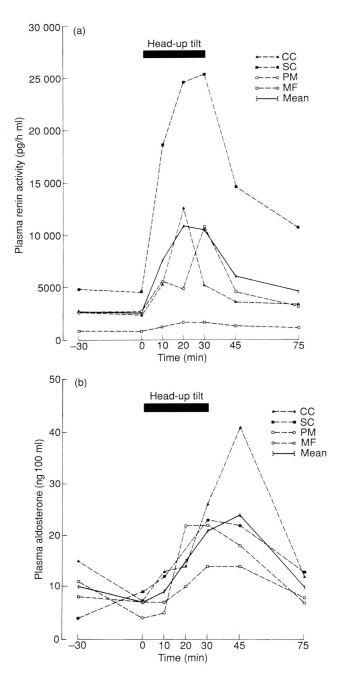

Fig. 51.8. (a) Plasma renin activity levels in four chronic tetraplegic patients before, during, and after head-up tilt to 45°. In three patients there was pronounced hypotension and a marked rise in plasma renin activity levels. Patient MF had minimal changes in blood pressure during head-up tilt and the smallest rise in plasma renin activity. (From Mathias *et al.* (1975).) (b) Plasma aldosterone levels before, during, and after head-up tilt to 45° in the same four patients as in (a). The rise in plasma aldosterone levels is later in timing to that of plasma renin activity. (From Mathias *et al.* (1975).)

observed in these with high lesions and in wheelchairs. Urine volume is usually reduced, often to extremely low levels, which occasionally raises the question of whether there may be obstruction to the urinary outflow tract. Oliguria may be due to a combination of

causes; these include a fall in blood pressure, thus reducing renal plasma flow and glomerular filtration rate, and an elevation in levels of the antidiuretic hormone, vasopressin. In high spinal lesions there is an exaggerated rise in vasopressin levels during head-up tilt as compared to normal subjects (Chapter 24).

During head-up postural change there is often a rapid rise in heart rate, which is inversely related to the fall in blood pressure. This is likely to be due to withdrawal of vagal tone in response to unloading of baroreceptor afferents, as it is markedly attenuated, although not abolished, by atropine. Propranolol also reduces the heart rate rise during tilt, suggesting that β-adrenoceptor stimulation also partially contributes. In the majority of patients, heart rate does not usually rise above 100 beats/min even during a marked fall in blood pressure. This therefore is different from the situation in patients with an intact sympathetic nervous system, who are in 'shock' with a similarly low level of blood pressure.

The clinical problems resulting from postural hypotension in high spinal lesions are not usually as severe and prolonged as those in patients with primary autonomic failure. Clinical observations indicate that the symptoms of postural hypotension are often diminished with frequent postural change to the head-up position, along with elevation of the head end of the bed at night. The activation of the renin–angiotensin–aldosterone axis, with both early and longer-acting effects resulting from vasoconstriction and plasma volume expansion, probably helps buffer the fall in blood pressure during head-up postural change. Another possibility is an improved ability to autoregulate cerebral blood flow, which such patients often can do at lower perfusion pressures than normal subjects. Whether changes in other circulating and locally produced hormones acting on the cerebral vasculature also contribute is not known.

A variety of physical methods has been used to prevent postural hypotension; these include abdominal binders and thigh cuffs, that prevent pooling. Activation of spinal sympathetic reflexes, by induction of muscle spasms or tapping of the anterior abdominal wall suprapubically to activate the urinary bladder, may be of value in some patients by causing autonomic dysreflexia and thus elevating blood pressure.

A range of drugs, as used in patients with autonomic failure (Chapter 36), may alleviate postural hypotension in high spinal-cord lesions. Such spinal patients, unlike patients with autonomic failure, are, however, prone to paroxysms of hypertension, which may be severe and exacerbated by such drugs. Usually, the need for drugs is for limited periods, when postural hypotension is a particular problem, as in the early stages of rehabilitation and after prolonged recumbency. If neither of these factors is responsible, other causes of orthostatic hypotension (especially non-neurogenic causes) need to be sought (Chapter 20). Ephedrine, in a dose of 15 mg half an hour before postural change, is often of value. Its ability to act directly on adrenoceptors and indirectly by releasing noradrenaline is probably the basis of its efficacy. Dihydroergotamine and other α-adrenoceptor agonists may have a role, especially if they have short-lived effects. Indomethacin, a prostaglandin synthetase inhibitor, also elevates basal blood pressure and reduces the blood pressure fall during postural change but has potential side-effects. In the majority of patients, however, drugs are not needed.

Valsalva manoeuvre

In high spinal lesions the responses to the Valsalva manoeuvre are abnormal because the baroreceptor reflex is impaired due to the dis-

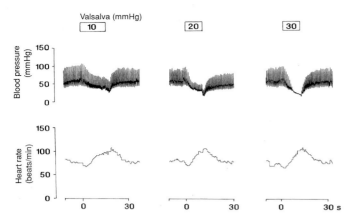

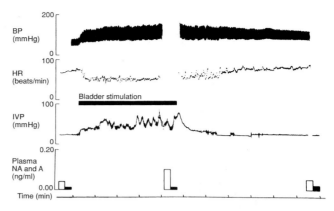

Fig. 51.9. Blood pressure and heart rate responses to the Valsalva manoeuvre in a tetraplegic patient. With increasing degrees of intrathoracic pressure there is a progressively greater fall in blood pressure in phase II. There is virtually no blood pressure recorded when intrathoracic pressure is raised to 30 mmHg. Blood pressure has been measured non-invasively with the Finapres. (van Lieshout *et al.* (1991).)

Fig. 51.10. Blood pressure (BP), heart rate (HR), intravesical pressure (IVP), and plasma noradrenaline (NA) and adrenaline (A) levels in a tetraplegic patient before, during, and after bladder stimulation induced by suprapubic percussion of the anterior abdominal wall. The rise in BP is accompanied by a fall in heart rate as a result of increased vagal activity in response to the rise in blood pressure. Level of plasma NA (open histograms), but not A (filled histograms) rise, suggesting an increase in sympathetic neural activity independently of adrenomedullary activation. (From Mathias and Frankel (1986).)

ruption of sympathetic efferent pathways through the cervical and thoracic spinal cord. When intrathoracic pressure is elevated there is a fall in blood pressure, despite a fairly modest increase in intrathoracic pressure that is often difficult to achieve and maintain because of the inability to activate intercostal muscles. There is no recovery in blood pressure while the intrathoracic pressure is elevated. Heart rate rises with the fall in blood pressure because the cardiac vagi respond to the fall in blood pressure. On reducing the elevated intrathoracic pressure, there is a gradual recovery of blood pressure with a reduction in heart rate that does not fall below the basal level.

The blood pressure may fall to extremely low levels during the Valsalva manoeuvre if intrathoracic pressure is elevated to 20 or 30 mmHg, as demonstrated in a tetraplegic who suffered severe dizziness while singing, which raised her intrathoracic pressure (van Lieshout *et al.* 1991) (Fig. 51.9). This ability to lower blood pressure has also been used to the benefit of patients, to prevent hypertension during urological surgery by increasing positive pressure during assisted ventilation.

Pressor stimuli originating above the lesion

Pressor stimuli dependent on sympathetic activation that either originate in, or are modulated by, the brain do not raise blood pressure in patients with complete cervical cord transaction. Stimuli such as mental arithmetic, a loud noise, and cutaneous stimulation by either pain or cold in areas above the lesion have no effect in tetraplegics, unlike in normal subjects in whom they elevate blood pressure. The lack of response to these stimuli provides evidence of severance of sympathetic pathways descending within the cervical spinal cord.

Pressor stimuli originating below the lesion: 'autonomic dysreflexia'

The reverse, an exaggerated rise in blood pressure, occurs in high spinal lesions when stimuli originate below the level of the lesion. Stimulation of the skin, abdominal and pelvic viscera, or skeletal muscles, can cause a paroxysmal rise in blood pressure (Fig. 51.10), which usually is accompanied by a fall in heart rate because of

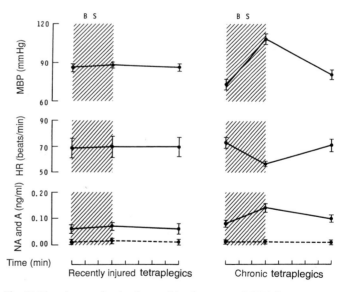

Fig. 51.11. Average levels of mean blood pressure (MBP), heart rate (HR), and plasma noradrenaline (NA, continuous line) and adrenaline (A, interrupted line) in recently injured and chronic tetraplegics, before, during, and after bladder stimulation (BS). The bars indicate ± SEM. No changes occur in the recently injured tetraplegics, unlike the chronic tetraplegics in whom MBP and plasma NA levels rise and HR falls. There are no changes in plasma A levels. (From Mathias *et al.* (1979*a*).)

increased vagal activity. In recently injured tetraplegics in spinal shock there is often no change in blood pressure or heart rate during such stimulation (Fig. 51.11). This differs markedly from the chronic stage when there is increased activity in a number of target organs supplied by the sympathetic and parasympathetic nerves. These effects, in combination, contribute to the syndrome of autonomic dysreflexia (Table 51.2). Detailed observations were made by Head and Riddoch (1917) who described sweating around and above the

Table 51.2. Clinical manifestations of autonomic dysreflexia

Paraesthesiae in neck, shoulders, and arms

Fullness in head

Hot ears

Throbbing headache, especially in the occipital and frontal regions

Tightness in chest and dyspnoea

Hypertension and bradycardia

Occasionally cardiac dysrythmias

Pupillary dilatation

Above lesion—pallor initially, followed by flushing of face and neck and sweating in areas above and around the lesion

Below lesion—cold peripheries; piloerection

Contraction of urinary bladder and large bowel[a]

Penile erection and seminal fluid emission[a]

[a]May occur as part of the 'mass reflex'.

level of the lesion, with evacuation of the urinary bladder and rectum, penile erection, and seminal fluid emission, together with skeletal muscle spasms—components of the 'mass reflex' in response to cutaneous stimulation below the lesion or during bladder and bowel evacuation. The cardiovascular changes, however, were not described until 1947, when Guttmann and Whitteridge reported their observations during urinary bladder stimulation. The cardiovascular responses to stimuli below the lesion include a rise in both systolic and diastolic blood pressure. There is a marked reduction in peripheral blood flow (Fig. 51.12) which may result in cold limbs, thus accounting for poikilothermia spinalis, one of the original terms used to describe autonomic dysreflexia. In addition to constriction of resistance vessels, there is also a rise in occluded venous pressure,

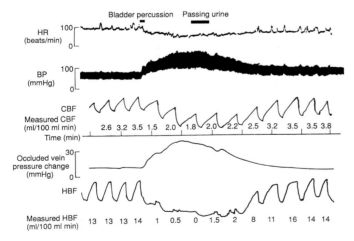

Fig. 51.12. The effects of bladder percussion and micturition on heart rate (HR), blood pressure (BP), calf blood flow (CBF), occluded vein pressure, and hand blood flow (HBF) in a chronic tetraplegic with a physiologically complete transaction of the cervical spinal cord. The rise in blood pressure is accompanied by a fall in heart rate (after an initial transient rise), a marked reduction in both calf and hand blood flow, and a rise in occluded vein pressure. (From Corbett et al. (1971).)

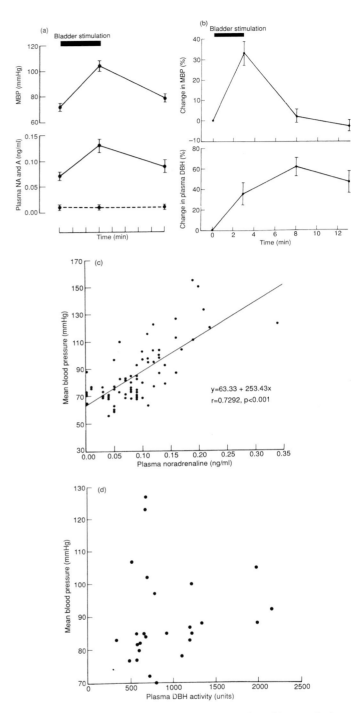

Fig. 51.13. (a), (b) Changes in mean blood pressure (MBP) in tetraplegic patients before, during, and after bladder stimulation. (a) Plasma noradrenaline (NA, continuous line) levels rise with the blood pressure and fall as the pressor effects wane. There is no change in plasma adrenaline (A, dashed line) levels. (b) Levels of plasma dopamine β-hydroxylase (DBH) rise slowly and remain elevated for a longer period. The bars indicate ± SEM. (C) There is a strong relationship between mean blood pressure and plasma noradrenaline levels, which is not observed for (d) plasma dopamine β-hydroxylase. In short-term studies, plasma noradrenaline levels appear to be a better indicator of sympathoneural activation than plasma dopamine β-hydroxylase levels. (From Mathias (1976a and Mathias et al. (1976a) and b).)

indicating contraction of capacitance vessels. There is an elevation in both stroke volume and cardiac output, suggestive of activation of spinal cardiac reflexes. These changes occur soon after stimulation, the rapidity indicating that they are of neurogenic origin and likely to be due to reflex sympathetic activity through the isolated spinal cord. Biochemical evidence of increased sympathoneural activity has been obtained from levels of plasma noradrenaline, which are closely correlated with the blood pressure changes (Fig. 51.13a,c). Plasma dopamine beta hydroxylase levels rise later (Fig. 51.13b) and are not related to the rise in blood pressure (Mathias *et al.* 1976b) (Fig. 51.13d). Plasma adrenaline levels do not change, indicating that adrenomedullary secretion does not contribute to the elevation in blood pressure. However, plasma noradrenaline levels, even at the height of hypertension and despite their increasing by two- or three-fold, are only moderately above the resting basal levels of normal subjects. This differs markedly from the extremely high levels of plasma catecholamines often found in patients with a phaeochromocytoma (Chapter 20). During autonomic dysreflexia, levels of other vasoconstrictor substances in plasma, such as renin (and by inference angiotensin II levels), aldosterone, vasopressin, and atrial natriuretic peptide remain unchanged or fall (Mathias *et al.* 1981; Krum *et al.* 1992). Whether levels of other vasoconstrictor peptides, such as neuropeptide Y (NPY) and endothelin, rise in man is not known. These are, however, more likely to play a local role than through circulating levels. In spinal animal models, plasma NPY levels do not rise during autonomic dysreflexia (Santajuliana *et al.* 1995); however, there is evidence that NPY spillover may increase markedly in certain regions, including the hepato-mesenteric vascular bed, without plasma levels changing substantially (Morris *et al.* 1997). The sympathetic skin response in complete tetraplegia is present in the feet during urinary bladder contraction but this does not occur with incomplete lesions (Previnaire *et al.* 1993); also, sweating does not occur in the feet during autonomic dysreflexia (Guttmann and Whitteridge 1947) and reasons for the dissociation are unclear.

The rise in blood pressure and the widespread involvement of the vasculature below the lesion, despite a modest and often localized stimulus only involving a few segments, suggest the spread of neuronal impulses intraspinally and/or extraspinally. In tetraplegics, microneurography indicates only a moderate and transient rise in

muscle sympathetic nerve activity during autonomic dysreflexia (Stjernberg *et al.* 1986) with no association between the cardiac cycle and muscle sympathetic nerve discharge as occurs normally (Fig. 51.14). There is evidence of hyperactivity of target organs innervated by the autonomic nervous system; as has been demonstrated in the dorsal foot vein of tetraplegics in response to local intravenous noradrenaline (Arnold *et al.* 1995). The exaggerated blood pressure response to various stimuli suggests supersensitivity of adrenoceptors, or that other mechanisms are responsible for the enhanced vascular response. Overall, the result of the physiological and pharmacological studies, in conjunction with the neurohormonal observations, suggest that the term 'autonomic hyper-reflexia' is erroneous and should not be used. Recent data, however, indicate a marked (15-fold) increase in noradrenaline spillover in the leg during bladder stimulation, suggesting that in high lesions greater quantities of noradrenaline may be released per impulse than previously recorded (Karlsson 1997) (Fig. 51.15).

Increased pressor responses to stimuli do not occur in patients with lesions below the fifth thoracic segment (Fig. 51.16), indicating that the sympathetic neural outflow above that level is of major importance in blood pressure homeostasis. It is likely that in the lesions below T5 there is sparing of the neural control of the large splanchnic circulatory bed. In high lesions, stimuli causing autonomic dysreflexia unmask primary cutaneovascular, viscerovascular, and somatovascular reflexes; these primary effects appear to be modulated by the brain in both normal subjects and in patients with lesions below T5, thus preventing hypertension. Indirect evidence for the role of descending cerebral pathways in preventing autonomic dysreflexia has emerged from measurement of the sympathetic skin response that tests integrity of sympathetic cholinergic pathways. In complete tetraplegics the response was absent in the hands and feet; however, in incomplete tetraplegics autonomic dysreflexia occurs only in those with an absent response, while in those with a response dysreflexia did not occur (Curt *et al.* 1996).

In high lesions, the heart rate may rise transiently with the elevation in blood pressure, presumably because of sympathetic stimulation of the heart as a result of spinal cardiac reflexes. There is usually a subsequent fall in heart rate because of stimulation of sinoaortic baroreceptors and increased vagal efferent activity. This may help dampen the rise in blood pressure during autonomic dysreflexia, as parasympathetic blockade with atropine or other anticholinergic agents that prevents this reflexly induced fall in heart rate often results in an even greater rise in blood pressure. During autonomic dysreflexia there is often facial vasodilatation accompanied by sweating, which may be profuse above the level of the lesion (Fig. 51.17). Sweating below the level of the lesion may be minimal. The precise mechanisms responsible are not known.

Autonomic dysreflexia is of major clinical importance. Mild episodes probably occur intermittently through the day, often are not noticed, and may be of little consequence. Hypertension, especially linked to bladder contractions and voiding, may not be accompanied by symptoms (silent autonomic dyreflexia; Linsenmeyer *et al.* 1996). When autonomic dysreflexia is prolonged there may be considerable morbidity, as a result of excessive sweating over the head and neck, and a throbbing headache. The latter is often, but not always, related to the level of blood pressure and may be dependent on distension of pain-sensitive cranial blood vessels. With recurrent

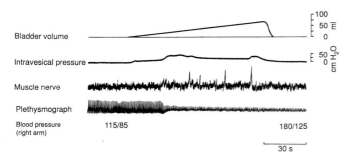

Fig. 51.14. Mean voltage neurogram record of sympathetic activity in a peroneal muscle nerve fascicle obtained while filling the urinary bladder with carbon dioxide (CO_2) at 50 cm³/min in a patient with a C5 lesion. There is an increase in intravesical volume and pressure associated with marked cutaneous vasoconstriction, as indicated by the photoelectrical pulse plethysmograph. Blood pressure is markedly elevated despite only a moderate increase in sympathetic nerve activity. (From Stjernberg *et al.* (1986).)

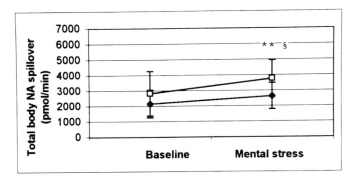

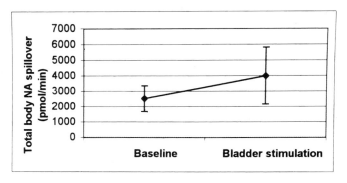

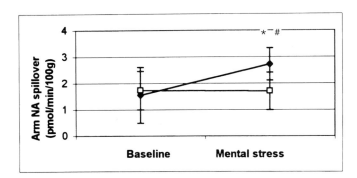

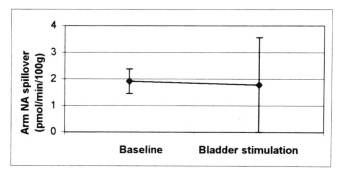

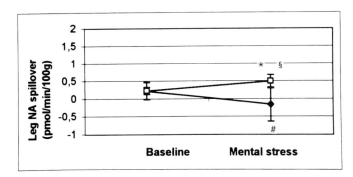

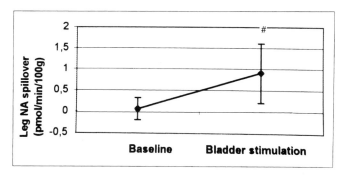

Fig. 51.15. Total body, arm and leg noradrenaline (NA) spillover (upper middle and lower panels, respectively) during mental stress (left panels) and bladder stimulation (right panels) in patients with high spinal-cord injuries (filled symbols) and in control subjects (open symbols; only in left panel). With mental stress, total and leg NA spillover increases in the controls, with an increase in arm NA spillover only in the spinal are indicated by * P < 0.05 and ** P < 0.01 and patients. With bladder stimulation (only in the spinal injured), leg NA spillover only increases. Significant differences between groups between baseline and stimulation by patients in patients and 8 controls (§). Values are means with 95% confidence interval. (From Karlsson 1997).)

episodes of dysreflexia, headache may be particularly severe, despite later but only modest elevations in blood pressure. This may be due to increased sensitivity of afferent nerves on blood vessels caused by the formation or release of substances including substance P, calcitonin-gene-related peptide, and prostaglandins. Other complications of the vasospasm and hypertension accompanying autonomic dysreflexia include myocardial failure and neurological deficits such as epileptic seizures, visual defects, and cerebral haemorrhage. These may result in extensive and permanent neurological deficits or death. Whether these cardiovascular abnormalities may become an even greater problem as patients grow older, and they become more vulnerable to cardiac and vascular damage, remains to be determined.

The key factor in the management of autonomic dysreflexia is prevention. It is necessary to determine the provoking cause and to rectify it (Table 51.3). To lower blood pressure rapidly, head-up tilt (which causes venous pooling) may be used initially, although occasionally a fall in blood pressure may induce autonomic dysreflexia and in particular hyperhidrosis (Khurana 1987). Various drugs are helpful, and their actions are related to the postulated mechanisms responsible for autonomic dysreflexia (Table 51.4). Preventing afferent stimulation, for instance by the use of a local anaesthetic, such as lignocaine in the urinary bladder, can be effective. Drugs which act partially (reserpine) or entirely (spinal anaesthetics) on the spinal cord are particularly useful especially in severe episodes of dysreflexia. The ganglionic blocker, hexamethonium, was used

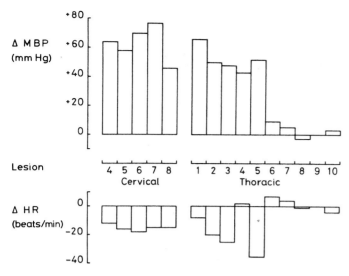

Fig. 51.16. Changes in mean blood pressure (Δ MBP) and heart rate (Δ HR) in patients with spinal cord lesions at different levels (cervical and thoracic) after bladder stimulation induced by suprapubic percussion of the anterior abdominal wall. In the cervical and high thoracic lesions there is a marked elevation in blood pressure and a fall in heart rate. In patients with lesions below T5 there are minimal cardiovascular changes. (From Mathias and Frankel (1986).)

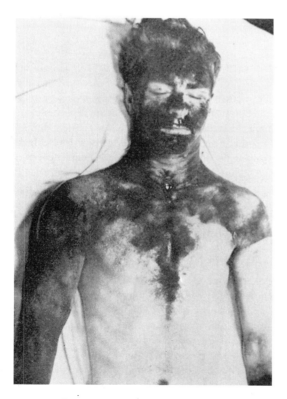

Fig. 51.17. Distribution of sweating, indicated by darker areas covered by quinizarine dye, in a tetraplegic patient during bladder distension. The band over the left arm indicates the site of the sphygmomanometer cuff. (From Guttmann (1976).)

Table 51.3. Causes of autonomic dysreflexia

Abdominal or pelvic visceral stimulation

Ureter
    Calculus
Urinary bladder
    Distension by blocked catheter or discoordinated bladder
    Infection
    Irritation by calculus, catheter, or bladder washout
Rectum and anus
    Enemas
    Faecal retention
    Anal fissure
Gastrointestinal organs
    Gastric dilatation
    Gastric ulceration
    Cholecystitis or cholelithiasis
Uterus
    Contraction during pregnancy
    Menstruation, occasionally

Cutaneous stimulation

Pressure sores
Infected ingrowing toenails
Burns

Skeletal muscle spasms

Especially in limbs with contractures

Miscellaneous

    Intrathecal neostigmine
    Electroejaculatory procedures
    Ejaculation
    Vaginal dilatation
    Urethra—insertion of catheter or abscess
    Fractures of bones

Table 51.4. Some of the drugs used in the management of autonomic dysreflexia classified according to their major site of action on the reflex arc and target organs

Afferent		Topical lignocaine
Spinal cord		Clonidine[a]
		Reserpine[a]
		Spinal anaesthetics
Efferent	Sympathetic ganglia	Hexamethonium
	Sympathetic nerve terminals	Guanethidine
	α-adrenoceptors	Phenoxybenzamine
Target organs	Blood vessels	Glyceryl trinitrate
		Nifedipine
	Sweat glands	Pro-Banthine®

[a]Clonidine and reserpine have multiple effects, some of which are peripheral.

successfully in the past but, like other drugs that reduce sympathetic efferent activity, is likely to cause profound postural hypotension. The α2-adrenoceptor agonist, clonidine, does not lower supine blood pressure but reduces hypertension during autonomic dysreflexia

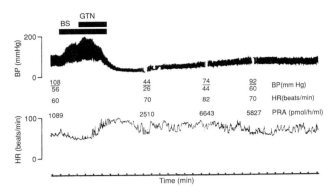

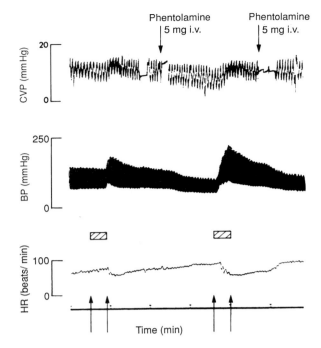

Fig. 51.18. Blood pressure (BP) and heart rate (HR) in a tetraplegic in the supine position before, during, and after bladder stimulation (BS) by suprapubic percussion of the anterior abdominal wall, which induces hypertension. Sublingual glyceryl trinitrate (GTN) (0.5 mg for 3.5 min) rapidly reverses the hypertension, elevates the heart rate, and then causes substantial hypotension. Levels of plasma renin activity (PRA) rise as a result of the fall in blood pressure. (From Mathias and Frankel (1988).)

(Mathias *et al.* 1979*c*). Drugs acting directly on blood vessels, such as glyceryl trinitrate and calcium-channel blockers, such as nifedipine (Thyberg *et al.* 1994), are also effective and have the advantage of being given sublingually. They also have the potential to cause severe hypotension (Fig. 51.18).

The α-adrenoceptor blockers theoretically should be highly effective in autonomic dysreflexia. Phenoxybenzamine, and the selective blockers prazosin and terazosin are useful in autonomic dysreflexia due to bladder outflow obstruction, as they relax the smooth muscle of the urinary sphincter (Chancellor *et al.* 1994). α-adrenoceptor blockers such as phentolamine may not prevent the paroxysmal surges in blood pressure during autonomic dysreflexia (Fig. 51.19). The reasons for this are unclear, but could include inadequate entry and disposition of the α-adrenoceptor blocker at postsynaptic sites, thus enabling the trans-synaptic actions of noradrenaline to continue. Furthermore, during autonomic dysreflexia there also may be secretion from sympathetic nerve endings of non-adrenergic substances, such as neuropeptide Y or adenosine triphosphate (ATP) which may cause vasoconstriction, not affected by α-adrenoceptor blockers. Preventing release, or depleting tissue levels of such substances, may explain the greater benefit provided by drugs such as reserpine and guanethidine in severe cases of dysreflexia, when other agents have failed.

In some patients, autonomic dysreflexia may be a major and recurring problem because of difficulty in either defining or resolving the precipitating cause. More unusual examples of the former are gastric ulceration or cholecystitis, which are difficult to detect because of lack of pain. A more common example, which may easily be missed, is an anal fissure. Despite recognizing the cause, it may be extremely difficult to resolve problems which include severe skeletal muscle spasms or recurrent urinary bladder infection. Long-term drug therapy for autonomic dysreflexia in such patients is often only partially successful and may result in undesirable side-effects. In severe cases, surgical procedures on the spinal cord, such as rhizotomy and cordotomy, or peripheral procedures, such as sacral and hypogastric neurotomy, may need to be considered. Non-surgical

Fig. 51.19. Central venous blood pressure (CVP), blood pressure (BP), and heart rate (HR) in a tetraplegic patient undergoing electroejaculation with stimuli given per rectum over the seminal vesicles during the times indicated by arrows and hatched areas. The α-adrenoceptor blocker phentolamine, even after a total close of 10 mg, did not suppress the paroxysmal rise in blood pressure during stimulation when reassessed latter (not shown in figure).

approaches, such as a subarachnoid block with alcohol or phenol, have also been utilized. However, these procedures usually abolish spinal reflex activity and result in flaccidity of skeletal muscles and bladder and bowel atony, with their attendant disadvantages.

Autonomic dysreflexia can be a particular problem during surgery, especially if the urinary bladder or the large bowel is involved. In these patients either spinal anaesthesia or a general anaesthetic, such as halothane, along with an increase in positive pressure ventilation, is often successful in controlling the hypertension (Fig. 51.20). Short-acting ganglionic blockers, such as trimethaphan, have been used successfully during surgery. The management of autonomic dysreflexia during pregnancy is discussed later.

Tracheal stimulation and intubation

Recently injured tetraplegics with high cervical lesions involving spinal segments that supply the phrenic nerves are dependent on artificial respiration because of diaphragmatic paralysis. In these patients bradycardia and cardiac arrest may occur during tracheal suction, especially when they are hypoxic (Fig. 51.21). The bradycardia is effectively prevented by atropine, which confirms the role of vagal efferent pathways in the response. The mechanisms by which tracheal suction and hypoxia contribute to bradycardia in these patients are outlined in Table 51.5. These stimuli activate vagal and glossopharyngeal afferents that increase vagal efferent activity. This is opposed by a number of factors, including the pulmonary inflation vagal reflex, which normally raises heart rate, as is observed in spon-

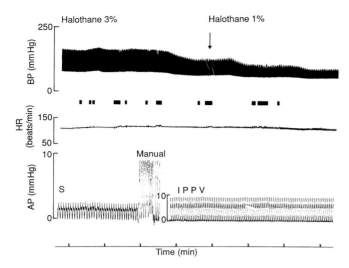

Fig. 51.20. Changes in blood pressure (BP) and heart rate (HR) of a chronic tetraplegic patient undergoing transurethral resection. The dark blocks indicate where resection and diathermy were performed. Airway pressure (AP) is also indicated when the patient was breathing spontaneously, was manually ventilated, and no intermittent positive pressure ventilation (IPPV). The blood pressure has been satisfactorily controlled on 3 per cent halothane. Increasing airway pressure reduces blood pressure and enables the use of a lower concentration of halothane (1 per cent), which successfully maintains the blood pressure during operative procedures which would otherwise greatly elevate it. (From Welply *et al.* (1975).)

Table 51.5. The major mechanisms contributing to bradycardia and cardiac arrest in recently injured tetraplegics in spinal shock during tracheal suction and hypoxia

	Tracheal suction	**Hypoxia**
Normal	Increased sympathetic nervous activity causes tachycardia and raises blood pressure	Bradycardia is the primary response opposed by the pulmonary (inflation) vagal reflex, resulting in tachycardia
Tetraplegics	No increase in sympathetic nervous activity, therefore no rise in heart rate or blood pressure. Vagal afferent stimulation may lead to unopposed vagal efferent activity	The primary response, bradycardia, is not opposed by the pulmonary (inflation) vagal reflex, because of disconnection from respirator or 'fixed' respiratory rate

Increased vagal cardiac tone
↓
Bradycardia and cardiac arrest

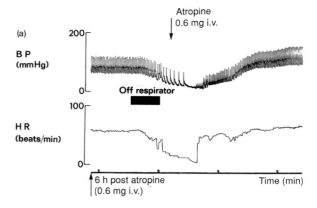

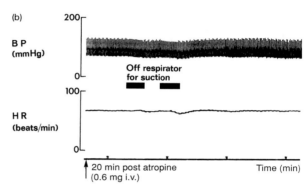

Fig. 51.21. (a) The effect of disconnecting the respirator (as required for aspirating the airways) on the blood pressure (BP) and heart rate (HR) of a recently injured tetraplegic patient (C4/5 lesion) in spinal shock, 6 h after the last dose of intravenous atropine. Sinus bradycardia and cardiac arrest (also observed on the electrocardiograph) were reversed by reconnection, intravenous atropine, and external cardiac massage. (From Frankel *et al.* (1975).) (b) The effect of tracheal suction, 20 min after atrophine. Disconnection from the respirator and tracheal suction did not lower either heart rate or blood pressure. (From Mathias (1976*b*).)

involved. Reconnecting the patient to the respirator will activate the pulmonary inflation vagal reflex, and the addition of oxygen will reverse hypoxia. External cardiac massage may be needed, along with intravenous atropine. Precipitant factors often include respiratory infection and pulmonary emboli. Both cause hypoxia, which initially may be difficult to reverse. Such patients may need maintenance atropine, in a dose of 0.3 or 0.6 mg either subcutaneously or intramuscularly at 4-hourly intervals. Parasympathomimetic agents such as neostigmine and carbachol, which reverse bladder and bowel atony in spinal shock, should be avoided or used with caution. Heart rate may be increased also by the use of β-adrenoceptor agonists, but drugs such as isoprenaline also have actions on vasodilatatory β_2–adrenoceptors, which may lower blood pressure further, as in chronic tetraplegics (Chapter 20). Temporary demand pacemakers have also been used.

In chronic tetraplegics, bradycardia and cardiac arrest may also occur when the trachea is stimulated while respiration is prevented, despite the potential presence of opposing sympathetic cardiac

taneously breathing tetraplegics when exposed either to hypoxia or to tracheal suction (Fig. 51.22). Other factors include the inability to activate sympathetic nerves, which are normally stimulated by tracheal suction or hypoxia.

The management of bradycardia and cardiac arrest during tracheal suction is directly related to knowledge of the mechanisms

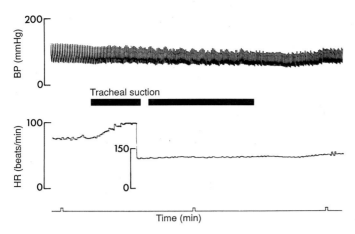

Fig. 51.22. Effect of tracheal suction on blood pressure (BP) and heart rate (HR) of a chronic tetraplegic patient 7 months after injury when he had recovered spontaneous respiration and isolated reflex spinal cord sympathetic activity. Tracheal suction performed through an indwelling tracheostomy tube caused hyperventilation, tachycardia, and a fall in blood pressure. The heart rate scale alters as shown. (From Mathias (1976*b*).)

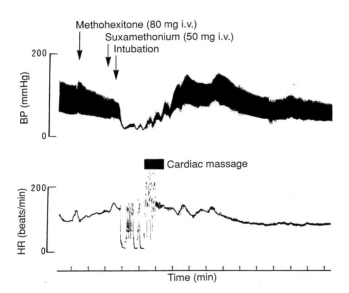

Fig. 51.23. The effect of endotracheal intubation on blood pressure (BP) and heart rate (HR) of a chronic tetraplegic patient being anaesthetized for urological surgery. Intubation was followed by cardiac arrest which was reversed by oxygen and external cardiac massage. (From Welply *et al.* (1975).)

reflexes operating at a spinal level. This may occur during endotracheal intubation after the use of skeletal muscle relaxants such as suxamethonium (Fig. 51.23). The mechanisms of this vagal reflex appear to be similar to those described in recently injured tetraplegics, with afferent vagal stimulation causing an increase in vagal efferent activity that is not opposed by the pulmonary inflation reflex because of respiratory paralysis. An important practical point is to administer an adequate amount of atropine prior to intubation, especially in patients who are at greater risk from autonomic dysreflexia and increased cardiac vagal activity, such as during urological surgery.

Food ingestion

In tetraplegics, unlike patients with chronic primary autonomic failure (Chapter 29), ingestion of either a balanced meal, an equivalent liquid meal (Baliga *et al.* 1997), or an isocaloric solution of glucose does not result in a substantial fall in supine blood pressure. The modest fall in blood pressure is accompanied by an elevation in heart rate. Levels of forearm venous plasma noradrenaline do not change, excluding a generalized increase in sympathetic nerve activity. The mechanisms responsible for preventing a substantial fall in blood pressure in tetraplegics are unclear; these could include the stimulation of reflexes from the gastrointestinal tract and mesentery (Chapter 29).

Hypoglycaemia

In normal individuals, hypoglycaemia results in a marked rise in plasma adrenaline levels and a modest rise in plasma noradrenaline levels. The clinical manifestations include anxiety, tremulousness, hunger, sweating, and tachycardia. There is little change in mean blood pressure as systolic blood pressure often rises and there is a small fall in diastolic blood pressure. Microneurography studies indicate that both muscle and skin sympathetic nerve activity increase during insulin hypoglycaemia, indicating that the response in normal individuals is not entirely due to adrenal stimulation and release of adrenaline. Similar or even greater increases in integrated muscle sympathetic nerve activity occur in adrenalectomized patients, in whom there is no rise in plasma adrenaline levels (see Chapter 29). In tetraplegics, insulin-induced hypoglycaemia does not raise levels of plasma adrenaline or noradrenaline (Fig. 51.24). There is a fall in sys-

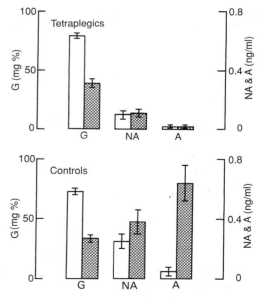

Fig. 51.24. Levels of blood glucose (G), plasma noradrenaline (NA), and adrenaline (A) before (blank histograms) and during (hatched histograms) insulin-induced hypoglycaemia in chronic tetraplegics (upper panel) and normal subjects (controls, lower panel). In the controls hypoglycaemia caused a small rise in plasma noradrenaline and a marked elevation in plasma adrenaline levels. A similar degree of hypoglycaemia did not change the low plasma noradrenaline and adrenaline levels in the tetraplegics. The bars indicate ± SEM. (From Mathias *et al.* (1979*b*).)

tolic blood pressure, along with a rise in heart rate. There are no symptoms of hypoglycaemia except for sedation, which is readily reversed with intravenous hypertonic glucose. If rapidly injected, however, this may cause a marked fall in blood pressure, as has been observed in patients with primary autonomic failure (Chapter 29). The symptoms accompanying hypoglycaemia in normal individuals, therefore, appear to be largely dependent upon an elevation in adrenaline levels and intact sympathetic nervous pathways. In tetraplegics and high thoracic lesions, the lack of warning signs accompanying neuroglycopenia are similar to observations made in some patients with diabetes mellitus and complicating autonomic neuropathy, or patients on non-selective β-adrenergic blockers.

Cardiovascular responses to pharmacological stimuli

Centrally acting agents—clonidine

Clonidine is an α_2–adrenoceptor agonist which has a number of actions that include cerebral effects, predominantly on the brainstem. In normal individuals this results in a withdrawal of sympathetic tone and a fall in blood pressure. Effects on the medullary vagal centres result in a fall in heart rate. In tetraplegics, intravenous clonidine (150 μg) transiently raises blood pressure, consistent with its peripheral agonist effects on postsynaptic α_1 and α_2 adrenoceptors. Neither intravenous (150 μg) nor oral (300 μg) clonidine lowers supine basal levels of blood pressure in tetraplegics (Fig. 51.25a) because of the disruption of descending sympathetic pathways. The heart rate, however, falls, in keeping with its vagal effects. Clonidine has additional effects, either on sympathetic neurones within the spinal cord or on peripheral presynaptic α_2–adrenoceptors which inhibit noradrenaline release. These may explain its partial ability to prevent hypertension during autonomic dysreflexia, as demonstrated during bladder stimulation (Fig. 51.25b; Mathias *et al.* 1979c). Clonidine is also able to reduce muscle spasticity and pain, as has been demonstrated also with intrathecal administration (Middleton *et al.* 1996). These actions may explain its value in the management of autonomic dysreflexia in high spinal-cord lesions.

Peripherally acting vasopressor agents

An increased pressor response to intravenously infused noradrenaline occurs in both recently injured and chronic tetraplegics (Fig. 51.26). This was originally considered to be a clinical manifestation of denervation hypersensitivity, as relating to Canon's law that denervated organs are supersensitive to their neurotransmitter. In classical denervation hypersensitivity, however, impairment of function of postganglionic sympathetic nerve terminals results in reduction in the neuronal uptake of noradrenaline. This inability to clear noradrenaline increases its synaptic concentration and results in a greater target organ response. In tetraplegics, however, there is histochemical evidence of intact adrenergic nerve terminals (Norberg and Normell 1974) and functional evidence during autonomic dysreflexia (as based on the rise in plasma noradrenaline, blood pressure, reflex increase in resistance and capacitance vessels, and increase noradrenaline spillover) of the integrity of postganglionic sympathetic nerves. Circulating levels of noradrenaline in tetraplegics and normal subjects are similar after identical intravenous infusions of noradrenaline, although the pressor responses are markedly different (Mathias *et al.* 1976c). Impaired clearance and higher levels of noradrenaline

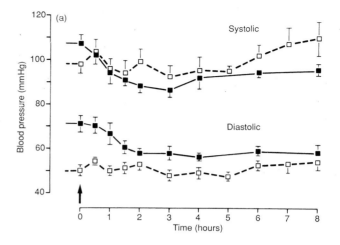

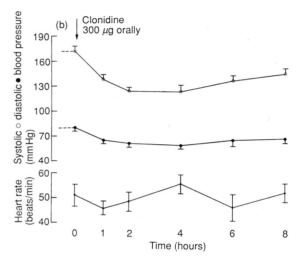

Fig. 51.25. (a) The effect of 300 μg of oral clonidine (at time 0, arrow) on systolic and diastolic blood pressure of normal subjects (filled squares, continuous line) and chronic tetraplegics (open squares, dashed line). There is a substantial fall in both systolic and diastolic blood pressure in the normal subjects but no fall in blood pressure in the tetraplegics. The bar indicate ± SEM. (From Reid *et al.* (1977).) (b) Systolic and diastolic blood pressure and heart rate recorded at the end of 3 min of bladder stimulation in a group of chronic tetraplegics before and after 300 μg of clonidine. There is a marked attenuation of the pressor response, with the largest reductions in the second and fourth hours. Effects persist even 8 hours after clonidine. The bars indicate ± SEM.

thus do not appear to account for the increased pressor responses in tetraplegics.

The lesion in tetraplegics and high thoracic lesions is effectively preganglionic, which is more proximal to the experimental lesions of immediately preganglionic nerves that also can cause an enhanced response to noradrenaline (decentralization hypersensitivity). This is thought to be due to an increase in receptor population, an improvement of the functional link between receptor activation and the final response, or both factors. Although tetraplegics have a low background level of sympathetic activity, this is punctuated by repeated episodes of autonomic dysreflexia, which ensure that sympathetic nerve terminals and receptors and target organs are intermittently

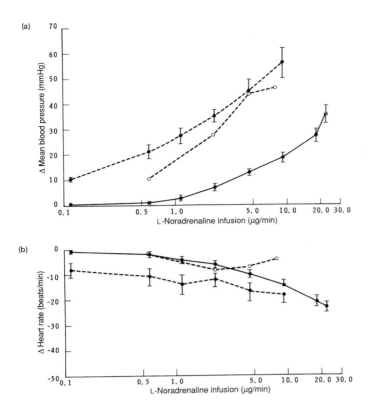

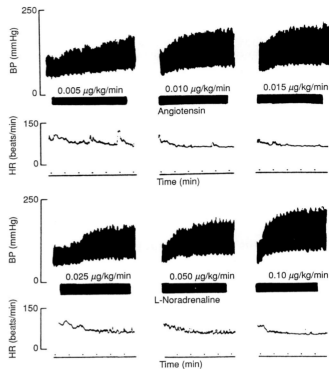

Fig. 51.26. Changes (Δ) in average mean blood pressure (a) and heart rate (b) during different dose infusion rates of noradrenaline in three recently injured tetraplegics (open circles, dashed line), five chronic tetraplegics (filled circles, dashed line), and 10 control subjects (filled circles, continuous line). The bars indicate ± SEM. There is an enhanced pressor response to noradrenaline in both groups of tetraplegics over the entire dose range studied. (From Mathias *et al.* (1976c, 1979a).)

Fig. 51.27. Blood pressure (BP) and heart rate (HR) effects of different dose infusion rates of angiotensin II (upper panels) and L-noradrenaline (lower panels) given intravenously to a chronic tetraplegic patient. These doses of angiotensin II and noradrenaline cause only small blood pressure changes in normal subjects. (From Mathias and Frankel (1986).)

kept active and stimulated. There is indirect evidence, based on *in vitro* studies of platelet α_2–adrenoceptor binding, that tetraplegics have a normal population of α-adrenoceptors (Davies *et al.* 1982). Microneurography studies, however, indicate a modest increase in muscle sympathetic nerve activity during autonomic dysreflexia when there is a pronounced vascular response (Stjernberg *et al.* 1986), suggesting that decentralization supersensitivity, for reasons that are currently unclear, may contribute to the enhanced pressor response to noradrenaline.

A further possibility includes the impairment of baroreflex pathways that descend through the cervical spinal cord and are normally concerned with buffering a rise in blood pressure. This would explain the elevated pressor response during autonomic dysreflexia and the clearly defined relationship between these hypertensive responses and the segmental level of the lesion at T5. In normal subjects it is likely that, despite a substantial rise in sympathoneural activity induced by a range of stimuli, blood pressure is maintained at near normal levels by efferent baroreflex activity, partly through the vagal efferents and predominantly by descending nerve tracts within the spinal cord, which selectively inhibit sympathetic vasoconstrictor activity and may even cause vasodilatation by mechanisms that are yet to be clearly defined in humans. The only intact efferent component of the baroreflex pathways in tetraplegics is the vagal outflow; this slows the

heart but is clearly inadequate in controlling the rise in blood pressure during autonomic dysreflexia. It is possible, therefore, that the absence of blood pressure restraining reflexes descending through the cervical and upper thoracic spinal cord down to the level of T5 may be a major factor accounting for the enhanced pressor responses to noradrenaline. This may also explain the observations that exaggerated pressor responses are not specific to α-adrenoceptor agonists but occur in response to agents with different structures and properties, ranging from phenylephrine to prostaglandin $F_{2\alpha}$, and angiotensin II. The low circulating levels of adrenaline and noradrenaline may not be major contributory factors, as there is a similar degree of pressor sensitivity to angiotensin II (Fig. 51.27), despite normal or elevated circulating levels of renin and angiotensin II. This argues strongly against receptor up-regulation alone being a factor.

The enhanced responses to pressor agents are of clinical importance, as the five to tenfold increase in sensitivity should be borne in mind if drugs with pressor actions are used in high spinal lesions.

Peripherally acting vasodepressor agents

Enhanced depressor responses to a range of vasodilatory substances also occur in high spinal-cord lesions. Bolus injections and intravenous infusion of isoprenaline lower blood pressure substantially (Chapter 20). Indirect evidence from *in vitro* β-adrenoceptor binding studies on lymphocytes exclude up-regulation of these receptors. In high lesions isoprenaline will stimulate both β_1– and β_2–adrenoceptors; it is likely that stimulation of the latter causes vasodilatation which would normally stimulate the baroreflex pathways, increase sympathetic activity, and prevent a substantial fall in blood pressure. This would not occur in high lesions and may account for the fall in blood pressure. The increase in heart rate, which is often exaggerated, is likely to be a combination of the vagal response to the fall in blood pressure and the direct β_1 effects of isoprenaline.

Enhanced vasodepressor responses occur to a variety of drugs, including intravenous prostaglandin E2 and sublingual glyceryl trinitrate and nifedipine. The last two may be used to advantage in high lesions, as they can be readily taken and can substantially lower blood pressure in autonomic dysreflexia. The risk of extreme hypotension should be kept in mind (Fig. 51.18).

Cutaneous circulation

The skin is innervated by the sympathetic nervous system and changes may occur both in recently injured and in chronic tetraplegics. Soon after injury there is often vasodilatation in the periphery, as the skin below the level of the lesion is often warmer and veins appear dilated. It is not clear whether this may lead to extravasation of fluid into subcutaneous tissue and contribute to skin breakdown and pressure sores, which is a major problem in recently injured patients. The vasodilatation may also involve mucosal tissues such as the nose, and result in nasal congestion, a problem seen in patients with high lesions who often have to breathe through their mouth. This has been referred to as Guttmann's sign, and is similar to the nasal vasodilatation after α-adrenoceptor blockade induced by either phenoxybenzamine or guanethidine, both previously used in the management of patients with hypertension.

The cutaneous Lewis or triple response varies in the different stages. In the stage of spinal shock, responses above and below the lesion are similar. This differs from the later phases, with return of isolated spinal-cord reflex activity, when stimulation of skin below the lesion results in cutaneous vasoconstriction, leading to skin pallor which may last for a prolonged period—hence the term 'dermatographia alba', as compared to 'dermatographia rubra' in the stage of spinal shock. In chronic high lesions, autonomic dysreflexia may result in marked constriction of cutaneous blood vessels (causing cold peripheries; poikilothermia spinalis) and activation of piloerector muscles (causing goose skin and pimples; cutis anserina) below the level of the lesion.

Thermoregulation

The autonomic nervous system plays an important role in the regulation of body temperature, which may be seriously deranged in tetraplegics.

Hypothermia

On exposure to cold a number of mechanisms are activated, which are dependent initially on appreciation of the temperature change and then on the ability to increase heat production and gain. Cold appreciation is dependent upon activation of both cutaneous and also central temperature receptors, which may explain why tetraplegics, although they have only a limited area of intact sensation, can still detect body cooling.

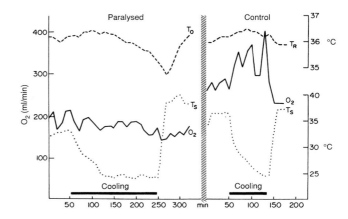

Fig. 51.28. The effect of body cooling on oesophageal (T_o), rectal (T_R), and skin (T_s) temperature and oxygen consumption (O_2) of a severely paralysed patient with poliomyelitis and a normal subject (control). The lack of shivering in the patient causes no rise in oxygen consumption and heat production which leads to a fall in central temperature, unlike the normal subject. (From Johnson and Spalding (1963).)

One of the major mechanisms responsible for heat production is shivering thermogenesis, which depends upon activation of skeletal muscles and shivering. In tetraplegics and those with high thoracic spinal cord lesions, a major proportion of skeletal muscle mass is not directly under voluntary control; this is a particular problem in spinal shock when there is skeletal muscle flaccidity. Hypothermia may therefore readily occur in such patients, as it does in other groups without autonomic lesions who have extensive paralysis either due to drugs or to poliomyelitis (Fig. 51.28). Tetraplegics and those with high thoracic lesions have the ability to shiver in innervated areas as the body temperature falls, but this often results only in a small increase in metabolism which, dependent upon the external temperature, may be inadequate for body temperature homeostasis. An additional problem in recently injured tetraplegics in spinal shock is cutaneous vasodilatation, and the inability to appropriately vasoconstrict. This enhances heat loss, lowers body temperature further, and can be a particular problem in causing hypothermia especially in temperate climates (Fig. 51.29). A low-reading rectal thermometer is essential in the assessment and management of hypothermia. The patient should be warmed, externally with care taken to prevent skin damage, and internally using warm drinks or infusion of warm saline. Drugs (including alcohol), which cause cutaneous vasodilatation and increase heat loss therefore should be strictly avoided.

Hyperthermia

Hyperthermia may occur particularly in tetraplegics and high spinal-cord lesions when environmental temperature is elevated, or in response to infection. Heat loss is dependent on two major mechanisms, vasodilatation and sweating, both of which are impaired in spinal lesions. Vasodilatation normally occurs during warming, and is dependent on a rise in central temperature. It may occur passively as a result of withdrawal of sympathetic vasoconstrictor tone, or actively. Both components are dependent on neural pathways within the cervical spinal cord, which are involved in high spinal-cord lesions (Fig. 51.30). Vasodilatation may also occur

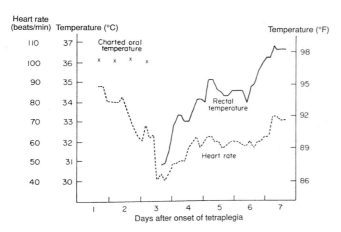

Fig. 51.29. Fall in central temperature (measured as rectal temperature) and heart rate in a recently injured tetraplegic in a temperate climate. Hypothermia is best monitored with a low-reading rectal thermometer and as indicated, may be missed if oral temperature is recorded. (From Pledger (1962).)

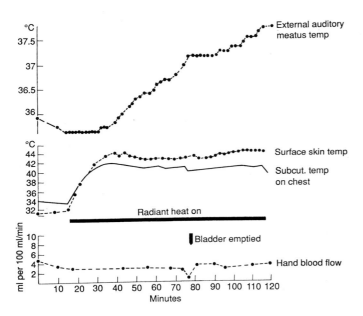

Fig. 51.30. Pronounced rise in both skin and core temperature (measured as external auditory meatus temperature) during application of radiant heat to the trunk of a tetraplegic patient. Hand blood flow does not rise, indicating lack of vasodilatation, as would occur normally during an elevation in temperature. (From Johnson (1965).)

following application of radiant or local heat to tetraplegics; this is more likely to be a direct effect than due to reflexes via the isolated spinal cord.

Sweating normally causes heat loss by evaporation, and is dependent upon a rise in central temperature and activation of sudomotor fibres within the sympathetic nervous system. Thermoregulatory sweating in large areas below the lesion is impaired in high spinal lesions, and is a further reason for these patients being prone to hyperthermia.

The maintenance of a suitable environmental temperature is of importance in the prevention of hyperthermia in high spinal lesions. When hyperthermia occurs, cooling with the aid of tepid sponging and increased air flow with a fan accelerates heat loss by a combination of evaporation, conduction, and convection. In severe cases, ice-cooled saline by intravenous infusion or urinary bladder irrigation and in extreme cases immersion of the whole body in an ice bath may be necessary. In hyperpyrexia associated with infection, drugs such as aspirin and paracetamol appear to be effective in lowering body temperature. The mechanisms by which they do this are unclear. Chlorpromazine is also effective, but has the potential to induce hypotension.

Gastrointestinal system

The autonomic nervous system richly innervates the gastrointestinal tract which is often affected especially in the early stages, after spinal-cord lesions.

Upper gastrointestinal bleeding

There is a high incidence of upper gastrointestinal bleeding in the early stages following spinal-cord injury. The incidence is greater in those with higher lesions. It is often unrelated to a previous history of peptic ulceration and may not be related to concomitant drug therapy, such as dexamethasone and analgesics. In such patients there is evidence of increased vagal activity, which may cause hyperacidity, along with high gastrin levels which also may contribute to gastric hypersecretion and ulceration.

The lesions may be either patchy or extensive and affect the oesophagus, stomach, or the duodenum. Erosions and ulceration may occur. Abdominal pain is usually absent. Shoulder-tip pain, accentuated by abdominal palpation, may indicate perforation. Autonomic dysreflexia may occur (Bar-On and Ohry 1995). There may be haematemesis or melaena. Fibre-optic endoscopy is probably the investigation of choice, the major limitation being the restriction to cervical spine mobility. Atropine may be needed to prevent vagal reflexes and bradycardia. The management consists of the administration of H_2 receptor antagonists (such as cimetidine or ranitidine), antacids, and fluid and blood replacement where relevant. The role of newer drugs such as omeprazole and orally active prostaglandin analogues, has not been clearly defined. Occasionally, surgery may be needed.

Paralytic ileus

This often occurs in spinal shock and may be accompanied by gastric dilatation. The mechanisms remain unclear as the motor innervation of the stomach and small intestines is by the vagus nerves, which are intact and often hyperactive in this phase. Paralytic ileus usually occurs a few days after injury and may be induced by solid food, which should therefore be avoided in the immediate period following a cervical or high thoracic spinal-cord injury.

Paralytic ileus results in meteorism which is a particular problem as it interferes with the movement of the diaphragm, often the only major functional muscle of respiration in these patients. It may be particularly prolonged in patients with intercurrent infection. The management consists of gastrointestinal aspiration to prevent further dilatation, the administration of intravenous fluids, and, if necessary, intravenous alimentation. Parasympathomimetic agents such as neostigmine are occasionally used to activate the bowel but carry the risk of potentiating bradycardia and cardiac arrest, especially in patients with high cervical lesions on artificial respiration. The dopamine antagonist, metoclopramide, which enhances gastric emptying, may be of value in some cases. It may be that newer drugs that increase gastrointestinal motility, such as the prodrug, cisapride and the cholecystokinin antagonist, loxeglumide, will be of value. Once spinal shock has subsided small intestine function often returns to normal. Tetraplegics and high thoracic lesions are, however, prone to paralytic ileus even in the chronic stage, especially after undergoing general anaesthesia and abdominal surgery.

Large bowel dysfunction

In spinal shock, paralysis of the sacral parasympathetic results in atony of the colon and rectum. Voluntary or reflexly induced defecation does not occur and this results in faecal retention. Digital evacuation is often necessary in the early stages.

After the stage of spinal shock, autonomous function of the lower bowel returns and is regulated at a spinal level, as it is abolished by intrathecal block with alcohol. The stimulus to bowel activity appears to be increased volume and distension, which then causes relaxation of the external anal sphincter and evacuation of contents. This stimulus is utilized in the reconditioning of lower bowel function. The diet should therefore include high residue foods together with mild laxatives and stool softeners, to ensure regular bowel evacuation. This is an important part of the management, as regular bowel movement prevents faecal retention which predisposes patients with high lesions to autonomic dysreflexia for a variety of reasons. These include distension of the lower bowel and the predisposition to haemorrhoids and anal fissures.

The urinary system

Function of the urinary bladder is dependent upon higher centres in the brain and the sympathetic and parasympathetic nerves, and is therefore affected in varying degrees in patients with spinal-cord lesions. In the chronic stage complications to the ureters and kidneys, such as infection, calculi, urinary reflux, hydroureters, and hydronephrosis, may lead to renal damage. resulting in chronic renal failure, which largely stems from this basic dysfunction.

In spinal shock there is usually complete paralysis of bladder function with retention of urine followed by distension and urinary overflow after excessive intravesical pressure has developed. This should be avoided, as it often impedes functional return of detrusor muscle activity once spinal shock has subsided. Bladder paralysis is invariable in most adult Europeans, but does not usually occur in children and adult Afro-Caribbeans. The management in spinal shock consists of drainage using an indwelling catheter, or preferably intermittent catheterization which causes fewer complications.

With the return of parasympathetic activity within the isolated sacral cord there is detrusor muscle contraction, which occurs in response to filling of the urinary bladder, or following stimuli such as tapping of the anterior abdominal wall suprapubically. This is the automatic reflex bladder, or neurogenic bladder. During detrusor contraction there is a need for simultaneous relaxation of the sphinc-

ters and pelvic floor to allow the free passage of urine. Training is needed to achieve co-ordination of these components of bladder function, and if this is successful male patients may be catheter-free, using a condom and receptacle to collect urine. In some patients, however, detrusor contraction is not accompanied by simultaneous relaxation of the bladder outlet, and in high lesions the resultant discoordinated bladder can cause marked autonomic dysreflexia. Retained urine often results in infection, which can involve the kidneys, especially when there is retrograde pressure in the urinary tract. In such patients an indwelling catheter, or various forms of urological and neurological surgery (Hohenfellner *et al.* 1996), may be needed to relieve the functional obstruction and prevent autonomic dysreflexia. The α-adrenoceptor blockers, phenoxybenzamine and prazosin, may be of value in some patients as the bladder outlet is relaxed. In low lesions there may be a flaccid bladder even in the chronic stage. Manual compression using Credé's manoeuvre is needed to ensure complete emptying, along with the other aids for urine collection.

In female patients, the bladder can be trained to empty in response to distension and external stimuli. Because of the lack of suitable collecting systems there may be incontinence, which is often not helped by an indwelling catheter. In some, an ileal conduit may be the most practical outcome.

Reproductive system

In the male reproduction and sexual function is dependent on the interrelationship between parasympathetic and sympathetic nerve function and therefore is usually impaired. Few changes occur in the female with spinal-cord injuries.

The male

Penile erection is dependent largely upon the sacral parasympathetic nerves with ejaculation dependent upon the sympathetic nerves. In spinal shock there is an absence of both erectile and ejaculatory function. In some patients, however, passive penile enlargement and priapism may occur, probably due to paralytic dilatation resulting in engorgement of the corpora cavernosa. Following the return of isolated spinal-cord reflex activity, penile erection may occur if the glans penis is stimulated, or as part of autonomic dysreflexia. Ejaculation, however, seldom occurs per urethra and is usually retrograde, as the associated contraction of muscles at the bladder neck which prevents seminal fluid flowing back into the bladder does not usually occur. In spinal-cord injuries, therefore, procreation in the male is largely dependent on the collection of seminal fluid for artificial insemination. The original technique involved intrathecal neostigmine which caused skeletal muscle depression followed by penile erection and ejaculation. In high lesions, side-effects such as vomiting and severe autonomic dysreflexia often occurred, and in one patient this resulted in cerebral haemorrhage and death. In addition to vibrator techniques, electroejaculation also is used, although this may result in severe hypertension, and careful monitoring of blood pressure is necessary in those with high lesions, especially when seminal emission occurs. Many of the drugs that are often used to lower blood pressure in autonomic dysreflexia are not the ideal ones to use during such procedures as they interrupt sympathetic pathways and have the potential to interfere with ejaculation.

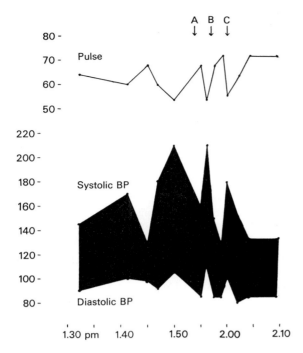

Fig. 51.31. Blood pressure and pulse rate in a paraplegic patient with a high thoracic lesion (T5) during (A) application of forceps, (B) completion of delivery, and (C) placental delivery. The hypertension is closely followed by bradycardia. (From Guttmann *et al.* (1965).)

The female

In women transient disruption of the menstrual cycle is often observed after spinal lesions, as occurs during other traumatic conditions or illnesses. There is usually a return to normal menstrual periods within a year. Successful pregnancies have been reported in both tetraplegics and paraplegics. In those with high lesions a particular problem is severe autonomic dysreflexia and paroxysmal hypertension (Fig. 51.31) which may be accompanied by cardiac dysrhythmias, especially during uterine contractions. Such patients are particularly prone to epileptic seizures and cerebral haemorrhage and it is essential to lower their blood pressure. Anticonvulsants such as phenytoin may be needed. Spinal anaesthesia appears to be a satisfactory method of preventing the hypertension without interfering with uterine contraction. This often allows progression of a normal delivery and avoids a Caesarean section.

References

Arnold, J. M., Feng, Q. P., Delaney, G. A., and Teasell, R. W. (1995). Autonomic dysreflexia in tetraplegic patients: evidence for alpha-adrenoceptor hyper-responsiveness. *Clin. Auton Res.* 5, 267–70.

Baliga, R. R., Catz, A. B., Watson, L. P., Short, D. J., Frankel, H. L., and Mathias, C. J. (1997). Cardiovascular and hormonal responses to food ingestion in humans with spinal cord transection. *Clin. Auton Res.* 7, 137–41.

Bar-On, Z. and Ohry, A. (1995). The acute abdomen in spinal cord injury individuals. *Paraplegia* 33, 704–6.

Chancellor, M. B., Erhard, M. J., Hirsch, I. H., and Stass, W. E. (1994). Prospective evaluation of terazosin for the treatment of autonomic dysreflexia. *J. Urol.* 151, 111–13.

Corbett, J. L., Frankel, H. L., and Harris, P. J. (1971). Cardio-vascular reflex responses to cutaneous and visceral stimuli in spinal man. *J. Physiol.* 215, 395.

Curt, A., Weinhardt, C., and Dietz, V. (1996). Significance of sympathetic skin response in the assessment of autonomic failure in patients with spinal injury. *J. autonom. nerv. Sys.* 61, 175–80.

Curt, A., Nitsche, B., Rodic, B., Schurch, B., and Dietz, V. (1997). Assessment of autonomic dysreflexia in patients with spinal cord injury. *J. Neurol. Neurosurg. Psychiat.* 62, 473–7.

Davies, I. B., Mathias, C. J., Sudera, D., and Sever, P. S. (1982). Agonist regulation of alpha-adrenergic receptor responses in man. *J. Cardiovasc. Pharmacol.* 4, s139–44.

Frankel, H. L., Michaelis, L. S., Golding, D. R., and Beral, V. (1972). The blood pressure in paraplegia-1. *Paraplegia* 10, 193–8.

Frankel, H. L., Mathias, C. J., and Spalding, J. M. K. (1975). Mechanisms of reflex cardiac arrest in tetraplegic patients. *Lancet* ii, 1183–5.

Guttmann, L. (1976). *Spinal cord injuries. Comprehensive management and research* (2nd edn). Blackwell Scientific, Oxford.

Guttmann, L. and Whitteridge, D. (1947). Effects of bladder distension on autonomic mechanisms after spinal cord injury. *Brain* 70, 361–404.

Guttmann, L., Frankel, H. L., and Paeslack, V. (1965). Cardiac irregularities during labour in paraplegic women. *Paraplegia* 3, 144–51.

Head, H. and Riddoch, G. (1917). The autonomic bladder, excessive sweating and some other reflex conditions in gross injuries of the spinal cord. *Brain* 40, 188–263.

Hohenfellner, M., Fahle, H., Dahms, S., Linn, J. F., Hutschenreiter, G., and Thuroff, J. W. (1996). Continent reconstruction of detrusor hyperreflexia by sacral bladder denervation combined with continent vesicostomy. *Urology* 47, (6), 930–1.

Inoue, K., Miyake, S., Kumashiro, M., Ogata, H., Ueta, T., and Akatsu, T. (1991). Power spectral analysis of blood pressure variability in traumatic quadriplegic humans. *Am. J. Physiol.* H842–4.

Johnson, R. H. (1965). Neurological studies in temperature regulation. *Ann. Roy. Coll. Surg.* 36, 339–52.

Johnson, R. H. and Spalding, J. M. K. (1963). Whole body metabolism of a paralysed man during surface cooling. *J. Physiol.* 166, 24P.

Karlsson, A.-K. (1997). Metabolism and sympathetic function in spinal cord injured subjects. PhD Thesis, University of Gothenburg, Sweden.

Khurana, R. K. (1987). Orthostatic hypotension-induced autonomic dysreflexia. *Neurology* 37, 1221–4.

Koh, J., Brown, T. E., Beighton, L. A., Ha, C. Y., and Eckberg, D. L. (1994). Human autonomic rhythms: vagal cardiac mechanisms in tetraplegic subjects. *J. Physiol.*, London 474, 483–95.

Kooner, J. S., da Costa, D. F., Frankel, H. L., Bannister, R., Peart, W. S., and Mathias, C. J. (1987). Recumbency induces hypertension, diuresis and natriuresis in autonomic failure, but diuresis alone in tetraplegia. *J. Hypertension* 5, (Suppl. 5), 327–9.

Krum, H., Louis, W. J., Brown, D. J., Clarke, S. J., Fleming, J. A., and Howes, L. G. (1992). Cardiovascular and vasoactive hormone responses to bladder distension in spinal and normal man. *Paraplegia* 30, 348–54.

Linsenmeyer, T. A, Campagnolo, D. I., and Chou, I. H. (1996). Silent autonomic dysreflexia during voiding in men with spinal cord injuries. *J. Urol.* 155, (2), 519–22.

Mathias, C. J. (1976a). Neurological disturbances of the cardiovascular system. D. Phil. thesis, University of Oxford.

Mathias, C. J. (1976b). Bradycardia and cardiac arrest during tracheal suction mechanisms in tetraplegic patients. *Eur. J. Intensive Care Med.* 2, 147–56.

Mathias, C. J. (1995). Orthostatic hypotension causes, mechanisms and influencing factors. *Neurology* 45, (suppl 5) 56–11.

Mathias, C. J., Frankel, H. L. (1986). The neurological and hormonal control of blood vessels and heart in spinal man. *J. Autonom. Nerv. Syst. Suppl.* 457–64.

Mathias, C. J. and Frankel, H. L. (1988). Cardiovascular control in spinal man. *Ann. Rev. Physiol.* 50, 577–92.

Mathias, C. J. and Frankel, H. L. (1992). The cardiovascular system in tetraplegia and paraplegia. Ins. *Handbook of Clinical Neurology*, vol 17,

Spinal Cord Trauma, (ed. H. L. Frankel) pp. 435–56. Elsevier Science Publishers B. V., Netherlands.

Mathias, C. J., Christensen, N. J., Corbett, J. L., Frankel, H. L., Goodwin, T. J., and Peart, W. S. (1975). Plasma catecholamines, plasma renin activity and plasma aldosterone in tetraplegic man, horizontal and tilted. *Clin. Sci. Mol. Med.* 49, 291–9.

Mathias, C. J., Christensen, N. J., Corbett, J. L., Frankel, H. L., and Spalding, J. M. K. (1976a). Plasma catecholamines during paroxysmal neurogenic hypertension in quadriplegic man, *Circulation Res.* 39, 204–8.

Mathias, C. J., Smith A. D., Frankel, H. L., and Spalding, J. M. K. (1976b). Release of dopamine B-hydroxylase during hypertension from sympathetic over-activity in man. *Cardiovascular Res.* 10, 176–81.

Mathias, C. J., Frankel, H. L., Christensen, N. J., and Spalding, J. M. K. (1976c). Enhanced pressor response to noradrenaline in patients with cervical spinal cord transaction. *Brain* 99, 757–70.

Mathias, C. J., Christensen, N. J., Frankel, H. L., and Spalding, J. M. K. (1979a). Cardiovascular control in recently injured tetraplegics in spinal shock. *Q. J. Med.*, NS 48, 273–87.

Mathias, C. J., Frankel, H. L., Turner, R. C., and Christensen, J. N. (1979b). Physiological responses to insulin hypoglycaemia in spinal man. *Paraplegia* 17, 319–26.

Mathias, C. J., Reid, J. L., Wing, L. M. H., Frankel, H. L., and Christensen, N. J. (1979c). Antihypertensive effects of clonidine in tetraplegic subjects devoid of central sympathetic control. *Clin. Sci.* 57, 425–8s.

Mathias, C. J., Frankel, H. L., Davies, I. B., James, V. H. T, and Peart, W. S. (1981). Renin and aldosterone release during sympathetic stimulation in tetraplegia. *Clin. Sci.* 60, 399–604.

Middleton, J. W., Siddall, P. J, Walker, S., Molloy, A. R., and Rutkowski, S. B. (1996). Intrathecal clonidine and baclofen in the management of spasticity and neuropathic pain following spinal cord injury: a case study. *Arch. Phys. Med. Rehabil.* 77, 824–6.

Morris, M. J., Cox, H. S., Lambert, G. W., et al. (1997). Region-specific neuropeptide Y overflows at rest and during sympathetic activation in humans. *Hypertension.* 29, 137–43.

Nitsche, B., Perschak, H., Curt, A., and Dietz, V. (1996). Loss of circadian blood pressure variability in complete tetraplegia. *J. Hum. Hypertens.* 10, 311–17.

Norberg, K. A. and Normell, L. A. (1974). Histochemical demonstration of sympathetic adrenergic denervation in human skin. *Acta Neurol. Scand.* 50, 261.

Pledger, H. G. (1962). Disorders of temperature regulation in acute traumatic paraplegia. *J. Bone Joint Surg.* 44B, 110–13.

Previnaire, J. G., Soler, J. M., and Hanson, P. (1993). Skin potential recordings during cystometry in spinal cord injured patients. *Paraplegia* 31, 13–21.

Reid, J. L., Wing, L. M. H., Mathias, C. J., Frankel, H. L., and Neill, E. (1977). The central hypotensive effect of clonidine: studies in tetraplegic subjects. *Clin. Pharmacol. Therapeut.* 21, 375–81.

Santajuliana, D., Zukowska-Grojec, Z., and Osborn, J. W. (1995). Contribution of alpha- and beta-adrenoceptors and neuropeptide Y to autonomic dysreflexia. *Clin. Auton Res.* 5, 91–7.

Stjernberg, L., Blumberg, H., and Wallin, B. G. (1986). Sympathetic activity in man after spinal cord injury: outflow to muscle below the lesion. *Brain* 109, 695–715.

Sutters, M., Wakefield, C., O'Neil, K., et al. (1992). The cardiovascular, endocrine and renal response of tetraplegic and paraplegic subjects to dietary sodium restriction. *J. Physiol., London* 457, 515–23.

Thyberg, M., Ertzgaard, P., Gylling, M., and Granerus, G. (1994). Effect of nifedipine on cystometry-induced elevation of blood pressure in patients with a reflex urinary bladder after a high level spinal cord injury. *Paraplegia* 32, 308–13.

van Lieshout, J. J., lmholz, B. P. M., Wesseling, K. H., Speelman, J. D., and Wieling, W. (1991). Singing-induced hypotension: a complication of high spinal cord lesion. *Neth. J. Med.* 38, 75–9.

Welply, N. C., Mathias, C. J., and Frankel, H. L. (1975). Circulatory reflexes in tetraplegics during artificial ventilation and general anaesthesia. *Paraplegia* 13, 172–82.

52. Autonomic and cerebrovascular aspects of migraine: pathophysiology and treatment

Lars Lykke Thomsen and Jes Olesen

Introduction

There are two main types of migraine—migraine with aura and migraine without aura. In migraine with aura, the attacks are initiated by 'marching' neurological symptoms—the aura—which typically affects one ore more of the following in the order of frequency: vision, speech, sensation, and strength, either alone or in combination. Apart from these aura symptoms, the attacks are the same as in migraine without aura and are characterized by severe pulsating headaches, lasting 4–72 hours, often unilateral and accompanied by nausea and hypersensitivity to light and sounds. Migraine headache is a very common complaint affecting up to 16 per cent of the adult population . The burden on society, in terms of work days lost, health care costs, and the amount of suffering by affected individuals, is enormous (Rasmussen 1995). The mechanisms of migraine are complex and still not fully understood. However, an impressive advance in basic and clinical headache research over the past two decades has markedly improved our understanding. As a consequence, the therapeutic strategies have become more specific. In fact migraine became one of the first neurological conditions to be treated successfully with a receptor-selective drug (the 5-HT$_{1D}$ receptor agonist, sumatriptan). Studies of the cephalic vascular system and its regulation have markedly contributed towards this development. This regulation is complex and involves autonomic, trigeminovascular, endothelial, and humoral factors (see Chapter 10). The present review focuses on these aspects of migraine pathophysiology. In addition links are drawn between autonomic and cerebrovascular aspects of migraine and the mechanism of action of specific anti-migraine therapy and potential targets for new drug development in migraine.

Blood flow and large artery dynamics in migraine

Cerebral blood flow in migraine

Clinical studies of regional cerebral blood flow (rCBF) in migraine with aura have shown a hypoperfusion, usually not reaching ischaemic thresholds, in the posterior part of the brain at the onset of the aura. This hypoperfusion gradually spreads forward to contiguous areas not respecting the territories of supply of the major arteries. The hypoperfusion lasts throughout the aura phase and well into the headache phase, after which hyperperfusion develops (Fig. 52.1). The relation between the usual unilateral aura symptoms and unilateral rCBF changes suggests that in the majority of patients the aura symptoms originate from the hemisphere affected by hypoperfusion (see

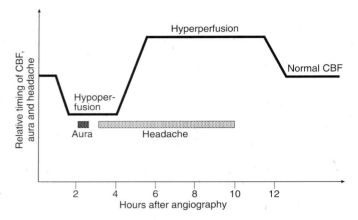

Fig. 52.1. Temporal relation between CBF changes, migraine aura, and migraine headache. No causal relation seems likely. Thus, hypoperfusion often outlasts the aura and the headache often starts during the hypoperfusion and disappears before end of hyperperfusion. (From Olesen *et al.* (1990), with permission.)

Olesen 1991). The characteristic spreading rCBF changes suggest that the migraine aura may be due to a so-called cortical spreading depression (Lauritzen 1994). This phenomenon consists of a depolarization of neurones and glial cells that spreads slowly across the cortical surface and which is associated with blood-flow changes similar to rCBF changes during migraine with aura (Table 52.1). Thus, the basis of the migraine aura seems to be neuronal in nature and rCBF changes seem to be secondary phenomena. In addition the timing between rCBF changes and headache in migraine with aura suggests that these events are not causally related.

Several previous SPECT and PET studies suggest that the cortical perfusion is unchanged during attacks of migraine without aura and also at the very beginning of provoked attacks (Olesen 1991). An interesting recent study applying positron emission tomography (PET) did, however, show spreading cortical blood-flow changes in a patient with symptoms not typical for a migraine aura as the patient mentioned only vague visual problems (Woods *et al.* 1994). Based on the clinical description, it cannot be ruled out that the patient actually suffered an attack of migraine without aura and despite the prominence of studies suggesting normal rCBF during migraine without aura more studies seem necessary before this question can be regarded as settled.

A recent PET scan study showed an ipsilateral centre of increased blood flow in the brainstem which persisted after successful treatment of headache with sumatriptan. The findings were made in nine

Table 52.1. Similarities between migraine aura and spreading depression (modified from Olesen 1993)

Factor	Migraine	Spreading depression
Site of origin	Primary visual cortex	High neuron density
Way of spread	Contiguous cortical	Contiguous cortical
Excitation/depression	Yes	Yes
Rate of spread	2–6 mm/min	2–6 mm/min
Unilateral	Yes	Yes
Repeated waves	Yes	Yes
Hypoperfusion lasting	Hours	Hours
Initial hyperperfusion	?	Yes
Autoregulation	Preserved	Preserved
CO_2 reactivity	Impaired	Impaired

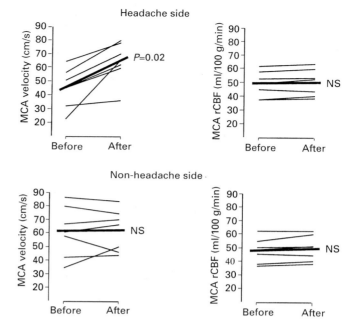

Fig. 52.2. Middle cerebral artery (MCA) blood velocity and perfusion (rCBF) during unilateral migraine headache. Responses before and after treatment with sumatriptan (2 mg intravenously). Sumatriptan induced a reversal of a decreased MCA velocity on the headache side whereas rCBF was unchanged. At the same time headaches disappeared (not shown on figures). These findings suggests that the mechanism of action of sumatriptan involves contraction of pathologically dilated large intracranial arteries. (From Friberg *et al.* (1991), with permission.)

patients studied within 6 hours of onset of right-sided migraine without aura. These changes were absent in a headache-free interval 3 days to 4 months later (Diener and May 1996).

Cranial arteries during migraine pain

Whereas blood-flow changes and therefore changes of arteriolar diameter seem unrelated to migraine pain, dilatation of the large cranial arteries has long been suspected to be a mechanism of migraine pain.

In a recent study, high-frequency ultrasound was used to demonstrate dilatation of the superficial temporal artery on the headache side during unilateral migraine attacks (Iversen *et al.* 1990). This dilatation was, however, small (9 per cent) and relative to a generalized vasoconstriction. Unfortunately, the diameter of the intracranial arteries is difficult to measure directly *in vivo*. However, the ultrasound technique, transcranial Doppler (TCD), provides measurements of the velocity of circulating blood in the large intracranial arteries at the base of the brain. Since changes in blood velocity in situations of unchanged blood flow are inversely related to changes in the cross-sectional vessel area, the TCD method provides an indirect way of estimating large intracranial artery diameter changes. Friberg and colleagues used a combination of TCD and SPECT, and measured middle cerebral artery (MCA) blood velocity and rCBF simultaneously in the supply area of the MCA during unilateral migraine headache. TCD recordings showed reduced velocity on the headache side as compared to the non-headache side. No such difference was found in rCBF in the MCA territory, a finding which suggests that the MCA was dilated on the headache side. In addition to this finding, evidence was provided showing that the 5-HT_1 receptor agonist sumatriptan (2 mg intravenously), returned blood velocity to normal without affecting rCBF, and at the same time ameliorated the headache (Friberg *et al.* 1991) (Fig. 52.2). Not all TCD studies have confirmed the presence of ipsilateral large artery dilatation (reviewed by Thomsen *et al.* 1995a). However, in a recent study focusing exclusively on MCA side-to-side asymmetry in patients suffering from

half-sided migraine without aura, reduced velocity was again demonstrated on the headache side (Thomsen *et al.* 1995a). Although these studies suggest an association between migraine pain and dilatation of the large cranial arteries, this does not necessarily imply that the pain is elicited by simple mechanical force caused by arterial dilatation. The magnitude of cranial arterial dilatation found in previous studies is most likely too small (9 per cent) (Iversen *et al.* 1990; Thomsen *et al.* 1995a) to be the only cause of pain. A likely possibility is a combination of arterial dilatation and sensitization of perivascular sensory nerve fibres or central pain processing.

Regulation of vascular tone in migraine

Due to this vascular involvement, a possible dysregulation of vascular tone in migraine has long been a subject of considerable interest. Based on cardiovascular tests, vasomotor reactions to temperature changes, and responses to pharmacological tests, as well as changes in biochemical parameters, hypo- as well as hyperfunctioning of both the sympathetic and parasympathetic nervous system has been suggested (Thomsen and Olesen 1995). Based on experimentally induced migraine attacks, a key role of the vasodilator molecule, nitric oxide, has been suggested and based on an animal model of so-called neurogenic inflammation and clinical studies of plasma levels of vasoactive neuropetides during migraine headache involvement of the trigeminovascular system has been suggested.

Cardiovascular reflexes

A number of studies have focused on sympathetically mediated cardiovascular reflexes, as elicited by the orthostatic test, the cold pressor test, and the isometric work test. An extensive series of studies has been published by Havanka-Kanniainen and colleagues. They found no evidence of disturbances in young migraineurs outside the attack (11–22 years old) as compared to a control group. Significant abnormalities suggesting sympathetic hypofunction were, however, found interictally in older migraineurs (aged 23–50 years) (Havanka-Kanniainen et al. 1986). No difference was found between these responses in migraineurs suffering from migraine with and without aura. During attacks a decreased blood pressure response to an isometric work test was found to be more pronounced than between attacks. Based on decreased RR variation during normal and deep breathing, and a decreased Valsalva ratio in migraineurs the same authors concluded that parasympathetic hypofunction was present in migraine. Gotoh and collaborators (1984) compared responses to a Valsalva manoeuvre, an orthostatic test, and Achner's test (reflex bradycardia induced by pressure on the eyeballs) interictally in migraine patients suffering from migraine either with or without aura to age-matched healthy controls. In addition, a noradrenaline bolus injection and eye installation tests were evaluated. Sympathetic hypofunction, with denervation hypersensitivity and parasympathetic hyperfunction was suggested. In contrast to this suggested sympathetic hypofunction other studies using similar cardiovascular tests have shown either sympathetic hyperfunction or normal sympathetic function. Furthermore, normal parasympathetic function has also been described, based on cardiovascular tests. In our own experience migraine is not associated with disturbed cardiovascular tests reflecting sympathetic function, whereas a mild parasympathetic hypofunction seems to be present (Thomsen and Olesen 1995).

Arterial and arteriolar vasomotor reactivity

Reduced vasodilatation in the forehead and hands of migraineurs after heating has been reported. In another study an increase of digital blood volume during heating was only absent in male migraineurs. In contrast, a peripherally applied cold stimulus failed to induce decreased hand blood flow in migraineurs. Finally, normal peripheral vasomotor reactivity in migraineurs has also been described (Thomsen and Olesen 1995).

Local autonomic control regarding the cranial arterial bed is obviously more relevant than studies of systemic vascular reactivity, but is more difficult to investigate. Using transcranial Doppler, a recent study showed no differences in MCA blood velocity responses in migraineurs studied during tests of cardiovascular sympathetic function both during and between attacks (Thomsen et al. 1995b). This suggests normal MCA reactivity during increased sympathetic drive. In the temporal region, extracranial blood-flow responses to an orthostatic test have been studied during and between migraine attacks. This study revealed no statistical difference between the attack and the attack-free state, apart from a slightly decreased response on the headache side as compared to the non- headache side during attack (Jensen 1987).

Cerebral blood-flow responses to functional tests such as speech, reading, listening, and arm work have been studied during attacks of migraine with aura. These activation procedures were not accompanied by the usual increase in regional cerebral blood flow (rCBF) in low-flow areas, whereas a normal, focal rCBF increase was observed in the non-affected parts of the brain. It is most likely, but not definitely established, that autoregulation is normal during attacks of both migraine with and without aura (Olesen 1991). Several studies have focused on cerebrovascular reactivity to alterations in $PaCO_2$. During attacks of migraine with aura, $PaCO_2$ reactivity seems to be impaired or abolished, whereas $PaCO_2$ reactivity seems to be normal during attacks of migraine without aura. Interictally an exaggerated PCO_2 reactivity during hyperventilation has recently been reported but only in migraine with aura (Thomsen and Olesen 1995). The interictal response to CO_2 inhalation may, however, be exaggerated both in migraine with and without aura, and more studies are needed to establish whether interictal differences in cerebrovascular reactivity between migraine with and without aura exists.

Pupillometry

Autonomic function may be studied by pupillometry. Such results generally suggest sympathetic or parasympathetic hypofunction in migraine. Interictally the mydriatic response to tyramine, phenylephrine, guanethidine and adrenaline was enhanced in adult migraineurs but not in children. Furthermore, pupillometric data have suggested α-receptor supersensitivity of the iris (see Thomsen and Olesen 1995).

Central sympathetic function and conclusions on functional studies of the autonomic nervous system in migraine

It has been suggested that the contingent negative variation (CNV)—a slow cerebral potential elicited by a reaction task with a warning and an imperative stimulus—is modulated by catecholamine afferents to the frontal cortex. If this is so, studies of CNV in migraine may indicate a central sympathetic involvement (Maertens de Noordhout et al. 1986). However, at present this possibility remains hypothetical. As mentioned, blood-flow changes in certain areas of the brainstem may be present during attacks (Diener and May 1996). This may be a visualization of a dysfunction of the locus ceruleus in migraine as previously suggested (Lance 1993).

Thus it may be concluded that brainstem activity involving the locus ceruleus which utilizes noradrenaline as a transmitter and which is involved in antinociception and extra- and intracranial vascular control may be present in migraine. However, a clear dysfunction of the sympathetic nervous system still remains to be shown. If sympathetic dysfunction is involved, most studies suggest hypofunction. However, considering that several studies, applying different methods, have been inconclusive and that the response of cranial arteries is normal during increased sympathetic activity, it seems unlikely that a sympathetic dysfunction plays any major role. Mild parasympathetic hypofunction with denervationsupersensitivity may be present in migraine. The origin of such disturbances are unknown and it remain to be demonstrated whether large cranial artery parasympathetic responses are abnormal and which transmitters or modulators may be involved.

Vasoactive neurotransmitters in migraine

5-HT and catecholamines

Plasma levels and urinary excretion of catecholamines and their metabolites have often been studied, but with contradicting results (Lance 1993; Thomsen and Olesen 1995). Indirect evidence points towards a role for the vasoactive amine 5-hydroxytryptamine (5-HT) in migraine. In humans 5-HT is found in the brain, the pineal gland, the blood, platelets, and blood vessels, including the circle of Willis. There is a close interaction between the central 5-HT system and the central noradrenergic system, but it is unknown whether this interaction plays a role in migraine. During attacks of migraine without aura the platelet content of 5-HT is decreased, but not during attacks of migraine with aura. 5-HT in platelet-free plasma, on the other hand, shows similar changes in both migraine with and without aura. Thus, interictally migraineurs have lower 5-HT and higher 5-hydroxyindoleacetic acid (5-HIAA, the main metabolite of 5-HT) compared to controls. During attacks, the plasma level of 5-HT increases significantly as compared to outside of attack, whereas 5-HIAA levels fall. This could imply a release of 5-HT from platelets during attack and/or an increased metabolic turnover of 5-HT outside of attack (Ferrari and Saxena 1995).

Neuropeptides and trigeminovascular mechanisms

Neuropeptide Y (NPY), vasoactive intestinal polypeptide (VIP), and substance P in blood from the external and internal jugular vein were normal during migraine attacks. However, increased levels of calcitonin-gene-related peptide (CGRP) in blood from the external jugular vein has been demonstrated during migraine attacks (Table 52.2) (Goadsby *et al.* 1990). Antidromic activity in perivascular nerve endings of trigeminal origin releases neurotransmitters, which in turn induce vasodilatation and plasma extravasation as part of a so-called neurogenic inflammation (Chapter 10). A series of experimental studies in rats has shown alterations in vascular permeability and ultrastructural changes in the dura mater associated with stimulation of the trigeminal ganglion (Moskowitz 1993; Chapter 10). Trigeminal ganglion stimulation has been shown to be associated with a release of CGRP and substance P in the rat and in humans. It remains to be demonstrated whether neurogenic inflammation takes place during migraine attacks.

Table 52.2. CGRP and substance P during migraine headache.

	CGRP	SP
Migraine with aura		
Site		
External jugular vein	92 ($\pm$11)*	5 ($\pm$2)
Cubital fosa	40 ($\pm$6)	5 ($\pm$3)
Control values	<40	<4
Migraine without aura		
Site		
External jugular vein	86 ($\pm$4)*	6 ($\pm$2)
Cubital fosa	43 ($\pm$6)	4 ($\pm$1)
Control values	<40	<4

*, $P > 0.001$. (Modified from Goadsby *et al.* 1990)

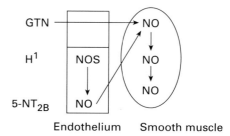

Fig. 52.3. Endothelium-derived relaxation. Nitric oxide (NO) is synthesized (via nitric oxide synthase, NOS) and released from the endothelium upon receptor stimulation (here illustrated by the histamine H_1 and 5-HT$_{2B}$ receptors). NO diffuses to adjacent smooth muscle and activates guanylate cyclase, hence causing increased cyclic guanosine monophosphate (cGMP). Glyceryl trinitrate (GTN) is a nitric oxide donor that induces migraine in susceptible individuals and activates the same pathway. Also, activation of H_1 and 5-HT$_{2B}$ receptors causes migraine headache in susceptible subjects.

Nitric oxide

Nitric oxide is not only a transmitter in parasympathetic perivascular nerves, it is also the main endothelium-derived relaxant factor (EDRF) (Fig. 52.3). Nitric oxide is liberated from the endothelium upon stimulation of several receptors and also by shear stress phenomena. Endothelial receptor stimulation may occur from the luminal side and perhaps also from the abluminal side. Thus, relevant transmitters may be released from perivascular nerve endings in the adventitia, diffuse to the endothelium, and stimulate the release of nitric oxide. Nitric oxide is a gas that easily crosses membranes. It thus enters smooth muscle cells and causes relaxation via activation of soluble guanylate cyclase hence causing accumulation of cyclic GMP. Glyceryl trinitrate (GTN) – which has been systematically validated as an experimental headache-inducing substance – is a nitric oxide donor, and hyperpersensitivity to nitric oxide has been shown indirectly in migraineurs by means of intravenous infusion of GTN. Interestingly, increased sensitivity to GTN in migraine has been shown both for the induction of pain (Fig. 52.4) and for dilatation of the middle cerebral artery (Fig. 52.5) (Olesen *et al.* 1995).

The nitric oxide pathway and the triggering of migraine pain

Not only has hypersensitivity to pain and arterial dilatation induced by GTN been demonstrated in migraine but this NO donor also triggers delayed genuine migraine attacks in migraineurs which are almost identical to spontaneous attacks. Based on these observations, hypotheses have been made stating that release of NO provides a common final pathway for several substances that trigger migraine pain (Olesen *et al.* 1995). Beside the NO donor, GTN, other substances which have been shown to reliably cause more headache than placebo in single-dose experiments include histamine, reserpine, and *meta*-chloro-phenylpiperazine (m-CPP). Interestingly, migraineurs have been described to be hypersensitive to these substances regarding headache development, which in migraineurs resembles migraine attacks, in controlled trials (Olesen *et al.* 1995). In a recent double-blind controlled trial, migraineurs were randomized to pre-treatment with either mepyramine or placebo before histamine infusion. Half of

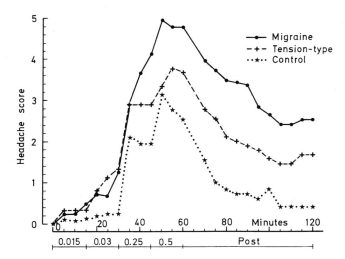

Fig. 52.4. Mean headache intensity over time during four doses of glyceryl trinitrate (GTN) in migraine patients, tension-type headache sufferers, and control subjects. Headache increased significantly above baseline after 35 minutes in all three groups. During doses above 0.015 μg/kg/min migraine patients experienced significantly more headache than controls ($P < 0.05$). In migraine patients the headache remained during the study period, whereas 60 min after the end of GTN infusion headache in both controls and tension-type headache patients was no different from baseline ($P < 0.001$ Kruskal Wallis, multiple range test $P < 0.05$). (From Olesen *et al.* (1993).)

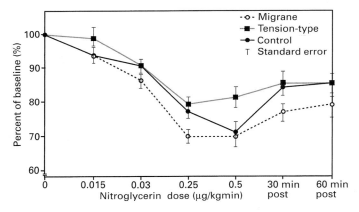

Fig. 52.5. Middle cerebral artery responses during four different doses of nitroglycerin. Comparison between responses in migraineurs (n = 17), tension-type headache sufferers (n = 9), and control subjects (n = 17). Migraineurs showed the most pronounced response ($p < 0.05$, ANOVA). A decrease in blood velocity indicates an increase in vessel area because cerebral blood flow is unchanged during GTN infusion. (From Thomsen *et al.* (1993).)

the placebo pre-treated patients developed a migraine attack. The mepyramine pretreated patients only developed a very mild headache, if any. Activation of endothelial H_1-receptors induces the formation of endogenous nitric oxide (Fig 52.3). Thus, as with GTN, the increased sensitivity to histamine in migraineurs may also be explained by hypersensitivity to activation of the NO pathway.

In migraineurs, reserpine has been shown to cause headache with some features of migraine. Reserpine depletes not only platelets but also presynaptic nerve terminals of their content of monoamines. Substances released include 5-HT. The 5-HT_{2B} (formerly called 5-HT_{1C} and 5-HT_{2C}) receptor has recently been suggested to play a crucial role in the initiation of spontaneous migraine attacks. 5-HT caused an endothelium-dependent relaxing response in a number of vessels from different species, and this effect was mediated via the 5-HT_{2B} receptor. The vascular response to 5-HT_{2B} activation, at least in the pig, is primarily a consequence of the release of NO (Fig. 52.3). Interestingly, in this context m-CPP is a direct agonist at the 5-HT_{2B} receptor and, therefore, is likely to cause vascular headache via NO synthesis. Thus, NO may be a common denominator for headaches induced by GTN, histamine, reserpine, and m-CPP. In addition, the 5HT_{2B} receptor may provide a link between the suggested biochemical changes in 5-HT metabolism during spontaneous migraine attacks and the nitric oxide pathway in migraine. In theory, formation of NO relevant for the triggering of spontaneous migraine may be elicited by fluctuations in numerous neurotransmitters, both in the blood and/or the brain, as part of pathological reactions such as spreading depression, activation of the trigeminovascular system with liberation of, for example, substance P, fever, and inflammation, via interleukins and histamine, etc. (Olesen *et al.* 1995).

Therapeutic implications

Mechanisms of action of acute migraine therapy

Traditionally the mechanism of action of acute migraine therapy (except generally acting analgesics) has been ascribed to constriction of pathologically dilated cranial arteries. Thus, intravenous administration of the effective anti-migraine drug, ergotamine, was long ago shown to reduce temporal artery pulsations in parallel with a decrease in headache intensity. It has been suggested recently that one important action of ergotamine may be the inhibition of antidromic release of trigeminal neuropeptides as part of a neurogenic inflammation (Moskowitz 1993). Ergotamine interacts with 5-HT, dopamine and noradrenaline receptors. Thus, elucidation of a specific receptor involvement requires more specific pharmacological tools. So far the most specific and highly effective acute migraine treatment available is the 5-HT_{1D} receptor agonist, sumatriptan. Several mechanisms of action of sumatriptan have been proposed. A direct pain-modulating effect in the central nervous system is unlikely since sumatriptan is soluble in water and crosses the blood-brain barrier very slowly. One possibility is that constriction of dilated large intracranial arteries provides the causative mechanism (Friberg *et al.* 1991). However, as with ergotamine, another possible mechanism of action is blockade of the release of sensory neuropeptides as part of a neurogenic inflammation (Moskowitz 1993). Since these neuropeptides also induce vasodilatation, the observed vasoconstrictive effect may be a secondary phenomenon. At the molecular level it is possible that sumatriptan interferes with the synthesis of nitric oxide. Thus, a recent experimental study suggests that sumatriptan possesses inhibitory actions on the enzyme nitric oxide synthase (NOS) at least in guinea-pig cerebral vessels (Rüdinger and I. Jansen-Olesen, pers. comm.).

Interaction with the nitric oxide cascade provides a possible mechanism of action of existing prophylactic migraine therapy

Regarding drugs with established prophylactic effect in migraine, their mechanism of action has for long been an enigma. These drugs include β-adrenergic blocking drugs without partial agonist activity (i.e. propranolol, metroprolol, atenol, nadolol, and timolol), antiserotonergic drugs (i.e. methysergide, pizotifen), and calcium antagonists (i.e. flunarizine and verapamil). Many observations suggest that all of these drugs interact with the NO-triggered cascade of reactions. Thus, calcium antagonists block the effect of pers. comm. activity in non-adrenergic non-cholinergic perivascular nerves by inhibiting calcium ion channels and therefore the activation of neuronal NOS (Toda, pers. comm.). Methysergide and pizotifen are 5-HT antagonists that do not discriminate between the 5-HT$_1$ and the 5-HT$_2$ receptors. It has recently been suggested that their effect is via 5-HT$_{2B}$ (formerly 5-HT$_{2C}$) receptor antagonism. 5-HT$_{2B}$ receptor stimulation liberates NO (Fig. 52.3). Thus, amine antagonists may well exert their action by reducing NO production. Propranolol blocks isoprenaline-induced relaxation of rat thoracic aorta in an endothelium-dependent fashion. The response is also blocked by the NOS inhibitor L-NOARG. The prophylactic effect of β-adrenergic blockers in migraine may thus result from blockade of β-adrenoceptor-induced NO production. Propranolol also antagonizes the 5-HT$_{2B}$ receptor on the endothelium. This is another mechanism whereby it may reduce endothelial NO production. In contrast to propranolol, pindolol which is ineffective in migraine, lacks affinity to the 5-HT$_{2B}$ receptor (Olesen et al. 1995).

Novel targets for drug development in migraine

Based on the elevated plasma levels of CGRP during migraine attacks, CGRP antagonists may be of importance as future antimigraine drugs. In addition, the central role of NO in migraine pain is also likely to offer future therapeutic possibilities. Thus, drugs which directly counteract the NO-activated cascade (NOS inhibitors, nitric oxide scavengers, guanylate cyclase inhibitors, etc.) may be effective in migraine. A recent study suggests that the non-specific NOS inhibitor L-N^G-methylarginine hydrochloride (546C88) is effective in the acute treatment of migraine headache (Lassen et al. 1997). The more specific these drug become the more effective they are likely to be, and the fewer side-effects they are likely to induce. Thus, a further understanding of the molecular mechanisms of migraine seems near and new therapies are likely to evolve.

References

Diener, H. C. and May, A. (1996). Positron emission tomography studies in acute migraine attacks. In *Migraine pharmacology and genetics* (ed. M. Sandler, M. Ferrari, and S. Harnett), pp. 109–14. Chapman & Hall, London.

Ferrari, M. D. and Saxena, P. (1995). 5-HT$_1$ receptors in migraine pathophysiology and treatment. *Eur. J. Neurology*, 2, 5–21.

Friberg, L., Olesen, J., Iversen, H. K., and Sperling, B. (1991). Migraine pain associated with middle cerebral artery dilatation: reversal by sumatriptan. *Lancet* 338, 13–17.

Goadsby, P. J., Edvinsson, L., and Ekman, R. (1990). Vasoactive peptide release in the extracerebral circulation of humans during migraine headache. *Ann. Neurol.* 28, 183–7.

Gotoh, F., Komatsumota, S., Araki, N., and Gomi, S. (1984). Noradrenergic nervous activity in migraine. *Arch. Neurol.* 41, 951–5.

Havanka-Kanniainen, H., Tolonen, U., and Myllyla, V. V. (1986). Autonomic dysfunction in adult migraineurs. *Headache* 26, 425–30.

Iversen, H. K., Nielsen, T. H., Olesen, J., and Tfelt-Hansen, P. (1990). Arterial responses during migraine headache. *Lancet* 336, 837–9.

Jensen, K. (1987). Subcutaneous blood flow in the temporal region of migraine patients. *Acta Neurol. Scand.* 72, 561–70.

Lance, J. W. (1993). *Mechanism and management of headache*, (5th edn). Butterworth-Heinemann, Oxford.

Lassen, L. H., Ashina, M., Christiansen, I., Ulrich, V., and Olesen, J. (1997). Nitric oxide synthase inhibition in migraine. *Lancet* 349, 401–2.

Lauritzen, M. (1994). Pathophysiology of the migraine aura. The spreading depression theory. *Brain* 117, 199–210.

Maertens de Noordhout, A., Timsit-Berthier, M., and Schoenen, J. (1986) Contigent negative variation in headache. *Ann. Neurol.* 19, 78–80.

Moskowitz, M. A. (1993). Neurogenic inflammation in the pathophysiology and treatment of migraine. *Neurology* 43 (Suppl. 3), S16–S20.

Olesen, J. (1991) Cerebral and extracranial circulatory disturbances in migraine: pathophysiological implications. *Cerebrovasc. Brain Metab. Rev.* 3, 1–28.

Olesen, J. (1993). Hemodynamics. In *The headaches*, (ed. J. Olesen, P. Tfelt-Hansen, and K. M. A. Welch), pp. 209–22. Raven Press, New York.

Oleson, J., Friberg, L., Oslen, T. S. et al. (1990). Timing and topography of cerebral blood flow and headache during migraine attacks. *Ann. Neurol.* 28, 791–8.

Oleson, J., Iversen, H. K., and Thomsen, L. L. (1993). Nitric oxide supersentivity: a possible molecular mechanism of migraine pain. *Neuroreport* 4, 1027–30.

Olesen, J., Thomsen, L. L., Lassen, L. H., and Jansen-Olesen, I. (1995). The nitric oxide hypothesis of migraine and other vascular headaches. *Cephalalgia* 15, 94–100.

Rasmussen, B. K. (1995). Epidemiology of headache. Thesis. *Cephalalgia* 15, 45–68.

Thomsen, L. L. and Olesen, J. (1995). The autonomic nervous system and the regulation of arterial tone in migraine. *Clin. Auton. Res.* 5, 243–50.

Thomsen, L. L., Iversen, H. K., Brinck, T. A., and Olesen, J. (1993). Arterial supersensitivity to nitric oxide (nitroglycerin) in migraine sufferes. *Cephalagia* 13, 395–9.

Thomsen, L. L., Iversen, H. K., and Olesen, J. (1995a). Cerebral blood flow velocities are reduced during attacks of unilateral migraine without aura. *Cephalalgia* 15, 109–16.

Thomsen, L. L, Iversen, H. K., Boesen, F., and Olesen J. (1995b). Transcranial Doppler and cardiovascular responses during cardiovascular autonomic tests in migraineurs during and outside of attacks. *Brain* 118, 1319–27.

Woods, R. P., Iacoboni, M., and Mazziotta, J. C. (1994). Bilateral spreading cerebral hypoperfusion during spontaneous migraine headache. *New Engl. J. Med.* 331, 1689–92.

53. Pain and the sympathetic nervous system

G. D. Schott

Introduction

In recent years there have been continuing doubts as to the role of the sympathetic nervous system in mechanisms of pain. These doubts are reflected even in the nomenclature of those pain states customarily associated with sympathetic dysfunction. Thus in 1994 the International Association for the Study of Pain (IASP) abandoned the inclusion of sympathetic dependency that had been included in the former definitions of these conditions published 8 years previously. New terminology was introduced as a result of consensus rather than greater understanding, and reflex sympathetic dystrophy and causalgia became renamed 'complex regional pain syndromes (CRPS)' types I and II, respectively (Merskey and Bogduk 1994). Whether this classification will become widely accepted remains unclear, and many authors continue to use the older and more familiar terms as well as various systems of scoring (e.g. Veldman *et al.* 1993). Confusion still exists, however, for both sympathetically maintained and sympathetically independent pain in the same patient are recognized, and even intermediate forms of dependency have been reported. Perhaps the most realistic, although flippant and scientifically meaningless, definition is that of 'a "funny" pain in a "funny-looking" limb' (Jadad *et al.* 1995), a term that many clinicians will recognize as unfortunately valid.

Re-appraisal of nomenclature reflects, amongst other aspects, a re-appraisal of the contribution of the sympathetic nervous system, and while the first part of this chapter deals with the classical views on the sympathetic nervous system and pain, the second part summarizes why the role of the sympathetic nervous system has become increasingly uncertain and why long-held views are being challenged. Discussion is confined to clinical aspects of this subject.

Classical views on the role of the sympathetic nervous system and pain

The concept of the involvement of the sympathetic system in pain can be attributed to the observations of the famous French surgeon, René Leriche. Although causalgia was first described by Weir Mitchell and colleagues during the time of the American Civil War (Mitchell *et al.* 1864), Mitchell knew nothing of the sympathetic nervous system. It was Leriche who observed that patients with causalgia often showed vasomotor changes similar to those seen in peripheral vascular disease, and that both conditions were alleviated by sympathectomy (Leriche 1916). Subsequently it was noted by Evans, Homan, and others during the early decades of this century that even the

more minor forms of these pain states, which to some extent resembled causalgia but in which major nerve injury was absent, appeared to improve with interruption of the sympathetic supply (reviewed by Bonica 1979). Hence the two classical components became established: certain pain states are sometimes accompanied by vasomotor, temperature, and trophic changes reminiscent of sympathetically mediated phenomena; and interrupting the sympathetic supply appears to alleviate the pain.

The clinical features include pain that is characteristically burning in quality and which gave rise to Weir Mitchell's term of causalgia. The pain is usually spontaneous and continuous, but may also be evoked by mechanical and thermal stimuli and be accompanied by allodynia (pain induced by normally innocuous stimuli such as contact), hyperalgesia, and hyperpathia. In all these conditions there are numerous other features which may also be present in various combinations (Table 53.1). As mentioned above, the classification of these pain states has been unsatisfactory, but they can be usefully separated into their extreme forms: causalgia (CRPS type II) and reflex sympathetic dystrophy (CRPS type I).

Causalgia (CRPS type II)

This condition, reviewed by Bonica (1979), is the most extreme form of the disorder and, by definition, follows damage to a major peripheral nerve. The pain occurred in perhaps 2–5 per cent of the cases of peripheral nerve injury sustained in the Second World War, com-

Table 53.1. Various features that may accompany pain

Skin erythematous, cyanosed, pale, or blotchy
Excessive, reduced, or absent sweating
Inappropriate warmth or coldness
Swelling or atrophy of skin
Loss of skin wrinkles or glossiness
Excess or loss of hair
Nails ridged, curved, thin, brittle, or clubbed
Subcutaneous atrophy or thickening
Dupuytren's and other contractures
Joint stiffness, acute or chronic arthritis
Osteoporosis—spotty, localized or widespread
Muscle wasting and weakness
Involuntary movements—tremor, dystonia, spasms

pared with less than 1 per cent in the Vietnam War. Nerve injuries can of course occur in non-combat situations, such as following brachial plexus traction injuries from motor-cycle accidents, and surgical and other iatrogenic nerve injuries.

The onset of the pain is usually immediately after nerve injury, although occasionally some delay occurs, with only 5 per cent of patients developing pain after more than 1 month. Those injuries particularly likely to be associated with the development of causalgia are lesions of the median or sciatic nerve or brachial plexus; incomplete lesions are more likely to cause causalgia than complete ones. Apart from the burning component of the pain, there may be other pains which are variously described as crushing, throbbing, or stabbing, and the pain is frequently very intense. The pain is often experienced in the periphery of the limb, is rather poorly localized, and occasionally it can spread widely, including the contralateral, mirror extremity. The pain tends to be worsened by stress of any sort, as well as by additional sensory stimuli such as noise or bright light. Although there are occasional reports of spontaneous remission over time, sometimes years, it is more common for the pain to persist indefinitely.

Reflex sympathetic dystrophy (RSD)(CRPS type I)

The clinical features are similar to those seen in causalgia but, by definition, the cause is not damage to a major peripheral nerve, and often the pain is not as severe. Indeed, Evans, who first used the term 'reflex sympathetic dystrophy', stated that pain could be absent, and patients without pain continue to be reported (Veldman et al. 1993). The classical features have been summarized on many occasions in the past (Bonica 1979), and in recent years both brief and more extensive reviews have appeared (Jänig and Schmidt 1992; Paice 1995; Jänig and Stanton-Hicks 1996).

The causes of RSD are numerous, although in about 50 per cent of cases the aetiology remains unknown. Of great importance, however, is that a full evaluation of the patient is made and a correct diagnosis established whenever possible. Attention has been drawn both to patients who had received extensive treatment for RSD before relevant peripheral nerve lesions were identified (Thimineur and Saberski 1996), and to patients whose pain was considered to have a psychogenic cause rather than being attributable to RSD (Ochoa 1994).

The most common cause of RSD is any sort of comparatively minor peripheral injury to an extremity, such as a simple sprain, a Colles' fracture, an otherwise uneventful surgical procedure as for Dupuytren's contracture, a knock, or an impact from a falling object. The traumatic episode, although comparatively mild and not associated with major nerve damage, sometimes appears particularly painful. The acute pain often fails to subside as expected or recurs days or even weeks afterwards. Many other causes have been described; these include virtually any disorder affecting the peripheral nervous system from disease (e.g. herpes zoster), accident (e.g. electric shock) or immobilization, and disorders affecting the central nervous system, including stroke, multiple sclerosis, or spinal trauma. RSD can also be associated with systemic illness such as pulmonary disease, and can occur after myocardial infarction and cardiac surgery. In the latter situations, but particularly following strokes, a focal form of RSD may occur—the shoulder–hand syndrome. Here there is pain and limitation of shoulder movements and an ipsilateral painful, swollen, and immobile hand. An analogous situation can develop in the lower limb. RSD may also occur not only in association with cerebral tumour and epilepsy, but particularly when there is concurrent use of phenobarbitone.

Transient forms of RSD may occur, particularly in pregnancy, when it especially affects the hip, and RSD can flit from one area to another (migratory osteoporosis). It has also been recognized that RSD occurs in children more frequently than was previously thought and is often underdiagnosed. It tends to affect the lower extremity and is more common in girls. It has been reported that children may best be managed by a multidisciplinary approach including physical forms of therapy in addition to use of sympathetic blocks, antidepressants, and other techniques (Wilder et al. 1992).

There is controversy as to whether certain individuals are more likely to develop RSD and perhaps causalgia. Patients with underlying diabetes and hyperlipidaemia have been studied, although with indefinite conclusions. Occasional familial cases have been reported, but the distribution of HLA tissue types is probably no different in patients compared with the normal population. While considerable psychiatric disturbances may result from these pain states, a review of the literature failed to find evidence that an individual's personality trait predisposes them to the development of these disorders (Lynch 1992).

Many forms of RSD, in particular the shoulder–hand syndrome, as well as some cases of causalgia, have been described as going through a process involving three phases, each lasting several weeks or months. However, these phases are very variable in their degree and duration and one phase may merge into another. In the early stages there are typically pain and pseudo-inflammatory changes, with hot, swollen extremities; there is then partial resolution with early atrophic changes, and finally there is the third stage of atrophic or dystrophic changes affecting the soft tissues with severe contractures, possibly ankylosis, and immobilization.

Although the frequency of development of RSD is unknown, the incidence of RSD following trauma must be extremely small. The shoulder–hand syndrome following myocardial infarction was estimated to occur in 10–15 per cent of cases some 30 years ago, but the frequency is perhaps 1–2 per cent at present, possibly due to earlier mobilization and greater awareness of the problem.

In both causalgia and RSD, numerous other features may coexist (Table 53.1). There is no correlation between the pain and these accompanying features, which are unpredictable. For example, an affected limb in a patient may exhibit either excessive or absent sweating, and may be puffy or atrophic, hot and red, or cold and cyanosed. Such variability and inconsistency were recognized many years ago and add to the difficulties in characterizing these disorders.

An additional feature sometimes seen is the development not only of spread but of bilateral phenomena after unilateral involvement. Both causalgia and RSD affecting one extremity can produce bilateral, mirror involvement, although, unfortunately, clinical descriptions of patients showing such phenomena often lack detail. Perhaps 20–30 per cent of patients with unilateral disease, particularly the shoulder–hand syndrome, are said to develop bilateral involvement, and investigations demonstrate subclinical involvement even more frequently. Indeed, some but not all authors have reported subclinical bilateral involvement, as determined by isotope scanning, in all the patients studied, abnormalities being more marked on the affected side. Even if not an important clinical aspect, the phenomenon is of significance in suggesting that central mechanisms may be very important in these conditions.

Investigations

These conditions have been investigated in an enormous number of ways. Most of the techniques are largely of relevance in research and there is no investigation that enables the diagnosis of causalgia or RSD to be confirmed. In clinical practice the diagnosis is empirical, and the main purpose of investigation is to reveal an underlying cause that requires assessment and treatment. Fractures, tumours, infections, and other skeletal disorders need to be identified, and it is always wise to X-ray the painful part, sometimes when appropriate including the contralateral part on the same plate when changes such as osteoporosis are being sought. Isotope bone scanning may be useful in identifying bony lesions such as an osteoid osteoma which, being painful, can produce a 'complex regional pain syndrome' curable by surgery, and occasionally CT, and particularly MRI, scanning may reveal important structural lesions. MRI scanning can also be used to demonstrate soft-tissue changes in these conditions.

However, investigations often prove unhelpful. For example, plain radiographs of the affected part may be normal in some patients and in others show the focal or more widespread osteoporosis (Sudeck's atrophy). The osteoporosis is typically periarticular, but spares the joint space itself. However, such changes may be seen in other conditions, including after immobilization, and give little clue as to the underlying processes. Isotope bone scanning, including immediate, early static, and late phase images, was thought could show characteristic features, but again has not proved to provide diagnostically helpful information; furthermore the scan appearances in early RSD are indistinguishable from those after sympathectomy (Mailis *et al.* 1994). Scanning has demonstrated that frequent spontaneous changes in bone blood flow can occur not only diurnally but also over weeks and months in an individual patient (Sherman *et al.* 1994). Such data indicate that explanations of underlying mechanisms and the results of experimental studies need to take into account not only the variability but also the temporal aspects of these phenomena.

Laboratory measurements are normal in causalgia and RSD. Thus the blood count, erythrocyte sedimentation rate, plasma proteins, and bone profile and tests for collagen, vascular, rheumatological, and autoimmune diseases are normal. A small increase in urinary hydroxyproline may occur, reflecting increased bone turnover, but is a non-specific feature. An abnormal laboratory test should therefore lead to a search for an alternative cause for the pain. Routine neurophysiological studies are usually unhelpful, except of course where there is underlying nerve damage.

As discussed below, the response of pain to sympathetic blockade cannot be used as a diagnostic aid. Moreover, pain relief after sympathetic blockade does not preclude a serious underlying cause, such a response, for instance, being reported in the treatment of malignant disease.

Treatment

The mainstay of treatment of causalgia and RSD (CRPS types II and I) has been sympathetic blockade (reviewed by Bonica 1979; Gybels and Sweet 1989). Sympathetic nerve blocks using local anaesthetic that produce pain relief have been considered diagnostic procedures, and are often used as a prelude to more permanent procedures. Blocks can be carried out for the upper limb, face, and upper trunk by blocking the stellate ganglion, or for the lower limb by lumbar sympathetic block. Intercostal and coeliac axis blocks may be undertaken for the trunk, and the latter, in particular, is a well-established method for obtaining pain relief for conditions such as carcinoma of the pancreas.

The problem with upper- and lower-limb blocks is to achieve a long-term therapeutic effect. Repeated blocks may be tried, although the success rate in causalgia may be only 18–25 per cent (Bonica 1979). In patients in whom repeated blocks are effective, and ideally after negative placebo blocks, permanent pain relief can be attempted either by chemical sympathetic blockade using phenol or alcohol, or by surgical sympathectomy. Unfortunately, effective temporary blocks do not assure that a permanent procedure will result in long-term pain relief. The success rate of sympathectomy in patients with causalgia from wartime injuries is said to range from 62 to 100 per cent, although not all reports are as optimistic. Many other procedures for obtaining sympathetic blockade have been reported, including temporary blockade of the stellate ganglion using morphine, and radio-frequency and ultrasound lesioning of the stellate ganglion.

All these procedures carry risks, and numerous complications of sympathetic nerve blocks have been described, although their incidence is not known. Some complications are trivial and short-lived, others are serious, permanent, or even fatal. In addition, chemical and surgical sympathectomy may be followed by post-sympathectomy neuralgia (sympathalgia) which is discussed below, and blocks using substances such as phenol or alcohol may result in a long-term chemical neuritis.

Another approach, introduced by Hannington-Kiff (1974), is the technique of regional intravenous chemical sympathetic denervation by means of guanethidine (for a review of the use and side-effects of this technique, see Yasuda and Schroeder 1994). This drug is infused into the limb which has been temporarily isolated from the systemic circulation using the Bier's block technique. Guanethidine is taken up into the adrenergic nerve terminals where it causes release and subsequently depletion of noradrenaline. Guanethidine is tissue bound and so does not usually enter the circulation in quantities sufficient to cause systemic effects. The injection is often temporarily very painful as the noradrenaline is released, and usually local anaesthetic is administered together with the adrenergic agent. Sometimes dramatic pain relief is said to occur even while the pressure cuff is still inflated, and weakness that may be present also disappears rapidly.

Regional intravenous guanethidine infusion is now a frequently undertaken procedure, but how many blocks and at what interval they should be carried out has not been established. Patients who have received as many as 39 blocks have been reported. The frequency of side-effects is unknown; they are often, but not always, brief and comparatively minor. Such side-effects include, in particular, postural hypotension, syncope, dizziness, and bradycardia, and other side-effects include temporary pain during the infusion, exacerbation of the original pain, an odd taste, retrosternal discomfort and chest pain, nasal congestion, skin rash, phlebitis, transient headache, mild ptosis, and temporary impotence. Oral guanethidine and phenoxybenzamine have been used, with doubtful efficacy and with a tendency to produce marked postural hypotension.

In the past few years a test procedure to determine whether a patient's pain is sympathetically dependent has been devised. The technique, described first by Arnér and colleagues (Arnér 1991) consists of increasing doses of intravenous phentolamine preceded by an infusion of lactated Ringer's solution to minimize hypotension (for details, see Raja *et al.* 1991). Transient pain relief achieved by phentolamine, an α-adrenergic antagonist, has been considered to identify those patients whose pain is maintained by the sympathetic nervous system, similar to the transient pain relief that may follow local anaesthetic sympathetic blockade. The intravenous phentolamine test is considered easier and safer than sympathetic blockade, though side-effects including nasal stuffiness, hypotension, cardiac arrhythmias, wheezing, and dizziness have been reported.

Many other methods of treatment, ranging from subarachnoid clonidine and morphine to psychotherapy, have been reported. These methods include regional intravenous infusion of steroids or ketanserin and parenteral calcitonin. Oral α- and β-blockers, anticonvulsants, analgesics, antidepressants, anti-inflammatory drugs, steroids, calcium-channel blockers, anticholinesterases, and griseofulvin have been tried, as have physical methods including spinal cord and transcutaneous electric nerve stimulation and acupuncture. The most recent drugs to be tried are the bisphosphonates (Schott 1997). These drugs are of interest as they have effects on bone including osteoporosis and also may alleviate pain within a few days; double-blind studies are awaited. If pain relief is achieved, even for a short period, it is essential that vigorous physiotherapy and mobilization are carried out immediately.

Unfortunately, few if any of these various techniques have been evaluated objectively, an aspect discussed below. Furthermore, diagnosis of the underlying condition is often elusive, groups of patients tend to include heterogeneous conditions, and follow-up is usually short. Hence it is very difficult to assess the value of any specific therapy and, in practice, patients are usually treated in a 'trial-and-error' fashion with sympathetic blockade being usually one of the first measures tried. Although there has been a consensus, difficult to prove, that early treatment provides the best outcome, this view has also been refuted. It should be noted that none of the substances discussed above is licensed for use in relief of pain, and the legal responsibility for using them lies with the doctor.

Evidence challenging the role of the sympathetic nervous system in pain

A century after the clinical features of causalgia were recognized, the involvement of the sympathetic nervous system in underlying pain mechanisms has not been clarified. I suggest that this is because the sympathetic system may not be solely or directly involved, and in the following section some evidence that challenges sympathetic involvement is summarized.

The lack of correlation of the clinical features with known sympathetic effects

From Table 53.1 it is evident that patients with pain can exhibit a very wide variety of clinical features which are inconsistent between different patients. This makes it difficult to envisage that, even after similar injuries, a single mechanism could account for the variability and unpredictability of the phenomena encountered. Furthermore, one injury in a patient may cause RSD yet another injury in the same patient may not, and even in the same patient the condition can change rapidly from one state to another. Although emotional stress and extraneous stimuli may worsen some patients' pain, conditions such as thyrotoxicosis, in which the sympathetic nervous system is hyperactive, are not painful. Conversely, diseases solely affecting the central and peripheral autonomic system neither result in pain nor loss of pain appreciation, and RSD may occur in a limb devoid of sympathetic function (Kimber *et al.* 1997).

Even in patients whose pain is improved after sympathetic blockade, there is no correlation between pain relief and the sympatholytic effects produced by the block in respect of time of onset, duration, or degree (for references see, for example, Schott 1994; Baron and Maier 1996). It appears illogical, however, to undertake a sympathetic block in those patients whose limbs are hot and swollen and presumably already vasodilated.

Studies in patients with RSD demonstrate that, contrary to the frequently reiterated supposition, the sympathetic outflow is not increased. Microneurographic studies indicate that physiologically the sympathetic outflow is normal (for references see Baron and Maier 1996), even when the limb is vasoconstricted (Casale and Elam 1992). Indeed, the sympathetic outflow may be diminished, as judged by the reduced concentration of noradrenaline and its breakdown product in venous blood draining the affected painful part, first reported by Drummond *et al.* (1991), and by the impairment of peripheral vasoconstrictor responses demonstrated by Kurvers *et al.* (1994).

Do the clinical features masquerade as sympathetic phenomena?

There is evidence suggesting that those clinical features that appear to be mediated by the sympathetic system might instead be attributable to the effects of substances emitted peripherally from small-diameter afferent as well as from sympathetic efferent nerve fibres. Such substances include CGRP and substance P, as well as catecholamines, ATP, histamine, neurokinins, and 5-HT. The presence of these substances in the periphery would not only sensitize peripheral nociceptors, especially if these were already damaged, but low-threshold, large-diameter and silent primary afferents could also become sensitized. Pain, allodynia, and perhaps mechanical and thermal hyperalgesia could thus develop through a variety of peripheral mechanisms (discussed by Ochoa 1994). Furthermore, some of these substances are potent vasodilators, some are vasoconstrictors, and some produce inflammatory changes which could contribute to the swelling and trophic phenomena often observed (reviewed by Dray 1996). The overall clinical effects, some of which confusingly mimic sympathetic phenomena, would necessarily be variable and unpredictable and depend on numerous factors, including the different neurotransmitters and neuromodulators present and the extent of any vascular and somatic and autonomic nerve damage. It is to be expected, therefore, that the clinical phenomena observed in these conditions would also be variable and unpredictable.

Lack of evidence that sympathetic blockade alleviates pain

It has long been held that patients' pain may be alleviated by interrupting the sympathetic outflow to the affected part. Since pain relief after sympathetic blockade is always uncertain and unpredictable, and the duration of any relief is also unpredictable, it is surprising that only in recent years has the efficacy of sympathetic blockade begin to be assessed critically. There are several reasons why methods of sympathetic blockade have been used for so long without critical evaluation: the impossibility of undertaking appropriate trials during wartime when causalgia was most commonly seen; the frequent reliance on anecdotal information rather than careful clinical studies; the lack of appreciation in former years of placebo effects; inadequate trials in often small numbers of people; the heterogeneous conditions seen amongst groups of patients studied; often brief follow-up periods; and doubtless the reluctance to conceive that views on the subject might reflect dogma rather than the result from objective assessment.

At present there is little evidence from controlled trials that blocking the sympathetic system alleviates pain in causalgia and RSD, and this dearth of evidence applies to all the methods used. Surgical sympathectomy is comparatively rarely undertaken now because of the absence of reliable, proven efficacy, the development of drug therapies and less invasive procedures, and the surgical risks and post-sympathectomy phenomena that may occur. Controlled trials are, of course, not feasible. Unfortunately there is no evidence whether prior effective sympathetic blocks are necessarily predictors of satisfactory outcome, although it is logical and usually (but not always) accepted that repeated placebo-controlled temporary blocks should alleviate pain before considering chemical or surgical sympathectomy.

It is astonishing that only recently has the efficacy of sympathetic blocks been assessed, with the result that after reviewing the available literature Carr et al. (1996) concluded that the benefit of sympathetic blockade with local anaesthetic was no greater than could be accounted for by placebo. A similar conclusion was reached by Jadad et al. (1995) in respect of the use of regional intravenous guanethidine blocks, which had been used for 20 years before objective evidence of their benefit was sought. The recently introduced use of intravenous phentolamine has also been questioned in respect of its reliability in relation to placebo effects (for references, see Ochoa 1994).

It can thus be seen that currently there is little to support the efficacy and hence use of sympathetic interruption in alleviating pain in causalgia and RSD (Schott 1998). It should be emphasized, however, that these studies report groups of patients and furthermore there are numerous anecdotal accounts of these techniques improving pain. It thus remains unclear whether individual patients with particular disorders or with particular accompanying clinical features may be helped by placebo-controlled procedures. It could also be argued that pain relief achieved by means of a placebo may be justified. The lack of objective data establishing the benefit of sympathetic blockade nevertheless challenges the theoretical basis for sympathetic involvement in pain.

Damage to the sympathetic system can produce pain

It is disconcerting that pain can be *caused* both by lesions and, in certain situations, by stimulation of the sympathetic nervous system (reviewed by Schott 1994). It is beyond doubt that lesions of the sympathetic nerves can cause pain in those disorders in which visceral afferents are necessarily involved (for review, see Cervero, 1994). However, pain may also occur in other instances when the sympathetic system has been damaged. For example, pain in the legs has been reported after lower aortic surgery; pain in the face and neck may follow cervical sympathectomy and may also occur with carotid artery disease (occlusion, fibromuscular dysplasia, dissection, after angiography and endarterectomy) and malignant cervical lymphadenopathy. Facial pain from involvement of parasympathetic fibres has been reported with lung tumours and hiatus hernia. The frequency of such pains is unknown but appears to be uncommon.

After chemical or surgical sympathectomy, pain may unpredictably ensue in 7–18 per cent of cases (Kramis *et al.* 1996). This post-sympathectomy pain, sympathalgia, tends to occur 1 or 2 weeks after sympathectomy, and after lumbar sympathectomy tends to affect the anterior thighs where there is aching pain, particularly at night, and also hyperpathia. There is often surrounding sweating. Sympathalgia tends to recover spontaneously and there have been uncontrolled reports of the benefits of anticonvulsants, including carbamazepine and phenytoin, as well as calcium-channel blockers.

Experimental stimulation of the sympathetic supply can induce pain (for references, see Schott 1994). There are rare reports of pain being induced by stimulation of the stellate ganglion and chain, producing pain in the face, axilla, and chest; stimulation of the coeliac plexus can produce pain in the abdomen; stimulation of the L1 ganglion can produce pain in the lower abdomen; and stimulation of the lumbar sympathetic plexus can produce pain in the leg. Pain on sympathetic stimulation of the sympathetic outflow can also be induced in the limbs of patients with pre-existing pain from localized damage.

It is evident therefore that, while disorders affecting the pure autonomic nervous system are not painful, both pathological and iatrogenic lesions and also stimulation of the sympathetic nervous system can occasionally cause pain. Yet, despite lack of evidence from controlled trials, anecdotal reports over decades indicate that sympathetic blockade may in some cases alleviate pain. Can the paradox be reconciled?

The role of visceral afferents?

The author has suggested that afferent fibres in the sympathetic outflow might be implicated (Schott 1994). These fellow-travelling afferents would necessarily be involved in those diseases which result in lesions of the sympathetic nerves, such as tumours, vascular disease, and trauma including surgery, as well as small-fibre neuropathies. These afferents, however, would not be involved in system disorders which purely affect the autonomic nervous system and indeed, as predicted, pain is not associated with such disorders.

Furthermore, procedures that interrupt the sympathetic outflow would necessarily also interrupt afferents contained within these nerves and could account for any pain relief that might occur. This particularly occurs in pain associated with conditions such as carcinoma of the pancreas and angina subserved by visceral afferents. In the periphery the blood vessels have both extensive afferent and autonomic innervations; whether some pain-subserving afferents from the periphery travel proximally together with perivascular autonomic nerves remains unclear.

Future directions

In the century that has elapsed since Weir Mitchell's original reports, the cause of pain in disorders which comprise causalgia (CRPS type

II), reflex sympathetic dystrophy (CRPS type I), and related conditions remains elusive. Many theories have been postulated but none has been able to account for all the facts. For example, it has been suggested that involvement of sympathetic fibres leads to denervation supersensitivity, and Arnold *et al.* (1993) demonstrated increased peripheral venous responsiveness to catecholamines in patients with RSD. Furthermore, α_1-adrenoreceptors have an increased density in the hyperalgesic skin of patients with RSD (Drummond *et al.* 1996). However, denervation sensitivity, could not account for a number of features, including the immediate onset and persistence of pain after injury that occurs in some patients, long before denervation supersensitivity could have occurred. Furthermore peripheral mechanisms alone cannot account either for those patients in whom spreading and bilateral pain states develop, or for those patients in whom other phenomena such as dystonia and tremor coexist (Bhatia *et al.* 1993). At least in such patients the central nervous system must be implicated (Schott 1986).

In recent years perhaps the most important outcome of many studies has been the realization that several previous conclusions appear to have been incomplete or erroneous: the sympathetic nervous system is not hyperactive in these pain states; a number of the clinical features are unlikely to be related primarily to dysfunction of the sympathetic nervous system, indicating that other explanations need to be sought; many studies have been inappropriately restricted to investigating sympathetically mediated mechanisms; and the effectiveness of interrupting the sympathetic system for alleviating pain, at least in groups of patients, has not so far been established, despite the very widespread and long-term use of such procedures. Whether afferents travelling within sympathetic nerves are relevant remains to be assessed. Unfortunately, although a variety of animal models have been developed, the applicability of these models to human pain disorders remains uncertain.

It appears that mediating these diverse pain states are likely to be a number of very different underlying mechanisms, and it seems improbable that any single mechanism could account for all these conditions. Careful clinical and laboratory studies of a few individual patients with very similar clinical features may prove more rewarding than studies of large numbers of patients with heterogeneous disorders.

References

Arnér, S. (1991). Intravenous phentolamine test: diagnostic and prognostic use in reflex sympathetic dystrophy. *Pain* 46, 17–22.

Arnold, J. M. O., Teasell, R. W., MacLeod, A. P., Brown, J. E., and Carruthers, S. G. (1993). Increased venous alpha-adrenoreceptor responsiveness in patients with reflex sympathetic dystrophy. *Ann. Int. Med.* 118, 619–22.

Baron, R. and Maier, C. (1996). Reflex sympathetic dystrophy: skin blood flow, sympathetic vasoconstrictor reflexes and pain before and after surgical sympathectomy. *Pain* 67, 317–26.

Bhatia, K. P., Bhatt, M. H., and Marsden, C. D. (1993). The causalgia–dystonia syndrome. *Brain* 116, 843–51.

Bonica, J. J. (1979). Causalgia and other reflex sympathetic dystrophies. In *Proceedings of the Second World Congress on Pain, Advances in Pain Research and Therapy*, Vol. 3, (ed. J. J. Bonica, J. C Liebeskind, and D. G. Albe-Fessard), pp. 141–66. Raven Press, New York.

Carr, D. B., Cepeda, M. S., and Lau, J. (1996). What is the evidence for the therapeutic role of local anesthetic sympathetic blockade in RSD or causalgia? An attempted meta-analysis. [Abstract]. *Eighth World Congress on Pain, Vancouver, August 17–22, 1996.* p. 406. IASP Press, Seattle.

Casale, R. and Elam, M. (1992). Normal sympathetic nerve activity in a reflex sympathetic dystrophy with marked skin vasoconstriction. *J. Autonom. Nerv. Syst.* 41, 215–20.

Cervero, F. (1994). Sensory innervation of the viscera: peripheral basis of visceral pain. *Physiol. Rev.* 74, 95–138.

Dray, A. (1996). Neurogenic mechanisms and neuropeptides in chronic pain. *Prog. Brain Res.* 110, 85–94.

Drummond, P. D., Finch, P. M., and Smythe, G. A. (1991). Reflex sympathetic dystrophy: the significance of differing plasma catecholamine concentrations in affected and unaffected limbs. *Brain* 114, 2025–36.

Drummond, P. D., Skipworth S., and Finch, P. M. (1996). Alpha 1–adrenoreceptors in normal and hyperalgesic human skin. *Clin. Sci.* 91, 73–7.

Gybels, J. M. and Sweet, W. H. (1989). *Neurosurgical treatment of persistent pain.* Vol. 11, pp. 257–81. Karger, Basel.

Hannington-Kiff, J.G. (1974). Intravenous regional sympathetic block with guanethidine. *Lancet* i, 1019–20.

Jadad, A. R., Carroll, D., Glynn, C. J., and McQuay, H. J. (1995). Intravenous regional sympathetic blockade for pain relief in reflex sympathetic dystrophy; a systematic review and a randomized, double-blind crossover study. *J. Pain Symptom Manage.* 10, 13–20.

Jänig, W. and Schmidt, R. F. (ed.) (1992). *Reflex sympathetic dystrophy. Pathophysiological mechanisms and clinical implications.* VCH, Weinheim.

Jänig, W. and Stanton-Hicks, M. (ed.) (1996). *Reflex sympathetic dystrophy: a reappraisal. Progress in Pain Research and Management,* Vol. 6. IASP Press, Seattle.

Kimber J. R., Smith, G. D. P., and Mathias, C. J. (1997). Reflex sympathetic dystrophy in a patient with peripheral sympathetic denervation. *Eur. J. Neurol.* 4, 315–17.

Kramis, R. C., Roberts, W. J., and Gillette, R. G. (1996). Post-sympathectomy neuralgia: hypotheses on peripheral and central neuronal mechanisms. *Pain* 64, 1–9.

Kurvers, H. A. J. M., Jacobs, M. J. H. M., Beuk, R. J. *et al.* (1994). Reflex sympathetic dystrophy: result of autonomic denervation? *Clin. Sci.* 87, 663–9.

Leriche, R. (1916). De la causalgie envisagée comme une névrite du sympathique et de son traitement par la dénudation et l'excision des plexus nerveux péri-artériels. *Presse Med.* 24, 178–80.

Lynch, M. E. (1992). Psychological aspects of reflex sympathetic dystrophy: a review of the adult and paediatric literature. *Pain* 49, 337–47.

Mailis, A., Meindok, H., Papagapiou, M., and Pham, D. (1994). Alterations of the three-phase bone scan after sympathectomy. *Clin. J. Pain* 10, 146–55.

Merskey, H. and Bogduk, N. (ed.) (1994). *Classification of chronic pain: descriptions of chronic pain syndromes and definitions of pain terms,* (2nd edn), pp. 40–2. IASP Press, Seattle.

Mitchell, S. W., Morehouse, G. R., and Keen, W. W. (1864). *Gunshot wounds and other injuries of nerves.* Lippincott, Philadephia.

Ochoa, J. L. (1994). Pain mechanisms in neuropathy. *Curr. Opin. Neurol.* 7, 407–14.

Paice, E. (1995). Reflex sympathetic dystrophy. *BMJ* 310, 1645–8.

Raja, S. N., Treede, R.-D., Davis, K. D., and Campbell, J. N. (1991). Systemic alpha-adrenergic blockade with phentolamine: a diagnostic test for sympathetically maintained pain. *Anesthesiology* 74, 691–8.

Schott, G. D. (1986). Mechanisms of causalgia and related clinical conditions. The role of the central and the sympathetic nervous systems. *Brain* 109, 717–38.

Schott, G. D. (1994). Visceral afferents: their contribution to 'sympathetic dependent' pain. *Brain* 117, 397–413.

Schott, G. D. (1997). Bisphosphonates for pain relief in reflex sympathetic dystrophy? *Lancet* 350, 1117.

Schoot, G. D. (1998). Interrupting the sympathetic outflow in cansalgia and reflex sympathetic dystrophy. A futile procedure for many patients. *BMJ* 316, 792–3.

Sherman, R. A., Karstetter, K. W., Damiano, M., and Evans, C. B. (1994). Stability of temperature asymmetries in reflex sympathetic dystrophy over time and changes in pain. *Clin. J. Pain* 10, 71–7.

Thimineur, M. A. and Saberski, L. (1996). Complex regional pain syndrome Type I (RSD) or peripheral mononeuropathy? A discussion of three cases. *Clin. J. Pain* 12, 145–50.

Veldman, P. H. J. M., Reynen, H. M., Arntz, I. E., and Goris, R. J. A. (1993). Signs and symptoms of reflex sympathetic dystrophy: prospective study of 829 patients. *Lancet* 342, 1012–16.

Wilder, R. T., Berde, C. B., Wolohan, M., Vieyra, M. A., Masek, B. J., and Micheli, L. J. (1992). Reflex sympathetic dystrophy in children. *J. Bone Joint Surg. Am.* 74–A, 910–19.

Yasuda, J. M. and Schroeder, D. J. (1994). Guanethidine for reflex sympathetic dystrophy. *Ann. Pharmocother.* 28, 338–41.

54. Drugs, chemicals, and toxins that alter autonomic function

Anne L. Tonkin and Derek B. Frewin

Introduction

Many drugs, chemicals, and toxins are capable of interacting with the autonomic nervous system to alter autonomic function in humans (Fig. 54.1). While acute exposure may cause autonomic overactivity, the chronic effect of most such compounds is a reduction in autonomic activity. This chapter will focus primarily on drugs and other chemicals that reduce autonomic activity, either directly by inhibiting the activity of autonomic nerve fibres and/or receptors or indirectly by causing an autonomic neuropathy. It will conclude with a discussion of compounds, including naturally occurring toxins and venoms, that cause an abnormal increased in autonomic activity.

Compounds that reduce autonomic activity directly

Therapeutic drugs

Drugs having pharmacodynamic effects that depend on direct antagonism of autonomic neurotransmission are very widely used in clini-

cal cardiovascular medicine. Such drug groups include antagonists at α- or β-adrenoceptors, centrally acting antihypertensive drugs, and ganglion blockers, all of which have been clinically important at various times, particularly in the management of hypertension. In general, their effects on autonomic function are well known and underpin their therapeutic efficacy. These drugs are described fully in pharmacological textbooks and will not be discussed in detail here.

It is also important to recognize those drugs that have antagonist activity within the autonomic nervous system in addition to their primary pharmacodynamic effect, often causing anticholinergic or α-antagonist adverse effects. Common examples are listed in Table 54.1.

In practice, the drugs that most commonly lead to clinical presentations suggesting autonomic dysfunction are those that have widespread use amongst the elderly. Both sympathetic and parasympathetic inhibition are more likely to cause clinically significant sequelae in the elderly than in younger individuals. Some important examples are discussed here.

Sympathetic inhibitors

The clinical effects of sympathetic inhibition depend upon the balance of α- and β-adrenoceptors affected by the particular drug.

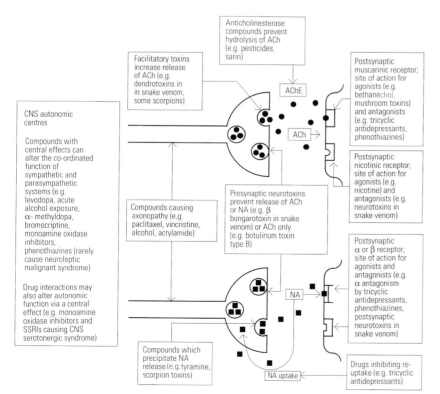

Fig. 54.1. Schematic representation of a cholinergic (upper) and noradrenergic (lower) autonomic synapse showing potential sites of action of drugs and toxins that influence autonomic function.

Drugs with peripheral α-antagonist properties (such as the phenothiazines, tricyclic antidepressants, and antihistamines) commonly cause orthostatic hypotension, particularly when more than one of these drugs are used in combination in an elderly individual. A less common but very important complication of α-receptor antagonism is the exacerbation of urinary incontinence. This is seen most commonly in elderly women and may have significant consequences, including institutionalization if the causative agent is not identified and removed.

β-Blocker drugs are well known to have negative inotropic effects, leading occasionally to significant exacerbations of cardiac failure. In addition, they have negative chronotropic effects, the latter being a particular risk when a β-blocker is administered in conjunction with other drugs that slow atrioventricular nodal conduction, such as digoxin or verapamil. Such a combination may cause clinically significant atrioventricular conduction delay, even in individuals with normal baseline ECGs. Exacerbation of symptoms of obstructive airways disease is also well recognized as a complication of the use of β-blockers in susceptible people.

Local administration of drugs with autonomic effects may also cause systemic symptoms. A well-recognized example of this phenomenon is the local instillation of timolol to the eye for the treatment of glaucoma, with subsequent exacerbation of bronchospasm or cardiac insufficiency due to its systemic β-adrenoceptor antagonist effect.

Parasympathetic inhibitors

Parasympathetic inhibition, particularly due to peripheral muscarinic receptor antagonism, occurs during treatment with many therapeutic drug groups (Table 54.1). Protriptyline and amitriptyline are the most potent antimuscarinic receptor antagonists amongst the tricyclic antidepressants, and should be considered as possible contributors to presentations such as urinary retention or constipation. An advantage of the newer antidepressant drugs, such as fluoxetine and venlafaxine, is that they do not have clinically important antagonistic effects at α- and muscarinic receptors. Class I antiarrhythmic agents such as quinidine and disopyramide also have significant antimuscarinic effects.

Anticholinergic drugs are sometimes given specifically to produce muscarinic antagonism. Examples are the use of benztropine in the management of Parkinson's disease or the movement disorders associated with antipsychotic use, and the use of oxybutynin in the management of bladder detrusor muscle instability. In all of these cases the drug is administered systemically and can be expected to have widespread autonomic effects. These include blurred vision due to cycloplegia, which is more symptomatic in young people with preserved lens accommodation, dry mouth, severe constipation, and urinary retention, particularly in the elderly male with prostatic hypertrophy. At very high doses, gastric emptying and gastric secretion may also be inhibited, leading to epigastric discomfort.

Centrally acting drugs

Many centrally acting drugs have autonomic effects, the pathogenesis of which remains poorly understood. Levodopa and dopamine D_2 receptor agonists, such as bromocriptine and pergolide, can cause severe orthostatic hypotension, particularly in the early phase of therapy. This effect is presumed to be related directly to a D_2 agonist action which reduces sympathetic outflow from the vasomotor centres of the brainstem. Other centrally acting drugs with similar clinical effects include the centrally acting antihypertensive drugs such as α-methyldopa and clonidine, and the non-specific monoamine oxidase inhibitors.

Other compounds

A wide variety of naturally occurring and synthetic compounds also interact with neurotransmission, thereby influencing autonomic function.

Table 54.1 Drugs with autonomic antagonist effects unrelated to their main therapeutic use

Autonomic effect	Drug/drug group	Clinical manifestations
α-Adrenoceptor antagonism	Phenothiazines Tricyclic antidepressants Antihistamines Quinidine	Orthostatic hypotension Nasal stuffiness Urinary incontinence (especially elderly women)
β-Adrenoceptor antagonism	Sotalol	Bronchospasm Negative inotropic and chronotropic effects
Muscarinic receptor antagonism	Phenothiazines Tricyclic antidepressants Antihistamines Quinidine, disopyramide	Urinary obstruction (especially elderly men) Dry mouth and eyes Blurred vision Sinus tachycardia Constipation Confusion
Central autonomic effects	Levodopa Dopamine agonists Monoamine oxidase inhibitors	Orthostatic hypotension

Nicotine

Nicotine has a variety of pharmacological actions and may be a source of toxicity apart from the effects of the by-products of tobacco smoking, the usual form of exposure. Nicotine binds to nicotinic receptors in autonomic ganglia, as well as at neuromuscular junctions and in the central nervous system. Acute autonomic effects include increased heart rate, blood pressure, and cutaneous vasoconstriction. Exposure to toxic doses (e.g. in tobacco workers or those exposed to nicotine-containing pesticides) can result in ganglionic paralysis with bradycardia, hypotension, coma, and eventual respiratory muscle paralysis. The role of nicotine in the pathogenesis of the known toxic effects of long-term tobacco smoking is unclear.

Anticholinesterase compounds

Compounds with anticholinesterase activity, such as organophosphorous esters and carbamate compounds, are commonly used in agriculture as insecticides. Acute ingestion by humans causes increased activity at autonomic ganglia and parasympathetic terminals (discussed later). In some circumstances, however, they may reduce autonomic function. Such a situation is observed after acute exposure to sarin gas, a highly toxic organophosphorous compound originally developed during the Second World War and more recently used in terrorist attacks (Morita *et al.* 1995). The autonomic effects of sarin were long-lasting (up to weeks) in some individuals, and observations on workers involved in handling similar compounds during the Second World War have indicated that autonomic dysfunction may persist for years after acute exposure. Long-term chronic exposure to organophosphorous ester insecticides may also produce persistent autonomic dysfunction, although the literature in this area is controversial. Organophosphorous compounds bind to acetylcholinesterase for a much longer period than the more recently developed carbamate compounds, and there is little evidence of prolonged toxicity with the latter group.

Herbal remedies

Many freely available proprietary herbal remedies contain alkaloids such as atropine and scopolamine and there have been case reports of anticholinergic poisoning resulting in confusion, dry mouth, tachycardia, and dilated pupils (Chan *et al.* 1994).

Illicit drugs

The first report of amphetamine-induced suppression of vasomotor outflow was published in 1996 (Smit *et al.* 1996), although this phenomenon has been observed previously in animal models. The clinical presentation occurred 10 hours after ingestion, and included pronounced drowsiness and severe orthostatic hypotension which was due, on formal baroreflex function testing, to suppression of vasomotor outflow with preservation of normal vagal function. Spontaneous recovery occurred over 3 days. This is a potential differential diagnosis in cases of acute autonomic neuropathy.

Contamination of illicit drugs may also lead to acute autonomic dysfunction. During the period 1996–97 a number of cases of acute anticholinergic poisoning were reported in individuals who had self-administered material sold as street 'heroin', but which had been mixed with scopolamine. The clinical picture of hallucinations, tachycardia, pupillary dilatation, dry skin and mucous membranes, and urinary retention responds rapidly to treatment with the anticholinesterase compound, physostigmine.

Snake venoms

Much progress has been made over recent years in understanding the molecular structure and mechanisms of toxicity of snake venoms (reviewed by Rees and Bilwes 1993). Apart from the therapeutic implications of these investigations, neurotoxins derived from snake venoms are becoming scientifically important as laboratory probes for the study of neural mechanisms. There is great variability in the neurotoxic components of venoms from various species of snake, but some generalizations can be made. Postsynaptic neurotoxins (also called α-neurotoxins) have an action similar to curare in that they bind to the nicotinic acetylcholine receptor on the postsynaptic membrane of the neuromuscular junction, causing flaccid paralysis. Nicotinic receptors in autonomic ganglia are less affected by α-neurotoxins, but are blocked by κ-neurotoxins, such as κ-bungarotoxin and κ-flavitoxin, both of which produce complete and long-lasting autonomic blockade at low doses. Other snake venom toxins are known to bind to biogenic amine receptors, including those for noradrenaline, dopamine, and serotonin. A different mechanism of autonomic inhibition is exemplified by β-bungarotoxin, a presynaptic neurotoxin, which irreversibly inhibits neurotransmitter release, probably by interfering with the function of a voltage-sensitive potassium channel.

Compounds that reduce autonomic activity by causing autonomic neuropathy

Drug- or toxin-induced autonomic neuropathy is an important potential diagnosis in the assessment of patients with evidence of subacute or chronic autonomic dysfunction. It is important to note that many neurotoxic compounds have selective effects on particular components of the nervous system, and not all compounds that cause peripheral neuropathy affect the autonomic system. An example is arsenic, which causes a primarily sensory neuropathy and has not been reported to cause autonomic dysfunction. Other examples include lead neurotoxicity, which commonly causes motor neuropathy and central nervous system effects (encephalopathy, behavioural changes) with little, if any, effect on autonomic function.

In specific clinical situations, damage to the autonomic nervous system is induced for therapeutic purposes by introduction of neurolytic agents into specific regions. Agents such as phenol are used for this purpose, and the resulting autonomic dysfunction includes the intended effect (e.g. in sympathectomy for peripheral vascular disease or hyperhidrosis) in addition to any unintended sequelae. More commonly, autonomic neuropathy is an unintended complication of exposure to drugs or chemicals in a therapeutic or occupational context.

Therapeutic exposure

Cytotoxic agents used in cancer chemotherapy

Vinca alkaloids

Vincristine and vinblastine are used in the chemotherapy of haematological malignancies such as lymphomas and leukaemias. Vincristine, and to a lesser extent, vinblastine, frequently cause a dose-dependent peripheral sensory neuropathy due to axonal degeneration. Both drugs bind to the protein tubulin, preventing its polymerization into microtubules that form the spindle apparatus essential for mitosis in both normal and malignant cells. In neurones, these microtubules appear to be involved in the rapid transport of essential proteins from the cell body to the axon, and interruption of the transport process results in axonal degeneration. In this form of neuropathy, longer fibres are more susceptible to damage, thus explaining the distal distribution of sensory loss and the particular susceptibility of the vagus nerve to damage.

There is controversy over how frequently this neurotoxic effect extends to autonomic neuropathy, although there have been many case reports of orthostatic hypotension, constipation, paralytic ileus, and urinary retention following treatment with vinca alkaloids, suggesting both sympathetic and parasympathetic involvement. Studies using formal tests of autonomic function have had varying results. Early data suggested that vincristine therapy was associated with abnormalities of both sympathetic and parasympathetic efferent activity. More recently, similar results were obtained in children in whom there was a transient suppression of heart rate variability during vincristine administration (Hirvonen *et al.* 1989) and in adults receiving vincristine (mean cumulative dose 9 mg) or vinblastine (mean 46 mg), a majority of whom showed abnormalities of BP control on tilt and during isometric handgrip (Roca *et al.* 1985). In contrast, a prospective study of 10 patients receiving a mean cumulative dose of 15.2 mg of vincristine, which caused peripheral sensorimotor neuropathy in all of them, showed no effect on Valsalva ratio, heart rate variability with deep breathing, or systolic blood pressure response to head-up tilt (Lahtinen *et al.* 1989). The clinical significance of vinca alkaloid-induced autonomic neuropathy remains controversial, and the cause of the apparently autonomic symptoms described in the case reports remains in some doubt.

Doxorubicin

Doxorubicin may rarely have toxic effects on peripheral neurones, particularly those in the dorsal root ganglia and autonomic ganglia. The toxicity takes the form of a neuronopathy and results in degeneration of the entire neurone, including its axonal processes.

Cisplatin

Although cisplatin frequently causes a predominantly sensory peripheral neuropathy, it appears that it only rarely affects the autonomic nervous system (Warner 1995). The only prospective clinical study in this area assessed 28 patients receiving cisplatin, vinblastine, and bleomycin and showed that two of them had abnormal heart rate responses to both the Valsalva manoeuvre and deep breathing, indicating parasympathetic dysfunction (Hansen 1990). Whether or not these patients, most of whom also had peripheral sensory neuropathy, were affected by cisplatin, vinblastine, or the combination of the two could not be determined.

Cytosine arabinoside

Peripheral nervous system disturbances caused by cytosine arabinoside are rare, but there has been one case report of a patient with acute leukaemia who developed Horner's syndrome and a severe, ultimately fatal, demyelinating peripheral neuropathy after receiving high doses (Nevill *et al.* 1989).

Paclitaxel (Taxol®)

Paclitaxel, a recently introduced chemotherapeutic agent with activity against breast and ovarian cancer, causes a peripheral sensory neuropathy, probably by preventing the normal dissociation of axonal microtubles. This action interferes with fast axonal transport, which appears to require repeated association and dissociation of microtubules. Recently, paclitaxel has also been reported to cause acute severe orthostatic hypotension (Jerian *et al.* 1993) associated with abnormalities in heart rate response to the Valsalva and deep breathing manoeuvres (parasympathetic dysfunction) and a loss of the normal pressor response to isometric hand grip (sympathetic dysfunction). Paralytic ileus and orthostatic hypotension appear to be the most common manifestations of paclitaxel-induced autonomic neuropathy, and patients with diabetes mellitus may be more susceptible to this complication (Warner 1995).

Other therapeutic drugs

Perhexiline maleate

Perhexiline, used as a last-line agent in the management of refractory angina, is known to cause a peripheral sensorimotor neuropathy. In a few of these cases the neurotoxicity extends to the autonomic nervous system, causing postural hypotension and abnormal heart rate control.

Amiodarone

Chronic treatment of cardiac arrhythmias with amiodarone causes peripheral neuropathy (predominantly sensory) in a small proportion of patients. In some of these there may also be autonomic dysfunction, manifested as orthostatic hypotension, although the evidence for this to date is not definitive.

Pentamidine

Pentamidine, commonly used in the management of *Pneumocystis carinii* pneumonia secondary to AIDS, has been associated with acute autonomic insufficiency manifested as severe orthostatic hypotension with a fixed heart rate, and complete loss of heart rate responsiveness to deep breathing and the Valsalva manoeuvre (Siddiqui and Ford 1995).

Gold

Gold therapy, often given for rheumatoid arthritis, may rarely cause autonomic dysfunction manifested by sweating and orthostatic hypotension which recovers a few months after cessation of gold (Fam 1988).

Occupational exposure

Organic solvents

Carbon disulphide

There is emerging evidence that long-term exposure over years to decades to low levels of carbon disulphide, for example in the viscose/rayon industry, may cause autonomic effects. Average cumulative exposure of 213 p.p.m.-years over 20 years resulted in parasympathetic dysfunction on formal testing (Ruijten *et al.* 1993), although the effects were very small and not associated with any clinical sequelae.

Styrene

Styrene monomer, an aromatic solvent used in the manufacture of polystyrene, resins, rubber, plastic, and fibreglass products, is known to cause acute neurotoxic effects following high-intensity exposure. The effect, if any, of low-level exposure is unclear. Very little is known regarding the possible mechanism of neurotoxicity, although some animal data suggest that dopamine metabolism may be a target.

Other organic solvents

Parasympathetic function (measured as changes in heart rate variability and heart rate responses to deep breathing and the Valsalva manoeuvre) appears to be disturbed in some workers exposed to a variety of organic solvents, including hydrocarbons, alcohols, ketones, esters, and ethers (Matikainen and Juntunen 1985). However, a study of printers with long-term exposure to toluene has shown no increase in the prevalence of peripheral neuropathy and no significant changes in autonomic function (Juntunen *et al.* 1985).

Acrylamide

Acrylamide, which is widely used in paper manufacture, water treatment, building construction, and laboratory research, is known to cause a distal symmetrical axonopathy which affects somatic and autonomic nerves. The underlying mechanism of toxicity may be interference with fast axonal transport. As is the case for other causes of axonal degeneration (including alcohol and other toxins), longer fibres are most susceptible to damage. In the autonomic nervous system the vagus nerve is the initial site of dysfunction, so that heart rate control and gastrointestinal function are impaired before blood pressure regulation becomes involved. Autonomic disturbances are uncommon in humans but have been studied extensively in experimental animals, in which damage to sympathetic vasomotor nerves as well as parasympathetic fibres has been demonstrated, both neurophysiologically and histologically.

Heavy metals

Chronic exposure to lead is known to cause a peripheral neuropathy with axonal degeneration, particularly affecting motor fibres. Whether or not the autonomic nervous system is also involved is controversial. Workers with mixed exposure to lead, zinc, and copper have been studied using heart rate variability techniques (Murata and Araki 1991) and were found to have reduced median nerve conduction velocities in addition to reduced RR variability, particularly in relation to respiratory variation (mediated by the vagus nerve). Lead exposure more commonly causes a predominantly motor peripheral neuropathy.

Other forms of exposure

Alcohol

Alcohol ingestion has both acute and chronic effects on autonomic function in humans. Acute exposure of healthy volunteers to alcohol reduces parasympathetic modulation of heart rate, measured by power spectral parameters of heart rate variability (Murata *et al.*

1994). The mechanism of this effect is uncertain, but may involve alterations in central cardiovascular control centres rather than a direct effect on vagal function.

Chronic alcohol abuse causes an axonal neuropathy, affecting both somatic (sensory and motor) and autonomic, predominantly vagal, function. Approximately 25 per cent of chronic alcohol abusers have detectable abnormalities in the parasympathetic control of heart rate (Monforte *et al.* 1995), while sympathetic function may become affected at a later stage, resulting in orthostatic hypotension and anhidrosis. Sympathetically-mediated blood pressure responses to pressor stimuli, including the cold pressor test and sustained isometric exercise, as well as phase IV of the Valsalva manoeuvre, are reduced in alcoholics compared with age-matched controls (Chida *et al.* 1994). Both somatic and autonomic nerve damage appear to be correlated to total lifetime ethanol intake (Monforte *et al.* 1995), and in some cases abstinence may result in an improvement over months to years. Long-term follow-up of chronic alcohol abusers suggests that the presence of autonomic abnormalities on clinical testing is associated with an increased mortality.

Pesticides

Most insecticides in common use in agricultural, industrial, or domestic settings are neurotoxic to the target organisms. In general they are not species-selective, and can also affect mammalian nervous systems, the outcome depending on the level of exposure in relation to body size. Organochlorine insecticides (such as DDT) affect sensory and motor nerves with few, if any, autonomic effects after acute or chronic exposure.

Organophosphorous compounds (discussed earlier in relation to their acute anticholinesterase activity) may also cause various subacute or chronic neuropathies. These have been reported following a single high-intensity exposure, as in the case of the use of organophosphorous-based chemical weapons in warfare, or during chronic exposure, for example in manufacturing processes.

Much interest in recent years has centred around the possible contribution of organophosphorous compounds to the peripheral neuropathies that have been demonstrated in veterans of the Persian Gulf war. While peripheral sensory abnormalities have been demonstrated in some studies, there is little information concerning autonomic involvement. A recent epidemiological study examining potential risk factors for clusters of symptoms reported by veterans found that the 'arthro-myo-neuropathy' form of the Gulf War syndrome (which includes peripheral paraesthesias) was related to the use of insect repellent containing 75 per cent *N,N*-diethyl-*m*-toluamide in ethanol, and to a history of adverse reactions to pyridostigmine, which was administered as prophylaxis against organophosphate exposure. None of the symptom clusters identified in this study included prominent autonomic features (Haley and Kurt 1997), but thus far no studies have specifically examined autonomic function in exposed veterans.

Botulinum toxin

Although rare, poisoning with botulinum toxin (type B) is an important differential diagnosis for the presentation of acute autonomic neuropathy, particularly when there is predominant parasympathetic dysfunction. The toxin acts on cholinergic synapses to prevent the calcium-mediated release of acetylcholine from the presynaptic terminal. Its effects are seen primarily at neuromuscular junctions and, to a lesser extent, at autonomic ganglia where the effect is to block autonomic transmission acutely.

Other drugs and toxins

Two case reports are available to indicate that systemic absorption of podophyllin, which is usually used topically for skin lesions, can result in axonal sensorimotor and autonomic neuropathy. In one case, full recovery had not yet occurred at the time of death 3 months after ingestion, and sural nerve biopsy showed signs of axonal degeneration (Chapon *et al.* 1991).

Compounds that increase autonomic activity

Excessive autonomic activity is frequently seen in individuals with denervation hypersensitivity (e.g. due to pre-existing autonomic neuropathy) during treatment with autonomic agonists. Examples include the use of sympathetic α-adrenoceptor agonists in orthostatic hypotension, and the parasympathomimetic agent, bethanechol, in the management of bladder atony. The effects are predictable from the pharmacological action of the agonist. In other situations, a toxic compound may cause abnormally increased autonomic activity in an individual with previously normal autonomic function.

Parasympathetic stimulation

Therapeutic drugs

A case has been described in which significant cholinergic toxicity was induced by the use of bethanechol in a patient with diabetic autonomic neuropathy. The patient suffered shivering, salivation, dyspnoea, profuse sweating and pinpoint pupils, requiring treatment with atropine (Caraco *et al.* 1990). Denervation hypersensitivity was presumed to be the underlying mechanism for the exaggerated response to usual therapeutic doses.

Other compounds

Similar muscarinic stimulatory effects are seen after poisoning with wild mushroom species that contain neurotoxins with muscarinic agonist activity. The effects occur rapidly and, predictably, include lacrimation, salivation, nausea, vomiting, abdominal pain, bronchospasm, headache, miosis, blurred vision, bradycardia, and hypotension. A similar clinical picture is seen acutely following anticholinesterase poisoning with agricultural chemicals such as organophosphorous compounds, which inhibit acetylcholinesterase. The inhibition results in the typical picture of increased secretions, bronchoconstriction, miosis, abdominal cramps, and bradycardia (all related to muscarinic receptor stimulation) and hypertension, muscle fasciculations, tremor and eventual muscle paralysis (due to nicotinic receptor stimulation at autonomic ganglia and at neuromuscular junctions).

Less common causes of this constellation of features include acute exposure to sarin gas, a highly toxic organophosphorous compound originally developed during the Second World War and more recently used in terrorist attacks (Morita *et al.* 1995). Snake venom toxins known as fasciculins also have anticholinesterase activity, both

at neuromuscular junctions, where they produce a prolonged muscular contraction, and at autonomic ganglia, where they increase autonomic transmission. These toxins have a synergistic effect with dendrotoxins, also found in some snake venoms, which act presynaptically to increase the release of acetylcholine (Rees and Bilwes 1993). Some scorpion toxins have a similar effect, probably by binding to neuronal voltage-sensitive potassium channels and increasing the spontaneous release of acetylcholine.

Sympathetic stimulation

Psychoactive drugs

Hyperactivity of the sympathetic division of the autonomic nervous system is seen occasionally as a consequence of exposure to psychoactive drugs, both therapeutic and illicit. Neuroleptic malignant syndrome is a syndrome thought to be mediated by changes in central dopaminergic transmission causing increased sympathetic outflow manifested as hyperthermia, muscle rigidity, and unstable blood pressure and heart rate. It occurs in fewer than 1 per cent of patients receiving antipsychotic drugs, but can be fatal if untreated. A similar clinical picture, with occasional fatalities, occurs in some individuals who ingest the so-called 'designer drug' Ecstasy (3,4-methylenedioxymethamphetamine [MDMA]) and other amphetamine derivatives.

An interaction between antidepressant drugs, which inhibit noradrenaline and/or serotonin reuptake from the synapse, and tyramine, which releases catecholamines from storage vesicles, can result in a marked increase in neurotransmitter concentrations within sympathetic synapses. Clinically there is marked sympathetic hyperactivity with sweating, tachycardia, and severe hypertension, which may lead to intracranial haemorrhage. A similar picture can be seen following the use of the combination of a monoamine oxidase inhibitor and a serotonin uptake inhibitor (such as fluoxetine). Known as the 'CNS serotonergic syndrome', it comprises general CNS overactivity, muscle spasms, hyperthermia, and autonomic instability, resulting in hyper- or hypotension, tachycardia, and profuse sweating. Fatalities have been reported. The mechanism is believed to be an increase in serotonergic activity, particularly involving 5-HT$_{1A}$ receptors in the brainstem and spinal cord.

Ketamine

The neurolept anaesthetic/analgesic agent, ketamine, has an interesting combination of stimulatory and inhibitory cardiovascular and respiratory effects. In isolated organ experiments, in the absence of an intact autonomic nervous system, it has a direct negative inotropic effect on the myocardium. However, in the intact animal or human, this is counterbalanced by a central stimulatory effect, probably mediated by increased sympathetic outflow, which results in an elevation in blood pressure, heart rate and cardiac output, and bronchodilatation.

Venoms and toxins

Some venomous creatures, including snakes and scorpions, cause prominent sympathetic hyperactivity, resulting in the potentially fatal clinical syndrome sometimes known as 'autonomic storm'. In the case of stings from some scorpion species which are common in India and the Middle East, the major problem is uncontrolled catecholamine release from sympathetic nerve endings and the adrenals, with acute hypertension and hypertensive encephalopathy, best treated with prazosin. In many instances the precise mechanism of action remains unknown. Some snake and scorpion venoms are known to contain dendrotoxin, which can augment sympathetic activity by stimulating catecholamine release from nerve endings in a similar manner to their effect on cholinergic transmission (discussed earlier).

Concluding remarks

While the mechanisms of action of drugs which interact reversibly with autonomic nerve fibres or receptors as part of their pharmacodynamic activity are well known, much remains to be established about the effect of drugs and other compounds causing autonomic neuropathy. Drugs, chemicals, and toxins should always be considered as a possible cause of autonomic neuropathy in patients presenting with the clinical manifestations of either sympathetic or parasympathetic dysfunction, or both.

References

Caraco, Y., Arnon, R., and Raz, I. (1990). Bethanecol-induced cholinergic toxicity in diabetic neuropathy. *Ann. Pharmacother.* 24, 327.

Chan, J. C. N., Chan, T. Y. K., Chan, K. L., Leung, N. W., Tomlinson, B., and Critchley, J. A. (1994). Anticholinergic poisoning from Chinese herbal medicines. *Aust. N. Z. J. Med.* 24, 317–18.

Chapon, F., Dupuy, B., Gosset, S. *et al.* (1991). Accidental poisoning with podophyllin: a case with study of peripheral nerve. *Rev. Neurol., Paris* 147, 240–3.

Chida, K., Takasu, T., Mori, N., Tokunaga, K., Komatsu, K., and Kawamura, H. (1994). Sympathetic dysfunction mediating cardiovascular regulation in alcoholic neuropathy. *Funct. Neurol.* 9, 65–73.

Fam, A. (1988). Gold neurotoxicity and myokymia. *J. Rheumatol.* 15, 528–9.

Haley, R. W. and Kurt, T. L., (1997). Self-reported exposure to neurotoxic chemical combinations in the Gulf War. A cross-sectional epidemiologic study. *J. Am. Med Ass.* 277, 231–327.

Hansen, S. W. (1990). Autonomic neuropathy after treatment with cisplatin, vinblastine, and bleomycin for germ cell cancer. *BMJ.* 300, 511–12.

Hirvonen, H. E., Salmi, T. T., Heinonen, E., Antila, K. J., and Valimaki, I. A. (1989). Vincristine treatment of acute lymphoblastic leukaemia induces transient autonomic cardioneuropathy. *Cancer* 64, 801–5.

Jerian, S. M., Sarosy, G. A., Link, C. J., Fingert, H. J., Reed, E., and Dohn, E. C. (1993). Incapacitating autonomic neuropathy precipitated by taxol. *Gynecol. Oncol.* 51, 277–80.

Juntunen, J., Matikainen, E., Antti-Poika, M., Suoranta, H., and Valle M. (1985). Nervous system effects of long-term occupational exposure to toluene. *Acta Neurol. Scand.* 72, 512–17.

Lahtinen, R., Koponen, A., Mustonen, J. *et al.* (1989). Discordance in the development of peripheral and autonomic neuropathy during vincristine therapy. *Eur. J. Haematol.* 43, 357–8.

Matikainen, E., and Juntunen, J. (1985). Autonomic nervous system dysfunction in workers exposed to organic solvents. *J. Neurol. Neurosurg. Psychiat.* 48, 1021–4.

Monforte, R., Estruch, R., Valls-Sole, J., Nicolas, J., Villalta, J., and Urbano-Marquez, (1995). Autonomic and peripheral neuropathies in patients with chronic alcoholism. A dose-related toxic effect of alcohol. *Arch. Neurol.* 52, 45–51.

Morita, H., Yanagisawa, N., Nakajima, T. *et al.* (1995). Sarin poisoning in Matsumoto, Japan. *Lancet* 346, 290–2.

Murata, K. and Araki, S. (1991). Autonomic nervous system dysfunction in workers exposed to lead, zinc, and copper in relation to peripheral nerve conduction: a study of R–R interval variability. *Am. J. Ind. Med.* 20, 663–71.

Murata, K., Araki, S., Yokoyama, K., and Ono, Y. (1994). Autonomic neurotoxicity of alcohol assessed by heart rate variability. *J. Autonom. Nerv. Syst.* 48, 105–11.

Nevill, T. J., Benstead, T. J., McCormick, C. W., and Hayne, O. A. (1989). Horner's syndrome and demyelinating peripheral neuropathy caused by high-dose cytosine arabinoside. *Am. J. Hematol.* 32, 314–15.

Rees, B. and Bilwes, A. (1993). Three-dimensional structures of neurotoxins and cardiotoxins. *Chem. Res. Toxicol.* 6, 385–406.

Roca, E., Bruera, E., Politi, P.M., *et al.* (1985). Vinca alkaloid-induced cardiovascular autonomic neuropathy. *Cancer Treat. Rep.* 69, 149–51.

Ruijten, M. W. M. M, Salle, H. J. A., and Verberk M. M. (1993). Verification of effects on the nervous system of low level occupational exposure to CS_2. *Br. J. Ind. Med.* 50, 301–7.

Siddiqui, M. A. and Ford, P. A. (1995). Acute severe autonomic insufficiency during pentamidine therapy. *Southern Med. J.* 88, 1087–8.

Smit, A. A. J., Wieling, W., Voogel, A. J., Koster, R. W., and van Zwieten, P. A. (1996). Orthostatic hypotension due to suppression of vasomotor outflow after emphetamine intoxication. *Mayo Clin. Proc.* 71, 1067–70.

Warner, E. (1995). Neurotoxicity of cisplatin and taxol. *Int. J. Gynecol. Cancer* 5, 161–9.

55. Ageing and the autonomic nervous system

Lewis A. Lipsitz

Introduction

Normal human ageing is associated with changes in the autonomic control of several bodily functions, particularly those served by cardiovascular and thermoregulatory systems. Since the autonomic nervous system functions to enable an organism to adapt rapidly to stress, these age-related changes may impair an older person's adaptive capacity. As a result, elderly people may develop clinical manifestations of autonomic insufficiency in response to physiological stresses. Common clinical manifestations of autonomic dysfunction in elderly patients include postural hypotension, postprandial hypotension, hypothermia, and heat stroke. These are rarely problematic in healthy elderly individuals under the usual demands of life, but may become clinically significant during exposure to a variety of external influences, such as medications, changes in fluid intake, or relatively hot or cold environmental temperatures. Other geriatric problems such as constipation, urinary incontinence, and sexual dysfunction may mimic autonomic insufficiency, but are usually caused by conditions outside of the autonomic nervous system. For example, sexual dysfunction in old age is more likely due to vascular disease, diabetes, depression, or medications, than it is to age-associated autonomic dysfunction. By recognizing this, clinicians can identify and treat the underlying disease and potentially improve the quality of life of their elderly patients.

Several methodological problems confound the interpretation of research data in the area of ageing and autonomic function. Research findings are often influenced by the presence of occult disease, making it inappropriate to attribute them to normal ageing. Furthermore, since clinical tests of autonomic function rely on reflex responses to specific stimuli, the actual level of abnormality is difficult to ascertain unless subjects of different ages receive identical stimuli. This may be difficult to achieve if, for example, the level of blood pressure, sympathetic arousal, intrathoracic pressure, core body temperature, or co-operation with a test differs as a function of age. In addition, most previous human studies have not been controlled adequately for body composition, physical exercise, and diet. Many of the reported autonomic nervous system changes with advancing age are probably due to a sedentary life style and decrease in lean body mass, rather than ageing *per se*.

Animal studies also must be interpreted with caution because of considerable differences in autonomic responses among different animal species. Some studies do not compare mature and senescent animals but, rather, look at the differences between young and mature animals. This approach may lead to confusion between true age-related changes and those that occur as a result of growth and development. Despite these complexities, accumulated evidence suggests that some deterioration in selected areas of autonomic nervous system function occurs with normal ageing.

This chapter will review age-related physiological changes in the autonomic nervous system that impair an older person's ability to adapt to stress, as well as common pathological conditions in advanced age that further impair autonomic function. The chapter will focus on those functions most commonly thought to be associated with autonomic changes in elderly individuals, namely thermoregulation, blood pressure regulation, control of respiration, gastrointestinal, urinary tract, and sexual function.

Temperature regulation

Thermoregulation requires sensory systems that detect temperature, central connections in the anterior hypothalamus, efferent autonomic pathways to the sweat glands and vasculature, metabolic processes that generate heat, and behavioural responses that enable an individual to adjust the temperature in their external environment. Efferent autonomic signals are transmitted primarily via the sympathetic nervous system from the brain to receptors in the sweat glands and vasculature, which function to preserve or dissipate heat. Impairment of thermoregulation in elderly persons—either due to autonomic dysfunction or complications of diseases and medications—increase their vulnerability to hypo- or hyperthermia (Wongsurawat *et al.* 1990). The sections that follow summarize age- and disease-related alterations in heat generation, conservation, and dissipation; temperature perception; and behavioural responses to ambient temperature changes. This material ends with a brief review of the common geriatric problems of hypothermia and heat stroke.

Heat generation

Basal metabolic rate

Ageing is accompanied by a gradual decrease in basal metabolic rate (BMR), due in large part to a reduction in skeletal muscle mass. The reduction in BMR is evident at thermoneutral temperatures and in response to cold environments (Collins *et al.* 1981a). Ageing is also associated with a blunted thermic response to feeding (Schwartz *et al.* 1990). Deconditioned sedentary individuals with muscle atrophy, and malnourished patients with inadequate energy stores, may not be able to generate sufficient heat to protect them from hypothermia when exposed to the cold.

Shivering

Shivering is an important mechanism of muscular heat production that is mediated through central hypothalamic pathways. Healthy elderly individuals exhibit delayed and less intense shivering on exposure to cold (Collins *et al.* 1981*a*). The mechanism of this alteration in shivering response is not known.

Heat conservation via vasoconstriction

Peripheral vasoconstriction in response to cold exposure is an important mechanism of heat conservation. Elderly individuals demonstrate considerable variability in their capacity to respond to cold exposure. However, in general, older people exhibit delayed and reduced cutaneous vasoconstriction after cold exposure (Collins *et al.* 1981*a*; Khan *et al.* 1992; Richardson *et al.* 1992).

Heat dissipation via vasodilatation and sweating

Sweating and vasodilatation normally occur in response to elevations in environmental temperature to prevent an excessive rise in core body temperature. Skin atrophy, which accompanies normal ageing, results in a loss of sweat glands. This may reduce the sweating response to heat. The elderly have a higher core temperature threshold for the onset of sweating and vasodilatation (Ryan and Lipsitz 1995). Some studies have shown that the age-related impairment in sweating is localized to certain regions, such as the thigh (Inoue *et al.* 1991).

Vasodilatory responses to radiant heat on the forearm have been investigated using Doppler skin blood flow velocity measurements (Richardson 1989). Young subjects demonstrate an increase in forearm cutaneous blood flow in response to local heat, while elderly subjects have an attenuated response. It is not clear whether this is secondary to reduced vasodilatation or less recruitment of capillary vessels. When the effect of age, cholesterol, and plasma glucose on cutaneous blood-flow response to ambient heat was investigated, age was the most important variable (Richardson 1989).

Temperature perception

Young individuals are able to discriminate temperature differences of 1–2 °C. In contrast, many elderly people are unable to detect differences in temperature closer than 2–4 °C (Collins *et al.* 1981*b*). Alterations in temperature perception with ageing may result in part from changes in the peripheral temperature receptors. These receptors are highly dependent on oxygen and therefore may be affected by diminished peripheral blood flow. Also, age-related alterations in skin collagen and elastic tissue may influence receptor function. The potential role of the hypothalamus on temperature perception and behaviour is not well elucidated.

Behavioural responses to ambient temperature

Elderly individuals with poor temperature discrimination also have less ability to regulate their ambient temperature. This was demonstrated in a study by Collins *et al.* (Collins *et al.* 1981*b*) in which subjects were asked to regulate room temperature by adjusting a thermostat. Elderly individuals with poor temperature discrimination lacked precision in adjusting the temperature, possibly due to impaired perception of ambient room temperature. This notion is supported by reports that elderly persons are less uncomfortable than the young when exposed to a cold environment, and require a more intense thermal stimulus to elicit a behavioural response (Taylor *et al.* 1995).

Clinical syndromes

Hypothermia

Hypothermia is defined as a decrease in core body temperature (oesophageal, rectal, or tympanic) below 35 °C or 95 °F. In UK surveys in 1975, 3.6 per cent of individuals over 65 admitted to the hospital were hypothermic. Unfortunately, prevalence data on hypothermia can be difficult to interpret as much of it relies on death certificate information which may underreport the incidence of hypothermia. In addition, many hospital emergency rooms may lack low-reading thermometers and therefore fail to detect hypothermia.

Elderly people in warm climates are also at risk of hypothermia (Kramer *et al.* 1989). In Israel, despite a warm climate, one-third of patients identified as hypothermic developed the condition during the warm season (Kramer *et al.* 1989). Disorders that contribute to the development of hypothermia are listed in Table 55.1. These conditions may predispose elderly people to hypothermia even under relatively mild cold stress. Diseases such as Parkinson's disease and severe arthritis can immobilize the older person and thereby impair

Table 55.1. Causes of hypothermia

Cold exposure
Medications
Phenothiazines
Narcotics
Vasodilators
Barbiturates
Alcohol
Inflammatory skin conditions
Paget's disease
Endocrine Disorders
Hypothyroidism
Hypopituitarism
Adrenal insufficiency
Diabetes mellitus
Hypoglycaemia
Sepsis
Malnutrition/starvation
Cardiovascular diseases
Congestive heart failure
Myocardial infarction
Uraemia
Hepatic failure
Neurological diseases
Stroke
Parkinson's disease
Hypothalamic tumours or strokes
Wernicke's encephalopathy
Spinal cord lesions

heat production. Malnutrition—by itself or in association with dementia, poor living conditions, cancer, or other conditions—can result in a lowered basal metabolic rate and reduced heat production. Neuroleptic medications impair central heat regulation. Sepsis is frequently observed among elderly patients admitted with hypothermia. It appears that underlying medical conditions predisposing to hypothermia are more common than autonomic dysfunction *per se*. Mortality in elderly persons with hypothermia is high and ranges from 30–80 per cent. Mortality from hypothermia in association with myxoedema is particularly high.

Heat stroke

Heat stroke also appears to be more prevalent in the elderly. This may be attributable to poor temperature perception and a lack of protective behavioural responses, or impairments in sweating and vasodilatation. Co-morbidity, such as dementia and neuroleptic medications, also impair the elderly person's capacity to detect and respond appropriately to elevated ambient temperatures.

Associated conditions

Abnormalities in temperature regulation are frequently seen in individuals with other symptoms of autonomic dysfunction. Postural hypotension may be more common in elderly people with a history of hypothermia. Temperature dysregulation may be due to a number of autonomic nervous system diseases that commonly occur in elderly persons. These include diabetes, multiple systems atrophy, Parkinson's disease, and other conditions that are reviewed extensively in other chapters.

Blood-pressure regulation

One of the most important, and most widely studied function of the autonomic nervous system is the maintenance of an adequate blood pressure to assure vital organ perfusion. Blood pressure is the product of heart rate, stroke volume, and systemic vascular resistance. These physiological parameters are regulated on a beat-to-beat basis by the baroreflex and both sympathetic and parasympathetic limbs of the autonomic nervous system. Normal human ageing is associated with several changes in autonomic regulation of blood pressure. The superimposition of cardiovascular diseases and the medications used to treat them in elderly patients, often leads to further decrements in autonomic function that manifest as hypotension and syncope. This section will review physiological and pathological changes in autonomic cardiovascular regulation associated with ageing, and the common geriatric syndromes that often result.

Baroreflex mechanisms

The baroreflex maintains a normal blood pressure by increasing heart rate and vascular resistance in response to transient reductions in stretch of arterial baroreceptors, and by decreasing these parameters in response to an increase in stretch of baroreceptors. Normal human ageing is associated with a reduction in baroreflex sensitivity. This is evident in the blunted cardioacceleratory response to stimuli such as upright posture, nitroprusside infusion, and lower-body negative pressure which lower arterial pressure, as well as a reduced bradycardic response to drugs such as phenylephrine that elevate

pressure. Furthermore, it is manifest by an increase in blood-pressure variability, often with potentially dangerous blood pressure reductions during hypotensive stresses such as upright posture or meal digestion.

Age-associated elevations in blood pressure have been considered to be both a possible cause and consequence of baroreflex impairment. Both normal ageing and hypertension exert independent effects on baroreflex sensitivity. It has been suggested that the decrease in arterial distensibility that accompanies ageing and hypertension results in diminished baroreceptor stretch, less tonic inhibition of the brainstem vasomotor centre, and increased sympathetic outflow. Increased sympathetic outflow results in increased circulating noradrenaline which, in turn, may result in further vasoconstriction, blood pressure elevation, and baroreflex impairment. This hypothesis is supported by elevated basal plasma noradrenaline levels and muscle sympathetic nerve activity, as well as a heightened plasma noradrenaline response to baroreceptor unloading in aged subjects. Furthermore, in healthy young subjects, carotid artery distensibility correlates with baroreflex sensitivity (Bonyhay *et al.* 1996). The relationship between ageing, hypertension, carotid stiffness, and baroreflex function remains to be fully elucidated.

The baroreflex may be impaired at any of multiple sites along its arc, including carotid and cardiopulmonary pressure receptors, afferent neuronal pathways, the brainstem (nucleus tractus solitarius) and higher regulatory centres, efferent sympathetic and parasympathetic neurones, postsynaptic cardiac β-receptors, or intracellular signal transduction G-proteins. Several lines of evidence discussed below localize the defect to the β-receptor and signal transduction pathways within myocardial cells.

Sympathetic nervous system
Basal sympathetic nerve activity

Much of our current knowledge about age-related changes in sympathetic nervous system function is derived from studies of circulating catecholamine levels, norepinephrine kinetics, and microneurographic recordings from sympathetic nerves to skeletal muscle. Significant evidence suggests that basal plasma noradrenaline levels increase with age.

Age-related elevations in plasma noradrenaline may be due to many factors, including increased appearance at the synapse, increased spillover into the systemic circulation, decreased reuptake by presynaptic neurones, decreased local metabolism, and decreased systemic clearance. To determine whether elevations in plasma noradrenaline levels reflect heightened sympathetic nervous system activity, or merely decreased clearance, recent investigations have used radiotracer methods to examine noradrenaline kinetics. Using tritiated noradrenaline infusions and a two-compartment model to estimate noradrenaline disposition, Veith *et al.* (1986) demonstrated a 32 per cent increase in arterialized noradrenaline appearance, and 19 per cent decrease in clearance in healthy elderly subjects compared to young.

Recent studies of sympathetic nervous system activity measured by microelectrode recordings from the peroneal nerve in healthy subjects demonstrate an age-related increase in muscle sympathetic nerve activity (Ng *et al.* 1993). Sympathetic nerve activity is higher in males than in females. Furthermore, venous plasma noradrenaline levels appear to correlate with muscle sympathetic nerve activity. These data lend further support to the notion that healthy ageing is associated with elevated basal sympathetic nervous system activity. It is not known whether this is related to arterial stiffness that may attenuate the stretch of baroreceptors in the carotid arteries and aortic arch, or whether it is due to alterations in central sympathetic outflow.

In contrast to noradrenaline, adrenaline is released directly into the bloodstream from the adrenal medulla in response to sympathetic stimulation, and is then transported via the circulation to target organs. Adrenaline is removed through non-neuronal uptake and metabolism. Plasma adrenaline levels are probably not affected by ageing.

Circadian rhythm of catecholamine levels

Catecholamines exhibit diurnal variation which is preserved during ageing. Plasma noradrenaline levels are highest during the late morning to early afternoon and fall gradually during the night. Elderly subjects have higher noradrenaline levels during a 24-hour period than young subjects. This elevation is most pronounced during the night and is associated with increased nocturnal wakefulness and less stage IV sleep in elderly subjects (Prinz *et al.* 1979).

Stimulated catecholamine levels

Postural stress induced by active standing and head-up tilt results in an exaggerated increase in plasma noradrenaline in old subjects compared to young. Furthermore, the time required for plasma noradrenaline levels to return to baseline is prolonged in elderly subjects (Young *et al.* 1980). The prolongation of noradrenaline response to sympathetic nervous system stimulation may falsely elevate supine resting levels if subjects are not given a sufficient length of time to achieve truly basal conditions. Plasma noradrenaline responses to isometric exercise, the cold pressor test, psychological stimuli, and graded levels of cardiac work, are all increased in old compared with young healthy subjects (Ryan and Lipsitz 1995).

β-Adrenergic activity

The fact that plasma noradrenaline levels are heightened and prolonged during hypotensive stress, but heart rate responses are blunted in elderly subjects, suggests that ageing results in impaired β-mediated adrenoceptor responses to sympathetic activation. This notion is further supported by the findings that infusions of β-adrenergic agonists result in smaller increases in heart rate, left ventricular ejection fraction, cardiac output, and vasodilatation in older compared to younger men (Lakatta 1993).

β₁-Adrenoceptors

In normal individuals stimulation of β_1-receptors using intravenous infusions of sympathetic agonists such as isoproterenol results in cardioacceleration. The dose of isoproterenol required to raise the heart rate is increased with ageing in humans and animals. The normal increase in heart rate induced by isoproterenol may also be due to a reflex cardioacceleratory response to the vasodilatation produced by simultaneous activation of β_2-receptors. Evidence discussed below indicates that β_2-adrenoceptor function is impaired with senescence.

In the heart the blunted cardioacceleratory response to β-adrenergic stimulation has been attributed to multiple molecular and biochemical changes in β-receptor-coupling and postreceptor events. The number of β-receptors on cardiac myocytes is unchanged with advancing age, but the affinity of β-receptors for agonists is reduced. Postreceptor changes with ageing include a decrease in the activity of G_s-proteins and the adenylate cyclase catalytic unit, and a decrease in cAMP-dependent phosphokinase-induced protein phosphorylation (Lakatta 1993). As a result of these changes, G-protein-mediated signal transduction is impaired. Although a recent study suggests that exercise training by treadmill running may increase β-adrenergic signal transduction in senescent rats (Scarpace *et al.* 1994), endurance exercise does not appear to improve the cardiac response to β-adrenergic stimulation in elderly humans (Stratton *et al.* 1992).

The decrease in cardiac contractile response to β-drenergic stimulation has been studied in rat ventricular myocytes, where it appears to be related to decreased influx of calcium ions via sarcolemmal calcium channels, and a reduction in the amplitude of the cytosolic calcium transient. These changes are similar to those seen in receptor desensitization due to prolonged exposure of myocardial tissue to β-adrenergic agonists. Thus, age-associated alterations in β-adrenergic response may be due to desensitization of the adenylate cyclase system in response to chronic elevations of plasma catecholamine levels (Lakatta 1993).

β₂-Adrenoceptors

Several studies suggest that β_2-mediated vasodilatation is also impaired in elderly individuals. In order to study β_2-adrenergic effects in isolation from baroreflex responses to systemic vasodilators, Pan *et al.* (1986) infused isoproterenol directly into the dorsal hand vein of healthy young and old subjects. Isoproterenol-mediated vascular relaxation was impaired in elderly individuals. In contrast, nitroglycerine-mediated relaxation was normal in both young and elderly subjects. Since nitrate-induced vasodilatation was intact, the impairment in β-agonist response was probably not due to structural alterations in the vessel wall. This finding supports an age-related decline in β_2-mediated vasodilatation in the elderly. As nitroglycerine acts independently of cAMP, the defect may lie at the level of cAMP production.

α-Adrenergic activity

Although current evidence suggests that β-adrenergic responsiveness decreases with normal ageing, age-related changes in the α-adrenergic system are not as well delineated. The data currently available suggest that α-receptors show less functional alteration than β-receptors during normal ageing.

In vitro studies of isolated human arteries and veins suggest that the α-mediated response to noradrenaline does not change with ageing (Ryan and Lipsitz 1995). This result is supported by the *in vivo* observation of preserved α_2-mediated phenylephrine-induced vasoconstriction of the dorsal hand vein (Pan *et al.* 1986). However, a recent study by Hogikyan and Supiano (1994) showed the α_1-adrenergic vasoconstrictor response to noradrenaline infusion to be reduced in the forearm of healthy elderly subjects. The fact that this impairment was reversed by suppression of sympathetic nervous system activity with guanadrel (Hogikyan and Supiano 1994), suggests that it is due to receptor desensitization in response to heightened sympathetic nervous system activity. This remarkable observation indicates that some of the autonomic nervous system changes associated with ageing may be reversible.

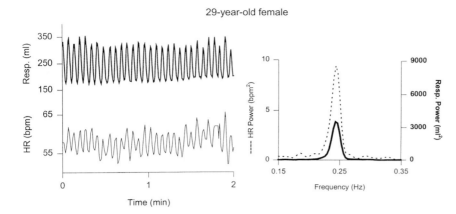

29-year-old female

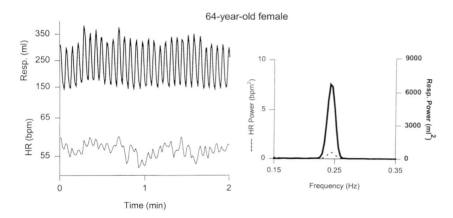

64-year-old female

Fig. 55.1. The age-related reduction in respiratory control of heart rate. Two minutes of continuous respiration (resp) during paced breathing at 15 breaths per minute (0.25 Hz), the simultaneous heart rate (HR), and the corresponding frequency spectra (right graphs) for HR (dashed line) and respiration (bold line) are shown for a healthy 29 year-old woman (top) and healthy 64-year-old woman (bottom). Note the reduction in amplitude of HR variation, despite similar respiratory amplitudes in the older woman compared to the young. This is reflected in the frequency spectra where HR power (amplitude squared) is markedly reduced in the older woman, despite somewhat greater respiratory power compared to that of the younger subject.

Parasympathetic nervous system

Age-related alterations in the parasympathetic nervous system are difficult to evaluate. Most of the currently available clinical evidence for a decline in parasympathetic function with ageing is derived from studies of heart rate (HR) variability. Previous studies demonstrating age-related reductions in overall HR variability in response to respiration, cough, and the Valsalva manoeuvre suggest that ageing is associated with impaired vagal control of HR (Fig. 55.1). Elderly patients with unexplained syncope have even greater impairments in HR responses to cough and deep breathing than elderly subjects without syncope (Maddens *et al.* 1987).

The ratio of RR intervals during expiration and inspiration is a standard method of evaluating autonomic function and reflects primarily parasympathetic influences on the heart rate. The expiration : inspiration RR interval is reduced with ageing. However, many physiological changes associated with ageing may influence this finding. Impaired baroreflex function, decreased cardiac responsiveness to sympathetic and parasympathetic input, and changes in lung and chest wall compliance—which affect intrathoracic pressures and venous return to the heart during deep breathing—may all influence heart rate variability. Furthermore, the reflex responses to respiratory manoeuvres are dependent on the extent of BP change, and therefore may vary from one individual to the next, depending on the performance of the test and the associated BP response. Therefore, RR variability during respiration cannot be considered a pure test of parasympathetic function.

Recently, the technique of frequency domain (spectral) analysis has been used to quantify the relative contributions of sympathetic and parasympathetic nervous systems to heart rate or interbeat interval variability. The power spectrum produced by this technique can be divided into low- and high-frequency components. Previous pharmacological blocking studies using β-blockade and/or atropine suggest that the low-frequency oscillations (0.06–0.12 Hz) represent baroreflex-mediated sympathetic and parasympathetic influences on heart period variability, while the high-frequency portion of the power spectrum (0.15–0.5 Hz) represents the respiratory sinus arrhythmia and is under parasympathetic control (Pagani *et al.* 1986). Frequency domain analysis techniques have confirmed that healthy ageing is associated with reductions in both baroreflex and parasympathetic modulation of heart rate, with a relatively greater loss of the high-frequency parasympathetic component (Lipsitz *et al.* 1990). Furthermore, there may be gender differences in heart rate variability, with relatively greater high-frequency variability in healthy women compared to men across all ages (Ryan *et al.* 1994). Given the known inverse relationship between heart rate variability and cardiovascular mortality, this finding may reflect healthier cardiovascular function in women compared to men.

It is important to recognize that frequency domain analyses yield different results depending on whether heart rate or interbeat interval (RR) is used as the unit of measure. RR interval is linearly related to cardiac vagal outflow, while heart rate is inversely related to RR interval and reflects minute-to-minute systemic haemodynamic

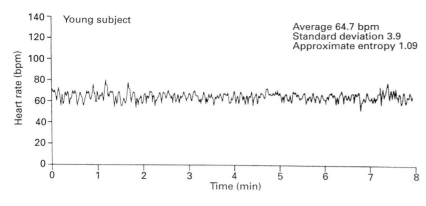

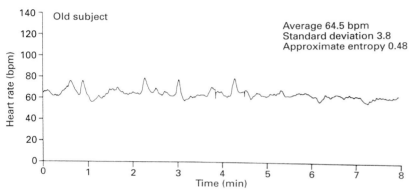

Fig. 55.2. Eight-minute heart rate time series during quiet supine rest for a 22-year-old female subject (top panel) and a 73-year-old male subject (bottom panel). 'Approximate entropy' (ApEn) is a measure of irregularity that quantifies the likelihood that a series of data points that are a certain distance apart for a given number of observations remain within the same distance on next incremental comparisons. A greater likelihood of remaining the same distance apart (i.e. greater regularity) produces smaller ApEn values. A completely random sequence of beats has the highest ApEn value, while a regular sequence (e.g. a sine wave) has the lowest. Despite the nearly identical mean heart rates and standard deviations (SD) of the two time series shown, the irregularity of the signal from the older subject is markedly reduced. (Adapted with permission from Lipsitz and Goldberger (1992).)

adjustments to physiological stimuli. Therefore, RR interval spectra are probably best suited for the evaluation of parasympathetic influences on the heart.

The age-related attenuation of autonomic, neurohumoral, and other influences on the heart results not only in a reduction in heart rate variability, but also in a marked change in the dynamics of beat-to-beat heart rate fluctuations. As shown in Fig. 55.2, the highly irregular, complex dynamics of heart rate variability that is characteristic of healthy young individuals is lost with healthy ageing, resulting in a more regular and predictable heart rate time series. This loss of complexity in heart rate dynamics appears to be generalizable to the fluctuating output of many different physiological processes as they age (Lipsitz and Goldberger 1992). For example, measurements of continuous blood pressure, electroencephalographic waves, frequently sampled thyrotrophin or luteinizing hormone levels, and centre-of-pressure changes during quiet stance all show more regular, less complex behaviour with ageing. This apparent loss of dynamic range in physiological functions may be due to fewer regulatory influences as an individual ages, thus leading to an impaired capacity to adapt to stress (Lipsitz and Goldberger 1992).

Cardiac ventricular function

The maintenance of a normal blood pressure also depends on the ability to generate an adequate cardiac output. Cardiac output tends to decrease with normal ageing, both at rest and with exercise. This is due not only to a reduction in heart rate response to β-adrenergic stimulation, as mentioned above, but also to changes in systolic and diastolic myocardial performance that influence stroke volume.

Diastolic function

As a result of several structural and functional changes in the myocardium, the aged heart stiffens and early diastolic ventricular filling becomes impaired. These changes include an increase in cross-linking of myocardial collagen and prolongation of ventricular relaxation time. The latter may be due in part to reduction in the active uptake of calcium into the sarcoplasmic reticulum after ventricular contraction, as a consequence of reduced oxygen tension in the coronary circulation, decreased oxidative phosphorylation, and cumulative mitochondrial peroxidation.

The age-related impairment in early ventricular filling makes the heart dependent on adequate preload to fill the ventricle, as well as on atrial contraction during late diastole to maintain stroke volume. Thus, orthostatic hypotension and syncope occur commonly in older people as a result of volume contraction or venous pooling which reduce cardiac preload, or at the onset of atrial fibrillation when the atrial contribution to cardiac output is suddenly lost.

Systolic function

With ageing there is preservation of myocardial contractile strength, but a decrease in left ventricular ejection fraction in response to exertion. This is due to both reduced β-adrenergic responsiveness, as well as an increase in afterload. Afterload, which represents opposition to left ventricular ejection, increases progressively with ageing due to stiffening of the ascending aorta, and narrowing of the peripheral vasculature. These changes result in an increase in systolic blood pressure. They also decrease the maximum cardiac output during exercise.

The cardiac response to exercise differs between healthy young and old subjects. While the young increase cardiac output via increases in heart rate and decreases in end systolic volume (greater contractility), the healthy elderly do so by increasing end diastolic volume (cardiac dilatation) (Rodeheffer *et al.* 1984). Thus, the elderly rely on the Frank–Starling relationship to achieve an increase in stroke volume during exercise. A similar mechanism can be demonstrated in young subjects in the presence of β-adrenergic blockade, suggesting that the age effect is due to reduced β-adrenergic responsiveness.

Recent data suggest that the decrease in maximal cardiac output during exercise observed in the elderly, may in large part be related to a sedentary life style and consequent cardiovascular deconditioning. A six-month training programme of endurance exercise training has been shown to enhance end-diastolic volume and contractility, thereby increasing ejection fraction, stroke volume, and cardiac output at peak exercise in elderly men (Stratton *et al.* 1994). Thus, the elderly may be able to compensate for age-associated physiological changes, by using alternate mechanisms (such as the Frank–Starling relationship) to maintain cardiac function at times of stress.

Intravascular volume regulation

An adequate blood pressure also depends on the maintenance of intravascular volume. Ageing is associated with a progressive decline in plasma renin, angiotensin II, and aldosterone levels, and elevations in atrial natriuretic peptide, all of which promote salt wasting by the kidney. Furthermore, healthy elderly individuals do not experience the same sense of thirst as younger subjects when they become hyperosmolar during water deprivation (Phillips *et al.* 1984). Thus, dehydration and hypotension may develop rapidly during conditions such as an acute illness, preparation for a medical procedure, or exposure to a warm climate, when insensible fluid losses are increased and/or access to oral fluids is limited. The interaction between volume contraction and impaired diastolic function may threaten cardiac output, and result in hypotension and organ ischaemia.

Regulation of organ blood flow

Age-related changes in vascular response to sympathetic nervous system activity have been described above. However, the regulation of blood flow to various circulatory beds also depends on complex interactions at the cellular level between the endothelium, local vasoactive peptides, neuroendocrine influences, and mechanical factors, few of which have been studied as a function of ageing in humans. In angiographically normal coronary arteries (Egashira *et al.* 1993) and the brachial artery (Gerhard *et al.* 1996), the endothelium-dependent vasodilatory response to acetylcholine or methacholine is reduced with ageing. In contrast, endothelium-independent vasodilation by nitroprusside is not affected by ageing.

Normal human ageing is also associated with a reduction in cerebral blood flow, which is further compromised by the presence of risk factors for cerebrovascular disease (Meyer and Shaw 1984). Although it is not clear whether the decline in cerebral blood flow is due to reduced supply or demand, it is likely that elderly individuals, particularly those with cerebrovascular disease, have a resting cerebral blood flow that is closer to the threshold for cerebral ischaemia. Consequently, relatively small, short-term reductions in blood pressure may produce cerebral ischaemic symptoms.

The brain normally maintains a constant blood flow over a wide range of perfusion pressures through the process of autoregulation. During reductions in blood pressure, resistance vessels in the brain dilate to restore blood flow to normal. Although the effects of ageing on cerebral autoregulation have received very little attention, limited data suggest that the autoregulation of cerebral blood flow is preserved into old age. However, patients with symptomatic postural hypotension appear to have a reduction in cerebral blood flow in response to decreased perfusion pressure (Wollner *et al.* 1979).

Clinical manifestations of impaired autonomic control of blood pressure

Two of the most common age-associated manifestations of autonomic nervous system impairment are postural and postprandial hypotension, defined as a 20 mmHg or greater decline in systolic blood pressure upon assumption of the upright posture, or within 1 hour of eating a meal, respectively. These are two distinct conditions which may or may not occur together in the same patient. Both are related to a reduction in venous blood return to the heart due to blood pooling in the lower extremities or splanchnic circulation, and inadequate baroreflex compensation. Several of the physiological abnormalities that may predispose normal elderly people to hypotension are summarized in Table 55.2. The onset of diseases in old age, such as diabetes, cerebrovascular disease, Parkinson's disease, malignancy, and amyloidosis, as well as the medications used to treat them, may have additional adverse effects on autonomic function (Table 55.3). Therefore, hypotensive syndromes in old age may be considered due to physiological changes that accompany usual ageing, and pathological conditions that become more prevalent with advancing age. In addition, several reflexes may precipitate hypotension in elderly people. These three classifications of the hypotensive syndromes are summarized in Table 55.4.

Postural hypotension

Postural hypotension is observed in less than 7 per cent of healthy normotensive elderly people, and in as many as 30 per cent of those over age 75 with multiple pathological conditions, particularly hypertension. The reported prevalence differs according to the population studied, the subject's position (supine to sitting or standing), and the time when measurements are taken (standing blood pressure is generally lower 1 minute after posture change than at 3 minutes). Furthermore, postural blood pressure changes may vary greatly during the day, and between days in frail elderly people. The postural

Table 55.2. Age-related physiological changes predisposing to hypotension

1. Decreased baroreflex sensitivity
   - (a) Diminished heart-rate response to hypotensive stimuli
   - (b) Impaired α-adrenergic vascular responsiveness
2. Impaired defence of intravascular volume
   - (a) Reduced secretion of renin, angiotensin, and aldosterone
   - (b) Increased atrial natriuretic peptide, supine and upright
   - (c) Decreased plasma vasopressin response to orthostasis
   - (d) Reduced thirst after water deprivation
3. Impaired early cardiac ventricular filling (diastolic dysfunction)

Table 55.3. Disease related causes of postural and postprandial hypotension

Central nervous system disorders
    Multiple system atrophy
    Brainstem lesions
    Multiple cerebral infarction
    Parkinson's disease
    Myelopathy

Peripheral and autonomic neuropathies
    Pure autonomic failure
    Diabetes
    Amyloidosis
    Tabes dorsalis
    Alcoholic and nutritional
    Paraneoplastic syndromes

Prolonged immobility

Medications
    Phenothiazines and other neuroleptics
    Monamine oxidase-B inhibitors
    Tricyclic antidepressants
    Antihypertensives and diuretics
    Levodopa
    Vasodilators
    β-Blockers
    Calcium-channel blockers
    Angiotensin-converting enzyme inhibitors

decline in blood pressure is greatest when supine blood pressure is highest. This usually occurs early in the morning after an overnight rest.

In a study of 911 long-stay nursing home residents whose supine and 1- and 3-minute standing blood pressures were taken four times during the day (before and after breakfast, and before and after lunch) by trained nurses using random zero sphigmomanometers, we defined three patterns of postural hypotension: isolated (occurring once, 18 per cent of subjects), variable (2–3 times, 20 per cent), and persistent (four or more times, 13 per cent) (Ooi *et al.* 1997). The presence of postural hypotension was associated with elevated supine systolic blood pressure before breakfast, dizziness or lightheadedness

upon standing, male gender, medication for Parkinson's disease, time of day (before breakfast), greater independence in activities of daily living, and low body mass index. Therefore, ambulatory residents with hypertension, or those taking anti-parkinsonian medications, may be at greatest risk of falls due to hypotension, particularly in the early morning when they first get out of bed.

Although postural hypotension is a cardinal feature of autonomic dysfunction in a young individual—often heralding the onset of autonomic failure—in the older person it is more likely to result from co-morbidity and medication usage (Table 55.3) than from a syndrome of pure autonomic failure.

On assumption of the upright posture, approximately 500 ml of blood pools in the lower extremities and splanchnic circulation, thereby reducing venous return to the heart. The consequent unloading of cardiopulmonary and carotid baroreceptors reduces tonic inhibitory input to brainstem vasomotor centres in the nucleus tractus solitarius and results in efferent sympathetic activation and parasympathetic withdrawal. Within 10 seconds of standing, the healthy young subject demonstrates a brisk heart rate response due to vagal inhibition. The systolic blood pressure falls transiently for 10–20 seconds, but is restored rapidly by sympathetically mediated cardioacceleration and vasoconstriction. Blood pressure may continue to fall if there is an excessive reduction in blood volume which is not counteracted by these normal physiological responses.

In the aged individual, the early baroreflex-mediated cardioacceleration observed in young people is blunted. This is probably due to defective cardiac β-receptor responsiveness discussed above. Despite the lack of heart rate acceleration on standing, most normotensive elderly persons are probably protected from postural hypotension by α-mediated vasoconstriction. However, when vasoconstriction is compromised by vasodilator medications or intravascular volume is reduced by diuretics, many elderly individuals lack the physiological reserve to guard against hypotension. These individuals have age-related impairments in cardioacceleration and heightened plasma noradrenaline responses to postural stress (Table 55.4); they are often asymptomatic, with no other evidence of autonomic dysfunction, and may be described as having 'physiological postural hypotension'.

In contrast, elderly persons with severe symptomatic postural hypotension have a 'pathological' condition due to specific diseases that impair autonomic function (Tables 55.3 and 55.4). These patients have symptoms of autonomic insufficiency and subnormal

Table 55.4. Mechanisms of hypotension in the elderly

Physiological (impaired adaptive capacity)		Pathological (disease-related)		Reflex (health and CV disease)	
1. Associated with HTN		1. Blunted noradrenaline response to posture or meals		1. Sudden bradycardia and/or hypotension	
2. Increased noradrenaline response to posture change				2. Causes:	
3. Precipitants of hypotension:		2. Causes:		• Carotid sinus hypersensitivity	
• hypovolemia		• CNS: strokes, MSA, Parkinson's		• Neurally mediated syncope	
• preload reduction		• PNS: DM, alcohol, amyloid		• Micturition, cough, swallow syncope	
• inactivity		• Pure autonomic failure			
• other drugs		• Salt-wasting: renal disease, Addison's disease.			

CV, cardiovascular; HTN, hypotension; CNS, central nervous system; MSA, multiple system atrophy; PNS, peripheral nervous system; DM, diabetes mellitus; EtOH, alcohol.

plasma noradrenaline responses to upright posture. They are chronically disabled by postural symptoms, in contrast to individuals with physiological postural hypotension who become symptomatic only during periods of excessive haemodynamic stress.

Postprandial hypotension

The epidemiology of postprandial hypotension is unknown, but it is particularly common in the nursing home population, and in elderly patients with unexplained syncope (Jansen and Lipsitz 1995). Like postural hypotension, postprandial hypotension is a condition commonly seen in patients with autonomic failure as well as in multiply impaired and healthy elderly people (see Chapter 29). In ways similar to postural hypotension, postprandial hypotension may also be viewed as a consequence of either age-related physiological changes or pathological abnormalities in autonomic function. Although the mechanisms of postprandial hypotension are unknown, asymptomatic elderly persons with the 'physiological' variant appear to have inadequate cardiovascular compensation for splanchnic blood pooling during food digestion. This is evident in the moderate decline in blood pressure after a meal and a blunted heart rate increase that is unable to compensate for reduced blood pressure. These individuals may become symptomatic if hypotensive medications are taken before a meal, or in the setting of volume contraction.

Elderly patients with pathological postprandial hypotension have marked, symptomatic reductions in blood pressure that may result in syncope. These patients demonstrate an initial increase in plasma noradrenaline following a meal, but a subsequent inappropriate decline at the time when blood pressure is falling.

Previous studies that have examined the potential role of various gut peptides, including insulin, in the pathophysiology of postprandial hypotension, have failed to find significant associations (Jansen and Lipsitz 1995). In autonomic failure, caffeine and somatostatin analogues may be beneficial in preventing postprandial hypotension. These agents may work by preventing splanchnic vasodilation, although the exact mechanisms are not fully understood. There is some evidence that walking after a meal may restore blood pressure to its baseline, and thus prevent postprandial hypotension.

Reflex causes of hypotension

Hypotension may also result from neurally mediated (vasovagal) syncope; the sudden triggering of vagal reflexes during micturition, defecation, or swallowing; or the stimulation of a hypersensitive carotid sinus reflex (Table 55.4). One probable mechanism of neurally mediated syncope is provocation of the Bezold–Jarisch reflex by marked sympathetic stimulation of a relatively empty cardiac ventricle, during upright posture. Stimulation of vagal C fibres in the ventricular wall by vigorous cardiac contraction results in reflex hypotension and bradycardia. This reflex may be less common in elderly patients due to age-related reductions in sympathetic and vagal control of heart rate.

In contrast, ageing is associated with an increased prevalence of carotid sinus hypersensitivity, probably due to dropout of sinus node pacemaker cells and the onset of ischaemic heart disease, rather than enhanced vagal outflow. However, the frequently observed hypotensive and bradycardic response to a Valsalva manoeuvre while straining to overcome faecal impaction during defecation, or to overcome prostatic obstruction in men during micturition, suggests that vagal reflexes remain an important cause of hypotension, even in advanced age.

Control of respiration

Autonomic control of pulmonary and circulatory systems are closely linked, so that adjustments in heart rate, cardiac output, blood pressure, and organ flow can be made in response to changing demands for oxygen. Ageing is associated with a reduction in the partial pressure of oxygen in the blood, primarily due to a mismatch of ventilation and perfusion in the dependent portions of the lungs. This results from a reduction in lung compliance which causes airways to close prematurely at higher lung volumes (increased closing volume), within the range of vital capacity. It has been thought that the relative hypoxaemia in advanced age is offset by a reduced tissue demand for oxygen (reduced maximal oxygen uptake or VO_{2max}). However, much of the reduction in VO_{2max} is attributable to reduced muscle mass, and is reversible with endurance exercise training.

Chemoreceptors located in brainstem respiratory centres adjust respiratory amplitude and frequency on a moment-to-moment basis, in order to assure adequate oxygen availability and carbon dioxide clearance from the blood. Longer-term changes in oxygen supply and demand are matched by finely tuned adjustments in the sensitivity (gain) of chemoreceptors. With advancing age, there is a decline in chemosensitivity to oxygen and carbon dioxide tension, resulting in relative hypoventilation in response to hypoxaemia or hypercarpnia. Thus, older individuals may be more vulnerable to vital organ ischaemia during stresses such as surgery, acute pulmonary infections, or high altitude, when oxygen availability is reduced.

Gastrointestinal function

Many of the common gastrointestinal symptoms experienced by elderly people, including heartburn, constipation, diarrhoea, and faecal incontinence, suggest that ageing is associated with impaired autonomic control of the gastrointestinal tract. However, in the absence of disease, ageing is associated with only minor alterations in gastrointestinal function. Early studies of elderly people demonstrated frequent nonpropulsive tertiary contractions of the oesophagus, impaired lower oesophageal sphincter relaxation, and delayed oesophageal emptying. This constellation of findings was called 'presbyoesophagus' because the abnormalities were thought to be due to ageing. However, many of the subjects of previous studies had medical and neurological conditions, including diabetes mellitus, that may have been responsible for these findings. More recent studies in healthy elderly people have revealed a small decrease in the amplitude of oesophageal contractions, a slight increase in the frequency of simultaneous contractions in the upper and lower oesophagus, and a decrease in the regularity of peristaltic waves after a swallow. These physiological changes may be due to a decrease in myenteric ganglion cells per unit area and thickening of the smooth muscle layer of the oesophagus. In healthy elderly people, however, these changes are usually asymptomatic.

In the stomach, basal and maximal gastric acid output decreases with normal ageing, probably as a result of gastric mucosal atrophy and drop-out of parietal cells. There may also be a minor delay in liquid emptying from the stomach. The role of the autonomic nervous system in these changes is not known.

There have been very few human studies of age-related changes in small and large bowel function. Although there is a significant slowing of colonic transit time in senescent rats due to decreased responsiveness to neurotransmitters and progressive denervation, both small- and large-intestinal motility are probably unchanged with normal human ageing. Constipation in elderly people is probably related more to a decrease in faecal water content and laxative abuse than to age-related changes in intestinal transit time. In the anorectal area, an increase in resting sphinctor tone and decrease in maximal contractile pressure have been observed in some healthy elders. Resting tone may be influenced by increases in collagenous connective tissue that replaces anal smooth muscle, while muscle loss may account for a reduction in the generation of anal squeeze pressure.

Urinary tract function

Alterations in lower urinary tract function that mimic autonomic insufficiency, particularly urinary incontinence, become increasingly prevalent with ageing. However, urinary symptoms are due primarily to age-associated diseases that affect autonomic nervous system control of the urinary tract, rather than ageing *per se*. Little is known about the effects of healthy human ageing on voiding function. Current evidence suggests that there are functional and structural changes in the lower urinary tract outside of the autonomic nervous system, that may predispose elderly people to urinary incontinence (Resnick 1995). These include declines in bladder capacity, contractility, and the ability to postpone voiding in both sexes, and decreases in urethral length and closing pressure in women. The prevalence of involuntary bladder contractions and the post-voiding residual bladder volume increase with age. Ultrastructurally, bladders of healthy elderly people with normal contractility show a normal configuration of muscle cells and cell junctions, but dominant dense bands and depleted caveolae in muscle cell membranes. In contrast, aged bladders with impaired contractility have widespread degeneration of muscle cells and axons superimposed on the 'dense band pattern'. These histopathological changes may be responsible for the age-related change in bladder contractility.

One of the most common causes of established incontinence in elderly people is detrusor overactivity. This may be associated with central nervous system disease (e.g. stroke), normal ageing, or local urinary tract abnormalities (e.g. prostatic obstruction). Ultrastructurally, the bladder demonstrates replacement of normal muscle junctions with 'protrusion junctions', that may facilitate propagation of heightened smooth muscle activity, causing involuntary bladder contractions. The role of the autonomic nervous system in these changes is not clear.

Sexual function

Normal sexual function is dependent on the complex integration of endocrine, autonomic, and vascular systems. The sympathetic nervous system innervates blood vessels in the reproductive organs; erectile tissue in the penis, clitoris, and bulbs of the vestibule; and smooth muscle in the seminal vesicles, prostate, vagina, and uterus. The parasympathetic nervous system also innervates erectile tissue in the penis and clitoris, as well as smooth muscle in the urethra, seminal vesicles, prostate, vagina, and uterus. In addition, parasympathetic nerves innervate glandular tissue and secretory epithelium in these structures. Although sexual dysfunction becomes more common with advancing age, ageing *per se* is not associated with impairments in autonomic control of genital function. Diseases such as diabetes, peripheral vascular disease, neuropathies, spinal-cord lesions, and uraemia, as well as alcohol and drugs, are most frequently implicated.

In women, reproductive capacity ends in mid-life at the time of menopause, and levels of 17-β-oestradiol, the predominant circulating oestrogen during reproductive life, decline. This subsequently predisposes women to the development of pathological conditions such as cardiovascular disease and osteoporosis. Men do not experience as abrupt a change in reproductive function as do women, but undergo gradual alterations in sex steroid metabolism that predispose them to prostate enlargement and bone loss. In men, normal ageing probably results in a modest degree of primary testicular failure, characterized by a decrease in testicular size. The age-related decline in testicular function is highly variable and its clinical implications have not been well established. It may contribute to a decline in the frequency of sexual activity, but probably plays a secondary role to social, psychological, and medical factors that have the greatest influence on sexual dysfunction in late life. Although both healthy men and women may experience changes in sexual performance with advancing age, their capacity to enjoy sexual activity remains intact.

References

Bonyhay, I., Jokkel, G., and Kollai, M. (1996). Relation between baroreflex sensitivity and carotid artery elasticity in healthy humans. *Am. J. Physiol.* 271, H1139–H1144.

Collins, K. J., Easton, J. C., and Exton-Smith, A. N. (1981*a*). Shivering thermogenesis and vasomotor responses with convective cooling in the elderly. *J. Physiol.*, London 320, 76.

Collins, K. J., Exton-Smith, A. N., and Dore, C. (1981*b*). Urban hypothermia: preferred temperature and thermal perception in old age. *BMJ* 282, 175–7.

Egashira, K., Inou, T., Hirooka, Y. *et al.* (1993). Effects of age on endothelium-dependent vasodilation of resistance coronary artery by acetylcholine in humans. *Circulation* 88, 77–81.

Gerhard, M., Roddy, M. A., Creager, S. J., and Creager, M. A. (1996). Ageing progressively impairs endothelium-dependent vasodilation in forearm resistance vessels of humans. *Hypertension* 27, 849–53.

Hogikyan, R. V. and Supiano, M. A. (1994). Arterial α-adrenergic responsiveness is decreased and SNS activity is increased in older humans. *Am. J. Physiol.* 266, E717–E724.

Inoue, Y., Nakao, M., Araki, T., and Murakami, H. (1991). Regional differences in the sweating responses of older and younger men. *J. Appl. Physiol.* 71, 2453–9.

Jansen, R. W. M. M. and Lipsitz, L. A. (1995). Postprandial hypotension: epidemiology, pathophysiology, and clinical management. *Ann. Int. Med.* 122, 286–95.

Khan, F., Spence, V. A., and Belch, J. J. F. (1992). Cutaneous vascular responses and thermoregulation in relation to age. *Clin. Sci.* 82, 521–8.

Kramer, M. R., Vandijk, J., and Rosin, A. J. (1989). Mortality in elderly patients with thermoregulatory failure. *Arch. Int. Med.* 149, 1521–3.

Lakatta, E. G. (1993). Deficient neuroendocrine regulation of the cardiovascular system with advancing age in healthy humans. *Circulation* 87, 631–6.

Lipsitz, L. A. and Goldberger, A. L. (1992). Loss of 'complexity' and ageing. Potential applications of fractals and chaos theory to senescence. *J. Am. Med. Ass.* **267**, 1806–9.

Lipsitz, L. A., Mietus, J., Moody, G. B., and Goldberger, A. L. (1990). Spectral characteristics of heart rate variability before and during postural tilt. Relations to ageing and risk of syncope. *Circulation* **81**, 1803–10.

Maddens, M. E., Lipsitz, L. A., Wei, J. Y., Pluchino, F. C., and Mark, R. (1987). Impaired heart rate responses to cough and deep breathing in elderly patients with unexplained syncope. *Am. J. Cardiol.* **60**, 1368–72.

Meyer, J. S. and Shaw, T. G. (1984). Cerebral blood flow in ageing. In *Clinical neurology of ageing*, (ed. M.L. Albert), pp. 178–96. Oxford University Press, New York.

Ng, A. V., Callister, R., Johnson, D. G., and Seals, D. R. (1993). Age and gender influence muscle sympathetic nerve activity at rest in healthy humans. *Hypertension* **21**, 498–503.

Ooi, W. L., Barrett, S., Hossain, M., Kelley-Gagnon, M. and Lipsitz, L. A. (1997). Patterns of orthostatic blood pressure change and their clinical correlates in a frail, elderly population. *J. Am. Med. Ass.* **277**, 1299–304.

Pagani, M., Lombardi, F., Guzzetti, S. *et al.* (1986). Power spectral analysis of heart rate and arterial pressure variabilities as a marker of sympatho-vagal interaction in man and conscious dog. *Cir. Res.* **59**, 178–93.

Pan, H. Y.-M., Hoffman, B. B., Pershe, R. A., and Blaschke, T. F. (1986). Decline in beta adrenergic receptor-mediated vascular relaxation with ageing in man. *J. Pharmacol. Exp. Ther.* **239**, 802–7.

Phillips, P. A., Phil, D., Rolls, B. J. *et al.* (1984). Reduced thirst after water deprivation in healthy elderly men. *New Engl. J. Med.*, **311**, 753–59.

Prinz, P. N., Halter, J., Benedetti, C. *et al.* (1979). Circadian variation of plasma catecholamines in young and old men: relation to rapid eye movement and slow wave sleep. *J. Clin. Endocrinol. Metab.* **49**, 300–4.

Resnick, N. (1995). Urinary Incontinence. *Lancet* **346**, 94–9.

Richardson, D. (1989). Effects of age on cutaneous circulatory response to direct heat on the forearm. *J. Gerontol.* **44**, M189–M194.

Richardson, D., Tyra, J., and McCray, A. (1992). Attenuation of the cutaneous vasoconstrictor response to cold in elderly men. *J. Gerontol.* **47**, M211–M214.

Rodeheffer, R. J., Gerstenblith, G., Becker, L. C., Fleg, J. L., Weisfeldt, M. L., and Lakatta, E. G. (1984). Exercise cardiac output is maintained with advancing age in healthy human subjects: cardiac dilatation and increased stroke volume compensate for a diminished heart-rate. *Circulation* **69**, 203–13.

Ryan, S. M. and Lipsitz, L. A. (1995). Age-related changes in the autonomic nervous system. In *Disorders of the autonomic nervous system*, (ed. D. Robertson and I. Biaggioni), pp. 61–82. Harwood Academic Publishers, Luxembourg.

Ryan, S. M., Goldberger, A. L., Pincus, S. M., Meitus, J., and Lipsitz, L. A. (1994). Gender- and age-related differences in heart-rate dynamics: are women more complex than men? *J. Am. Coll. Cardiol.* **24**, 1700–7.

Scarpace, P. J., Shu, Y., and Tumer, N. (1994). Influence of exercise training on myocardial β-adrenergic signal transduction: differential regulation with age. *J. Appl. Physiol.* **77**, 737–41.

Schwartz, R. S., Jaeger, L.,F., and Veith, R. C., (1990). The thermic effect of feeding in older men: the importance of the sympathetic nervous system. *Metabolism* **39**, 733–7.

Stratton, J. R., Cerqueira, M. D., Schwartz, R. S. *et al.* (1992). Differences in cardiovascular responses to isoproterenol in relation to age and exercise training in healthy men. *Circulation* **86**, 504–12.

Stratton, J. R., Levy, W. C., Cerqueira, M. D., Schwartz, R. S., and Abrass, I. B. (1994). Cardiovascular responses to exercise. Effects of ageing and exercise training in healthy men. *Circulation* **89**, 1648–55.

Taylor, N. A., Allsopp, N. K., and Parkes, D. G. (1995). Preferred room temperature of young vs aged males: the influence of thermal sensation, thermal comfort, and affect. *J. Gerontol.* **50**, M216–M221.

Veith, R. C., Featherstone, J. A., Linares, O. A., and Halter, J. B. (1986). Age differences in plasma norepinephrine kinetics in humans. *J. Gerontol.* **41**, 319–24.

Wollner, L., McCarthy, S. T., Soper, N. D. W., and Macy, D. J. (1979). Failure of cerebral autoregulation as a cause of brain dysfunction in the elderly. *BMJ* **1**, 1117–18.

Wongsurawat, N., Davis, B. B., and Morley, J. E. (1990). Thermoregulatory failure in the elderly. *J. Am. Geriatr. Soc.* **38**, 899–906.

Young, J. B., Rowe, J. W., Pallotta, J. A., Sparrow, D., and Landsberg, L. (1980). Enhanced plasma norepinephrine response to upright posture and oral glucose administration in elderly human subjects. *Metabolism* **29**, 532–9.

Index